ENCYCLOPEDIA OF

HEALTH
SERVICES
RESEARCH

Editorial Board

ENCYCLOPEDIA OF

HEALTH SERVICES RESEARCH

VOLUME TWO

ROSS M. MULLNER EDITOR
University of Illinois at Chicago

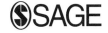

Los Angeles | London | New Delhi
Singapore | Washington DC

A SAGE Reference Publication

For information:

 SAGE Publications, Inc.
2455 Teller Road
Thousand Oaks, California 91320
E-mail: order@sagepub.com

SAGE Publications Ltd.
1 Oliver's Yard
55 City Road
London, EC1Y 1SP
United Kingdom

SAGE Publications India Pvt. Ltd.
B 1/I 1 Mohan Cooperative Industrial Area
Mathura Road, New Delhi 110 044
India

SAGE Publications Asia-Pacific Pte. Ltd.
33 Pekin Street #02-01
Far East Square
Singapore 048763

Printed in the United States of America.

Library of Congress Cataloging-in-Publication Data

Encyclopedia of health services research/edited by Ross M. Mullner.
    p. cm.
Includes bibliographical references and index.
ISBN 978-1-4129-5179-1 (cloth: alk. paper)
  1. Public health—Research—Encyclopedias. 2. Medical care—Research—Encyclopedias.
I. Mullner, Ross M.
[DNLM: 1. Health Services Research—Encyclopedias—English. W 13 E554 2009]

RA440.85.E63 2009
362.103—dc22   2008052885

This book is printed on acid-free paper.

09 10 11 12 13 10 9 8 7 6 5 4 3 2 1

Publisher:	Rolf A. Janke
Acquisitions Editor:	Jim Brace-Thompson
Editorial Assistant:	Michele Thompson
Developmental Editor:	Carole Maurer
Reference Systems Manager:	Leticia M. Gutierrez
Reference Systems Coordinator:	Laura Notton
Production Editor:	Kate Schroeder
Copy Editor:	QuADS Prepress (P) Ltd.
Typesetter:	C&M Digitals (P) Ltd.
Proofreader:	Kevin Gleason, Anne Rogers
Indexer:	Mary Fran Prottsman
Cover Designer:	Glenn Vogel
Marketing Manager:	Amberlyn McKay

Contents

List of Entries

AARP
Abt Associates
Academic Medical Centers
AcademyHealth
Access, Models of
Access to Healthcare
Accreditation
Activities of Daily Living (ADL)
Acute and Chronic Diseases
Aday, Lu Ann
Administrative Costs
Adverse Drug Events
Adverse Selection
Agency for Healthcare Research and Quality
    (AHRQ)
Aiken, Linda H.
Allied Health Professionals
Altman, Drew E.
Ambulatory Care
American Academy of Family Physicians (AAFP)
American Academy of Pediatrics (AAP)
American Association of Colleges of Nursing
    (AACN)
American Association of Preferred Provider
    Organizations (AAPPO)
American College of Healthcare Executives
    (ACHE)
American Enterprise Institute for Public Policy
    Research (AEI)
American Health Care Association (AHCA)
American Health Planning Association (AHPA)
American Hospital Association (AHA)
American Medical Association (AMA)
American Nurses Association (ANA)
American Osteopathic Association (AOA)
American Public Health Association (APHA)
American Society of Health Economists (ASHE)
America's Health Insurance Plans (AHIP)
Andersen, Ronald M.

Anderson, Odin W.
Antitrust Law
Arrow, Kenneth J.
Association for the Accreditation of Human
    Research Protection Programs (AAHRPP)
Association of American Medical Colleges
    (AAMC)
Association of University Programs in Health
    Administration (AUPHA)

Benchmarking
Berwick, Donald M.
Bioterrorism
Blue Cross and Blue Shield
Brook, Robert H.
Brookings Institution

Canadian Association for Health Services and
    Policy Research (CAHSPR)
Canadian Health Services Research Foundation
    (CHSRF)
Canadian Institute of Health Services and Policy
    Research (IHSPR)
Cancer Care
Capitation
Carve-Outs
Case Management
Case-Mix Adjustment
Cato Institute
Causal Analysis
Center for Studying Health System Change
Centers for Disease Control and Prevention
    (CDC)
Centers for Medicare and Medicaid Services
    (CMS)
Certificate of Need (CON)
Charity Care
Chassin, Mark R.
Child Care

Primary-Care Physicians
Project HOPE
Prospective Payment
Provider-Based Research Networks (PBRNs)
Public Health
Public Health Policy Advocacy
Public Policy

Quality-Adjusted Life Years (QALYs)
Quality Enhancement Research Initiative
  (QUERI) of the Veterans Health
  Administration (VHA)
Quality Improvement Organizations (QIOs)
Quality Indicators
Quality Management
Quality of Healthcare
Quality of Life, Health-Related (HRQOL)
Quality of Well-Being Scale (QWB)

RAND Corporation
RAND Health Insurance Experiment
Randomized Controlled Trials (RCTs)
Rationing Healthcare
Regulation
Reinhardt, Uwe E.
Relman, Arnold S.
Resource-Based Relative Value Scale (RBRVS)
Rice, Dorothy P.
Risk
Robert Wood Johnson Foundation (RWJF)
Roemer, Milton I.
Roos, Leslie L.
Roos, Noralou P.
Rorem, C. Rufus
Rosenbaum, Sara
RTI International
Rural Health

Sackett, David L.
Safety Net
Satisfaction Surveys
Scott, W. Richard
Selective Contracting
Severity Adjustment
Shapiro, Sam
Sheps, Cecil G.
Shortell, Stephen M.
Short-Form Health Surveys (SF-36, -12, -8)

Single-Payer System
Skilled-Nursing Facilities
Starfield, Barbara
Starr, Paul
State-Based Health Insurance Initiatives
State Children's Health Insurance Program
  (SCHIP)
Stevens, Rosemary A.
Structure-Process-Outcome Quality Measures
Substance Abuse and Mental Health Services
  Administration (SAMHSA)
Supplier-Induced Demand

Tarlov, Alvin R.
Tax Subsidy of Employer-Sponsored Health
  Insurance
Technology Assessment
Telemedicine
Terrorism. *See* Bioterrorism
Thompson, John Devereaux
Timeliness of Healthcare
Tobacco Use
Transportation
TRICARE, Military Health System

Uncompensated Healthcare
Uninsured Individuals
United Kingdom's National Health Service (NHS)
United Kingdom's National Institute for Health
  and Clinical Excellence (NICE)
University HealthSystem Consortium (UHC)
Urban Institute
U.S. Department of Veterans Affairs (VA)
U.S. Food and Drug Administration (FDA)
U.S. Government Accountability
  Office (GAO)
U.S. National Health Expenditures

Volume-Outcome Relationship
Vulnerable Populations

Ware, John E.
Wennberg, John E.
White, Kerr L.
Wilensky, Gail R.
Williams, Alan H.
Women's Health Issues
World Health Organization (WHO)

L

LEAPFROG GROUP

The Leapfrog Group is an initiative that was started by large employers that purchase healthcare. Leapfrog works to create breakthroughs in the safety, quality, and affordability of healthcare. It is supported through its membership base, as well as the Business Roundtable (BRT), the Robert Wood Johnson Foundation (RWJF), and others. The mission of the Leapfrog Group is to facilitate enormous leaps forward in the safety, quality, and affordability of healthcare by supporting informed healthcare decisions of purchasers and consumers and by promoting healthcare that is high in value by realigning incentives and rewards.

Background

In 1998, a consortium of large employers began to discuss how they could collaborate and use their purchasing power to influence the quality and affordability of healthcare. These employers realized that billions of dollars were being spent on healthcare without any evaluation of its quality or its providers. A 2000 national Institute of Medicine (IOM) report, *To Err Is Human: Building a Safer Health System,* estimated that as many as 98,000 hospital patients die each year from preventable medical errors. The report recommended that large employers could use their market leverage to influence the quality and safety of healthcare. The founders of Leapfrog recognized that significant "leaps" forward could be taken to improve patient safety and quality by rewarding hospitals that implemented substantial changes. In 2000, BRT set aside funding, and the Leapfrog Group was officially created.

The Leapfrog Group has a growing consortium that includes many of the nation's largest corporations and other large purchasers of healthcare that provide benefits to more than 37 million individuals across the country. Member organizations of Leapfrog agree to make their healthcare-purchasing decisions with the goal of encouraging quality improvement among the providers and consumers involved. Leapfrog estimates that if all hospitals in the nation implemented its first three leaps of recommended safety and quality practices, more than 65,000 lives could be saved, more than 907,000 medical errors could be prevented, and about $41.5 billion could be saved annually.

Initiatives

The Leapfrog Group is well-known for its Hospital Quality and Safety Survey, which is conducted annually and completed by hospitals on a voluntary basis. The survey measures hospital performance on the use of computer physician order entry, evidence-based hospital referral, intensive care unit staffing by physicians experienced in critical care medicine, and the Leapfrog safe practices score. Leapfrog's survey goals are based on the following criteria: There is substantial scientific evidence that the safety and quality practices can significantly reduce preventable medical errors; the implementation of these practices is feasible;

consumers can readily benefit from these practices; and health plans, purchasers, and consumers can readily distinguish if these practices are present or absent in selecting their healthcare provider.

In 2008, the survey integrated the first set of hospital efficiency measures using standardized measures from the Joint Commission. The survey also serves as the basis for Leapfrog's Hospital Rewards Program, a pay-for-performance program that assesses the value of patient care by measuring performance along two dimensions— the quality of the care hospitals provide and how efficiently they deliver it.

To fuel the drive toward value-driven health care, Leapfrog developed the Incentive and Reward Compendium, a free database that categorizes and describes financial programs—such as those that reward providers with quality bonuses—and non-financial programs—such as those that reward providers with public recognition. These programs aim to affect hospitals, physicians, health plans, and/or consumers.

Bridges to Excellence and The Leapfrog Group have also formed a partnership to use the strengths of each organization to develop and implement programs that reward healthcare providers. Leapfrog lends its expertise in performance measures and public reporting, while Bridges to Excellence contributes its knowledge of implementing programs that reward healthcare providers for quality improvement.

Purchasing Principles

Leapfrog works to create improvements in the quality of healthcare by building transparency through its voluntary survey, providing incentives and rewards to hospitals that improve the quality of care they provide to patients, and creating consistency and leverage for change by collaborating with other organizations to develop quality and safety initiatives. Leapfrog's member organizations agree to follow four principles when making healthcare-purchasing decisions for their employees: increase awareness and inform enrollees about healthcare safety, quality, and affordability and the importance of comparing among healthcare providers; reward and recognize healthcare providers for making significant advances in the safety, quality, and affordability of healthcare;

hold health plans accountable for implementing the purchasing principles of Leapfrog; and build the support of consultants and brokers to use Leapfrog's principles with their clients.

To promote these purchasing principles, the Leapfrog Hospital Rewards Program, a pay-for-performance program, was launched in 2005 to drive improvements in hospital quality and efficiency for five clinical conditions by rewarding hospitals that demonstrated excellence in sustaining improvements. The five clinical conditions are (1) coronary artery bypass graft, (2) percutaneous coronary intervention, (3) acute myocardial infarction, (4) community-acquired pneumonia, and (5) deliveries/neonatal care. The efficiency measure applies a regional price adjuster to the average reimbursement a hospital receives for a given condition.

Current Issues

Beginning in June 2001, the Leapfrog Group began collecting data on hospitals by surveying urban and suburban hospitals in six geographic regions, which has now grown to 33 regions. The survey of the 33 regions covers more than 1,300 hospitals. These hospitals represent about 58% of all hospital beds in the nation, and they serve over half of the population of the nation. Free access to the ratings of these hospitals can be found at Leapfrog's Web site.

The Leapfrog Group continues to advocate for change by improving the quality and safety of patient care through its member organizations' purchasing power. Leapfrog's efforts have become a driving force in transforming the nation's healthcare system to ensure high-quality care and purchasing based on value.

Jared Lane K. Maeda and Kat Song

See also Health Report Cards; Joint Commission; Medical Errors; National Quality Forum (NQF); Outcomes Movement; Pay-for-Performance; Quality of Healthcare; Robert Wood Johnson Foundation (RWJF)

Further Readings

Birckmeyer, John D., and Justin B. Dimick. "Potential Benefits of the New Leapfrog Standards: Effect of Process and Outcome Measures," *Surgery* 135(6): 576–78, June 2004.

Delbanco, Suzanne. "Employers Flex Their Muscles as Health Care Purchasers," *Surgical Clinics of North America* 87(4): 883–87, August 2007.

Galvin, Robert S., Suzanne Delbanco, Arnold Milstein, et al. "Has the Leapfrog Group Had an Impact on the Health Care Market?" *Health Affairs* 24(1): 228–33, January–February 2005.

Kohn, Linda T., Janet M. Corrigan, and Molla S. Donaldson, (eds.), Committee on Quality of Health Care in America. *To Err Is Human: Building a Safer Health System.* Washington, DC: National Academy Press 2000.

Milstein, Arnold, Robert S. Galvin, Suzanne Delbanco, et al. "Improving the Safety of Health Care: The Leapfrog Initiative," *Effective Clinical Practice* 3(6): 313–16, November–December 2000.

Pronovost, Peter, David A. Thompson, and Christine G. Holzmueller. "Impact of the Leapfrog Group's Intensive Care Unit Physician Staffing Standard," *Journal of Critical Care* 22(2): 89–96, June 2007.

Sandrick, Karen. "One Giant Leap for Quality. When Boards Get Behind Quality Initiatives, Patient Care Benefits," *Trustee* 58(3): 22–24, 26, March 2005.

Web Sites

Leapfrog Group: http://www.leapfroggroup.org
Leapfrog Hospital and Quality and Safety Survey: http://www.leapfroggroup.org/cp
Leapfrog Pay-for-Performance Initiatives: http://www.leapfroggroup.org/for_hospitals/fh-incentives_and_rewards

LEE, PHILIP R.

Philip R. Lee is an academic who has served as a senior federal health policy official in two administrations. He also is a frequent advisor to federal, state, and local health policy makers.

Born in San Francisco, Lee grew up in Palo Alto, California, and is one of five children, all of whom became practicing physicians. Lee earned a medical degree from Stanford University in 1948. He joined the U.S. Navy and served as a medical officer from 1949 to 1951. From 1951 to 1956, Lee was a fellow at the New York University's Medical Center and Goldwater Hospital. He completed a fellowship at Mayo Clinic from 1953 to 1955 and earned a master's degree from University of Minnesota in 1955. From there, Lee rejoined the faculty at New York University until he returned to Palo Alto in 1956. There, he worked as an internist at the Palo Alto Medical Clinic, which was founded by his father, Russell Lee, in 1930.

As a practicing physician during the 1960s, Lee joined a group called the Chowder and Marching Society, headed by Lester Breslow. The society met monthly and presented papers on various health policy topics. Also during this time, Lee was one of the founders of the Bay Area Committee for Medical Aid for the Aged. Additionally, he became actively involved in the King-Anderson Bill, which later became Medicare Part A. It was during this time that he became interested in governmental policies and practices.

In 1963, Lee left his medical practice and joined the federal government, becoming the director of health services in the Office of Technical Cooperation and Research in the Agency for International Development (AID). While in that position, he assisted in developing the first federal policies on family planning, malaria control, environmental sanitation, medical education, and the Food for Peace program. Additionally, he worked to better coordinate AID with the U.S. Public Health Service.

From 1965 to 1969, Lee served as the first assistant secretary in the U.S. Department of Health, Education and Welfare (now split into the Department of Education and the Department of Health and Human Services) under President Lyndon B. Johnson. In his position, Lee was involved in a wide range of policy issues, including bioethics, biomedical research, environmental health, family planning, and the education of health professionals. One of his main tasks was to implement the Medicare program, which was passed in 1965.

From 1969 to 1972, Lee served as the chancellor of the University of California, San Francisco (UCSF), where he helped increase the enrollment of minority students, particularly in the health professions. In 1972, while he was a professor in the School of Medicine, he founded the Institute for Health Policy Studies, which was the first of its kind in the nation. Lee served as the director of the institute until 1993, when he retired from UCSF to accept the appointment of Assistant Secretary for Health in the Department of Health and Human

Services under President Bill Clinton from 1993 to 1997. Additionally, Lee served in several other capacities. He was the first president of the San Francisco Health Commission. He served on the Board of Trustees of the Carnegie Corporation and the Mayo Foundation. And he headed the federal Physician Payment Review Commission (PPRC) from 1986 to 1993.

Lee has been honored for his many accomplishments. He received the David Rogers Award from the Association of American Medical Colleges (AAMC) in 1998, the National Academy of Sciences, Institute of Medicine's Gustav O. Lienhard Award in 2000, the American Public Health Association's Sedgwick Medal in 2000, the Henrik Blum Award from the California Public Health Association in 2001, and the National Hero Award in 2002. In 2007, the health policy institute he founded at the University of California, San Francisco, was renamed the Philip R. Lee Institute for Health Policy Studies in his honor.

Lee is the author or coauthor of more than 150 articles and four books. One of his books, *The Nation's Health,* is in its seventh edition. Although he is retired, Lee is currently working on policy issues such as diversity in medical education, financing national health insurance, and evidence- and population-based healthcare.

Amie Lulinski Norris

See also Cohen, Wilbur J.; Diversity in Healthcare Management; Medicare; Public Health; Public Policy

Further Readings

Boufford, Jo, and Philip R. Lee. *Health Policies for the 21st Century: Challenges and Recommendations for the U.S. Department of Health and Human Services.* New York: Milbank Memorial Fund, 2001.

Lee, Philip R., Carroll L. Estes, and Fatima M. Rodriguez, eds. *The Nation's Health.* 7th ed. Sudbury, MA: Jones and Bartlett, 2003.

Rockefellar, Nancy M. Interview with Philip R. Lee, M.D. *Diversity Series* 4A–4B. San Francisco: University of California, Department of Anthropology, History, and Social Medicine, UCSF Oral History Program, 2006.

Silverman, Milton, and Philip R. Lee. *Pills, Profits, and Politics.* Berkeley: University of California Press, 1974.

Web Sites

Philip R. Lee Institute for Health Policy Studies, University of California, San Francisco (UCSF): http://ihps.medschool.ucsf.edu

LEWIN GROUP

The Lewin Group is a nationally recognized healthcare and human services management consulting firm. The Lewin Group provides policy-focused empirical research, hands-on technical assistance, and evaluation services to federal, state, and local governments, foundations, associations, hospitals and health systems, insurers and health plans, and medical technology companies.

Background

Founded by Lawrence S. Lewin in 1970, the Lewin Group, which is located in Falls Church, Virginia, recently was acquired by Ingenix, Inc., a leading health information technology company. Lewin's strategic and analytical services aim to help clients improve policy and expand knowledge of healthcare through the integration of evidence-based practices; enact, run, and evaluate programs to enhance delivery and financing of healthcare and human services; deal with shifts in healthcare practice, technology, and regulation; optimize performance, quality, coverage, and health outcomes; and create strategies for institutions, communities, governments, and people to make healthcare and human services systems more effective. Lewin's consultants are drawn from industry, government, academia, and the health professions. Many are national authorities whose strategies for health and human services system improvements come from a personal experience with imperatives for change.

Lewin's policy research work includes both long-term studies and quick-turnaround policy analyses. Federal and state clients and others count on the Lewin Group for their in-depth experience and innovative, analytic approaches.

Modeling Health Reform

The Lewin Group has been a leader in the health reform and coverage arena and is one of the few independent sources of information on the financial impacts of health coverage expansion and national and state health reform initiatives. The Health Benefits Simulation Model (HBSM), developed by The Lewin Group, is a well-vetted, proprietary microsimulation model of the U.S. healthcare system. The model, based on the Medical Expenditures Panel Survey data and surveys of employers and health plans, provides a comprehensive representation of public and private insurance coverage and health spending. These data enable The Lewin Group to simulate the effect of a wide range of health reform initiatives on major stakeholder groups, including employers, state and federal governments, families, and providers. The model has been used by Republicans and Democrats to analyze a broad range of health reform proposals at both the state and the federal level, including The Lewin Group's independent analysis of the Clinton health reform proposal of 1993, comparative analysis of the proposed health plans of President George W. Bush and Senator John F. Kerry (D-MA) during the 2004 presidential campaign, President Bush's health insurance proposal of 2007, and the Healthy Americans Act introduced by Senator Ron Wyden (D-OR). The Lewin Group has developed comparisons of alternative coverage expansions for organizations such as the Robert Wood Johnson Foundation (RWJF) and the Commonwealth Fund. Lewin also has modeled a wide range of health reform models for individual states, including tax credits, the single-payer model, and individual mandate proposals.

Cost-of-Illness Studies

The Lewin Group's cost-of-illness studies provide information on both the direct medical costs associated with a disease and the indirect costs, such as lost productivity and premature deaths. These costs are estimated from the perspective of society, healthcare payers, and consumers.

Lewin recently completed a study on the national cost of diabetes for the American Diabetes Association. The study estimated the national economic burden of diabetes at $174 billion in 2007, approximately $116 billion in additional healthcare expenditures attributed to diabetes and $58 billion in lost productivity from absenteeism, reduced productivity, permanent disability, and premature mortality.

In addition, Lewin continues to estimate the economic cost of drug abuse in the United States for the Office of National Drug Control Policy. Lewin has also studied the economic burden of alcohol abuse for the National Institutes of Health (NIH) and is updating these estimates for the Centers for Disease Control and Prevention (CDC) 2008 report. Other studies being conducted include the prevalence and cost of 17 digestive conditions for the American Gastroenterological Association; the cost of obesity, alcohol abuse, and tobacco use for the U.S. Department of Defense/TRICARE Management Activity; the cost of skin disease for the Society for Investigative Dermatology; and the cost of Chronic Fatigue Syndrome for the CDC.

Long-Term Care

Lewin's Center on Long Term Care brings together experts from across the organization to promote systems change for individuals who have long-term care needs due to chronic conditions or disability. The Lewin Group's staff provides policy development support and technical assistance for the U.S. Administration on Aging's (AoA) efforts to reform the nation's long-term care system so that older adults and individuals with disabilities can live independent lives in their communities. The organization also assists states and local communities to understand the implications of the aging baby boom population and its impact on the range of government services, from transportation to housing and healthcare.

Lewin also recently conducted a study documenting the significant number of older adults, particularly among the "oldest old" (persons 85 and older), who have elected to stay in their homes and in residential alternatives rather than move to nursing homes. The findings speculate on the impact this shift will have on the future demand for long-term care. Through the Centers for Medicare and Medicaid Services (CMS)–sponsored National Direct Service Workforce Resource Center, Lewin additionally supported efforts to improve the recruitment and retention of direct-service workers, who help people with disabilities and older adults to live independently.

Healthcare Workforce: Supply and Demand

An adequate supply of healthcare workers is integral to achieving the nation's goal of ensuring access to quality and affordable healthcare. The Lewin Group is helping healthcare stakeholders understand the implications of demographic trends; changes in the healthcare operating environment; and policies and programs on efforts to train, recruit, and retain health workers. Lewin uses a quantitative approach to help decision makers in the public and private sectors deal effectively with health worker supply and demand and related issues, such as workforce management and program design. The Lewin Group has also worked with the Health Resources and Services Administration (HRSA), states, professional associations, health systems, insurers, and others to develop models that project supply and demand for physicians, nurses, and other health workers.

Lisa Chimento

See also Cost of Healthcare; Diabetes; Disability; Healthcare Reform; Health Insurance Coverage; Health Workforce; Long-Term Care; State-Based Health Insurance Initiatives

Further Readings

Bureau of Health Professions. *Physician Supply and Demand: Projections to 2020.* Rockville, MD: Health Resources and Services Administration, Bureau of Health Professions, 2006.

Dall, Timothy M., Sarah Edge Mann, Yiduo Zhang, et al. "Economic Costs of Diabetes in the U.S. in 2007," *Diabetes Care* 31(3): 1–20, March 2008.

Dall, Timothy M., Yidue Zhang, Yaozhu J. Chen, et al. "Cost Associated With Being Overweight and With Obesity, High Alcohol Consumption, and Tobacco Use Within the Military Health System's TRICARE Prime-Enrolled Population," *American Journal of Health Promotion* 22(2): 120–39, November 2007.

Mark, Tami L., Rosanna M. Coffey, Rita Vandivort-Warren, et al. "U.S. Spending for Mental Health and Substance Abuse Treatment, 1991–2001," *Health Affairs* Web Exclusive W5–W133, 2005.

Office of National Drug Control Policy. *The Economic Costs of Drug Abuse in the United States: 1992–2002.* Washington, DC: Executive Office of the President, 2004.

Reynolds, Kenneth J., Suzanne D. Vernon, Ellen Bouchery, et al. "The Economic Impact of Chronic Fatigue Syndrome," *Cost Effectiveness and Resource Allocation* 2(4): 1–9, 2004.

Sheils, John, and Randall Haught. "The Cost of Tax-Exempt Health Benefits in 2004," *Health Affairs* Web Exclusive W4–W106, 2004.

Web Sites

Lewin Group: http://www.lewin.com

LICENSING

Healthcare professionals are licensed by the government to protect the healthcare consumer and to ensure a minimum standard of quality of care. Most healthcare professionals cannot practice unless they are licensed. The licensing of healthcare professionals in the United States is carried out at the state government level, and it limits who can and who cannot provide care. The federal government, however, also plays a role in the regulation of healthcare providers by coordinating state licensure programs through a centralized database known as the National Practitioner Data Bank (NPDB), which contains disciplinary actions of providers, and by imposing requirements on providers who receive federal reimbursement (e.g., Medicare, Medicaid).

Background

The government sanction of medical practice dates back thousands of years in India and China. In the Western world, King Henry VIII of England in 1518 established a charter to grant licenses to qualified physicians. In the United States, the American Medical Association (AMA) played a pivotal role in the 19th century supporting state enactment of licensure laws for physicians. Between 1874 and 1915, licensing requirements for medical practice were passed in all states in the nation. Often, as one state passed licensing requirements, poor-quality physicians would move to another unregulated state to practice. However, eventually, as all states required licensing, many poorly trained and unqualified physicians left the profession, which ultimately resulted in better quality of care and increased status of the profession.

The push by the AMA for state licensure served as a model for the licensing of other healthcare professionals. By the 1920s, most states enacted licensing programs for dentists, pharmacists, nurses, and other healthcare providers. Most allied health professionals, including dental hygienists, physical therapists, and emergency medical technicians, were required to receive licensing by 1960. The health professions have generally advocated for state licensure in addition to standardized education and training.

Role of State Licensing Boards

State licensing boards serve as gatekeepers to control the entry of clinical practice. The role of the state boards is to confirm a provider's training and education and to administer a prerequisite examination before allowing providers to engage in clinical practice. The state boards issue licenses to providers who pass the examinations, renew licenses, and enforce the basic standards of the profession. Members of state boards generally consist of individuals in the profession and sometimes include consumer representatives. The state boards may function independently or as part of a state's department of health. State licensing boards operate under statutes and regulations and have oversight by the state legislature. The boards also maintain procedural rules.

The licensing of providers usually entails two components. First, they must have graduated from a school that has been certified in the state desired to practice in as well as pass a state-administered examination. Second, they must also provide the state board with basic information about themselves. The education requirement has allowed for state oversight of education curricula.

The renewal of a license is generally based on not having any disciplinary action against a provider since the period of the individual's last review and fulfilling a certain number of continuing-education units. If a provider, however, has had a disciplinary action against it, it must be given due process that entails a fair proceeding to contest the charges before the state board revokes or suspends its license. The provider must be properly informed of the charges and be given a fair hearing. An appeal board may determine if proper procedures were followed if a discipline is sanctioned, and the provider may appeal to the courts. Although disciplinary actions are made public, they are usually not widely publicized.

Issues of Licensing

The state licensure of healthcare providers raises several issues. Since licensure is carried out at the state level, there are wide variations in professional standards as well as in the enforcement of those standards. The coordination by states and the federal government on the NPDB is also precarious. Providers with disciplinary action against them may be able to evade enforcement officials and seek licensure to practice in another state.

The use of professional peers on state licensing boards is also an area of contention. Although professional peers have the credentials necessary to evaluate other providers in their profession, serious questions have been raised about the objectivity of such a review process and whether this is really a form of professional self-regulation. There are concerns that professional peer board members may be more interested in maintaining the reputation of their profession or may impose barriers to the entry of new providers to control competition. Furthermore, consumer advocates argue that the low level of enforcement by state licensing boards is indicative of the boards serving the interests of the profession over those of the public.

Future Implications

Licensing continues to play an important role as the cornerstone of ensuring quality in healthcare. However, there remain some concerns over whether licensing is best carried out at the state or federal level and whether the professions are able to adequately regulate themselves. Also, there are questions over whether patients are better protected by government oversight or through economic market forces. For the time being, state licensing remains the foundation for regulating the clinical practice of most healthcare professionals.

Jared Lane K. Maeda

See also American Medical Association (AMA); Malpractice; National Practitioner Data Bank; Nurses; Patient Safety; Physicians; Quality of Healthcare; Regulation

Further Readings

American Medical Association. *State Medical Licensure Requirements and Statistics.* Chicago: American Medical Association, 2007.

Ameringer, Carl F. *State Medical Boards and the Politics of Public Protection.* Baltimore: Johns Hopkins University Press, 1999.

Field, Robert I. *Health Care Regulation in America: Complexity, Confrontation, and Compromise.* New York: Oxford University Press, 2007.

Pawlson, L. Gregory, and Margaret E. O'Kane. "Professionalism, Regulation, and the Market: Impact on Accountability for Quality Care," *Health Affairs* 21(3): 200–207, May–June 2002.

Sacks, Terence J. *Careers in Medicine.* 3d ed. New York: McGraw-Hill, 2006.

Shryock, Richard H. *Medical Licensing in America, 1650–1965.* Baltimore: Johns Hopkins University Press, 1967.

Web Sites

American Medical Association (AMA): http://www.ama-assn.org

Council on Licensure, Enforcement and Regulation (CLEAR): http://www.clearhq.org

Federation of State Medical Boards (FSMB): http://www.fsmb.org

National Council of State Boards of Nursing (NCSBN): http://www.ncsbn.org

National Practitioner Data Bank (NPDB): http://www.npdb-hipdb.hrsa.gov

LIFE EXPECTANCY

Life expectancy is the average number of years that an individual of a given age is expected to live. Life expectancy may be determined by race, gender, or other characteristics using age-specific death rates or life tables for the population with that characteristic. Life expectancy at birth is often cited, but it can be given for any age group.

For example, in 2005, the life expectancy at birth for the total U. S. population was 77.8 years; for those 65 years of age, it was 83.7 years; and for those 75 years of age, it was 87.0 years.

Health services researchers use life expectancy as a broad indicator of the overall health of a given population. They often compare the life expectancy and health expenditures of nations with various health delivery systems. Although the United States has a higher life expectancy than the global average, it is only slightly higher than the average for developed nations. The United States ranks 48th highest in life expectancy, surpassed by nations such as Japan, Sweden, Switzerland, Australia, and Canada.

History

The English statistician John Graunt constructed the first life table, a statistical table that uses age-specific death rates to determine a group's average life expectancy. Graunt, who is considered the founder of the science of demography and vital statistics, was interested in studying the effects of epidemics on populations. He analyzed the *Bills of Mortality,* which recorded the weekly count of births and deaths in London parishes. In 1662, he published the results of his findings in *Natural and Political Observations Made Upon the Bills of Mortality.*

Edward Wigglesworth constructed the first life table in America in 1793. Wigglesworth used mortality data reported in 1789 from Massachusetts, Maine, and New Hampshire. He estimated the average life expectancy at birth was about 35 years.

Actuaries have been constructing and using life tables for decades to determine the premium rates for life insurance policies based on the average life expectancy of enrollees. Actuaries at the Social Security Administration (SSA) also use life tables to monitor Social Security enrollees. And the National Center for Health Statistics (NCHS) uses life tables to monitor mortality trends in the nation's population.

Recently, the concept of life expectancy has been modified to focus on healthy life expectancy, sometimes called health-adjusted life expectancy (HALE), which extends life expectancy measures by accounting for the health states of populations. In 2000, the World Health Organization (WHO)

reported for the first time healthy life expectancy for its 191 member countries.

Reasons for Increased Life Expectancy

During the 20th century, life expectancy in the United States rose dramatically. In 1900, the average life expectancy at birth for the nation's total population was 47.3 years; by 1999, it had increased to 76.7 years. This increase in lifespan is attributable to many advances in the nation's public health. In 1999, the Centers for Disease Control and Prevention (CDC) identified a number of factors that contributed to the dramatic increase in life expectancy, including vaccinations, control of infectious diseases, safer and healthier foods, healthier mothers and babies, safer workplaces, motor vehicle safety, decline in deaths from coronary heart disease and stroke, and recognition of tobacco use as a major health hazard.

Public health vaccination campaigns in the nation have eliminated many deadly diseases. Because of vaccinations, once common deadly diseases, such as diphtheria, tetanus, poliomyelitis, measles, mumps, and rubella, have been virtually eliminated. And smallpox has been totally eradicated.

Public health efforts led to the establishment of local and state health departments across the nation. These health departments initiated environmental and sanitation programs, such as clean drinking water, sewage disposal, garbage disposal, mosquito control, and educational programs, which decreased exposure to infectious diseases.

Safer and healthier foods were developed. Better food processing has resulted in fewer deaths because of microbial contamination. In addition, foods have become more nutritious; many are fortified to eliminate major nutritional deficiency diseases such as rickets, goiter, and pellagra.

Mother and infant deaths have been greatly reduced by better hygiene and nutrition programs. In addition, there was greater access to healthcare, family planning programs, antibiotics, and technological advances in maternal and neonatal medicine.

Work-related deaths, injuries, and health problems have greatly declined as a result of more safety measures and greater regulation. Once common diseases such as coal workers' pneumoconiosis (black lung) and silicosis have come under better control.

Engineering improvements in both vehicles and highways and changes in personal behavior, such as the use of safety belts, child safety seats, or motorcycle helmets, and decreased drinking and driving, has resulted in a large reduction in motor vehicle-related deaths.

The discovery of the major underlying risk factors of heart disease and stroke—smoking, diet, exercise, and blood pressure control—has resulted in smoking cessation and blood pressure control programs. There was also improved access to early detection and better medical treatment.

Since the 1964 Surgeon General's report on the health risks of smoking, smoking among adults has decreased, and millions of smoking-related deaths have been prevented. Public health anti-smoking campaigns have resulted in greater public awareness of the major health-related problems caused by smoking.

Future Implications

While the average life expectancy in the United States has risen to nearly 78 years, it seems unlikely that it will continue to increase at a fast pace in the future. Much of the past increase in life expectancy was due to decreases in infant mortality and infectious diseases, and other factors. In the future, any increase in life expectancy will likely be small incremental gains of perhaps a month or two per year. Some future years may even see a slight decrease in life expectancy due to factors such as increased diabetes and obesity.

Xinjian Du

See also Acute and Chronic Diseases; Comparing Health Systems; Epidemiology; Health Disparities; Mortality; Mortality, Major Causes in the United States; Public Health

Further Readings

Carey, James R. *Longevity: The Biology and Demography of Life Span*. Princeton, NJ: Princeton University Press, 2003.

Centers for Disease Control and Prevention. "Ten Great Public Health Achievements: United States, 1900–

1999," *Journal of the American Medical Association* 281(16): 1481–84, April 28, 1999.

Day, Peter, Jamie Pearce, and Danny Dorling, "Twelve Worlds: A Geo-Demographic Comparison of Global Inequalities in Mortality," *Journal of Epidemiology and Community Health* 62(11): 1002–1010, November 2008.

Perenboom, R. J. M., L. M. van Herten, H. C. Boshuizen, et al. "Life Expectancy Without Chronic Morbidity: Trends in Gender and Socioeconomic Disparities," *Public Health Reports* 120(1): 46–54, January–February 2005.

Web Sites

National Center for Health Statistics (NCHS): http://www.cdc.gov/nchs

National Institute on Aging (NIA): http://www.nia.nih.gov

Social Security Online: http://www.ssa.gov/OACT/STATS/table4c6.html

World Health Organization (WHO): http://www.who.int

LOMAS, JONATHAN

Jonathan Lomas was a faculty member in the department of clinical epidemiology and biostatistics at McMaster University in Hamilton, Ontario, Canada, from 1982 to 1997; Professor of Health Policy Analysis from 1992 to 1997; and inaugural Chief Executive Officer of the Canadian Health Services Research Foundation (CHSRF) from 1997 to 2007. Although Lomas's undergraduate training was in experimental psychology at Oxford University, his landmark contributions have been as a scholar in the field of health policy analysis and as an innovator in improving the relevance and use of health services research in health system decision making.

Lomas's scholarly contributions touched on all three "levels of health policy" (as he called them)—clinical policy, administrative/organizational policy, and public policy, but it was his research in the domain of clinical policy that first brought him widespread attention. His most widely cited scholarly article, "Do Practice Guidelines Guide Practice? The Effect of a Consensus Statement on the Practice of Physicians," was published in the prestigious *New England Journal of Medicine* in 1989. His research on administrative and public policy addressed highly topical policy issues such as the regionalization of health services delivery in Canada. His writing about innovative models for priority setting in health services research ("On Being a Good Listener . . ." *Milbank Quarterly,* 2003) and about conducting research in close partnership with health systems decision makers ("Using 'Linkage and Exchange' to Move Research Into Policy at a Canadian Foundation," *Health Affairs,* 2000) has been highly influential among research-funding organizations.

Under Lomas's leadership, the CHSRF designed its research programs (i.e., the Capacity for Applied and Developmental Research and Evaluation [CADRE] program) to build a critical mass of applied health services and nursing researchers in Canada and to create a supportive environment for these researchers to engage with decision makers. It also designed training and support programs for decision makers, such as the Executive Training for Research Application (EXTRA) program, and a widely emulated 1:3:25 rule for organizing research reports. Its program designs and "linkage and exchange" philosophy have served as a point of reference for many large and small organizations seeking to improve the use of research in decision making in Canada and internationally.

Lomas is also known for cofounding McMaster University's Centre for Health Economics and Policy Analysis, his scholarly work with the Population Health Programme of the Canadian Institute for Advanced Research (1988–2004), and his service contributions in Canada (Federal, Provincial, Territorial Advisory Committee to Deputy Ministers on Health Services, 1994–1996; Ontario Premier's Council on Health, Well-Being and Social Justice, 1991–1994; Interim Governing Council and Institute Advisory Board of the Canadian Institute of Health Research, 1999–2004) and the United States (member of the board of directors of the Association for Health Services Research and its successor AcademyHealth, 1999–2005).

He also made an impact through consultancies for the World Health Organization (WHO) and other international agencies in Australia, Indonesia, Myanmar, the Philippines, South Korea, Sri Lanka, and Thailand. He was a visiting scholar at the University of Gadjah Mada in Indonesia (1990), the University of Sydney and the Department of Health of the New South Wales Government in Australia (1996–1997), the Dutch national research and development agency ZonMw (2004), and the Ministry of Health in New Zealand (2007). In recognition of his scholarly and professional impact, the University of Montreal awarded him an honorary doctorate degree in 2005, and he was elected a fellow of the Royal Society of Canada and the Canadian Academy of Health Sciences in 2006.

John N. Lavis

See also AcademyHealth; Canadian Health Services Research Foundation (CHSRF); Canadian Institute of Health Services and Policy Research (IHSPR); Clinical Practice Guidelines; Epidemiology; Health Services Research in Canada; Public Health; Public Policy

Further Readings

Lomas, J., G. M. Anderson, K. Domnick-Pierre, et al. "Do Practice Guidelines Guide Practice? The Effect of a Consensus Statement on the Practice of Physicians," *New England Journal of Medicine* 321(19): 1306–1311, November 9, 1989.

Lomas, Jonathan. "Using 'Linkage and Exchange' to Move Research and Policy at a Canadian Foundation," *Health Affairs* 19(3): 236–40, May–June, 2000.

Lomas, Jonathan. "Health Services Research: More Lessons From Kaiser Permanente and Veterans' Affairs Healthcare System," *British Medical Journal* 327(7427): 1301–1302, December 6, 2003.

Lomas, Jonathan. "The In-Between World of Knowledge Brokering," *British Medical Journal* 334(7585): 129–32, January 20, 2007.

Lomas, Jonathan, Naomi Fulop, Diane Gagnon, et al. "On Being a Good Listener: Setting Priorities for Applied Health Services Research," *Milbank Quarterly* 81(3): 363–88, September 2003.

Web Sites

AcademyHealth: http://www.academyhealth.org
Canadian Health Services Research Foundation (CHSRF): http://www.chsrf.ca

LONG-TERM CARE

Long-term care (LTC) includes a wide variety of health and support services that are provided to the frail, the elderly, and individuals with chronic disease conditions and disabilities. LTC is largely personal, custodial, and unskilled care provided to those who cannot care for themselves for extended periods of time. The majority of those receiving LTC are the frail elderly who suffer from multiple chronic diseases. In the United States, about 60% of all individuals 65 years of age or older require at least some type of LTC services during their lifetime, and over 40% need care in a nursing home for some period of time. In 2006, there were 37.3 million people in the nation 65 years of age or older, or about one in every eight Americans. By 2030, the number is expected to grow to 71.5 million people, or about one in every five Americans. Although the family is the primary source of LTC, the increasing size of the nation's older population coupled with decreasing family size and high divorce rates will invariably increase the demand for paid LTC services.

The need for LTC services for people suffering from chronic disabilities is often estimated using the criteria of Activity of Daily Living (ADL) or the Limitations of the Instrumental Activities of Daily Living (IADL). The ADL criteria include bathing, dressing, getting in or out of bed, getting around inside, toileting, and eating; and the IADL criteria are light housework, laundry, meal preparation, grocery shopping, getting around outside, managing money, taking medications, and telephoning. According to the National Institute on Aging, in 2006, about 20% of all Medicare enrollees, including 5% who were institutionalized, had limitations in one or more ADLs. However, only about half of those individuals were estimated to be receiving personal care. The majority of those (65%) who received personal care obtained it from unpaid caregivers (i.e., spouse, adult children, other family members, and friends), about 26% received personal care from both unpaid and paid caregivers, and the remaining 8% received personal care from only paid caregivers.

Projected Demand for Paid Care

The demand for paid LTC services is expected to increase sharply in the future because of the growth in the nation's older population. A simulation study conducted by the Urban Institute in 2007 estimates that between 2000 and 2040 the number of older adults with chronic disabilities in the nation will more than double, increasing from about 10 million to about 21 million individuals. Although the study projected an overall declining rate of old-age disability during the period, the total number of individuals with disabilities will more than double simply because of the enormous size of the older population by 2040. This trend is troubling because at the same time that it will be occurring, family size is likely to decline, and there will be rising divorce rates and an increase in female employment rates. As a result, the demand for paid LTC services is projected to increase sharply in the future. The study estimates that the number of old people receiving paid home care will increase from 2.2 million to 5.2 million and the number of older nursing home residents will increase from 1.2 million to 2.7 million individuals.

Financing Long-Term Care

Meeting the projected need for LTC will be a daunting task for both the private and the public sectors, considering that LTC services for older adults already represent a substantial share of the nation's total healthcare spending. In 2005, nursing home and home health care accounted for slightly over 10% of national personal health expenditures, or about $169 billion. This amount does not include care provided by family or friends on an unpaid basis (often called "informal care"). It only includes the costs of care from paid providers.

The largest share, 48%, of the nation's LTC costs are paid for by Medicaid, a jointly funded state and federal program; state and local governments pay for 19%; and the private sector (through out-of-pocket and insurance premiums) pays 31% of the total LTC costs. However, the federal government pays for LTC through its portion of the Medicaid program and also through the Medicare program. These two sources pay for 50% of the nation's LTC costs, making the federal government the single largest payer for LTC.

Medicare Coverage

Since the implementation of Medicare's hospital prospective payment system in 1983, which encouraged the nation's hospitals to shorten patient length of stays and discharge patients as quickly as possible, nursing homes have seen an increasing number of individuals requiring post-acute rehabilitation. Specifically, Medicare Part A will pay for their care at a skilled-nursing facility (SNF) only if the care occurs within 30 days of a hospitalization of 3 or more days and is certified as medically necessary. Covered services are similar to those for inpatient hospital stays but also include rehabilitation services and medical equipment. However, Medicare does not cover nursing facility care if the individual does not require skilled nursing or skilled rehabilitation services. Although the number of SNF days provided by Medicare is limited to 100 days per benefit period, the average length of stay in an SNF is usually less than 2 weeks. Under Medicare, no copayment is required for up to 20 days; a copayment is required for Days 21 to 100; and after 100 days, the individual pays the total cost.

While SNF care may be viewed as an extension of hospital inpatient care rather than true LTC, home health care has increasingly been transformed into a source of long-term personal assistance for Medicare beneficiaries, especially those with severe functional limitations and cognitive impairment. Both Medicare Part A and B cover part-time or intermittent skilled nursing care and home health aide services, and some therapies that are ordered by a physician and provided by a Medicare-certified home health agency. Specifically, Part A covers the first 100 visits following a 3-day hospital stay or an SNF stay, and Part B covers any visits thereafter. Home health care under Part A and B has no copayment and no deductible.

Medicare Part A covers hospice care for individuals with a terminal illness, generally individuals who are not expected to live more than 6 months. Although Medicare does not consider hospice care to be an LTC service, an increasing number of hospice patients are living well beyond 6 months, and hospices are becoming more like an LTC setting for those with terminal illnesses who are bed-stricken. Hospice services include drugs for symptom control and pain relief, medical and support services from a Medicare-approved hospice provider, and other services not otherwise covered by Medicare (e.g., grief counseling). Hospice care is usually provided in a patient's home (which may include a nursing home if that is where the patient lives) or a hospice care facility. However, Medicare does cover some short-term hospital and inpatient respite care provided to a hospice patient to allow the usual caregiver to rest.

Medicaid Coverage

Although the number of short stays has increased, the majority of nursing home residents require long-term custodial care. Most nursing home care is paid for by Medicaid and by the resident's own resources. According to the National Center for Health Statistics 2004 National Nursing Home Survey, Medicaid paid for at least some of their care for 65% of all nursing home residents, private/other sources paid for 22%, and Medicare paid for 13%.

During the past decade, a growing number of older individuals have opted to reside in community residential facilities, such as assisted living facilities, board and care, and continuing-care retirement communities, instead of being placed into nursing homes. Currently, an estimated 1 million individuals live in residential facilities, largely financed from their own resources. The public sector has taken note of this trend. States, which have been concerned about the increasing number of Medicaid residents in nursing homes, have started using Medicaid to fund those living at home and in the community through Home and Community-Based Service (HCBS) waiver programs. The primary purpose of such programs is to keep those at risk of being institutionalized in nursing homes at home or in the community. The program provides family members with supplementary services including adult day care services to help them continue to provide care. Some states are also trying to relocate nursing home residents back in the community. As a result of these and other changes, the percentage of total Medicaid spending on nursing homes was reduced to 44% in 2006, and the percentage of spending for home health and personal care increased to 41%.

Dual Eligible Beneficiaries

Some Medicare enrollees also are Medicaid recipients, and they are called *dual eligibles*. For those who are dual eligibles, Medicare covers its set of medical services, while Medicaid pays for the individual's Medicare premiums and cost sharing, and—for those below certain income and asset thresholds—LTC services. The dual eligibles tend to be older, sicker, poorer, and they use more expensive medical services. The dual eligibles have an important impact on LTC spending. Since Medicare covers SNF care, some dual-eligible patients are discharged from hospitals to SNF for LTC services. After Medicare stops paying for their care, the dual eligibles rely on Medicaid to pay for their LTC services. In some cases, noninstitutional options may have been more appropriate, which may have provided better outcomes for the individual and lower costs for both Medicare and Medicaid. Efforts are now being made to better coordinate and integrate LTC services between Medicare and Medicaid.

Private Coverage

Medicare and Medicaid are not ideal providers of LTC. For the most part, Medicare was designed to provide acute care not LTC, and the Medicaid program was designed to provide medical care to the deserving poor in certain limited categories, particularly women and children. Specifically, Medicare only pays for medically necessary SNF or home health care. While Medicare pays for about 18% of LTC, it only pays under specific circumstances. If the type of care needed does not meet Medicare's rules, it does not pay. In terms of Medicaid, individuals with assets and financial resources often do not qualify for Medicaid unless they use up their resources by paying for care and become poor. Furthermore, states apply strict preadmission screening to deter people from being institutionalized in nursing homes.

Because of the many problems associated with Medicare and Medicaid, most people who need LTC end up paying for some or all of their care using their own assets and financial resources. However, LTC is very expensive. For example, based on national averages for 2006, a semiprivate room in a nursing home costs $171 per day, a private room in a nursing home costs $194 per day, a stay in an assisted living facility (one-bedroom unit) costs $2,691 per month, the use of a home health aide service costs $25 per hour, the use of a homemaker service costs $17 per hour, and a stay in an adult day healthcare center costs $56 per day.

To pay the costs of LTC, some people purchase LTC insurance. Currently, about 10% of the nation's population purchase LTC insurance. The average annual premium costs for a policy purchased in 2005, across all age groups of buyers and all types of insurance policies, was just over $1,900. This represents a comprehensive policy (covering both nursing facilities and at-home care) that provides an average of 5.5 years worth of benefits, with a daily benefit payment of $143. Most policies purchased also included some form of automatic inflation protection.

Other insurance also pays for some limited LTC services. Most Medicare enrollees purchase a Medicare supplemental insurance plan, or Medigap insurance, which is sold by private health insurance companies to cover some of the "gaps" in expenses that are not covered by Medicare. In addition to covering some of the costs of Medicare's copayments and deductibles, some Medigap policies also provide additional benefits such as at-home recovery care.

A reverse mortgage may also be an option for some individuals who need LTC and expect to live in their current home for several years. A reverse mortgage is a special type of home equity loan, where home owners 62 years of age or older receive a loan against their home that does not have to be paid back as long as they live in their home. The home owner receives a lump-sum payment, a monthly payment, or a line of credit against the value of the home without selling it.

Public Policy: Acts Related to Long-Term Care

A number of federal acts are directly related to LTC. Some of the major acts include the Deficit Reduction Act of 2005, the Older Americans Act of 2001, the Millennium Health Care and Benefits Act of 1999, and the Balanced Budget Act of 1997. Each act is discussed below.

Deficit Reduction Act of 2005

The Deficit Reduction Act of 2005 refined the eligibility requirement for state Medicaid recipients by tightening standards for citizenship and immigration documentation and by changing the rules concerning LTC eligibility. Specifically, the period for determining community spouse income and assets was lengthened from 36 to 60 months, individuals whose homes exceeded $500,000 in value were disqualified, and the states were required to impose partial months of ineligibility. The act also contained a provision allowing for the expansion of a National LTC Partnership program to all states. The goal of the program is to encourage individuals to purchase private LTC insurance. In the program, individuals who exhaust their LTC insurance benefits can retain a greater amount of their assets and still qualify for state Medicaid, without having to "spend down." Specifically, purchasers would be allowed to keep a dollar of assets for every dollar they receive in benefits from the program. The ability to retain additional assets, yet still use Medicaid as a "safety net" if private coverage does not suffice, is an incentive for more individuals to purchase at least a moderate amount of private coverage.

Older Americans Act of 2001

The Older Americans Act of 2001 is one of the most significant laws affecting LTC. It changed the bias toward institutionalizing LTC. In passing the act, the U.S. Congress recognized the family's role in providing LTC. The act has the goal of retaining the family as caregivers of the elderly who desire to be cared for in the home. It provides funding, through state and local Aging Network agencies, to help families and older individuals remain independent within their communities. While there are no specific financial eligibility criteria for Older Americans Act services, they are generally targeted at low-income, frail seniors over age 60 and minority elders and seniors living in rural areas.

Millennium Health Care and Benefits Act of 1999

The Millennium Health Care and Benefits Act of 1999 expanded the Veterans Health Administration's (VHA) programs to increase access to nursing home care and other extended care services to veterans who do not have service-related disabilities but who are unable to pay the costs of necessary care. For those who qualify, the benefits can provide financial assistance for some LTC costs. Copayments may apply depending on the veteran's income level. The VHA also has a Housebound and Aid and Attendance Allowance Program that provides cash grants to eligible disabled veterans and surviving spouses in lieu of formally provided homemaker, personal-care, and other services needed for assistance in activities of daily living and other help at home.

Balanced Budget Act of 1997

Several provisions of the Balanced Budget Act of 1997 addressed the explosive growth of Medicare's home health care expenses in the early 1990s. Home health care, which in 1989 accounted for only 2.5% of all Medicare Part A expenditures, exceeded 15% of the total in 1996. To stem the growth, the act moved home health care to a prospective payment system, and it discouraged hospital ownership of home healthcare agencies. The act dramatically reduced Medicare's home health care expenditures and utilization; expenditures in the following 2 years after the act's passage declined by 52%, the percentage of Medicare beneficiaries receiving home health care services for the first time declined by about 20%, and the use among those who availed of these services declined by 39%.

Future Implications

The projected future growth in the nation's older population will seriously challenge both the private and the public sectors. With declining family size and high divorce rates, the need for paid LTC services will greatly increase in the future. Many future retirees will likely not have the necessary financial resources to afford the LTC they need. The future strain on the Medicare and Medicaid programs will be enormous. To address these issues, policymakers must develop new innovative ways of financing and providing LTC, which politicians will support and the general public will accept.

Kyusuk Chung

See also Chronic Care Model; Continuum of Care; Disability; Long-Term Care Costs in the United States; Medicaid; Medicare; Nursing Homes; Skilled-Nursing Facilities

Further Readings

Buelow, Janet R. *Listening to the Voices of Long-Term Care*. Lanham, MD: University Press of America, 2007.

Gibson, Mary Jo, and Donald L. Redfoot. *Comparing Long-Term Care in Germany and the United States: What Can We Learn From Each Other?* Washington, DC: AARP Public Policy Institute, 2007.

Golant, Stephen M., and Joan Hyde, eds. *The Assisted Living Residence: A Vision for the Future*. Baltimore: Johns Hopkins University Press, 2008.

Jurkowski, Elaine Theresa. *Policy and Program Planning for Older Americans: Realities and Visions*. New York: Springer, 2008.

Morris, Michael, and Johnette Hartnett. *Disability, Long-Term Care, and Health Care in the 21st Century*. New York: Nova Science, 2009.

Presho, Margaret, ed. *Managing Long Term Conditions: A Social Model for Community Practice*. Hoboken, NJ: Wiley-Blackwell, 2008.

Pruchno, Rachael A., and Michael A. Smyer, eds. *Challenges of an Aging Society: Ethical Dilemmas, Political Issues*. Baltimore: Johns Hopkins University Press, 2007.

Sullivan-Marx, Eileen, and Deanna Gray-Miceli, eds. *Leadership and Management Skills for Long-Term Care*. New York: Springer, 2008.

Web Sites

AARP: http://www.aarp.org

American Society on Aging (ASA): http://www.asaging.org

National Clearinghouse for Long-Term Care Information: http://www.longtermcare.gov

National Council on Aging (NCOA): http://www.ncoa.org

National Institute on Aging (NIA): http://www.nia.nih.gov

LONG-TERM CARE COSTS IN THE UNITED STATES

Long-term care (LTC) is often viewed as a service involving only the elderly. In reality, individuals of all ages, including children, nonelderly adults, as well as older persons, use LTC services. Approximately 37% of LTC recipients are under 65 years of age. Individuals in these three age groups can be further subdivided into classes, including those individuals facing physical challenges, persons with persistent and severe mental illness, children with developmental disabilities, adults with intellectual disabilities, persons with some type of dementia, and individuals with some combination of these challenges.

In 2005, expenditures in the United States for LTC services such as nursing home care, assisted living, and home health totaled over $200 billion. Roughly 72% of those expenditures came from the public coffers, largely the Medicaid or Medicare programs, with payments from private insurance (7.2%), other private spending (2.7%), and out-of-pocket expenditures by individuals accounting for most of the rest of spending on formal LTC services.

Indeed, LTC is an area of healthcare where consumers or their families pay a relatively substantial proportion of the costs of formal care. Historically, for the health services used by the elderly, only expenditures for prescription medications have been more heavily funded by out-of-pocket expenditures. In 2005, out-of-pocket expenditures for LTC financed 18% ($37 billion) of the costs of all LTC services.

Costs are quite high for those paying for LTC from personal funds, especially when one considers the average income of those frail and vulnerable individuals in need of it. In 2006, the estimated average annual cost of a private room in a nursing home was just over $70,000. For those who could afford it, a private room in an assisted living facility might cost more than $30,000 a year for room, board, oversight, and basic services, such as medication assistance, with the potential for substantial additional costs for special services, such as more extensive personal care, medications, and therapies. With an hourly cost of an estimated $25 per hour for a home health aide, an individual receiving only 4 hours of personal care assistance per day would spend more than $36,000 a year for such help.

While much attention is focused on public expenditures for care, it is important to emphasize that no matter which group of LTC recipients we

discuss, informal caregivers provide the vast majority of care. Family and friends provide an estimated 80% of all LTC. Informal caregivers typically provide many hours of care each week, and the average duration of caregiving is over 4 years—and usually longer for caregivers of persons with Alzheimer's disease. Nearly half of these caregivers place their own economic status and retirement at risk by reducing or losing employment and income to provide care. The value of unpaid care is difficult to determine, but in 2006, the AARP Policy Institute estimated that the value of unpaid LTC was $354 billion annually, which substantially exceeded the total expenditures on formal services.

Long-Term Care and the Elderly

The variety of individuals receiving LTC and the variety of settings in which it can be provided make it difficult to succinctly summarize all aspects of its costs. The remainder of this entry focuses on LTC costs for the frail elderly, who constitute more than 60% of those needing LTC services. Special attention is given to the projected LTC costs associated with aging among the baby boomer generation.

High mortality rates and lower life expectancy during the 19th and early 20th centuries kept the issue of LTC off the policy agenda. Life expectancy at birth in 1900 in the United States was only 47 years, and children with profound disabilities and individuals with developmental disabilities had an even more limited life expectancy. The few persons who survived into old age in America were cared for either by their families at home or in the local "poor farms" or "almshouses" supported by local or county governments or charitable organizations. Many of those with persistent and severe mental illness also faced institutional care or relegation to poor farms. But, by 2004, life expectancy at birth was almost 78 years, life expectancy for someone aged 65 years had increased to 84, and life expectancy for someone at 75 years of age had increased to nearly 87.

In the mid 20th century came the passage of the Medicare and Medicaid programs. That legislation placed LTC costs firmly on the policy agendas of the states and the federal government. The Medicaid program, which is jointly funded by the states and the federal government, pays for the vast majority of LTC costs. In 2005, Medicaid paid just over $100 billion for nursing home and home care services, almost 49% of the total costs of these services, compared with just over $42 billion (20%) paid by Medicare for these same types of services.

A major concern of some policymakers has been the transfer of assets by the elderly to younger family members to qualify for Medicaid LTC services. However, the U.S. Government Accountability Office (GAO) analysis of the 2002 Health and Retirement Study data indicated that those elderly most likely to need LTC services had a median annual income of less than $14,000 and median nonhousing assets of less than $4,000. Recapture of transferred assets in such a population is not likely to have a significant impact on Medicaid expenditures for LTC.

One of the current policy debates surrounding LTC costs is *rebalancing*. Since the implementation of Medicaid, public funding for LTC has almost exclusively supported the provision of LTC in institutional settings (nursing homes). At the same time, almost all consumers would prefer to receive LTC in a community setting, and public funding agencies want to reduce expenditures for the most expensive type of LTC, nursing homes. Rebalancing is typically thought of as requiring an increase in the proportion of funding going to community-based care while reducing the proportion of funds going to nursing home care. Another alternative, of course, is simply expanding expenditures for LTC and targeting these additional funds for use in other forms of residential LTC and for home- and community-based services.

Rebalancing is currently far from complete. In 2005, almost two thirds of LTC expenditures went to support nursing home care for individuals with severe physical and cognitive impairment. Despite this, the inadequacy of nursing home reimbursement is apparent. The majority of nursing homes are understaffed and thus at risk of being unable to meet the needs of their residents.

Another policy option that many hoped would help reduce the public costs of LTC was LTC insurance. However, LTC insurance has not seen the growth in the number of policyholders needed before it can serve as a substitute for a significant proportion of Medicaid payments to nursing homes. The elderly find it difficult to afford LTC insurance, and younger individuals have shown little interest in paying premiums now for benefits that they may need in 30 to 40 years.

Dealing With the Baby Boomers

No discussion of LTC costs in this country can be complete without a discussion of what many see as the looming explosion in LTC needs and expenditures as the baby boomer generation ages. Baby boomers include those individuals born between 1946 and 1964. Based on estimates from the Urban Institute's simulations, the number of older adults with disabilities will increase from 10 million to 21 million from 2000 to 2040. The number of elderly receiving paid home care will increase from 2.2 million to 5.3 million, while the number of nursing home residents will grow from 1.2 to 2.7 million. All this will occur at the same time that the number of middle-aged or younger individuals who might serve as informal or formal caregivers will fall because of long-term reductions in the nation's birth rate.

As the more than 70 million baby boomers age, some estimates indicate that Medicaid costs will grow from 3% of the U.S. gross domestic product (GDP) in 2000 to approximately 11% of GDP by 2080. Some researchers argue relatively persuasively that reduced disability in the elderly population could dramatically reduce these projected expenditure levels.

These population dynamics and cost projections have raised serious concern among many analysts and policymakers. The federal government's response to these concerns, at this point, has largely been an attempt to increase individual responsibility by encouraging the purchase of LTC insurance and increased personal savings for LTC costs. The Centers for Medicare and Medicaid Services (CMS) informational campaign for Medicare recipients, titled "Own Your Own Future," is only one example of this approach.

As the baby boomers age, the nation will be faced with a series of difficult decisions. How much of the cost of LTC is the responsibility of society, and how much is the responsibility of the individual? What reallocations of social and personal resources will be necessary to meet the challenges presented by the projected explosion in the number of frail elders who will need LTC? What is an equitable distribution of total LTC spending?

How can we balance spending for the elderly's LTC needs with other pressing social priorities?

However, we might do well to remember that at each stage of its life course the baby boomer generation has presented unprecedented challenges to our society. First, this generation needed expanded public school services; then they needed expanded higher education; and then they needed jobs. At each point, our society successfully reallocated or generated the resources to meet those needs. One can only wonder how this looming challenge will differ from those earlier trials.

Charles D. Phillips and Catherine Hawes

See also Centers for Medicare and Medicaid Services (CMS); Cost of Healthcare; Life Expectancy; Long-Term Care; Medicaid; Medicare; Nursing Homes; Payment Mechanisms

Further Readings

Gibson, Mary Jo, and Ari N. Houser. *Valuing the Invaluable: A New Look at the Economic Value of Family Caregiving.* Washington, DC: AARP, 2006.

Johnson, Richard W., Desmond Toohey, and Joshua M. Weiner. *Meeting the Long-Term Care Needs of the Baby Boomers: How Changing Families Will Affect Paid Helpers and Institutions.* The Retirement Project, Discussion Paper 07–04. Washington, DC: Urban Institute, 2007.

Komisar, Harriet L., and Lee Shirey Thompson. *National Spending on Long-Term Care.* Fact Sheet, Long-Term Care Financing Project. Washington DC: Georgetown University, 2007.

Koitz, Dave, Mellissa D. Bobb, and Ben Page. *The Looming Budgetary Impact of Society's Aging.* Congressional Budget Office Long-Range Fiscal Policy Brief, No. 2. Washington, DC: Congressional Budget Office, July 3, 2002.

Manton, Kenneth G., Gene R. Lowrimore, Arthur D. Ulian, et al. "Labor Force Participation and Human Capital Increases in an Aging Population and Implications for U.S. Research Investment," *Proceedings of the National Academy of Sciences* 104(26): 10802–10807, June 26, 2007.

Miller, Edward Allan, and Vincent Mor. *Out of the Shadows: Envisioning a Brighter Future for Long-Term Care in America.* Providence, RI: Brown University, Center for Gerontology and Health Care Research, 2006.

National Alliance for Caregiving and AARP. *Caregiving in the U.S.* Washington, DC: National Alliance for Caregiving and AARP, 2004.

U.S. Government Accountability Office. *Medicaid: Transfers of Assets by Elderly Individuals to Obtain Long-Term Care Coverage.* GAO-05-968. Washington, DC: Government Accountability Office, 2005.

Web Sites

AARP: http://www.aarp.org

Centers for Medicare and Medicaid Services (CMS): http://www.cms.hhs.gov

Congressional Budget Office (CBO): http://www.cbo.gov

Urban Institute (UI): http://www.urban.org

U.S. Government Accountability Office (GAO): http://www.gao.gov

LUFT, HAROLD S.

Harold S. Luft is a leading health services researcher. He is perhaps best known for his work on how health maintenance organizations (HMOs) achieve cost savings compared with fee-for-service medicine and his discovery of the volume-quality relationship in healthcare—the inverse relationship between the volume of hospital procedures performed and in-hospital patient mortality for certain surgeries and medical conditions.

Luft is the former Caldwell B. Esselstyn Professor of Health Policy and Health Economics and director of the Institute for Health Policy Studies at the University of California, San Francisco (UCSF). In 2008, he became the director of the Palo Alto Medical Foundation Research Institute.

Born in 1947 in Newark, New Jersey, Luft received his bachelor's degree, master's degree, and doctorate from Harvard University, where he specialized in health sector economics and public finance. Prior to joining UCSF in 1978, he was an assistant professor in the Health Services Research Program at Stanford University.

Luft has undertaken research in a variety of areas, including the applications of cost-benefit analysis, the relationship between hospital volumes and patient outcomes, the regionalization of hospital services, HMOs, risk assessment and risk adjustment, quality and outcomes of care, and healthcare reform in various states and communities. He also has studied the role of large databases and informatics tools to improve healthcare.

Throughout his long career, Luft has authored or coauthored five books and almost 200 scientific journal articles. His most recent book, *Total Cure: Rebuilding the American Healthcare System,* proposes a fundamental restructuring of the nation's financing and delivery of healthcare. He also has served on many editorial boards, including the journal *Inquiry,* and was the coeditor-in-chief of *Health Services Research* from 1997 to 2006.

Luft has received many awards and recognitions for his outstanding contributions to the field. He was awarded the Investigator Award in Health Policy Research from the Robert Wood Johnson Foundation (RWJF) in 2004; the Distinguished Investigator Award from the Association of Health Services Research in 1999; and the William B. Graham Prize for Health Services Research, sponsored by the Association of University Programs in Health Administration (AUPHA) and the Baxter Allegiance Foundation, in 1998. He also was a fellow of the Center for Advanced Study in Behavioral Sciences, the National Science Foundation, and the Carnegie Foundation and a Graduate Prize Fellow at Harvard University.

Luft is a member of the National Academy of Sciences, Institute of Medicine (IOM). He was a member of and chaired the National Advisory Council of the Agency for Health Care Policy and Research (now the Agency for Healthcare Research and Quality). He is a research associate at the National Bureau of Economic Research (NBER). In addition, Luft has served on the board of AcademyHealth. And he also has been a consultant to a number of federal agencies, including the Health Care Financing Administration (HCFA) (now the Centers for Medicare and Medicaid Services [CMS]), the National Institute of Mental Health (NIMH), the U.S Commission on Civil Rights, and the U.S. General Accounting Office (GAO) (now the U.S. General Accountability Office).

Luft has also been pivotally involved in multidisciplinary postdoctoral training for more than 35 years. He served as the codirector or associate director for three training programs sponsored jointly by UCSF and the University of California, Berkeley.

Ross M. Mullner

See also Health Economics; Health Maintenance Organizations (HMO); Managed Care; National Health Insurance; Public Policy; Quality of Healthcare; Volume-Outcome Relationship

Further Readings

Luft, Harold S. "Assessing the Evidence on HMO Performance," *Milbank Memorial Fund Quarterly* 58(4): 501–36, 1980.

Luft, Harold S. "Health Maintenance Organizations and the Rationing of Medical Care," *Milbank Memorial Fund Quarterly* 60(2): 268–306, 1982.

Luft, Harold S. *Total Cure: Rebuilding the American Healthcare System.* Cambridge, MA: Harvard University Press, 2008.

Luft, Harold S. "Universal Health Care Coverage: A Potential Hybrid Solution," *Journal of the American Medical Association* 297(10): 1115–18, March 14, 2007.

Luft Harold S., John P. Bunker, and Alain C. Enthoven. "Should Operations Be Regionalized? The Empirical Relation Between Surgical Volume and Mortality," *New England Journal of Medicine* 301(25): 1364–69, December 20, 1979.

Luft, Harold S., Sandra S. Hunt, and Susan C. Maerki. "The Volume-Outcome Relationship: Practice-Makes-Perfect or Selective-Referral Patterns?" *Health Services Research* 22(2): 157–82, June 1987.

Web Sites

Palo Alto Medical Foundation (PAMF) Research Institute: http://www.pamf.org/research

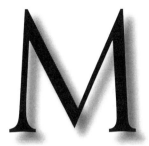

Malpractice

Malpractice is defined as professional negligence that results in injury or harm to an individual. Although the term *malpractice* can be applied to other professions, the most common reference is in the area of medicine or healthcare. The Joint Commission defines malpractice as "improper or unethical conduct or unreasonable lack of skill by a holder of a professional or official position." Malpractice arises from the branch of law called tort law or civil law, where a remedy can be provided for the action. This is different from criminal law or penal law, where causes of action lead to prosecution. When malpractice occurs in healthcare delivery, it is referred to as *medical malpractice,* although it can involve any healthcare provider or facility.

This entry focuses first on the elements necessary to establish a claim of medical malpractice. Then, it discusses the incidence of malpractice. Last, this entry addresses the limitations that may occur as a result of medical malpractice claims.

Elements of Malpractice

To make a claim that medical malpractice has occurred, a claimant must establish four elements: (1) duty, (2) breach of duty, (3) causation, and (4) damages. All four of these elements must exist and must be proven for a medical malpractice claim to be satisfied. Unlike criminal actions, where the standard is "beyond a reasonable doubt," in civil actions such as malpractice, the standard of proof is "the preponderance of evidence, which means more likely than not," or 51 on a scale of 100.

Duty

The *duty of care* is a legal obligation that requires that an individual adhere to a reasonable standard of care when performing acts that could cause harm to another. Although the law does not necessarily define the duty of care, its meaning may develop through common law or local customs. For example, physicians generally are said to have a duty of care by virtue of the physician–patient relationship. This relationship may be established when a patient first makes an appointment to receive care and treatment, or it may be established when a physician is consulted to render emergency care and treatment. Hospital or other healthcare facility personnel are said to have a duty of care because they are either employees or contractors for an agent that agrees to deliver services to a patient. Pharmacists also have a duty of care when they can reasonably foresee that their actions or inactions could reasonably cause harm to clients. Although all healthcare employees generally are expected to honor the duty of care for patients under their care, there have been cases where employees have successfully argued that they did not have a duty of care because provision of care would have violated their own ethical principles.

In healthcare, the duty a professional owes to an individual under his or her care is based on *standards of care.* Standards of care address the reasonableness of care and hold a professional accountable to deliver care as would a reasonable person with similar training and skills in similar circumstances. This is known as the *reasonable-person standard.*

Standards of care may be defined in a number of ways. For an individual holding a license to practice a profession, the standard may be defined through the elements articulated in a scope of professional practice. This is generally one of the ways by which standards of care can be established for physicians, dentists, nurses, physical and occupational therapists, and other similarly credentialed individuals. Standards of care also may be established by state laws, by accrediting and professional associations, and through organizational policies and procedures that govern how care is to be rendered.

Depending on the locale, standards of care may follow national standards or be based on local customs and practices. If a national standard is applied, this means that the reasonable-person standard would be based on what similarly trained individuals with similar skills would do under the same conditions anywhere in the United States. On the other hand, if a local standard is applied, the standard would reflect what similarly trained individuals would be expected to do in communities that have the characteristics of the community where the care was rendered. Since most healthcare professionals are expected to be educated to deliver care anywhere, it is more common to find a national standard of care applied.

In determining the applicable standard of care for specific actions of a professional, there is an expectation that if a professional carries out a task *requiring* special knowledge and skill, she or he will be evaluated as if she or he *possessed* the requisite knowledge and skill to perform the task. For example, if a resident physician performs a procedure such as insertion of a chest tube and causes the patient harm, that resident will be judged by the standards that govern the insertion of a chest tube by a fully trained physician in the appropriate medical specialty. If those reasonable-person standards are not met, the resident will be deemed to have deviated from acceptable standards of practice.

The issue of "reasonable person" often emerges when more than one group of professionals possess the knowledge and training to carry out a specific role. This can occur, for example, when advanced-practice nurses, physician's assistants, or other similarly credentialed individuals perform functions that had previously been only in the scope of physician practice. In these cases, the other professionals will be held to the same standard as that expected of the physician.

Breach of Duty

A *breach of duty* occurs when the care rendered is unreasonable or fails to meet the reasonable-person standard of care previously described. In medical malpractice, an expert witness is generally called upon to help establish the applicable standard of care and then to testify as to whether the healthcare professional met or breached the standard established.

There are three common legal terms that relate to the manner in which a professional might fail to meet the applicable standard: (1) nonfeasance, (2) misfeasance, and (3) malfeasance. *Nonfeasance* refers to the failure to do something that was expected. For example, if the applicable standard of care for a particular hospital indicates that a medical patient's vital signs are to be taken every 4 hours, failure to take them at that interval as a minimum would constitute nonfeasance. Similarly, if a patient had laboratory tests ordered and the laboratory, although able, failed to collect the necessary specimens, that would also be considered nonfeasance. Nonfeasance is also referred to as an *error of omission.* Failure to act or nonfeasance, in itself, however, does not constitute malpractice.

Misfeasance occurs when there are errors due to mistakes or carelessness. Medical errors such as wrong-site surgery, administration of medication or treatments to the wrong patient, failure to adequately respond to information about changes in a patient's medical condition, or prescribing medications that may be contraindicated based on a patient's other medications or medical history are examples of mistakes or carelessness. These types of errors are also referred to as *errors of commission.* In its report *To Err Is Human: Building a Safer Health System,* the national Institute of Medicine (IOM) identifies the types of errors that commonly occur in healthcare and establishes strategies to improve communication between healthcare workers as an approach to reducing these errors. In addition, the Joint Commission has identified strategies to improve institutional responses to *sentinel events,* those instances of misfeasance that lead to death or serious injury. Although most of the breaches of standards of care that lead to claims of malpractice come from errors and mistakes that are deemed misfeasance, not all misfeasance will lead to sustainable claims of malpractice.

Malfeasance is intentional wrongdoing. It occurs when an individual or group does something that is legally or morally wrong. An example of intentional wrongdoing in healthcare might be filling a patient's prescription for an expensive medication with a placebo yet charging the patient or the health insurance company for the medication that was ordered. At a time when the cost and quality of healthcare are under intense scrutiny, it has been argued that health insurance company actions denying access to needed costly services for subscribers is also a form of malfeasance. Although malfeasance can result in allegations of malpractice, the intentional wrongdoing often makes this a criminal offense.

Causation

The third element that is necessary to establish a claim of malpractice is that the breach of duty or failure to meet the prescribed standard of care must be the direct cause of injury to the patient. This is often the most difficult element to prove in a lawsuit that arises out of an act of negligence. To satisfy this element, the plaintiff or injured party must prove that but for the actions of the healthcare provider, the injury sustained would not have occurred. Causation is attributed based on the concept of probability. To satisfy this element, an expert witness must be able to state to a degree of reasonable probability (51%) that the injury was caused by the breach of standard of care.

Major discrepancies can exist between the plaintiff's and the healthcare professional defendant's positions about causation even if there is agreement that the professional did not meet the applicable standard of care. For example, a nurse providing care to a mother in labor may have incorrectly read the fetal monitor strips. Although the nurse did not recognize some of the changes on the strip, this error may not be deemed to have caused an injury when the infant was born with a congenital malformation. However, an expert witness for the plaintiff might allege that the failure to correctly read the fetal monitor strips led to a delay in the delivery of the infant, which further compromised the infant's condition at birth.

Sometimes there are areas of disagreement about causation depending on the types of healthcare providers involved and the applicable scopes of practice. For example, if a nurse saw that a patient was not responding to a particular treatment or medication and communicated that to the physician and the physician delayed getting to the hospital to care for the patient, it may not be possible to attribute responsibility to the nurse for the delay. However, if the nurse saw that the patient was not responding to treatment and communicated it only in the medical record, without making the physician aware of the problem, then he or she could be judged with a reasonable degree of medical probability to have caused the injury that occurred to the patient as the result of delayed medical care.

Damages

The final element that must be satisfied in a case alleging malpractice is that damages have occurred. To recover damages, a plaintiff must establish that he or she suffered physical, financial, or emotional injury as the result of the healthcare professional's deviation from the acceptable standard of care. If a plaintiff is able to establish that all the elements of malpractice have been satisfied and a judge or jury agrees with this determination, a monetary settlement is imposed to compensate for the injuries sustained.

There are three types of damages that may be awarded to a plaintiff: (1) economic, (2) noneconomic, and (3) punitive. Economic damages are the result of actual costs or financial losses sustained by the plaintiff or his or her family because of the negligence. These may include the cost of additional or subsequent care associated with any residual impairment, lost wages of the individual or of a family member who has had to provide care to the injured individual, and estimations of future care costs.

Noneconomic damages are those damages that the law assumes to accumulate from the consequences of the negligent act. The plaintiff can be compensated for emotional stress, interference with his or her enjoyment of life, and what has been called pain and suffering. Although some jurisdictions have made efforts to limit awards for noneconomic damages, they still constitute a significant amount of the damage recovery for a plaintiff.

Punitive damages are what are called punishing damages: Punitive damages are awarded to punish a wrongdoing that is outrageous in character. One of the legal terms used when a request is made for punitive damages is that the act represented a *reckless disregard* for the safety and well-being of the injured party or that the care rendered was incompetent. Two examples of acts that could lead to the award of punitive damages are providing healthcare when impaired by drugs or alcohol or failure to provide care for a patient despite repeated requests to be physically present. Hospitals can also be charged with punitive damages when they continue to grant privileges to a staff member who has acted in the manner described above. In addition, hospitals have been charged punitive damages for holding themselves out to the community as offering a particular type of service but not delivering it in a way that meets the appropriate standard of care. For example, if a hospital says that it does open-heart surgery but does not have trained and available support staff, an award of punitive damages could result from the injury or death of a surgical patient because of the inappropriate staffing. Although punitive damages are often requested in malpractice cases, they are infrequently awarded. However, when they are awarded, they can be significantly higher than the total of the economic and noneconomic damages awarded. In some jurisdictions, health malpractice insurance companies are prohibited from covering the cost to a defendant related to the award of punitive damages.

Incidence of Malpractice

Although the actual number of claims for malpractice is unknown, there are data that suggest that patient injuries occur too frequently. In 1999, a national IOM report estimated that as many as 98,000 individuals die in the nation's hospitals each year as a result of medical errors. This number

was similar to that reported in earlier studies. A 1984 Harvard research study found that 1% of a representative sample of all patients hospitalized in New York State experienced injuries and one quarter of that number died. If the New York findings were extrapolated nationwide, the numbers would represent more than 234,000 patient injuries and 80,000 deaths per year from negligence. A 2006 follow-up of the 1999 national IOM study found that 1.5 million people were harmed due to medication errors alone. More than half of these errors occurred in long-term care facilities with the remainder divided between outpatient facilities treating Medicare recipients and hospitals.

Despite the number of injuries and deaths reported, fewer than 1% of physicians nationwide have had claims made against them for malpractice. Although this number is rising, the scope of the involvement of physicians and other professionals remains small. About one half of all cases brought to trial in 2002 in the 75 largest counties in the United States involved cases against surgeons, and one third were against nonsurgeon physicians. In the same report, 90% of plaintiffs alleged death or permanent disability.

Although there are significant errors that can and do occur in the delivery of healthcare, the rate of success in winning a malpractice claim in court is low. Although almost 52% of other civil torts are settled in favor of the plaintiffs, in medical malpractice cases that number drops to 27%.

Resulting Limitations

A major concern with medical malpractice is that the increasing numbers of claims, the costs associated with defending them, and the sizes of the awards when the claims are successful have led to limitations in access to healthcare. The loss of access is not related to the inability of patients to pay for care but rather to decisions by professionals to leave practice completely, leave specialty practice, or limit the types of medical conditions that they are willing to treat. In the past several years, for example, many obstetrician-gynecologists are limiting their practices to gynecology only, and neurosurgeons and other subspecialists are limiting the sizes of their practices or are refusing to perform complex surgical procedures. In many cases, these decisions are made due to the high cost of malpractice insurance coverage. In other cases, the decisions are made due to the high cost of emotional investments in refuting claims that the professionals believe are unjustified.

Rising medical malpractice insurance premiums coupled with the growing number of uninsured or underinsured individuals nationally may be a prescription for disaster. Many individuals who lack adequate health insurance coverage have limited access to care and do not appropriately manage their chronic medical conditions, nor do they receive preventive care. When they do seek needed care, often their disease conditions are more advanced and complex, hence healthcare providers are at increased risk of making errors. It is these errors that lead to future claims of malpractice and a cycle that many believe is out of control.

Linda F. Samson

See also American Hospital Association (AHA); American Medical Association (AMA); Clinical Practice Guidelines; Cost of Healthcare; Institute of Medicine (IOM); Joint Commission; Medical Errors; Quality of Healthcare

Further Readings

Anderson, Richard E., ed. *Medical Malpractice: A Physician's Sourcebook*. Totowa, NJ: Humana Press, 2004.

Aspden, Phillip, Julie Wolcott, J. Lyle Bootman, et al., eds. *Preventing Medication Errors*. Washington, DC: National Academy Press, 2006.

Baker, Tom. *The Medical Malpractice Myth*. Chicago: University of Chicago Press, 2005.

Gorombei, D. A., P. Crowell, and L. Plate. "Medical Malpractice Tort Reform," *Journal of Legal Nurse Consulting* 18(1): 20–23, 2007.

Helm, Ann, ed. *Nursing Malpractice: Sidestepping Legal Minefields*. Philadelphia: Lippincott, Williams and Wilkins, 2003.

Kohn, Linda T., Janet M. Corrigan, and Molla S. Donaldson, eds. *To Err Is Human: Building a Safer Health System*. Washington, DC: National Academy Press, 1999.

Sage, William M., and Rogan Kersh, eds. *Medical Malpractice and the U.S. Health Care System*. New York: Cambridge University Press, 2006.

Sloan, Frank A., Penny B. Githens, Ellen Wright Clayton, et al. *Suing for Medical Malpractice*. Chicago: University of Chicago Press, 1993.

Stubenrauch, James M. "Malpractice vs. Negligence," *American Journal of Nursing* 107(7): 63, July 2007.

Thorpe, Kenneth E. "The Medical Malpractice 'Crisis': Recent Trends and the Impact of State Tort Reforms," *Health Affairs* Web Exclusive, January 21, 2004, http://www.content.healthaffairs.org/cgi/content/full/hlthaff.w4.20v1/DC1

Vidmar, Neil. *Medical Malpractice and the American Jury: Confronting the Myths About Jury Incompetence, Deep Pockets, and Outrageous Damage Awards*. Ann Arbor: University of Michigan Press, 1997.

Web Sites

American Hospital Association (AHA): http://www.aha.org
American Medical Association (AMA): http://www.ama-assn.org
American Trial Lawyers Association (ATLA): http://www.theatla.com
Health Care Choices: http://www.healthcarechoices.org/profile.htm
Joint Commission: http://www.jointcommission.org
National Practitioner Data Bank (NPDB): http://www.npdb-hipdb.hrsa.gov
Physician Insurers Association of America (PIAA): http://www.piaa.us
U.S. Department of Justice: http://www.ojp.usdoj.gov/bjs/abstract/mmtvlc01.htm

MANAGED CARE

Managed care is a complex system that involves the active coordination of and arrangement for the provision of health services and the coverage of health benefits. The term *managed care* was coined in the 1980s to name the array of emerging health insurance products that were evolving in response to skyrocketing healthcare costs. To differentiate these new products from traditional insurance, commercial insurers adopted the generic term *managed care* to describe health benefit products that attempted to control the cost of care by restricting the choice of providers or the use of medical services. Today, it encompasses a broad spectrum of organizational structures and benefit plans such as (a) health maintenance organizations (HMOs), (b) preferred provider organizations (PPOs), (c) point of service plans (POS), (d) individual practice associations (IPAs), (e) exclusive provider organizations (EPOs), and (f) consumer-directed healthcare (CDH).

The exact nature of managed care is constantly evolving in response to the changing demands of consumers, employers, and regulators. There are three key components of managed care: (1) the network or contractual relationship with healthcare providers, (2) the oversight or coordination of medical care, and (3) the structure of the covered healthcare benefits and copayments. Early managed-care plans were nothing more than networks of providers who agreed to accept lower reimbursements to be included in a plan's network of preferred providers: hence, preferred provider organizations or PPOs. There were benefits or financial penalties if the insured did or did not use a preferred provider. Later on, managed-care organizations added medical-management initiatives such as preauthorization of services and mandatory second opinions. In response to rising political pressures, medical management has evolved away from prior authorization to focus more on care coordination and disease management. Recently, financial incentives and disincentives have taken the forefront in efforts to influence healthcare costs, taking the form of CDH. CDH uses an array of benefit designs with higher copayments, higher deductibles, or both to empower consumers to more effectively manage their healthcare.

Contracting and Networks

Provider contracting was the easiest and therefore the first component of managed care to be implemented. Insurers began requiring providers who wanted to be included in their network of preferred providers to agree to negotiated discounts off their standard rates. Prior to the advent of PPOs, most hospital services were being reimbursed at 100% of the billed charges. These fees were loosely based on cost plus some percentage above the estimated cost. This methodology actually encouraged higher charges and contributed to the rapid escalation of healthcare costs.

Physicians and other healthcare providers had been reimbursed at billed charges or community-average rate, known as *usual, customary, and reasonable* (UCR). Early PPOs simply negotiated a lower reimbursement, usually taking an additional 10% or 20% off the billed or UCR fees.

Whereas the discounting of fees yielded some initial cost relief, it did not change the inherent dynamics; each insurer developed different contracting strategies to try to affect hospital costs. Most hospitals preferred a variant of fee-for-service. Thus, the most common arrangement was a greater discount off the billed charges. Under some contracts, facilities would agree to a flat, daily rate (per diem). Initially, these rates were all-inclusive for all levels of care. Eventually, per diem contracts became more sophisticated, and the rates were negotiated based on the complexity of the service provided, with higher rates for more complex services such as intensive care units, maternity, pediatrics, and so on. As technology and costs advanced, per diem contracts began to include carve-outs for high-cost devices (e.g., implantable pacemakers) and medications.

Another method of facility reimbursement—developed and implemented by Medicare in the mid-1980s—was based on Diagnostic Related Groupings (DRGs). Facilities received a fixed reimbursement for all anticipated services based on the expected average cost of care for a patient with a specific discharge diagnosis. DRG payments fundamentally changed the dynamics of hospital reimbursement. Once hospitals were no longer reimbursed on a cost-plus basis, they began to address the different factors that influenced the cost of care in their facilities. Hospitals instituted utilization reviews of patient stays to identify and address the excessive length of hospitalizations. Hospitals also implemented pharmacy and therapeutic committees to identify opportunities to lower medication and medical-device costs. These efforts led to shorter lengths of hospitalization; increased use of lower-cost, generic, and therapeutically equivalent medications; and greater standardization of implantable medical devices and appliances.

A few hospital systems were so confident in their ability to manage costs that they began taking the risk of *global capitation* for the inpatient and outpatient care they provided. Some hospitals established their own health plans; others negotiated full-risk contracts with insurers. Although few of these contracts and health plans remain, the collective efforts of hospitals to manage their cost of care have resulted in shorter lengths of hospitalization and a more efficient use of resources.

Although relatively rare, organ-transplant services were an early focus of managed-care organizations due to their high cost, wide variation in cost, and variation in the outcomes for similar transplant services across the country. Often, the higher-cost facilities were achieving less favorable outcomes with lower survival rates. In an effort to achieve better outcomes for lower costs, insurers began limiting coverage for transplants to preferred facilities. These preferred facilities were often referred to as *centers of excellence*. Eventually, preferential contracting for centers of excellence expanded to include other complex medical procedures as well as some high-volume or high-cost cardiac procedures.

To encourage patients to seek care at these preferred centers of excellence, insurers would usually cover patients' additional travel and housing expenses. In addition, health coverage plans were often designed to waive or limit patient cost sharing if services were obtained at the insurers' preferred centers. Initially, each insurer developed his or her own list of centers of excellence based on individual criteria. However, as the process spread, specialty medical societies and academic medical centers became involved in developing criteria and tracking outcomes. This lead to increased accountability and more transparency.

Medical Management and Care Coordination

A 1986 RAND Corporation Report suggested that one third of medical procedures were unnecessary. This perception of overuse became an early focus of managed care. Initial efforts to influence the care provided included (a) mandatory second opinions for elective surgery, (b) prior authorization for elective procedures and diagnostic tests such as CT scans, and (c) limiting the networks of medical specialists. Prior authorization programs were implemented to reduce the use of high-cost, frequently ordered procedures and to ensure that patients were referred to in-network preferred facilities and providers.

In addition to prior authorization of elective hospitalizations, hospitalizations were reviewed against external criteria and benchmarks. The clinical criteria for determining the medical need for ongoing hospitalization that were developed by InterQual, Inc. were the most commonly used criteria by hospitals and were adopted by the Medicare program in 1999. InterQual's criteria did not set an expected length of stay for a hospitalization; rather, they assessed whether a patient needed to remain at a particular level of care (e.g., intensive care or hospitalization) based on the treatment and services the patient was receiving.

Health plans tended to use the inpatient care guidelines developed by Milliman and Robertson, Inc. (now Milliman, Inc.) in the late 1980s. The Milliman care guidelines assigned an expected length of stay for each hospitalization based on an optimal outcome. The guidelines were evidence based and reviewed by expert panels of physicians. The Milliman care guidelines specified the expected progression of hospitalized care for specific medical and surgical procedures. Before the Milliman guidelines were introduced into a market, the actual length of hospital stays was usually significantly longer than the optimal length specified by the guidelines. Initially, extended hospitalization due to a delay in care would result in denial or carving out of hospital days—that is, nonpayment of hospital charges for the excess days; within 6 to 12 months, hospitalization lengths of stay shortened, approaching the guideline targets. Initially, denial of payment for hospital days accounted for a small portion of the resultant savings (5–10%). Most of the savings came from shorter hospitalizations due to the changes in practice patterns brought on by the clinical guidelines.

Once physicians and hospitals modified their practice patterns to conform to the guidelines, the denial of payment was minimal (2–3%), and there was marginal subsequent decrease in hospitalization lengths of stay. This lack of ongoing improvement often called into question the need for continuing inpatient utilization management programs. This tension intensified in the late 1990s when public and political perceptions of managed care soured. As a result, many insurers scaled back their inpatient utilization management programs.

Outpatient utilization management programs, although effective, did not result in such clear-cut savings. The major impact was not through denial of services, which averaged 2% to 4%, but rather was due to a reduction in the number of services requested by providers due to their perception of oversight, the *sentinel effect*. In the inpatient setting, the sentinel effect was demonstrated by the shorter length of hospitalization. In the outpatient setting, it was more difficult to measure the impact: As the sentinel effect resulted in a reduction in the services requested, it was measurement of a nonevent. The impact of the sentinel effect was believed to be 2 to 3 times greater than the effect of the actual denials. However, as most insurers did not have detailed authorization statistics to measure the impact of changes in the utilization management programs, their effectiveness was often underestimated.

Even with the streamlining and automation of these programs, they often cost 1% to 1.5% of premiums. Ignoring the sentinel effect savings of 4% to 9% and accounting only for the savings from denials, the net savings from these utilization management programs was in the 1% to 3% range, which was often thought to be too little to justify the administrative costs and the negative marketing impacts. In response to a public and political backlash against managed care in the late 1990s, many insurers reduced or eliminated their utilization management programs, choosing instead to influence use through increased financial cost sharing and deductibles. By eliminating their utilization management programs, insurers also took themselves out of the unenviable role of trying to control healthcare costs by managing the demand for services. Instead, insurers attempted to influence healthcare costs through higher copayments, greater cost sharing, and higher deductibles.

By increasing consumers' out-of-pocket costs for healthcare services, insurers and employers hoped to slow the rise in healthcare costs by discouraging unnecessary care. However, there is concern that higher deductibles and cost sharing may have a negative impact on health outcomes by discouraging early intervention and preventive care. For commercial and Medicare populations, there is greater emphasis on managing use through financial disincentives and cost sharing than through robust utilization management programs, one notable exception being in the area of managed Medicaid.

Disease and Care Management

In the 1970s and 1980s, some academic medical centers, large medical groups, and staff- or group-model HMOs had multidisciplinary specialty clinics that focused on a single condition or disease (diabetes, cystic fibrosis, anticoagulation, etc.). These programs were predominantly disease focused and institution based and were developed to streamline the operational aspects of a clinic visit.

Health plans and insurers developed *disease management* programs in the early 1990s to lower hospitalizations and emergency room visits for high-use patients with specific diseases, hence the name *disease management*. Individuals were identified for enrollment in disease management programs by retrospective claims reviews or by provider referrals.

Nurse case managers, pharmacists, and physicians would review hospital medical claims and pharmacy records to identify opportunities for intervention to prevent repeat hospitalizations. A key focus of these programs was educating patients and their families so that they could better understand and manage their illness. These programs would emphasize the (a) importance of following treatment recommendations, (b) early recognition of exacerbations and complications, and (c) methods for preventive intervention.

Numerous studies documented the lack of standardization of care and the slow adoption of national treatment guidelines by physicians. Disease management programs were one method used by managed care to disseminate and encourage the use of evidence-based guidelines. By adopting and promoting national guidelines to patients and physicians, disease management programs attempted to improve health outcomes through greater compliance with the recommended treatment guidelines. Managed-care organizations could identify individuals who met the criteria for inclusion in a disease management program from medical claims data, hospital admissions records, emergency department visits, and pharmacy claims. Once the individuals were identified, nurse case managers and pharmacists would review their medical histories and claims data to assess if their care was in compliance with the guideline recommendations. If changes in treatment protocols were needed, a nurse, pharmacist or physician would contact the individual's treating physician to obtain additional information and review the recommended guidelines. If necessary, a nurse case manager or a physician could also contact the physician to discuss additional intervention, such as a consultation with a specialist or more frequent physician visits. Initially, disease management programs for asthma and congestive heart failure were very successful in encouraging adoption of the guidelines, improving outcomes, and reducing costs.

Disease management programs continued to evolve, increasing the number of diseases covered, the scope of the interventions, and the comprehensiveness of the interventions. Disease management programs became more proactive in identifying candidates for their programs by using sophisticated predictive-modeling software in their analysis of medical claims, pharmacy, and laboratory data. Predictive modeling allowed disease management programs to identify individuals who were at greater risk for complications from their illness and to initiate interventions to prevent costly treatments for complications and hospitalizations.

During the past decade, traditional disease management programs have expanded beyond a single-disease focus to encompass the individual's overall healthcare needs. As a result, the term *disease management* has transitioned to *care management* to signify these changes. The options for intervention have also greatly expanded. Current care management programs provide a wide array of education options, from quarterly newsletters to comprehensive Web-based educational offerings. Interventions may be as simple as prescription refill reminders or may include ongoing home-based monitoring of symptoms and an expanding array of biometric information such as blood pressure, weight, and blood oxygen saturation. By identifying early changes in their conditions, individuals, nurse case managers, and physicians can intervene early and prevent or minimize exacerbations of the conditions.

Whereas the scope of care management programs has expanded, the emphasis has remained on improving health outcomes through greater standardization of care in compliance with evidence-based medical guidelines. A RAND Corporation study, in 2003, estimated that patients with chronic illness received only 55% of the care recommended by the established national guidelines. Another

study, conducted by the Dartmouth Atlas Project, suggests that 30% of U.S. healthcare costs could be saved by increased standardization of care, emphasizing preventive care, and focusing on managing chronic disease.

Medicaid Managed Care

One area in which managed care has continued to grow is Medicaid. Since the early 1990s, state Medicaid programs have turned increasingly to managed care to improve access to care and to contain costs. Many states have enrolled sizable portions of their Medicaid beneficiary populations in some form of managed care. As Medicaid programs provide health coverage to individuals and families with low incomes, the copayments and beneficiary out-of-pocket expenses are minimal. Unlike commercial programs in which managed-care organizations have attempted to substitute financial cost sharing to control costs, Medicaid managed care has continued to emphasize utilization management and disease management programs to achieve savings. Although the nature and composition of these utilization management programs vary greatly by state and by company, the majority of their cost savings result from reduced inpatient use and pharmacy expenses.

Future Implications

Over the past 30 years, managed care has undergone a dramatic evolution. The term *managed care* now represents such a broad array of products, services, and interventions that it nearly defies explicit definition. Managed care can broadly be described as any strategy of organizing healthcare delivery to influence cost. Another way to define managed care is to describe what it is not—unmanaged care: unrestricted healthcare coverage that allows the beneficiary to see any healthcare provider for any service at any time without any financial consequences.

As healthcare costs continued to rise, the government, payers, and individuals sought solutions and alternatives. Managed care offered consumers expanded coverage and lower out-of-pocket expenses with some restrictions on access and limitations on use. It offered employers price moderation and insulated consumers from the true financial costs of their healthcare. Managed care's expansion of coverage for preventive services, well-child examinations, prenatal care, immunizations, pharmacy services, and disease care management programs went from being new and innovative programs to basic requirements of health insurance coverage.

In part as a result of managed care's success in expanding covered benefits, controlling healthcare costs, and financially insulating consumers from the cost of their care, there was a backlash against any constraints or restrictions on individuals' healthcare desires: In the face of managed care's successes, people questioned whether such restrictions were necessary or appropriate. Managed care became the scapegoat for rising healthcare costs and Americans' reluctant recognition that societal resources for healthcare were not unlimited.

In response to political and marketplace pressures, managed care developed new strategies and products that imposed fewer restrictions and gave consumers greater control along with greater financial responsibility for their health care. These consumer-directed products substituted the individual's willingness to pay for managed care's medical-necessity criteria. For a price, this approach removed managed-care programs from the process of making decisions about whom individuals could see or what care was medically necessary and allowed unimpeded access to care. Individuals with sufficient financial means can access all the care that they desire; conversely, a greater number of Americans are deciding what healthcare they get based on what they can afford.

Although CDH has been a politically successful strategy, rising healthcare costs continue to erode health insurance coverage. The proportion of employers offering health insurance coverage has declined to 60% in 2006 from 69% in 2000. Employers that continue to offer health coverage are requiring employees to pay a higher portion of health insurance costs through higher premium contributions, increased copayments, and larger deductibles. All these changes are leading to a rising number of uninsured individuals as people are unable or unwilling to pay these higher out-of-pocket costs. With the demand for healthcare services in the United States continuing to grow faster than our ability to pay for them, it is clear that the future will require trade-offs: Will healthcare coverage be affordable and accessible or will there be restrictions and limitations? Are individuals entitled to all the healthcare services they want? Should everyone be guaranteed the healthcare they need? Regardless of the payment mechanism—single payer, nationalized health system, or the current model—some form of managed care will likely remain.

Bruce A. Weiss

See also Carve-Outs; Case Management; Consumer-Directed Health Plans (CDHPs); Disease Management; Health Maintenance Organizations (HMOs); Medicaid; Preferred Provider Organizations (PPOs); Primary Care Case Management (PCCM)

Further Readings

Bloche, M. Gregg. "Consumer-Directed Health Care," *New England Journal of Medicine* 355(17): 1756–59, October 26, 2006.
Committee on the Quality of Health Care in America, Institute of Medicine. *Crossing the Quality Chasm: A New Health System for the 21st Century.* Washington, DC: National Academy Press, 2001.
Enthoven, Alain C. "The History and Principles of Managed Competition," *Health Affairs* 12(Suppl.): 24–48, 1993.
Iglehart, John K. "The American Health Care System: Managed Care," *New England Journal of Medicine* 327(10): 742–47, September 3, 1992.
Marquis, M. Susan, Jeannette A. Rogowski, and Jose J. Escarce. "The Managed Care Backlash: Did Consumers Vote With Their Feet?" *Inquiry* 41(4): 376–90, Winter 2004–2005.
McGlynn, Elizabeth A., Steven M. Asch, John Adams, et al. "The Quality of Health Care Delivered to Adults in the United States," *New England Journal of Medicine* 348(26): 2635–45, June 26, 2003.
Newhouse, Joseph P. "Consumer-Directed Health Plans and the RAND Health Insurance Experiment," *Health Affairs* 23(6): 107–113, November–December 2004.
Robinson, James C. "The End of Managed Care," *Journal of the American Medical Association* 285(20): 2622–28, May 23, 2001.
Starr, P. *The Social Transformation of American Medicine: The Rise of a Sovereign Profession and the Making of a Vast Industry.* New York: Basic Books, 1983.

Web Sites

Dartmouth Atlas Working Group:
   http://www.dartmouthatlas.org
Disease Management Association of America (DMAA):
   http://www.dmaa.org
Henry J. Kaiser Family Foundation (KFF):
   http://www.kff.org
InterQual, Inc.: http://www.interqual.com
Managed Care Museum:
   http://www.managedcaremuseum.com
Milliman, Inc.: http://www.milliman.com
RAND Corporation: http://www.rand.org

MARKET FAILURE

A market failure exists in the healthcare market when the allocation of goods or services is not efficient—an *allocative inefficiency.* Efficiency is measured by the concept of *Pareto efficiency,* a situation where goods or services have been allocated among members of society in such a way that they cannot be reallocated so as to improve the welfare of at least one member without reducing the welfare of others. A *perfectly competitive market* is a hypothetical ideal market in which there are (a) a large number of buyers and sellers in the market, (b) free entry into and exit out of the market, (c) homogeneity of the goods or services, and (d) perfect knowledge. A perfectly competitive market is an efficient market and the yardstick against which economists and others measure whether a *market failure* exists. A market failure is problematic because it results in a market transaction that is socially inefficient—that is, where the market price does not equal the marginal cost and where potential welfare gains to trade exist but are not achieved. In this entry, the common types of market failure in healthcare are explained, and then potential solutions to these failures are discussed.

Types of Market Failure

The healthcare market exhibits a number of properties that deviate from a socially efficient market. The most significant characteristics of the healthcare market that result in a market failure include (a) the presence of *market power,* (b) information

problem of *uncertainty,* (c) *asymmetric* information, and (d) the existence of positive and negative *externalities.*

Market Power

Market power exists when an individual firm has the ability to influence the market price of a good or service with the result that the price exceeds the marginal cost of the good or service. Market power violates the assumption that a sufficiently large number of sellers exists to guarantee that each individual seller is a *price taker* in a perfectly competitive market. Market power includes situations ranging from imperfect competition, in which multiple sellers compete against each other and each has some influence over the price, to a monopolistic market, in which there is only one seller and this seller has control over the entire market. The presence of market power leads to market failure because of *deadweight loss*—that is, a loss to society due to a market price that is greater than and a market quantity that is less than the market price and quantity in an efficient market.

A classic example of a monopoly in the healthcare market is the market for a drug that is covered by a patent. With a patented drug, only one manufacturer has the legal right to produce the drug until the patent expires, creating a monopoly market until the patent's expiration. As a monopolist, the manufacturer will charge a price that exceeds the efficient price (i.e., the price that would exist in a perfectly competitive market) and sell a quantity of the drug that is less than the efficient quantity.

More commonly, firms may have *monopoly power,* a situation in which there are multiple sellers of a good or service but one seller can increase its price and still maintain at least some of its market share. Both physicians and hospitals exercise varying degrees of monopoly power. A physician could increase his or her fee for an office visit, for example, and still keep some patients. Whereas some patients may decide to go to a different physician after the fee increase, other patients will remain at the physician's practice. This ability to increase fees without losing all the firm's business is market power. Again, because an efficient market means that sellers are price takers, this is a clear violation of a perfectly competitive assumption.

Uncertainty

Uncertainty about an individual's future demand for medical care is an information problem that leads to a market failure in the healthcare market. The unpredictability of illness creates uncertainty regarding when healthcare will be needed, what services will be required, and how much the care will cost. Uncertainty creates a market failure because consumers (i.e., patients) do not know the type or quantity of services that they will need and producers (i.e., providers) do not know the type or quantity of services that they will need to provide.

Uncertainty abounds in healthcare. The occurrence of illness is largely unpredictable. Once an individual becomes ill, the diagnosis is not always known with certainty. Clinical symptoms such as fever, cough, abdominal pain, and shortness of breath are symptomatic of many illnesses. The optimal treatment also may not be certain. Many illnesses can be treated in multiple ways, and the outcomes are not perfectly tied to these treatments. Individuals would like to insure against all these types of uncertainty; however, a market does not exist for all of them.

Asymmetric Information

A second information problem in the healthcare market is asymmetric information. Asymmetric information is a situation where one party in a relationship has more information or more accurate information than another party. This inequality of information violates the perfectly competitive assumption that all parties involved in a transaction have perfect information. Asymmetric information leads to a market failure if demand and supply are interdependent rather than independent.

In healthcare, a market failure stems from asymmetric information in situations where consumers do not have the expertise to independently determine their own demand for healthcare services or monitor the quality of the services provided. Consumers may lack sufficient knowledge to diagnose their illness, evaluate the different courses of treatment, and select the optimal treatment. Hence, the provider influences the consumer's demand thereby creating interdependence between demand and supply.

In addition, consumers have less information about the quality of their healthcare providers than the providers have about their own quality. For primary care and other frequently purchased services (e.g., care for chronic conditions), consumers have the opportunity to learn about the quality of the provider over time, through experience or trial and error. For services that individuals make use of infrequently or only need once (e.g., a kidney transplant), asymmetric information is a more important issue. The consumer cannot learn about the quality of a provider through experience and, therefore, is unable to monitor the quality of the care delivered.

Because of specialized medical training, a provider usually has more information than the patient about his or her diagnosis and the necessary treatment. The provider acts as an agent of the patient, thereby diagnosing the patient's illness, recommending a treatment, and often, providing the recommended treatment. Through this principal-agent relationship, the patient delegates some decision-making power to the provider, thereby allowing the provider to influence his or her demand. Even if a provider shares with the patient all available information about his or her illness, treatment options, and expected outcomes, it may still be difficult or even impossible for the individual consumer to make the optimal decision without the provider's recommendation, given the complexity and quantity of medical information that must be assimilated for complicated health problems.

Externalities

An externality exists when the decision of a consumer or producer incurs costs or benefits for other consumers or producers. An externality is negative when an individual's or a firm's decision creates a cost for others; it is positive when an individual's or a firm's decision creates a benefit for others. An externality results in a market failure because the market price fails to take into account the social costs and benefits that are realized by individuals or firms other than the consumer or producer.

Externalities in healthcare may affect production or consumption. An example of a *positive consumption externality* is obtaining a flu vaccination. By obtaining a flu shot, an individual directly benefits by protecting himself or herself from contracting the flu. And other members of society benefit from the individual who obtained the flu shot, as well, because it reduces their risk of contracting the flu. An individual's decision on whether to obtain a flu shot is based on his or her marginal cost compared with his or her marginal benefit from receiving the vaccination. The individual does not consider the downstream consequences of his or her decision (i.e., whether the risk to others of contracting the flu is reduced by him or her receiving a flu shot). When individuals bear the full cost of a decision in the presence of a positive consumption externality, too few goods or services will be purchased in the market—that is, too few people will purchase a flu shot—even though other members of society also benefit from the decision. A classic example of a *negative consumption externality* is smoking: An individual's decision to smoke in a public place has a negative impact on others through secondhand smoke.

On the production side, research is a common *positive production externality.* An individual or firm producing scientific research affects the welfare of others in society by creating knowledge that could benefit the broader community. When the full costs of research are wholly borne by the individual scientist or institution, however, too little research will be undertaken. An example of a *negative production externality* is a hospital that incinerates used surgical supplies containing PVC, which turns into the toxic chemical dioxin when burned. The firm passes a social cost onto other individuals by increasing their risk of cancer, but this cost is not borne by the firm itself.

Solutions

The government may intervene in situations where the market cannot achieve an efficient allocation on its own. The government has several mechanisms by which to intervene and improve the market. However, government involvement is not necessarily the optimal action; many believe that it should only step in if the marginal benefits from the intervention exceed the marginal costs of the intervention, after factoring in spillover effects on other markets and individuals. In addition, as technology and other innovations evolve over time, new markets may develop to facilitate more efficient allocations.

Health Insurance

Health insurance is a mechanism that mitigates market failure associated with uncertainty. Health insurance protects an individual against financial losses associated with healthcare costs due to an illness or injury that cannot be predicted either in terms of occurrence or magnitude. For groups in which private coverage is not accessible, the government may function as the insurance provider. Public insurance programs, such as Medicare and Medicaid, ensure that the highest-risk individuals who do not have access to employer-provided health insurance offerings can obtain insurance coverage. At the same time, health insurance also introduces additional market problems, including *moral hazard* and *adverse selection.*

Taxes

To solve the problems of externalities—where the marginal private benefits do not equal the marginal social benefits or where the marginal private costs do not equal the marginal social costs—taxes and subsidies (i.e., negative taxes) can be used. Taxes are used when the marginal private costs are less than the marginal social costs, and subsidies are used when the marginal private benefits are less than the marginal social benefits.

Taxes alter the economic incentives of the buyer and seller: Taxes make it more costly to produce the externality, causing the quantity of the externality to decrease. The tax should equal the additional cost levied on the parties harmed by the externality, and the funds raised should be used to compensate those individuals. Although taxes force the creator of the externality to internalize the costs of their actions, taxes are not a perfect solution for several reasons. First, they allow the externality to continue; hence, individuals will still be harmed by the externality but will theoretically be compensated for their loss. Second, it is difficult to assess the actual cost of the externality that is imposed on others, so the tax is only an approximation of the real cost. Third, taxes generate monitoring costs to ensure that the parties creating the externality pay the tax.

Regulation

Direct government involvement is another solution to many market failures. With no regulation, pharmaceutical companies might invest less in research and development—and ultimately develop fewer new drugs that society would benefit from—because other companies could act as free riders and replicate the inventor's products without incurring the research and development costs required to bring a new product to market. Patent protections, therefore, encourage pharmaceutical companies to invest more in research and development by providing a protected period of time when the developing company will be the sole provider of its drug.

Regulation also more clearly defines and enforces property rights when they are ambiguous in the market. By assigning property rights, regulations determine whether one party has the right to produce an externality or another party has the right to not consume the externality. Smoking bans in public places—restaurants or bars, for example—implicitly assign the right to clean air to the nonsmoker and remove the right to smoke in these places, thereby prohibiting smokers from passing along secondhand smoke to others. As with taxes, it is important to assess the marginal costs and benefits of regulations. Smoking bans decrease the likelihood of illnesses such as lung cancer but may impose a cost on other parties (e.g., restaurants and bars) if the net effect is fewer patrons, smaller tabs per patron, or both.

Antitrust policies prevent the existence of monopolies, the most extreme type of market power. If a monopoly or oligopoly is beneficial to a market because of economies of scale, however, the government may allow its formation but may regulate prices.

Licensing of health professionals and healthcare organizations is a regulatory strategy to mitigate a market failure related to the lack of information on the quality of providers. Licensing and certification ensures a minimum quality level but restricts the quantity of providers and limits competition from other types of providers through restrictions on the scope of practice.

The Availability of Information

New technology and other innovations can improve the availability of information. New diagnostic technologies can improve the certainty of a diagnosis, and the Internet has created a venue for consumers to freely access information on healthcare providers. For example, the Centers for Medicare and Medicaid Services (CMS) now publish information on the Internet on hospital processes of care, outcomes of care, and patient satisfaction to allow consumers to compare the quality of care provided across the nation's hospitals.

New technological advances such as those made through the widespread adoption of the Internet will continue to improve the availability of information, which may be the most consequential change. Yet, distilling the vast amount of medical information available on the Internet, selecting the most valid and credible information, then assimilating it to a level that is useful to the individual consumer is no small feat. An Internet search through Google on diabetes treatment or diabetes care, for example, turned up 2.5 million results.

Although the Internet has armed consumers with more information to help diagnose their illnesses, determine alternative courses of treatment, judge the potential health outcomes, and judge provider quality, healthcare providers nevertheless remain the experts in delivering healthcare. Comparative information on healthcare quality—about which providers give the best care and have the best risk- and severity-adjusted outcomes—remains limited. Although several Web sites provide comparative information on some hospital-based healthcare outcomes, most quality comparisons continue to rely on either intermediate outcomes or proxies of quality—such as the occurrence of malpractice judgments, patient satisfaction data, and process outcomes—rather than health and healthcare outcomes. Further work is needed to determine how to accurately measure and compare health and healthcare outcomes across the continuum of providers (e.g., hospitals, physicians, nursing homes) and report the findings in a manner that is both easily accessible and comprehensible to consumers.

Two external forces may also increase information transparency. First, a shift to high-deductible health insurance plans increases the need for consumer-targeted information in the public domain on both quality and prices so that consumers can assess both the quality and out-of-pocket costs of alternative treatments. Second, medical travel—travel for medical care outside one's home country—may also increase the availability and comparability of information on quality and prices for some services. Non-U.S. healthcare providers catering to international patients, including U.S. patients, now publish on the Internet inclusive prices for the common surgical procedures provided at their facilities. (In the United States, although prices have been relatively transparent for a small set of elective procedures traditionally not covered by health insurance [e.g., Botox and LASIK surgery], it has generally been very difficult if not impossible to obtain, in advance, the price that an uninsured individual will pay out of pocket for a surgical procedure or hospitalization.) These two forces may ultimately drive providers to disseminate information on prices and quality and, ultimately, compel the government to facilitate the collection and dissemination of comparative information.

Tricia J. Johnson

See also Adverse Selection; Economic Spillover; Healthcare Markets; Health Economics; Health Insurance; Moral Hazard; Regulation; Supplier-Induced Demand

Further Readings

Arrow, Kenneth J. "Uncertainty and the Welfare Economics of Medical Care," *American Economic Review* 53(5): 941–73, December 1963.

Glied, Sherry A. "Health Insurance and Market Failure Since Arrow," *Journal of Health Politics, Policy and Law* 26(5): 957–65, October 2001.

Haas-Wilson, Deborah. "Arrow and the Information Market Failure in Health Care: The Changing Content and Sources of Health Care Information," *Journal of Health Politics, Policy and Law* 26(5): 1031–1044, October 2001.

Hammer, Peter J., Deborah Haas-Wilson, and William M. Sage. "Kenneth Arrow and the Changing Economics of Health Care: 'Why Arrow? Why Now?'" *Journal of Health Politics, Policy and Law* 26(5): 835–49, October 2001.

Kuttner, Robert. "Market-Based Failure: A Second Opinion on U.S. Health Care Costs," *New England Journal of Medicine* 358(6): 549–51, February 7, 2008.

Reinhardt, Uwe E. "Can Efficiency in Health Care Be Left to the Market?" *Journal of Health Politics, Policy and Law* 26(5): 967–92, October 2001.

Rice, Thomas H. *The Economics of Health Reconsidered.* 2d ed. Chicago: Health Administration Press, 2003.

Sloan, Frank A. "Arrow's Concept of the Health Care Consumer: A Forty-Year Retrospective," *Journal of Health Politics, Policy and Law* 26(5): 899–911, October 2001.

Web Sites

American Economics Association (AEA): http://www.vanderbilt.edu/AEA

American Society of Health Economists (ASHE): http://healtheconomics.us

International Health Economics Association (iHEA): http://www.healtheconomics.org

National Bureau of Economic Research (NBER): http://www.nber.org

World Health Organization (WHO): http://www.who.int

MARMOR, THEODORE R.

Theodore (Ted) R. Marmor is Professor Emeritus of Public Policy and Political Science at Yale University, where he taught from 1979 to 2007. Currently he is an adjunct professor of public policy at the John F. Kennedy School of Government at Harvard University. His specialization is the contemporary welfare state in North America and Europe, with particular expertise on healthcare policy. His research on healthcare has yielded a national and international reputation as the most recognized academician in healthcare policy and politics. Marmor's first book, *The Politics of Medicare* (1970), is a classic in the field. The second edition of *The Politics of Medicare* (2000) traces developments in healthcare policy since the enactment of Medicare in 1965. In the decades since Medicare was enacted, Marmor has been a prominent analyst of health policy and advocate of universal healthcare.

Born in New York City on February 24, 1939, he received his bachelor's degree from Harvard University in 1960; attended Wadham College, Oxford from 1961 to 1962; and then returned to Harvard, earning his doctoral degree in 1966. Marmor began his academic career as an assistant professor of political science and was promoted to associate professor at the University of Wisconsin during 1967 to 1970, then joined the faculty at the University of Minnesota (1970–1973) and later the University of Chicago (1973–1979) before going to Yale University in 1979.

In 1966, Marmor was special assistant to Wilbur Cohen, the Secretary of Health, Education, and Welfare; he served as associate dean at the School of Public Affairs during his tenure at the University of Minnesota; and at Yale University, he chaired the board of its Center for Health Services. He was a member of President Carter's Commission on the National Agenda for the 1980s and a senior policy advisor to Democratic presidential candidate Walter Mondale during the 1984 election campaign. Marmor has testified before congressional committees about healthcare reform, social security, and welfare policy in addition to acting as an expert witness in health-related judicial proceedings, including the constitutionality of the Canada Health Act, disputes over Medicare, and U.S. asbestos litigation.

Marmor serves on the editorial boards of the *Journal of Comparative Policy Analysis: Research and Practice*; the *Journal of Health Services Research and Policy*; the *International Journal of Health Planning and Management*; and the *Journal of Health Politics, Policy, and Law*. He was a centennial visiting professor at the London School of Economics (2000–2003) and has been a fellow or visiting fellow with the Australian National University, the Canadian Institute for Advanced Research, All Souls College at Oxford University, and the Netherlands Institute for Advanced Study. During 1993 to 2003, he was director of the Robert Wood Johnson Foundation Post-doctoral Program (Medical Care and Social Sciences).

Marmor has authored or coauthored 13 books, nearly 200 scholarly articles and book chapters, and more than 100 op-ed pieces in magazines and newspapers here and abroad. His scholarship has appeared in many prestigious journals, including the *American Political Science Review*, the *Michigan Law Review*, the *American Journal of Obstetrics and Gynecology*, the *New England Journal of Medicine*, the *Journal of Health Politics, Policy, and Law*, and the *Canadian Medical Association Journal*.

Raymond Tatalovich

See also Cohen, Wilbur J.; Equity, Efficiency, and Effectiveness in Healthcare; Healthcare Reform; Medicaid; Medicare; Public Health Policy Advocacy; Public Policy; Regulation

Further Readings

Marmor, Theodore R. *America's Misunderstood Welfare State: Persistent Myths, Enduring Realities*, with Jerry L. Mashaw and Philip L. Harvey. New York: Basic Books, 1990.

Marmor, Theodore R. *Understanding Health Care Reform*. New Haven, CT: Yale University Press, 1994.

Marmor, Theodore R. *The Politics of Medicare*. 2d ed. New York: Aldine de Gruyter, 2000.

Web Sites

Yale School of Management: http://mba.yale.edu

MATHEMATICA POLICY RESEARCH (MPR)

Mathematica Policy Research, Inc. (MPR), established in 1968 as a division of Mathematica, Inc., is a policy research organization that specializes in data collection and evaluation and policy analysis. The company provides research expertise, survey design and implementation techniques, information technology, and policy assessments to a wide variety of clients, including government agencies, universities, and foundations. For the past 40 years, MPR has helped to inform, shape, and enrich public policy.

Organizational Structure

MPR was incorporated under its current name in 1975, and it became an employee-owned entity in 1986. Headquartered in Princeton, New Jersey, the organization also has offices in Washington, D.C.; Cambridge, Massachusetts; and Ann Arbor, Michigan. The organization has partnered with the Robert Wood Johnson Foundation (RWJF) to establish the Center for Studying Health System Change (HSC), which is a wholly owned subsidiary of Mathematica, Inc. The HSC and MPR share administrative resources and collaborate on key studies and research projects.

Two major divisions of MPR are the surveys and information services division and the research division. The surveys and information services division gives clients the tools, technology, and customized surveys that help them gather appropriate and meaningful facts and figures. The research division builds on these efforts, providing findings and scientific evidence that policymakers can use in their decision making.

In the surveys and information services division, staff members help clients (a) identify the best data collection methods, (b) design custom survey instruments for small and large samples, (c) recognize the special needs of data collection in diverse populations, (d) conduct statistical analysis and modeling, and (e) use advanced technology for surveying and data management. MPR takes into account factors that may cause bias and skew survey results such as language barriers and subject disabilities. The organization also employs Internet technology and Web-based techniques to enhance its surveys.

The research division conducts research for the public and private sectors, strengthening an evidence-based approach to shaping policy agendas. The division is responsible for (a) developing experiments and demonstrations; (b) quantitatively evaluating programs by looking at econometric and statistical analyses of their effects, benefits and costs, quality, and value of output; and (c) qualitatively evaluating implementation and operations, using process and case study analyses. Researchers also predict the effects of proposed changes through the use of microsimulation and provide ongoing support to bolster research infrastructure. Through the expertise of systems analysts, social psychologists, economists, sociologists, demographers, and education specialists, the division is focused on conducting policy analyses to better understand the implications of policy choices in key research areas. The organization strives to communicate and disseminate its findings to policymakers and the general public.

Main Research Areas

MPR has conducted studies on programs and policy in the following areas: education, labor, welfare, nutrition, disability, early childhood, and healthcare. The organization focuses on these areas because they remain central to local, state, and federal policy.

Education

MPR provides research and evaluation of education efforts ranging from early-childhood schooling, to kindergarten through 12th grade, and beyond. It examines elementary reading and mathematics curricula, teacher quality, interventions for at-risk youth, after-school initiatives, college access and preparation, charter schools, school choice programs, education technology, school and student performance competencies, and career-focused education. The organization is also committed to improving education research overall by strengthening research methods and reviews. The organization administers the What Works Clearinghouse, a tool established by the U.S. Department of Education's Institute of Education Services that collects, reviews, and reports on studies of education programs, practices, and products. It is also involved with the evaluations of the Teach for America, No Child Left Behind, Head Start, and Upward Bound programs.

Labor

By examining the factors that affect the workforce, MPR helps to inform career training and placement interventions as well as employment policies. The organization focuses on research aimed at expanding opportunities for at-risk youth, disadvantaged adults, young people living in poverty, experienced workers who have lost their jobs, people who are involved in criminal activity and the criminal justice system, and others who face barriers to entering the workforce.

Welfare

MPR is involved in many projects that evaluate welfare reform efforts at the state and national levels. For example, it has examined initiatives— designed to help Technical Assistance for Needy Families (TANF) recipients—that look at interventions aimed at strengthening families, father involvement and support, healthy relationships, and abstinence education for teens. The organization evaluates welfare-to-work initiatives, efforts to increase job opportunities, long-term dependency on multiple public aid programs, and cost projections for federal and state programs. These research efforts help educate policymakers and program administrators seeking to improve the systems.

Nutrition

The organization's researchers study nutrition issues such as access to food, public food and nutrition assistance programs, emergency food assistance networks, and growing trends in obesity. For more than 30 years, the organization has extensively examined the Food Stamp Program and the Special Supplemental Nutrition Program for Women, Infants, and Children (WIC), helping policymakers assess reform efforts and continue to make revisions. In addition, its researchers have studied school nutrition programs, including school lunch and breakfast programs, as well as initiatives to improve children's diets and eating habits. With its findings, MPR informs ongoing efforts to improve the dietary status of all Americans.

Disability

For people living with disabilities and chronic diseases, advances in medicine and technology lead to more opportunities and increased independence; such changes may have important public policy implications at the state and national levels. The organization conducts research on programs such as Social Security and Medicaid, and it also gathers data on children with disabilities and their families. In addition, the organization looks at job programs for disabled adults. Mathematica's Center for Studying Disability Policy (CSDP) works with disability organizations and advocacy groups to enhance policy changes; it focuses on assessing service delivery, financing, resources, and disincentives. These efforts help leaders develop public policy to meet the changing needs of this special population.

Early Childhood

MPR studies and evaluates interventions aimed at improving the well-being of young children. These programs include (a) Head Start, (b) the Family and Child Experiences Survey (FACES),

(c) affordable day-care programs, (d) preschool curricula, and (e) initiatives serving low-income families.

Healthcare

In addition to its work relating to chronic disease and disability, MPR conducts a wide range of studies on health and the healthcare system. Researchers analyze costs, financing, insurance mechanisms, and coverage. MPR has also explored the effectiveness and quality of public- and private-sector services and the delivery of care. Specific projects include assessing the success of Medicaid, the State Children's Health Insurance Program (SCHIP), and private coverage options at increasing access to care for low-income families. The organization's work is also concerned with public health initiatives such as chronic-disease management programs and infectious-disease control measures. It evaluates programs that are designed to address mental health parity and health systems quality, and it also examines the role of advanced technology in improving health outcomes. Last, it provides leadership and policy advocates with the tools to promote sound and informed policy agendas.

Future Implications

MPR continues to provide policymakers and the general public with key information. Over the past few years, it has worked increasingly with international clients and begun addressing issues at a global level. Moving forward, the organization will ensure quality data collection, evaluation, and analysis for the United States and beyond.

Kathryn Langley

See also Center for Studying Health System Change; Health Insurance; Health Surveys; Medicaid; Medicare; Public Health; Public Policy

Further Readings

Del Grosso, Patricia, Amy Brown, Heather Zaveri, et al. *Oral Health Promotion, Prevention, and Treatment Strategies for Head Start Families: Early Findings From the Oral Health Initiative Evaluation.* Vol. 1: *Final Interim Report.* Princeton, NJ: Mathematica Policy Research, 2007.

Mathematica Policy Research. *Establishing Evidence, Elevating Standards, Enriching Policy: 40 Years.* Princeton, NJ: Mathematica Policy Research, 2008.

Rosenbach, Margo, Carol Irvin, Angelia Merrill, et al. *National Evaluation of the State Children's Health Insurance Program: A Decade of Expanding Coverage and Improving Access: Final Report.* Princeton, NJ: Mathematica Policy Research, 2007.

Web Sites

Center for Studying Health System Change (HSC): http://www.hschange.com

Mathematica Policy Research (MPR): http://www.mathematica-mpr.com

MAYNARD, ALAN

Alan Maynard is a well-known, highly respected health economist in the United Kingdom. Maynard has been instrumental in initiating policies for the UK National Health Service (NHS). Specifically, he proposed the establishment of the General Practitioner Fund Holding, from which physicians are given budgets to fund their activities as well as secondary care for their patients. He also proposed that the NHS only pay for pharmaceutical drugs that their manufacturers could demonstrate to be cost-effective and efficient. This proposal ultimately led to the formation of the National Institute of Clinical Excellence (NICE).

Maynard is a professor of health economics and the director of the York Health Policy Group in the Department of Health Sciences at the University of York. He is also an adjunct professor at the University of Technology in Sydney, Australia.

Maynard was educated at the University of Newcastle-upon-Tyne, earning first-class honors in economics in 1967. He received a bachelor's degree from the University of York in 1968. He did his postgraduate work at the University of York; while there, he was introduced to the field of public expenditure, which ignited his interest in healthcare. He taught economics as an assistant lecturer and then lecturer at the University of Exeter from 1968 to 1971. From there, he returned to the University of York as a lecturer in economics. In 1977, he became senior lecturer at York, where he founded the Graduate Program in Health Economics, serving as its director until 1983. In 1983, he became a professor of economics and the founding director of the Centre for Health Economics at York. From 1995 to 1996, he served as the secretary and chief executive of the Nuffield Provincial Hospitals Trust, a foundation that funds research in health policy. In 1996, he returned to the University of York as a professor of health economics and the director of the York Health Policy Group.

Maynard was made an honorary member of the Faculty of Public Health Medicine of the Royal Colleges of Physicians in 1993. He was elected president of the International Health Economic Association (iHEA) in 1999. He was named a fellow at the Academy of Medical Sciences for the United Kingdom in 2000. In 2002, he was named adjunct professor at the Centre for Health Economics in Research and Evaluation at the University of Technology in Sydney, Australia. He has been awarded honorary doctorate degrees from the Universities of Aberdeen (2003) and Northumbria (2006).

He is the founding editor of *Health Economics* and has written more than 250 scholarly articles and 10 books. He also is a member of the editorial boards of the *British Journal of Obstetrics and Gynaecology, Pharmacoeconomics, Health Manpower Management,* and the *Drug and Alcohol Review.*

In addition to Maynard's academic experience, he has served the NHS as a member of the York Health Authority (1983–1991), nonexecutive director of the York National Health Service Hospital (1991–1997), and has been the chair of the hospital since 1997.

Maynard has provided consultant services for the UK Department for International Development, the World Health Organization (WHO), and the World Bank on healthcare issues in Cyprus, Greece, Thailand, Brazil, Mexico, China, Botswana, South Africa, Bolivia, Chile, Lithuania, Latvia, Hungary, Russia, Malawi, Serbia, Kyrgyzstan, and Ukraine.

Currently, Maynard is working on improving the performance of health technology assessment and workforce productivity. In the next 10 years, he hopes to see proper routine measurement and management of patient-reported outcome measures.

Amie Lulinski Norris

See also Health Economics; International Health Economics Association (iHEA); Pharmacoeconomics; United Kingdom's National Health Service (NHS); United Kingdom's National Institute for Health and Clinical Excellence (NICE)

Further Readings

Maynard, Alan. *The Public-Private Mix for Health.* Abingdon, UK: Radcliffe, 2005.

Maynard, Alan. "European Health Policy Challenges," *Health Economics* 14(Suppl. 4): S255–63, September 2005.

Maynard, Alan. "Is Doctors' Self Interest Undermining the National Health Service?" *British Medical Journal* 334(7587): 234, February 3, 2007.

Maynard, Alan, Karen Bloor, and Nick Freemantle. "Challenges for the National Institute for Clinical Excellence," *British Medical Journal* 329(7459): 227–29, July 24, 2004.

Scott, Anthony, Alan Maynard, and Robert Elliott, eds. *Advances in Health Economics.* New York: Wiley, 2003.

Web Site

University of York, Department of Health Sciences: http://www.york.ac.uk/healthsciences/gsp/staff/amaynd.htm

MCNERNEY, WALTER J.

In his 45-year career, Walter J. McNerney (1925–2005) had a profound impact on the nation's healthcare system. McNerney played a pivotal role in the creation of the federal Medicare program, he was a leading educator in hospital administration, and he was the president of the national Blue Cross and Blue Shield Association.

Born in 1925 in New Haven, Connecticut, McNerney earned a bachelor's degree in industrial administration from Yale University in 1947. After graduation, he taught advanced mathematics at the Hopkins School, a private college-preparatory school in New Haven. He left New Haven to attend the University of Minnesota, where he earned a master's degree in hospital administration in 1950. Over the next several years, he held various administrative positions in hospitals in Providence, Rhode Island, and Pittsburgh, Pennsylvania.

McNerney joined the faculty of the University of Michigan in 1955, where he founded and headed the university's hospital administration program in the School of Business. While at the university, he developed the program's curriculum, taught hundreds of students, and conducted one of the largest, most comprehensive research projects ever undertaken in healthcare. The landmark project detailed the availability, use, quality, finance, and politics of healthcare across the state of Michigan. The results of the project were published in *Hospital and Medical Economics,* a massive two-volume set.

In 1961, McNerney left the University of Michigan to become the president of the national Blue Cross Association. As president, he oversaw the merger with the Blue Shield Association and the subsequent creation of the national Blue Cross and Blue Shield Association. McNerney was instrumental in getting the independent Blue Cross and Blue Shield plans to offer health maintenance organizations (HMOs) and managed-care plans, because he thought that the implementation of managed care was inevitable.

In 1963, he founded the journal *Inquiry.* Today, *Inquiry* is one of the top three peer-reviewed scholarly publications in the field of health services research.

McNerney was a leading advisor to President Lyndon B. Johnson. In partnership with the administration's Wilbur J. Cohen, he developed the blueprint for the Medicare program that, together with Medicaid, was signed into law in 1965. Under President Richard M. Nixon, McNerney also served as chairman of the task force on Medicaid. The panel's final report called for an overhaul of the federal-state apportionment of costs and responsibilities, issues that remain contentious to this day.

After retiring from the Blue Cross and Blue Shield Association in 1981, McNerney went back to academe, becoming the Herman Smith Professor of Health Policy at the Kellogg School of Business at Northwestern University. While teaching at the university, he continued to consult with numerous organizations. He retired in 1998 after suffering a stroke. In 2005, McNerney died at his Winnetka, Illinois home, at the age of 80.

During his long and illustrious career at the University of Michigan, the Blue Cross and Blue Shield Association, and Northwestern University, McNerney mentored hundreds of students as well as junior and senior managers. He served on numerous government and private-sector committees and advisory bodies. He frequently testified before various congressional committees. He worked tirelessly with community organizations and charitable foundations. He wrote 3 books and more than 75 articles on various aspects of healthcare. His areas of expertise included healthcare insurance, management, financing, education, leadership, philanthropy, strategy, and policy. Because of his large number of areas of expertise and wide general knowledge, many considered McNerney a 20th-century Renaissance man.

Tara Moore

See also Association of University Programs in Health Administration (AUPHA); Blue Cross and Blue Shield; Cohen, Wilbur J.; Health Insurance; Medicaid; Medicare; Public Policy

Further Readings

Berman, Howard. "Walter J. McNerney: Remembrances," *Inquiry* 42(3): 201–207, Fall 2005.
Conrad, Douglas A. "Memories of Walter J. McNerney: His Contributions to Health Administration and to Health Administration Education," *Journal of Health Administration Education* 23(4): 331–34, Fall 2006.
Cunningham, Robert, III and Robert M. Cunningham, Jr. *The Blues: A History of the Blue Cross and Blue Shield System.* De Kalb: Northern Illinois University Press, 1997.
McNerney, Walter J. *Health Care Coalitions: New Substance or More Cosmetics?* (The Michael M. Davis Lecture). Chicago: Graduate School of Business, Center for Health Administration Studies, University of Chicago, 1982.
McNerney, Walter J. "In Our New Competitive World, Is the Health Field Headed for Investor-Owned Takeover? Is It for Better or Worse?" (The Andrew Pattullo Lecture). *Journal of Health Administration Education* 14: 77–91, 1996.
McNerney, Walter J., and Study Staff, University of Michigan. *Hospital and Medical Economics: A Study of Population, Services, Costs, Methods of Payment, and Controls.* 2 vols. Chicago: Hospital Research and Educational Trust, 1962.

Web Site

Blue Cross and Blue Shield Association (BCBSA): http://www.bcbs.com/about/history

MEASUREMENT IN HEALTH SERVICES RESEARCH

Measurement in health services research often involves assessing a person's well-being through self-report instruments. Whereas the presence of disease and its effects on mortality can be directly ascertained through clinical observation, the assessment of well-being requires the development of self-report instruments. The measurement of well-being and other internal states (e.g., depression) involves an individual's responses to items that represent various manifestations (e.g., symptoms, attitudes, and beliefs) that collectively reflect the main features of the constructs. The use of measurement in health services research has grown since the 1960s due to policy initiatives such as President Lyndon B. Johnson's "War on Poverty" that necessitated self-report measures to guide program planning and monitor program effectiveness. With support from the National Center for Health Services Research (NCHSR), development and use of multi-item scales has increased dramatically across the spectrum of health services. As a result of contributions from many different disciplines, an array of measures of health status and health outcomes have been developed to evaluate whether healthcare is achieving its mission of reducing disease, disability, and pain and improving health-related quality of life.

Overview

For health service measures to achieve their intended purpose, they must be developed on the basis of a sound theoretical framework and a thorough understanding of the constructs being measured, and rigorous procedures must be used during instrument validation. Sophisticated statistical procedures for data analysis cannot compensate for measures that lack sufficient reliability, validity, and sensitivity. For the responses to individual items or questions to translate into meaningful measures, consideration should be given not only to the underlying theory and the empirical evidence but also to the measurement model being used. Presently, the most common approach in health services research for obtaining meaningful scores on measurement instruments is the *classical test theory* (CTT) approach in which raw item scores are mathematically manipulated, usually by summing across the item scores to obtain a total score. Similarly, the prevalent *instrument validation strategies* are derived from the CTT procedures for instrument development. However, there are alternative measurement models, including the Rasch model and item response theory (IRT), that provide viable alternatives to CTT and are starting to gain acceptance in health services research.

Classical Test Theory

For more than 80 years, CTT has been the basis for the development and evaluation of health services instruments. Under this framework, no distributional assumptions about scores are made. Like modern test theories, CTT does make the assumption that the trait being measured is unidimensional. Perhaps due to its simplicity and relatively weak assumptions, CTT continues to be the prevalent measurement model in health services research. Whereas CTT has played an important role in measuring the diverse panoply of health conditions, the major limitations associated with it have been well-documented in the psychometric literature: (a) sample dependence, (b) test dependence, (c) all items are not created equal, (d) scores are nonlinear and noninterval, and (e) lack of efficiency.

Sample Dependence

Under CTT, item parameters (e.g., item difficulty and other item statistics) are sample dependent. This means that items may have greater difficulty estimates or reflect high severity when they are administered to respondents at the low end of the score continuum but have smaller difficulty estimates or reflect less severity with respondents at the high end of the score continuum. That item statistics depend on the sample with which they are estimated means that these statistics have limited value, except when the sample is similar to

the ultimate patient population for which future instruments will be constructed. Unfortunately, such similarity is rare because instrument validation studies most often rely on samples of convenience, and over time, a population's level of the construct being measured may change.

Test Dependence

The test score, which is often used as a descriptor of a respondent on a given construct, is test dependent. If the level of "difficulty" of the items in the test instrument is changed, as might be done in the context of computer-adaptive tests, then the test scores are no longer on the same mathematical metric. Therefore, they are not a useful variable for comparing respondents to each other or to performance standards.

All Items Are Not Created Equal

The creation of raw scores by summing item responses assumes that the items are equivalent with respect to their position on the construct. In general, this is not a valid assumption.

Scores Are Nonlinear and Noninterval

Ideally, measures derived from health services instruments should be linearly related to the construct being measured. Furthermore, the magnitude of change represented by a single unit on the measurement continuum should remain constant across the measurement spectrum. Regardless of a score's range or whether it is converted to a standard metric, raw scores do not possess the property of linear interval measurement. Noninterval measurement can have serious implications regarding the sensitivity of CTT-based instruments. Research comparing CTT-based scores to Rasch-based measures indicates that the raw scores tend to overestimate trait levels at the low end of the measurement spectrum and underestimate trait levels at the high end.

Lack of Efficiency

In the 1980s, with healthcare practitioners and researchers demanding more measures, the need arose for greater efficiency without a loss of reliability and validity. The CTT model is less than ideal for efficiency because it achieves greater test reliability by increasing the number of items.

Rasch and IRT Measurement Models

Although the early work in IRT took place at the same time as that of the Rasch model, the Danish mathematician and statistician Georg Rasch (1901–1980) was the first to formalize his measurement model. Common to the Rasch and other IRT models is the idea that underlying a respondent's performance on a set of items, questions, performance tasks, or even rating scales is a set of human characteristics known as *latent traits*. These traits, broadly or narrowly defined, are not directly observable. Instead, they must be inferred from an individual's responses to the items or questions comprising the measurement instrument. The IRT measurement model provides an estimate of a given trait by specifying a probabilistic relationship between the items and their characteristics and the estimated trial level. In the Rasch model, this probabilistic relationship is stated most simply for dichotomous items.

There are three features of the Rasch model that are of particular note. First, the use of a probabilistic model allows instrument developers to compare the actual and expected response patterns for a set of items, thereby providing a mechanism for assessing the *model fit*. If the responses are generally consistent with the *model expectations*, the measure is judged to fit the Rasch model and, therefore, has the desired properties of conjoint additivity and sample-free and test-free measurement. Second, the direct comparison between *person measures* and item parameters is possible because both are measured on the same scale: the logit or "log odds ratio" scale. The ability to distinguish person measures and item parameters has important implications with respect to the assessment of change and the evaluation of an instrument's generalizability across cultures. Third, the use of logarithms permits the "bent ruler" of raw scores to have linear and equal-interval properties. Logarithms are useful in transforming curvilinear functions into linear relationships. In the 19th century, the German experimental psychologist Gustav Fechner (1801–1887) was the first to realize that the relationship between stimuli and responses when measuring human characteristics is not linear but rather logarithmic. This suggests that the logarithmic scale both has desirable measurement properties and is well suited for measuring many human characteristics.

Multiparameter IRT Models

Other IRT models include additional item parameters. Whereas the Rasch model makes the assumption that discrimination is equal for all items, multiparameter models typically estimate an *item discrimination parameter*. In educational testing, a *guessing parameter* also may be included. Whereas its *difficulty* refers to the location of the item on the measurement continuum, its *discrimination* refers to the steepness or the slope of the item's characteristic curve (ICC). Items with steep ICCs indicate that a unit change in a person's measure corresponds to a large change in the probability of endorsing the item. Conversely, low discrimination indicates that a unit change on the measure corresponds to a relatively small change in the probability of item endorsement. The guessing parameter is quantified as the probability of item endorsement at the lower asymptote of the ICC.

Research has demonstrated that the Rasch model has properties, associated with additive conjoint measurement, that are required by parametric statistics and advantageous for accurate assessment of change over time. If the data fit the model reasonably well, the Rasch model—compared with CTT and other IRT models—makes the clearest justification that interval- and even ratio-level measurement is obtainable with the survey instruments.

Application of Rasch Measurement

Although Rasch and IRT have their roots in educational testing, these measurement models have been adapted for use in health services research. Some of the earliest health-related applications of Rasch and IRT were in the field of rehabilitation. The initial efforts generally involved the use of the Rasch model. This may be due, in part, to the fact that the Rasch model has lower sample size requirements, compared with multiparameter models, to obtain stable item parameters and accurate person measures. This makes it more suitable for the measurement of highly select populations such as persons with specific types of physical impairments.

Rehabilitation emphasizes monitoring and assessing a person's abilities with respect to physical functioning and the performance of the activities of daily living (ADL). Rehabilitation researchers quickly recognized the limitations in raw scores and the potential of Rasch measurement to produce precise, equal-interval measures. The use of the Rasch model to provide unambiguous measures of the change resulting from rehabilitation made it an attractive alternative to the estimation of change using raw scores, which has long been known to have serious problems. The application of modern measurement models quickly spread to other areas of health research, including health services research.

Measurement of Change

In health services research, the analysis of change is a difficult issue, which may be complicated or confounded by the properties of the measurement instruments. Because of its linear, interval-scaling properties, Rasch measurement enables the assessment and adjustment of measures over time—when the meanings of items may have changed due to differing interpretations of the items and differing use of the rating scale from time one to time two. For the research purpose of interpreting the outcomes, the development of linear, interval, clinical measures makes it possible to move past the reliance on statistical significance, with numbers that are difficult to interpret clinically, to the assessments of outcomes that have clear clinical criteria. Having clinical milestones on the ruler enables the use of much simpler and more easily interpretable numbers that tell the practitioner and researcher (a) how many patients got better in each group, (b) how many patients are borderline and require careful watching, and (c) how many patients are still severe and require a stronger or a different intervention.

Assessing the Cross-Cultural Stability of Item Parameters

To assess individual change, it is important to establish the stability of item parameters over time. It is also critical to determine if measures are

equivalent between culturally defined groups. Measurement equivalence is necessary to make accurate quantitative comparisons across culturally or linguistically defined groups. During the past decade, numerous journal articles have been published concerning the cross-cultural and linguistic equivalence of health and health outcome measures using modern measurement methods. The ability of the Rasch and other IRT measurement models to separate person measures and item parameters and the use of differential item functioning (DIF) analysis have undoubtedly contributed to the growth of this area. Compared with test developers in the fields of education and psychology, health outcome researchers have been slow to acknowledge the presence of DIF in their instruments. However, the incorporation of Rasch and IRT methods in health services research in recent years has led investigators to examine DIF on several measures across a variety of culturally and linguistically defined groups. DIF by country or language has been identified on measures of functional status, disease activity, pain, substance abuse, and health-related quality of life. The presence of DIF does not necessarily indicate that the item(s) producing DIF are biased. DIF may reveal the presence of real group differences. For instance, males and females frequently differ in their presentation of depressive symptoms; likewise, adolescents and adults may differ in their patterns of substance use and symptoms of substance dependence and abuse.

Whereas the Rasch and IRT models provide a mechanism for detecting and adjusting for DIF, it is also important to generate theories and hypotheses that explain the causes of DIF. Rather than simply purging items that fail to fit the measurement model or controlling for DIF through the use of anchoring and equating procedures, understanding the causes of these problems can add greatly to the researchers' ability to write better items. It is also important to note that although DIF is extremely useful in detecting *item* bias, *measures* may be biased or nonequivalent in other ways. For instance, a construct can be defined differently across different cultures (*construct bias*), and there may also be differences in the sample characteristics and administration procedures (*method bias*). Thus, whereas DIF represents an important tool in establishing cross-cultural equivalence, it must be integrated into a larger process of establishing cross-cultural validity.

Computerized Adaptive Testing

Healthcare providers are under increasing pressure from consumers as well as public and private funders to demonstrate that they can provide evidence-based interventions that achieve reliable outcomes. To make matters more complicated, public and private funders have been demanding more detailed assessment (e.g., to diagnostic criteria or a standard for a given area) or other evidence of the standardization of care. Of course, they are also concerned about how the scores translate into diagnosis, placement, and treatment-planning recommendations, particularly for specialty and costly services. Although these efforts hold promise, they also have associated costs: Longer assessments may lead to patient fatigue or agitation; the staff time to learn, administer, interpret, and report on the standardized assessment consumes resources and is costly for the treatment agencies.

Computerized adaptive testing (CAT), coupled with modern psychometric methods and *item banking,* represents a promising solution to the measurement problems encountered with the traditional fixed-form instruments. The combined use of CAT, Rasch, and IRT measurement models plus item banking provides comprehensive and precise measurement with a limited burden to respondents.

CAT algorithms are designed to select and administer a subset of items in a process likened to a binary search. The selected items are tailored to the person's level on the measured construct, and the unnecessary items are eliminated from the assessment process with a minimal loss of measurement precision. This results in a reduced respondent burden and enhanced content specificity. Conversely, item banking increases the content coverage and minimizes the presence of measurement floor and ceiling effects. In addition, CAT is more practical and reliable over a wide range of score levels. Evidence of the efficacy of CAT has revealed several practical advantages, including (a) substantial reductions (50–90%) in the respondent burden, (b) the virtual elimination of ceiling and floor effects, and (c) gains in precision. Though CAT offers significant benefits, the development of

a working CAT requires considerable time and resources, particularly with respect to item bank development and maintenance. A well-developed CAT, however, if it gains widespread acceptance in the field, has the potential to replace the plethora of instruments that now exist for the measurement of health constructs. A CAT item bank can contain enough items to exhaustively represent the construct of interest and produce scores on a single standardized ruler.

Future Implications

The tools for achieving high-quality, valid, and precise measurement in health services research are now readily available. The use of Rasch models is increasing, and they can be applied to a wide range of new applications. These measurement models will likely continue to be adopted toward the ultimate goal of improving each individual's health and well-being.

Barth B. Riley, Kendon J. Conrad,
and Karon Cook

See also Disease; General Health Questionnaire; Health; Health Surveys; Quality of Well-Being Scale; Satisfaction Surveys; Short-Form Health Surveys (SF-36, -12, -8); Ware, John E.

Further Readings

Allen, Mary J., and Wendy M. Yen. *Introduction to Measurement Theory.* Long Grove, IL: Waveland Press, 2002.

Bond, Trevor G., and Christine M. Fox. *Applying the Rasch Model: Fundamental Measurement in the Human Sciences.* 2d ed. Toledo, OH: University of Toledo, 2007.

Conrad, Kendon J., and Everett V. Smith. "International Conference on Objective Measurement Applications of Rasch Analysis in Health Care," *Medical Care* 42(1 Suppl.): 4–6, January 2004.

Embretson, Susan E., and Steven P. Reise. *Item Response Theory for Psychologists.* Mahwah, NJ: Lawrence Erlbaum, 2000.

McDowell, Ian. *Measuring Health: A Guide to Rating Scales and Questionnaires.* 3d ed. New York: Oxford University Press, 2006.

Velozo, Craig A., Ying Wang, Leigh Lehman, et al. "Utilizing Rasch Measurement Models to Develop a

Computer Adaptive Self-Report of Walking, Climbing, and Running," *Disability and Rehabilitation* 30(6): 458–67, 2008.

Wilson, Mark R. *Constructing Measures: An Item Response Modeling Approach.* Mahwah, NJ: Lawrence Erlbaum, 2005.

Web Sites

American Statistical Association (ASA): http://www.amstat.org

Council of American Survey Research Organizations (CASRO): http://www.casro.org

Institute for Objective Measurement (IOM): http://www.rasch.org

MECHANIC, DAVID

David Mechanic is the René Dubos Professor of Behavioral Sciences and the director of the Institute for Health, Health Care Policy, and Aging Research (IHHCPAR) at Rutgers University. He is a preeminent medical sociologist whose research and writing deal with the social aspects of health and healthcare.

Mechanic earned his bachelor's degree from the City College of New York (1956) and his master's (1957) and doctorate (1959) degrees in sociology from Stanford University. In 1960, he joined the faculty of the University of Wisconsin–Madison where he was the chair of the Department of Sociology (1973–1979) and the director of the Center for Medical Sociology and Health Services Research (1972–1979). In 1979, he moved to Rutgers University where he was dean of the Faculty of Arts and Sciences (1980–1984) and, in 1985, became the founding director of IHHCPAR, which he continues to direct. Mechanic also serves as the director of the Robert Wood Johnson Foundation's Investigator Awards in Health Policy Research Program.

Mechanic has been an extraordinary and pioneering leader in the social and behavioral sciences of health, health services, and health and mental health policy over the past 40 years. His work has been innovative in a number of research areas. Mechanic developed the field of illness behavior—that is, the study of how people perceive, evaluate, and selectively act in response to symptoms. His conceptualization of the appraisal and meaning processes that accompany illness as affected by socialization and situational cues has influenced generations of work on the use of health services.

One of Mechanic's distinctive qualities has been his vision in identifying trends and defining new research areas and perspectives in healthcare policy. In his classic study on the social adaptation to stress, he developed an alternative theory to the then pervasive psychodynamic perspective. His model, showing how adaptation was influenced largely by active instrumental initiatives structured by social context and communication patterns, became the dominant research paradigm in the study of stress, coping, and social support.

Mechanic was one of the first researchers to recognize the possibilities yet also the worrisome issues related to managed care. His early articles on the rationing of healthcare established a framework for examining alternative allocation mechanisms. His work on the dynamics of physician payment in capitation and fee-for-service practices in the United Kingdom and the United States anticipated future studies of payment mechanisms. Other major contributions are noteworthy for examining risk selection, population health, policy challenges in addressing racial disparities, and trust relationships between clients and physicians.

Mechanic's recent work explores why reaching consensus and implementing significant reform in the American healthcare system is so problematic. He reasons that until the political will and concerted efforts for change favor the healthcare needs of the population and not the benefit to individuals and organizations who profit from healthcare, reform will remain elusive.

Mechanic has received many notable awards, including the Health Services Research Prize from the Association of University Programs in Health Administration (AUPHA) and the Baxter Allegiance Foundation; the Distinguished Investigator Award from the Association for Health Services Research; the Rema Lapouse Award and the first Carl Taube Award from the American Public Health Association (APHA); and the Distinguished Career Award for the Practice of Sociology, the

Distinguished Medical Sociologist Award, and the Lifetime Achievement Award in Mental Health from the American Sociological Association (ASA). He received the Benjamin Rush Award (with Lecture) from the American Psychiatric Association (APA) and gave the Inaugural Lecture of the Award in the Behavioral and Social Sciences honoring Matilda White Riley at the National Institutes of Health (NIH). Mechanic was elected to the National Academy of Sciences (NAS), and he was also the first sociologist elected to the national Institute of Medicine (IOM).

Carol A. Boyer

See also Access to Healthcare; Health Disparities; Managed Care; Medical Sociology; Mental Health; Public Health; Public Policy; Rationing Healthcare

Further Readings

Mechanic, David. *The Truth About Health Care: Why Reform Is Not Working in America*. New Brunswick, NJ: Rutgers University Press, 2006.

Mechanic, David. "Barriers to Help-Seeking, Detection, and Adequate Treatment for Anxiety and Mood Disorders: Implications for Health Care Policy," *Journal of Clinical Psychiatry* 68(Suppl. 2): 20–26, February 2007.

Mechanic, David. "Mental Health Services Then and Now," *Health Affairs* 26(6): 1548–50, November–December 2007.

Mechanic, David. "Population Health: Challenges for Science and Society," *Milbank Quarterly* 85(3): 533–59, 2007.

Mechanic, David. *Mental Health and Social Policy: Beyond Managed Care*. 5th ed. Boston: Allyn and Bacon, 2008.

Mechanic, David, and Scott Bilder. "Treatment of People with Mental Illness: A Decade Long Perspective," *Health Affairs* 23(4): 84–95, July–August 2004.

Mechanic, David, Lynn Rogut, David Colby, et al., eds. *Policy Challenges in Modern Health Care*. New Brunswick, NJ: Rutgers University Press, 2005.

Web Site

Institute for Health, Health Care Policy, and Aging Research (IHHCPAR): http://www.ihhcpar.rutgers.edu

MEDICAID

Medicaid is a federal and state entitlement program that provides medical benefits to low-income and low-resource individuals and families who meet federal and state eligibility requirements. The Medicaid program is the largest source of medical funding for poor people in the United States. Medicaid is overseen by the Centers for Medicare and Medicaid Services (CMS) in the U.S. Department of Health and Human Services (HHS), but the program is primarily administered at the state level. The federal government provides financial assistance to states, with a greater share of financial support going to states with lower average per capita incomes. Although states vary widely in their program requirements and the services offered, there are certain groups and services that must be covered, including care for children, pregnant women, and disabled individuals. The State Children's Health Insurance Program (SCHIP) and the Program for All-Inclusive Care for the Elderly (PACE) are two special programs within Medicaid designed to cover uninsured children and to provide home- and community-based care to the elderly, respectively.

Background

Medicaid was initially planned as an addition to programs that provided cash assistance to vulnerable groups such as the elderly, disabled, and children and families. Medicaid was signed into law in 1965, as Title XIX of the Social Security Act. It was designed to be a joint program between the states and the federal government to provide medical assistance to qualified needy individuals. This program is primarily coordinated by state agencies with additional funding provided by the federal government.

Medicaid has grown significantly in recent years due to (a) increased use of services; (b) expanded coverage to larger and growing populations; (c) increased costs associated with medical care, drugs, and technology; and (d) an increased need for acute and long-term care. In 2006, total federal and state Medicaid costs reached $303.8 billion, and the program covered close to 59 million people or 20% of the population in fiscal year (FY)

2005. Medicaid costs are expected to rise significantly in the coming years: Estimates place Medicaid costs in FY2009 at $445 billion.

Who Medicaid Covers

To receive Medicaid, individuals or families must fit in a certain designated group. Although there is wide variation among the states, there are certain groups they must cover to receive federal funds. States must provide coverage to those already receiving federal income assistance, such as families eligible for coverage through Aid to Families With Dependent Children (AFDC). Although AFDC was replaced in the 1996 welfare reform bill with Temporary Aid for Needy Families (TANF), Medicaid generally covers anyone who would have been eligible under the AFDC guidelines of 1996. States must also cover individuals falling into one of the other seven *categorically needy* eligibility groups. Many of the designations for coverage require incomes at or below the federal poverty level; for reference, for 2007, 100% of the federal poverty level for a family of four was $20,650 per year or $1720.83 per month. (There are different poverty levels for families in Hawai'i Alaska, and Washington, D.C.) However, having a low income is not sufficient to receive coverage through Medicaid: One must also fit in one of the designated eligibility groups. Furthermore, low-income persons with a certain amount of other assets usually would not be eligible for Medicaid until they "spend down" or deplete their assets to fit in a *medically needy* category (see below).

The categorically needy include (a) families eligible for AFDC (as of 1996), (b) pregnant women and children under 6 years old with a family income at or below 133% of the federal poverty level, (c) children aged 6 to 19 with a family income up to 100% of the federal poverty level, (d) caretakers of children under age 18 (or age 19 if the child is still in school), (e) Social Security Income recipients, (f) individuals receiving adoption or foster care assistance through Title IV of the Social Security Act, (g) people living in medical institutions meeting certain Social Security income requirements, and (h) certain Medicare beneficiaries.

In addition to the categorically needy groups, 34 states and the District of Columbia offer coverage to those fitting in designated medically needy groups. This category allows states to offer coverage to individuals who otherwise would not be covered under Medicaid. The conditions for the medically needy groups can be more restrictive than those for the categorically needy, but people are able to spend down to reach their state's medically needy level. If a state does choose to have a medically needy category, there are certain groups that the federal government requires the state to cover: (a) pregnant women for 60 days post-delivery, (b) children under 18, (c) certain newborns for the 1st year of life, and (d) some blind people. Additional groups that states may choose to cover include (a) children under 21 who are full-time students, (b) caretaker relatives, (c) people over age 65, (d) blind people, (e) disabled people, and (f) others who would be eligible if they were not already enrolled in a health maintenance organization (HMO).

There is a third group of people that receive benefits from Medicaid, and they fall in another category known as "special groups." For example, Medicaid will pay the Medicare premiums, deductible, and coinsurance fees for Medicare recipients who have incomes less than 135% of the federal poverty level. Medicaid will also pay Medicare Part A premiums for Qualified Working Disabled Individuals, who are disabled people who lose Medicare because they are working. These individuals must meet certain income requirements as well and have an income less than 200% of the federal poverty level. The Ticket to Work and Work Incentives Acts of 1999 allow states to expand their Medicaid eligibility to working disabled people. Disabled individuals between the ages of 18 and 65 can be offered Medicaid coverage, even if they exceed Social Security income guidelines, if they are able to and choose to work. If an individual's disabling condition improves, he or she may still be eligible for coverage but may have to share part of the cost of medical care. Certain states offer coverage for special medical conditions as well, but this varies widely by state. For example, 10 states and the District of Columbia offer Medicaid coverage to uninsured tuberculosis patients (for tuberculosis treatment only), and all 50 states offer Medicaid coverage for a specific period of time for women with breast or cervical cancer. All 50 states provide long-term care services for Medicaid-eligible people who qualify for individual care.

Under the Personal Responsibility and Work Opportunity Reconciliation Act of 1996, also known as the *welfare reform bill,* legal resident aliens who entered the United States after 1996 are ineligible for Medicaid coverage for the first 5 years they are in the country. However, states have the ability to modify this requirement if they choose to cover legal resident aliens earlier. All states must provide and cover emergency services for legal aliens.

Program of All-Inclusive Care for the Elderly

PACE was designed to provide an alternative to institutional care for those over 55 years of age requiring skilled nursing care. Working in PACE teams, caseworkers manage and coordinate all the necessary care and services for these individuals, usually provided through adult day-care centers, home health care, and outpatient hospital care. The program helps individuals maintain a more independent lifestyle and still receive the care they need. The providers are paid exclusively through PACE, and they are not able to implement any limits or costs to the patients.

State Children's Health Insurance Plan

Title XXI of the Social Security Act enacted SCHIP and allows states to incorporate SCHIP as part of Medicaid or as an independent program. SCHIP provides additional federal funds for states to cover uninsured children through Medicaid. SCHIP reaches a group of children that would not have otherwise been eligible for Medicaid coverage by covering those up to age 19 whose parents' income is too high for Medicaid but too low to afford private insurance. SCHIP usually covers families with an income at or below 200% of the federal poverty level. All state SCHIP programs must include free immunizations and well-baby visits; other services may have a copay. The immigration status of the parents usually does not matter in regard to medical coverage for their children: As long as the child is a U.S. citizen, he or she will be covered by Medicaid.

Approximately 25% of all the children in the United States, and 50% of all the low-income children, receive their health coverage through Medicaid or SCHIP. Since SCHIP was authorized in 1997, the rate of uninsured children has dropped from 23% in 1997 to 14% in 2005. Children who are covered report similar access to primary and preventive care as children covered by private insurance (but lower access to dental care). Since SCHIP began, improved health outcomes for covered children have been reported, such as fewer emergency room visits for asthma and improved school performance.

What Medicaid Covers

There are certain services that states must provide coverage for, as mandated by the federal government. For people who fall in the categorically needy groups, states must provide coverage for (a) inpatient and outpatient hospital visits; (b) laboratory tests and X rays; (c) pediatric and family nurse practitioners; (d) nursing facility services for individuals over age 21; (e) regular screening up to age 21 as part of Early and Periodic Screening, Diagnosis, and Treatment (EPSDT); (f) family planning care and supplies; (g) rural health clinic care; (h) physician services; (i) dental services; (j) home health services for individuals eligible for nursing care, including home health aides and medical supplies; (k) nurse midwife services; (l) prenatal care; and (m) postpartum care for 60 days. For states with medically needy categories, the following services must be covered: (a) prenatal care and delivery, (b) postpartum care for certain groups under age 18, and (c) home health services for certain groups.

States have the option of providing additional services that are listed under Medicaid law and may also provide some services to certain groups of medically needy individuals. For some of these optional services, states are eligible for federal funding. Examples of additional services for which states can receive federal support are (a) diagnostic services, (b) clinic services, (c) care centers for mentally retarded individuals, (d) prescription drugs and prosthetic devices, (e) optometrist services and eyeglasses, (f) nursing services for individuals under age 21, (g) transportation services to and from medical care, (h) rehabilitation services and physical therapy, and (i) home- and community-based care for individuals with chronic conditions.

How Medicaid Works

Medicaid is overseen by the CMS in the HHS. The federal government provides some guidelines for who will be covered and how, but the requirements and programs vary widely by state, and states take the primary role in administering their statewide Medicaid programs. Medicaid is funded through federal and state funds, and the federal government pays different shares for different states. The share from the federal government is determined by the Federal Medical Assistance Percentage (FMAP), which uses a formula comparing the state's average per capita income with the national average per capita income. This federal-funding share is inversely associated with the state's per capita income. Thus, in a state with a lower per capita income, the federal government will pay a larger share of Medicaid, and in states with higher per capita incomes, the federal government will pay a smaller share. The government share, or FMAP, must be between 50% and 83% of Medicaid costs. In 2008, the federal minimum FMAP was 50% with the highest share, paid to Mississippi, at 76.29%. The FMAP for Washington, D.C. was recently raised permanently from 50% to 70%. For children covered under SCHIP, the federal government pays a higher share, averaging about 70% for all states. The federal government reimburses 100% for care through the Indian Health Service (IHS), a branch of the HHS. It also provides extra financial support to the 12 states that provide the highest rates of emergency care to undocumented immigrants.

There has been recent growth in the use of managed care in Medicaid as an alternative method of both payment and delivery of services. States can apply for waivers from the government in designing and implementing Medicaid managed-care programs. Two sections of the Social Security Act describe waivers available to states in this area: (1) Section 1915(b) allows states to design "innovative healthcare delivery or reimbursement systems" and (2) Section 1115 allows states to carry out demonstration projects to test programs designed to cover uninsured individuals without significantly raising costs. In 2006, approximately 65% of Medicaid recipients were enrolled in managed-care programs, up from only 14% in 1993.

The state is responsible for paying the providers who offer services to Medicaid recipients and accept Medicaid payments. Providers are usually paid through fee-for-service methods or prepayment programs such as the managed-care programs mentioned above. It is also the responsibility of states to ensure that there are enough providers in certain geographic areas who accept Medicaid. For hospitals that treat a disproportionate number of Medicaid recipients and other low-income or uninsured people, the state must make additional payments through a system known as the Disproportionate Share Hospital Adjustment. Some Medicaid beneficiaries may pay a small copayment for services, but there are certain groups that the federal government excludes from having to pay any share of medical costs. These special groups include (a) pregnant women, (b) children under the age of 18, (c) hospital or nursing home patients who would otherwise pay for their own care, and (d) anyone receiving emergency care or family planning services.

States have the power to determine the amount and duration of services they will cover, such as the number of days in the hospital or the number of doctor visits. However, federal law stipulates that these limits be fair and not discriminate on any basis. For example, states cannot limit coverage for medically necessary services for children, such as those considered part of EPSDT.

Like the waivers for managed-care programs and the inclusion of extra groups, states can also apply for waivers to cover additional services such as community- or home-based services for individuals who would otherwise require institutionalization. However, to receive a waiver the state must offer evidence that the plan or service addition is cost-effective.

In administering the state Medicaid program, each state is responsible for (a) setting the rates of payment; (b) establishing eligibility guidelines; (c) determining the types and durations of eligible services; (d) informing recipients about participating providers; and (e) ensuring that recipients receive timely, quality, and appropriate medical care. In addition, the state legislature is able to change state Medicaid policies.

The Cost of Medicaid

Total Medicaid costs for 2006, including both the federal and state expenditures, reached approximately $303.8 billion. Of this figure, 57.8% was for acute care, 36.6% for long-term care, and 5.6% for disproportionate-share hospital payments.

Considering the approximately 59 million Medicaid recipients, the overall average cost per person is about $4,662, but the costs vary considerably among certain groups. For example, children constitute about 50% of all Medicaid recipients and are covered at an average cost of about $1,617 per child. Adults make up about 26% of Medicaid recipients at an average cost of $2,102 per person. Care for elderly and disabled Medicaid recipients costs the most by far: the elderly make up 10.3% of Medicaid recipients and cost an average of $11,839 per person; disabled individuals covered by Medicaid (14.1% of all recipients) cost an average of $13,524 per person.

In the coming years, long-term care will continue to be a large and growing expense for Medicaid. In 2006, Medicaid paid $48.6 billion for nursing facilities, accounting for 41% of the total costs in these areas. The program paid an additional $45.4 billion for home health and personal care.

Dual Eligibility

Under certain circumstances, individuals can be dually eligible for both Medicare and Medicaid. Medicare beneficiaries whose incomes and resources are low enough to qualify in one of Medicaid's eligible categories can receive Medicaid assistance in addition to their Medicare coverage. In these cases, Medicaid supplements Medicare coverage, and additional services not covered by Medicare may be covered (e.g., nursing home care beyond Medicare's 100-day limit). The two main groups of Medicare recipients who are eligible for assistance from Medicaid with Medicare premiums and copayments are known as (1) Qualified Medicare Beneficiaries (QMBs) and (2) Specified Low-Income Medicare Beneficiaries (SLMBs). QMBs are Medicare recipients with incomes less than 100% of the federal poverty level; for these individuals, Medicaid pays their Medicare Part A and Part B premiums, coinsurance, and deductibles. For SLMBs, an income less than 120% of the federal poverty level is sufficient to meet the

eligibility requirement, and Medicaid will pay their Part A and Part B premiums. A third group—working disabled people who have incomes less than 200% of the federal poverty level and who have lost Medicare because they have returned to work—are known as Qualified Disabled and Working Individuals; they are eligible to buy Medicare Parts A and B, and Medicaid will pay their Medicare Part A premiums. A final group of qualified individuals—those who have Medicare and are between 120% and 175% of the federal poverty level—are also eligible to receive Medicaid assistance in paying their Part B premiums. With Medicare Part D recently enacted, Medicaid will no longer provide prescription drug benefits for dually eligible Medicare recipients. It must be noted that in all these cases of dually eligible people, Medicare will always pay first because Medicaid is the payer of last resort. Nationwide, about 6.5 million Medicare recipients receive supplemental assistance from Medicaid.

Future Implications

In the future, managed care will likely become a more popular method as states seek to provide and pay for care for Medicaid recipients and, at the same time, control costs. Medicaid costs will continue to rise as the population ages, long-term care use becomes more frequent, eligible populations grow, and the cost of medical care increases.

Emily Rosenthal

See also Centers for Medicare and Medicaid Services (CMS); Coinsurance, Copays, and Deductibles; Cost of Healthcare; Fee-for-Service; Health Maintenance Organizations (HMOs); Long-Term Care; Medicare; State Children's Health Insurance Program (SCHIP)

Further Readings

Engel, Jonathan. *Poor People's Medicine: Medicaid and American Charity Care Since 1965*. Durham, NC: Duke University Press, 2006.

Grogan, Colleen M., and Michael K. Gusmano. *Healthy Voices, Unhealthy Silence: Advocacy and Health Policy for the Poor*. Washington, DC: Georgetown University Press, 2007.

Hoffman, Earl Dirk, Jr., Barbara S. Klees, and Catherine A. Curtis. "Overview of the Medicare and Medicaid

Programs," *Health Care Financing Review, Statistical Supplement.* pp. 1–281, 283–304, 2005.

Ketler, Sophia R., ed. *Medicaid: Services, Costs, and Future.* New York: Nova Science, 2008.

Smith, David G., and Judith Moore. *Medicaid Politics and Policy, 1965–2007.* New Brunswick, NJ: Transaction Publishers, 2008.

Social Security Act. Available from Social Security Online. http://www.socialsecurity.gov/OP_Home/ssact/ssact.htm

Stevens, Robert, and Rosemary Stevens. *Welfare Medicine in America: A Case Study of Medicaid.* New Brunswick, NJ: Transaction Publishers, 2003.

Web Sites

Center for Health Care Strategies (CHCS): http://www.chcs.org

Centers for Medicare and Medicaid Services (CMS): http://www.cms.hhs.gov

Kaiser Family Foundation, State Health Facts: http://www.statehealthfacts.org/comparetable.jsp?ind=188&cat=4

National Academy for State Health Policy (NASHP): http://www.nashp.org

National Association of State Medicaid Directors (NASMD): http://www.nasmd.org

National Conference of State Legislatures (NCSL): http://www.ncsl.org

MEDICAL ERRORS

Until the 2000 report by the national Institute of Medicine (IOM) *To Err Is Human: Building a Safer Health System,* medical errors were a relatively low priority in the U.S. healthcare system. Medical errors were regarded as uncommon. Physicians and other healthcare providers generally attributed them to "a few bad apples" and the occasional slip. However, data pointing to the pervasiveness of the problem were already available, leading the IOM to estimate that between 44,000 and 98,000 Americans die each year as a result of medical errors.

Since that report, medical errors and patient safety have become a major focus of health services research and policy making, providing a key role for the former in shaping the latter, as both government and nongovernmental organizations develop regulations and guidelines for reducing errors to improve patient safety and the quality of care. There has also been a major shift from blaming the individuals who make errors to recognizing that the individuals function within systems and that those systems critically influence individual performance.

Definitions and Concepts

Key definitions and concepts—many adapted from systems-based research on error prevention in other industries—underlie the current efforts to understand and prevent medical errors. An error is defined by the IOM as either the failure of a planned action to be completed as intended or the use of a wrong plan to achieve an aim. The former is referred to as an *error of execution* and the latter as an *error of planning.* This formulation is based on the work of James Reason and others who extensively studied accidents in aviation and other industries.

Errors of execution are due either to *slips* or *lapses.* A slip is an observable error of execution, such as when a surgeon inadvertently cuts the wrong tissue. A lapse is unobservable, as when an internist forgets to order antibiotics for a patient with pneumonia after intending to do so. In both cases the physician knew what the right thing was to do and intended to do it. In contrast, errors of planning are mistakes in that the actions proceeded as planned but the plan was wrong.

Errors may be classified as *biomedical* or *contextual,* the former occurring because of inattention to processes occurring within the boundary of the skin and the latter from inattention to processes expressed outside that boundary—that is, processes that form the context of a patient's illness. Failing to prescribe a medication that effectively treats a serious condition is a biomedical error. Prescribing a medication that a patient cannot afford when a less costly effective medication is available is a contextual error. In both instances, the patient does not obtain the necessary therapy: in the first, from a failure to attend correctly to the patient's disease and, in the second, from inattention to the context surrounding the disease.

Fortunately, not all errors result in an *adverse event,* the term for an injury that is caused by medical mismanagement. Neglecting to wash one's hands prior to examining a postsurgical wound is an error, for instance, but in most cases this does not result in a wound infection because of the patients' inherent capacity to fight off infection. Conversely, adverse events may occur despite flawless care: A patient's surgical wound may become infected despite excellent sterile technique. Harm that is specifically attributable to error is termed a *preventable adverse event.*

Occasionally, preventable adverse events are due to *negligence*—when the care provided falls below the standard expected of a reasonable and knowledgeable practitioner under the circumstances, as established in a court of law. Most preventable adverse events, however, are considered to be the end result of conditions in the organization that preceded the actual incident.

James Reason distinguished *active* from *latent* errors. Latent errors may include the faulty design of instruments or technologies, poorly installed or functioning equipment, or a dysfunctional work environment where communication or work conditions are not suitable to meet the demands of the job. They may be difficult to detect, but they form the backdrop for the observed, or active, error. The point where an active error occurs is also referred to as the *sharp end* of the system, as in the slip of a surgeon's knife, whereas the latent preconditions for the error are referred to as the *blunt end,* as in the faulty lighting or poor staffing that diminishes an operator's technical performance at the time of the preventable adverse event.

The structured process for identifying contributing factors such as latent errors leading up to an incident is often described as *root cause analysis,* or *systems analysis.* A critical incident may be a near miss or close call, in which an error or series of errors did not produce an injury only because of chance. It may also be a *severe adverse event,* sometimes termed a *sentinel event,* in which severe injury or death to a patient occurred. Reason has described what he calls the "Swiss cheese" model: the view that "holes" may be identified in every layer of an organization's systems of operation. In organizations that lack a culture of safety, where teams may not work well together, or equipment is poorly functional, the holes may be sufficiently large and numerous that it is not uncommon for them to "line up," leading to error chains that result in a high incidence of preventable adverse events.

The Scope of the Problem

Safety is defined as freedom from accidental injury. Because of the high prevalence of preventable adverse events that injure patients, healthcare is unfortunately not as safe as it could be. Early awareness of the magnitude of the problem emerged in 1991 from the Harvard Medical Practice Study of approximately 30,000 randomly examined discharges from 51 hospitals in New York State in 1984. That study found that 3.7% of the hospitalizations were prolonged or resulted in disability because of an adverse event. More than half (58%) of these adverse events were deemed preventable, and 27.6% met the legal criteria for negligence. Nearly one fifth (19%) of the adverse events were medication related, 14% were due to wound infections, and technical complications accounted for 13%. Overall, 13.6% of adverse events were fatal.

Similar findings emerged from a subsequent corroborative study published in 2000 and are based on an analysis of 15,000 hospital discharge records from Colorado and Utah in 1992. The investigators selected a representative rather than a random sample of hospitals, and the records were reviewed by only one rather than two physicians but with greater standardization of the review process. Adverse events were found to be slightly less common at 2.9%; however, the proportions deemed preventable and negligent were nearly the same as those found in New York at 53% and 29.2%, respectively.

The most significant difference between the two studies was the incidence of adverse events that were fatal: The rate of 6.6% in Colorado and Utah was about half the number in New York. Variations in study design, margin of error, and actual differences in error rates in the two studies could all contribute to the discrepant findings. Extrapolating from these numbers to the more than 33 million hospital admissions in the nation in 1997, and excluding unpreventable adverse events from the analysis, produced the widely quoted estimate that medical errors may cause 44,000 to 98,000 preventable deaths per year.

Smaller studies and the recognition that several categories of errors are missed using exclusively hospital-based discharge data has led many to believe that the estimates of preventable adverse events and fatal incidents, as serious as they are, nevertheless *underrepresent* the true magnitude of the problem. In an analysis of more than 1,000 intensive-care units (ICUs) and surgical patients admitted to a teaching hospital, preventable adverse events were identified in 45.8% of the cases, with 17.7% leading to disability or death. The chance of an adverse event increased by about 6% per day of hospitalization.

Furthermore, because most methods for identifying errors and their adverse effects are limited to assessments of the medical record, they miss contextual errors, which are rarely documented. For instance, the failure to take into account a patient's lack of transportation to a Coumadin clinic when prescribing the blood thinner for atrial fibrillation may lead to a preventable bleed, but the medical record will show only that the patient did not adhere to an apparently correct plan of care. Identifying such errors requires case analysis, direct observation, or standardized patients to simulate the conditions under which they might occur.

Preventable Adverse Drug Events

Medication errors are the most studied medical errors because of the extensive charting associated with medication administration and the ever-increasing volume of medications administered each year. Medication errors may occur during (a) prescribing, (b) dispensing, (c) administering, (d) monitoring, and (e) the systems management control process. The latter includes failures to identify drug interactions or to coordinate the administration of medications with other aspects of care (e.g., holding anticoagulation medication before a surgical procedure). When a medication causes an injury it is called an *adverse drug event* (ADE). When such an event is due to medication error it is termed a *preventable adverse drug event*.

At least 1.5 million preventable adverse drug events occur each year in the United States as a result of medication errors. Of these, about 22% occur in hospitals, 31% in outpatient Medicare patients, and 47% in long-term care nursing homes. These data exclude (a) all outpatients under 65 years of age who are not enrolled in the Medicare program, (b) errors patients made taking their own medications, and (c) errors of omission when healthcare providers neglected to prescribe

medications with established benefit (e.g., beta blockers for postmyocardial infarction).

A compendium of data on medication errors and preventable adverse drug events is contained in the 2007 national IOM publication *Preventing Medication Errors*. Prescribing and administration errors are the most common. In hospitals, between 0.1 and 0.3 medication orders are incorrect per patient per day. Medications are incorrectly administered 11% of the time, not counting "wrong time" errors. On average, one administration error, such as the wrong dosage or the wrong rate of administration, occurs per patient per day.

Not all healthcare facilities have the same error rate. In studying 36 facilities, medication administration error rates ranged from 0% to 26%. Error rates have been linked to incomplete or illegible prescriptions and, at the blunt end of the system, to hiring practices that lead to high patient-to-nurse ratios with high nurse workloads.

The morbidity and costs of preventable adverse drug events are high. A 1997 study conservatively estimated that 400,000 inpatient adverse drug events occur in the United States per year at a cost of $5,857 per incident. Adjusting for the rise in healthcare costs and inflation, the additional hospital costs incurred per inpatient preventable adverse drug event in 2008 was $12,403 with avoidable healthcare expenses totaling $5 billion. Based on a 2000 study of the ambulatory costs of Medicare patients (again making similar adjustments), just in this subset of the nation's population, outpatient preventable adverse drug event costs in 2008 are $3,406 per incident and $1.5 billion nationally. Note that none of these estimates take into account lost earnings, losses related to not being able to carry out the activities of daily living (ADL) such as self-care, and the effects of pain and suffering. The calculations also do not include the costs related to preventable adverse drug events when patients do not take their medications correctly or due to overuse and underuse errors by healthcare providers when prescribing.

Disclosures of Errors

Physicians have long feared disclosing medical errors to patients because of concerns that they are more likely to be sued. Employers and insurers shared similar concerns and did not encourage disclosure. However, recent evidence clearly shows that physicians who exhibit transparency and say they are sorry for the medical error are, in fact, substantially less likely to be sued. Furthermore, the legal penalties for deception—for withholding information or misleading patients—have become a further incentive for truth telling.

Several ethical tenets commonly applied to the physician–patient relationship also mandate full disclosure of adverse events. First, adverse events often have consequences that require medical intervention. Patients can only participate in decision making regarding subsequent care if they are fully informed of the circumstances necessitating further intervention. In this respect, disclosure is an essential component of autonomy and informed consent.

Second, truth telling is considered essential to respect for persons. When patients entrust themselves to physicians, they expect full transparency, even with regard to near misses. In studies where patients have been given hypothetical scenarios involving even minor incidents related to their care, 98% say that they would want to know what happened. Furthermore, they have indicated that they would be more likely to sue their physicians if they later discovered that information had been withheld or covered up. Hence deception— independent of the actual physical harm that occurred—is regarded by patients, almost universally, as a harm in itself.

Third, full disclosure is essential to justice and fairness. Although they may, in fact, be less likely to sue, patients have the right to seek compensation for injuries when they occur, if they so choose.

Error Reporting

In addition to the legal and ethical imperatives for candor with patients about errors related to their care, disclosure of all such incidents internally and to regulatory bodies through formalized reporting systems is critical to accountability and quality improvement. There are a number of obstacles, however, to effective error reporting systems. Physicians may fear negative repercussions, including malpractice litigation, disciplinary action, or loss of hospital privileges. They may be hesitant to personally acknowledge errors in a profession that emphasizes perfectionism. They may be skeptical that their reports, which are often time-consuming to file, will be used to improve care. At the institutional level, organizations also face concerns about how they are regarded and practical issues about how best to use the data. A major challenge, then, is creating reporting systems that (a) are easy to access, (b) provide certain legal protections to reporters and institutions, and (c) use the data to improve the processes of care.

Reporting systems for medical errors and adverse events can be mandatory or voluntary. Also, reporting can come directly from the provider, or reports may be submitted by the organization. Finally, reporting can be to an external monitor, such as a state or federal entity, or remain internal to the organization with periodic external audits. Each has its advantages and disadvantages. For instance, direct reporting by practitioners to a national database provides frontline information and bypasses the employer, which may be reassuring to a reporter who is reluctant to notify management each time an error occurs. On the other hand, internal tracking of errors enables organizations to identify system problems and make the necessary changes.

Since the mid-1980s, a growing number of individual states have had adverse event reporting systems of various kinds. The number of reports filed has ranged from fewer than 20 in a year in some cases to tens of thousands in others, indicating the severity of the problem of underreporting. States have also varied greatly in the information made available to the public. Patient confidentiality is always maintained, but whether the names of physicians, hospitals, and health systems or the numbers of adverse events per site are released and whether the data are freely accessible on the Internet all vary. Synthesis and analysis of data, particularly across states, has been almost uniformly poor.

At the federal level, the U.S. Food and Drug Administration (FDA) is an example of a national reporting program for adverse events linked to medications and other medical products. All malfunctions, serious injuries, and deaths must be reported by either the facility or the manufacturer, depending on the circumstances. However, these problems are generally not due to provider or systems errors at the organizational level. The focus is on identifying product defects or risks associated with products through postmarketing surveillance.

To address the unmet need for a comprehensive reporting system that is easily accessible, provides legal protections, and has analytic and response capabilities, the U.S. Congress passed the Patient Safety and Quality Improvement Act of 2005, which established Patient Safety Organizations (PSOs) to collect and process confidential information reported by healthcare providers. The law gives full confidentiality protection to reporters and limits the use of the information in legal proceedings. Both public and private entities—for-profit or not-for-profit (excluding insurance organizations)—may apply to become PSOs if they are capable of meeting the complex requirements to qualify. The act also created a network of patient safety databases (NPSDs) for centralizing data to establish national as well as regional statistics related to errors, adverse events, and the effect of safety improvement initiatives.

Internationally, concerns about medical errors, adverse events, and the strategies for reporting them have developed in parallel. Australia, Canada, and the United Kingdom have all initiated reporting systems. The World Health Organization (WHO) has created the World Alliance for Patient Safety, following a resolution in 2002. Its charge includes a broad range of safety initiatives, such as data collection on adverse events related to healthcare delivery in developing countries, as well as guidelines for adverse event reporting.

Despite these efforts, physicians indicate that medical-error-reporting systems are still inadequate. A survey of U.S. physicians found that they were more likely to discuss errors with their colleagues than make a formal report. Only a third of physicians felt that reporting systems at their organizations were adequate. Few had confidence in the process. Nevertheless, 83% indicated that they had, at some point, filed a formal report of an error. Major areas where physicians wanted to see improvement were in assurances that (a) reports remain confidential and nondiscoverable, (b) the data will guide system improvements, (c) there will be no penalties or other negative repercussions, and (d) the process will take less than 2 minutes to complete.

Although physicians have concerns about the reporting process, interest in the problem of errors and how to prevent them is high. Most physicians now believe that reporting errors is necessary to improve patient safety, and most feel that they are not getting adequate information about how to prevent them. Increasingly, physicians are embracing a culture of safety.

Progress in Reducing Errors

There has been a major shift in attitudes toward medical errors and the need to protect patients from preventable harm. In the peer-reviewed medical literature, articles addressing issues of patient safety more than tripled during the 5 years following the 2000 IOM report, compared with the previous 5 years. The number of federally funded patient safety research awards increased nearly 30-fold. Starting in 2001, the U.S. Congress has appropriated $50 million annually to fund many of these studies.

What has been the impact of such investments? Evidence that healthcare has become substantially safer is not yet strong. There have been discrete studies showing improvements in certain areas. For instance, hospitals with tight infection control procedures have documented a reduction in hospital-acquired infections, and fatalities related to the accidental injection of concentrated potassium chloride have been prevented by removing the product from nursing unit shelves. There may be many other such examples of a positive effect. Underdeveloped error tracking systems have confounded efforts to assess progress.

A number of organizations, along with the government, have committed to the patient safety movement, setting specific goals and strategies for preventing medical errors. The Agency for Healthcare Research and Quality's (AHRQ's) Center for Quality Improvement and Safety leads the federal government's efforts to (a) set standards and measures called *patient safety indicators;* (b) educate healthcare providers, administrators, and the general public; and (c) guide the research agenda. The Joint Commission has played a key role in enforcing change by requiring hospitals to follow specific error prevention strategies, such as (a) improved patient identification, (b) surgical-site verification, and (c) standards for communicating information. Private–public partnerships—such as the Institute for Health Improvement's (IHI's) 100,000 lives campaign, which enlisted thousands of hospitals to adopt proven methods of reducing avoidable deaths—have been cosponsored by the federal AHRQ, the Centers for Disease Control and Prevention (CDC), and the Centers for Medicare and Medicaid Services (CMS), exemplifying a broad-based commitment to make healthcare safe. Building on that momentum, the IHI and its partners embarked on a "5 million lives" campaign to protect patients over a period of 2 years from 5 million incidents of medical harm. The movement to eliminate medical errors is still young but maturing rapidly.

Saul J. Weiner

See also Agency for Healthcare Research and Quality (AHRQ); Health Report Cards; Institute for Healthcare Improvement (IHI); International Classification for Patient Safety (ICPS); Joint Commission; Patient Safety; Pay For Performance; Quality of Healthcare

Further Readings

Aspden, Philip, and the Committee on Identifying and Preventing Medication Errors. *Preventing Medication Errors.* Washington, DC: National Academies Press, 2007.

Dhillon, B. S. *Reliability Technology, Human Error, and Quality in Health Care.* Boca Raton, FL: CRC Press, 2008.

Kohn, Linda T., Janet M. Corrigan, Molla S. Donaldson, and the Committee on Quality of Health Care in America. *To Err Is Human: Building a Safer Health System.* Washington, DC: National Academy Press, 2000.

Moller, Aage R. *A New Epidemic: Harm in Health Care: How to Make Rational Decisions About Medical and Surgical Treatment.* New York: Nova Biomedical Books, 2007.

Peters, George A., and Barbara J. Peters. *Medical Error and Patient Safety: Human Factors in Medicine.* Boca Raton, FL: CRC Press, 2008.

Reason, James. "Human Error: Models and Management," *British Medical Journal* 320(7237): 768–70, March 18, 2000.

Vance, James E. *A Guide to Patient Safety in the Medical Practice.* Chicago: American Medical Association, 2008.

Wachter, Robert M. *Understanding Patient Safety.* New York: McGraw-Hill Medical, 2008.

Web Sites

Agency for Healthcare Research and Quality (AHRQ): http://www.ahrq.gov/qual

Health Grades: http://www.healthgrades.com

Institute for Healthcare Improvement (IHI): http://www.ihi.org/ihi

Institute for Safe Medication Practices (ISMP): http://www.ismp.org

Joint Commission: http://www.jointcommission.org

U.S. Food and Drug Administration (FDA): http://www.fda.gov

MEDICAL GROUP PRACTICE

Medical group practice, a form of medical practice that dates back to the 1800s, can be defined in a number of ways. The Medical Group Management Association (MGMA), an organization representing group practice executives, administrators, and managers, and the American Medical Association (AMA), the nation's largest physician association, consider medical group practices to have the following elements: (a) a formal or legal arrangement; (b) three or more physicians; and (c) shared business and clinical operations, facilities, staff, and equipment.

Recent federal health legislation regarding physician self-referral, known as the Stark legislation (named for U.S. Congressman Fortney "Pete" Stark), has defined medical group practice in a slightly different manner. First, the federal legal definition is broader in scope, including groups with two or more physicians. At the same time, this definition applies more stringent criteria that stipulate that (a) all physicians in the group must provide a full range of patient care services appropriate to their specialties and be responsible for the bulk of the care provided through the group; (b) group income and expenses must be distributed according to an established plan; and (c) decision making in the group must be centralized with respect to functions such as governance, budgets, billing, and use.

Regardless of how they are defined, the ways medical group practices look and act vary considerably. Medical group practices may be composed of physicians with the same specialty or physicians with different specialties. And they can include other types of medical professionals such as dentists and podiatrists. These groups may be embedded within larger health systems. They may work out of a single location or many locations. Medical group practices may or may not be physician owned. These practices can range in size from a few physicians to thousands of primary-care and specialty-care providers. One of the best-known medical group practices in the nation is the Mayo Clinic, which is based in Rochester, Minnesota, and employs more than 3,300 physicians, scientists, and researchers at multiple sites across the country.

Importance

Medical group practices are important to the study of health services research because they represent an increasingly common vehicle for the delivery of medical care. They also, theoretically, hold much potential for improving the quality and efficiency of the delivery of medical services.

The number of medical group practices and the number of physicians practicing in them has grown over time. The AMA reported that there were just over 4,000 medical group practices in 1965 but nearly 20,000 in 1996, representing approximately 11% and 32% of all physicians in the nation. More recently, the Agency for Healthcare Research and Quality (AHRQ) supported a collaborative study between the MGMA and the University of Minnesota School of Public Health that sought to establish a nationally representative database of medical group practices. This effort resulted in the estimate that the number of medical group practices had grown to nearly 37,000 in 2003 and that the physicians in them represented almost 67% of all office-based physicians in the nation. Based on these findings, medical group practices deliver a large proportion of the medical care in the nation.

One reason for the establishment and continuation of medical group practices is that increased medical specialization and technical complexity require the integration of multiple physicians into a single practice to provide appropriate and necessary patient care services. Medical group practices are also an attractive employment option for many physicians because they may provide certain advantages over solo practice. For example,

medical group practices often provide malpractice coverage, the sharing of on-call duties, and the intellectual challenge and stimulation of working with colleagues from a variety of disciplines and specialties.

Medical group practices are thought to contribute to the efficient and high-quality delivery of medical care in a number of ways. Some medical group practices provide a wide and complex range of services on-site. Medical group practices may contain costs through centralized purchasing, uniform coding and billing, and the sharing of auxiliary medical and administrative staff. These practice groups may be able to enhance access to care through extended office hours. A medical group practice's organizational culture—including factors such as the extent to which the group's physicians share information, are innovative and collegial, and subscribe to a group identity—is also thought to affect healthcare costs and quality.

Future Implications

Medical group practices are an increasingly important feature in the healthcare delivery system in the United States. As a result, it is increasingly important and necessary when conducting health services research to consider their impact on the quality, effectiveness, and efficiency of the delivery of medical care. However, given the large number of medical group practices and the wide variation in the ways they are organized, the influences of this type of practice may be difficult to disentangle from other causal factors in an already complex system of healthcare delivery. These factors can include (a) a physician's training, (b) the medical group's payment structure, (c) its organizational culture, (d) the influences of partners and colleagues, (e) the rules and standards established by the health maintenance organizations (HMOs) and health insurance companies with which the group is contracted, (f) patient expectations, and (g) community standards. As knowledge of medical group practices and their operations continues to grow, health services researchers will be able to make vital improvements in the delivery of healthcare.

Penny L. Havlicek

See also Access to Healthcare; American Medical Association (AMA); Equity, Efficiency, and Effectiveness in Healthcare; Forces Changing Healthcare; Health Workforce; Managed Care; Physicians; Quality of Healthcare

Further Readings

Casalino, Lawrence P., Kelly J. Devers, Timothy K. Lake, et al. "Benefits of and Barriers to Large Medical Group Practices in the United States," *Archives of Internal Medicine* 163(16): 1958–64, September 8, 2003.

Medical Group Management Association. *Performance and Practices of Successful Medical Groups: 2008 Report Based on 2007 Data.* Englewood, CO: Medical Group Management Association, 2008.

Reiboldt, J. Max, Craig W. Hunter, P. Todd DeWeese, et al. *Integration Strategies for the Medical Practice.* 2d ed. Chicago: American Medical Association Press, 2006.

Tollen, Laura. *Physician Organization in Relation to Quality and Efficiency of Care: A Synthesis of Recent Literature.* New York: Commonwealth Fund, 2008.

Web Sites

American Medical Association (AMA): http://www.ama-assn.org

American Medical Group Association (AMGA): http://www.amga.org

Medical Group Management Association (MGMA): http://www.mgma.com

MEDICALIZATION

Medicalization is a process through which human problems come to be defined as medical problems. In brief, society considers certain behaviors to be deviant. But "deviance" is not inherent in the behavior; instead, it is the result of social judgments that shift over time in response to the ideas expounded by the social institution prevailing at the time. For example, deviant behavior was seen as sinful when religion was the predominant social institution and in a position to define the nature of human problems. As confidence in empirical explanations began to take hold, the view that

deviance is a matter of *sinfulness* gave way to the view that deviant behavior is a violation of social norms and laws, that is, *badness.* Medicalization signifies the most recent shift, transforming the definition of deviance again, this time from badness to *sickness.*

The Power to Define Sickness

The concept of medicalization was introduced during the second half of the 20th century when Americans were registering rising distrust in and disillusionment with the values being expounded by the leaders of most social institutions. Hence, the times were conducive to rejecting a socially defined view of deviance in favor of a medical-based perspective. Critics argued, and many observers agreed, that the prerogative to determine what is and what is not a medical problem gives physicians tremendous power. The question of whether this is more socially beneficial or detrimental remains unsettled.

Talcott Parsons (1902–1979), an American, Harvard University sociologist, is credited with initiating discussion of the vital social role played by physicians in differentiating between true sickness and malingering. He based this proposition on the premise that social stability and continuity require that all members of society fulfill their respective social roles. Because the "sick" role offers the benefit of excusing a person from normal responsibilities, it is important to ensure that people do not take inappropriate advantage. By identifying what constitutes real illness, physicians are in a position to grant patients a temporary exemption from their normal role responsibilities. By labeling symptoms as true illness, physicians are granting the patient a period of "legitimated deviance." Physicians then go on to restore the sick person to full health so that he or she can carry out the normal role expectations. Because physicians are willing to accept this weighty burden, Parsons maintained that they should be generously rewarded.

Parsons's model of the sick role depicted recovery from acute illness as the only acceptable resolution to a period of legitimated deviance. Detractors pointed out that this portrayal meant that those who did not or could not get well were doomed to being permanently labeled as deviants.

A number of observers have made the point that having the power to determine whether the symptoms patients present with are, in fact, indicative of a disease gives physicians undue power to act as moral arbiters. From time to time, the discovery of a newly identified disease reinvigorates the charge that physicians have too much power and that patients' complaints are too often dismissed as illegitimate. The discovery of Lyme disease provides a vivid illustration. According to media reports, it was only through the efforts of one courageous woman that the disease was finally identified. Because her symptoms were so common (i.e., headaches, body rashes, and flu-like conditions), she was diagnosed with various conditions from poison ivy to hysteria by the many physicians she visited. The media reported that the physicians denied the existence of this particular patient's disease because it did not fit a recognized diagnostic label. Not only was she repeatedly told that she was a hypochondriac, she was denied the benefits of the sick role as well as treatment.

The story, which received much media attention at the time, had the effect of bringing numerous patients to physicians' offices with similarly vague symptoms insisting that they, too, had Lyme disease. When physicians did not find evidence of the disease, many of these patients became convinced that callous physicians were unwilling to treat them, fueling the view that medicine's power was certainly excessive and probably socially dysfunctional.

The question whether physicians should have the final say in determining whether a particular set of symptoms is indicative of the existence of disease—the essence of medicalization—continues to be contentious, particularly as groups of people who share some experience that they believe has caused them to experience a particular set of symptoms insist that physicians identify those symptoms as a disease or syndrome. Understanding the ramifications associated with the sick role helps explain the persistent efforts on the part of many of those afflicted with various human problems to portray them as illnesses.

Physicians and the Promotion of Medicalization

Whether physicians are actively engaged in promoting and sustaining medicalization is another point of debate. A number of commentators have taken the position that the medical profession has, in some instances, purposefully engaged in expanding its scope of control. Michel Foucault, for example, noted that early practitioners of psychiatry were particularly zealous in their efforts to define the limits of acceptable social behavior. Thomas Szasz stated that psychiatrists were finding evidence of mental illness in people who were simply rejecting the roles that society imposed on them. He maintained that psychiatrists were guilty of trying to convince such people that their behavior indicated that they were "sick," and they required medication to help them fit in the role or roles, often undesirable ones, that society had prescribed.

Similarly, the idea that women who resisted the limited range of social positions and roles dictated by society from the post–World War II period through the rebellious 1960s were likely to be the objects of such labels and treatment is, at least in some circles, now a matter of conventional wisdom. Feminists argue that the medical profession continues today to impose its definition of the feminine ideal: They say that plastic surgeons are defining our standards of beauty, both facial and in body shape, and that other physicians are ready to prescribe a wide range of pharmaceuticals—including weight-loss medications, mood-altering drugs, sleep aids, energy boosters, and so on—more to women than to men. The fact that some women demand such treatments they attribute to a distorted set of social values which are promoted by a wide range of self-interested parties who benefit from the medicalization of such common conditions as aging-related changes.

Physicians' motivations for actively promoting medicalization, to the extent that they may have been doing so, have not yet been examined closely. Whether physicians are motivated by the promise of increased income, as the representatives of managed-care organizations have argued; or by greater social prestige and authority, as some social scientists maintain; or are truly interested in improving the lot of people who are not only plagued by pain and suffering but stigmatized as well, which is the position taken by spokespeople for the medical profession, has not been the subject of much debate or investigation.

Eliot Freidson is one the few social scientists whose observations addressed the issue directly. He argued that physicians are not so much motivated by the possibility of increased income as by the opportunity to gain professional recognition and possibly have their names attached to the discovery of a new disease or syndrome. He proceeded from the observation that medicine had been very successful in its efforts to define the scope of and monopolize medical work through medical licensure. That, he pointed out, effectively prevents other health practitioners from ministering to patients' complaints using treatments other than those approved by the medical profession. Freidson coined the term *professional dominance*. He argued that physicians behave in a dominant fashion in their interactions with anyone over whom they can impose their authority, from patients to other healthcare workers. Feminists embraced Freidson's observations on the role physicians assigned to nurses—who are overwhelmingly female—as handmaidens to physicians

It is worth noting that critics of medicine's power were most vocal during the same years that society was registering especially high regard for the medical profession: during the post–World War II years until the end of the 1970s. Throughout this period, prestige surveys consistently accorded medicine the top rank compared with other occupations. Surveys documenting the level of trust society was willing to accord particular social institutions consistently found that medicine inspired more trust than other social institutions. The decline in trust in the profession of medicine coincided with the rise of managed care during the 1980s. The spokespeople for managed-care organizations presented themselves as interested in protecting patients from physicians who, they said, were more interested in their own pocketbooks than their patients' welfare. Thereby, in a few short years, the corporate sector succeeded at what social critics had been striving to accomplish for several decades.

The charge that physicians engage in medicalization lost much of its condemnatory power in this atmosphere, given that a wide range of other failings were also being attributed to the profession. Yet patients have generally said, and continue to say, that their own physicians are wonderful but that they are the exception.

Medicalization and the Role of Other Interested Parties

The criticism aimed at the medical profession that it promotes the medicalization of routine human problems has not had an ameliorating effect because the list of additional agents interested in promoting medicalization continues to expand. Many members of the public afflicted with certain conditions have been active in their efforts to aid, abet, and pressure medicine to define those conditions as sickness. One practical reason why patients would want to do this is that having a condition defined as an illness results in medical insurance coverage. Another reason is that there are certain conditions that members of the public want very much to see labeled as sickness to avoid the stigma attached to the alternative: Sickness indicates that the cause of the problem is biological and not the result of weakness of character—that is, it is sickness not badness.

Attention deficit disorder, hyperactivity, and hyperkinesis are illustrative of this phenomenon. Some parents and teachers initially identified socially disruptive behaviors as problematic and requested medications that will reduce the incidence of such behavior. Physicians must, of course, agree to diagnose the condition as an illness and prescribe medications designed to control the behavior. The thrust of the criticism is that the diagnosis is being too liberally applied. An important question that does not generally arise is whether diagnosing and medicating the child as having a "minimal brain dysfunction"—that is, a sickness—is more or less damaging than determining that the child is a social deviant who willfully misbehaves and deserves to be punished—that is, that the child is bad.

Further evidence that the medicalization of children's behavior is not waning is apparent in the discovery of new syndromes: "school refusal behavior," for example, (i.e., skipping school), which has recently been identified by some psychiatrists as a sign of an anxiety disorder requiring medical treatment.

Posttraumatic stress disorder (PTSD) is another example of a more or less successful effort to have particular behaviors recognized as illness rather than badness. The designation allows those having difficulty readjusting to civil society after wartime service in the military to receive the benefits that go along with the sick role—from the psychological and emotional benefits that come with the extension of sympathy, to the greater understanding and tolerance of absence from work due to a range of physical and psychological problems.

There are also instances of a less successful transition from badness to sickness as reflected, for example, in the social attitude toward alcoholism. Many individuals who have this problem have been unwavering in their efforts to have society accept the view that alcoholism is a disease. The Yale School of Alcoholism Studies (which emerged in the 1930s), now the Rutgers Center of Alcohol Studies (as of 1962)—neither of which has operated under the auspices of medical practitioners—have provided the main impetus for dissemination of this definition. Physicians, generally, have been less eager to define alcoholism as a disease; in part, no doubt, because alcoholism does not lend itself to a traditional medical approach to either prevention or cure. Medical treatment of the health problems brought on by alcoholism, though, is uncontested.

The role played by the public health community must be included in the discussion of medicalization because of its stance on the value of punishment versus therapeutic intervention in controlling certain behaviors. Members of the public health community not only oppose the use of legal sanctions to reduce the prevalence of deviant behavior, they also oppose treating people who engage in destructive and risky behavior on an individual basis. They hold that control of such behavior would be better addressed through population-based solutions. Public health practitioners have argued that the morbidity and mortality associated with violence, intravenous drug abuse, and other forms of substance abuse should be viewed in much the same way as other man-made diseases—smoking-related illnesses, for instance—and treated accordingly. They point out that intervention at the level of treating the individual who is suffering the consequences of engaging in risky behaviors comes too late. They maintain that more benign approaches, particularly public education, would be far more effective.

There are also instances of medicalization being *imposed* on the medical profession, as illustrated by the legal mandate governing how physicians deal with child abuse. Physicians are required to report suspected cases of child abuse when they examine children brought to their offices or, more likely, the emergency room. Medical treatment of the child is not at issue. However, some physicians resist reporting this form of deviance arguing that the children are likely to suffer further abuse when the abuser is threatened with legal sanctions and the removal of the child from the home.

Demedicalization

There is one well-known case of demedicalization—homosexuality. The first edition of the *Diagnostic and Statistical Manual of Mental Disorders* (DSM) published by the American Psychiatric Association (APA) in 1952, listed homosexuality as a "Sociopathic Personality Disorder." It continued to be listed as a form of "sexual deviation" over the next two decades even as the challenge from homosexual activists, both within and outside the APA, gained momentum. In 1973, the APA Board of Trustees voted to adopt a new definition. As of that time, only those homosexuals who are disturbed by their condition are to be considered candidates for treatment. Many in the gay community welcomed the change. Others pointed out that there was no counterpart for the designation of "Homosexual-Conflict Disorder" for heterosexuals, as in "Heterosexual-Conflict Disorder." Society has become more accepting of homosexuality and homosexual unions since the early 1970s. Whether the APA's decision contributed to the shift in social attitudes is not clear.

New Forces Promoting Medicalization

Although the term *medicalization* is now less likely to be invoked, the process appears to be proceeding at an accelerating rate along two related paths. One is the treatment of conditions that research indicates will lead to illness in the future and that can be identified using objective indicators of physical status. The second revolves around the possibility of enhancing the performance of persons who are healthy.

Turning to the first path, medicine has been more aggressive in recent years in lowering the cutoff that separates what is a normal reading from what requires attention for a range of physical indicators such as hypertension, cholesterol level, and diabetes. Physicians often strongly recommend lifestyle changes, primarily more exercise and changes in diet. Although this may be a form of medicalization, it is not one that provides the benefits long associated with the sick role. In fact, it requires a certain amount of sacrifice in giving up familiar patterns of behavior that are not considered deviant. Whether society comes to define self-indulgent eating habits and avoidance of exercise as deviant and requiring some form of intervention (e.g., increased regulation or taxation) besides physicians' admonitions remains to be seen. The shift in social attitudes toward drinking and driving provides a good example of society's power to redefine what is acceptable versus unacceptable behavior, without physicians taking the leading role.

Whether the health problems that result when patients will not or cannot make the behavioral changes that are intended to lower readings on their blood pressure, low density lipids, and blood sugar should be defined as syndromes is a matter of debate in the medical community. Obesity is a case in point. From the medical profession's perspective, defining what is and what is not a disease revolves around questions of ethics and a consensus regarding best practices, not issues of social deviance. To illustrate, the American Academy of Family Practice (AAFP) declared, in 2004, that obesity is a disease; the American Medical Association (AMA), however, maintains that it is clearly a major health problem but not a disease. Those who favor defining obesity as a disease say that this will cause it to be taken more seriously. Those who are opposed say that doing so will have the effect of diminishing personal and social responsibility.

Ethics and best practices are also at issue in how medicine should treat such touchy problems as gender allocation surgery at birth, gender-based selection of fetuses, treating women who have lost interest in sex with testosterone creams, and so on. There is no denying the fact that members of the public are demanding a wide range of interventions and that there are growing numbers of willing providers. To illustrate, according to the American Society for Aesthetic Plastic Surgery (ASAPS), 11.5 million cosmetic procedures were performed in the United States in 2005. This is a 444% increase from 1997 to 2005. There were 3.29 million Botox injections, making it the most popular procedure. By some estimates, this procedure has become a $15 billion business.

Now that patients are increasingly directly involved in requesting treatment for what they perceive to be unwelcome and avoidable physical problems, direct-to-consumer advertising by pharmaceutical companies is a new force in convincing the public that their problems are actually syndromes that can be successfully treated with prescription drugs. Some physicians say that they feel pressured to prescribe medications when there is no evidence that a person is afflicted with the illness featured in the ads. Even when patients do experience some of the symptoms being described in the ads, physicians often maintain that waiting to see whether the symptoms diminish is preferable to reaching at once for pharmaceuticals.

The second newly evolving medicalization path revolves around the "heal or enhance" debate, which has been limited to revelations about athletes, until recently, but is increasingly affecting the general public. Some physicians take the position that anything that helps patients is within the legitimate scope of medical practice. Others argue that *restoring* function should not be confused with *enhancing* function. The worry is that it is becoming more and more difficult to draw the line between ethical and unethical practices. Is it ethical to prescribe stimulants that can help enhance grades? Is it ethical to prescribe Alzheimer's medications to enhance memory? Is "cosmetic neurology"—described by its main promoter as the modulation of "motor, cognitive, and affective systems"—an acceptable medical practice? The demand for such enhancements is clearly growing where competitive pressure is greatest—that is, in professional athletics and advanced educational training.

It is difficult to imagine what might replace the medicalization process that shifts badness to sickness, especially as it is increasingly accompanied by the promise of an unrestrained potential to redefine a wide range of human problems as medical problems, which people might then rid themselves of simply by taking a pill.

Grace Budrys

See also Diagnostic and Statistical Manual of Mental Disorders (DSM); Direct-to-Consumer Advertising (DTCA); Disease; Health; International Classification of Diseases (ICD); Medical Sociology; Physicians; Public Health

Further Readings

Conrad, Peter. *The Medicalization of Society: On the Transformation of Human Conditions Into Treatable Disorders.* Baltimore: Johns Hopkins University Press, 2007.

Foucault, Michel. *Madness and Civilization: A History of Insanity in the Age of Reason.* New York: Vintage Press, 1965.

Freidson, Eliot. *Professional Dominance.* New York: Atherton, 1970.

Hadler, Martin, "'Fibromyalgia' and the Medicalization of Misery," *Journal of Rheumatology* 30(8): 1668–70, August 2003.

Kuczynski, Alex. *Beauty Junkies: Inside Our $15 Billion Obsession With Cosmetic Surgery.* New York: Doubleday, 2006.

Parsons, Talcott. *The Social System.* Glencoe, IL: Free Press, 1951.

Szasz, Thomas S. *The Medicalization of Everyday Life: Selected Essays.* Syracuse, NY: Syracuse University Press, 2007.

Wolpe, Paul Root. "Treatment, Enhancement, and the Ethics of Neurotherapeutics," *Brain and Cognition* 50(3): 387–95, December 2002.

Web Sites

American Academy of Child and Adolescent Psychiatry (AACAP): http://www.aacap.org

American Society for Aesthetic Plastic Surgery (ASAPS): http://www.surgery.org

National Institute of Drug Abuse (NIDA): http://www.nida.nih.gov

MEDICAL SOCIOLOGY

Medical sociology is a large, substantive area within the general field of sociology. Using a sociological perspective, theories, and research methods, medical sociology is concerned with the social causes and consequences of health and disease. Some of the major areas that medical sociology studies include (a) the social aspects of health and disease, particularly health and illness behavior and the role of the sick; (b) the social behavior of healthcare professionals and their patients, particularly physician–patient interaction; (c) the social functions of healthcare organizations and institutions, particularly hospitals and healthcare networks; (d) the social patterns of health services; and (e) the international comparisons of healthcare delivery systems, particularly comparing the healthcare system of the United States with that of Canada and the United Kingdom.

History

Although a number of medical sociology articles appeared in the late 19th and early 20th centuries, the field is generally regarded as beginning in 1951 with the publication of Talcott Parsons's book *The Social System*. In his book, Parsons (1902–1979), the influential American, Harvard University sociologist, presented a functionalist theory of the "sick" role. He argued that patients who (a) do not intentionally cause their own illness, (b) seek help from a physician, and (c) strive to get well are entitled to relief from their normal role responsibilities—a period of legitimated deviance. Those who do not follow these rules are engaging in deviant behavior and must be socially sanctioned. Otherwise, Parsons argued, society risks social instability. As for physicians, Parsons said that they bear heavy responsibility for insuring that patients do not take advantage of the sick role. Accordingly, they deserve a high level of social reward in the form of status and income.

Although Parsons's theory of the sick role has become a basic concept in medical sociology, other sociologists have strongly criticized it. They point out that the theory (a) fails to address the wide variations in the way people view sickness and define sick-role behavior; (b) does not take into consideration various types of diseases, such as chronic diseases and mental illness; (c) is based on a traditional, one-to-one interaction between a patient and a physician, which frequently does not occur; and (d) is based on a middle-class pattern of behavior that fails to consider the sick role of lower socioeconomic classes.

In the 1970s, medical sociology changed dramatically. Many medical sociologists suddenly reversed their position and embraced a *critical theoretical perspective*. They argued that physicians act in a *dominant* fashion in their interactions with patients and other healthcare workers. This assessment captured society's growing skepticism regarding physicians' social position, but it did not have much practical impact on physicians.

That changed during the 1980s with the emergence of managed care. Managed-care spokespeople announced that they would not only eliminate the inefficiencies associated with nonprofit-organizational management but also protect patients from physicians who were primarily motivated by profit. The medical-sociological critique was no longer daring. A backlash against managed care did not come until the mid-1990s, and by that time social confidence in medicine, if not in one's own physician, had been badly damaged.

System Goals

In retrospect, the medical-sociological contribution to understanding healthcare delivery was most clearly identified with the discipline of sociology during the 1950s and 1960s when the work was primarily theoretical. It is clear that medical-sociological observations reflected concern about the quality of healthcare. The fact that medicine was delivered in private offices with little professional oversight meant that social control over quality was a basic social concern. During the 1970s, medical sociologists did the underlying work on access or the availability of healthcare. This body of work constitutes a major methodological contribution. By the 1980s, cost containment rose to the forefront pushing medical-sociological work aside in preference to medical economics.

Availability of Data and Interdisciplinary Research

The introduction of computers during the 1980s had a radical effect on medical sociology and other disciplines involved in health services research. Internet technology permitted the government to collect and report statistics in a timely manner and make them publicly available. This, combined with the fact that healthcare had become a central social concern, meant that an increasing number of institutions, as opposed to individuals, were interested in analyzing health statistics for the purpose of influencing policy. Organizations began employing researchers, who were expected to work as members of interdisciplinary teams and produce clearly written position papers free from exclusive disciplinary jargon. Many medical sociologists now define themselves as health services researchers or population health researchers.

Current Status and Future Direction

Today, medical sociology is a mature, objective, and independent field of study and work. There are a large number of professional medical sociologists conducting research and teaching in many countries, including the United States, Canada, Australia, Germany, Japan, and the United Kingdom. Medical sociology is the third largest section in the American Sociology Association, and it is the largest section in the British and German sociological associations. Most college and university sociology departments in the United States offer introductory courses in medical sociology, and several universities have well-established doctoral degree programs in medical sociology. Through the decades, medical-sociology concepts and research methodologies grounded in mainstream sociology have become integrated into the larger health research enterprise. The reverse is also true: Medical sociology continues to expand but is doing so in recognition of advances outside the discipline.

Grace Budrys

See also Access, Models of; Anderson, Odin W.; Computers; Disease; Health; Healthcare Organization Theory; Health Surveys; Medicalization

Further Readings

Bloom, Samuel W. *The Word as Scalpel: A History of Medical Sociology*. New York: Oxford University Press, 2002.

Brown, Phil, ed. *Perspectives in Medical Sociology*. 4th ed. Long Grove, IL: Waveland Press, 2008.

Cockerham, William C. *Medical Sociology*. 10th ed. Upper Saddle River, NJ: Pearson/Prentice Hall, 2007.

Parsons, Talcott. *The Social System*. Glencoe, IL: Free Press, 1951.

Timmermans, Stefan, and Steven S. Haas. "Towards a Sociology of Disease," *Sociology of Health and Illness* 30(5): 659–76, July 2008.

Wainwright, David, ed. *A Sociology of Health*. Thousand Oaks, CA: Sage, 2008.

Web Sites

European Society of Health and Medical Sociology
(ESHMS): http://www.eshms.org

Medical Sociology Section, American Sociological
Association (ASA): http://dept.kent.edu/sociology/
asamedsoc

Medical Sociology Study Group, British Sociological
Association (BSA): http://www.britsoc.co.uk/medsoc

MEDICAL TRAVEL

Medical travel refers to persons traveling outside
their home region in pursuit of healthcare that is
more accessible, of higher quality, or of lower
cost. It is a narrower term than *medical tourism*
(also *health tourism*), which refers to consumers
seeking health services of all kinds outside their
home region—including spa treatments and other
wellness services—as well as the industries that
cater to these consumers. The *medical tourism
industry* includes care providers and also related
services such as intermediaries, concierges, travel
specialists, and providers of room and board for
medical travelers. Medical travel is distinct from
travel medicine, which refers to preventive medical care provided to consumers in preparation for
their planned travel (e.g., vaccinations for diseases
occurring in the destination area).

Reasons for Medical Travel

There are many reasons why patients travel for
medical care; most can be categorized into three
main areas: (1) access, (2) cost, and (3) quality.
Patients travel for access reasons if they are seeking care that they cannot receive in their own
community. Access may be subcategorized according to (a) patients who are seeking care that is not
provided in their home region versus (b) patients
who may be able to receive comparable care at
home but not in a timely fashion, and so they are
seeking more expeditious care elsewhere. Seeking
care unavailable in one's own community is probably the oldest form of medical travel; stories of
epic journeys to find a mystical healer or rare
elixir are relatively common and date back many
centuries. A more modern example can be found
in the patients from the United States who have

traveled to India to receive hip-resurfacing treatments, because the treatment was viewed as superior to hip replacement surgery but the procedure
was not yet approved in the United States. The
other subcategory—more expeditious access—
includes patients who live in countries with
nationalized healthcare systems who may face
months-long wait times for treatment at home and
who can receive immediate care in other countries
with the same or very similar procedures. (Seeking
more expeditious care can be viewed as an unfair
or selfish practice by others from the same community, who sometimes refer to the practice as
line jumping.)

Patients also travel for care in pursuit of lower
costs. Elective procedures—that is, those not covered by insurance plans (e.g., cosmetic surgery)—
can involve significant out-of-pocket expenses, and
so these procedures are an important driver of cost-
based medical travel. The financial motivations for
comparison shopping can be even more substantial
for uninsured and underinsured patients who have
the financial resources to pursue care outside their
communities' safety nets. Such patients, particularly those in need of major medical procedures,
have substantial financial incentive to seek out the
most cost-efficient care they can find, given their
comfort level with travel as well as the perceived
competency and safety of the procedures and care
providers. Hospitals in developing countries, which
have much lower operating costs, can provide some
procedures for 20% or less of the amount that providers in the United States would charge. This can
save uninsured patients tens or even hundreds of
thousands of dollars, enough to make medical
travel options enticing for a substantial proportion
of patients needing high-end care. Given the size of
this cost differential, some insurers have also begun
providing plans—for U.S. employers with workers
in states bordering Mexico—that require medical
travel for nonurgent care.

The final category, quality, may similarly be
broken down into several subcategories. One
such segment comprises wealthy individuals from
developing countries where there are few or no
modern healthcare systems. In addition to traveling to other countries for major procedures, such
patients may also travel to receive a better standard of routine care. A second important segment
is patients pursuing cutting-edge healthcare—in

particular, high-tech procedures that may only be available from a finite number of providers in the world and are perceived to be superior to the more readily available treatment options. Inbound medical travel to major academic medical centers in the United States typically falls in this latter category.

Because medical travelers often pay up front and in cash, most health systems regard these patients as a particularly desirable clientele. Some developing countries, in particular, have come to view medical travelers as an important foundation for other types of economic development. Patients who come to a country for care may tend to stay longer in that country than other kinds of tourists do and, as a result, spend additional money in the local economy. Like tourists of other types, once medical travelers have visited a country for the first time, they are also more likely to return. For these reasons, the governments of some countries have established organized efforts to attract these patients to their private healthcare systems.

Accreditation

Although access, cost, and quality all pose measurement challenges, the quality of healthcare is a particularly complex and difficult construct on which to compare care providers internationally. Different countries, and sometimes different regions within a country, often have very different approaches to quality assurance and credentialing, making meaningful comparisons across providers very difficult. Providers who want to attract an international patient base need to demonstrate quality via universally acceptable means, which has led to substantial interest in pursuing internationally recognizable accreditations. The most widely used hospital accreditation provider is Joint Commission International, an international program offered by the Joint Commission, based in the United States. Other providers, such as the International Organization for Standardization, also offer accreditation programs primarily for institutional, international, health services providers. Surgeons and other physicians can achieve similar accreditation status by maintaining board certification in countries in which their international patients either reside or feel confident.

Future Implications

The forecasts of future growth in medical travel vary considerably but, in general, predict that it will continue to expand at a pace exceeding the broader growth in medical services worldwide. As healthcare costs continue to escalate, as pressures for greater transparency in quality and cost facilitate performance comparisons, and as experiences with medical travel become more familiar, the range of and the opting for costly, nonurgent medical services on a global scale will grow. Further advances in technologies that support telemediated services will also facilitate the remote provision of precare and aftercare, which may also foster the expansion of medical travel options in the coming years.

Andrew N. Garman, Arnold Milstein, and Matthew M. Anderson

See also Access to Healthcare; Accreditation; Comparing Health Systems; Cost of Healthcare; International Health Systems; Joint Commission; Quality of Healthcare

Further Readings

Bookman, Milica Z., and Karla R. Bookman. *Medical Tourism in Developing Countries.* New York: Palgrave-Macmillan, 2007.

Burkett, Levi. "Medical Tourism: Concerns, Benefits, and the American Legal Perspective," *Journal of Legal Medicine* 28(2): 223–45, April–June 2007.

Drager, Nick, and Cesar Vieira, eds. *Trade in Health Services: Global, Regional, and Country Perspectives.* Washington, DC: Pan-American Health Organization, 2002.

Forgione, Dana A., and Pamela C. Smith. "Medical Tourism and Its Impact on the U.S. Health Care System," *Journal of Health Care Finance* 34(1): 27–35, Fall 2007.

Herrick, D. "Medical Tourism: Global Competition in Health Care." Washington, DC: National Center for Policy Analysis, November 2007.

Milstein, Arnold, and Mark Smith. "Will the Surgical World Become Flat?" *Health Affairs* 26(1): 137–41, 2007.

Ramirez de Arellano, Annette B. "Patients Without Borders: The Emergence of Medical Tourism," *International Journal of Health Services* 37(1): 193–98, 2007.

U.S. Senate, Special Committee on Aging. *The Globalization of Health Care: Can Medical Tourism Reduce Health Care Costs?* Hearings Before the Special Committee on Aging, U.S. Senate. 109th Cong., 2d sess. (June 27, 2006): Serial No. 109–126. Washington, DC: Government Printing Office, 2006.

Web Sites

American Medical Association (AMA): http://www.ama-assn.org
HealthCare Tourism International: http://www.healthcaretrip.org
International Organization for Standardization (ISO): http://www.iso.org
Joint Commission International (JCI): http://www.jointcommissioninternational.org
Pan-American Health Organization (PAHO): http://www.paho.org
Travel Industry Association (TIA): http://www.tia.org
U.S. Office of Trade and Tourism Industries (OTTI): http://tinet.ita.doc.gov
World Health Organization (WHO): http://www.who.int

MEDICARE

Medicare is a health insurance program for (a) people aged 65 or older, (b) people under age 65 with certain disabilities, and (c) people at any age with end-stage renal disease (ESRD). It is the nation's largest health insurance program, covering nearly 44 million Americans. The Medicare program is administered by the Centers for Medicare and Medicaid Services (CMS), and beneficiaries may apply for Medicare benefits 3 months before they reach 65 years of age. Almost 9 million individuals, or approximately 20% of Medicare beneficiaries, receive their care through the Medicare Advantage program, and more than 90% of beneficiaries receive prescription drug coverage of some type. Medicare spending is a large component of the federal budget and national health spending: In 2006, Medicare benefit payments totaled $374 billion and accounted for 12% of the federal budget. The spending on Medicare benefits is about 20% of the nation's total healthcare expenditures.

History

President Lyndon B. Johnson signed the Medicare program into law in 1965 as Title XVIII of the Social Security Act. The Medicare program was originally designed to provide health insurance to the aged.

Prior to its enactment, there were several key moments in history that led up to the Medicare legislation. In 1935, the first federal government health insurance bill was introduced in the U.S. Congress. Later, in 1945, President Harry S Truman became the first sitting president to officially endorse the idea of national health insurance. In 1961, President John F. Kennedy recommended to the U.S. Congress a health insurance program for the elderly under Social Security, and in 1965 President Lyndon B. Johnson signed Medicare into law.

Throughout the history of Medicare, there have been several major reforms to the program. When first implemented in 1966, Medicare primarily covered persons over the age of 65. In 1973, Medicare eligibility was extended to people with disabilities and those with ESRD. In 1976, health maintenance organizations (HMOs) began to be offered as a Medicare option. In 1983, the Medicare program began reimbursing hospitals based on a prospective payment system. In 1997, the Medicare+Choice program was enacted and is known today as Medicare Part C or the Medicare Advantage plans. In 2003, President George W. Bush signed the Medicare Modernization Act (MMA) into law, establishing a voluntary, outpatient prescription drug benefit program—known as Medicare Part D—that became available to Medicare beneficiaries in 2006. Under this law, Medicare Advantage was also established, allowing private insurance companies to offer choices in coverage to Medicare beneficiaries.

Medicare's Parts

Medicare consists of four parts: A, B, C, and D. The original Medicare plan included Medicare Part A (hospital) and Part B (medical). Medicare Part C is also called the Medicare Advantage plans (HMOs and preferred provider organizations [PPOs]). Medicare Part D is for prescription drug coverage. Medicare Parts B, C, and D are optional. Most individuals either have Parts A and

B, Part D and a Medigap (Medicare Supplemental Insurance) policy, or Part C (which combines Parts A and B) and Part D.

Eligible individuals do not have to be retired to get Medicare. Unlike Social Security, working people can still receive full Medicare benefits at age 65. People who are already receiving Social Security benefits are automatically enrolled in Medicare without an additional application.

Medicare Part A

Most people do not pay for Medicare Part A because they contributed to the Medicare Trust Fund for 40 quarters. Medicare Part A is largely financed through hospital insurance taxes; it provides basic protection against the costs of inpatient hospital and other institutional-provider care. Officially, this program is called the Hospital Insurance Benefits for the Aged and Disabled, although it includes much more than just hospital benefits. Medicare Part A not only helps pay for inpatient hospital stays, but it also covers skilled nursing care, home health care, and hospice care. Unofficially, this program is sometimes called basic Medicare or hospital insurance because the authorization for the program is Part A of Title XVIII of the Social Security Act.

Whereas most people do not pay a premium for Medicare Part A, they are responsible for a deductible for inpatient hospital stays. The deductible is the amount a person with Medicare must pay for healthcare before Medicare begins to pay. There was a deductible of $1,024 in 2008 for hospital stays of up to 60 days, and additional costs for longer stays. The costs are different for other Medicare Part A services. Skilled-nursing facility coinsurance, for example, is $128 per day for days 21 through 100 for each benefit period.

Medicare Part B

Medicare Part B is a voluntary program that covers the costs of physician and other healthcare practitioner services, items, and supplies not covered under the basic program. It is financed through monthly premiums from enrollees and contributions from the federal government.

This program is more formally known as the Supplementary Medical Insurance Benefits for the Aged and Disabled, but it is often also called supplementary Medicare or the medical insurance program. Medicare Part B is medical insurance that helps cover physicians' services and outpatient care such as preventive services, including screening tests and vaccinations, diagnostic tests, some therapies, and durable medical equipment, such as wheelchairs and walkers.

In addition to the monthly premium for Medicare Part B, there is also a deductible; in 2008, this was $135. This means that in 2008, a person with Medicare was responsible for the first $135 of his or her Medicare approved Part B medical services before Medicare Part B started paying for care. The deductible amount can change each year. People with the original Medicare plan also are responsible for some copayments or coinsurance for Medicare Part B services. The amount depends on the service but is 20% in most cases.

Medicare Part C

A third Medicare program, Medicare Part C, expands managed-care options for beneficiaries who are entitled to Part A and are enrolled in Part B. Medicare Part C was created under the Balanced Budget Act of 1997 and is also called Medicare Advantage. This program was formerly known as Medicare+Choice. Since January 1, 1999, beneficiaries have had the option of choosing to receive their health benefits through the traditional Medicare fee-for-service program or to select a managed-care plan certified under Medicare Advantage. The payments Medicare makes to a Medicare Advantage plan replace the amount that Medicare would otherwise have paid under Parts A and B.

There are several types of Medicare Advantage plans. A Medicare Advantage organization (MAO) is a public or privately owned entity organized and licensed by a state as a risk-bearing entity (with the exception of provider-sponsored organizations receiving waivers) and is certified by the CMS as meeting the Medicare Advantage contract requirements. A Medicare Advantage plan has health benefits coverage—offered by an MAO under a policy or contract—that includes a specific set of health benefits offered at a uniform premium and uniform level of cost sharing to all Medicare beneficiaries residing in the service area (or segment of the service area) of the plan. A Medicare Advantage plan may also provide a prescription drug benefit. In 2008, 9.7 million beneficiaries were enrolled in Medicare Advantage plans with the majority (70%) in HMO plans.

Medicare Part D

Most recently, the Medicare program was expanded by the MMA of 2003 to include a prescription drug benefit under a new Medicare Part D of the Social Security Act. Beneficiaries entitled to Part A and enrolled in Part B, enrollees in Medicare Advantage and private fee-for-service plans, and enrollees in Medicare Savings Account Plans are all eligible for the prescription drug benefit. The prescription drug benefit became available to eligible individuals on January 1, 2006.

Premiums and Enrollment

Most people do not have to pay a monthly charge (premium) for Medicare Part A because they or their spouse paid Medicare or Federal Insurance Contributions Act (FICA) taxes while they were working. This is the tax withheld from a person's salary, or that an individual pays from their self-employment income, that funds the Social Security and Medicare programs. When people pay these taxes on their earnings, it is called Medicare-covered employment. If a person and his or her spouse did not pay Medicare taxes while they were working or did not work long enough (usually 10 years or 40 quarters in most cases) to qualify for premium-free Part A, he or she may still be able to get Medicare Part A by paying a monthly premium. In 2008, the Part A premium was $233 for people having 30 to 39 quarters of Medicare-covered employment, or $423 for those who are not otherwise eligible for premium-free hospital insurance and have fewer than 30 quarters of Medicare-covered employment.

Qualifying beneficiaries can choose whether or not to enroll in Medicare Part B medical insurance. Those who enroll are responsible for a monthly premium for Medicare Part B, which was $96.40 in 2008. Starting January 1, 2007, some people with higher annual incomes—more than $80,000 if filing an individual federal income tax return or more than $160,000 if married, filing jointly—pay a higher Medicare Part B premium. These amounts change each year. The majority of beneficiaries pay only the standard Medicare Part B premium.

People can sign up for Medicare Part B at anytime during a 7-month period that begins 3 months before the month they become eligible for Medicare. This is called the initial enrollment period (IEP). People who do not take Medicare Part B when they are first eligible may have to wait to sign up during a general enrollment period (GEP). This period runs from January 1 through March 31 of each year, with coverage effective July 1 of that year. Most people who do not take Medicare Part B when they are first eligible will also have to pay a premium penalty of 10% for each full 12-month period they could have had Medicare Part B but did not sign up for it, except in certain situations. In most cases, individuals will have to pay this penalty for as long as they have Medicare Part B.

Most people covered by a group health plan based on current employment (their own or their spouse's) can delay enrolling in Medicare Part B without a penalty. These individuals get a special enrollment period. They can enroll in Medicare Part B at anytime while they are still covered by their employer or union group health plan based on current employment, or during the 8 months following the month the employment ends or the group health plan coverage ends, whichever is first. Most people who sign up for Medicare Part B during a special enrollment period do not pay higher premiums.

People who choose Medicare Part B usually have the premium automatically taken out of their monthly Social Security or Railroad Retirement payment. Federal government retirees may be able to have the premium deducted from their retirement check.

People can choose to get Medicare healthcare coverage in several ways. Which Medicare plan people choose may affect their costs, benefits, and convenience, and their physician, hospital, and pharmacy choices. Nonetheless, no matter how people choose to get their Medicare healthcare, they are still enrolled in the Medicare program.

The original Medicare plan is available nationwide; it is also known as "fee-for-service." People in the original Medicare plan may go to any physician, specialist, hospital, or other healthcare provider who accepts Medicare. However, there are other plans besides the original Medicare plan that people can choose to get their Medicare health coverage.

Medigap Insurance

A Medigap policy is a health insurance policy sold by private insurance companies to fill the "gaps" in coverage under the original Medicare plan, including the deductibles, coinsurance, and copayments mentioned above. Some Medigap policies also provide benefits that Medicare does not include such as emergency healthcare when traveling outside the United States. The insurance companies that sell these policies must follow federal and state laws that protect people with Medicare. The Medigap policy must be clearly identified as Medicare Supplement Insurance.

A Medigap policy only works with the original Medicare plan. If an individual joins a Medicare Advantage plan or other Medicare plan, then the Medigap policy cannot pay any deductibles, copayments, or other cost sharing under the Medicare plan. In all states except Massachusetts, Minnesota, and Wisconsin, a Medigap policy must be one of 12 standardized plans (A–L) so that people can compare them easily. Each plan has a different set of benefits. The benefits in any Medigap plan A to L are the same for any insurance company. It is important for individuals to compare Medigap policies because the costs vary.

In most Medicare Advantage plans, members usually get all their Medicare-covered healthcare through that plan. The plan may offer extra benefits such as Medicare prescription drug coverage as well as coverage for vision, hearing, dental, or health and wellness programs. If a plan offers a network of healthcare providers and hospitals, people may very often have to use only that panel of providers. However, it is important to note that people who join a Medicare Advantage plan are still in the Medicare program and still receive all their regular Part A and Part B services. Additionally, beneficiaries in a Medicare Advantage plan still have Medicare rights and protections.

Medicare Prescription Drug Benefits

All people with Medicare now have the option to join a plan that covers prescription drugs. Anyone who has Medicare Part A, or Part B, or both Part A and Part B is eligible to join a Medicare drug plan and must enroll in a plan to get Medicare prescription drug coverage. However, people who live outside the United States or who are incarcerated may not enroll and are not eligible for coverage. The CMS contract with private companies offering Medicare prescription drug plans to negotiate discounted prices on behalf of their enrollees. People may also receive Medicare drug coverage through a Medicare Advantage plan or other Medicare plan, if they are enrolled in one. Some employers and unions may provide Medicare prescription drug coverage through employer/ union group plans to their retirees. The drug benefit is offered through stand-alone prescription drug plans (PDPs) and Medicare Advantage prescription drug (MA-PD) plans, such as HMOs that cover all Medicare benefits, including drugs.

Generally, there are two types of enrollment periods when people can sign up for Medicare prescription drug coverage: (1) the IEP is for 7 months starting 3 months before the month they become entitled to Medicare; (2) the annual coordinated election period is from November 15 to December 31 each year. During this period, a person who is not enrolled in a Medicare drug plan can choose to enroll.

People who do not enroll when they are first eligible may have to pay a penalty to enroll later. Most people who wait until after the end of their IEP to join a Medicare drug plan will have their premiums go up 1% of the national base premium for every month they waited to enroll. These individuals will usually have to pay this penalty as long as they have Medicare prescription drug coverage.

The costs of prescription drug benefits vary depending on the plan. Plans must provide a standard level of coverage, but they may offer more coverage or additional drugs, usually at a higher monthly premium. In most cases, for coverage in 2008, people paid a monthly premium that varied for different plans, a deductible, and a copayment or coinsurance. Once a Medicare beneficiary spent $4,050 out of pocket for covered drug costs during 2008, they paid 5% of their drug costs for the rest of the calendar year. This is called *catastrophic coverage*, and it could take effect even sooner in some plans. All these amounts can change each year.

Medicare Part D plans vary in benefit design, covered drugs, and utilization management tools, such as prior authorization, quantity limits, and step therapy. The CMS established minimum requirements for Medicare Part D plan formularies to help ensure that plans do not offer formularies that discriminate against or discourage the enrollment of certain types of beneficiaries. Enrollment in Medicare drug plans is voluntary, with the exception of dual-eligible (people in both Medicare and Medicaid) and certain low-income beneficiaries who are automatically enrolled in a prescription drug plan if they do not choose a plan on their own.

Many people with limited income and resources will get extra help paying for prescription drugs. The extra help is available to people with Medicare who have an income below 150% of the federal poverty level and limited resources. Resources also are counted for the person and a spouse, if living together. The resource limits in 2007 were $11,710 for an individual and $23,410 for a married couple.

Future Implications

The Medicare program continues to fulfill the vision of President Johnson's Great Society by furnishing healthcare services for the elderly as well as for persons with disabilities and ESRD. The program serves tens of millions of Americans each year by providing essential healthcare coverage. However, there is growing concern over Medicare's rising costs and questions about the ability of the program to sustain itself over time. The public policy debate concerning the direction and solvency of the nation's Medicare program will be an increasingly important topic of discussion in the future.

Raymond J. Swisher

See also Centers for Medicare and Medicaid Services (CMS); Health Insurance; Managed Care; Medicaid; Medicare Part D Prescription Drug Benefit; Medicare Payment Advisory Commission (MedPAC)

Further Readings

Bishop, Harold M., Jenny M. Burke, Paul T. Clark, et al. *CCH Medicare Explained*. Riverwoods, IL: CCH, 2008.

Cassel, Christine K. *Medicare Matters: What Geriatric Medicine Can Teach American Health Care: With a New Preface*. Berkeley: University of California Press/Milbank Memorial Fund, 2007.

Marmor, Theodore R. *The Politics of Medicare*. 2d ed. New York: Aldine de Gruyter, 2000.

Medicare Payment Advisory Commission. *Report to Congress: Promoting Greater Efficiency in Medicare*. Washington, DC: Medicare Payment Advisory Commission, 2007.

Moon, Marilyn. *Medicare: A Policy Primer*. Washington, DC: Urban Institute Press, 2006.

Pauly, Mark V. *Markets Without Magic: How Competition Might Save Medicare*. Washington, DC: AEI Press, 2008.

Peltz, Marlene C., ed. *Medicare and Medicaid: Critical Issues and Developments*. New York: Nova Science, 2007.

U.S. Department of Health and Human Services Centers for Medicare and Medicaid Services. *Medicare and You*. Baltimore: Centers for Medicare and Medicaid Services, 2008.

Web Sites

Centers for Medicare and Medicaid Services (CMS): http://www.cms.hhs.gov

Commonwealth Fund: http://www.commonwealthfund.org

Henry J. Kaiser Family Foundation (KFF): http://www.kff.org

Medicare: http://www.medicare.gov

My Medicare Matters, National Council on Aging: http://www.mymedicarematters.org

Robert Wood Johnson Foundation (RWJF): http://www.rwjf.org

MEDICARE PART D PRESCRIPTION DRUG BENEFIT

On December 8, 2003, President George W. Bush signed into law the Medicare Prescription Drug, Improvement, and Modernization Act of 2003, or MMA. This legislation was the most significant expansion of the nation's Medicare program since its inception in 1965. The MMA provides seniors and individuals with disabilities with voluntary prescription drug coverage, referred to as Medicare

Part D. The new coverage began on January 1, 2006. Until the MMA, Medicare did not provide coverage for outpatient prescription drugs.

The Medicare prescription drug benefit is voluntary insurance that covers both brand name and generic prescription drugs at participating pharmacies. All Medicare beneficiaries are eligible for this coverage, regardless of income level and financial resources, health status, or current prescription expenses. Individuals enrolled in Medicare Part A (hospital insurance), Medicare Part B (medical insurance), or both Part A and Part B are eligible for Medicare Part D. To obtain prescription drug coverage, a Medicare beneficiary must enroll in a Medicare prescription drug plan.

The Centers for Medicare and Medicaid Services (CMS), the U.S. federal agency that administers the Medicare program, contract with private companies offering Medicare prescription drug plans and negotiate discounted prices on behalf of Medicare beneficiaries. Individuals may also receive Medicare drug coverage through Medicare Advantage plans or another Medicare plan, if they are enrolled in one. Some employers and unions may also provide Medicare prescription drug coverage to their retirees through employer/union group plans.

Enrollment

Generally, there are three periods of time when individuals can sign up for Medicare prescription drug coverage. The IEP is 7 months long, starting 3 months before the month of becoming entitled to Medicare. Second, there is an annual coordinated election period from November 15 through December 31 each year. During the annual coordinated election period, individuals who are not enrolled in a Medicare drug plan may enroll, and individuals who are already in a Medicare drug plan may drop or switch plans. The change will be effective from January 1 of the following year. Third, there are special situations that entitle individuals to a special enrollment period, such as an involuntary loss of *creditable prescription drug coverage* or a change of permanent residence out of the plan's service area.

In most cases, if an individual does not join a plan during the IEP, his or her premium will increase 1% of the national base premium for every full month he or she waits to enroll.

(The national base premium was $27.35, for 2007). The individual will have to pay this penalty, in addition to the premium, for as long as he or she has Medicare prescription drug coverage. Moreover, one may have to wait until the next annual coordinated election period, November 15 to December 31, to enroll. The enrollment will be effective from January 1 of the following year. However, if a person has other drug coverage that is at least as good as the Medicare prescription drug coverage, called creditable prescription drug coverage, the penalty will not apply.

Coverage and Costs

Medicare drug plans are not all the same. Plans vary based on costs, which drugs are covered, and which pharmacies are in the network. Like other insurance, if an individual joins a Medicare drug plan, in most cases he or she will pay monthly premiums, which vary by plan, and a yearly deductible. They will also pay a part of the costs of the prescriptions, including a copayment or coinsurance. Costs will vary depending on the specific Medicare drug plan. Some plans offer more coverage and additional drugs for a higher monthly premium.

There may be a point during the year when a Medicare beneficiary will be paying 100% coinsurance, called the *coverage gap*. However, there are some Medicare drug plans that do not have a coverage gap or that pay for some drugs during the gap. Once the total out-of-pocket costs paid by a beneficiary reach a set amount ($3,850, in 2007), the plan will pay all but 5% or a small copayment for the rest of the year. This is called *catastrophic coverage*. All plans must offer this catastrophic coverage. The CMS sets the standard premium, deductible, and copayment amounts every year. These are minimum requirements for drug plans offering basic coverage.

As already noted, all individuals with Medicare can get prescription drug coverage. This is true regardless of their income level and financial resources, health status, or how much they pay for prescriptions. Moreover, many individuals with limited income and resources will get extra help paying for their prescription drugs. Individuals with the lowest incomes will pay no premiums or deductibles and only have a small or no copayments. And individuals with slightly higher incomes will have a reduced deductible and pay a little more out-of-pocket (15%) coinsurance.

Covered Drugs and Participating Pharmacies

Medicare Part D–covered drugs are defined as (a) drugs available only by prescription, used and sold in the United States, and used for a medically accepted indication; (b) biological products; (c) insulin; and (d) vaccines. The definition also includes medical supplies associated with the injection of insulin (i.e., syringes, needles, alcohol swabs, and gauze). Certain drugs or classes of drugs, or their medical uses, are excluded by law from Medicare Part D coverage.

Not all Medicare Part D–covered drugs are included by each drug plan. Each plan has a *formulary* or list of covered drugs. Plans' formularies must include a range of drugs to ensure that individuals with different medical conditions can get the treatment they need. A plan's formulary may not include every drug that a beneficiary takes. However, in most cases, a similar drug that is safe and effective will be available.

Medicare requires plans to have convenient pharmacies for individuals to choose from. Each company offering a Medicare drug plan will have a directory of pharmacies that work with the plan. Generally, a beneficiary must use one of the pharmacies listed in this directory for the plan to cover their prescriptions. However, some plans will allow individuals to use a pharmacy that is not in the plan's network for a higher cost. Plans cannot require the use of mail-order pharmacies, but they may offer them as an option, many times at a reduced cost to the beneficiary.

Future Implications

The CMS estimate that 39 million individuals—more than 90% of all Medicare beneficiaries—have prescription drug coverage. Of these individuals, approximately 24 million have coverage through the Medicare Part D program. As the population ages and more individuals join the Medicare program, Medicare Part D prescription drug coverage will become an increasingly important part of the nation's healthcare delivery system.

Todd Stankewicz

See also Centers for Medicare and Medicaid Services (CMS); Cost of Healthcare; Health Insurance; Medicare; Pharmaceutical Industry; Pharmacoeconomics; Prescription and Generic Drug Use

Further Readings

Fincham, Jack E. *The Medicare Part D Drug Program: Making the Most of the Benefit.* Sudbury, MA: Jones and Bartlett, 2007.

IMS Health. *Medicare Part D: The First Year.* Plymouth Meeting, PA: IMS Health, 2007.

McAdams, David, and Michael Schwarz. "Perverse Incentives in the Medicare Prescription Drug Benefit." *Inquiry* 44(2): 157–66, 2007.

Stuart, Bruce C., Becky A. Briesacher, Jalpa A. Doshi, et al. "Will Part D Produce Savings in Part A and Part B? The Impact of Prescription Drug Coverage on Medicare Program Expenditures." *Inquiry* 44(2): 146–56, 2007.

Web Sites

AARP: http://www.aarpmedicarerx.com

Center for Medicare Advocacy: http://www.medicareadvocacy.org/FAQ_PartD.htm

Medicare: http://www.medicare.gov

National Council on Aging: http://www.mymedicarematters.org

Pharmaceutical Research and Manufacturers of America (PhRMA): http://www.phrma.org

MEDICARE PAYMENT ADVISORY COMMISSION (MEDPAC)

The Medicare Payment Advisory Commission (MedPAC) is a small, independent, federal agency that advises the U.S. Congress on issues affecting the Medicare program. Established by the Balanced Budget Act of 1997, the commission monitors the Medicare program, reviews its policies, conducts studies, and makes recommendations to Congress. MedPAC combines the functions of two prior government agencies: the Prospective Payment Assessment Commission (ProPAC) and the Physician Payment Review Commission (PPRC).

Commissioners and Staff Members

MedPAC is composed of 17 commissioners and approximately 35 professional staff members. The commissioners, who are appointed by the U.S. Comptroller General and the head of the U.S. General Accountability Office (GAO), serve 3-year terms (subject to renewal) on a part-time basis. Appointments are staggered to maintain continuity: Every year approximately five or six commissioners end their appointments and new commissioners are appointed. The commissioners come from various geographic regions, and they bring a wide array of experience and expertise. Currently, the commissioners include actuaries, lawyers, physicians, and policymakers.

The commission's professional staff members include an executive director as well as various policy analysts, research assistants, administrative staff, and consultants. Its staff members prepare analyses of proposed regulations, write issue briefs, and contribute to the preparation of congressional testimony. Furthermore, they provide technical support to the staffs of congressional committees through memos and briefings.

Purpose

The commission's statutory mandate is quite broad. In addition to advising the U.S. Congress on payments to private health plans participating in the Medicare program and to providers in Medicare's traditional fee-for-service program, the commission also analyzes access to care, quality of care, and other issues affecting Medicare.

Public Meetings

The commission holds seven formal public meetings per year in Washington, D.C. At these meetings, the commission's professional staff members present their research and research regarding policy issues for the commissioners to discuss, and the commission's reports and specific recommendations to the U.S. Congress are approved. Time for public comment is always provided. Each meeting's agenda and briefs, as well as the transcripts from the meetings, are posted on the commission's Web site.

Commissioners and professional staff members also seek input on Medicare issues through informal meetings with individuals interested in the program, including staff members from various congressional committees and the Centers for Medicare and Medicaid Services (CMS), healthcare researchers, medical providers, various beneficiary advocates, and professional associations.

Publications

MedPAC publishes a variety of documents, including reports, data books, congressional testimony, contractor reports, comment letters, Medicare basics, and payment basics. Its specific recommendations to the U.S. Congress and supporting analyses are published in two annual reports, which are issued in March and June of each year. These have included consideration of Medicare payment policy and promoting greater efficiency in Medicare. At the request of Congress, the commission also publishes reports on a variety of other Medicare-related subjects.

The commission publishes a yearly data book that provides statistical information on a variety of Medicare topics (e.g., national healthcare and Medicare spending, Medicare beneficiary demographics, and dual-eligible beneficiaries). It is frequently called on to testify before Congress and to submit reports on various Medicare issues. MedPAC publishes various reports that have been produced under contract for them by outside authors. The commission often submits formal comments on proposed regulations issued by the Secretary of the Department of Health and Human Services (HHS) and on various Medicare-related reports to Congress. It also publishes Medicare Basics for the public (e.g., Medicare benefit design, Medicare Advantage benchmarks, and payment compared with the average Medicare fee-for-service spending) and Medicare Payment Basics (e.g., ambulatory surgical centers payment system and clinical laboratory services payment system), both of which provide brief overviews of various Medicare topics.

All its publications are available on the commission's Web site.

Future Implications

MedPAC is in a unique position to influence policy making for the nation's Medicare program. In the past few years, the commission's recommendations have had substantial impact, and the U.S.

Congress feels obligated to weigh its recommendations carefully. The commission's reports and testimony make important contributions to federal legislation. In the future, with the growing number of elderly people and the rising costs of Medicare, the commission's recommendations will continue to be highly valued.

Vikrant Vats

See also Centers for Medicare and Medicaid Services (CMS); Health Insurance; Medicare; Payment Mechanisms; Public Policy; Regulation; U.S. Government Accountability Office (GAO)

Further Readings

Lubell, Jennifer. "MedPAC: Can't We All Get Along. Agency Examines Ways Docs, Hospitals Compete," *Modern Healthcare* 37(36): 8–9, September 10, 2007.
Medicare Payment Advisory Commission. *A Data Book: Healthcare Spending and the Medicare Program.* Washington, DC: Medicare Payment Advisory Commission, 2007.
Medicare Payment Advisory Commission. *Report to the Congress: Promoting Greater Efficiency in Medicare.* Washington, DC: Medicare Payment Advisory Commission, 2007.
Medicare Payment Advisory Commission. *Report to the Congress: Medicare Payment Policy.* Washington, DC: Medicare Payment Advisory Commission, 2008.
Neigh, Janet E. "MedPAC Examining Medicare Hospice Benefit Reimbursement System," *Caring* 27(1): 60–61, January 2008.

Web Sites

Centers for Medicare and Medicaid Services (CMS): http://www.cms.hhs.gov
Medicare Payment Advisory Commission (MedPAC): http://www.medpac.gov
U.S. Government Accountability Office (GAO): http://www.gao.gov
U.S. House of Representatives: http://www.house.gov
U.S. Senate: http://www.senate.gov

MENTAL HEALTH

More than 50 years ago, the World Health Organization (WHO) defined mental health as a complete state of mental and physical well-being, and not simply the absence of disease. This definition emphasizes the positive features of mental well-being. Good mental health is associated with positive family, community, and school or work involvement, as well as with a supportive group of friends.

In contrast, mental illness usually is associated with the absence of one or more of these positive involvements. Mental illness can be characterized by problems in one's thinking, emotions, behaviors, or any combination of these three. The American Psychiatric Association (APA) has developed a classification system for mental disorders based on these characteristics, published as the *Diagnostic and Statistical Manual of Mental Disorders (DSM)*.

The most common mental disorders among adults in the United States are depression and anxiety, each of which affects about 10% of the population. Much less common are bipolar disorder—a combination of depression and mania, which affects about 4% of adults—and schizophrenia, which affects about 1% of the adult population. Both can lead to disabilities, and both bipolar disorder and schizophrenia are known to have a genetic basis, at least in some population groups.

About 25% of adults have a mental disorder within a 1-year period, and about 50% will have a mental disorder in their lifetime. About 6% of adults become seriously disabled as a result of mental illness. Less is known about the rates of specific mental illnesses in children and adolescents. However, about 20% of youths suffer from one or more disorders, and 9% to 13% of them are seriously disabled. Soon, national data will be available on the rates of specific disorders in this population.

Historical Overview

Because mental illness has not been well understood in the past, the history of mental illness and care is characterized by misunderstanding and exclusion. These can lead to stigmatization, by which a person or a family is blamed for the mental illness and deliberately excluded from social groups, community activities, and work. Only recently has mental illness been truly recognized as a treatable illness from which one can recover.

In the American colonial period, people who had mental illness were called "the insane" and were cared for by their families or in local almshouses. Around the time of the American Revolution, a system of state mental hospitals was constructed. The first of these facilities, Eastern State Hospital, was built near Williamsburg, Virginia, shortly before the Revolution. Usually, these facilities were located in rural areas because it was thought that persons with mental illness would benefit from good air and the quiet atmosphere of a rural setting.

After World War I, it became clear that a large number of potential recruits had been excluded from military service because of mental illness. It also became clear that battle fatigue, suffered by soldiers who had experienced combat, was a form of mental illness. As a result, in the early 1930s, the Veterans Administration created a system of general hospitals that also provided psychiatric care. In the early 1940s, a system of general hospitals in local communities was created, many of which offered psychiatric care, and in the 1950s, a large number of private psychiatric hospitals were founded, principally in urban areas.

In 1949, President Harry S. Truman signed legislation creating the National Institute of Mental Health (NIMH). In 1954, the drug chlorpromazine (sold under the trade names of Largactil and Thorazine) was approved in the United States for psychiatric treatment. It was hailed as a wonder drug to treat severe mental illness. With the advent of drug therapy, the nation's state mental hospitals began to empty, a process later called *deinstitutionalization*. However, many of the former inpatients of the mental hospitals became homeless, were placed in nursing homes, or were even incarcerated in jails or prisons.

In 1963, President John F. Kennedy signed federal legislation creating a national system of community mental health centers, which would be available throughout the nation. It was estimated that 1,500 of these facilities would be required to serve the entire American population. More than 800 facilities were built before President Ronald Reagan ended federal funding for the program in 1981.

From 1980 to the end of the 20th century, the mental healthcare field strove to provide effective care in local communities for public clients who had mental illnesses that led to serious disabilities. Although effective programs were developed for both adults and youths, these programs were not broadly implemented. In 1992, President George H. W. Bush signed federal legislation creating the Substance Abuse and Mental Health Services Administration (SAMHSA) with the mission of improving both mental health and substance use care throughout the nation.

With the dawning of the 21st century, a new awareness has developed that effective care is available, that one can recover from mental illness, and that one who has had a mental illness can lead a happy and productive life in the community. This new approach has been heralded by representatives of the mental healthcare community and broadly embraced by many Americans.

Many successes in mental health have been achieved, in large measure due to the development and growth of an effective mental health consumer movement in parallel with the rapid growth of the family movement. Many American communities have access to (a) an affiliate of Mental Health America, representing consumers; (b) an affiliate of the National Alliance for Mental Illness, representing both families and consumers; and (c) the Federation of Families for Children's Mental Health, representing both families and children.

Recent Reports

Several recent reports will likely have a major effect on the future of mental healthcare in the United States.

More than 200 years after the first U.S. Surgeon General took office in 1798, the first-ever *Mental Health: A Report of the Surgeon General* was issued in 1999. This report examined the scientific foundation for current mental illness care practices and identified opportunities for care improvement. Significantly, the scientific foundations of mental health clinical and services research was found to be quite robust. The report identified the integration of mental health with general healthcare as the step forward needed most in the near term, with the goal that the two systems become one and treat both mind and body at the same time.

In 2002, slightly more than 25 years after President Jimmy Carter convened the first President's Commission on Mental Health,

President George W. Bush convened the President's New Freedom Commission on Mental Health. The new commission met for a year and then issued a report titled *Achieving the Promise: Transforming Mental Health Care in America* in 2003. The report identified six major goals for the improvement of mental healthcare in America: (1) Americans understand that mental health is essential to overall health; (2) mental healthcare is consumer and family driven; (3) disparities in mental health services are eliminated; (4) early mental health screening, assessment, and referral to services are common practice; (5) excellent mental healthcare is delivered and research is accelerated; and (6) technology is used to access mental healthcare and information.

In 2005, the prestigious national Institute of Medicine (IOM) issued a study titled *Improving the Quality of Health Care for Mental and Substance Use Conditions*. This landmark study provided a plan for achieving the goals outlined by the President's New Freedom Commission on Mental Health. A new set of "care rules" was identified to improve care quality. These rules promoted (a) better provider-consumer information exchange, (b) more stable care relationships, and (c) a more central role for consumer input regarding care. Care quality was determined to relate to six factors: (1) safety, (2) efficiency, (3) effectiveness, (4) equitability, (5) timeliness, and (6) person-centeredness. (For the latter, IOM identified the consumer's input as the "true north" of the healthcare system.) Finally, four key strategies were recommended to bring about necessary system changes: (1) financing reform, (2) training of providers, (3) implementation of care that has a sound scientific basis, and (4) better use of information technology and performance measures. As with each of the earlier reports, it was strongly recommended that the integration of mental health and general healthcare be a high priority.

Who Receives Care?

At least half of those who experience a mental disorder each year do not receive any care at all. Among the 10% to 12% of the American population who do receive mental healthcare, about half (5–6%) actually see a mental health specialist. These specialists include psychiatrists, psychologists, social workers, psychiatric nurses, marriage or family therapists, and clinical mental health counselors. Typically, these providers see clients either in the practitioner's office or in an outpatient clinic or community mental health center.

The remaining 5% to 6% of the American population who receive care for mental illness are seen only by a general, medical physician. This pattern is particularly pronounced for children, who likely are seen only by their pediatricians, and for elderly persons, who likely are seen only by their personal physicians. Most primary-care physicians are not adequately trained to recognize and treat the full spectrum of mental illnesses.

About one fourth of those who experience a mental disorder each year suffer from a serious mental illness such as schizophrenia and suffer the greatest consequences in their loss of community participation. Many of these people are homeless and jobless because of their illnesses. Frequently, they receive their only mental healthcare through a state mental health agency, sometimes in a state mental hospital or local, outpatient, mental health clinic.

Each year, many other Americans have a range of mental health problems with symptoms that are not severe enough to qualify as mental illnesses. Only a very small percentage of this group seeks or receives care. Often, when care is sought, the first point of contact is a company employee assistance program, many of which offer both mental health and substance use care services, or a school or college health service.

If so many youths and adults have mental illnesses, why do so few receive care? In a word, stigma, which can lead to the rejection of care for fear that other family members, neighbors, fellow employees, and friends will find out. Many people interpret seeking care as a sign of weakness and fear that it will have negative effects in the future, such as diminished job prospects or the loss of friends. Stigma can also manifest through negative managerial, boardroom, and legislative decisions about funding for mental healthcare. It is well-known, for example, that insurance benefits for mental illnesses provide less annual and lifetime coverage than for physical disorders. This differential has spawned major efforts by national mental health leaders to seek parity for mental health benefits in both private and public insurance plans. In its most extreme forms, stigma manifests as discrimination against people with mental illness.

Some progress has been made in addressing the stigma of mental illness. Depression, anxiety, and even schizophrenia show up on some television shows as part of a character's story line. Well-known national figures have disclosed their own illnesses: Tipper Gore, the wife of the former vice president Al Gore, and Mike Wallace, a longtime anchor on the popular investigative television newsmagazine show *60 Minutes,* both have discussed their bouts with depression. And the popular author Danielle Steel has written a gripping account of the bipolar disorder suffered by her eldest son. National organizations have also mobilized to combat stigma. As a result, the stigma associated with mental illness has diminished, but it has not yet been extinguished.

Recent Improvements in Care

In the past quarter century, there have been changes in the way Americans view mental health and the way mental illness is treated. Many of these changes are positive steps, though others have introduced new societal problems. The main changes are discussed briefly below.

Care Has Moved From Institutions to the Community

There are about 250,000 fewer psychiatric beds today compared with 25 years ago. Community-based care has expanded dramatically. Yet many persons have been left behind. Witness the dramatic growth in mental illness among the homeless as well as among the less affluent segments of American society.

Care Is Better Integrated Into Overall Support Systems

It is now widely understood that those with the most severe mental illnesses require care systems that span mental health, overall health, rehabilitation, and social support services in the community. At the heart of such systems are case managers who work to achieve better community integration for their clients. Yet many of these systems lack

essential components, particularly in the most rural areas and the poorest urban areas.

Care Includes a Broad Range of Modern, Psychotropic Medications

Medications are now available for virtually all the major mental illnesses. Yet many people do not receive modern medications because they lack the financial resources to pay for them. Even when more effective, modern formulations are available, older medications—some developed as long ago as 50 years—are used because they cost less. Some newer medications have also given rise to concerns about secondary effects, particularly metabolic changes that can lead to diabetes and heart disease.

Care Has Become More Consumer and Family Centered

A quarter century ago, mental healthcare providers made virtually all the decisions about the nature of mental healthcare and its duration. Now, consumers and family members help define the objectives and the content of care. Yet a chasm frequently exists—between the provider and consumer perspectives and between the consumer and family perspectives—that can diminish the effectiveness of care.

Debate Over Forced Treatment Continues

In the past, this debate focused on inpatient commitment. Now, it focuses on outpatient commitment in community settings. Some community members and professionals favor outpatient commitment or court-determined and directed outpatient care if clients do not follow recommended treatment practices. Many consumers oppose it as an infringement on personal rights. This debate has fostered the development of creative alternatives. For example, *advance directives* are similar to a living will in that a person makes his or her wishes known in advance and appoints a personal representative to reflect these views of patient care in subsequent proceedings. It may be useful to view forced outpatient commitment as a measure of system failure in that it generally occurs only when prior care has not been adequate.

*Disparities in Mental
Healthcare Have Been Identified*

It has been known for decades that racial, ethnic, gender, and age disparities exist in the occurrence of mental illnesses and in mental healthcare services. Yet it is only recently that these disparities have been recognized as national policy concerns. As a result, mental health providers and systems will need to learn to adapt themselves to a broader diversity of clients and develop a heightened level of sensitivity to cultural and biological differences.

*Integration of Mental and
Physical Healthcare Services Has Begun*

Until as recently as a decade ago, mental healthcare and physical healthcare systems operated in separate, parallel worlds. With approximately 5% to 6% of the American population receiving mental healthcare only from general physicians, there is an urgent need to open a dialogue on better ways to integrate the two fields. It is now realized, for example, that financial incentives, training, and new system configurations will be needed. A similar dialogue has started between the mental health and substance use care fields.

Other issues also will need to be addressed. As more effective community care systems are built in the short-term future, they will need to consider (a) the role that the faith-based community can play in prevention and early intervention, (b) the potential role of private-public partnerships, (c) the need for effective linkages with the human service community, and (d) the need for effective outreach to those who are disenfranchised or subjected to discrimination. Moreover, the new community systems must have the capacity to respond to disasters, which can have major effects on mental health and well-being similar to those experienced after the 9/11 terrorist attacks in New York and Washington, D.C.

In the distant future, several other trends can be anticipated to emerge or strengthen. One trend that is likely to affect mental healthcare is the move toward consumer- and family-centered care. Consumers and family members will seek and receive more responsibility for health and healthcare. Already, consumer-operated and peer-supported mental health services have become more common, with individuals and family members allowed and expected to take on a greater role in the direct management of mental disease.

The use of new technologies will likely become an even more important vehicle for delivering mental healthcare. Currently, telecommunication, computer, and Internet technologies are being linked to offer "care at a distance." Several thousand Web sites now offer interpersonal psychotherapy, expanding the scope of mental health care services, much as the telephone expanded healthcare providers' ability to help their patients in the past. Rapid advances also are being made in voice-activated automatic-response systems and in the application of artificial-intelligence systems to real-world problems. As a result, it is now possible to receive care and guidance through a computer program without human intervention. Other automated systems are being developed to monitor—at home, in real time—and report physical symptoms to healthcare providers. As these noninterpersonal technologies become more pervasive, new concerns are likely to arise about how and when human intervention in the mental healthcare process is appropriate or even essential.

Also very promising will be the development of new genetic treatments over the next 5 to 10 years for biologically based mental disorders. To date, virtually no genetic interventions are recommended or implemented in the mental health field. Now that the basic human genome has been mapped, this situation may change radically as genetic interventions are developed for mental disorders that have a genetic basis.

Ronald W. Manderscheid

See also Access to Healthcare; Ambulatory Care; *Diagnostic and Statistical Manual of Mental Disorders (DSM)*; Disability; Disease; Epidemiology; Mental Health Epidemiology; Public Health

Further Readings

American Psychiatric Association. *Diagnostic and Statistical Manual of Mental Disorders*. 4th ed. Washington, DC: American Psychiatric Association, 2000.

Center for Mental Health Services. *Mental Health, United States, 2004*. Edited by R. W. Manderscheid and J. T. Berry HHS Pub. No. (SMA)-06–4195. Rockville, MD: Substance Abuse and Mental Health Services Administration, 2006.

Committee on Crossing the Quality Chasm: Adaptation to Mental Health and Addiction Disorders. *Improving the Quality of Health Care for Mental and Substance-Use Conditions: Quality Chasm Series.* Washington, DC: National Academies Press, 2006.

New Freedom Commission on Mental Health. *Achieving the Promise: Transforming Mental Health Care in America. Final Report.* HHS Pub. No. (SMA)-03–3832. Rockville, MD: U.S. Department of Health and Human Services, 2003.

U.S. Department of Health and Human Services. *Mental Health: A Report of the Surgeon General.* Rockville, MD: U.S. Department of Health and Human Services, Substance Abuse and Mental Health Services Administration, Center for Mental Health Services, National Institutes of Health, National Institute of Mental Health, 1999.

Web Sites

American Psychiatric Association (APA): http://www.psych.org

Centers for Disease Control and Prevention (CDC), Mental Health Work Group: http://www.cdc.gov/mentalhealth

Federation of Families for Children's Mental Health (FFCMH): http://www.ffcmh.org

Mental Health America (MHA): http://www.nmha.org

National Alliance for Mental Illness (NAMI): http://www.nami.org

National Institute of Mental Health (NIMH): http://www.nimh.nih.gov

New Freedom Commission on Mental Health: http://www.mentalhealthcommission.gov

Substance Abuse and Mental Health Services Administration (SAMHSA): http://www.samhsa.gov

MENTAL HEALTH EPIDEMIOLOGY

Mental health epidemiology is the study of the prevalence and incidence of mental health disorders. This entry defines basic epidemiology concepts and describes the historical development of mental health epidemiology in the United States. In conclusion, it outlines some of the promising new directions mental health epidemiology will likely take in the future.

Only in the past 30 years have public health and health services researchers been able to combine statistical sampling methods, interviewer scales, and appropriate analytical tools and collect detailed information on specific medical diagnoses that can be generalized to a defined national population. This combination of resources has enabled researchers to measure the magnitude of mental health disorders in the United States's population. In general terms, researchers now estimate that about one quarter of the nation's adult population has a diagnosable mental disorder in any 1-year period of time and that the lifetime expectation is that about 1 in 2 adults will suffer from these disorders. For children and adolescents, the 1-year figure is about 1 in 5. For any other medical disorder (e.g., heart disease, diabetes, hepatitis), these figures would be considered signs of a public health crisis.

Some Basic Concepts of Epidemiology

To understand epidemiology, several key concepts are critical. Two important basic concepts are the *prevalence* and the *incidence* of disease. Prevalence refers to the *total* number of disease cases in a period of time for a defined population. This period of time can be 1 day in length, called *point prevalence,* or 1 year in length, called *period prevalence.* Incidence refers to the number of *new* disease cases occurring during a period of time for a defined population, either *point incidence* or *period incidence,* as differentiated above.

A major goal of epidemiology is to measure both the prevalence and the incidence of a disease. By definition, the ratio of incidence to prevalence will always be 1 or less. The higher this ratio, the greater the turnover in the diseased population. For example, depression has both a high incidence and a high prevalence, which means that there is considerable turnover in the population with this disease and that many persons with this disease recover in a relatively short period of time. In contrast, schizophrenia has a very low prevalence and even lower incidence. This means that there is a very low turnover in this population and that persons with this disease have it for a long period of time.

To measure a disease's period prevalence, measures of the number of disease cases at Time 1 and Time 2 are required. Period prevalence is the sum of these two figures (i.e., point prevalence plus incidence). Remember that the period prevalence is always equal to or greater than the period incidence. By extension, it should be noted that point prevalence can be viewed as the sum of the disease cases at the beginning of a day plus the number of new incident cases over the course of the day.

Period incidence also requires measurement at two time points. Period incidence means that a person does not have the disease at Time 1 but develops the disease between Time 1 and Time 2. By extension, point incidence means that a person did not have the disease at the beginning of the day but developed the disease over the course of the day.

Frequently, sociodemographic factors such as age, gender, race or ethnicity, and place of residence are examined in relation to a disease. From such analyses, for example, Hollingshead and Redlich were able to determine that the prevalence of mental illness was 8 times as large in the lowest social class as compared with the highest social class.

Early Work in Mental Health Epidemiology

Beginning in 1840, the U.S. superintendent of the census began to collect information, as part of the nation's decennial census of population, on the number of persons living in households who were "insane or idiotic." Similar data were collected on persons residing in state mental hospitals. The sum of these two numbers provides a very primitive, early estimate of the prevalence of mental illness in the United States. This procedure was continued until 1900 with progressive refinement in the diagnostic categories.

After that time, specific questions on mental illness were no longer asked of the household population, but data were collected more frequently on state mental hospitals. Over time, the data collected from state mental hospitals, *treated prevalence,* became the surrogate for total community prevalence—that is, the sum of the community and hospital figures. These hospital data were reported by the U.S. Public Health Service in a publication series called *Patients in Mental Institutions.* As additional types of hospitals—Veterans Administration Medical Centers, general community hospitals, and private psychiatric hospitals—were developed in the 1930s and later, their figures were also added to these data collections.

Beginning of the Modern Era

The beginning of the modern era of mental health epidemiology can be traced to a famous study conducted in Stirling County, New York, in 1952. At that time, Stirling County was rural, with a total population of about 20,000 persons. More than 1,000 male and female adult heads of households were interviewed for the study, and the American Psychiatric Association's new *Diagnostic and Statistical Manual of Mental Disorders (DSM-1)* was used for the first time. Two psychiatrists reviewed the interview ratings. The purpose of the study was to examine the relationship between sociocultural disintegration and specific mental disorders. Lifetime prevalence was estimated at 57% for all *DSM-1* disorders measured, and current prevalence was estimated to be 90% of the lifetime rate.

An equally famous study from this period is the Midtown Manhattan Study conducted in 1954. The study population included 175,000 adults between the ages of 20 and 59 who resided in Midtown Manhattan. Of this number, 1,660 were interviewed. Two psychiatrists reviewed the ratings. The purpose of the study was to examine the relationship between stress indicators and mental impairment. Unlike the Stirling County Study, the Midtown Manhattan Study developed an overall measure of mental disorders and ratings for several symptom groups rather than ratings for specific disorders. Current prevalence was estimated at 81.5% for mild to incapacitated impairment. No lifetime prevalence figure was provided.

Both of these studies contributed significantly to the understanding of how to conduct mental health epidemiological fieldwork. However, both also had considerable limitations. Both were surveys conducted in small geographical areas, and both were focused on the noninstitutionalized population. Persons with mental illness who resided in psychiatric hospitals at the time of the studies were not counted.

It should be noted that the newly formed National Institute of Mental Health (NIMH) was developing *psychiatric case registers* at about the same time the Stirling County and Midtown Manhattan studies were being conducted. A psychiatric case register is a continuous recording of all persons who present for mental health treatment from a defined geographical area, together with detailed treatment data. A case register is a very valuable tool for understanding the precise patterns of care provided to persons with specific disorders. The most notable of these psychiatric case registers were for the states of Maryland and Hawaii and for Monroe County, New York. The two state case registers were discontinued at the end of the 1960s, and the Monroe County case register was discontinued at the end of the 1980s.

A Landmark National Study

From the time of the Stirling County and Midtown Manhattan studies until the early 1980s, work was underway at NIMH and in the mental health research field to improve the measurement of specific mental disorders using interview techniques. At the same time, the specification of mental disorders was refined with the release of the second and third generation of the *Diagnostic and Statistical Manual of Mental Disorders* (*DSM-II* and *DSM-III*). From these efforts came the Diagnostic Interview Schedule (DIS). The DIS was the first field survey instrument that could be administered solely by a lay interviewer and from which specific mental illness diagnoses could be derived, with further clinical review.

The DIS became the basic survey instrument for the epidemiological catchment area (ECA) project conducted in 1983 under the leadership of NIMH. This survey project was conducted among persons 18 years of age and older in five geographic areas across the nation: (1) New Haven, Connecticut; (2) Baltimore, Maryland; (3) St. Louis, Missouri; (4) Durham, North Carolina; and (5) Los Angeles, California. The purpose of the study was to produce lifetime and annual prevalence estimates for specific mental disorders and to produce estimates of the incidence of these disorders for a 1-year period. The national estimates were produced using the 1980 population figures, even though the data were collected in 1983. Annual period prevalence was estimated to be 28.1% for all disorders, and separate estimates were provided for specific disorders. A very important finding from this study was that only about 15% of the adult population received any mental healthcare, and only 6% received care from a mental health provider such as a psychiatrist or psychologist.

The ECA project was widely acclaimed at the time it was reported to the field, and its results were used broadly for policy, clinical, and financial analysis. To the present time, this study has provided the only annual incidence figures for specific diagnoses that have ever been collected on a national basis. Problems of individual recall were noted in the lifetime prevalence figures; hence, they have received relatively little attention by the field.

Current Generation of Work

Almost a decade after the ECA fieldwork was completed, a new study, the National Comorbidity Survey (NCS) was undertaken between 1990 and 1992 on a national probability sample of more than 8,000 persons, 15 to 54 years of age, from the household population. NIMH supported this new study. This effort was the very first to assess mental illness in a national probability sample. It was also the first effort to use the World Health Organization's Composite International Diagnostic Instrument (CIDI), based on the *DSM-III-R* and administered by lay interviewers. Fourteen different psychiatric disorders were assessed. Annual prevalence figures were similar to those reported from the ECA, with almost 30% of respondents having a mental illness. Lifetime prevalence was reported to be almost 50%. Equally important, more than half of all the persons with a lifetime disorder had a history of three or more comorbid disorders. Of those with a disorder in the past year, less than 20% received any care; for those with a lifetime disorder, the percentage receiving any treatment was less than 40%.

A broad range of mental health issues have been explored by researchers using NCS data, which are publicly available; numerous scientific articles have been published from it. However, NCS did not include a scale for schizophrenia, and it did not collect incidence data.

In 2001 and 2002, the same set of NCS respondents was reinterviewed. NIMH and the Center for Mental Health Services supported this effort. The reinterview study is called NCS-2. This study was conducted to examine the course of mental disorders, as well as the relationship between primary mental disorders and secondary substance use disorders. From this study, the framework of the "window of opportunity" has been developed.

This framework points to opportunities to intervene between the onset of a primary mental disorder and the onset of a secondary substance use disorder to prevent the latter.

At the same time, an NCS-R (Replication) prevalence survey was carried out on a new national probability sample of 10,000 respondents, 18 years of age and older, using a revised CIDI based on *DSM-IV*. More than 32% of the respondents had a disorder in a 1-year period, and more than 57% had a lifetime disorder.

Currently, the results from a parallel study of 10,000 adolescents, called the NCS-A (Adolescents), are being analyzed. Once reported, this study will be the first national effort to collect detailed prevalence information on a national probability sample of adolescents, 12 to 17 years of age.

Some Related National Work

In 2006, funding was provided by the Center for Mental Health Services to add mental health questions to the Behavioral Risk Factor Surveillance System (BRFSS), operated by the U.S. Centers for Disease Control and Prevention (CDC). The BRFSS is composed of 51 parallel, state telephone surveys of samples of adults and is conducted each year. The mental health questions added to the BRFSS were the first eight items from the Physician Health Questionnaire (PHQ-8), which provide a measure of depression. Unlike all earlier mental health epidemiology efforts, the BRFSS is capable of producing direct state estimates in addition to national estimates. In this first effort, 38 states added the mental health questions. Initial results will be available from the Center for Mental Health Services.

In 2007, the BRFSS work was extended by adding the K-6, a measure developed in the NCS to assess whether an adult respondent has serious mental illness. These results will be released in 2008.

Promising New Directions

As indicated above, mental health epidemiology in the United States has steadily progressed from small, local studies using inconsistent nonstandardized measures to sophisticated, national probability samples using internationally recognized and validated research instruments. The field of

mental health epidemiology is also developing the capacity to make accurate, state-level estimates, which will be very useful for state and local health planners, various departments of state government, and state policymakers.

The future will likely hold many changes for the field of epidemiology in general and for mental health epidemiology in particular. Some of the anticipated changes are outlined below.

Electronic Health and Personal Health Records

A process is already underway to implement electronic health records (EHRs) and personal health records (PHRs) in the United States. Comprehensive EHRs will contain detailed continuous information on a person's health status and the healthcare he or she receives. PHRs will translate this information into action steps that consumers will be able to take to improve their health status and the quality of their care, as well as to engage in self-care activities.

The EHRs and PHRs will provide an entirely new source of data for mental health epidemiology. These electronic files will be universal. They will be continuous records. And they will contain detailed information on the full range of a person's comorbidities. The implication is that traditional epidemiological-survey data collections will be replaced by continuous data collection from these electronic files.

To facilitate this outcome, it will be essential to ensure that very high-quality information is entered into these EHRs and PHRs, using the very best instruments available. The VistA EHR developed by the U.S. Department of Veteran Affairs for military veterans has already demonstrated how this might be accomplished. More effort needs to be spent on ensuring comparable data standards in EHRs and PHRs for items and scales measuring mental health epidemiology.

Improved Knowledge Base

Two types of scientific advances hold considerable promise for the future of mental health epidemiology. First, with the decoding of the human genome and the development of large-scale population samples of DNA, it will be possible to determine genomic patterns for persons with particular disorders. Some mental disorders, such as schizophrenia and depression, are already known to have genetic components, at least in specific population subgroups. As this knowledge is developed, it will need to be incorporated into mental health epidemiology.

Second, major efforts are currently underway to develop what is called *personal medicine*. Stated simply, this is an effort to match care uniquely to a particular individual. Hence, rather than a general drug formulary for a psychotropic medication, the formula would be prepared specifically for each individual. Clearly, how each patient responds to a medication could be used to develop an entirely new classification system for mental disorders: Instead of relying on a series of questions to identify a particular disorder, drug responsiveness could be used for this purpose.

Enlightened Consumers

As the mental health consumer movement continues to evolve in the United States, consumers will be able (a) to better recognize the signs and symptoms of mental illness, (b) to understand and evaluate the quality of care they receive, and (c) to engage in self-help activities. This is all part of a major transformation effort to promote true recovery and independence. As this evolution progresses, consumers and the providers who serve them may become less willing to participate in national or state mental health epidemiology survey efforts. They will also want to know and understand how the results from such research can be applied directly to their own care and recovery. Hence, future research efforts will need to include new components that address these concerns and interests.

Stigma and Privacy

The mental health field has two preeminent concerns that need to be addressed on an ongoing basis. The first is stigma based on the ideas that (a) people feign mental illness and are really laggards, (b) mental health treatment doesn't work, and (c) mental health treatment is too expensive. Although these contentions are not true, they color any debate about mental health issues from the U.S. Congress to a local community group. A 1-year

prevalence of 25% may not be taken seriously as a public health crisis because of stigma and because of unfounded beliefs about persons with mental illness and the care they receive.

Major national efforts are underway to combat stigma against persons with mental illness. These efforts take the form of educational campaigns, discussions with family members and consumers, and engaging people in mental health initiatives. With an annual prevalence of 25% and a lifetime prevalence of 50%, virtually every family in the nation has one or more members who experience mental illness.

The second and related issue is privacy or confidentiality. Because of work and social discrimination, persons with mental illness are very reluctant to share information about their illness or care. These wishes for privacy need to be respected, and strong standards of confidentiality need to be enforced. And healthcare providers, insurers, employers, and other institutions all need to be held to a very high and strict standard in this area.

Those engaged in mental health epidemiology need to recognize these issues and address them head-on. To address stigma, they need to consider mental illness in the general context of all illnesses. Past research on comorbidity is a very positive movement in this direction. With regard to confidentiality, researchers need to ensure that epidemiological data are not released inappropriately, particularly as the nation moves into the era of EHRs and PHRs.

Ronald W. Manderscheid

See also *Diagnostic and Statistical Manual of Mental Disorders (DSM)*; Disease; Epidemiology; Forces Changing Healthcare; Mental Health; National Institutes of Health (NIH); Public Health

Further Readings

Center for Mental Health Services. *Mental Health, United States, 2004.* Edited by R. W. Manderscheid and J. T. Berry. HHS Pub. No. (SMA)-06–4195. Rockville, MD: Substance Abuse and Mental Health Services Administration, 2006.

Eaton, William W., and Larry G. Kessler, eds. *Epidemiology Field Methods in Psychiatry.* New York: Academic Press, 1985.

Hollingshead, August B., and Frederick C. Redlich. *Social Class and Mental Illness: A Community Study.* New York: Wiley, 1958.

Oakes, J. Michael, and Jay S. Kaufman, eds. *Methods in Social Epidemiology.* San Francisco: Jossey-Bass, 2006.

Prince, Martin, Robert Stewart, Tamsin Ford, et al., eds. *Practical Psychiatric Epidemiology.* New York: Oxford University Press, 2003.

Susser, Erza, Sharon Schwartz, Alfredo Morabia, et al. *Psychiatric Epidemiology: Searching for the Causes of Mental Disorders.* New York: Oxford University Press, 2006.

Tsuang, Ming T., and Mauiricio Tohen, eds. *Textbook in Psychiatric Epidemiology.* 2d ed. New York: Wiley-Liss, 2002.

Web Sites

American College of Epidemiology: http://acepidemiology.org

American Psychiatric Association (APA): http://www.psych.org

American Public Health Association (APHA): http://www.apha.org

Centers for Disease Control and Prevention (CDC): http://www.cdc.gov/brfss

National Comorbidity Survey and Replication: http://www.hcp.med.harvard.edu/ncs

National Institute of Mental Health (NIMH): http://www.nimh.nih.gov

Office of the National Coordinator on Health Information Technology: http://www.hhs.gov/healthit

Society for Epidemiologic Research: http://www.epiresearch.org

Substance Abuse and Mental Health Services Administration (SAMHSA): http://www.samhsa.gov

META-ANALYSIS

Meta-analysis, a tool developed to summarize the findings from randomized clinical trials (RCTs), can be used by many scientific fields, including health services research, to statistically combine data from many individual studies. A meta-analysis adds up the results for each participant in the experimental group and in the control group of all the relevant studies and presents an easily understood summary; it also provides a visual depiction of the outcome, a *forest diagram,* in which the results of each study are shown, making it obvious if all the studies agree or not. For example, if some studies find that an intervention or experimental group is worse than the control group, and other studies find it better, the disagreement can be seen at a glance.

The term *meta-analysis* was coined by the American statistician Gene V. Glass while he was a faculty member at the University of Colorado at Boulder in 1976. However, the practice actually originated before 1976 as many meta-analyses were published earlier. The use of meta-analysis in clinical medicine was systematically developed in the United Kingdom by the Cochrane Collaboration, an international group of thousands of volunteers founded in 1993 and named after the British epidemiologist Archibald "Archie" L. Cochrane (1909–1988). The Cochrane Collaboration is an international, not-for-profit organization that produces and maintains systematic reviews of healthcare interventions, doing their meta-analysis in a standard way. These meta-analyses are published electronically in the Cochrane Database of Systematic Reviews, which are published many times a year and can be easily updated.

Meta-analysis consists of (a) a systematic search of the literature, identifying studies by predefined criteria; (b) extracting numerical results from each study for the experimental and control subjects, on various outcomes and their difference; plus (c) the calculation of parameters reflecting their statistical confidence (e.g., standard deviation and sample size).

The Meta-Analytic Method

To conduct a meta-analysis, a researcher conducts a literature search to find all the studies that meet certain predefined qualitative and quantitative inclusion or exclusion criteria. This is often computer based, with each search term and database used listed. As computer searches often miss important articles and reports, hand searches are also necessary, including searching the bibliography in each journal article to identify other applicable studies. If possible, the translations of the relevant foreign-language articles should be acquired.

It is vital that all studies in the meta-analysis meet reasonable criteria; otherwise there is the potential for bias. Meta-analysis is no better than the studies that go into it. If there is bias in even a few studies, it will translate into bias in the meta-analytic summary. Sometimes, one will see a meta-analysis with rather exacting criteria for the selection of studies. This may defeat the purpose of a meta-analysis because having very exhaustive inclusion criteria excludes studies that do not fit with the researcher's preconceptions. For this reason, the Cochrane Collaboration always includes a list of excluded studies. The criteria for study inclusion should be simple and straightforward and capture all the well-controlled studies in a field. One can then examine some of the minor methodological differences across studies by *sensitivity analysis* and *meta-regression* to see if they do make a difference.

It is not appropriate to statistically evaluate a participant's measure twice, as if it were for different subjects. Each participant should be counted only once. To demonstrate this *double publication redundancy,* investigators may initially report on the first 20 subjects and, in another article, report on a total of 60 subjects that include the original 20 subjects. Clearly, the same participants counted twice or more will amplify any finding. In addition, bias is introduced when undue weight is given to the findings of groups reporting their data in multiple publications as opposed to those reporting their findings in only one source.

Some researchers perform multiple statistical analyses and stress the most favorable outcome. For meta-analysis, predefined systematic numerical information should be extracted from each study.

The Statistics of Meta-Analysis

Effect Size

The *effect size* is the magnitude of the difference between the intervention or experimental groups and the control groups, regardless of the sample size. This is different from the *statistical significance,* which is defined as the probability that such a finding may happen by chance, leading to the rejection of the null hypothesis. Statistical significance is dependent, in part, on the sample size, so studies with a large number of subjects may yield a highly significant result. The effect size of a *continuous variable* is frequently expressed as the mean, or average, of the experimental group minus the mean of the control group divided by their pooled standard deviation.

Many outcomes are inherently qualitative, for example, living versus dead or having a disease versus not having a disease. For qualitative or *discontinuous* data, the effect size for an intervention-control comparison is primarily expressed as the difference between the percentages with and without an event in the experimental group and the control group using indices such as *odds ratios, risk ratios,* or *risk differences* to provide a measure of the differences. Inherently qualitative outcomes should be dealt with as such. Here, researchers would generally prefer using a continuous variable, but sometimes it is useful to supplement with a dichotomous variable. Dichotomizing data should be done using predefined criteria. An advantage of dichotomous data is that information from each individual subject can often be extracted (i.e., the results stem from real participants) from the observations of individual subjects rather than conducted on summary statistical parameters. This approach is inherently meaningful to researchers, whereas a change of abstract continuous units may not be.

The statistical methods for analyzing qualitative data are essentially a *stratified* or *fold contingency table.* Epidemiologists have been using these statistical methods for many years.

Studies often present a vast amount of data obtained through the use of various rating scales, measurement instruments, and statistical techniques, which makes it difficult to compare the results as they are expressed in a wide variety of units. In meta-analytic statistics, the control group mean or average is subtracted from the intervention or experimental group mean and then divided by the pooled group standard deviation, a process that is similar to the notion of *percentage change scores.* As a result, the data are expressed in uniform units. This allows researchers to focus their attention on the hypothesis they are examining rather than be distracted by the many different units among studies.

Statistical Methods

Most meta-analysis uses standard statistical techniques for continuous data and the Mantel-Haenszel model, or some variant thereof, for discontinuous data. Because continuous data possess more power than discrete data, continuous data are preferred, when available, to derive the effect size. The sample size, mean, and standard deviations can be easily extracted from RCTs as well as many other types of published studies. Unfortunately, many reports provide the sample size and means for the assorted groups but do not report the standard deviations (or standard error of the mean) that are needed for effect size calculations. Standard deviation or its equivalent should always be reported. Sometimes, standard deviations can be computed from the results of the statistical test presented. Part of meta-analysis is the calculation of variance in standard units. Meta-analyses can be done with fixed (assuming each study to have a fixed effect size) or random models (not assuming this). Generally, random models put more emphasis on the smaller studies.

Consistent Results

One of the major objectives of meta-analysis is to demonstrate, when studies are combined, that the findings are consistently homogenous. When consistent findings are present, some studies will be clearly statistically significant whereas others may have strong nonsignificant trends in the same direction, which summates the essential agreement, because the results are similar.

Sensitivity Analysis and Meta-Regression

The pattern and consistency of results across all studies is vital. For example, if there are several small-sample, positive RCTs and many large-sample, negative trials, it is likely that the smaller studies were deviations or wishful thinking. If the results between individual studies are highly dissonant, it is erroneous to conclude that the overall effect is statistically significant. Rather, the prudent conclusion is that some studies show intervention effects and others do not, which requires the researcher to explain this discrepancy. It is preferable to appraise studies by a priori criteria for methodological precision and then examine if there is a similar effect size in the more rather than less rigorous studies.

There are many arbitrary assumptions that can go into a meta-analysis, involving how to classify studies and the exact criteria for inclusion. It is important to perform a *sensitivity analysis* by analyzing the same data set with different assumptions, often with 5 to 10 alternate examinations. The blinding and randomization or other methodologies protect against bias. Sensitivity analysis is recalculation of the meta-analysis under different assumptions. Frequently researchers will drop a certain type of study to determine if the other studies produce the same results as the total, thereby demonstrating that the overall results are not an artifact of a given type of study. A sensitivity analysis can be done by using a different choice in deciding which studies to include, or a different outcome measure. However, the problem with dropping studies is the loss of statistical power.

A *metaregression* differs in that it includes all the studies but examines whether there is a systematic difference between one or another *moderator variable*. The moderator variables could be continuous or dichotomous (i.e., the meta-analytic equivalent of analysis of variance or analysis of covariance). The moderator variables are not randomly assigned nor are they usually blinded. Many biases could affect moderator variables. The same cautions that apply when imputing cause from statistical correlation analysis apply to a meta-regression as it is an exploratory technique.

The Graphic Inspection of Results

The quintessence of meta-analysis is the inspection of the data. Thus, this method generates a visual or numeric illustration of each study in the context of all the others. A review of the actual data gives the analytical reader a feel for the data. When the results from several studies are converted into similar units, a simple inspection of a graph or table quickly displays which trials have dissimilar outcomes from the majority. Such disparate outcomes can also be examined by a variety of statistical parameters. For example, a researcher can calculate a statistical *index of homogeneity*, whereby he or she can remove the most discrepant study from the analysis, recalculate, and in so doing reveal that all but one study in the data set are homogenous. If two studies are discrepant, then the researcher can remove both from the study and again recalculate the parameters of statistical homogeneity, and so on. When there are a number of blinded studies, the interpretation of efficacy is usually straightforward, particularly when the results are not statistically significant. A few biased studies mixed in with valid studies might produce a significant difference. In interpreting the results of the meta-analysis, it is important to examine the effect size and its significance, as well as the consistency of the results. The confidence interval or standard deviation and sample size provide a bridge to inspect uncertainty in the same units.

Meta-Analysis Versus Narrative Reviews

Narrative reviews of scientific findings are often based on clinical wisdom and can be highly subjective: The author of a narrative review may accept the results of studies without any critical assessment. The author may summarize several highly publicized references in support of a certain position, even reporting redundant data, but the reader may discover that many of the quoted studies are inadequately controlled. The author selectively chooses what studies to mention and selects what aspects to mention or omit, as well as giving his or her opinion as to what the bottom line is. Additionally, limited evidence from controlled studies failing to find a big difference is often interpreted as finding the opposite result. But an area that is not studied does not imply the opposite of the hypothesis, only insufficient studies. Ideally, the researcher should carefully consider each individual study before coming to any conclusions. However, when there are many controlled studies, the individual researcher often cannot remember all the results. Thus, a meta-analysis can often provide a more meaningful summary than a narrative review.

The File Drawer Problem

One of the most important drawbacks in meta-analysis is the "file drawer" problem. Researchers have found that positive findings are much more likely to be published than negative findings. And positive findings are more likely to be printed in more prestigious journals. Estimates can be made according to assumptions about such a pattern. An example of such estimates is the *funnel plot,* which is often included in a meta-analysis. However, such plots are no better than the assumptions underlying them. To minimize this bias, researchers recommend including all reasonable-quality studies as well as search reports of symposia, meeting presentations, relevant Web sites, exhibits, and other available unpublished data; they also recommend contacting investigators and funding sources for data and, if necessary, obtaining data using the Freedom of Information Act.

One safeguard is to calculate the number of participants whose negative results (hypothetically hidden in a file drawer) would convert a positive meta-analysis to a negative one (the fail-safe number). It seems likely that the file drawer issue is also a problem for narrative reviews as they generally do not seek to consider all relevant studies.

Omnibus Methods

Meta-analysis does not simply count the number of studies that display a significant difference, average their means not weighted by sample size, or add up the *p values*. These methods, which are referred to as omnibus or vote-counting methods, have many methodological problems. The results obtained by adding *p* values can be excessively influenced by a few disparate studies, as shown by various researchers using simulation models.

Implications

A large literature on meta-analysis has developed over the years, documenting the extensive experience and the methodological and statistical issues associated with it. The most important aspect of a meta-analysis, no matter how technically excellent, is no better than the soundness of the judgment that goes into the selection of the studies and their interpretation so that they make sense mechanistically.

Although meta-analysis has been traditionally used to summarize RCTs and genetic studies, it can also be used to summarize various health services research studies, case-controlled studies, observational studies, or even uncontrolled studies that use a common methodology. Knowledge of the data provides some empirical benchmarks to help distinguish empirical findings from the results of dogma, wishful thinking, or political pressures.

John M. Davis, Chunbo Li, and Stefan Leucht

See also Benchmarking; Causal Analysis; Cochrane, Archibald L.; Cohort Studies; Cross-Sectional Studies; Evidence-Based Medicine (EBM); Measurement in Health Services Research; Randomized Controlled Trials (RCTs)

Further Readings

Egger, Matthias, George Davey Smith, and Douglas G. Altman, eds. *Systematic Reviews in Health Care: Meta-Analysis in Context*. 2d ed. London: BMJ, 2003.

Higgins, Julian P. T., Simon G. Thompson, Jonathan J. Deeks, et al. "Measuring Inconsistency in Meta-Analysis," *British Medical Journal* 327(7414): 557–60, September 6, 2003.

Lipsey, Mark W., and David B. Wilson. *Practical Meta-Analysis*. Thousand Oaks, CA: Sage, 2001.

Petitti, Diana B. *Meta-Analysis, Decision Analysis, and Cost-Effectiveness Analysis: Methods for Quantitative Synthesis in Medicine*. 2d ed. New York: Oxford University Press, 2000.

Stangl, Dalene K. and Donald A. Berry, eds. *Meta-Analysis in Medicine and Health Policy*. New York: Marcel Dekker, 2000.

Sutton, Alexander J., and Julian P. T. Higgins. "Recent Developments in Meta-Analysis," *Statistics in Medicine* 27(5): 625–50, February 28, 2008.

Web Site

Cochrane Collaboration: http://www.cochrane.org

MIDWEST BUSINESS GROUP ON HEALTH

The Chicago-based Midwest Business Group on Health (MBGH) is a leading regional healthcare coalition of major private and public employers. The MBGH works with its member employers to help them control and lower their healthcare costs and obtain more value for their healthcare benefit dollars. As an organization, the coalition offers its members a wide variety of health benefit, educational seminars; networking opportunities; initiatives and demonstration projects; and group purchasing programs. The MBGH is also a member of the National Business Coalition on Health (NBCH).

Background

Established in January 1980 by a small group of large, Midwest employers, the nonprofit MGBH has grown to include more than 80 major employers responsible for more than 2 million covered lives in 11 states. These employers collectively spend more than $2.5 billion annually on their employees' healthcare benefits. Over the years, the coalition's mission has also broadened and expanded. Initially, it was mainly concerned with ways to lower and control the costs of healthcare; today, it also addresses the quality, safety, and value of healthcare.

Membership

The MBGH is primarily funded through employer membership dues. Membership is for a 12-month period with dues based on the employer's number of U.S. workers. Public and nonprofit employers receive a 50% discount off their membership dues. Specifically, the coalition has four membership categories: (1) business members, which are for-profit organizations (e.g., Bank of America, Caterpillar, and Ford Motor Company); (2) provider members, which are community-based healthcare provider organizations such as hospital systems (e.g., Advocate Health Care, Alexian Brothers Hospital Network, and Carle Clinic Association); (3) nonprofit and government members, which include academic, research, and government organizations (e.g., the Federal Reserve Bank of Chicago, the state of Illinois, and the University of Chicago); and (4) associate members, which include providers of healthcare and medical products or consulting and management services (e.g., Abbott Laboratories, Deloitte, and Johnson and Johnson Health Services).

Organizational Structure

The MBGH is governed by a board of directors, which consists of the president, chief executive officer, and secretary of the coalition and 18 board members. The board members are elected from the various member employers. A professional staff of six individuals—the president, vice president, director of projects and communications, director of operations, membership and administration coordinator, and projects coordinator—manages the coalition.

Products and Services

The MBGH provides three types of services to its member employers: (1) learning network programs, (2) health benefit purchasing groups, and (3) health benefits and quality initiatives. These services help member employers connect and learn from each other as well as obtain various products and services.

The coalition's learning network programs include the following: (a) monthly learning network meetings; (b) an annual conference; (c) employer, health, roundtable discussions; (d) health system user groups; (e) benchmark survey services; and (f) monthly, Medicare, employer forum telephone calls. The employer, health, roundtable discussions address pharmacy benefits, consumer-directed health plans (CDHPs) and consumerism, union benefits, and wellness and health management issues.

To help its member employers obtain competitive rates, superior services, performance evaluations, and performance guarantees, the MBGH has established an affiliate, the Midwest Health Purchasers Foundation (MHPF), which provides various health benefit purchasing groups. The foundation helps coalition member employers (a) enroll their workers in several Chicago health maintenance organizations (HMOs), (b) obtain pharmacy services (e.g., retail, mail, and specialty drugs), (c) obtain health promotion and risk management services, (d) obtain disease management services (e.g., acute-care counseling, and high-cost case management), (e) obtain audit services to examine the performance of third-party administrators (TPAs) and health plans, (f) manage Medicare Part D services, and (g) implement and manage incentive programs and products.

The MBGH undertakes a large number of health benefit and quality initiatives. Specifically, the coalition develops and supports various initiatives that test healthcare measurement tools and improve community health. Some of its recent initiatives include (a) an employee self-report tool that analyzes the impact of chronic disease on productivity; (b) measuring the costs of overuse, underuse, and misuse of healthcare and the role of purchasers in addressing these problems;

(c) determining what information consumers want to know about their physicians; and (d) studies of employer adoption of value-based benefit strategies and the correlation of benefit incentives to changes in employee behavior.

In 2003, the MBGH's initiative on the cost of overuse, underuse, and misuse of healthcare gained national attention with its estimate that about 30% of all direct healthcare outlays are the result of poor quality of care. In 2007, the MBGH, working with two pharmacist associations, initiated Taking Control of Your Health, a diabetes management demonstration project. The project uses specially trained pharmacists to conduct individual meetings with employees to help educate, motivate, and empower them to better manage their diabetes. In 2008, the coalition received a grant from the National Business Group on Health (NBGH) to expand the program.

Amy L. Sulkin

See also Cost Containment Strategies; Cost of Healthcare; Employee Health Benefits; Health Insurance; Health Insurance Coverage; Leapfrog Group; National Business Group on Health (NBGH); Pacific Business Group on Health (PBGH)

Further Readings

Butterfoss, Frances Dunn. *Coalitions and Partnerships in Community Health*. San Francisco: Jossey-Bass, 2007.

Camillus, Joseph A., and Meredith B. Rosenthal. "Health Care Coalitions: From Joint Purchasing to Local Health Reform," *Inquiry* 45(2): 142–52, Summer 2008.

Midwest Business Group on Health. *Reducing the Costs of Poor-Quality Health Care Through Responsible Purchasing Leadership*. Chicago: Midwest Business Group on Health, 2003.

Midwest Business Group on Health. *Employers' Readiness to Adopt Value-Based Benefit Strategies*. Chicago: Midwest Business Group on Health, 2008.

Web Sites

Midwest Business Group on Health (MBGH): http://www.mbgh.org

National Business Coalition on Health (NBCH): http://www.nbch.org

MILBANK MEMORIAL FUND

For most of its history, the Milbank Memorial Fund has collaborated with decision makers in the public and private sectors to use the best available evidence and experience in making policy for healthcare and population health. Its founders, Elizabeth Milbank Anderson—who provided the endowment in increments between 1905 and 1921—and Albert G. Milbank—who led the board from 1905 until his death in 1949—dedicated the fund to devising effective policy to improve the well-being of people, especially those with low incomes.

History

The fund's history can be divided into five segments: (1) 1905 to 1920, (2) 1921 to 1936, (3) 1937 to 1961, (4) 1961 to 1989, and (5) 1990 to the present. From 1905 until Elizabeth Milbank Anderson's death in 1920, the Memorial Fund Association, as it was then called, worked with officials of government and charitable agencies that served the poor in New York City. Notable projects included constructing public baths on models devised by health officials in Europe; increasing children's access to health and related services; and demonstrating the feasibility of a "home hospital," residences, and health services for families, one or more members of which had tuberculosis.

Between 1921 and 1936, the fund and its allies in government and medicine addressed major issues in improving access to appropriate healthcare and related services. Its first chief executive, John A. Kingsbury, a veteran manager in city government and charitable organizations, organized multiyear demonstrations of new methods of integrating services provided by the government and charities in New York City, Syracuse, and rural Cattaraugus County, New York. The fund appointed a technical board of prominent health experts to advise and evaluate these projects. This board produced a periodic bulletin evaluating the work of the demonstrations and commissioned a book about each of them. The bulletin, published continuously since 1923, is now the *Milbank Quarterly*.

The fund addressed controversial issues of health policy between 1926 and 1935. In 1926, for example, it helped organize the consortium of foundations to finance a Committee on the Costs of Medical Care (CCMC). Research reports by the committee's staff are landmarks in the history of health services research. In 1932, however, most of the physician members of the CCMC refused to sign its final report because it recommended the prepayment of healthcare and the reorganization of physicians into large group practices dominated by specialists.

Kingsbury and his staff at the fund advocated including these recommendations, as well as funding to expand access to health services, in the Social Security Act of 1935. The fund seconded two employees to the staff of the cabinet-level committee that drafted what became the Social Security Act. This advocacy increased antagonism toward the fund among critics of the CCMC report in organized medicine. Several medical societies recommended that physicians advise mothers to boycott Borden's condensed milk—an ingredient in infant formula—because stock in that company accounted for a substantial percentage of the fund's assets. In 1935, the board of the fund fired Kingsbury but reaffirmed its commitment to increased access to health services.

During the next quarter century, the fund maintained this commitment but through projects and publications that avoided controversy. Its chief executive from 1937 to 1961, Frank Boudreau, was a public health physician who had joined the new social medicine movement as an official of the League of Nations. He led the fund in conducting and commissioning policy-related research on nutrition, fertility and birth control, and mental health. The fund convened annual conferences addressed and attended by researchers and policymakers. In the 1950s, fund staff helped inform policy on substituting community for institutional care of the mentally ill and facilitated the establishment of the Population Council.

The fund chose not to prioritize activities related to policy between 1961 and 1989. Alexander Robertson, chief executive from 1961 to 1967, managed a fellowship program in social medicine for young academic physicians from North and South America. His successor from 1967 to 1977, Leroy Burney, accorded priority to the reform of higher education for public health. The next chief executive, Robert H. Ebert—1978 to 1984 and 1988 to 1989—organized a fellowship program in clinical epidemiology; several of its alumni became leaders in the field subsequently called evidence-based health research and practice. Sidney Lee, 1984 to 1988, mounted projects to improve the health of migrant and seasonal workers and their families.

In the 1960s, the *Milbank Quarterly* became, and has remained, a highly regarded, international journal of research on health services and policy and on population health. The fund was designated an operating foundation under 1967 amendments to the Internal Revenue Code on the basis of the *Quarterly* and miscellaneous reports.

Since 1990, however, the fund has used its regulatory status as an operating foundation to collaborate with many decision makers in the public and private sectors to bring the best available evidence to bear on policy and practice. A new chairman, Samuel L. (Tony) Milbank (1990 to present), and two presidents, Daniel M. Fox (1990–2007) and Carmen Hooker (2007 to present), led this restoration of what had been the fund's mission during its first half century.

Future Implications

The fund currently prioritizes responsiveness to its constituents, who are mainly decision makers but also include researchers who are able to inform policy in the United States and other countries. The fund's largest program since the early 1990s has been its partnership with the Reforming States Group (RSG). The RSG is a voluntary association of senior officials of the legislative and executive branches of government from each of the states, from most Canadian provinces, and recently, from Australia, England, and Scotland. Its members assist one another to acquire and assess evidence and experience that could improve policy for healthcare and population health.

In addition to its work with the RSG, the fund and its constituents have recently addressed issues that include (a) public health law reform, (b) the adequacy of the income available to retirees over the next generation, (c) the importance of global health issues for American foreign and security policy, and (d) improving long-term and palliative care. The fund continues to publish the *Milbank Quarterly* and occasional reports and copublishes a book series with the University of California Press.

Daniel M. Fox

See also Committee on the Costs of Medical Care (CCMC); Health Insurance; Health Services Research Journals; Public Health; Public Policy

Further Readings

Ameringer, Carl F. *The Health Care Revolution: From Medical Monopoly to Market Competition.* Berkeley: Milbank Memorial Fund/University of California Press, 2008.

Cassel, Christine K. *Medicare Matters: What Geriatric Medicine Can Teach American Health Care.* Berkeley: Milbank Memorial Fund/University of California Press, 2007.

Daly, Jeanne. *Evidence-Based Medicine and the Search for a Science of Clinical Care.* Berkeley: Milbank Memorial Fund/University of California Press, 2005.

Fairchild, Amy L., Ronald Bayer, and James Colgrove. *Searching Eyes: Privacy, the State, and Disease Surveillance in America.* Berkeley: Milbank Memorial Fund/University of California Press, 2007.

Fox, Daniel M. "The Significance of the Milbank Memorial Fund for Policy: An Assessment at Its Centennial," *Milbank Quarterly* 84(1): 1–23, 2006.

Web Site

Milbank Memorial Fund: http://www.milbank.org

MINIMUM DATA SET (MDS) FOR NURSING HOME RESIDENT ASSESSMENT

The provision of appropriate care in nursing facilities requires comprehensive knowledge of residents' strengths, weaknesses, and problems. As one feature of the Omnibus Budget Reconciliation Act of 1987 (OBRA 87), the U.S. Congress sought to ensure the availability of such information by mandating a national resident assessment system, including a uniform set of items and definitions for assessing all residents in nursing facilities in the United States. The need for uniform resident assessment in long-term care had been long recognized. A 1986 study by the national Institute of Medicine (IOM) focused on how to improve nursing home regulation and identified uniform resident assessment as a cornerstone of any effort to improve quality. Indeed, this recommendation, along with a host of others in the Institute's report, formed the basis for many of the nursing home reform provisions in OBRA 87, requiring each certified nursing facility to conduct a comprehensive, accurate, standardized, reproducible assessment of each resident's functional capacities.

In 1988, the Health Care Financing Administration (HCFA) (now the Centers for Medicare and Medicaid Services [CMS]) contracted with the Research Triangle Institute, the Hebrew Rehabilitation Center for the Aged, Brown University, and the University of Michigan to develop and evaluate a uniform resident assessment system. The resident assessment instrument that emerged was designed as a minimum data set (MDS) of items, definitions, and response categories aimed at providing a comprehensive assessment. In addition, the resident assessment protocols (RAPs), which are part of the resident assessment instrument (RAI), provide guidelines for more in-depth assessment of 18 conditions that affect the functional well-being of nursing home residents (e.g., falls, urinary incontinence, cognition difficulties, and use of restraints).

Development of the Instrument

In developing the RAI, more than 60 prior assessment instruments that had been developed for screening, admission, and research purposes were reviewed for comprehensiveness and to identify common domains, items, definitions, responses, and scoring patterns. These were used to develop multiple instrument drafts, all of which underwent extensive review by literally hundreds of experts representing all the professions that work with nursing home residents. The resulting instrument contains more than 300 data elements, many of which measure the traditional domains of functioning, personal-care activities, and the amount of "hands-on" and supervision time associated with each

personal-care area, as well as basic demographic factors. Other domains covered in the MDS include (a) decision making; (b) behavioral problems; (c) symptoms, diagnoses, and conditions; (d) social interaction and regulations; (e) skin care needs; and (f) services received. Newest of all were data elements about the residents' life-long behavioral styles and preferences, as well as documentation of the existence and type of an advance directive.

Field Testing

As with all research instruments, extensive field testing and reliability testing were undertaken. Numerous sets of independent reliability trials were undertaken during the development processes. The results of these reliability studies clearly demonstrated that when MDS data are gathered in a research context, it is possible to obtain reliability levels that make the data useful for research purposes. The MDS items met traditional standards of good reliability in key areas of functional status such as cognition, activities of daily living (ADL) performance, continence, and disease diagnoses.

Development of reliable data on the functional status of nursing home residents is a task that largely defies traditional approaches to measurement. Nursing home residents are a special population and present special measurement challenges. Most nursing home residents have some level of cognitive impairment and exhibit behavior changes. The abilities and status of many nursing home residents with physical or cognitive impairments vary throughout the day and over time. Still others have communication difficulties that impede traditional research interview interactions. These characteristics seriously limit the effectiveness of simple "point in time" estimates of a resident's status, no matter how well standardized, and argue against relying on a single informant, which is the usual approach with research instruments. For these reasons, the assessment approach incorporated in the MDS relies on the input of multiple individuals who interact with the resident throughout the course of the day or night.

As part of an evaluation of the national implementation of the MDS, the quality-of-health status and the resident assessment information in the residents' charts before and after the implementation of the MDS was addressed. Research nurses extracted data from a sample of more than 2,000 nursing home residents in more than 250 randomly selected facilities in 1990 and again in 1993. The analyses revealed that, in 1990, accurate information was available in 68% of the items in the patients' records, whereas in 1993, that average had climbed to 84%. Although accuracy levels from records sampled from participating nursing homes varied considerably in the 10 states studied, in all cases there was an improvement in data accuracy associated with the introduction of the MDS.

The most recent reliability study of the MDS compared the assessments performed by *facility* nurses—on between 25 and 30 residents from more than 250 facilities located in 10 states—with those undertaken by *research* nurses uniformly trained by a team of researchers. Of the more than 100 items evaluated, almost all revealed high levels of reliability, although there was substantial inter-facility variation that suggests that some facilities departed from the standard approach. These findings are consistent with studies finding substantial disagreement between selected MDS items in residents' charts and research data collected about the same residents.

Clinical Scales

The utility of the MDS for clinical and research applications has been further enhanced by the development of concise and clinically meaningful scales summarizing the functioning of individual residents. For example, the Cognitive Performance Scale, which replicates the mini-mental-status exam at an accuracy of nearly 90%, has been developed from items in the MDS. Similarly, an ADL scale that captures the hierarchy of ADL performance has been formulated and a new measure of "social engagement" developed, which is one of the first efforts to quantify a qualitative aspect of the personal and social interactions of an individual in a nursing home. Other summary measures of items in the MDS include measures of mood, behavioral disruption, medical instability, and more refined aspects of cognitive and executive functioning, including qualitative features of dementia.

Computerized Data

To facilitate ongoing quality monitoring and case-mix reimbursement for both Medicare and state Medicaid programs, the Centers for Medicare and Medicaid Services (CMS) mandated the computerization of all MDS data in 1998. Since then, all MDS assessments are computerized and transmitted to a national repository maintained by CMS. These data are used (a) by state regulators charged with inspecting nursing homes to ensure compliance with the Medicare and Medicaid conditions of participation, (b) by Medicare and some state Medicaid programs to differentially pay facilities as a function of the acuity of their residents, and (c) to create quality measures that are publicly reported on national Web sites to assist individuals and their families in selecting a nursing home. Furthermore, nursing facility management—as a stimulus to guide and initiate internal quality improvement efforts—increasingly uses MDS data on residents' acuity, pattern of services use, and quality.

Use for Policy, Regulatory, and Quality Improvement

The MDS is being extensively used for policy, regulatory, and quality improvement purposes. The new measure of resident case-mix, which is being used to reimburse facilities differentially (Resource Utilization Groups–III), is based on the MDS. State regulators inspecting nursing homes also use the MDS in residents' charts to determine whether the residents assessed as potentially having selected care needs are getting the relevant services. Finally, drawing on the concepts of statistical quality improvement, quality indicators are being developed as benchmarks against which nursing homes can compare their quality of performance.

The impact of the nationally mandated MDS for U.S. nursing home resident assessment has been profound. The MDS has also been adopted in other nations. As of 2008, the MDS has been translated into 20 languages (e.g., French, Spanish, Italian, Swedish, German, Chinese, Japanese, and Korean). Canada and Iceland have adopted a version of the MDS as the basis for reforming their own nursing home programs and to institute case-mix reimbursement and quality management programs. Finland, Germany, Italy, and Switzerland have instituted experiments in large geographic areas. An international organization, the InterRAI, has been formed with the express purpose of sharing experiences in implementing the MDS as (a) a clinical-care-planning tool, (b) an administrative information system for management decisions, and (c) a basis for policy analysis of a nation's healthcare system.

Future Changes

The original, national Institute of Medicine (IOM) recommendations suggested that the MDS not be static. In keeping with that suggestion, CMS commissioned an early redesign of the initial instrument, and this was implemented in 1996. Nearly a decade later, CMS has announced that it will be introducing a major redesign of the MDS (Version 3.0) in 2009. This new instrument has the benefit of many years of additional research on the utility of various measures of quality, functional performance, and clinical-care needs. It also has benefited from considerable additional research focused on capturing the "voice" of the residents' experiences and quality of life. Changes from the earlier versions include a focus on directly interviewing the residents and an emphasis on their quality of life in addition to their quality of care. This means that facility staff will first attempt to directly ask residents questions about their experience in the home, with all the associated problems of response acquiescence, residents' unwillingness to complain, and cognitive impairment difficulties. Whereas earlier versions of the MDS appeared to underestimate the prevalence of psychosocial problems, it is likely that new difficulties will arise with the revised version. Nonetheless, in keeping with the spirit of the original recommendation, resident assessment instruments must be dynamic, reflecting the changing context of nursing home care and the case-mix of the patients served.

In many ways, the introduction of the MDS has catapulted the nursing home industry into the information age. It is possible, given the implementation of the MDS, that the goals of the IOM recommendations may be reached and that ongoing comprehensive assessment may actually have a positive impact on the quality of care for nursing home residents.

Vincent Mor

See also Activities of Daily Living (ADL); Centers for Medicare and Medicaid Services (CMS); Long-Term Care; Nursing Home Quality; Nursing Homes; Quality of Healthcare; Skilled-Nursing Facilities; Vulnerable Populations

Further Readings

Arling, Greg, Robert L. Kane, Christine Mueller, et al. "Explaining Direct Care Resource Use of Nursing Home Residents: Findings From Time Studies in Four States," *Health Services Research* 42(2): 827–46, April 2007.

Committee on Nursing Home Regulation, Institute of Medicine. *Improving the Quality of Care in Nursing Homes.* Washington, DC: National Academy Press, 1986.

Dellefield, Mary Ellen. "Implementation of the Resident Assessment Instrument/Minimum Data Set in the Nursing Home as Organization: Implications for Quality Improvement in RN Clinical Assessment," *Geriatric Nursing* 28(6): 377–86, November–December 2007.

Lee, Feng-Ping, Carol Leppa, and Karen Schepp. "Using the Minimum Data Set to Determine Predictors of Terminal Restlessness Among Nursing Home Residents," *Journal of Nursing Research* 14(4): 286–96, December 2006.

Mor, Vincent. "A Comprehensive Clinical Assessment Tool to Inform Policy and Practice: Applications of the Minimum Data Set," *Medical Care* 42(4): III50–III59, April 2004.

Mor, Vincent, Katherine Berg, Joseph Angelelli, et al. "The Quality of Quality Measurement in U.S. Nursing Homes," Special issue 2, *Gerontologist* 43 37–46, April, 2003.

Zimmerman, David R. "Improving Nursing Home Quality of Care Through Outcome Data: The MDS Quality Indicators," *International Journal of Geriatric Psychiatry* 18(3): 205–257, March 2003.

Web Sites

Centers for Medicare and Medicaid Services (CMS), Nursing Home Quality Initiatives: http://www.cms.hhs.gov/NursingHomeQualityInits/20_NHQIMDS20.asp
InterRAI: http://www.interrai.org

MORAL HAZARD

Moral hazard arises in implicit and contractual relationships in which one party behaves differently because of the relationship, and these actions improve one party's utility but have a negative consequence for the other party. In healthcare, moral hazard is most commonly associated with insurance, where the purchase of health insurance induces an increase in the likelihood of a loss covered by the insurance policy, the size of the loss, or both the likelihood and size of the loss.

Asymmetric Information

Moral hazard arises because of asymmetric information between the two parties. When one party, the *agent,* has more information than another party, the *principal,* in a relationship, the agent can take actions that are not observable to the principal and that benefit the agent but are costly to the principal. If the information and actions were perfectly observable to both parties, the agent would be unlikely to take these actions. For example, an individual without auto insurance may take many precautions to prevent his or her car from being stolen: He or she may only park the car in security-monitored parking lots, install a security system, and make certain that no valuables are left in plain sight in the car. If this individual purchases an auto insurance policy that fully insures against theft, the individual may not take any of these precautions—he or she may park in high crime areas, not use a car security system, and leave valuables in plain sight in the car—because the individual knows that the insurance company will reimburse him or her if the car is stolen. As the insurance company cannot monitor how the individual safeguards the car against theft, these actions benefit the individual; it takes less time and effort not to use these safeguards, but by not taking these actions, he or she increases the chance that the car will be broken into or stolen. In economic terms, this increases both the likelihood of a loss occurring and the size of the loss, if a loss occurs.

Although both moral hazard and *adverse selection* arise because of asymmetric information between parties, moral hazard is a "hidden action" taken by the agent, which is not observable by the principal. Adverse selection, on the other hand, is known as a "hidden type" or "hidden information" problem where the principal cannot observe the characteristics of the agent before entering into an implicit or explicit contract, and the agent makes decisions about the relationship that benefit him or her but are costly to the principal.

Health Insurance

Moral hazard in health insurance can occur in two basic ways. *Ex ante* moral hazard occurs when an insured individual takes less preventive care than he or she would take if the individual did not have insurance, and these preventive-care efforts would reduce the likelihood or size of a loss covered by the insurance policy. The second type of moral hazard occurs *ex post,* when an individual demands more healthcare services when covered by an insurance policy than he or she would demand if the individual paid the full cost of healthcare. The evidence that ex post moral hazard exists in health insurance is quite strong. Although there has been less evidence in support of ex ante moral hazard, it is gaining attention in the health insurance market.

Ex ante moral hazard includes the actions taken by an insured individual prior to contracting an illness or disease that increase the probability of contracting the illness or increase the cost of medical care covered by health insurance once the illness is contracted. Examples of ex ante moral hazard include a lack of preventive care, for example, an unhealthy diet, sedentary lifestyle, and other health behaviors that increase the likelihood of obesity and chronic health conditions such as heart disease and diabetes. Through healthy-lifestyle behaviors such as a healthy diet and physical exercise, an individual can reduce the risk of these chronic conditions. The theory of ex ante moral hazard suggests that individuals who have insurance will invest in fewer healthy-lifestyle behaviors than those without health insurance because they do not bear the full cost of their unhealthy-lifestyle behaviors when covered by insurance.

Ex post moral hazard takes place after a loss occurs—in healthcare, this means after an individual becomes ill. Without health insurance coverage, an individual will purchase healthcare services up to the point where the marginal cost of these services is equal to the marginal private benefit obtained from these services. Health insurance coverage reduces the marginal cost of these services that is paid by the consumer. Therefore, with health insurance coverage, the consumer still purchases services up to the point where his or her private marginal cost of these services equals his or her marginal private benefit. However, in that the consumer's marginal private cost is reduced, the quantity of services consumed is higher. As the generosity of a health insurance policy increases, ex post moral hazard also increases, because the consumer bears a smaller proportion of the cost of care. In the most extreme case where an insurance policy fully covers the cost of medical care and the consumer has no out-of-pocket costs, the consumer uses medical care up to the point where he or she obtains almost no marginal benefit from these services, even though the full cost of care is still paid by the insurer.

Solutions

Health insurers use a combination of mechanisms targeted at the demand for care (i.e., mechanisms that are targeted at consumers or enrollees) and the supply of care (i.e., mechanisms targeted at healthcare providers) to mitigate ex post moral hazard. Demand-side mechanisms shift some of the risk originally borne by the insurer to the enrollee through deductibles and coinsurance. Shifting risk to the enrollee increases the marginal cost of care consumed by the enrollee. Although increasing enrollee cost sharing mitigates moral hazard, the trade-off is a reduction in risk spreading, which is an inherent purpose of health insurance.

Supply-side mechanisms are strategies that target providers, including financial incentives such as reimbursement strategies and nonfinancial incentives such as the use of gatekeeper primary care physicians, second opinions, prior authorization, and review of usage. The use of capitated per-member-per-month compensation rather than per-unit fee-for-service reimbursement is one solution that has been used to reduce moral hazard. Fee-for-service reimbursement aligns the financial incentives of the healthcare providers with the enrollees, incentivizing the delivery of more

services or more expensive services than necessary. A shift to capitation removes the financial incentive to provide more than necessary care. Instead, the provider is incentivized to provide efficient services to treat an illness, aligning the provider's incentives with the health insurer rather than the enrollee, thereby reducing the extent of ex post moral hazard.

Solutions to mitigate ex ante moral hazard need to incentivize enrollees to obtain preventive care by reducing the financial and nonfinancial costs of taking preventive actions or by increasing the marginal costs of failing to take preventive actions. Health insurers may fully cover the costs of immunizations, for example, to encourage enrollees to obtain them.

Future Implications

The U.S. federal government and private health insurers alike have been promoting *consumer-directed health plans* (CDHPs)—high-deductible health plans with health savings accounts—as a mechanism to control increasing healthcare costs. CDHPs directly target ex post moral hazard. These plans shift a greater proportion of the risk to the consumer and, by increasing the consumer's cost, require him or her to share the burden. CDHPs give the consumer an incentive to search for and obtain the most efficient healthcare services. For CDHPs to be successful, however, both prices and information on the quality of care must be transparent and publicly available so that consumers can compare across both treatments and healthcare providers to identify the most efficient method and provider of care. Although the nation's healthcare industry is improving the dissemination of information on the quality of healthcare through Web sites such as Hospital Compare, information is not yet easily available to all consumers. For example, not all consumers have access to or know how to use the Internet. Furthermore, solutions to mitigate moral hazard must be balanced with trade-offs that increase the risk borne by the individual consumer. The nation's healthcare industry is still searching for the optimal combination of risk spreading and moral hazard.

Tricia J. Johnson

See also Adverse Selection; Capitation; Consumer-Directed Health Plans (CDHPs); Healthcare Markets; Health Economics; Health Insurance; Payment Mechanisms; RAND Health Insurance Experiment

Further Readings

Arrow, Kenneth J. "Uncertainty and the Welfare Economics of Medical Care," *American Economic Review* 53(5): 941–73, December 1963.

Manning, Willard G., and M. Susan Marquis. "Health Insurance: The Tradeoff Between Risk Pooling and Moral Hazard," *Journal of Health Economics*, 15(5): 609–639, March 1996.

Newhouse, Joseph P. "Reconsidering the Moral Hazard-Risk Avoidance Tradeoff," *Journal of Health Economics* 25(5): 1005–1014, September 2006.

Pauly, Mark V. "The Economics of Moral Hazard: Comment," *American Economic Review* 58(3 pt. 1): 531–37, June 1968.

Zweifel, Peter, and Willard G. Manning. "Moral Hazard and Consumer Incentives in Health Care," in A. J. Culyer and J. P. Newhouse, eds. *Handbook of Health Economics*, Vol. 1A. Amsterdam: Elsevier, North-Holland, 2000.

Web Sites

Hospital Compare: http://www.hospitalcompare.hhs.gov
RAND Health Insurance Experiment:
   http://www.rand.org/health/projects/hie

MORBIDITY

The term *morbidity* comes from the Latin word *morbidus,* meaning a condition of being unhealthy or having a disease or an illness. Today, morbidity refers to an illness, disease, or disability. It also includes the burden caused by a health condition or the state of poor health. Morbidity is often measured using the incidence or prevalence rates of a disease in a population. Public health and health services researchers study the incidence rates of diseases to determine trends. For example, the incidence rate will show whether a specific disease is increasing or decreasing in a population. In contrast, the prevalence rate will show the overall burden of a disease, which may be used to determine the resources needed and consumed for treatment.

Overview

Morbidity or illness greatly affects an individual's as well as a population's quality of life. When trying to define or measure the factors that cause some individuals to be unhealthy, it is important to also understand the concept of health. The determinants of health have been acknowledged by the World Health Organization (WHO) to include (a) the social and economic environment, (b) the physical environment, and (c) the person's individual characteristics and behaviors. As the leading causes of illness and death have shifted from infectious diseases to chronic diseases, there has been much work to better understand the social determinants of health and the causes of morbidity. Some commonly used indicators of a population's health include the presence of child abuse, poverty, youth suicide, alcohol-related traffic fatalities, teenage drug use, depression; social networks and social capital.

Measures of Morbidity

Since the mid-1800s, conditions affecting health status began to be measured in a routine and systematized manner in the United States. As a result, incidence and prevalence rates have been used to measure the presence and rate of illnesses or conditions that interfere with a population's well-being. The *incidence rate* is also known as the cumulative incidence or the number of new cases of a disease or condition, and the *prevalence rate* refers to the number of existing cases of a disease or condition in a population.

The incidence rate can be calculated and used whenever a condition (physical or mental health related) has a defined diagnosis. Incidence rates can also provide a measure of the risk of acquiring a particular condition. An example of the incidence rate of diabetes in a city of 141,000 residents with 535 new cases of diabetes in 2008 would require the following calculation: 535/141,000 = 0.00379 or 3.8 per 1,000 population. Given that the incidence rate of diabetes was 0.4%, if an individual was a member of that population he or she had a 0.4% chance of getting diabetes. It should be cautioned that extrapolating population data to individuals can be misleading because individual risk factors and behaviors vary widely.

The second common measure of morbidity is prevalence. For example, if a researcher was interested in the prevalence of breast cancer among women in a given city with 141,000 residents and there were 5,076 cases of breast cancer during 2008, the prevalence rate would be calculated as follows: 5,076/141,000 = 0.036 or 36 per 1,000 population. Because prevalence also measures the total number of existing cases of a condition in a population, it can be used to determine the burden of that disease on society. In other words, knowing that 36 residents per 1,000 population, or 5,076 residents currently have breast cancer can give some guidance as to the demand for healthcare services as well as the public health programs that should be provided.

By examining the incidence and prevalence rates, the trends and patterns in the distribution of diseases can be studied. From this information, decisions can be made in terms of resource distribution and planning efforts for prevention and treatment.

In addition to the morbidity associated with specific conditions, it is important to be aware that in many populations, especially the elderly, there will be multiple morbidities (comorbidities) present at the same time. Thus, comorbidities must also be taken into account to understand the full burden of disease.

Measures of Disease Burden

Measures of morbidity, which generally include quality of life or years of life lost due to an increase in morbidity, are difficult to quantify. However, several measures of morbidity have been developed that combine the concepts of the number of years lived with the quality of those years. The two most commonly used measures are the disability-adjusted life year (DALY) and the quality-adjusted life year (QALY).

The DALY was developed by the Global Burden of Disease study by the WHO as a means of estimating the burden of disease in various parts of the world. This study not only looked at life expectancy tables but also factored in the burden of injuries, risk factors, and diseases. DALYs combine the effect of years of life lost prematurely and the disability of a population. As a result, mortality and morbidity are combined into a single measurement.

QALY is another method of measuring the burden of disease by taking into account not only the quantity of years lived but also the quality of life. Each year of perfect health is rated as 1.0 and death is rated as 0. QALYs are often used in cost-utility analyses to measure the effectiveness of specific medical interventions. Regarding the use of QALYs, there have been several debates as to whether some years should actually be rated with negative numbers, because some conditions might be viewed as worse than death. Furthermore, it is difficult to define what is "perfect health."

The Compression of Morbidity

Due to the increasing recognition of the growing burden of disease, there is now a greater emphasis on the *compression of morbidity,* that is, reducing the number of years that individuals are affected by chronic diseases. The goal of the compression of morbidity is to keep populations disease free for as long as possible. The objective of the compression of morbidity is to decrease the number of years that an individual suffers from disease at the same time maximizing his or her life span. It has been suggested that aging-related morbidity can be reduced through healthier lifestyles.

The Global Burden of Disease

In one of the most comprehensive research projects ever undertaken to look at the global burden of disease, the WHO identified the most important risk factors that are the causes of disability, disease, and death in the world today. Globally, the top 10 risks are (1) being underweight; (2) having unsafe sex; (3) having high blood pressure; (4) using tobacco; (5) consuming alcohol; (6) having unsafe water, sanitation, and hygiene; (7) having iron deficiency; (8) having indoor smoke from solid fuels; (9) having high cholesterol; and (10) being obese.

In developing countries, such as those in sub-Saharan Africa, being underweight is the major cause of disease burden; this condition also affects hundreds of millions of the poorest people throughout the world. On the other hand, in developed countries the leading risks of disease are tobacco use, alcohol consumption, high blood pressure, high cholesterol, and obesity. A disturbing finding from this report was the conclusion that the world is living more dangerously than ever before. In regard to health, this is because the poor have few choices in their lives, and those not limited by poverty who do have choices make the wrong choices concerning their health behaviors and activities.

Future Implications

Measuring and understanding the determinants of morbidity are key to ensuring the health and vitality of a population. As the leading causes of morbidity and mortality in developed countries shift from infectious to chronic diseases, appropriate health planning must be undertaken. Additionally, in developing countries, the urgent need to stem the rise in infectious diseases is paramount to decrease the burden of morbidity and improve the quality of life.

James C. Hagen

See also Acute and Chronic Diseases; Centers for Disease Control and Prevention (CDC); Disease; Emerging Diseases; Epidemiology; Infectious Diseases; Mortality; Quality-Adjusted Life Years (QALYs)

Further Readings

Fries, James F. "Frailty, Heart Disease, and Stroke: The Compression of Morbidity Paradigm," *American Journal of Preventive Medicine* 29(5 Suppl. 1): 164–68, December 2005.

Gordis, Leon. *Epidemiology.* 4th ed. Philadelphia: Saunders-Elsevier, in press.

Lopez, Alan D., Colin D. Mathers, Majid Ezzali, et al., eds. *Global Burden of Disease and Risk Factors.* Washington, DC: World Bank and Oxford University Press, 2006.

Michaud, Catherine M., Christopher J. L. Murray, and Barry R. Bloom. "Burden of Disease: Implications for Future Research," *Journal of the American Medical Association* 285(5): 535–39, February 7, 2001.

Mokdad, Ali H., James S. Marks, Donna F. Stroup, et al. "Actual Causes of Death in the United States, 2000," *Journal of the American Medical Association* 291(10): 1238–45, March 10, 2004.

Segui-Gomez, Maria, and Ellen J. MacKenzie. "Measuring the Public Health Impact of Injuries," *Epidemiologic Reviews* 25(1): 3–19, 2003.

Web Sites

Centers for Disease Control and Prevention (CDC): http://www.cdc.gov

National Center for Health Statistics (NCHS): http://www.cdc.gov/nchs

World Health Organization (WHO): http://www.who.int

MORTALITY

Mortality is simply defined as death, and it is the end result of life. A *mortality rate* is the proportion of deaths in a given place over a specified period of time. The numerator includes the number of persons who died in a given geographic area over a period of time, and the denominator is the total population in the same geographic area. The mortality rate is generally reported as a proportion of deaths per 1,000, 10,000, or 100,000 individuals. In health services research, mortality rates are often used as general indicators of the health and well-being of groups and populations.

Overview

Mortality rates are based on death data that come from *vital statistics registries*. Vital statistics include all the prominent life events: births, marriages, divorces, and deaths. The registration of all these life events is required in the United States, and state health departments compile vital statistics summaries on deaths. The primary source of death information in the United States is the standardized death certificate, which is kept by individual state health departments and is completed by physicians or coroners at the local level. The major components of the death certificate include personal identifiers, demographic information, and the manner and cause of death.

Mortality Rates and Ratios

There are many types of mortality rates and ratios, for example, the *crude mortality rate, age-standardized mortality rate, disease-specific mortality rate,* and *infant mortality rate.* Each type of mortality rate and ratio has its specific uses and limitations. The following are the most common types of mortality rates.

The Crude Mortality Rate

A crude mortality rate represents a rough estimate of mortality and is seldom used because it does not take into account the variations in a group's or population's age composition. The crude mortality rate is calculated by taking the total number of deaths during a 1-year period divided by the total population midyear for a specified geographic area. The rate is usually presented as deaths per 100,000 individuals. Crude mortality rates can sometimes be misleading. For example, a developed country may have a higher crude mortality rate than a developing country because of the increased number of elderly who may die in a given year. Therefore, mortality rates generally should be standardized to reflect this difference in population characteristics.

The Age-Standardized Mortality Rate

An age-standardized mortality rate is determined by taking the number of deaths in a specific age cohort occurring during 1 year divided by the midyear population of the specific age cohort. The derived rate is usually presented in terms of deaths per 1,000 or 100,000 individuals. Age-specific rates are refinements on the crude mortality rates. Note that, in putting a limitation on age, the same restriction must be applied to both the numerator and denominator, so that every individual in the denominator group will be at risk for entering the numerator group.

The Disease-Specific Mortality Rate

The disease-specific mortality rate is specified for a certain disease, such as tuberculosis or HIV/AIDS. The numerator in this rate is the number of deaths from a specific cause or disease and the denominator is the total population at midyear. Again, these rates are usually expressed in terms of annual mortality figures from a specific cause per 1,000 or 100,000 individuals.

The Case Fatality Rate

The case fatality rate is a measure of how severe a disease is and is usually reported as a percentage. The case fatality rate is calculated by taking the number of deaths from a specific cause after the onset of the disease (i.e., after diagnosis) during a specified period of time divided by the number of cases of the disease, multiplied by 100. This "rate" illustrates the percentage of individuals who die from a specified disease within a certain time after diagnosis.

The Proportional Mortality Ratio (PMR)

The PMR is a measure of the proportion of deaths from a specific disease compared with all deaths. The PMR is calculated by taking the total number of deaths from a certain disease over a specified period of time divided by the total number of deaths from all causes in the identical period of time. The PMR does not measure the risk of dying from a specific disease: The proportions change as a result of increases or decreases in the mortality rates of other diseases.

The Maternal Mortality Rate

The maternal mortality rate is calculated by dividing the number of deaths from childbearing causes during 1 year over the total number of live births during the identical year. This proportion is usually reported as deaths per 100,000. The maternal mortality rate measures the number of mothers who die giving birth.

The Infant Mortality Rate

The infant mortality rate is an overall measure of infant deaths. The numerator for this death rate is the number of children under the age of 1 who die over a 1-year period, and the denominator is the total number of live births during the same year. The result is typically multiplied by 1,000 to calculate a rate of infant deaths.

The Perinatal Mortality Rate

The perinatal mortality rate measures the number of infant deaths occurring around the period of birth. The perinatal mortality rate is calculated by taking the number of fetal deaths and the number of infants under 1 week of age who die during a period of a year divided by the total number of live births plus the total number of fetal deaths in the same year. This rate is typically expressed as deaths per 1,000.

The Neonatal Mortality Rate

The neonatal mortality rate is calculated by dividing the total number of children under 28 days old who die during a particular year by the number of live births during the same year. This rate is usually multiplied by a factor of 1,000.

The Fetal Mortality Rate

The fetal mortality rate is calculated by dividing the number of fetal (unborn infant) deaths during a particular year by the total number of live births plus fetal deaths during the identical year. This rate is usually multiplied by a factor of 1,000.

The Standardized Mortality Ratio (SMR)

The SMR is used to examine the differences in death rates between what is observed and what is expected. It is calculated by dividing the number of individuals who die per year by the number of individuals expected to die during the same year multiplied by 100. An SMR of less than 100 indicates that the observed deaths are less than what is expected, a value of 100 shows that the number of expected deaths is equal to the number of observed deaths, and an SMR of more than 100 demonstrates that observed deaths are greater than what is expected.

The Years of Potential Life Lost (YPLL)

The YPLL is a mortality index that has been used increasingly in recent years. It indicates the number of "years lost" as a result of an early death. It is calculated by first subtracting an individual's age at death from a standard age of life expectancy (generally, 65 years old). The smaller the subtrahend, the larger is the number of years of potential life lost. This calculation yields the YPLL for one individual. To calculate YPLL for the entire population, the YPLLs for all individuals are added together for a specific cause of death. YPLLs can be used to compare the causes of premature deaths.

Sources of Mortality Data

There are several sources of mortality data that are available to health services researchers. Information from death certificates is aggregated in comprehensive mortality databases and is reported by various federal agencies. Data may also be collected by agencies at the time of death for the purposes of issuing survivor benefits. Researchers may need this information on mortality and the cause of death to calculate a variety of mortality rates, to assess survival rates for a disease of interest, or to verify deaths in a multisite clinical trial.

The Morbidity and Mortality Weekly Report (MMWR)

The *MMWR* is published weekly by the U.S. Centers for Disease Control and Prevention (CDC). This publication originated from the National Quarantine Act, passed by the U.S. Congress in 1878, requiring American Consuls to file reports on conditions abroad and on vessels bound for U.S. ports. From these reports, the surgeon general of the U.S. Public Health Service (PHS) prepared weekly abstracts for transmission to PHS officers, collectors of customs, and state and local health authorities. The format, content, and sponsoring government agencies have changed over the years until, in 1961, the CDC published its first issue of *MMWR*. The *MMWR* is the only regular weekly periodical published in the United States that documents morbidity from all 50 states and 5 territories and mortality from 121 cities that represent one third of the nation's population.

The National Death Index (NDI)

The NDI was created in 1981 by the National Center for Health Statistics (NCHS) in response to a growing need for a national source of mortality data. The NDI is compiled from death certificate data received from all 50 state health departments. It is particularly useful to verify large numbers of deaths. The NDI is considered to be the gold standard of death databases; however, it is available only to researchers in medical and health sciences research for statistical purposes. There is a cost associated with the NDI data and suitable projects must be approved by NCHS, which necessitates additional time as the review and approval of projects may take several months.

The Death Master File (DMF)

The DMF is compiled and maintained by the U.S. Social Security Administration (SSA) and is only one of several mortality databases available to the public: For small studies, where the verification of only a few deaths is necessary, Web searches may be quickly and easily completed at no cost. SSA data depend on an individual having a Social Security number, and the death must have been reported to the SSA. The DMF contains only basic information on each decedent. However, once the verification of death has been confirmed, researchers can then procure the death certificates from the appropriate state agencies. The cause of death information also can be acquired from the SSA.

The Beneficiary Identification and Records Locator Subsystem (BIRLS)

The BIRLS is a death database maintained by the U.S. Department of Veterans Affairs (VA). This database was created in the 1970s as an update to a manual system designed to collect information for veterans' benefit programs. The majority of BIRLS records are of veterans whose survivors applied for death benefits. The inclusion of a veteran's death record depends on the submission of a copy of the individual's death certificate to the VA. This database has two major limitations: First, it only contains data on U.S. veterans, and second, it is only available to VA researchers.

The World Health Organization (WHO) Mortality Statistics

The WHO statistics include mortality information from WHO member states around the globe. WHO collects and distributes data on (a) mortality,

(b) estimates on causes of deaths and the global burden of disease, and (c) statistics on life expectancy. Mortality rates can be compared and contrasted across nations as much of the WHO data collected are universally standardized. For example, the cause of death information is reported for all countries using International Classification of Diseases (ICD) codes.

Future Implications

Mortality data play an important role in health services research studies because it provides a general indication of a population's health as well as the trends and patterns in the leading causes of death. As the demographics of populations shift, mortality data will continue to be used to examine the demand and need for specific healthcare services. Mortality rates are also used as one measure of the quality of care provided by healthcare institutions and systems.

Joseph D. Kubal

See also Centers for Disease Control and Prevention (CDC); Disease; Epidemiology; Health; Morbidity; Mortality, Major Causes in the United States; Public Health; Quality of Healthcare; World Health Organization (WHO)

Further Readings

Black, William C., David A. Haggstrom, and H. Gilbert Welch. "All-Cause Mortality in Randomized Trials of Cancer Screening," *Journal of the National Cancer Institute* 94(3): 167–73, February 2002.

Gordis, Leon. *Epidemiology.* 4th ed. Philadelphia: Saunders-Elsevier, 2008.

Manton, K. G., Igor Akushevich, and Julia Kravchenko. *Cancer Mortality and Morbidity Patterns in the U.S. Population: An Interdisciplinary Approach.* New York: Springer, 2009.

Mathers, Colin D., and Dejan Loncar. *Updated Projections of Global Mortality and Burden of Disease, 2002–2030: Data Sources, Methods, and Results.* Geneva, Switzerland: World Health Organization, 2005.

Zupan, Jelka, and Elisabeth Ahman. *Neonatal and Perinatal Mortality: Country, Regional, and Global Estimates.* Geneva, Switzerland: World Health Organization, 2006.

MORTALITY, MAJOR CAUSES IN THE UNITED STATES

For decades, heart disease, cancer, and stroke have been the top three leading causes of death in the United States. Deaths from heart disease, cancer, and stroke together account for almost 60% of all deaths in the nation. The prevalence of these three major diseases has important implications for the delivery, organization, and exploitation of healthcare services. It also guides public health policy and programmatic efforts at the national, state, and local levels. Mortality trends, risk factors, and the prevention of each disease are discussed below.

Heart Disease

Heart disease is the leading cause of mortality in the United States with about 700,000 deaths occurring annually, accounting for approximately 29% of all deaths in the nation. Heart disease, also known as cardiovascular disease, encompasses a number of abnormal conditions, including coronary heart disease (CHD) and hypertension (high blood pressure), that affect the heart and its blood vessels. CHD is the most common type; it leads to hardening and narrowing of the arteries, making it harder for blood to reach the heart. It can lead to angina (chest pain or discomfort), myocardial infarction (heart attack), congestive heart failure, or arrhythmia (abnormal heart beat).

Mortality Trends

Mortality rates for CHD rose in the United States during the period from 1949 to 1967 and have been declining since, particularly for acute myocardial infarction and chronic ischemic heart disease (CIHD). Death rates decreased steadily from 1968 to 1981, but the decrease has begun to slow. An increasing number of people survive their first heart attack.

The mortality declines have been attributed to prevention efforts as well as to improvements in medical care. There have been substantial decreases in the prevalence of some of the major cardiovascular risk factors such as smoking, elevated total cholesterol, and high blood pressure. Advances in medicine have led to a revolution in the treatments for established heart disease, with major breakthroughs in evidence-based medical and surgical techniques, including the use of coronary artery bypass grafting, coronary angioplasty, and stents. Despite overall declining trends, heart disease mortality is still a disparate burden on minority populations.

Risk Factors

Extensive research has identified both the major and contributing risk factors associated with an increased risk of developing CHD, but their exact significance and prevalence have not been precisely determined. Some of these risk factors are modifiable, whereas others are not. The risk of developing CHD is directly proportional to a person's number of risk factors as well as to the level of each risk factor.

Major nonmodifiable CHD risk factors include age, male gender, and heredity, including race. The children of parents with heart disease are more likely to develop the disease. African Americans, who tend to have more severe high blood pressure than Whites, have a higher risk of heart disease. The risk of heart disease is also higher among Mexican Americans, American Indians, native Hawaiians, and some Asian Americans than among Whites. Major modifiable risk factors include smoking, high blood cholesterol, high blood pressure, physical inactivity, obesity and being overweight, and having diabetes mellitus. Additional factors contributing to CHD risk include stress and excessive alcohol intake.

Prevention

Taking steps to prevent and control the known risk factors can reduce the occurrence of CHD.

Additionally, knowing the signs and symptoms of a heart attack, calling for emergency medical services, and immediately going to a hospital are crucial to positive outcomes. People who have had a heart attack can also work to reduce their risk of future attacks.

Despite our greater understanding of the risk factors of CHD, the prevalence of both obesity and diabetes in the U.S. population has increased over the past 25 years, with approximately 34% of adults aged 20 and over being obese. The rising prevalence of obesity and diabetes may reverse the decline in CHD-related deaths. Aggressive public health programs to control these risk factors are urgently needed.

Cancer

Cancer is the second leading cause of mortality in the United States with about 500,000 deaths occurring annually, accounting for approximately 23% of all deaths. Cancers, also called *malignant neoplasms,* include a large group of diseases in which abnormal cells divide without control and can invade healthy body tissues. Cancer cells can spread to other parts of the body through the blood and lymph systems. There are more than 100 different types of cancer. Lung cancer is the most common cause of cancer-related deaths in the United States for both men and women, resulting in approximately 157,000 deaths each year. Among men, prostate cancer mortality is second, followed by colon and rectum cancer. In women, lung cancer, breast cancer, and colon and rectum cancer are the leading types of fatal cancers. Among women, breast cancer is the most common cancer and the second most common cause of cancer death, with approximately 40,000 deaths per year.

Mortality Trends

Whereas the rates for other major chronic diseases have decreased substantially since 1950, cancer-related death rates showed a steady increase until the 1990s. The death rate from all cancers combined has decreased by 1.6% per year since 1993 for men and 0.8% per year since 1992 for women. The first decline in the number of cancer deaths occurred in 2003, when there were 369 fewer cancer-related deaths than in 2002. From 2003 to 2004, the number of recorded cancer deaths decreased by 1,160 in men and by 1,854 in women. Compared with the peak rates in 1990 for men and 1991 for women, the cancer death rate in 2003 was 16.3% lower for men and 8.5% lower for women.

Among men, most of the increase in cancer death rates prior to 1990 was attributable to lung cancer. Since 1990, the age-adjusted lung cancer death rate in men has been decreasing. Death rates from prostate and colorectal cancers have also decreased. Among women, lung cancer is currently the most common cause of cancer death, with the death rate more than twice what it was 25 years ago. Breast cancer death rates were constant from 1930 to 1990 but have since decreased by about 24%. The death rates for stomach and uterine cancers have decreased steadily since 1930; colorectal cancer death rates have been decreasing for more than 50 years.

Overall, *cancer incidence rates* are higher in men than in women. Among men, African Americans have the highest incidence followed by Whites, Hispanics, Asian Americans/Pacific Islanders, and American Indians/Alaskan Natives. Racial differences in cancer incidence among women are less pronounced; White women have the highest incidence rates followed by African Americans, Hispanics, American Indians/Alaskan Natives, and Asian Americans/Pacific Islanders.

Overall, *cancer death rates* are higher for men than for women in every racial and ethnic group. African American men and women have the highest rates of cancer mortality. Death rates for myeloma and cancers of the prostate, larynx, stomach, oral cavity, esophagus, liver, small intestine, colon and rectum, lung and bronchus, and pancreas are all higher in African American men than in White men. Death rates for African American women are also higher than for White women for myeloma and cancers of the stomach, cervix, esophagus, larynx, uterus, small intestine, pancreas, colon and rectum, liver, breast, urinary bladder, gallbladder, and oral cavity. Although cancer death rates are higher in African American men and women than for their White counterparts, the cancer death rate is declining faster for African Americans than for Whites.

Risk Factors

A number of cancer risk factors have been identified, including increasing age, family history of cancer, environmental factors, and lifestyle factors. As with heart disease, some of the risk factors are modifiable and others are not. Perhaps the most recognized and preventable cancer risk factor is tobacco use. Research clearly indicates that tobacco use is a major cause of cancer-related deaths. It has been estimated that cigarette smoking accounts for 85% of all lung cancers in smokers. Another risk factor is postmenopausal obesity, which is associated with breast cancer due to the conversion of adipose tissue to estrogen. A lack of vitamins B and D may also be a risk factor for breast, prostate, and colon cancers.

Prevention

To lower the risk of developing cancer, the American Cancer Society recommends (a) avoiding tobacco products, (b) consuming a diet rich in fruits and vegetables and low in saturated fats, and (c) exercising moderately and maintaining a healthy weight. Specifically, the society recommends eating five or more serving of fruits and vegetables a day, which may protect against cancers of the mouth and pharynx, esophagus, lung, stomach, and colon and rectum. It recommends that adults engage in at least moderate physical activity for 30 minutes or more on 5 or more days a week.

Stroke

Stroke is the third leading cause of mortality in the United States; about 160,000 stroke deaths occur annually, accounting for approximately 7% of all deaths. Stroke, sometimes referred to by the older term *cerebrovascular accident* (CVA), occurs due to interrupted blood flow to an area of the brain. This may be caused by an arterial blockage or rupture. Hence, stroke is classified into two major types: ischemic (blockage) or hemorrhagic (rupture). *Ischemic stroke* can occur due to thrombosis, embolism, or systemic hypoperfusion. *Hemorrhagic stroke* can result from intracerebral hemorrhage or subarachnoid hemorrhage. Approximately 80% of strokes are due to ischemic cerebral infarction and 20% to brain hemorrhage. A transient ischemic attack (TIA) is defined clinically by the temporary nature of the associated neurological symptoms, which last less than 24 hours by the classic definition. Recognition of a TIA is crucial because it is an important predictor of future ischemic events.

Regardless of the cause, an interrupted blood supply to the brain results in cell damage and neurological injury. Consequently, functions controlled by the affected area of the brain, such as speech, movement, and memory, may be lost. The outcome depends on the location and extent of the brain area damaged. A small stroke may result in only minor problems such as weakness of an arm or leg. Larger strokes may result in paralysis on one side of the body or loss of the ability to speak. Some people suffer transient loss of function and recover completely from strokes. More than two thirds of survivors, however, experience some type of residual disability as well as emotional problems.

Strokes can occur at any age. However, the risk of having a stroke more than doubles for each decade a person lives beyond the age of 55. Nearly 75% of all strokes occur in people over the age of 65. Stroke death rates are higher for African Americans than for Whites, even at younger ages.

Mortality Trends

Overall, stroke mortality declined steadily from 1950 through the mid-1970s, then increased. During 1979 to 1989, stroke mortality declined one third more rapidly than the other 10 leading causes of death. Recent data, however, suggest that there is a slowing of the decline in stroke mortality rates. For the period 1968 to 2005, the decrease in stroke mortality rates appears to be due to improving survival rates rather than from a decline in the incidence of stroke.

The constant morbidity rates combined with constant rates of high blood pressure highlight the need for improved prevention to reduce the number of strokes. For several decades, the southeastern United States has had the highest stroke mortality rate in the nation and has been described as the "stroke belt." It is not clear what factor or factors contribute to the higher incidence and mortality from stroke in this region.

Risk Factors

Some of the risk factors for stroke are non-modifiable, such as age, gender, and race. The risk of stroke increases with age. Males are more susceptible overall to having a stroke, but women aged 35 to 44 are also susceptible—possibly due to pregnancy and oral contraceptive use—as are women over age 85. One's family history, environment, and lifestyle also influence the risk of having a stroke.

Modifiable risk factors for stroke include high blood pressure, smoking, diabetes, asymptomatic carotid stenosis, atrial fibrillation, and hyperlipidemia. Blood pressure, especially systolic blood pressure, increases with age. Isolated high systolic blood pressure (more than 160 mmHg) is an important risk factor for stroke in the elderly. Smoking causes reduced blood vessel distensibility leading to increased arterial wall stiffness. Smoking is also associated with increased fibrinogen levels, increased platelet aggregation, decreased high-density lipoprotein (HDL) cholesterol levels, and increased hematocrit. Diabetes is a risk factor for atherogenesis and leads to obesity, high blood pressure, and hypercholesterolemia. Hyperlipidemia also contributes to atherogenesis and, hence, stroke. In older persons, congestive heart failure is an important risk factor for stroke. Other factors that may be risk factors for stroke include obesity, physical inactivity, poor nutrition, alcohol abuse, drug abuse, sickle-cell anemia, hormone replacement therapy, and oral contraceptive use.

Prevention

To prevent the occurrence of stroke, regular adult screening for high blood pressure at least every 2 years is recommended for appropriate management, evaluation, and treatment. Appropriate control of high blood pressure for patients with Type 1 or 2 diabetes significantly reduces their incidence of stroke, whereas blood glucose control has been proven to be less effective. The long-term use of anticoagulants such as aspirin and warfarin, especially for individuals with atrial fibrillation, has been shown to decrease stroke mortality. Patients with coronary disease and hyperlipidemia should be managed with statins to lower the risk of stroke. Last, patients who smoke should be encouraged to stop.

Intersecting Risk and Prevention Pathways

Although heart disease, cancer, and stroke are separate diseases, they have many overlapping risk factors and prevention pathways. Obesity, physical inactivity, and tobacco use as well as high blood cholesterol, high blood pressure, and diabetes are risk factors for heart disease, some cancers, and stroke. For example, cigarette smokers are more likely to develop heart disease than are nonsmokers, smokers have a much higher incidence of lung cancer than nonsmokers, and smoking approximately doubles a person's risk for stroke.

Responding to public health campaigns, millions of Americans have changed their eating habits, reducing saturated fat in their diets and lowering their serum cholesterol levels. Fewer adults are smoking cigarettes. More people with hypertension are being treated to control their high blood pressure. And millions of people exercise during their leisure time. These changes in lifestyle have significantly contributed to the decline in heart disease, cancer, and stroke deaths. At the same time, however, a large number of people continue to be physically inactive and are overeating, gaining weight, and becoming obese. In addition, these three diseases may all occur at any age from childhood to adulthood. And many adolescents and teenagers are engaging in unhealthy behaviors such as smoking.

Further reducing major risk factors such as high blood pressure, high blood cholesterol, tobacco use, diabetes, physical inactivity, and poor nutrition could eliminate much of the incidence of heart disease and stroke as well as some cancers. Determining effective prevention measures and therapy is increasingly important for both understanding past disease trends and planning future preventive and therapeutic strategies.

Memoona Hasnain and Grace Male

See also Cancer Care; Disease; Epidemiology; International Classification of Diseases (ICD); Life Expectancy; Mortality; Preventive Care; Public Health

Further Readings

Baker, Daryll M. *Stroke Prevention in Clinical Practice.* London: Springer, 2008.
Columbus, Frank H. *Trends in Cancer Prevention.* New York: Nova Science, 2007.

Edlow, Jonathan A. *Stroke*. Westport, CT: Greenwood Press, 2008.

Fang, Jing, Michael H. Alderman, Nora L. Keenan, et al. "Declining U.S. Stroke Hospitalization Since 1997: National Hospital Discharge Survey, 1988–2004," *Neuroepidemiology* 29(3–4), 243–49, 2007.

Heron, Minino A. "Deaths: Leading Causes for 2004," *National Vital Statistics Reports* 56(5): 1–95, November 20, 2007.

Jemal, Ahmedin, Rebecca Siegel, Elizabeth Ward, et al. "Cancer Statistics, 2008," *CA: A Cancer Journal for Clinicians* 58(2): 71–96, March–April 2008.

Marmot, Michael G., and Paul Elliott. *Coronary Heart Disease Epidemiology: From Aetiology to Public Health*. 2d ed. New York: Oxford University Press, 2005.

Pampel, Fred C., and Seth Pauley. *Progress Against Heart Disease*. Westport, CT: Praeger, 2004.

Tierney, Edward F., Edward W. Gregg, and K. M. Venkat Narayan. "Leading Causes of Death in the United States," *Journal of the American Medical Association* 295(4): 383, January 25, 2006.

Web Sites

American Cancer Society (ACS): http://www.cancer.org

American Heart Association (AHA): http://www.americanheart.org

National Cancer Institute (NCI): http://www.cancer.gov

National Center for Health Statistics (NCHS): http://www.cdc.gov/nchs

National Heart, Lung, and Blood Institute (NHLBI): http://www.nhlbi.nih.gov

National Institute of Neurological Disorders and Stroke (NINDS): http://www.ninds.nih.gov

National Stroke Association: http://www.stroke.org

MULTIHOSPITAL HEALTHCARE SYSTEMS

Multihospital healthcare systems are defined as two or more hospitals owned, leased, sponsored, or contract managed by a central organization. They are also sometimes referred to as *hospital chains*. In 2006, the American Hospital Association (AHA) reported a total of 369 multihospital healthcare systems in the United States. These systems contained 2,755 hospitals, nearly 56% of all U.S. hospitals. The vast majority of the systems, 299, or 81%, were not for profit. Of the remaining systems, 65 were investor-owned (for-profit) and 5 were government-owned organizations.

Horizontally and Vertically Integrated Systems

Multihospital healthcare systems are often differentiated as being either horizontally integrated or vertically integrated systems. The term *horizontally integrated system* refers to groups of similar organizations providing similar services (e.g., two or more community hospitals). The primary goal of developing a horizontally integrated system is generally to capture the market for a particular service within a specific geographic location. These types of multihospital systems tend to be in close geographic proximity to one another. *Vertically integrated systems* attempt to link different levels of healthcare services (e.g., primary care, acute care, and postacute care) together to move toward providing full service delivery. Such multihospital systems may include the ownership of managed-care organizations, for example, that can serve as feeders to the inpatient facilities. This type of multihospital system can be dispersed across a wide geographic area (e.g., in different states). Most multihospital healthcare systems in the United States are vertically integrated.

Reasons for System Integration

There are a number of reasons cited regarding the benefits—to an autonomous, freestanding hospital—of joining a multihospital healthcare system. One of the primary goals of integrating into multihospital systems is to achieve economies of scale and scope in delivering healthcare. In theory, when hospitals integrate into a system, they can take advantage of significant cost savings in organizational operation. These economies can be achieved in a variety of ways. First, multihospital systems may be able to reduce costs by receiving volume discounts on the purchase of services and supplies. Second, equipment and service costs can be reduced by eliminating overlap and duplication. Third, administration costs can be reduced by centralizing functions such as marketing, legal, human resource management, and planning.

A second perceived benefit of systems integration is the spreading of financial risk. In theory, members of multihospital systems are better able to absorb the financial impact of a turbulent healthcare environment than are freestanding hospitals.

Third, multihospital systems help hospitals provide better-coordinated patient care. In a vertically integrated system, for example, it may be possible to provide a full array of patient care services without having to refer the patient to an outside provider. Such a system can provide the continuum of care from primary care through inpatient care to postacute or long-term care.

A fourth factor cited as being a benefit of integration is increased administrative efficiency. By centralizing many administrative functions, it is possible to standardize many processes, including planning, marketing, human resource management, and quality improvement strategies.

Finally, all the benefits listed above can be enhanced through the development of an integrated, systemwide information system. The ability to have current, accurate information on all phases of the system's operation enhances its ability to both respond and be proactive to enhance success.

The empirical evidence on whether such benefits have actually been achieved is not clear. Although some multihospital systems report reductions in operational costs, in general, such claims of gains seem exaggerated. The most recent data available indicate, for example, that the average total cost per occupied hospital bed is higher in multihospital systems than in autonomous freestanding hospitals. Vertically integrated systems owning managed-care organizations do seem to have lower costs than systems without such ownership. This may indicate that a useful gatekeeper function is being performed by the systems' health maintenance organizations (HMOs).

The Veterans Administration

One of the largest vertically integrated multihospital systems in the nation is operated by the Veterans Administration (VA). Its mission is to provide a full array of healthcare services to U.S. military veterans. The veterans healthcare system is headed by the undersecretary of health and is funded by federal tax dollars. The fiscal year 2008 budget for the Veterans Health Administration (VHA), which runs hospitals and other health facilities, was in excess of $36 billion, which represents more than 40% of the VA's total annual budget. The VHA operates 153 medical centers and 724 community-based outpatient centers across the nation and employs more than a quarter of a million people.

The operation of the VA as a system is one example of successful integration. According to Phillip Longman, VA hospitals have moved from being some of the worst healthcare providers in the nation to some of the very best. The benefits derived from running the VA with systemwide standards of care, safety, and quality improvement have been substantial and have occurred in a relatively short time frame.

Future Implications

The general trend in the percentages of hospitals integrated into multihospital healthcare systems—over the 5 most recent years for which AHA data are available—indicates an increase. The percentage of hospitals in systems has risen from less than 46% to nearly 55% between 2001 and 2005.

Although the evidence is mixed on whether multihospital healthcare systems deliver the potential benefits noted earlier, it is apparent that they offer some advantages. As the healthcare environment continues to remain turbulent, autonomous freestanding hospitals will feel pressure to band together with other institutions to ensure their survival.

Ralph Bell

See also American Hospital Association (AHA); Competition in Healthcare; Healthcare Financial Management; Healthcare Markets; Healthcare Organization Theory; Health Economics; Hospitals; U.S. Department of Veterans Affairs (VA)

Further Readings

Bazzoli, Gloria J., Stephen M. Shortell, and Nicole L. Dubbs. "Rejoinder to Taxonomy of Health Networks and Systems: A Reassessment," *Health Services Research* 41(3 pt. 1): 629–39, June 2006.

Evans, Melanie, and Vince Galloro. "Growth Amid Signs of Strain: Our Annual Hospital Systems Survey Indicates a Strong Bottom Line Overall, but Operating Margins Beginning to Erode," *Modern Healthcare* 37(24): 24–8, June 11, 2007.

Ford, Eric W., and Jeremy C. Short. "The Impact of Health System Membership on Patient Safety Initiatives," *Health Care Management Review* 33(1): 13–20, January–March 2008.

Li, Pengxiang, James A. Bahensky, Mirou Jaana, et al. "Role of Multihospital System Membership in Electronic Medical Record Adoption," *Health Care Management Review* 33(2): 169–77, April–June 2008.

Longman, Phillip. *Best Care Anywhere: Why VA Health Care Is Better Than Yours.* Sausalito, CA: PoliPointPress, 2007.

Weil, Thomas P. *Health Networks: Can They Be the Solution?* Ann Arbor: University of Michigan Press, 2001.

Web Sites

American Hospital Association (AHA): http://www.aha.org

Center for Studying Health System Change (HSC): http://www.hschange.com

Federation of American Hospitals: http://www.americanhospitals.com

Healthcare Financial Management Association (HFMA): http://www.hfma.org

U.S. Department of Veterans Affairs (VA): http://www.va.gov

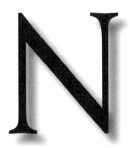

NATIONAL ALLIANCE FOR THE MENTALLY ILL (NAMI)

Founded in 1979 by family members of seriously compromised mental health consumers in Wisconsin, the National Alliance for the Mentally Ill (NAMI) is one of the nation's largest grassroots health organizations. With a national office in Arlington, Virginia, and state-based organizations in all 50 states, NAMI is well connected to communities across the country. NAMI organizations and their supporters strive not only to improve the quality of life of those who suffer from mental illness but also to eliminate mental illness all together. Although NAMI started out with the purpose of supporting consumers of mental healthcare, it now also supports family members of those who have mental illness. NAMI supporters include a variety of community leaders, educators, healthcare providers, researchers, advocates, and families. The organization is open to all who are interested in membership.

Education and Training

Education and training opportunities through NAMI are targeted to four major audiences: consumers, families and caregivers, the general public, and providers. Consumer education includes multimedia presentations, a NAMI support group, and the Peer-to-Peer program, which offers individualized information.

Education for families is delivered through the Family-to-Family program, which provides education for family members of those with mental illness and a multimedia presentation, *Hearts and Minds,* which aims to decrease heart disease among mental health consumers.

Trained consumers prepare and present programs for the general public to community groups through an educational speakers' bureau that demonstrates recovery and provides accurate education about mental illness. The general efforts include the multimedia presentation *In Our Own Voice.* Parents and Teachers as Allies is a program specific to educators that is provided by teachers who are trained mental health consumers and family members.

Education for providers includes the NAMI Provider Education course, taught by consumers, consumers' family members, and mental health professionals, which offers 10 weeks of training for mental health providers.

Advocacy Functions

NAMI's initial purpose was to protect the most disabled mentally ill individuals who could not advocate for themselves. Rather than focus solely on the patient, NAMI encourages a partnership between healthcare teams, consumers, and their families. Today, NAMI is advised by the Consumer Council and provides numerous avenues for consumer support.

The NAMI on Campus initiative provides student-led support to fellow students who either have mental illness or are affected by it in another way. Services include education for students, faculty, and college administrations; advocacy for students with mental illnesses; and promotion of early detection and treatment. Efforts to counter the effects of stigma against mental illness are of equal importance.

NAMI's Multicultural Action Center (MAC) was created in response to reports by the Surgeon General and the national Institute of Medicine (IOM) regarding the extreme toll that lack of quality treatment for mental health has taken on our country. The center seeks to secure culturally sensitive access to mental health services for all persons and their families, especially people of color, who are disproportionately represented among consumers who receive low-quality mental health services or none at all. Current priorities regarding policy changes for the center include health disparities; culturally competent services, including proper language fit between providers and consumers; research, particularly in the area of genetics, children and adolescents with mental illness, and depression; and the overrepresentation of mental illness in correctional systems. In connection with the group's Support Technical Assistance Resource (STAR) Center, MAC produces a newsletter called *Recovery for All*.

NAMI also conducts educational courses for consumers and families, including the Peer-to-Peer course for consumers, the NAMI-CARE (Consumers Advocating Recovery Through Empowerment) Mutual Support Program, and the *Hearts and Minds* multimedia program. It offers resources such as the NAMI Information Help Line and online communities for discussion of common interests. The Child and Adolescent Action Center provides discussion groups for teen consumers as well as for parents and caregivers of children and adolescents.

Internet Resources

Other services provided over the Internet include the following: legal support and guidance for consumers; resources for providers; mental health news and pertinent research updates; legislative alerts and updates; and FaithNet, a Web site representing the partnership between the faith community and NAMI.

Initiatives

Many public awareness initiatives are spearheaded by NAMI. Mental Illness Awareness Week, held during the 1st week of October, is intended to raise public awareness about the myths of mental illness and the benefits of treatment. NAMI Campaign for the Mind of America is a political initiative designed to create relationships at the local, state, and federal levels of government. These relationships are meant to promote policies that advance mental health through economic and scientific systems.

NAMI Action Centers focus on the specific needs of unique groups such as children and adolescents, multicultural populations, and clients of the criminal justice system. These action centers work to develop and promote education, advocacy, and research among these particular groups.

Policy Research

Mental healthcare policy is a priority for NAMI and is highlighted through specific areas of interest, including integration of consumers and family members in development of mental health services in all settings, equitable access to the most current and complete mental healthcare interventions, and insurance coverage for mental health services. The research activities and awareness initiatives supported by NAMI focus on positive policy change.

Publications

NAMI produces several publications for its members, including the quarterly *The Advocate*. It also provides many specialty publications that address the multifaceted needs of its members. The NAMI Child and Adolescent Action Center publishes *NAMI Beginnings*. And *Recovery for All* is published in connection with the STAR Center and MAC.

Events

NAMI hosts a series of annual *NAMI Walks* held at multiple sites with the purpose of raising funds and awareness of treatment needs of mental health consumers; in 2007, more than 69 walks were held throughout the country. Another large fund-raiser is the annual Washington, D.C., black tie affair, *Unmasking Mental Illness Science and Research Gala,* which helps to raise money for research efforts focused on identifying the etiology and treatment of mental illness.

Future Implications

NAMI remains committed to improving the lives of individuals suffering from mental illness as well as their families and communities. Through outreach, support, education, and research efforts, NAMI can help increase understanding of mental health and promote policy changes that affect this area.

Della Derscheid

See also Access to Healthcare; Community Mental Health Centers (CMHCs); *Diagnostic and Statistical Manual of Mental Disorders (DSM)*; Medical Sociology; Mental Health; Mental Health Epidemiology; Substance Abuse and Mental Health Services Administration (SAMHSA)

Further Readings

Cook, Linda J. "Striving to Help College Students With Mental Health Issues," *Journal of Psychosocial Nursing and Mental Health Services* 45(4): 40–44, April 2007.

Drapalski, Amy, Tina Marshall, Diana Seybolt, et al. "Unmet Needs of Families of Adults With Mental Illness and Preferences Regarding Family Services," *Psychiatric Services* 59(6): 655–62, June 2008.

Mohr, Wanda K., Joan E. Lafuze, and Brian D. Mohr. "Opening Caregiver Minds: National Alliance for the Mentally Ill's (NAMI) Provider Education Program," *Archives of Psychiatric Nursing* 14(5): 235–43, 2000.

"NAMI Publishes Report Cards on State Mental Health Systems," *Psychiatric Services* 57(4): 592, April 2006.

Web Sites

National Alliance on Mental Illness (NAMI): http://www.nami.org

National Institute of Mental Health (NIMH): http://www.nimh.nih.gov

Substance Abuse and Mental Health Services Administration (SAMHSA): http://www.samhsa.gov

NATIONAL ASSOCIATION OF HEALTH DATA ORGANIZATIONS (NAHDO)

The National Association of Health Data Organizations (NAHDO) is a national, nonprofit membership and educational association established to promote the uniformity and public availability of health data to inform healthcare cost, quality, and access decisions. Based in Salt Lake City, Utah, the association brings together the public and private sectors of the health information industry to improve and facilitate the collection and use of healthcare data for diverse audiences and applications.

Background

The Washington Business Group on Health (WBGH)—now the National Business Group on Health (NBGH)—and the Intergovernmental Health Policy Project (IHPP) at George Washington University established NAHDO in the spring of 1986. Representatives from state health data organizations in Arizona, Colorado, Iowa, Maryland, New Hampshire, New Jersey, and Tennessee met with WBGH and IHPP in Washington, D.C., to launch NAHDO. Shortly thereafter, the new association became a private, not-for-profit, national, educational membership organization.

In 1989, NAHDO's board of directors broadened the membership qualifications to include organizations and individuals from both the private for-profit and the not-for-profit sectors. Today, the association's membership includes state health data organizations, federal agencies, peer review organizations, software and hardware vendors, consulting groups, universities, representatives from state and regional hospital associations, managed-care organizations, health services research organizations, and the media.

NAHDO is governed by a board of directors representing states, healthcare organizations, corporations, and payers. The organization is funded through membership dues, meeting revenues, and grants. NAHDO's staff, the board of directors, and its members work as a community of professionals to overcome the political and technical challenges to healthcare transparency and performance reporting. Some segments of the healthcare industry still resist independent, objective public reporting on quality and cost. The association works with its members and other allies to improve the underlying data sources and promote consumers' use of the data.

Functions

NAHDO monitors the data collection and release policies of state and private health data organizations. Members and reporting data agencies and their national and local stakeholders use this information for planning purposes. The association also uses this information to advocate sustainable funding for statewide health data systems and to advise states about best practices in data collection and dissemination. The group provides technical assistance and guidance to states to establish statewide health data hospital inpatient and emergency department reporting systems, facility-based ambulatory-surgery reporting systems, health maintenance organizations, and health plan performance measurement systems, and recently, the group began to facilitate the establishment of all-payer, all-claims reporting systems for commercial and public health plans. The association also provides technical assistance to health data agencies to produce data products and comparative reports, including consumer quality reports and Web sites.

Partnerships

NAHDO is a leader in promoting and implementing national standards that support public health and quality reporting purposes. NAHDO's National Standards Consultant is a voting member of the National Uniform Billing Committee (NUBC), which maintains hospital content standards under the Health Insurance Portability and Accountability Act of 1996 (HIPAA), and a voting member of the American National Standards Institute X12N and Health Level 7 (HL7), both data standards maintenance organizations. NAHDO actively worked to add standard data fields to the core uniform billing standard (Uniform Bill 04), such as a "present-on-admission indicator" for each diagnosis and a standard race and ethnicity standard for electronic hospital transactions. The association and its standards consultant have produced the *Health Data Reporting Guide* for the national X12N standards for inpatient hospital encounters to be used by state agencies.

NAHDO represents state health data system interests in national forums, including the National Quality Forum (NQF), to promote measures that are relevant for state and public health agencies and provides testimony and comment to federal agencies and national entities, including the National Committee on Vital and Health Statistics. The association is a leader in the implementation of Web-based data query systems, and it provides technical assistance to states implementing Web-based reporting and promotes data dissemination policies that support interactive, dynamic Web-based data release. It also works with its members, state data system stewards, to make healthcare data available for public health programs and surveillance.

Activities and Meetings

NADHO has convened annual meetings of its members for more than 20 years, and it conducts special regional and topical workshops as well as online conferences called webinars. These meetings and webinars facilitate state-to-state information sharing and transfer of knowledge. The association's technical expertise also includes discussion forums, Listservs, and newsletters. Like most membership-based associations, NAHDO's success is directly linked to its members' involvement, expertise, and commitment to its mission.

Denise Love

See also Benchmarking; Data Privacy; Data Security; Data Sources in Conducting Health Services Research; Healthcare Cost and Utilization Project (HCUP); Health Informatics; Health Insurance Portability and Accountability Act of 1996 (HIPAA); Quality of Healthcare

Further Readings

Love, Denise, and Gulzar H. Shah. "Reflections on Organizational Issues in Developing, Implementing, and Maintaining State Web-Based Data Query

Systems," *Journal of Public Health Management and Practice* 12(2): 184–88, March–April 2006.

Love, Denise, Luis M. C. Paita, and William S. Custer. "Data Sharing and Dissemination Strategies for Fostering Competition in Health Care," *Health Services Research* 36(1 pt. 2): 277–90, April 2001.

Rudolph, Barbara A., Gulzar H. Shah, and Denise Love. "Small Numbers, Disclosure Risk, Security, and Reliability Issues in Web-Based Data Query," *Journal of Public Health Management and Practice* 12(2): 176–83, March–April 2006.

Web Sites

National Association of Health Data Organizations (NAHDO): http://nahdo.org

National Association for Public Health Statistics and Information Systems (NAPHSIS): http://www.naphsis.org

National Committee on Vital and Health Statistics (NCVHS): http://www.ncvhs.hhs.gov

NATIONAL ASSOCIATION OF STATE MEDICAID DIRECTORS (NASMD)

The National Association of State Medicaid Directors (NASMD) is a professional and bipartisan nonprofit organization composed of officials from Medicaid programs in the 50 states, the District of Columbia, and the U.S. territories. It is one of the nine affiliate organizations under the American Public Human Services Association (APHSA). Its focus is on improving the health and well-being of adults, children, and families by advocating for effective public human service policies. The NASMD, whose members include state directors and their senior staff, has operated as a focal point for communication between state programs and the federal government since 1979. It also works to provide an information network for the states on pertinent Medicaid policy and program issues. Its efforts help inform and influence legislative policy, federal and state regulations, health information technology, and Medicaid reform. The key issues addressed by the NASMD include the following: citizenship requirements, coordination of benefits, long-term care, and prescription drug coverage.

Organizational Structure

The structure of the NASMD includes a 12-member Executive Committee. In addition to a chair, vice chair, cochair, and immediate past chair, representatives from four geographic regions and the U.S. territories serve on this committee. Two members from each region—the Midwest, West, Northeast, and South—sit on the committee; whereas the U.S. territories have a single member. This group oversees administrative matters for the association, represents the NASMD in meetings with the Centers for Medicare and Medicaid Services (CMS), offers testimony before the U.S. Congress when appropriate, and provides overall policy guidance for the association.

Technical Advisory Groups

The association also has several Technical Advisory Groups (TAGs). These work groups are a joint effort of state programs and the CMS. They get together to discuss issues that may arise from Medicaid programs and operations. TAGs do not set policy; rather, they serve as a sounding board to develop strategies surrounding technical or operational concerns. If the TAG determines that the issue being dealt with might have significant policy implications, group members will defer to the Executive Committee or the full NASMD for consideration. TAG members communicate strategies and solutions to the states in their region, helping provide the necessary information and resources.

The NASMD currently has 10 TAGs, which cover issues such as welfare reform, long-term care, managed care, and prescription medications. The Eligibility Policy TAG helps state programs and the CMS to interpret and implement welfare reform laws as they affect eligibility for recipients; the Chronic Care TAG, formerly known as the Long-Term Care TAG, handles home- and community-based services, quality and cost-effectiveness of these services, and delivery-of-care methods; and the Fraud and Abuse Control TAG serves as a forum for all control activities, including effective methods of identifying fraud and excess and implementing legislation to strengthen control measures. The Managed Care TAG looks at the cost setting, quality assurance, and state and federal issues that may come to light in the development and implementation of managed-care programs.

Similarly, the Quality TAG offers ongoing information to state programs on the quality of services provided by managed-care programs. The Pharmacy TAG assists state programs with issues concerning prescription drugs, alternative medications, drug utilization, cost containment of medication coverage, and drug dispute authorizations; and the Systems TAG helps CMS and state programs to review the quality of their systems and data collection. The Payment Error Rate Measurement (PERM) TAG was initiated in 2007 to help address issues associated with this new program; the Medicaid and Mental Health TAG helps state programs to address mental health benefits and to identify challenges that arise in this area; and finally, the Coordination of Benefits/Third Party Liability TAG helps to develop better coordination and collection of third-party payments.

Centers

The NASMD also houses the Center for Workers with Disabilities, which helps states administer Medicaid Infrastructure grants. Specifically, the center assists states in developing Medicaid-Buy-In programs for employees with disabilities, and it provides technical guidance and support to states to increase the number of disabled individuals in the workforce. Like the NASMD, the Center for Workers with Disabilities serves as an information exchange between state programs, offering resources for program development, policy analysis, and technical assistance. It benefits from the resources of NASMD, especially when partnering with federal agencies, other state organizations, and policymakers.

The Medicaid and Mental Health Center is also affiliated with the National Association of State Medicaid Directors. This center collaborates with the Substance Abuse and Mental Health Services Administration (SAMHSA), the National Institute of Mental Health (NIMH), and the National Association of State Mental Health Program Directors (NASMHPD) to explore the relationship between Medicaid benefits and mental health needs. The center also collects information and resources on a broad array of services, including state regulation of residential facilities, mental health parity legislation, depression care, service utilization, reimbursement and cost-effectiveness,

and drug therapy effectiveness. While the center focuses on mental health services, it handles the dissemination of information and resources in the same way as NASMD and the Center for Workers with Disabilities.

Future Implications

The NASMD and the APHSA continue to support the changing needs of Medicaid administrators and professionals. State regulations and federal legislation remain dynamic, shifting to reflect new approaches to human services and public health policy. In response to policy reform and new laws, the NASMD created new TAGs and focused on specific key regulation issues. In this sense, the association will play an ongoing and vital role in helping state Medicaid programs and administrators, as well as federal agencies, politicians, and the general public, to provide needed support and resources.

Kathryn Langley

See also Centers for Medicare and Medicaid Services (CMS); Health Insurance; Medicaid; Nursing Homes; Public Policy; State-Based Health Insurance Initiatives; Vulnerable Populations

Further Readings

National Association of State Medicaid Directors. *Medicaid Reform Initiatives and Their Relationship to Health Centers.* Washington, DC: National Association of State Medicaid Directors, 2006.

National Association of State Medicaid Directors. *State Perspectives on Emerging Medicaid Long-Term Care Policies and Practices.* Washington, DC: National Association of State Medicaid Directors, 2007.

National Association of State Medicaid Directors. *State Perspectives: Medicaid Pharmacy Policies and Practices.* Washington, DC: National Association of State Medical Directors, 2007.

Web Sites

American Public Human Services Association (APHSA): http://www.aphsa.org

Centers for Medicare and Medicaid Services (CMS): http://www.cms.hhs.gov

National Association of State Medicaid Directors (NASMD): http://www.nasmd.org

NATIONAL BUSINESS GROUP ON HEALTH (NBGH)

The National Business Group on Health (NBGH) is a nonprofit healthcare coalition that represents large employers' views on national health policy issues and provides practical solutions to its members' healthcare concerns. Based in Washington, D.C., the NBGH's members include mainly large companies, which provide coverage to more than 50 million workers, retirees, and their families throughout the United States. Under the leadership of its president, the NBGH strives to attain transparency, increase the use of technology assessment to ensure access to beneficial new technologies, eliminate ineffective technologies, and make evidence-based practices the standard of healthcare.

Background

The NBGH (formerly known as the Washington Business Group on Health) was founded in 1974 to serve as a leading voice for large employers dedicated to finding innovative and progressive solutions to the nation's most important healthcare issues.

Mission

The main objective of the NBGH is to provide business solutions, be the national voice of large employers, link large employers with Washington, drive national policy on healthcare and productivity issues, and encourage hands-on membership involvement.

Membership

Over 290 companies are members of NBGH. Many of the members are Fortune 500 companies. Current members include such companies as American Express, the Boeing Company, Cisco Systems, DuPont Company, Ford Motor Company, IBM Corporation, Marriott International, Inc., NIKE, Inc., Time Warner, Wal-Mart Stores, Inc., and Xerox Corporation. Membership dues fund most of the coalition's activities; however, it does receive funds from the federal government, private foundations, and other health-related sources.

Governance, Staffing, and Organizational Structure

The NBGH is governed by a board of directors, which consists of approximately 20 individuals from member companies and the president of the coalition. NBGH's staff consists of approximately 33 individuals, including a president, five vice presidents, and 27 managers, analysts, and other employees. Staff members work in eight areas: (1) finance and administration; (2) membership and member services; (3) public policy; (4) Institute on the Costs and Health Effects of Obesity; (5) Institute on Health Care Costs and Solutions; (6) Global Health Benefits Institute; (7) the Center for Prevention and Health Services; and (8) the Institute on Health, Productivity and Human Capital.

Activities, Services, and Products

The NBGH provides many activities, services, and products for its members. The coalition holds a number of meetings throughout the year, including leadership meetings, employers' summits, and an annual national conference. It holds weekly webinars and monthly conference calls. The NBGH also conducts a number of surveys of its members and provides the results of its surveys to members so that they can benchmark their performance in various areas.

Many of the NBGH's activities center in a number of institutes, committees, and councils. Its institutes and committees include the following: Global Health Benefits Institute; Institute on Health Care Costs and Solutions; Institute on the Costs and Health Effects of Obesity; National Leadership Committee of Consumer Directed Health Care; and National Committee of Evidence-Based Benefit Design. The coalition's councils include the following: Public Policy Advisory Group; Council on Employee Health and Productivity; and Pharmaceutical Council.

The NBGH is engaged in a number of public policy initiatives. It provides its membership with timely information and analysis on health policy issues that have a direct impact on employers. The coalition also encourages its members to be actively involved in the political process by writing to members of the U.S. Congress and signing petitions. Additionally, the NBGH works to assist legislators and policymakers to understand how certain issues affect employer-sponsored healthcare.

The NBGH publishes newsletters, policy briefs, and reports. Many of these publications are available on the coalition's Web site. However, some publications are only available to member companies.

The NBGH presents several annual awards to its members and others, including the Award for Excellence and Innovation in Value Purchasing, the Best Employers for Healthy Lifestyles Award, and the Behavioral Health Award, to recognize individuals, employers, and programs.

Future Implications

The NBGH's membership continues to grow, as large businesses are confronted with increasing challenges in tackling complex healthcare issues. With its membership's pivotal involvement, the NBGH works to improve the health of tens of millions of individuals across the nation. The NBGH remains a leading voice in advocating for change in healthcare, and it will likely continue to play a key role in shaping the future of the nation's healthcare system.

Jared Lane K. Maeda

See also Cost of Healthcare; Evidence-Based Medicine; Forces Changing Healthcare; Health Insurance; Leapfrog Group; Midwest Business Group on Health; Quality of Healthcare; Technology Assessment

Further Readings

Darling, Helen. "Employment-Based Health Benefits and Public-Sector Coverage: Opportunity for Leadership," *Health Affairs* 25(6): 1475–86, November–December 2006.

Darling, Helen. "Evidence-Based Benefit Design. Interview by Ian Morrison," *Managed Care* 16(9 Suppl. 9): 21–3, September 2007.

Darling, Helen. "Interview With a Quality Leader: Helen Darling on Healthcare Business Coalitions, Purchasing, and Health Policy. Interview by Joann-Genovick-Richards and Jill Flateland." *Journal of Healthcare Quality* 27(2): 26–8, 36, March–April 2005.

Meyerhoff, Allen S., and David A. Crozier. "Health Care Coalitions: The Evolution of a Movement," *Health Affairs* 3(1): 120–28, Spring 1984.

National Business Group on Health. *A Toolkit for Action: The Imperative for Health Reform.* Washington, DC: National Business Group on Health, 2008.

Web Sites

Leapfrog Group: http://www.leapfroggroup.org

Midwest Business Group on Health (MBGH): http://www.mbgh.org

National Business Coalition on Health (NBCH): http://www.nbch.org

National Business Group on Health (NBGH): http://www.businessgrouphealth.org

National Labor Alliance of Health Care Coalitions (NLAHCC): http://www.nlahcc.org

NATIONAL CENTER FOR ASSISTED LIVING (NCAL)

The National Center for Assisted Living (NCAL) is the assisted living voice of the American Health Care Association (AHCA), the nation's largest association representing long-term care. The diversification of long-term care has brought rapid growth to the assisted living profession, and the center is an important resource for professionals in the field. Specifically, the Center serves the needs of the assisted living community through advocacy activities, education, networking, professional development, and quality initiatives.

Background

Located in Washington, D.C., the NCAL is an individual membership association. Through its national federation of state affiliates, the Center supports lobbying efforts at the state level. While the Center primarily focuses on federal issues, it also provides the support that state affiliates need to affect policy decisions regarding assisted living issues.

The Center's state affiliates actively represent assisted living providers' interests in state regulatory issues. In recent years, assisted living has received increasing attention at the federal level: the U.S. Congress, the Department of Labor, the General Accountability Office (GAO), and the Department of Health and Human Services have each examined various aspects of assisted living operations.

The NCAL and the AHCA have worked together to offer strong federal representation and have the largest long-term care federal relations in Washington, D.C. Both organizations are recognized as important sources of information and opinion by policymakers and regulators. Whether serving on a federal agency task force or testifying before the U.S. Congress, the Center ensures that its members' voices are heard.

Activities

The NCAL represents the assisted living community through various communications and by working directly with the media. The general public's perception of assisted living affects all the staff members of assisted living organizations and the environment in which providers operate. Whether delivered through news releases, direct media mailings, media interviews, or responses to media queries, the Center's research findings and position statements find their way into newspapers, magazines, and newsletters reaching the public and other critical audiences.

The Center publishes books, reports, and newsletters. One of its most widely read publications is *A Consumer's Guide to Assisted Living and Residential Care*, which is designed to help consumers select an assisted living facility that meets their needs. The book provides a description of services and includes a checklist and cost calculator.

The Center periodically publishes guidance resources for providers. For example, in 2007 it published *The Power of Ethical Marketing*, complimentary copies of which it distributed to all interested parties on request.

The Center publishes a number of monthly newsletters. Its *Assisted Living Focus* covers the latest business news, trends, regulatory activity, and legislative developments concerning long-term care and assisted living. This newsletter also provides examples of some of the best practices in assisted living residences across the nation. The *AHCA/NCAL Gazette* is a daily publication

designed to keep state association leaders informed of state and national news that affects long-term care professionals so that they can incorporate current national trends into their decision making at the state level. *AHCA Notes* is a monthly newsletter that updates the Center's members on long-term care trends as well as state and national regulatory and legislative activity. Additionally, the Center has an e-newsletter, *NCALconnections*, which is targeted at the association's leadership, state affiliates, and associate business members.

The Center also created and sponsors the National Assisted Living Week. Held each September, this annual event is designed to raise awareness of the assisted living profession and to encourage community support. Each year, the Center develops an original *National Assisted Living Week Planning Guide* as well as a product catalog for its members. Both are designed to promote high-quality services in assisted living residences nationwide.

The NCAL is committed to high-quality assisted living services and provides a number of tools and educational products designed for the assisted living professional. The Center actively supports Quality First, a covenant for healthy, affordable, and ethical long-term care, and adherence to its principles and goals. The Center also maintains a professional staff of experts who are available to answer member questions and who conduct original studies, surveys, and other timely research on assisted living.

Together, the NCAL and AHCA host an annual convention and offer a number of educational seminars that are designed to keep assisted living professionals apprised of the latest trends, innovations, theories, and legal developments that affect their operations. State affiliate associations also provide regional educational programs. The NCAL and the AHCA also collaborate to maintain the Mark A. Jerstad Information Resource Center, which contains a wide collection of materials about assisted living that can be accessed by members.

The NCAL's Web site is widely used. Its features include consumer and long-term care information, weekly electronic updates of issues and trends, regulatory issues, previews of and order forms for publications, other assisted living products, and "members only" information.

Katherine Lehman

See also Access to Healthcare; American Health Care Association (AHCA); Disability; Disease Management; Long-Term Care; Medicaid; Medicare; Vulnerable Populations

Further Readings

Carlson, Eric. *Critical Issues in Assisted Living: Who's In, Who's Out, and Who's Providing the Care.* Washington, DC: National Senior Citizens Law Center, 2005.

Golant, Stephen M., and Joan Hyde, eds. *The Assisted Living Residence: A Vision for the Future.* Baltimore: Johns Hopkins University Press, 2008.

National Center for Assisted Living. *Assisted Living State Regulatory Review.* Washington, DC: National Center for Assisted Living, 2008.

Pearce, Benjamin W. *Senior Living Communities: Operations Management and Marketing for Assisted Living, Congregate, and Continuing Care Retirement Communities.* 2d ed. Baltimore: Johns Hopkins University Press, 2007.

Web Sites

American Health Care Association (AHCA): http://www.ahcancal.org

National Center for Assisted Living (NCAL): http://www.ncal.org

NATIONAL CENTER FOR HEALTH STATISTICS (NCHS)

Located in Hyattsville, Maryland, the National Center for Health Statistics (NCHS) is the primary health statistics agency of the federal government. NCHS is part of the Centers for Disease Control and Prevention (CDC). Through cooperation with states and other partners, the CDC provides health surveillance to monitor and prevent outbreaks of disease, implement strategies to prevent disease, and maintain national health statistics.

The primary mission of NCHS is to compile statistical information to guide public health and health policymakers. Mandated by the U.S. Congress, NCHS addresses the entire spectrum of human health from birth through death. It investigates overall health status, lifestyles, and exposure to unhealthy influences affecting designated populations. Data are also gathered on the onset and diagnosis of illness and disability. For health policymakers, NCHS investigates the use and financing of healthcare and rehabilitative services. In addition to data collection and analysis, NCHS disseminates its data to interested health partners, conducts studies in statistical and survey research methodology, and provides technical assistance in access to or use of existing health-related data. It also has cooperative working programs with public and private agencies and organizations at the state, national, and international levels.

History

The first NCHS surveys on the nation's health were mandated through the federal National Health Survey Act (PL 84–652) enacted on July 3, 1956. The purpose of these surveys was to provide continuing study of the nation's health. These surveys also provided a means for the study of methods and techniques for obtaining statistical health information and disseminating the findings to those who could benefit from them.

In 1960, NCHS became an established organization within the U.S. Public Health Service (PHS) through the merging of the National Health Survey and the National Office of Vital Statistics. The PHS became responsible for vital statistics in 1946 as a result of the transfer of that responsibility from the U.S. Bureau of the Census.

NCHS was established in law and its mandate codified under Section 306 of the Public Health Services Act through the Health Services Research and Evaluation and Health Statistics Act of 1974 (PL 93–353). This act required NCHS to perform a variety of functions related to health in the United States. NCHS was called on to collect a wide range of statistical information on illness and disability nationwide. Data from birth, death, marriage, and divorce records were to be obtained annually. NCHS also had the role of supporting research, demonstrations, and evaluations regarding survey methods. Technical assistance was to be provided to state and local jurisdictions. Finally, this act established the National Committee on Vital and Health Statistics, which provided an expert advisory committee to the Secretary of the Department of Health and Human Services (HHS).

Authority was established in 1970 and then formally instituted through PL 95–623 in 1978 to create the Cooperative Health Statistics System. The purpose of this program was to coordinate as well as provide support and evaluation of the state and federal health statistics systems.

In 1989, with the establishment of the Agency for Health Care Policy and Research by PL 101–239 for the study of healthcare effectiveness and outcomes, the legislative authority of the National Center for Health Services Research (NCHSR) was eliminated. This law produced a number of amendments to NCHS's authority.

As the interest in obtaining more detailed data on racial and ethnic populations grew, the federal Disadvantaged Minority Health Improvement Act of 1990 (PL 101–527) mandated NCHS to obtain vital statistics, conduct national surveys, and establish a grants program for learning more about minority populations.

Data Sources and Surveys

NCHS employs a variety of methodologies and collaborations with public and private health partners to obtain accurate information regarding the health of the population, influences on health, and health outcomes. Data systems and surveys are employed, with some conducted annually and others periodically. Systems based on populations collect information through personal interviews with individuals, physicians, and facility administrators in healthcare organizations. They also obtain information through examinations, such as physical and dental examinations, laboratory tests, and nutritional assessments. Systems based on records look at hospital records, state vital registration and state death certificates for information. Many of NCHS's surveys are conducted via telephone interviews, including the National Immunization Survey (NIS), the National Asthma Survey (NAS), the National Survey of Children's Health (NSCH), and the Joint Canada/United States Survey of Health (JCUSH).

Population-based surveys include the National Health Interview Survey (NHIS), the National Health and Nutrition Examination Survey (NHANES), and the National Survey of Family Growth (NSFG). Record-based surveys include the

National Health Care Survey (NHCS) and the National Vital Statistics System. Many key surveys and data sources are detailed below.

National Health and Nutrition Examination Survey (NHANES)

The NHANES is a very comprehensive assessment that aims to get a picture of the health and nutritional status of the general population. Data are obtained on a nationally representative sample of approximately 5,000 people of all ages each year. Much focus has been placed on obtaining data on African Americans, Mexican Americans, adolescents, pregnant women, and people over age 60. While some of the data are obtained through home-based personal interviews, much of the information is collected through the use of specially designed Mobile Examination Centers that allow for quality control. These mobile centers travel to 15 sites in the nation each year, conducting physical medical examinations, standardized dental examinations, physiological measurements, and laboratory tests on blood and urine. The data collected include the prevalence of specific conditions or chronic diseases, blood pressure, serum cholesterol, body measurements, nutritional status and deficiencies, and exposure to environmental toxins.

NHANES also studies a number of diseases, medical conditions, and health indicators that affect the nation's population. These conditions include allergies, anemia, diabetes, eye disease, hearing loss, kidney disease, nutrition, obesity, oral health, osteoporosis, physical activity and fitness, vision, cardiovascular disease, cognitive functioning, environmental exposure, infectious diseases, reproductive history, sexually transmitted diseases, supplements, and medications. These data are considered the most authoritative source for standardized clinical, physical, and psychological information on the nation's population. Findings from the survey are used by a joint U.S. Department of Health and Human Services and U.S. Department of Agriculture program that monitors the diet and nutritional status of Americans to create food policies and dietary guidelines. Results are published in Series 11 of the *Vital and Health Statistics* series and *Advance Data from Vital and Health Statistics*.

National Health Care Survey (NHCS)

The NHCS is a record-based survey designed to collect data that can be used to analyze patient outcomes, the relationship between health and use of health services, and the use of healthcare services at the local level. The NHCS constitutes a family of surveys each of which relates to a specific setting. Currently, there are four surveys that study aspects of ambulatory- and hospital-care settings: the National Ambulatory Medical Care Survey (NAMCS), which samples visits to nonfederally employed physician's offices that primarily provide service in direct patient care; the National Hospital Ambulatory Medical Care Survey (NHAMCS), which is conducted in a national sample of hospital emergency and outpatient departments in the 50 states and the District of Columbia; the National Hospital Discharge Survey (NHDS), which obtains a representative sample of information on inpatients discharged from short-term hospital stays in general and children's general hospitals; and the National Survey of Ambulatory Surgery (NSAS), which provides the only national sample of information regarding ambulatory-surgery visits.

Two other surveys included in this family of surveys are the National Home and Hospice Care Survey (NHHCS) and the National Nursing Home Survey (NNHS), which address long-term care settings. The NHHCS collects information about licensed or certified agencies providing home and hospice care as well as their current patients and discharges. The NNHS provides a national sample of data about licensed or certified nursing homes, their residents, and their staff.

National Health Interview Survey (NHIS)

The NHIS is a major data collection project of NCHS. Beginning with the National Health Survey Act of 1956, continuing surveys and studies were established to gather current, accurate statistical information on illness and disability in the United States. These studies and surveys were specifically concerned with measuring the incidence, prevalence, and distribution and effects of disease, and the medical services rendered to treat them. The first survey from this act was initiated in 1957 and is now called the National Health Interview Survey. In 1960, NCHS began conducting the survey following the merging of the National Health Survey and the National Vital Statistics Division.

The NHIS is a population-based survey providing principal information on the status of health, illness, and disability of civilian, noninstitutionalized populations in the nation. The survey is conducted annually through interviews of approximately 50,000 households. Questions are based on current health topics, which may vary from year to year. For example, in 1986, topics focused on health insurance, vitamin use, dental care, and longest job worked. In 1990, the focus was on health promotion and disease prevention, assistive devices, podiatric services, and hearing impairments. Since 1987, questions on knowledge and attitudes about HIV/AIDS have been included each year. Data from the survey provide information on the incidence and prevalence of disease and the relationship between health and demographic and socioeconomic characteristics. Results of the survey are published in Series 10 of *Vital and Health Statistics* series and *Advance Data From Vital and Health Statistics*.

National Immunization Survey (NIS)

The NIS, sponsored by the National Immunization Program (NIP) and conducted jointly by NIP and NCHS, began in 1994. This survey monitors childhood immunization coverage levels among children in the nation. Estimates of vaccination coverage are generated for each of 78 Immunization Action Plans (IAP) which include the 50 states, the District of Columbia, and 27 large metropolitan areas; NIS also provides estimates at the national level. Newly licensed vaccinations recommended for use are included as well. The survey uses a random digital dialing telephone method, searching for households with children aged 19 to 35 months currently living in the nation. Parents or guardians are interviewed to provide names and dates of vaccines charted on the child's "shot card" that is kept in the home. Demographic and socioeconomic information is also collected. At the end of the interview, the interviewers ask permission to follow up by mail with the child's vaccination providers, which may include pediatricians, family physicians, and other health providers, for verification. Quarterly estimates of vaccination coverage are calculated, and data are used to evaluate progress toward national goals, such as the Healthy People 2010 initiative. The CDC also uses this data to identify states with the highest and lowest rates of immunization.

Longitudinal Studies of Aging (LSOAs)

The LSOAs is a collaborative effort between NCHS and the National Institute on Aging (NIA). Two cohorts of persons aged 70 years or older are studied for changes in health, functional status, living arrangements, and the use of health services as they move through the older ages of life. Four surveys are included in this project: the 1984 Supplement on Aging (SOA); the 1984–1990 Longitudinal Study of Aging (LSOA); the Second Supplement on Aging (SOA II); and the 1994–2000 Second Longitudinal Study of Aging (LSOA II). A recent addition is the 1994–2002 LSOA II Linked Mortality File, which includes all the participants of the LSOA II aged 70 and older. It provides follow-up mortality data, including fact, date, and cause of death, from the LSOA II participation from 1994–2000 through December 31, 2002.

National Survey of Family Growth (NSFG)

The NSFG, a population-based survey conducted through household interviews of women of childbearing age, monitors change in childbearing practices and measures reproductive health. More specifically, these data address family-planning practices and attitudes, factors influencing fertility, fecundity impairments, sexual activity, family formation, and aspects of maternal and child health. Cycles I and II of this survey began in 1973 and 1976, with interviews conducted with approximately 10,000 never-married women aged 15 to 44 years. The population sample was expanded with Cycles III and IV in 1982–1983 and 1988, respectively, to include a representation of all women aged 15 to 44 years regardless of marital status. At this time, new topics were also introduced to include beginning of sexual activity, first use of contraceptives, first use of family planning services, knowledge and experience of sexually transmitted diseases, and adoption. During Cycle IV in 1990, respondents were reinterviewed by telephone. Results are published in Series 23 of the *Vital and Health Statistics* series and *Advance Data From Vital and Health Statistics.*

National Vital Statistics System (NVSS)

The NVSS is a collaborative intergovernmental effort to obtain official vital statistics on the registration of births, deaths, marriages, and divorces at the state and local levels within the 50 states, two cities (Washington, D.C., and New York City), and five territories (Puerto Rico, the Virgin Islands, Guam, American Samoa, and the Commonwealth of the Northern Marina Islands). These data provide public health officials with important information for monitoring progress in achieving health goals. These data can tell public health officials, for example, the number and location of teen births in a given year, the risk factors for problematic pregnancies, the rate of infant mortality, the leading causes of death, and the life expectancy of a population. One very significant component of the NVSS is the National Death Index (NDI). In collaboration with state offices, NCHS is able to index death records that may be used for epidemiological studies or verifications of death for individuals being studied. Additional components of the NVSS include Linked Birth and Infant Death Data Set, the National Survey of Family Growth, the Matched Multiple Birth Data Set, the National Maternal and Infant Health Survey, and the National Mortality Follow-back Survey. Data from the NVSS are published in electronic form through the *Vital Statistics of the United States,* the *National Vital Statistics Reports,* and additional reports. In addition, electronic micro-data files containing individual vital records are accessible for public use.

Health Topics

NCHS also produces data covering a wide range of specific health topics. Summary data sheets are made available on its Web site for important current health concerns. The site provides portraits of health status for specific critical age groups, such as infants and toddlers, children, adolescents, and older adults. Information on health conditions such as cancer, injuries, obesity, and teenage pregnancy is available. Individual summary data sheets also address current health-related issues, including patient safety, health insurance and access to care, and racial and ethnic health disparities.

Utilization of Data

Numerous audiences make use of NCHS data. The U.S. Congress and health policymakers use the data to track initiatives, prioritize prevention and research programs, and evaluate outcomes. Epidemiologists, biomedical researchers, and health services researchers look for trends in diseases, uncover the relationship between risk factors and diseases, and monitor the use of health services. Pharmaceutical and food manufacturers, research firms, consulting firms, and trade associations make use of the data for their businesses. Public health professionals employ this information to determine preventable illnesses and evaluate intervention programs. Physicians use the data to evaluate health and risk factors in their patients, such as cholesterol, weight, blood pressure, and growth chart records for children. Media and advocacy groups rely on the data to help raise awareness of major health issues such as cancer, diabetes, heart disease, Alzheimer's disease, and health disparities.

International Activities

The NCHS works collaboratively with other countries and other agencies of the PHS to conduct comparative international research. Experts from the United States and other countries are brought together to focus on specific health issues of mutual interest. Some examples of global research include the examination of perinatal and infant mortality, health and healthcare of the elderly, and international comparability of health data.

Research and Survey Methodology

The NCHS also maintains an active program in statistical research and survey methods. The National Laboratory for Collaborative Research in Cognition and Survey Measurement, a major initiative started in 1985, applies cognitive methods in questionnaire survey research design. The NCHS develops and tests its data collection instruments in collaboration with other internal programs and through research contracts with academic scientists. Another area of interest for NCHS is determining analytical methods for their registration systems and sample surveys. Research is also conducted on the development of automated and graphical technology. Survey design research, where a program is developed to evaluate, redesign, and link many of the surveys so as to improve efficiency and analytical capability, remains an important area of focus.

Publications and Data Access

The NCHS uses multiple means to disseminate vital and health statistics and the results of its research to as broad a range of people as possible. In addition to publications, public use data files, and unpublished tabulations, efforts are made to reach various specialized groups of data users, health professionals, and the general public through journal articles, presentations, speeches, conferences, workshops, and consultations. Information services available through the NCHS also provide reference and referral services, maintain mailing lists for distribution of new publications, coordinate requests for presentations and exhibits, and issue a catalog of publications and electronic products.

Its Web site makes data on current important health concerns available. Published reports also are available both in print and online. Major publication series include *Health, United States, Vital and Health Statistics, Advance Data From Vital and Health Statistics, Vital Statistics of the United States,* and *Monthly Vital Statistics Report.* In addition, data files for public use are made available to researchers for analysis. Pretabulated tables of state-level data are prepared on specific interest health issues such as births and deaths. State and national data on a range of health topics are available through interactive data warehouses, examples of which include *Health Data for All Ages* and *Trends in Health and Aging.* At the Research Data Center, detailed data are available through secure access.

Future Implications

The NCHS plays a vital role in the collection, interpretation, and dissemination of important health data. Through its many surveys and studies, as well as its collaborative efforts with state, regional, community, and academic entities, the NCHS captures broad and in-depth information on individuals, health professionals, and health-care institutions. Further advances in technology will make this data, recommendations, and research findings even more accessible.

Barbara Nail-Chiwetalu

See also Centers for Disease Control and Prevention (CDC); Data Sources in Conducting Health Services Research; Health Indicators, Leading; Health Surveys; Morbidity; Mortality; Public Health; Public Policy

Further Readings

Adams, Patricia F., Jacqueline W. Lucas, and Patricia M. Barnes. *Summary Health Statistics for the U.S. Population: National Health Interview Survey 2006.* HHS Pub. No. 2008–1564. Hyattsville, MD: National Center for Health Statistics, 2008.

Bernstein, Amy B. *Health Care in America: Trends in Utilization.* HHS Pub. No. 2004–1031. Hyattsville, MD: National Center for Health Statistics, 2003.

Hueston, William J., Mark E. Geesey, and Vanessa Diaz. "Prenatal Care Initiation Among Pregnant Teens in the United States: An Analysis Over 25 Years," *Journal of Adolescent Health* 42(3): 243–8, March 2008.

Lochner, Kimberly, Robert A. Hummer, Stephanie Bartee, et al. "The Public-Use National Health Interview Survey Linked Mortality Files: Methods of Reidentification Risk Avoidance and Comparative Analysis," *American Journal of Epidemiology* 168(3): 336–44, August 1, 2008.

Web Sites

Centers for Disease Control and Prevention (CDC): http://www.cdc.gov

National Center for Health Statistics (NCHS): http://www.cdc.gov/nchs

NATIONAL CITIZENS' COALITION FOR NURSING HOME REFORM (NCCNHR)

The National Citizens' Coalition for Nursing Home Reform (NCCNHR) is a nonprofit membership organization that advocates for the rights, safety, and dignity of America's long-term care residents. Located in Washington, D.C., NCCNHR is a coalition of approximately 200 citizen advocacy organizations with members from 42 states in the United States as well as long-term care ombudsman from most states. These organizations and NCCNHR's approximately 1,000 individual members work to improve the quality of long-term care, largely focusing on nursing home care and assisted living but recently expanding to include home and community-based care.

Both its mission and structure make NCCNHR a unique organization. Most citizen advocacy groups in healthcare tend to focus on one disease or on conditions affecting a single organ system (e.g., American Cancer Society), or they focus on a specific group of citizens (e.g., AARP), attempting to address the entire spectrum of their health needs. In contrast, NCCNHR advocates for individuals receiving one type of healthcare—residential long-term care.

This national-level coalition of diverse citizen action groups had its beginning in 1975. Its founder, Elma L. Holder, was then working with the National Gray Panthers' Long-Term Care Action Project. She organized a conference in Washington, D.C., that included members of a dozen citizen advocacy groups who came together to speak with the nursing home industry concerning the need for fundamental change in their operations. At the conference, attendees discovered that they shared a variety of common interests. These interests and goals led them to form NCCNHR. Holder became NCCNHR's first executive director, a position she held for two decades, during which she transformed the organization from a small startup advocacy group to its current status as the primary voice of nursing home residents in national public policy.

Throughout its years of operation, NCCNHR has engaged in a wide variety of activities to improve nursing home care. It has trained members of the national service program Volunteers in Service to America (VISTA), operated a National Long-Term Care Ombudsman Resource Center, maintained an information clearinghouse on residential long-term care, issued reports on a range of topics, published books to inform consumers and policymakers, and educated members of the

U.S. Congress and officials in executive branch agencies who play major roles in long-term care public policy. It also provides important technical assistance and support to its member organizations that work for change at the state and local levels.

One of NCCNHR's greatest achievements was its involvement in the development, passage, and implementation of the Nursing Home Reform Act, part of the federal Omnibus Budget Reconciliation Act of 1987 (OBRA-87). NCCNHR was the motivating core of a coalition of consumer groups, unions, and provider associations that generated bipartisan support for the OBRA-87 reforms. OBRA-87 contained the seeds of a new model of nursing home care that included uniform resident assessment, increased attention to resident rights and quality of life, and a revised set of quality standards and enforcement remedies. OBRA-87 was a fundamental change in federal regulation, shifting the focus of regulators from paper compliance with regulations to the actual care and quality of life experienced by residents. Furthermore, with its focus on resident-centered care, it laid the foundation for the current movement for culture change in nursing homes.

As important as its role in the development and passage of federal legislation was, NCCNHR also deserves considerable credit for its dogged determination to ensure that all elements of OBRA-87 were implemented in their original form. While the nation's nursing home industry did not use all of its considerable political power to oppose OBRA-87's passage, the industry did commit itself to delaying the implementation of the enforcement remedies and attempting to have these measures watered down as they were translated into rules and regulatory procedures. During this period of conflict in the mid-1990s, NCCNHR was the unifying force that brought together citizen advocates, medical and gerontological professionals, and policymakers to fight against efforts to repeal segments of OBRA-87 or to render it toothless in its implementation.

In recent years, NCCNHR has expanded its emphasis from concerns about standards and enforcement to include more engagement with the nursing home industry and regulatory agencies in their quality improvement efforts. In part, this change reflects the nursing home industry's relative success in riding the wave of "healthcare excellence," which is so popular in current public policy circles. This approach to thinking about quality moves policymakers away from a purely punitive or regulatory approach. Instead, it places much more emphasis on collaborative quality improvement efforts involving government, consumers, and providers. As part of this effort, NCCNHR has embraced the culture change movement in nursing homes, voicing its support for such resident-centered approaches to care as the Pioneers, the Eden Alternative, the Wellspring Initiative, and the Green House Movement.

In terms of its organizational structure, NCCNHR is governed by a 20-person board, which includes a number of nursing home residents. Board members are elected by NCCNHR's member groups and meet quarterly to deal with policies, financing, and strategic planning. The Executive Director, approximately seven paid staff members, a few consultants, and volunteers conduct its Washington, D.C., operations. As with many groups advocating for vulnerable populations, maintaining adequate funding is NCCNHR's major organizational challenge. It has an annual budget of approximately $1.2 million. Over 40% of NCCNHR's current revenues come from a grant supporting its operation of the National Long Term Care Ombudsman Resource Center. Other grants and donations provide the remainder of NCCNHR's revenues.

Recently, NCCNHR changed its name. It is now the NCCNHR: the National Consumer Voice for Quality Long-Term Care. This new name reflects its broadened mission. Since its inception in 1975 it has, with scarce resources, successfully advocated for millions of frail and vulnerable Americans receiving nursing home care. Its current advocacy efforts include such public policy issues as nursing home staffing standards, poor working conditions in nursing homes, residents' rights and empowerment, the development of family councils for residents' families, reducing physical and chemical restraint use, the high costs of poor quality care, and the adequacy of quality assurance in assisted living and other forms of residential care.

Charles D. Phillips and Catherine Hawes

See also Long-Term Care; Medicaid; Nursing Home Quality; Nursing Homes; Public Policy; Quality of Healthcare; Vulnerable Populations

Further Readings

Burger, Sarah Greene. *Nursing Home Staffing: A Guide for Residents, Families, Friends, and Caregivers.* Washington, DC: National Citizens' Coalition for Nursing Home Reform, 2002.

Burger, Sarah Greene, Virginia Fraser, Sarah Hunt, et al. *Nursing Homes: Getting Good Care There.* 2d ed. Washington, DC: National Citizens' Coalition for Nursing Home Reform, 2001.

Harrington, Charlene, Helen Carrillo, and C. LaCava. *Nursing Facilities, Staffing, Residents, and Facility Deficiencies, 1999 Through 2005.* San Francisco: Department of Social and Behavioral Sciences, University of California, San Francisco, 2006.

Web Sites

National Citizens' Coalition for Nursing Home Reform (NCCNHR): http://nccnhr.org

National Long Term Care Ombudsman Resource Center (ORC): http://www.itcombudsman.org

Pioneer Network: http://www.pioneernetwork.net

Social Security Online, Omnibus Budget Reconciliation Act of 1987 (OBRA-87), Public Law 100–203, Subsection C: Nursing Home Reform: http://www.ssa.gov/OP_Home/comp2/comp2toc.html

NATIONAL COALITION ON HEALTH CARE (NCHC)

The National Coalition on Health Care (NCHC) is one of the nation's largest and most broadly representative alliances working to improve healthcare in America. The nonprofit and nonpartisan NCHC was founded in 1990 and comprises more than 70 organizations, employing or representing about 150 million Americans. The coalition works to bring large and small employers as well as consumer, labor, and religious groups, primary-care providers, and health and pension funds together. The core principles of NCHC include the following: bringing healthcare coverage to all, managing healthcare costs, improving healthcare quality and patient safety, increasing administrative simplification, and ensuring more equitable financing. The coalition's slogan states that the nation is capable of achieving better and affordable healthcare for everyone.

Overview

The NCHC is headquartered in Washington, D.C. The honorary cochairs of the organization include former presidents George H. W. Bush and Jimmy Carter. The present cochairs include the former governor of Iowa, Robert D. Ray and the former member of the U.S. Congress from Florida, Paul G. Rogers. In addition, 14 members serve on the Board of Directors; these individuals are prominent in the fields of politics, academia, and health and community services and in the business sector. The NCHC also has a staff comprising the president, executive director, senior vice president for policy and strategy, senior vice president for operations, and administrative staff. Additionally, the various members of the coalition include large and small businesses; labor, consumer, religious, and primary-care provider groups; distinguished leaders from academia, business, and government; and distinguished politicians.

Purpose and Principles

The NCHC seeks to focus public attention on the current problems and inequities in America's healthcare system. It strives to provide people with factual information, helping them to form educated opinions and bring about necessary change. In addition, the NCHC's health advocacy efforts are centered on three main issues: (1) the state of the quality of healthcare in the nation, (2) the rising costs of healthcare, and (3) the growing number of uninsured and underinsured Americans. These issues have been addressed by the coalition's national social marketing and education strategy campaign, which is focused on establishing a national policy that will ensure access to quality, appropriate, and affordable healthcare.

To accomplish the goals of improving the quality of care, lowering costs, and providing health insurance coverage to all Americans, the NCHC has identified five guiding principles that it feels are necessary for effective policy reform.

Healthcare Coverage for All

The NCHC advocates for mandatory health coverage for all. This goal can be accomplished in many ways, including efforts that involve the use of employer and individual mandates, Medicaid and State Children's Health Insurance Program (SCHIP) expansion, individual subsidies, and a number of related ideas as part of a multifaceted approach.

Cost Management

The NCHC supports the creation of an independent board, chartered and overseen by the U.S. Congress, that would be responsible for establishing and administering measures for calibrating rates and limitations to keep costs and insurance premiums in alignment with defined annual targets.

Improvement of Healthcare Quality and Safety

The NCHC recommends the establishment of a federal board to lead the development and coordination of a national effort to improve healthcare quality and set common treatment standards. In addition, the proposed board would oversee protocols for patient records, prescription ordering, billing standards, and privacy standards.

Equitable Financing

The NCHC's members suggest that health plans should be funded from a wide variety of sources, including general revenues, earmarked taxes and fees, employer contributions, individual contributions, and co-payments. The NCHC also advocates the use of sliding scale assistance for lower-income citizens.

Simplified Administration

The NCHC endorses the establishment and utilization of a core standard healthcare benefits package to create a consistent set of ground rules for patients, payers, and providers. The creation of a national information technology structure for healthcare should ultimately lead to decreased costs and medical errors.

Strategies

The NCHC uses different approaches to target and reach healthcare interest groups, community activists, the media, and the general public. The coalition began its work by identifying concerns and gaps in the public's knowledge. As a result, it has published a series of reports designed to furnish basic information about the changes and challenges in the nation's healthcare system.

One of NCHC's recent reports, *Prevention's Potential for Slowing the Growth of Medical Spending* (2007), deals with the preventive aspects of healthcare interventions. Using immunizations as an example, the report highlights the future cost savings of early prevention efforts. Previous reports released by the coalition have focused on cost, quality, and access to healthcare.

In addition to publishing reports, the NCHC furthers its advocacy campaign through involvement in public forums, congressional hearings, conferences, social events, and media appearances. Much of the coalition's work is available and accessible online at its Web site.

As a nonpartisan alliance, the NCHC briefs policymakers and shares its reports with politicians and bureaucrats in the administration. Local representatives that are coalition members also reach out to other organizations and opinion leaders at the state level. In the past, the coalition has also conducted a national advertising campaign in popular media outlets, including *The New York Times*, *The Washington Post*, *USA TODAY*, and *Roll Call*. Coalition members also place advertisements in their own internal publications and in the local media.

Fact Sheets

The NCHC has developed fact sheets on many issues, which are broadly classified into five categories: health insurance coverage, cost, quality, world healthcare data, and economic sheets. Several of the coalition's available economic fact sheets point out the impact of rapidly escalating healthcare costs and insurance premiums on workers and their families, business operations, small businesses, pension programs and beneficiaries, the federal budget, state governments, and local communities. Healthcare researchers, healthcare activists, and the general public can use these compiled resources. For example, the fact sheet on World Healthcare Data provides information on Canada, France, Germany, the United Kingdom, and Japan. These data offer a global view of different healthcare systems, their funding resources, and the costs associated with them.

Future Implications

The NCHC is a broad-based organization that advocates for a multitude of changes to the nation's healthcare system. It is important to note, however, that the coalition's members also include large national insurance companies and pharmaceutical corporations. While these members might represent a conflict of interest, the coalition continues its media campaigns and furthers its commitment to improving the quality of healthcare, decreasing healthcare costs, and increasing access to health insurance coverage.

Vikrant Vats

See also Access to Healthcare; Cost Containment Strategies; Cost of Healthcare; Health Insurance Coverage; Medical Errors; Patient Safety; Quality of Healthcare; Uninsured Individuals

Further Readings

National Coalition on Health Care. *Building a Better Health Care System: Specifications for Reform.* Washington, DC: National Coalition on Health Care, 2004.

Russell, Louis B. *Prevention's Potential for Slowing the Growth of Medical Spending.* Washington, DC: National Coalition on Health Care, 2007.

Schoeni, Patricia Q., ed. *Care in the ICU: Teaming Up to Improve Quality.* Washington, DC: National Coalition on Health Care, 2002.

Simmons, Henry E., and Mark A. Goldberg. *Charting the Cost of Inaction.* Washington, DC: National Coalition on Health Care, 2003.

Thorpe, Kenneth E. *Impacts of Health Care Reform: Projections of Costs and Savings.* Washington, DC: National Coalition on Health Care, 2005.

Web Sites

Institute for Healthcare Improvement (IHI): http://www.ihi.org

National Coalition on Health Care (NCHC): http://www.nchc.org

NATIONAL COMMISSION FOR QUALITY LONG-TERM CARE (NCQLTC)

The National Commission for Quality Long-Term Care (NCQLTC) is a nonpartisan and independent body charged with the responsibility for improving long-term care in the United States. The commission, which has been cochaired by former U.S. Senator Bob Kerrey and former Speaker of the House of Representatives Newt Gingrich, comprises appointed commissioners who reflect a diversity of backgrounds ranging from academic, government, quality improvement, and long-term care settings. The commission was created as an outgrowth of a long-term care industry–driven quality initiative titled "Quality First: A Covenant for Healthy, Affordable, and Ethical Long-Term Care," and it is overseen by The New School.

In 2004, three leading long-term care organizations called for an independent commission to evaluate the quality of long-term care in the nation, identify the factors that influence quality improvement, and recommend strategies to sustain quality improvement nationally. The commission was convened in October 2004 and was originally housed at the National Quality Forum. The three founding organizations—the Alliance for Quality Nursing Home Care (AQNHC), the American Association of Homes and Services for the Aging (AAHSA), and the American Health Care Association (AHCA)—provide funding for the commission's work. The commission functions independently, led by its executive director Doug Pace, and is currently located at The New School.

Background

The growing concern over the quality of long-term care prompted the three major long-term care organizations listed above to pledge to a 5-year voluntary initiative entitled "Quality First: A Covenant for Healthy, Affordable, and Ethical Long-Term Care" on July 16, 2002. This initiative was aimed at attaining excellence in the quality of care and services for older persons as well as increasing the public trust in the delivery of care and services. The reasoning behind this initiative was that, if quality could be reliably measured and the results made publicly available, providers would be motivated to improve their quality, and the public would be able to distinguish between good and poor performers.

At about the same time, the U.S. Department of Health and Human Services (HHS) launched its Nursing Home Quality Initiative (NHQI) and the Home Health Quality Initiative (HHQI). With the growing number of initiatives focused on long-term care, there was a need for an independent body to evaluate long-term care quality, identify the factors that influence improvements in quality of care, and make recommendations about national efforts that could result in sustained quality improvement.

Long-Term Care Reform

The nation's long-term care system is currently straining to meet the demands of a growing older population whose magnitude was never anticipated. Some of the challenges that the system is confronted with include individuals who face a loss of independence because of disability and who may also be confronted with a loss of home, income, and/or assets. Individuals may also face a loss of their family and choice among long-term care options. Often families have little of the information or training needed to support those with disabilities; direct care workers are generally paid low salaries and receive little respect from the medical community and general public. Provider organizations may be pressured to deliver high-quality care but face constraints with low reimbursements. In addition, regulatory agencies are unable to enforce regulations that should serve to protect individuals receiving long-term care due to staffing shortages; and policymakers are grappling with pressures to improve long-term care while balancing the budget.

Given the challenges of the nation's long-term care system, the commission is committed to finding solutions to the most pressing questions that affect the aging population. These questions include the following: How can long-term care be financed consistently with policies that ensure that all Americans have choices? How can long-term care workers be retained? What are the best approaches for improving and ensuring quality? Where can

Americans obtain credible information to compare their options for long-term care?

Although the nation's long-term care system faces significant challenges, there is much promise of finding feasible solutions. The commission has laid out a road map for long-term care reform with six key areas: culture transformation, empowering individuals and families, workforce, technology, regulation, and finance.

The commission believes that the culture of long-term care can be transformed through organizational innovations that improve an individual's quality of life and quality of care. Some promising initiatives that can facilitate this cultural transformation include resident-centered care and the provision of palliative and hospice care. Additionally, individuals and families can be empowered through a broader array of high-quality, affordable, and accessible long-term care services that are available in homes and communities. Family caregivers must also be given the tools, information, and support that will allow them to continue their role in caring for those with disabilities. The long-term care workforce must be supported to improve their working conditions and wages and be provided with greater opportunities for advancement. Technology should be used more effectively to promote higher quality of care and greater consumer independence. Furthermore, long-term care regulations must be accurate, timely, and consistently implemented to improve quality. Last, the commission believes that there should be a long-term care financing system that is fair and equitable and that every American should have access to the services they need to live independently for as long as possible.

Future Implications

The long-term care system is faced with daunting challenges in the way of meeting the needs of a growing elderly population. On December 3, 2007, the commission issued its final report that called for a national discussion about how the nation can create a new and better long-term care system. The report features recommendations in the areas of workforce, quality, and technology. In addition, it also discusses important steps that must be taken in identifying crucial features of a long-term care financing system.

Jared Lane K. Maeda and Douglas Pace

See also Access to Healthcare; Long-Term Care; Medicaid; Medicare; Nursing Home Quality; Nursing Homes; Quality Indicators; Quality of Healthcare

Further Readings

Bearing Point Management and Technology Consultants. *Essential but Not Sufficient: Information Technology in Long-Term Care as an Enabler of Consumer Independence and Quality Improvement.* Washington, DC: National Commission for Quality Long-Term Care, 2007.

Institute for the Future of Aging Services. *The Long-Term Care Workforce: Can the Crisis Be Fixed?* Washington, DC: National Commission for Quality Long-Term Care, 2007.

Miller, Edward Alan, and Vincent Mor. *Out of the Shadows: Envisioning a Brighter Future for Long-Term Care in America.* Washington, DC: National Commission for Quality Long-Term Care, 2006.

National Commission for Quality Long-Term Care. *From Isolation to Integration: Recommendations to Improve Quality in Long-Term Care.* Washington, DC: National Commission for Quality Long-Term Care, 2007.

Tumlinson, Anne, Scott Woods, and Avalere Health. *Long-Term Care in America: An Introduction.* Washington, DC: National Commission for Quality Long-Term Care, 2007.

Web Sites

National Commission for Quality Long-Term Care (NCQLTC): http://qualitylongtermcarecommission.org

NATIONAL COMMITTEE FOR QUALITY ASSURANCE (NCQA)

The National Committee for Quality Assurance (NCQA) is a major driving force in improving the quality of the nation's healthcare system. NCQA establishes standards of quality and service that health plans should provide to their members. Known for its Healthcare Effectiveness Data and Information Set (HEDIS) measures, NCQA provides voluntary accreditation of physicians, medical groups, and health plans. It strives to transform the quality of healthcare through measurement, transparency, and accountability.

Background

Located in Washington, D.C., the National Committee for Quality Assurance (NCQA) was founded in 1990 as a private, nonprofit organization. At the time, there were few nationwide efforts to systematically measure and improve quality. Since then, NCQA has been working vigorously with employers, providers, health plans, patients, and policymakers to build a consensus on healthcare quality. These efforts have focused on how to best measure and improve quality.

NCQA maintains a diverse set of programs to accomplish its mission of improving quality in healthcare. Specifically, it offers five accreditation programs, four certification programs, and four physician recognition programs that apply to health plans, medical groups, and individual physicians, all of which are voluntary. NCQA relies on the system of measure, analyze, improve, and repeat to address healthcare quality.

Quality Assessment

NCQA employs a variety of approaches to assess healthcare quality, including on- and off-site surveys, audits, satisfaction surveys, and performance measures. It uses these methods in its accreditation, certification, recognition, and performance programs that evaluate organizations, medical groups, and physicians. Through these programs, NCQA obtains relevant information on healthcare quality that is made available to consumers, employers, health plans, and physicians. The information gathered from these programs can be used by consumers and employers to make informed purchasing decisions regarding their healthcare as well as drive quality improvement efforts.

NCQA's seal is highly recognized as a symbol of quality. The organizations and individuals who participate in NCQA's programs earn the privilege of using the Committee's seal. Organizations that seek NCQA accreditation must pass a rigorous and comprehensive review and complete an annual performance survey. Health plans must meet more than 60 standards and report on performance in more than 40 areas to be accredited with additional criteria that continue to be added each year. Although the standards and requirements per assessment program vary, the participating organizations and individuals must be able to demonstrate that quality practice, clinical, and satisfaction thresholds are met. In 2008, NCQA started evaluating preferred provider organizations (PPOs) on the same standards, measures, and patient experience ratings that it uses to evaluate health maintenance organizations (HMOs) and point of service (POS) plans, to allow consumers and purchasers to reliably compare across different health plans.

Many of the nation's leading employers, federal and state government, and individual consumers rely on NCQA's accreditation to select among various health plans. Furthermore, in more than 30 states, health plans that are NCQA accredited are exempted from most or all of the requirements of annual state audits.

NCQA also offers a variety of educational programs and publications for providers and organizations to help meet quality goals. These programs include educational seminars, online continuing education programs, corporate training, and special events.

Performance Measurement

NCQA has played a significant role in refining performance measures. Performance measures allow for the direct comparison of health plans. In the mid-1990s, NCQA developed objective measures that resulted in a standardized measurement tool known as the Healthcare Effectiveness Data and Information Set (HEDIS), which is widely used by the industry. It has also developed other measures for various healthcare organizations.

HEDIS is a tool used by over 90% of the nation's health insurance plans to measure areas of patient care and service. This comprehensive tool surveys a broad area of healthcare that includes 71 measures over 8 domains of care. HEDIS measures cover the effectiveness of care; health plan stability; cost of care; access of care; use of services; informed choice; health plan information; and satisfaction of care. Some areas of HEDIS measurement include breast cancer screenings, beta-blocker treatment after a heart attack, antidepressant medication management, and comprehensive diabetes care.

The availability of HEDIS allows for an objective, standardized measurement and reporting that permits side-by-side comparison on the performance of health plans and comparison of performance to benchmarks. HEDIS also enables

health plans to target their areas of improvement. To stay current, the HEDIS measurement set is updated annually. Employers and patients use HEDIS data and accreditation information to make their purchasing decisions. Health maintenance organizations (HMOs) submit HEDIS data to participate in the Medicare Advantage program.

The early efforts of HEDIS included a narrow set of preventive process measures. Since then, HEDIS has grown to include a broad array of measures that include the underuse, overuse, value, processes, and outcomes of care. In 2008, HEDIS included measures that assess how many children under 2 years of age and enrolled in a Medicaid managed-care program have been tested for lead exposure. Another new measure examined if patients with aggravated chronic obstructive pulmonary disease (COPD) received prescriptions for bronchodilators and systemic corticosteroids at discharge from a hospital or emergency department.

As the HEDIS measures continue to evolve, NCQA ensures that the measures contain the features of relevance, soundness, and feasibility. NCQA also makes certain that the measures are valid, address focal areas, and are not onerous to implement.

NCQA has published *The State of Health Care Quality* since 1997, which gives an overall assessment of the U.S. healthcare system. This report is released just prior to the open-enrollment season when individuals choose their health plan for the following year. Over the past 5 years, the report has shown that health plans have made significant improvements across a broad range of quality measures.

Physician Recognition

NCQA's physician recognition programs help patients identify providers who consistently deliver evidence-based care. Employers have also begun to realize the value of the physician recognition program.

In collaboration with the American Diabetes Association and the American Heart Association/ American Stroke Association, NCQA has developed two physician recognition programs. These programs recognize physicians who deliver excellent care to patients with diabetes or cardiac-related illnesses. Physicians who participate in the recognition programs have also rapidly improved the care they deliver. Those who participated in the Diabetes Physician Recognition Program increased their rates of nephropathy screening, lipid screening, and blood pressure control by 50% to 100% within 5 years.

Another program, the Physician Practice Connection, recognizes physicians who have implemented practice systems, such as electronic medical records, that help them consistently deliver high-quality care. A new program will identify physicians who provide efficient and effective evidence-based care for patients with back pain.

Public Reporting

An educated consumer serves as a powerful driving force for improving healthcare. Thus, NCQA works to facilitate informed consumer choices by making available, free of charge, most of the information it collects on health plans, medical groups, and physicians to the media and individuals via the Internet. To reach as wide an audience as possible, NCQA also maintains a partnership with U.S. News & World Report to produce its annual list of "America's Best Health Plans."

NCQA also has a number of tools available to help consumers make informed decisions. The interactive Health Plan Report Card contains a searchable database that allows consumers to choose an appropriate health plan. The report card, which is based on the review of hundreds of health plans, includes a comprehensive evaluation of member satisfaction, clinical quality, and key systems and processes as well as accreditation information and performance ratings. NCQA also makes available an online directory of physicians in its recognition programs and a quality dividend calculator that can estimate the increased productivity and decrease in sick days that are the result of selecting a high-quality health plan. Quality Compass is another tool developed for consumers. This tool contains comprehensive health plan performance data, trend data, and health plan-specific HEDIS rates, in addition to regional and national averages. With Quality Compass, users can track quality improvement, analyze annual plan performance, develop custom reports, and conduct market analyses.

Public Policy

NCQA also maintains an active public policy department. The department works with legislators and policymakers to educate them on how to support healthcare policies that benefit the public. In addition, the NCQA works collaboratively with other organizations to advance policies that improve the efficiency and quality of the healthcare system.

Future Implications

The National Committee for Quality Assurance (NCQA) continues to stimulate significant improvements in healthcare quality through its quality assessment, performance measurement, and physician recognition programs. It is furthering its work by developing a broader set of performance measures and expanding the boundaries of quality. NCQA remains a leader for facilitating change in the nation's healthcare system by providing employers and consumers with the necessary tools and information to make informed choices.

Jared Lane K. Maeda

See also Healthcare Effectiveness Data and Information Set (HEDIS); Health Maintenance Organizations (HMOs); Health Report Cards; Managed Care; Outcomes Movement; Preferred Provider Organizations (PPO); Quality Indicators; Quality of Healthcare

Further Readings
McCormick, Danny, David U. Himmelstein, Steffie Woolhandler, et al. "Relationship Between Low Quality-of-Care Scores and HMOs' Subsequent Public Disclosure of Quality-of-Care Scores," *Journal of the American Medical Association* 288(12): 1484–90, September 25, 2002.

Mihalik, Gary J., Michael R. Scherer, and Robert K. Schrecter. "The High Price of Quality: A Cost Analysis of NCQA Accreditation," *Journal of Health Care Finance* 29(3): 38–47, Spring 2003.

National Committee for Quality Assurance. *The Essential Guide to Health Care Quality.* Washington, DC: National Committee for Quality Assurance, 2007

National Committee for Quality Assurance. *The State of Health Care Quality.* Washington, DC: National Committee for Quality Assurance, 2007.

Ohldin, Andrea, and Adrienne Mims. "The Search for Value in Health Care: A Review of the National Committee for Quality Assurance Efforts," *Journal of the National Medical Association* 94(5): 344–50, May 2002.

O'Kane, Margaret E. "Redefining Value in Health Care: A New Imperative," *Healthcare Financial Management* 60(8): 64–8, August 2006.

Reinke, Tom. "NCQA Shifts Focus on Physician Performance," *Managed Care* 16(3): 48, 53, March 2007.

Web Sites

National Committee for Quality Assurance (NCQA): http://ncqa.org
NCQA Health Plan Report Card: http://reportcard.ncqa.org

NATIONAL GUIDELINE CLEARINGHOUSE (NGC)

The National Guideline Clearinghouse (NGC) is a federally funded Web site devoted to maintaining a current database of clinical practice guidelines for physicians, other health professionals, and healthcare providers. Specifically, the mission of the NGC is to provide objective, detailed information on clinical practice guidelines and to further their dissemination, implementation, and use. The clearinghouse accomplishes its mission through a number of different components. It provides a searchable database of current clinical practice guidelines, each with an abstract and full-text version (or link to purchase). It offers guideline comparisons—either in the form of automatically generated side-by-side comparisons or novel documents written by the clearinghouse—comparing differences and similarities between guidelines on the same topic. Guidelines and guideline comparisons can be downloaded to personal digital assistants (PDAs) for easy, mobile viewing. The Web site contains an annotated bibliography section that offers a database of clinical-practice-guideline-related resources from peer-reviewed journals and other sources. Finally, it provides a Listserv for discussion of clinical-practice-guideline-related issues and questions.

Background

The initial construction of the NGC began in 1997. To gain input and support for the proposed clearinghouse, individuals in the U.S. Department of Health and Human Services (HHS) met with representatives from the American Medical Association (AMA), the American Association of Health Plans (AAHP), and the U.S. Agency for Health Care Policy and Research (now the Agency for Healthcare Research and Quality, or AHRQ). In December, 1998, the clearinghouse was launched, and it was officially unveiled in January, 1999.

When launched, the clearinghouse included approximately 200 clinical practice guidelines and other related material. By 2000, the number of guidelines had more than tripled to nearly 700. Similarly, the number of visitors to the Web site increased substantially. By the end of the 1st year of its operation, there were more than 17 million hits and 1 million sessions (a "hit" is looking at one page, while a "session" involves multiple concurrent hits).

Usage has continued to increase to approximately 38,000 visits a week. The average user visits about 10 pages and stays for around 6 minutes. Also, the clearinghouse is continuing to grow in size every week—it currently has over 4,000 guidelines available on the Web site.

Clinical Practice Guidelines

Clinical practice guidelines are commonly defined by the national Institute of Medicine (IOM) as "systematically developed statements to assist practitioner and patient decisions about appropriate healthcare for specific clinical circumstances." The number of clinical practice guidelines has greatly increased during the past two decades. This has primarily been due to research studies that showed that physician's practices and treatments vary greatly and to the increase in managed care. The belief is that using clinical practice guidelines can lead to more standardized practice and thus increased quality and cost-effectiveness.

Health Partners, a health insurance company based in Minnesota, found that among its physicians, more than 80 different treatments were being used for bladder infections. To address this type of substantial variation in treatments, clinical practice guidelines have been developed—in theory care can now be standardized to effective treatment plans. However, the situation is not that simple—in the NGC, there are 13 different guidelines relating to urinary tract infections (including bladder). Physicians must sift through these guidelines to see which one is applicable to their particular patients—since some guidelines may be age or gender specific or may be related to a specific subtype of the condition (chronic urinary tract infection, for example).

A different study looked at the cost-effectiveness of clinical practice guidelines. It found that, among coronary-care intensive-care unit patients, discharging patients according to the established guideline decreased the amount of time spent in the hospital without changing mortality rates or health status at follow-up. This saved an average of $1,000 per patient.

Development of Guidelines

Historically, one of the major problems with clinical practice guidelines has been the lack of a consistent set of rules used in their development and implementation. To address this problem, the NGC has implemented a number of requirements for inclusion into its database.

Guidelines submitted for inclusion must be current (within the past 5 years). They must include systematically developed statements that help physicians and others make decisions for their patients. They must be developed under the auspices of medical specialty associations; by relevant professional societies, public or private organizations, government agencies at the federal, state, or local level; or by healthcare organizations or plans. Finally, they must be available in English for free or for a fee. Among guidelines submitted to the clearinghouse for inclusion, only about 10% are rejected for not meeting the inclusion criteria.

Additional recommendations for guideline development have been discussed in various journal articles. The articles suggest making a formal cost analysis a part of guidelines, defining evidence and how it was selected, making data available for review, and the use of randomized controlled trials as part of the evidence.

Users of Guidelines

Information on who uses clinical practice guidelines varies based on a number of factors. Among family practitioners, about 60% were at least somewhat familiar with three relevant guidelines; 14% reported not being familiar with any of the three presented guidelines. The use of the guidelines varied based on the guideline, ranging from 44% to 64%. Additionally, staff-model health maintenance organization (HMO) physicians were very likely (100%) to use guidelines, especially as compared with those in private practice (23%).

As for those who use the NGC, it is difficult to know exactly, but most likely nurses and physicians are its greatest users. The majority of hits come during normal business hours, suggesting that healthcare providers may be using it at work or during their practice. It is also believed that younger physicians are using the clearinghouse more than older physicians, because younger physicians are more likely to be trained in information systems and feel more comfortable using the Internet in general.

Issues and Problems

While clinical practice guidelines seem like a good idea in theory, there are often issues and problems in their implementation. These problems include keeping the guidelines up to date with current knowledge, methodological problems with their development, the usefulness of the guidelines to patients with multiple comorbidities, and the problem of physician resistance to using the guidelines in their practices.

Keeping Guidelines Current

With constantly changing research and technology, clinical practice guidelines are also changing. This means that a physician or other healthcare provider may access a guideline, use its recommendations, and later find out that it is already out of date or inaccurate. In addition, depending on the nature of the guidelines, different review criteria might be required. For example, the treatment for ingrown toenails is less dynamic than cancer therapies; therefore, clinical practice guidelines relating to cancer treatment should be reviewed more frequently than those relating to more established treatments.

One review of 279 clinical practice guidelines found that a large majority (89%) of them failed to include a statement about when they should be reviewed or when they should expire. This becomes problematic because, as previously discussed, without a set date of review; these guidelines might continue to be reviewed long after they have been made current.

Additionally, the time at which a study is published can be a year or more after the data was initially taken. A guideline is partially based on studies, so it may take another year or two before a guideline is published. By the time the guideline is found in the NGC, it may be based on data that are 3 to 4 years old. Thus, when reviewing guidelines (especially ones without a set expiration date), physicians and other healthcare providers should note the dates of the supporting studies and any other dates provided in the guideline.

The NGC works to minimize this problem by requiring all guidelines to have been made current within the past 5 years. It automatically eliminates those that are older from its database, unless there is evidence that it has been or will soon be updated.

Guideline Methodology

Another problem is the consistency in methodology of the guideline development. In a study of 279 clinical practice guidelines, not one of the guidelines met all the criteria set forth by the authors. Most frequently, the guidelines lacked methodological standards such as not disclosing information about how data was obtained, extracted, selected for inclusion, and graded.

One additional problem is implicit value judgments used in the guidelines. Frequently, the authors of guidelines have to make a decision about what the patient is most likely to want. While these decisions may seem relatively obvious, not all patients may share the same values as the researchers. For example, one article cited an example of this problem with the use of aspirin instead of ticlopidine in the treatment of patients with transient ischemic attack (or mini stroke). Aspirin is cheap and available over the counter; however, ticlopidine produces a 15% lower risk of another attack. This lower risk, however, comes at a price—including

monetary, temporal (needing refills and trips to the pharmacy), and bodily (it requires periodic white blood cell counts). The assumption that the authors point out is frequently held by researchers is that the patient would rather take the cheaper over-the-counter aspirin than the more expensive, more effective ticlopidine. While this may be true for most patients, it may not be true in every case. Therefore, clinical practice guidelines should make explicit any implicit value judgments made in the development of the guidelines.

Comorbidities

Guidelines are often written with one medical condition in mind. However, many patients have comorbid conditions or multiple diseases. For example, 48% of Medicare beneficiaries have three or more chronic disease conditions. One study examined this problem explicitly by looking at relevant clinical practice guidelines for a hypothetical 78-year-old woman with five comorbid conditions: osteoporosis, osteoarthritis, Type 2 diabetes, hypertension, and chronic obstructive pulmonary disease (COPD). It found that strictly following all the guidelines would produce drug-disease and drug-drug and drug-food interactions. In addition, the patient would be taking 12 medications (19 doses) per day at five different times. The estimated cost of the drugs would be about $400 per month.

Strictly following clinical practice guidelines that only focus on one disease can be difficult. It is important to be aware of the limitations of the guidelines in treating patients with comorbidities. In addition, it may be beneficial for future guidelines to address and prioritize comorbidities.

Physician Resistance

Not all physicians are interested in using clinical practice guidelines or the NGC. Some physicians are reluctant because they feel that using guidelines is "cookbook medicine," which takes away their medical skills. Others are reluctant to use them in everyday practice because they feel comfortable with medical conditions they see on a regular basis; however, they might consult relevant guidelines for preparing presentations, treating complex cases, or in other special situations.

Specialists are most likely to consult clinical practice guidelines in their respective journals. So the NGC may not be as popular as it might, because physicians are already accessing guidelines from different sources. If they hold their own journal in the utmost regard, then they may have no interest in or need for searching for other guidelines from other sources.

Future Implications

Clinical practice guidelines can be beneficial if regularly used and properly developed. With the advent of new technology, it has become possible to centralize information—in this case, in the form of the NGC. The clearinghouse has grown dramatically over the past several years, and it will undoubtedly continue to grow. Additionally, as it grows, so will the number of people who will use it. Currently, there are thousands of visits per week, and this number will grow as knowledge of this database grows.

Clinical practice guidelines were originally developed to standardize practices to more evidence-based interventions and in an attempt to lower costs. It has been shown that these guidelines can accomplish both of these goals given the right conditions. For large change to be realized, guidelines must be appropriately developed (including cost analysis and statements of implicit judgment) and more widely used in practice.

Ultimately, the NGC is a valuable resource for physicians and other healthcare providers. It continues to provide a central access point for current clinical practice guidelines.

John Schrom

See also Agency for Healthcare Research and Quality (AHRQ); Clinical Decision Support; Clinical Practice Guidelines; Evidence-Based Medicine (EBM); Outcomes Movement; Quality of Healthcare; United Kingdom's National Institute for Health and Clinical Excellence (NICE)

Further Readings

Bowker, Richard, Monica Lakhanpaul, Maria Atkinson, et al., eds. *How to Write a Guideline From Start to Finish: A Handbook for Healthcare Professionals.* New York: Churchill Livingston Elsevier, 2008.

Cassey, Margaret Z. "Incorporating the National Guideline Clearinghouse into Evidence-Based Nursing Practice," *Nursing Economics* 25(5): 302–303, September–October 2007.

Fenton, Susan H., and Robert G. Badgett. "A Comparison of Primary Care Information in UpToDate and the National Guideline Clearinghouse," *Journal of the American Medical Library Association* 95(3): 255–59, July 2007.

Rao, Goutham. *Rational Medical Decision Making: A Case-Based Approach.* New York: McGraw-Hill Medical, 2007.

Skolnik, Neil S., Doron Schneider, Richard Neill, et al., eds. *Essential Practice Guidelines in Primary Care.* Totowa, NJ: Humana Press, 2007.

Web Sites

Agency for Healthcare Research and Quality (AHRQ): http://www.ahrq.gov

American Medical Association (AMA): http://www.ama-assn.org

National Guideline Clearinghouse (NGC): http://www.guidelines.gov

NATIONAL HEALTHCARE DISPARITIES REPORT (NHDR)

The *National Healthcare Disparities Report* (NHDR) is a comprehensive overview of the racial, ethnic, and socioeconomic disparities in the access to and quality of healthcare in the nation's general population; among priority populations including women, children, the elderly, racial and ethnic minority groups, low-income groups, and residents of rural areas; and for individuals with special healthcare needs, including the disabled, people in need of long-term care, and people requiring end-of-life care. The federal Healthcare Research and Quality Act of 1999 directed the Agency for Healthcare Research and Quality (AHRQ) to develop an annual NHDR to provide a summary of the state of healthcare disparities in the United States. The first NHDR was released in 2003. The 2004 report built on the first report by providing an updated national overview of disparities and added another critical goal: tracking the nation's progress toward eliminating healthcare disparities.

The 2005 report focused mainly on tracking progress toward eliminating disparities, while the 2006 and 2007 reports focused on healthcare access and quality improvements for different populations across the nation.

Overview

The NHDR is a vital step in the effort to improve healthcare in the United States. By tracking racial, ethnic, and socioeconomic disparities in healthcare access and quality over time, this can increase the general awareness about disparities and inspire action to reduce and/or eliminate them. The NHDR also offers data and analyses that can help researchers, policymakers, clinicians, administrators, and community leaders to monitor the trends, determine areas of greatest need, identify best practices for addressing those needs, and develop new and improved interventions to eliminate healthcare disparities. Additionally, communities and providers can use the NHDR methods and measures to determine the most serious disparities, create targeted interventions, and track progress against national standards.

Key Findings of the Reports

The 2003 Report

The 2003 NHDR presented seven key findings: (1) inequality in quality persists, (2) disparities come at a personal and societal price, (3) differential access to healthcare may lead to disparities in quality, (4) opportunities to provide preventive care are frequently missed, (5) knowledge of why disparities exist is limited, (6) improvement is possible, and (7) data limitations hinder targeted improvement efforts.

Specifically, the report confirmed that there were significant inequalities in healthcare quality in the nation along racial, ethnic, and socioeconomic lines. For example, the report showed that compared with Whites, minorities were more likely to be diagnosed with late-stage breast and colorectal cancer and patients of lower socioeconomic status were less likely to receive recommended diabetic services and were more likely to be hospitalized for diabetes and its complications.

Healthcare disparities were also found to be costly for individuals and for society as a whole. Disparities in quality of care can lead to missed diagnoses and poorly managed care, resulting in avoidable and expensive complications. For individuals, disparities in healthcare can cause disability, lost productivity, and morbidity. For society, treating conditions that have worsened as the result of poor care and/or poor management results in considerable financial costs, notably for taxpayers, who fund public healthcare programs.

Barriers to access to healthcare can also lead to adverse health outcomes. For example, individuals without health insurance coverage or a usual source of care are generally less likely to obtain preventive healthcare services and are more likely to delay seeking needed care. As a result, these individuals are more likely to seek medical care with their illness at later and less treatable stages.

Disparities among population groups were also found to exist in the use of evidence-based preventive services. For example, many racial and ethnic minorities and individuals of lower socioeconomic status were less likely to receive screening and treatment for cardiac risk factors and recommended immunizations.

Findings from the report suggested that targeted efforts could reduce healthcare disparities. For example, community-based cervical cancer screening and outreach programs may be the reason why Black women have higher screening rates for cervical cancer and no evidence of later-stage cervical cancer presentation despite the fact that in general Blacks and the poor are more likely to seek care with later-stage cancers and to have higher death rates.

The 2004 Report

The 2004 NHDR presented three key findings: (1) disparities are pervasive; (2) improvement is possible; and (3) gaps in information exist, particularly for specific medical conditions and populations.

Specifically, the report found that disparities were pervasive in the nation's healthcare system. Disparities affected healthcare across all dimensions of access and quality; across many medical conditions, levels and types of care, and healthcare settings; and within many subpopulations.

The report found that in both 2000 and 2001, Asians, when compared with Whites, received poorer quality of care for approximately 10% of the quality measures and had poorer access to care for approximately one third of the access measures. Also, Blacks, when compared with Whites, received poorer quality of care for approximately two thirds of the quality measures and had poorer access to care for approximately 40% of the access measures.

Several gaps identified in the 2003 NHDR were filled in the 2004 report. These included increased information on hospital care received by American Indians and Alaska Natives; healthcare delivered in community health centers; children with special healthcare needs; and a broader analysis that allowed for the separation of disparities related to race, ethnicity, and socioeconomic status.

The 2005 Report

The 2005 NHDR presented four key findings: (1) disparities still exist, (2) some disparities are diminishing, (3) opportunities for improvement still remain, (4) and information about disparities is improving.

Specifically, the report found that disparities still existed in nearly all aspects of healthcare. Minorities and the poor continued to receive lower-quality healthcare than comparison groups and also had worse access to care. The report found that for racial minorities, more disparities in quality of care were improving than were worsening. The persistence of disparities indicated that opportunities for improvement remained.

The 2006 Report

The 2006 NHDR presented four key findings: (1) disparities still remain; (2) some disparities are decreasing, while others continue to increase; (3) there remain opportunities to reduce disparities; and (4) information on disparities is getting better, but there are still gaps.

Specifically, the report found that minorities and the poor continued to receive poor-quality care and had poor access to care. The report also highlighted that for the poor, most disparities were getting worse. These gaps indicated that ample opportunity existed to continue to improve these deficient areas and also indicated the need for better data and measures.

The 2007 Report

The 2007 NHDR presented three key findings: (1) disparities in healthcare quality and access are not decreasing, although progress continues to be made; (2) the largest gaps in quality and access are not being reduced; and (3) lack of health insurance coverage continues to be a major barrier to reducing disparities.

Specifically, the report found that although overall progress continues to be made to improve healthcare quality, some of the largest gaps in quality persist. For example, the proportion of Blacks who receive hemodialysis has improved since 2001, and their current rate of treatment is not statistically different from Whites. However, despite the improvement, gaps in health still remain. Blacks were found to have a 10 times higher rate of new AIDS cases than Whites. The report also highlighted that the growing number of uninsured individuals significantly contributes to the problem of poor healthcare quality.

Future Implications

Moving forward, the improvement in available data and the recording of trends in access and the quality of healthcare will enable future NHDRs to identify and lead to decreases in inequities in health. By tracking outcomes and looking at the most vulnerable populations, these reports will continue to serve as important tools in eliminating health disparities.

Elizabeth A. Calhoun and Anna M. S. Duloy

See also Access to Healthcare; Agency for Healthcare Research and Quality (AHRQ); Cultural Competency; Ethnic and Racial Barriers to Healthcare; Health Disparities; Healthy People 2010; Vulnerable Populations

Further Readings

Agency for Healthcare Research and Quality. *National Healthcare Disparities Report*. Rockville, MD: Agency for Healthcare Research and Quality, 2003–2007.

Brady, Jeffrey, Karen Ho, and Carolyn M. Clancy, "The Quality and Disparities Reports: Why Is Progress So Slow?" *American Journal of Medical Quality* 23(5): 396–8, September–October 2008.

Kelley, Edward, Ernest Moy, Daniel Stryer, et al. "The National Healthcare Quality and Disparities Reports: An Overview," *Medical Care* 43(3 Suppl.): 13–18, March 2005.

Moy, Ernest, Elizabeth Dayton, and Carolyn M. Clancy, "Compiling the Evidence: The National Disparities Reports," *Health Affairs* 24(2): 376–87, March–April 2005.

Web Sites

Agency for Healthcare Research and Quality (AHRQ): http://www.ahrq.gov

Families USA: http://www.familiesusa.org

Henry J. Kaiser Family Foundation (KFF): http://www.kff.org

NATIONAL HEALTHCARE QUALITY REPORT (NHQR)

The National Healthcare Quality Report (NHQR) is a comprehensive source of information on trends in the quality of healthcare provided to the American people. It is published annually by the U.S. Agency for Healthcare Research and Quality (AHRQ). A key objective of the report is to inform the U.S. Congress and national healthcare policymakers on quality of care issues as well as to monitor the impact of federal and state changes in healthcare. The report is relevant to health services researchers because they investigate the link between healthcare quality, access, and costs, as well as how the translation of evidence into clinical practice and organizational actions affects outcomes of care.

Background

The idea behind reporting the quality of healthcare to the general public originated towards the end of the 20th century at a time when national discourse on health reform and strategies to improve performance in quality and safety of care had gained momentum. A strategic imperative of

reform called for accountability and transparency as important catalysts to fostering system changes. During the 1990s, a Clinton Presidential Advisory Commission on Consumer Protection and Quality in the Health Care Industry issued a report in 1998 calling for a national commitment from the public and private sectors to improve healthcare quality and reporting. By the end of the decade, the U.S. Congress enacted the Healthcare Research and Quality Act of 1999 directing the AHRQ to publish annual reports that addressed the quality information gap. Around the same period, the National Academy of Sciences, Institute of Medicine (IOM), released two seminal reports on healthcare quality (*To Err Is Human* and *Crossing the Quality Chasm*) that would shape the overall framework of the NHQR.

Framework

The NHQR is anchored on a framework that sets forth the concept of healthcare quality resulting from the dynamic interplay between the organizational delivery system domains and consumer domains of care. The organizational domains correspond to the traits of quality that exemplify effectiveness (giving care based on current scientific knowledge, avoiding overuse or underuse), safety (avoiding harm), timeliness (giving care when needed), and patient-centeredness (giving care that respects patient preferences and values). The consumer domains correspond to the traits of quality that result from obtaining care, which include staying healthy, getting better, managing chronic illness or disability, and coping with end-of-life issues. Thus, quality is indicated by a matrix of the four dimensions of organizational quality and four dimensions of consumer care to exemplify the interdependence between healthcare structures and how outcomes of consumer care influence system performance.

Content Focus

The U.S. Congress stipulates that the NHQR provide information on the relationship between quality, outcomes, access, utilization, and changes over time on frequently occurring clinical conditions, including the impact of federal and state policy changes. In this capacity, the NHQR differs from other national comparative quality reports because it provides a broad perspective on quality, by assessing progress and defining actions to improve performance across a wide range of provider settings, clinical conditions, and populations. Although the report was commissioned to inform Congress, it also seeks to enhance awareness among policy leaders, purchasers, providers, health professionals, researchers, and the lay public using a chart-book format that highlights key findings and themes to facilitate and encourage the use of data among this audience. Findings of quality outcomes are presented in chapters organized by the four domains of organizational quality, plus appendixes with data tables and measurement specifications for researchers and analysts. The report underscores four basic themes that point to what areas of quality are improving, where variability remains, where progress is strong, and where opportunities for improvement remain, using examples across states and regions by clinical conditions and patient characteristics. It also highlights progress on measures used in national quality initiatives such as Medicare's Quality Improvement Organizations (QIOs) and disease management programs. The NHQR is also published with a companion report, the National Healthcare Disparities Report (NHDR), which emphasizes trends in the quality of healthcare for racial and ethnic minority groups and other vulnerable populations.

Quality Measures

The NHRQ draws on a broad set of quality measures selected based on their importance (e.g., health effects on morbidity and mortality, financial impact), scientific soundness, and feasibility for collection. Quality measures are constructed using various public- and private-sector data sources collected from national and federal data systems, sample data from healthcare facilities and individual providers, population survey data, surveillance and vital statistics data, and health plan data from the Health Employer Data Information System (HEDIS). Each year, the report analyzes 200 to 300 measures, balanced across dimensions of organizational and consumer care, to present information on quality for frequently occurring medical conditions across different populations seeking care and treatment in acute-, ambulatory-, preventive-, nursing-, home health-, and managed-care settings.

Future Direction

While the NHQR is the broadest analysis of longitudinal data on national trends in the quality of healthcare, it remains a work in progress. The analysis of measures has gradually expanded since it was first published in 2003. A major challenge to maintaining its viability as a trustworthy source of information on trends in quality of care hinges on advancements in the field of quality measurement itself. National initiatives to expand measurement across the entire spectrum of medical conditions, populations, and provider settings are likely to remain public policy imperatives for reducing variation in the quality of healthcare for all Americans.

Iris Garcia-Caban

See also Agency for Healthcare Research and Quality (AHRQ); Medical Errors; National Healthcare Disparities Report (NHDR); Outcomes Movement; Patient Safety; Quality Improvement Organizations (QIOs); Quality Indicators; Quality of Healthcare

Further Readings

Agency for Healthcare Research and Quality. *2006 National Healthcare Quality Report*. Rockville, MD: U.S. Department of Health and Human Services, 2006.

Hurtado, Margarita P., Elaine K. Swift, and Janet M. Corrigan, eds. *Envisioning the National Health Care Quality Report*. Washington, DC: National Academies Press, 2001.

Kohn, Linda T., Janet Corrigan, and Molla S. Donaldson, eds. *To Err Is Human: Building a Safer Health System*. Washington, DC: National Academies Press, 2000.

Institute of Medicine, Committee on Quality of Health Care in America. *Crossing the Quality Chasm: A New Health System for the 21st Century*. Washington, DC: National Academies Press, 2001.

Web Sites

Agency for Healthcare Research and Quality (AHRQ): http://www.ahrq.gov

Joint Commission: http://www.jointcommission.org

National Healthcare Quality Report (NHRQ): http://nhqrnet.ahrq.gov/nhqr/jsp/nhqr.jsp

President's Advisory Commission on Consumer Protection and Quality in the Health Care Industry: http://www.hcqualitycommission.gov

NATIONAL HEALTH INSURANCE

National health insurance provides healthcare coverage for all of a country's population against the costs associated with illness and required healthcare. The term also refers to government-financed, guaranteed, and/or mandated health insurance for all citizens. The system, as a rule, is publicly funded from general tax revenues and does not include direct charges to patients such as deductibles or copayments. The various types of national health insurance systems may differ in terms of how they are structured and financed. Some form of national health insurance currently exists in Australia, in Canada, in China, in virtually all of Europe, in New Zealand, and in much of Africa and Asia.

Overview

National health insurance systems begin with the basic assumption that healthcare is an entitlement and a right of citizens and even, in many cases, of residents. It aims to insure all citizens for a comprehensive range of medical and hospital services, generally covering inpatient and outpatient services, physician services, prescription drugs, and many forms of rehabilitation. A national health insurance system places virtually all responsibility for both regulation and financing of healthcare with government. The government sets standards for a core set of benefits that must be included in the healthcare or medical programs, and it provides funding for these services. In a national health insurance system, some private insurance, which is relatively expensive, may be available to individuals who wish to use it as a supplement or, in some cases, as a substitute for the national program. As a supplement, this private insurance may cover those services that are not included in the basic health insurance scheme, such as prescription drugs, dental and vision services, and certain forms of institutional care. Overall, public sources cover the vast majority of healthcare that may be needed by an individual. In Canada, for example, the national health insurance system represents about 70% of total healthcare spending.

The major features of a national health insurance system include the following: It is universal, covering all citizens; it is comprehensive, covering all conventional medical care including inpatient and outpatient services; it is accessible, with no restrictions on services that are covered or extra charges to patients; it is portable within a country; and it is publicly administered and under the control of government or a nonprofit agency or organization.

In many national health insurance systems, private practitioners provide healthcare services and are paid on a fee-for-service basis. A fee schedule for all services is set each year through negotiations between the government, insurers, and providers. Annual fee increases are determined by the previous year's rate plus an allowance for inflation and increases due to advances in technology and innovation. There are similar negotiated fee schedules for diagnostic tests and referrals to specialists. Most physicians are self-employed in either solo or small-group practices, as are other practitioners such as dentists and pharmacists. In some national health insurance systems, physicians receive an annual salary as employees of the government.

For inpatient services, hospitals are not-for-profit and are overseen by boards of trustees or by a government regulatory agency. They receive an annual global budget, and these funds are expected to cover all care for all the patients in a given year. Institutional care outside the hospital is provided by facilities such as nursing homes and rehabilitation centers, which are reimbursed on a per diem basis.

In a national health insurance system, all citizens have the same public insurance coverage for physician and hospital care, which covers all medically necessary services. Patients have free choice of any provider in the system (which is virtually all physicians). While other industrialized countries, including the United States, rely on patient cost-sharing arrangements such as deductibles and copayments, most national health insurance systems have elected not to use these methods for cost containment. As a result, there are not direct costs to seeking care for those covered by a national health insurance system. Under this type of system, primary care is the foundation of healthcare, and patients are encouraged, though not required, to visit their primary-care physician rather than seeking a specialist directly. Eighty-five percent of Canadians, for example, have a primary-care physician whom they see on a regular basis. Specialists receive a larger fee for their services when a primary-care physician refers their patients to them. This practice encourages providers to direct patients to use their generalist appropriately.

In a healthcare system organized around national health insurance, every individual who is covered is issued an insurance or medical card. Consumers present this card when they visit the physician or the hospital; the provider, in turn, submits charges to the government or agency administering the system for reimbursement. For the basic set of medical services covered by public insurance, no further paperwork is required by either the patient or the physician. For care received in a hospital, the hospital is responsible for managing the resources allocated for each case to keep within its annual global budget. Additional paperwork may be required for supplemental services that are insured privately.

This basic public insurance for physician and hospital services includes only limited coverage for a variety of supplemental health benefits, and the majority of these supplemental services are paid for through private insurance or out-of-pocket payment by patients. Those services that are not fully covered by the public insurance scheme include prescription drugs, dental care, vision care, medical equipment and appliances, independent living arrangements for the disabled and the services of allied health professionals. While some public coverage for these services is available in limited cases, the rates of coverage vary on a case-by-case basis. In some countries, for example, the coverage and rates vary by geographic region or area. Because of this, supplemental health benefits are often funded through private health insurance or through additional allocations by regional or local governments. In many cases, these costs for additional or supplemental services have been rising, as they are not subject to the same price bargaining structures as physicians' fees and hospital costs.

National Health Insurance in Context

National health insurance can best be understood by examining the different methods for financing and organizing healthcare systems. There are three basic sets of institutional relationships in different healthcare systems: reimbursement, contractual, and integrated. The reimbursement system, which is usually combined with fee-for-service payments, is common in countries with a mix of public and private insurers and providers, including Canada, Germany, Japan, and the United States. The contract system is found in social insurance systems, as in the Netherlands, which has predominantly private, nonprofit providers. It involves an agreement between providers and third-party payers to impose limits on the total amount and distribution of spending. Contract agreements typically include global prospective budgets for hospitals and rules for reimbursement, including per diem or capitation payments. Integrated systems combine into one agency the funding for as well as the provision of health services. Health professionals are usually salaried employees, and agency budgets serve to control spending. Public integrated health systems are found in the United Kingdom and the Scandinavian countries.

In general, countries combine these relationships in the healthcare system through social insurance or public health services. Social insurance countries finance healthcare from general taxation or from compulsory payroll and employer contributions. Employment-based taxes often provide the financing for nonprofit "sickness funds" that then reimburse providers for services. There are two broad types of integrated public systems: those that are nationally integrated, such as the United Kingdom's National Health Service (NHS); and those that are organized at the local level through the counties, as in Scandinavia.

Similarities and Differences With the U.S. System

The United States does not have a comprehensive healthcare system that provides a core set of services to all citizens. Instead, some form of national health insurance is provided to the elderly through the nation's Medicare program, to low-income and disabled persons through the state-administered Medicaid program, to veterans through the Veterans Health Administration (VHA), and to low-income children through the State Children's Health Insurance Program (SCHIP). These American programs are remarkably similar to national health insurance programs in countries such as Australia, Canada, England, and New Zealand, in terms of their organization and financing. Some of the administrative or organizational relationships, such as the federal/state partnerships, are similar to those in Canada.

In Canada, as in the United States, most physicians operate in private practice. Unlike the U.S. model, however, all Canadian physicians are part of the same insurance program. The benefit of this model for the Canadian system is two-fold: a single fee schedule can be negotiated for all providers in each province; and the risks and benefits of participation are spread among all physicians.

Some, though not all, of the cost-control mechanisms used in many national health insurance systems are also common in U.S. public and private insurance programs. The most notable exception to this is the fact that the Canadian system does not use point-of-care patient cost-sharing mechanisms such as deductibles and copayments, as do most U.S. private insurers and, increasingly, Medicaid and Medicare plans. The global budgeting scheme used for payment to hospitals in Canada is different from the U.S. Medicare's Diagnosis Related Groups (DRGs) mechanism used to control the costs of an episode of hospital care. The global budget arrangement in Canada is perhaps somewhat more labor-intensive for the hospital because it requires overall planning for all patient encounters in a year rather than the immediate resource management for each individual episode of care required by DRGs.

U.S. managed-care organizations typically pay providers through a capitation arrangement, where payments are made on a per-patient basis. Rather than capitation, however, physicians in many national health insurance systems are paid on a fee-for-service basis for each patient encounter; these fees are negotiated in advance, however, and are much lower than in the United States, even under capitation schemes.

The most striking difference is the breadth of coverage offered by most national health insurance systems. Between 90% and 95% of citizens in these systems are insured by public health insurance, and in most cases the government will pay for care provided to patients regardless of whether they have an insurance card. As a result, physicians do not incur financial risk by caring for uninsured patients, as is the case in the United States.

Administrative Costs and Cost Controls

Estimates of administrative costs in national health insurance systems range from less than 1% to rates similar to those of U.S. private insurers, which is roughly 20%. These studies attempt to take into account additional sources of overhead not included in the lower estimates, such as the hidden costs of tax-based financing and patient-time costs. Notwithstanding such attempts to uncover real but hidden costs of national health insurance systems, administrative costs of these healthcare systems are significantly lower than those in the United States.

Two components at play in these systems appear to be key to achieving administrative efficiency. First, a macromanagement approach to cost control sets and enforces overall budgetary limits on hospitals and clinics. Being a single-payer system saves time and cost for both the coverage party, either the government or a not-for-profit agency, and the provider, by having a single billing system. Second, by setting global budgets, rather than itemizing charges and then billing for each encounter with each individual patient, the system reduces the amount of time and personnel needed for administration.

Waiting Lists

Waiting lists, or queues, are a concern for consumers in national health insurance systems and for American policymakers looking at these systems. Waiting times for certain procedures are longer in many of the national health insurance countries than they are in the United States. This issue is a source of anxiety for Canadian patients, for example, as well as a difficult planning concern for its policymakers. In response, the Canadian province of Ontario operates a waiting list management program, which uses guidelines that include indicators of severity and urgency to place patients in appropriate rank order. Studies suggest that those with more severe or urgent conditions do experience shorter waiting times.

It is difficult to get accurate data on the average waiting times for nonemergency procedures in Canada because there are separate waiting lists for each category of procedure, and there have been no organized efforts to collect data on waiting times until recently. These recent efforts include a survey of people in Canada and four other countries that shows that the average waiting time for elective surgery was more than 1 month, with 27% of people surveyed indicating that they had waited more than 4 months.

Some analyses also suggest that mortality rates for people waiting for coronary artery bypass graft are actually lower than expected mortality rates for cardiac patients generally, which indicates that the waiting list management system has been successful at identifying and rapidly treating those patients whose cardiac disease requires immediate attention.

Studies have found waiting times to be longer in Canada than in the United States for a variety of elective surgeries. For example, in a study of knee replacement comparing a large sample of American Medicare patients to Canadian patients, researchers found that the average waiting time was twice as long in Canada. The waiting period for the initial orthopedic consultation was 4 weeks, as compared with 2 weeks in the United States; the waiting period for the knee replacement surgery was 8 weeks, as compared with 3 weeks in the United States. The study found no differences in overall satisfaction with the surgery between the two groups.

The type of rationing embodied by waiting lists also applies to other types of high-technology healthcare services, such as the use of magnetic resonance imaging (MRI) machines. National health insurance systems usually set limits on the number of MRI machines that will be available, and it plans where they will be available geographically. In 2004 there were 4 times more MRI machines per million in the United States than in Canada (19.5 vs. 4.6). In this case, too, there does appear to be a rational process based on medical need and urgency that determines the patient's placement in the queue and ultimate receipt of services.

Waiting lists for elective procedures are often considered a source of cost control in Canada because they can reduce use and therefore spending, but they do not appear to be a large source of the overall spending differential with the United States. The procedures for which the waiting lists in Canada are the longest account for a very small proportion, approximately 3%, of overall spending in both the United States and Canada.

Costs and Benefits

Overall, it is very difficult to assess the costs and benefits of a national health insurance system as compared with a system that is a mix of public and private insurance or with one dominated by private health insurance. Some of the benefits of national health insurance include universal or near-universal coverage, predictable overall costs for the healthcare system, affordability for consumers, equity across user groups, efficiency in the allocation and use of resources, and provision of comprehensive care in inpatient and outpatient settings. The costs of this system include rationing of care, waiting lists, relatively high taxes for citizens, and restrictions on the types of care that will be covered. These costs and benefits will be assessed and balanced in different ways depending on the objectives government, consumers, and providers want to achieve.

From another perspective, it is almost impossible politically in most national health insurance systems to cut benefits, even with the cost pressures facing most systems. It would violate the principles of universality and solidarity that are associated with these systems. On the other hand, the national insurance model makes it possible to eliminate, or nearly eliminate, the administrative costs that are associated with multiple payers. The national health insurance model has considerable leverage in bargaining with providers.

As a result of affordable access to healthcare services for all citizens, Canadians enjoy very good health relative to people in other industrialized nations, including the United States. In a study comparing 13 of the world's major industrial countries using a total of 16 health indicators, Canada ranked 3rd on average, while the United States ranked 12th. The 13 countries included Australia, Belgium, Canada, Denmark, Finland, France,

Germany, Japan, the Netherlands, Spain, Sweden, the United Kingdom, and the United States. In other words, national health insurance systems appear to produce very positive health outcomes.

What many Americans find appealing about national health insurance systems such as those found in Australia, Canada, and the United Kingdom is that they eliminate insecurity about the availability of health insurance and the potential for financial ruin caused by illness. The systems also contain costs, with a smaller proportion of total economic activity devoted to healthcare, as compared with the current system in the United States.

Lessons to Be Learned

What can we learn from a national healthcare system, such as the Canadian system, whose fundamental philosophical and organizational principles are so different from our own? Perhaps more than one might at first glance think. As already noted, the United States already has various healthcare insurance programs that are universal in nature; these programs focus on specific groups of people and not the population as a whole, though.

The United States should evaluate what can be learned from national health insurance systems and the policy challenges they face in the context of a crisis of expectations. Americans want access to high-quality healthcare that offers choice among providers at relatively low costs without any type of rationing in the form of queues or waiting times. In other words, they want high-quality healthcare on demand and they want to be empowered to make their own selection of providers and treatments based on the best medical information available. Existing national health insurance systems provide some good examples and some promise that such expectations can be met under a national system. These systems, as a whole, have managed to insure all citizens for a comprehensive range of medical and hospital services, while also containing medical costs. However, there are fundamental philosophical barriers to adopting such a system in the United States, and this is where the crisis of expectations becomes most apparent. Canada, for example, has been successful in creating a relatively low-cost, easy-access healthcare system that includes a great deal of choice and only moderate

waiting times. But it has done so through governmental power and control. American consumers also want their healthcare system to be relatively free of government regulation. To this extent, national health insurance may be beyond the scope of possible reform options.

However, if Americans see that they could actually spend less on healthcare, this attitude may begin to change. For example, the United States now spends approximately the same percentage of its gross domestic product (GDP) on public health insurance programs as other industrialized countries, about 7%. The United States uses that percentage to cover a small portion of people, while the other countries are able to cover all their citizens with the same amount. The U.S. spends another 7%, or $800 billion, for private insurance, and the number of uninsured American has grown to 47.5 million.

Other dimensions of quality and patients' experiences help assess how desirable national health insurance may or may not be in the United States. Waiting times for U.S. patients with insurance are less than those for most Canadians who do not have life-threatening conditions. The longest waits and greatest anxiety are experienced by American patients who do not have health insurance coverage, although one solution to this well-documented disparity would be a system that afforded more complete coverage to all Americans.

Universal health insurance means providing insurance to all, not necessarily requiring that everyone share the same system. What is essential in this type of system is that health insurance provide coverage to all people in comparable terms. Since 1985, tension between consumers, providers, and third-party payers, including government, has been growing over which goals or objectives to maximize. The tensions are reflected in the vexing task of balancing cost containment, quality assurance, and freedom of choice for consumers and providers. Systems of national health insurance offer some important lessons for the United States on each of these critical dimensions.

Robert F. Rich

See also Access to Healthcare; Healthcare Reform; Health Services Research in Canada; International Health Systems; Public Policy; Rationing Healthcare; Single-Payer System; United Kingdom's National Health Service (NHS)

Further Readings

Boychuk, Gerard W. *National Health Insurance in the United States and Canada: Race, Territory, and the Roots of Difference.* Washington, DC: Georgetown University Press, 2008.

Canadian Institute for Health Information. *CIHI report shows increase in MRI and CT scanners, up more than 75% in the last decade.* Retrieved from http://secure.cihi.ca/cihiweb/dispPage.jsp?cw_page=media_13jan2005_e

Century Foundation. *The Basics: National Health Insurance: Lessons from Abroad.* New York: Century Foundation Press, 2008.

Funigiello, Philip J. *Chronic Politics: Health Care Security from FDR to George W. Bush.* Lawrence: University Press of Kansas, 2005.

Goodman, John C., Gerald L. Musgrave, and Devon M. Herrick. *Lives at Risk: Single-Payer National Health Insurance Around the World.* Lanham, MD: Rowman and Littlefield, 2004.

Gordon, Colon. *Dead on Arrival: The Politics of Health Care in Twentieth-Century America.* Princeton, NJ: Princeton University Press, 2003.

Hall, George M. *A Tide in the Affairs of Medicine: National Health Insurance as the Augury of Medicine.* St. Louis, MO: Warren H. Green, 2004.

Quadagno, Jill S. *One Nation, Uninsured: Why the U.S. has no National Health Insurance.* New York: Oxford University Press, 2005.

Web Sites

AARP: http://www.aarp.org

Physicians for a National Health Program (PNHP): http://www.pnhp.org

Universal Health Care Action Network (UHCAN): http://www.uhcan.org

World Health Organization (WHO): http://www.who.int

NATIONAL HEALTH POLICY FORUM (NHPF)

The National Health Policy Forum (NHPF), created in 1971, is a think tank that provides current research and information to senior staff in the U.S. Congress and executive agencies in an objective format and that offers an opportunity to discuss complex health issues in a private setting. It was founded based on a recognized need to provide accurate, unbiased information to senior congressional staff and administrators of executive agencies in Washington, D.C.

Health policy issues often contain many layers and require complex decisions for policymakers. The NHPF offers a nonpartisan exchange of information, thus providing policymakers with an opportunity to sort through the complex layers to make accurate and informed decisions. The forum itself does not take positions on specific health issues, but rather, provides objective information based on research and data to policymakers. It works to promote understanding of complex health issues and foster decision making. The NHPF is affiliated with George Washington University.

Organizational Structure

The NHPF consists of a staff of 19 people who produce resources for policymakers and the general public. The forum's employees have strong backgrounds in federal government, which provides an understanding of not only the governmental process, but also the exact types of issues and decisions faced by policymakers.

The forum's director is responsible for overseeing the activities of the staff. The director serves as a resource not only to the staff, but to policymakers and funding bodies as well. The director is responsible for the direction of the educational activities provided to federal policymakers. The forum's deputy director coordinates grant writing and reporting activities, daily operations, and programming.

In addition, the NHPF has a publications director, who serves as editor for all publications produced by the forum and guides production of print materials, visuals, and the forum's Web site. Research associates are assigned to conduct research and analysis of specific health issues. The health issues addressed by research associates range from healthcare provider issues, aging services, and long-term care to healthcare safety net and public health issues. Research associates conduct research, analyze the results, and write reports about their assigned health issues.

Activities and Services

The NHPF produces several types of resources including issue briefs, background papers, and short briefs about programs and practices called "the Basics." Materials categorized under this section aim to provide a basic introduction to a health topic. Issue briefs are short reports analyzing a variety of health-related topics and issues, whereas background papers provide a more in-depth examination of a major health issue, looking at the history, theory, and the various positions of a topic.

The NHPF also conducts meetings and workshops on a regular basis for researchers, policymakers, leaders in the healthcare industry, and consumers. Participants attend these events on an invitation-only basis. Forum meetings provide an opportunity for leaders and decision makers in health policy to come together to discuss health issues in an off-the-record setting. A specific health topic is designated for each forum session. An expert speaker or panel presents current information relevant to the designated topic. In addition to regularly scheduled forum sessions, senior congressional staff may request briefings on specific health issues. These briefings offer more in-depth analysis and discussion of a topic. The forum makes materials and handouts from these sessions available on its Web site.

The forum's Web site provides users with access to the same health policy information that is provided to policymakers. Information and materials including issue briefs, background papers, site visit reports, and meeting archives are grouped by content area. The Web site includes information about aging and long-term care, behavioral health, children's health, coverage and access, federalism, Medicaid, Medicare, pharmaceuticals, private markets, public health and preparedness, quality, research and technology, and welfare.

The NHPF also provides access to papers produced by the Health Insurance Reform Project (HIRP) on its Web site. The HIRP, another nonprofit, nonpartisan organization working as an independent voice in the health policy arena, strives to improve the health insurance and healthcare industries by monitoring trends and policy. While it is also affiliated with George Washington University, HIRP is separate from the forum.

The forum also coordinates site visits for federal policymakers. Site visits are held throughout the country to showcase innovative programs and to demonstrate how local health communities deal with specific issues. Recent site visits addressed topics relating to senior citizen health and housing, rural health systems, health records, access to care, and quality of care.

Funding

The NHPF is supported by grants and financial contributions from several foundations and corporations. While 98% of its funding comes from a number of private foundations such as the W. K. Kellogg Foundation and the Robert Wood Johnson Foundation, approximately 2% of its revenue comes from corporate contributions from health insurance companies, pharmaceutical companies, and other private corporations.

Kristin Hartsaw

See also Child Care; Long-Term Care; Medicaid; Medicare; Pharmaceutical Industry; Public Health; Public Policy; Technology Assessment

Further Readings

Merlis, Mark. *Medicare Advantage Payment Policy.* Washington, DC: National Health Policy Forum, 2007.
O'Shaughnessy, Carol V. *The Aging Services Network: Accomplishments and Challenges in Serving a Growing Elderly Population.* Washington, DC: National Health Policy Forum, 2008.
Ryan, Jennifer. *Completing the Recipe for Children's Health: New Variations on Key Ingredients.* Washington, DC: National Health Policy Forum, 2008.
Tucker, Leslie. *Pharmacogenomics: A Primer for Policymakers.* Washington, DC: National Health Policy Forum, 2008.

Web Site

National Health Policy Forum (NHPF): http://www.nhpf.org

NATIONAL HEALTH SERVICE CORPS (NHSC)

The National Health Service Corps (NHSC) is a federal program that recruits primary healthcare professionals to serve in designated Health Professional Shortage Areas (HPSAs). The Corps enlists primary-care physicians and other healthcare practitioners with scholarships and education loan repayment plans that require work in underserved areas of the nation. In FY2007, the program's budget was $125 million.

Background

The U.S. Congress created the NHSC in 1970 with the passage of the Emergency Health Personnel Act (PL 91–623) in response to the increasing geographic imbalance in access to primary care. By the end of the 1960s, rural areas suffered shortages of physicians as existing physicians retired and new ones preferred practicing in less remote areas. Innercity urban areas also were experiencing the loss of physicians and other healthcare professionals.

To identify areas of need, the federal government broadly defines and specifically identifies HPSAs. These areas have a shortage of primary-medical-care, dental, or mental health providers and may be geographic (a county or service area), demographic (low-income population), or institutional (comprehensive health center, federally qualified healthcare center, or other public facility). Specific shortage areas are designated by the Secretary of the Department of Health and Human Services (HHS). Currently, there are over 5,000 designated shortage areas in the nation. These shortage areas encompass about 50 million Americans, or 20% of the U.S. population.

Organizational Structure

The NHSC program is managed by the U.S. Department of Health and Human Services, Health Resources and Services Administration's Bureau of Health Professions (BHPr). The program has a national advisory council, which comprises 15 clinicians and healthcare administrators. The council identifies priorities, suggests and analyzes policy changes, and generally advises possible improvements in access to primary care through the program to the Secretary of the HHS and the Administrator of the Health Resources and Services Administration (HRSA).

Scholarship and Loan Programs

Under the NHSC Scholarship Program, student recruits agree to serve 1 year as a salaried professional in an approved underserved area after graduation for each year that they received the full tuition scholarship. After their commitment, scholarship recipients may enter private practice wherever they wish, but the hope is that they will stay in the underserved area. The scholarships are available to U.S. citizens studying to be allopathic or osteopathic physicians, dentists, nurse practitioners, physician assistants, nurse midwives, and other specific healthcare professionals.

The NHSC Loan Repayment Program, added in 1987, allows healthcare professionals to join the Corps and practice in an underserved area in exchange for repayment of a portion of their educational loans. Both newly graduated as well as seasoned professionals are eligible. The loan repayment program contracts require a minimum 2-year commitment to the placement site, and recipients may be able to extend the assignment to gain further loan repayment. Newly graduated or seasoned professionals are eligible, but must be U.S. citizens and be licensed and/or certified (depending on the profession). Specifically, eligible professionals include allopathic and osteopathic physicians, primary-care certified nurse practitioners, certified nurse-midwives, primary-care physician assistants, general-practice dentists, registered clinical dental hygienists, health service psychologists, licensed clinical social workers, psychiatric nurse specialists, marriage and family therapists, and licensed professional counselors.

Other Programs

The NHSC also recruits professionals to serve on a basis other than to repay obligations of a scholarship or for loan repayment. One such recruiting effort is the Rapid Response Program. Rapid responders, all primary-care professionals, serve as U.S. Public Health Service (USPHS) commissioned officers for 3 years in a medically underserved area and receive training to be part of a mobile team available in case of a large scale or national emergency.

Additionally, the NHSC also runs the Ambassador Program, which is composed of volunteers on college and university campuses or in communities. The Ambassador Program is composed of about 650 members. College Ambassadors help promote careers in primary care and inform, recruit, and support interested students. Community Ambassadors also help recruit clinicians and provide mentorship and support for Corps members.

Program Success

Since its inception, the NHSC has supported over 27,000 health professional recruits in every state, territory, and possession of the United States. In 2007, the program had 4,600 health professionals working in underserved urban and rural areas, with 50% serving in community health centers. They serve 5 million people. As part of its mission, the Corps hopes that its members will continue to practice in underserved communities once they have fulfilled their obligatory service. Records show that many Corps members do not stay at their original placement site, leaving the impression that access in underserved areas is not dramatically improved in the long term. However, further studies reveal that, although these professionals do not necessarily stay in their original placement site, many do go to other underserved areas to practice. Over 75% of those who repay their loans continue to work in underserved areas, while just over 60% of scholarship recipients remain.

Ruth Ann Althaus

See also Access to Healthcare; Health Professional Shortage Areas (HPSAs); Health Resources and Services Administration (HRSA); Primary Care; Public Health; Rural Health; Vulnerable Populations

Further Readings

Mullan, Fitzhugh. "The National Health Service Corps and Inner-City Hospitals," *New England Journal of Medicine* 336(22): 1601–1604, May 29, 1997.

Mullan, Fitzhugh. "The Muscular Samaritan: The National Health Service Corps in the New Century," *Health Affairs* 18(2): 168–75, March–April 1999.

Probst, Janice C., Michael E. Samuels, Terry V. Shaw, et al. "The National Health Service Corps and Medicaid Inpatient Care: Experience in a Southern State," *Southern Medical Journal* 96(8): 775–83, August 2003.

Web Sites

Association of American Medical Colleges (AAMC): http://www.aamc.org

National Association of Community Health Centers (NACHC): http://www.nachc.com

National Health Service Corps (NHSC): http://nhsc.bhpr.hrsa.gov

U.S. Public Health Service (USPHS): http://www.usphs.gov

NATIONAL INFORMATION CENTER ON HEALTH SERVICES RESEARCH AND HEALTH CARE TECHNOLOGY (NICHSR)

The National Information Center on Health Services Research and Health Care Technology (NICHSR) was established by the federal National Institute of Health Revitalization Act of 1993 (PL 103–43). A unit of the National Library of Medicine (NLM), the NICHSR has the broad mission of improving the collection, storage, analysis, retrieval, and dissemination of information on health services research, clinical practice guidelines, and healthcare technology, including the assessment of such technology. The NICHSR has a professional staff of six, including librarians and a health data standards specialist. It reports to the director of the NLM.

Goals

The overall goals of the NICHSR are as follows: (a) to make the results of health services research, including clinical practice guidelines and technology assessments, readily available to health practitioners, healthcare administrators, health policymakers, payers, and the information professionals who serve these groups; (b) to improve access to data and information needed by the creators of health services research; and (c) to contribute to the information infrastructure needed to foster patient record systems that can produce useful health services research data as a by-product of providing healthcare.

Health services research is a multidisciplinary field; its research domains include individuals, families, organizations, institutions, and communities. As a result, evidence from health services research is spread through a variety of sources, often making it difficult for health professionals, healthcare administrators, and health policymakers to find the information needed to guide their decision making. It is the role of the NICHSR to meet this need by coordinating the development and management of information resources and services at the NLM in the fields of health services research and public health.

Databases

An important aspect of this role is the selection of health services literature for the NLM's collection, including both published research and grey literature (e.g., material that is not found through conventional channels such as recent technical reports and working papers from research groups or committees). This function is coordinated jointly through the NICHSR, the Literature Selection Technical Review Committee (LSTRC), and the NLM's Technical Services Division. This bibliographic information used to reside in a separate database known as HealthSTAR, but in 2000, it was integrated with other NLM resources. It is now available in the following ways: (a) journal citations are added weekly to the NLM's PubMed; (b) books, book chapters, technical reports, and conference papers are added regularly to the NLM's online catalog, LocatorPlus; and (c) meeting abstracts from AcademyHealth (formerly the Academy for Health Services Research and Health Policy and the Association for Health Services Research) and Health Technology Assessment International (HTAi) (formerly known as the International Society of Technology Assessment in Health Care) are accessible through the NLM Gateway.

In addition to these resources, the NICHSR coordinates the development and maintenance of databases related to health services research. Available databases include the following: (a) HSTAT, a free, Web-based resource of full-text documents that provide health information and support healthcare decision making; (b) HSRProj, a database of citations to research-in-progress funded by federal and state agencies and foundation grants and contracts; and (c) Health Services and Sciences Research Resources (HSRR), a free searchable catalog of research databases, survey instruments, and software relevant to health services research, behavioral and social sciences, and public health. The HSRProj became available in 1995. It builds on a database developed by the staff of AcademyHealth and the Cecil G. Sheps Center for Health Services Research at the University of North Carolina at Chapel Hill. Finally, the NLM's Directory of Information Resources On-line, known as DIRLINE, has a special subfile covering health services research organizations, including those involved in technology assessment and development of clinical practice guidelines.

Recent Activities

In 2005, the NICHSR launched the HSR Information Central, a Web portal designed to centralize access to health services research information. The HSR Information Central was developed with input from the Agency for Healthcare Research and Quality (AHRQ), the National Cancer Institute (NCI), the Health Services Research and Development Service (HSR&D) at the Veterans Administration, and other organizations. A librarian evaluates each link on the HSR Information Central before it is added to the site, and users of the site are encouraged to submit additional Web links via the "Suggest-a-Link" form available at the site.

In addition to its online databases, the NICHSR and other NLM staff develop guides, fact sheets, bibliographies, and other products targeted to health services researchers. The NICHSR has developed classes and other training materials designed to assist health sciences librarians in providing health services research to their patrons. Core library recommendations have been developed for the areas of health services research methodology, health outcomes, health economics, and health policy. These lists include books, journals, and Web sites and are intended to guide individuals unfamiliar with the subject area. The NICHSR has also created online self-study courses, such as "Finding and Using Health Statistics," "Introduction to Health Care Technology Assessment," and "Health Economics Information Resources."

The NICHSR collaborates with NLM units and with members of the National Network of Libraries of Medicine to exhibit NLM products and services and to present training classes at national meetings of health services research–related organizations. The NICHSR, along with other NLM staff, is an active participant in Partners in Information Access for the Public Health Workforce. This initiative works to improve information for public health working professionals. Other partners include the Agency for Healthcare Research and Quality (AHRQ), the American Public Health Association (APHA), the Association of Schools of Public Health (ASPH), the Association of State and Territorial Health Officials (ASTHO), the Centers for Disease Control and Prevention (CDC), the Health Resources and Services Administration (HRSA), the Medical Library Association (MLA), the National Association of County and City Health Officials (NACCHO), the National Network of Libraries of Medicine (NN/LM), the Public Health Foundation (PHF), and the Society for Public Health Education (SOPHE). The NICHSR also works closely with the AHRQ and other organizations to improve the dissemination of the results of health services research.

Future Implications

The passage of the federal Health Insurance Portability and Accountability Act of 1996 (HIPAA) created new challenges for health services research, focusing on computer-based patient records, security, and privacy standards. Recent research and development efforts at the NICHSR have focused on the expansion of the Unified Medical Language Systems' Metathesaurus to improve its utility in creating and retrieving computer-based patient records, as well as the funding of extramural research and evaluation involving the creation and use of computer-based patient records.

Susan Jacobson and Catherine Selden

See also Agency for Healthcare Research and Quality (AHRQ); Health Communication; Healthcare Web Sites; Health Informatics; Health Services Research, Origins; Health Services Research Journals; National Institutes of Health (NIH); Technology Assessment

Further Readings

National Information Center on Health Services Research and Health Care Technology and AcademyHealth. *Health Outcomes Core Library Recommendations.* Bethesda, MD: National Information Center on Health Services Research and Health Care Technology, 2004.
National Information Center on Health Services Research and Health Care Technology. *Introduction to Health Services Research: A Self-Study Course.* Bethesda, MD: National Information Center on Health Services Research and Health Care Technology, 2007.
National Information Center on Health Services Research and Health Care Technology. *Finding and Using Health Statistics.* Bethesda, MD: National Information Center on Health Services Research and Health Care Technology, 2008.
Wilczynski, Nancy L., R. Brian Haynes, John N. Lavis, et al. "Optimal Search Strategies for Detecting Health Services Research Studies in MEDLINE," *Canada Medical Association Journal* 171(10): 1179–85, November 9, 2004.

Web Sites

National Information Center on Health Services Research and Health Care Technology (NICHSR): http://www.nlm.nih.gov/nichsr
National Library of Medicine (NLM): http://www.nlm.nih.gov
Partners in Information Access for the Public Health Workforce: http://phpartners.org

NATIONAL INSTITUTES OF HEALTH (NIH)

The National Institutes of Health (NIH) is the principal federal agency responsible for overseeing and financially supporting health-related and biomedical research. It funds and oversees research conducted within the United States as well as research conducted internationally. The primary goal of the NIH is to promote health and prevent disease through health-related research that provides significant insights and solutions to these problems. The NIH is regarded as one of the world's leading biomedical research centers and it is the hub of medical research activity in the nation. Researchers at the NIH are at the forefront of finding ways to prevent, treat, and cure diseases as well as find the causes of rare and common diseases. The NIH works to improve the health of people in the United States and save the lives of millions.

The NIH consists of 20 institutes and 7 centers, each with its own specific areas of research and resources of health information. The NIH is 1 of 11 U.S. Public Health Service Agencies of the U.S. Department of Health and Human Services (HHS). The NIH's headquarters and main campus are located in Bethesda, Maryland, with satellite sites across the nation. In 2007, NIH had a staff of more than 18,000 employees and a budget of nearly $28 billion. Additionally, more than 83% of the NIH's funds were awarded through competitive grants and contracts to over 325,000 researchers located at universities, medical schools, and research institutions throughout the nation and the world.

History

The political and historical context has contributed to the multifaceted organization of the NIH's institutes, centers, and offices and their myriad roles and responsibilities. The NIH began in 1887 with one research scientist, Joseph J. Kinyoun, working in a one-room laboratory within the Marine Hospital Service (MHS). As a physician he was authorized to create the Hygienic Laboratory located at Staten Island, New York. The Hygienic Laboratory was primarily used to conduct bacteriological research focusing on screening for infectious diseases such as cholera among merchant seamen and officers of the U.S. Navy. As a result, research activities were limited to biological investigations, and they did not address other factors affecting the public's health.

During the early 20th century, the general public increasingly believed in the usefulness of science to advance the health of Americans, which provided numerous opportunities to expand the roles and responsibilities of the Hygienic Laboratory. A series of legislative events prompted the transformation of the Hygienic Laboratory into a federal agency responsible for the nation's health.

In 1930, the Hygienic Laboratory was officially renamed the National Institute of Health, and it was authorized to provide research training fellowships through the passage of the Ransdell Act (PL 71–251). The U.S. Congress passed the Public Health Service Act (PL 78–410) in 1944, which gave the U.S. Surgeon General of the Public Health Service (PHS) increasing authority to fund research

studies and designated the newly established National Cancer Institute (NCI) as an Institute of the NIH. Accordingly, the NIH gradually began to enlarge its facilities and research funding mechanisms. The NCI was already authorized by the U.S. Congress in 1937 through the National Cancer Institute Act (PL 75–244) to provide research funds to nonfederal workers and to sponsor research training fellowships outside of the organization. As the other institutes were established, between 1948 and 2000, the thriving NCI grants and research training programs continued to expand. Funding for the NIH grew tremendously during this time period, from $2.5 million in 1944 to more than $1 billion in 1966. And NIH funding has continued to expand.

Overview

Over the decades, the significant work of the NIH has resulted in numerous important discoveries and medical treatments that have saved the lives of many, increased the life expectancy of the nation's population, and improved the quality of life of individuals. The NIH has been able to translate research findings into interventions that have benefited the general public, patients, and their families. Furthermore, the outcomes of the NIH's research have resulted in decreased death rates from heart disease, stroke, HIV/AIDS, and sudden infant death syndrome (SIDS); the increased survival rate of childhood cancer patients; and prevention of the spread of infectious diseases through vaccinations.

In addition to conducting cutting-edge research that has transformed medical science, the NIH also provides funding and training opportunities. All its institutes support research, funding, and training opportunities for research scientists in a variety of settings such as hospitals, universities, and laboratories. The NIH centers also provide and coordinate resources that facilitate intensive research training and development of a strong national research infrastructure. Under the guidance of the Office of the Director, the 27 institutes and centers aim to meet the four stated overarching goals of the NIH: (1) to foster fundamental creative discoveries, innovative research strategies, and their applications as a basis to advance the nation's capacity to protect and improve health significantly; (2) to develop, maintain, and renew scientific human and physical resources that will ensure the nation's capability to prevent disease; (3) to expand the knowledge base in medical and associated sciences in order to enhance the nation's economic well-being and ensure a continued high return on the public investment in research; and (4) to exemplify and promote the highest level of scientific integrity, public accountability, and social responsibility in the conduct of science. The establishment of these institutes reflects the direction of present scientific discoveries and societal needs. Specifically, the NIH concentrates its research agenda and educational efforts on input from expert researchers and clinicians, patient advocacy and grassroots organizations, and representatives from the U.S. Congress.

With federal funds, the NIH supports intramural and extramural research studies in which both types of studies undergo a careful process of scientific review before investigation, and they follow strict guidelines throughout the research process. Intramural research activities are conducted in NIH laboratories and at the NIH Clinical Center at its main campus in Bethesda. Seven major NIH Inter-Institute Scientific Interest Groups are organized by the NIH Office of Intramural Research and offer training opportunities and expert guidance for junior researchers. The NIH Office of Extramural Research (OER) develops and implements NIH grants, policies, and guidelines primarily for university investigators. The NIH awards funds to external organizations to help accomplish its program goals through research grants, cooperative agreements, and contracts.

In FY2006, approximately 50,000 research grants were awarded through the OER. Grant applications and cooperative agreements are subject to a system of two separate peer reviews. One is a scientific assessment, and the second is an evaluation of the first assessment as well as resource funding allocations.

Contracts are reviewed under a separate process including a request for proposals (RFP) based on the needs of the specific institute. RFPs are reviewed by peer reviewers and NIH staff reviewers. The offers that are deemed the most beneficial to the public are awarded contracts. The peer review system constructs a foundation of decision making based on scientific integrity and responsibility regarding the federal stewardship of funds.

Institutes

The NIH comprises 20 different institutes that work to accomplish its overarching goals. Each institute is briefly discussed below.

National Cancer Institute

The National Cancer Institute (NCI) was established in 1937 to conduct and support research concerning the cause, diagnosis, prevention, and treatment of cancer and to regularly provide federal cancer statistics. Of all the institutes at the NIH, the NCI has the largest budget, at nearly $4.7 billion. The NCI publishes a large number of articles, books, and other material on various types of cancer, treatment options, clinical trials, coping with cancer, testing for cancer, nutrition, and cancer risk factors.

National Eye Institute

The National Eye Institute (NEI) was established in 1968 to conduct and support vision research to prevent and treat visual impairment and blindness. The NEI conducts public educational programs through its National Eye Health Education Program. The NEI publications include information about eye diseases and disorders and eye care resources.

National Heart, Lung, and Blood Institute

The National Heart, Lung, and Blood Institute (NHLBI), established in 1948, fosters and furthers research on cardiovascular diseases as well as sleep disorders. The NHLBI publications include health assessment and educational resources for patients, clinicians, and researchers.

National Human Genome Research Institute

The National Human Genome Research Institute (NHGRI) was established in 1989 to represent the work of the NIH on the International Human Genome Project (IHGP). After the successful completion of the IHGP in 2003, the NHGRI continues to conduct and support human genome research. The NHGRI educational resources include a Human Genome Project CD and genetics and genomics education resources for the public.

National Institute on Aging

The National Institute on Aging (NIA), created in 1974, is focused on better understanding the aging process through scientific research. Currently, the NIA funds external research studies on the biology of aging, behavioral research, neuroscience, and geriatrics and gerontology. The NIA's publications include information related to healthy aging, medications, safety, Alzheimer's disease, health conditions related to aging, and care giving.

National Institute on Alcohol Abuse and Alcoholism

The National Institute on Alcohol Abuse and Alcoholism (NIAAA) was established in 1970 to conduct and support research on the causal factors, diagnosis, prevention, and treatment of alcohol-related conditions. The NIAAA's publications include the journal *Alcohol Research and Health,* professional education materials for researchers and clinicians, and pamphlets and brochures on alcohol-related topics for the public.

National Institute of Allergy and Infectious Diseases

National Institute of Allergy and Infectious Diseases (NIAID), which focuses on research on infectious, immunologic, and allergic diseases, was established in 1948. The NIAID strategic plan for the 21st century includes further investigation of allergic diseases and asthma, autoimmune diseases (e.g., Type 1 diabetes, rheumatoid arthritis, and multiple sclerosis), HIV/AIDS, tuberculosis, malaria, influenza, hepatitis, and bioterrorism.

National Institute of Arthritis and Musculoskeletal and Skin Diseases

The National Institute of Arthritis and Musculoskeletal and Skin Diseases (NIAMS), created in 1986, examines and supports research on the causal factors, diagnosis, prevention, and treatment of arthritis and musculoskeletal and skin diseases. The NIAMS' Information Clearinghouse provides health information for professionals and the general public.

National Institute of Biomedical Imaging and Bioengineering

The National Institute of Biomedical Imaging and Bioengineering (NIBIB) is the most recently established institute. Since 2000, it has worked to foster the study of biomedical technology and engineering. Currently, the NIBIB supports external research studies on biomaterials, biomedical informatics, biomedical and medical imaging, nanotechnology, nuclear medicine, tissue engineering, and ultrasound.

National Institute of Child Health and Human Development

The National Institute of Child Health and Human Development (NICHD) was established in 1962 to conduct and support the study of infants, children, and their families and human development across the lifespan. The NICHD currently supports external research studies on developmental biology and perinatal medicine, reproductive health, child development, and pediatric and maternal HIV/AIDS. It also sponsors health campaigns to target problems such as autism, obesity, and sudden infant death syndrome (SIDS).

National Institute on Deafness and Other Communication Disorders

Since its inception in 1988, the National Institute on Deafness and Other Communication Disorders (NIDCD) has focused on the study of communication disorders. Currently, the NIDCD is conducting research studies on human communication and genetics, sensory and signal transduction mechanisms, and physiological and developmental studies of the inner ear.

National Institute of Dental and Craniofacial Research

The National Institute of Dental and Craniofacial Research (NIDCR) was established in 1948 to conduct and support research on the causal factors, diagnosis, prevention, and treatment of craniofacial-oral-dental diseases and disorders. The NIDCR is currently conducting research studies on genomics and proteomics, as well as the repair and regeneration of tissues related to craniofacial-oral-dental diseases and disorders.

National Institute of Diabetes and Digestive and Kidney Diseases

The National Institute of Diabetes and Digestive and Kidney Diseases (NIDDK), established in 1948, supports and conducts research on the study of diabetes as well as endocrine, metabolic, digestive, kidney, urologic, and hematologic diseases. The NIDDK clearinghouse provides publications for patients and researchers on diabetes and digestive, kidney, and urologic diseases.

National Institute on Drug Abuse

Established in 1973, the National Institute on Drug Abuse (NIDA) works to advance research on the causal factors, diagnosis, prevention, and treatment of drug abuse and addiction. The NIDA provides a vast array of prevention and treatment resources to healthcare providers, researchers, parents, and teachers, as well as to students and young adults. Currently, the NIDA supports external research studies on treatment for drug disorders, drug abuse aspects of HIV/AIDS, genetics and genomics of drug addiction, and prescription drug abuse.

National Institute of Environmental Health Sciences

The National Institute of Environmental Health Sciences (NIEHS) was created in 1969 to conduct and support the study of environmental factors and causes related to health and illness. The NIEHS 2006–2011 Strategic Plan includes goals to increase the understanding of environmental influences related to human biology and to expand clinical research programs on environmental exposures.

National Institute of General Medical Sciences

The National Institute of General Medical Sciences (NIGMS), active since 1962, focuses on the study of biomedical sciences for understanding the pathways of disease diagnosis, prevention, and treatment. The NIGMS funds studies on bioinformatics and computational biology; cell biology and biophysics; structural genomics and proteomics technology; genetics and developmental biology; and pharmacology, physiology, and biological chemistry.

National Institute of Mental Health

The National Institute of Mental Health (NIMH) is charged with advancing research on the causal factors, diagnosis, prevention, and treatment of mental illness. It was established in 1949. Currently, the NIMH funds external research studies on basic neuroscience and behavioral science, adult and pediatric mental disorders, biobehavioral processes related to HIV/AIDS transmission and infection, and mental health interventions.

National Institute of Neurological Disorders and Stroke

The National Institute of Neurological Disorders and Stroke (NINDS), created in 1950, conducts and fosters research on the causal factors, diagnosis, prevention, and treatment of neurological disease and stroke. The NINDS areas of neuroscience research include, but are not limited to, the structure and functioning of the nervous system through examining neural circuits, neural environment, neurodegeneration, and neurogenetics.

National Institute of Nursing Research

Since 1986, the National Institute of Nursing Research (NINR) has focused its efforts on nursing research among individuals, families, communities, and populations. Currently, the NINR areas of research emphasis include improving health promotion and quality of life, eliminating health disparities, and advancing end-of-life research.

National Library of Medicine

The National Library of Medicine (NLM), established in 1956, strives to advance the study of biomedical informatics and communications. The NLM is located at the NIH headquarters in Bethesda, Maryland, and serves as the world's largest medical library. The NLM's online databases, such as PubMed/Medline, include biomedical publications from thousands of journals; MedlinePlus serves as a resource for health information for professionals and the general public.

Centers

In addition to its 20 institutes, the NIH houses 7 research centers. Each center is briefly discussed below.

Center for Information Technology

The Center for Information Technology (CIT) has been working to develop computer systems, provide computer facilities, and conduct computational research since its creation in 1964. The CIT supports NIH's institutes with information technology, computing, and telecommunications services. For example, the CIT's Division of Computational Bioscience applies technologies to biomedical applications such as biomedical informatics and medical imaging.

Center for Scientific Review

The Center for Scientific Review (CSR), which was established in 1946, recruits and organizes expert peer reviewers into study sections to evaluate the research grant applications sent to the NIH. These external experts are recruited nationally and represent the areas of expertise needed to effectively decide on funding of the most promising research activities.

John E. Fogarty International Center

The John E. Fogarty International Center (FIC) was established in 1968 to promote and support research on global health. Currently, the FIC funds research studies in the developing world on brain disorders, maternal and child health, and infectious diseases, such as HIV/AIDS and tuberculosis. It also supports international research partnerships.

National Center for Complementary and Alternative Medicine

In 1999, the NIH created the National Center for Complementary and Alternative Medicine (NCCAM) to focus on complementary and alternative medical (CAM) practices and training efforts. Currently, the NCCAM areas of research emphasis include mind-body medicine practices, pharmaceutical and pharmacokinetic properties of CAM products, energy medicine, traditional/ indigenous practices, and ethical and social issues related to the use of CAM.

National Center on Minority Health and Health Disparities

The National Center on Minority Health and Health Disparities (NCMHD), established in 1993, conducts and supports research to improve minority health and eliminate health disparities. Currently, the NCMHD provides loan repayment funds for researchers working in minority health and health disparities research, as well as for those who are developing external research training programs and centers.

National Center for Research Resources

The National Center for Research Resources (NCRR), created in 1962, provides researchers with biomedical resources as well as technological support to develop successful clinical research environments. Currently, the NCRR focuses on providing support in biomedical technology, clinical research, comparative medicine, and research infrastructure.

NIH Clinical Center

Originally established as a research hospital facility in 1953, the NIH Clinical Center (CC) supports clinical research conducted by all the NIH institutes and centers. Admission to the CC is selective and based on NIH study objectives. The CC also provides numerous training opportunities to researchers through lectures and computer-based training as well as fellowship programs.

Future Implications

For more than a century, the NIH has been responsible for improving the nation's health through biomedical and behavioral research. The NIH continues its important work of discovering new knowledge to improve the nation's health through its ambitious research agenda. Additionally, through its institutes and centers, the NIH strives to provide resources and expertise in the broad spectrum of clinical medicine and public health. The NIH furthers its goals by sponsoring research, fellowships, training, and infrastructure development. Through the translation of biomedical research discoveries into means of disease prevention and improvements in clinical outcomes, reduction in the individual and societal burden of disease is being achieved.

Michelle Choi Wu

See also Acute and Chronic Diseases; Centers for Disease Control and Prevention (CDC); Cohort Studies; Community-Based Participatory Research (CBPR); Health Disparities; Mortality, Major Causes in the United States; National Information Center on Health Services Research and Health Care Technology (NICHSR); Randomized Controlled Trials (RCT)

Further Readings

Hannaway, Caroline, ed. *Biomedicine in the Twentieth Century: Practices, Policies, and Politics.* Washington, DC: IOS Press, 2008.

Robinson, Judith. *Noble Conspirator: Florence S. Mahoney and the Rise of the National Institutes of Health.* Washington, DC: Francis Press, 2001.

Varmus, Harold. *The Art and Politics of Science.* New York: W. W. Norton, 2009.

Zerhouni, Elias A. "The NIH Roadmap," *Science* 302(5642): 63–72, October 3, 2003.

Zerhouni, Elias A. "Translational and Clinical Science: Time for a New Vision," *New England Journal of Medicine* 353(15): 1621–23, October 13, 2005.

Zerhouni, Elias A., "NIH in the Post-Doubling Era: Realities and Strategies," *Science* 314(5802): 1088–1090, November 17, 2006.

Zerhouni, Elias A., and Barbara Alving. "Clinical and Translational Science Awards: A Framework for a National Research Agenda," *Translational Research* 148(1): 4–5, July 2006.

Web Sites

National Institutes of Health (NIH): http://www.nih.gov

National Institutes of Health, Clinical Trials: http://clinicaltrials.gov

National Institutes of Health, Institutes, Centers, & Offices: http://www.nih.gov/icd

National Institutes of Health, Office of Extramural Research: http://grants.nih.gov/grants/oer.htm

National Institutes of Health, Research and Training Opportunities: http://www.training.nih.gov

NATIONAL MEDICAL ASSOCIATION (NMA)

The National Medical Association (NMA) promotes the collective interests of physicians and patients of African descent and other minority and underserved populations in the United States. The association carries out this mission by serving as the collective voice of Black physicians. It is a leading force for parity in medicine, the elimination of health disparities, and the promotion of optimal health.

History

The National Medical Association was founded in the fall of 1895 at the Cotton States and International Exposition in Atlanta, Georgia, after a group of Black physicians were denied admission into the American Medical Association (AMA). In a climate of segregation, the National Medical Association was founded to provide an organization for Black physicians and health professionals. Robert F. Boyd of Nashville, Tennessee, served as the association's first president.

The main priority for the first National Medical Association's agenda was how to improve the health of the nation's Black population, which exceeded 10 million in 1912, and increase the number of Black physicians to adequately serve the health of that population. The association's members worked on these priorities by opening hospitals with an emphasis on physician training and by studying the major diseases contracted by Blacks, such as tuberculosis, hookworm, and pellagra.

In 1909, the first issue of the *Journal of the National Medical Association* was published. Charles V. Roman served as the journal's first editor. From its beginning, the journal focused on scholarly research and findings regarding the treatment, management, and prevention of illness and disease.

In the 1940s, the National Medical Association continued its efforts to eliminate discrimination in the nation's hospitals and medical schools. In 1951, the association was responsible for several segregated medical schools located in the South and nearby states beginning to admit Black students. Within a 10-year period, the number of Black students attending these medical schools doubled. By the 1960s, 14 of the 26 southern medical schools admitted Black students.

In 1957, the first Imhotep National Conference on Hospital Integration was held. This annual meeting was sponsored by the National Medical Association, the National Association for the Advancement of Colored People (NAACP), the National Urban League, and the Medico-Chirurgical Society of the District of Columbia (an affiliate of the National Medical Association). This conference was successfully used as a platform to disseminate strategies to foster the elimination of segregation in healthcare.

During the turbulent 1960s, the National Medical Association was a viable force in the nation's civil rights movement. The association advocated for civil rights by coordinating sit-ins, marches, and picket lines and by lobbying to pass a federal civil rights act. It supported Martin Luther King Jr.'s efforts to register voters in Selma, Alabama, which ultimately led to the passage of the Civil Rights Act of 1965. The passage of this act was instrumental in giving Blacks hope of improving their health status by outlawing discrimination in government-funded health programs. In particular, the act assured them access to healthcare through Medicare and Medicaid programs, and the professional staffs and patient populations at hospitals were desegregated.

Activities

Currently, the National Medical Association represents more than 30,000 Black physicians and their patients. The association continues to publish the *Journal of the National Medical Association* monthly, the quarterly *Healthy Living* newsletter, targeted to physicians and patients, and the e-newsletter *NMA News*. It also publishes the *Convention Daily News*, which is available at the association's Annual Convention and Scientific Assembly, where about 1,000 scientific sessions are held.

The association offers many continuing medical education (CME) courses at its national assembly as well as at regional, state, and local society meetings offered in its 33 state and 98 local affiliated medical societies. All its courses are accredited by the Accreditation Council for Continuing Medical Education.

The National Medical Association sponsors a wide range of externally funded programs. These include the Smoking Cessation Program, the National Diabetes Education Program (cosponsored with the U.S. Department of Health and Human Services' National Diabetes Education Program [NDEP]), the Clinical Trials Project Impact program to increase minority physicians and consumer awareness and participation in clinical trials, and the Black Bag Mentoring program to facilitate African American residents' and students' access to practicing physicians.

In 2004, the association formed The W. Montague Cobb/National Medical Association Health Institute. The focus of the institute is to identify, develop, and implement solutions that will reduce racial and ethnic health disparities and improve the health of all Americans. The institute has four centers: (1) the Multicultural Health Center; (2) the Research, Surveillance and Professional Education Center; (3) the Community/Public Media Information Center; (4) and the Mobilization and Advocacy Center.

The association holds an annual National Colloquium on African American Health to foster its advocacy mission by offering programs to train healthcare leaders to address and eliminate health disparities of Blacks, other minorities, the poor, and the medically underserved.

The National Medical Association's advocacy efforts are continued through its International Affairs Committee, which serves as a resource to assist and enhance association members' participation in medical missions around the world. In addition, association members' spouses formed the Auxiliary to the National Medical Association. The auxiliary's current efforts consist of developing and promoting a National Auxiliary Program on Health, Education, and Legislation.

The association also supports the Student National Medical Association (SNMA). Started in 1964 by medical students from Howard University College of Medicine and Meharry Medical College, the Student Medical Association currently has over 5,000 members, including medical students, pre-medical students, residents, and physicians. Its primary focus is the needs and concerns of medical students of color, although its efforts include encouraging elementary, high school, and college students to consider and prepare for medical and scientific careers. The National Medical Association also provides a Career Center to assist in the employment and recruitment of minorities into medical professions.

Ophelia T. Morey

See also Diversity in Healthcare Management; Ethnic and Racial Barriers to Healthcare; Health Disparities; Health Workforce; National Healthcare Disparities Report (NHDR); Physicians; Vulnerable Populations

Further Readings

Braithwaite, Ronald L., and Sandra E Taylor. *Health Issues in the Black Community.* 2d ed. San Francisco: Jossey-Bass, 2001.

Committee on Institutional and Policy-Level Strategies for Increasing the Diversity of the U.S. Healthcare Workforce, Institute of Medicine. *In the Nation's Compelling Interest: Ensuring Diversity in the Health Care Workforce.* Washington, DC: National Academies Press, 2004.

Hansen, Axel C. "African Americans in Medicine," *Journal of the National Medical Association* 94(4): 266–71, April 2002.

LaVeist, Thomas A. *Minority Populations and Health: An Introduction to Health Disparities in the United States.* San Francisco: Jossey-Bass, 2005.

Liebschutz, Jane M., Godwin O. Darko, Erin P. Finley, et al. "In the Minority: Black Physicians in Residency and their Experiences," *Journal of the National Medical Association* 98(9): 1441–8, September 2006.

Satcher, David, Rubens J. Pamies, and Nancy N., Woelfl, eds. *Multicultural Medicine and Health Disparities.* New York: McGraw-Hill, 2006.

Schlueter, Eric M. "The Bridge to Diversity: The Role of the National Medical Association and the African-American Physician," *Journal of the National Medical Association* 98(9): 1515–17, 2006.

Wilson, Donald E., and Jeanette M. Kaczmarek. "The History of African-American Physicians and Medicine in the United States," *Journal of the Association for Academic Minority Physicians* 4(3): 93–98, February 1993.

Web Sites

Auxiliary to the National Medical Association (ANMA): http://www.anmanet.org

National Medical Association (NMA): http://www.nmanet.org

Student National Medical Association (SNMA): http://www.snma.org

NATIONAL PATIENT SAFETY GOALS (NPSG)

The Joint Commission's National Patient Safety Goals (NPSG) address problematic areas in healthcare by using evidence- and expert-based solutions. The NPSG are composed of implementation expectations and requirements for Joint Commission–accredited organizations. Where possible, the goals focus on systemwide improvements. The goals are program specific and apply variously to ambulatory care, office-based surgery, behavioral healthcare, critical-access hospitals, disease-specific care, home care, hospitals, laboratories, long-term care, integrated delivery systems, managed-care organizations, and preferred provider organizations (PPOs). All Joint Commission–accredited healthcare organizations are expected to implement the goals or approved alternatives to the services the organization provides in order to obtain or maintain their accreditation. The first goals were approved in 2002 and have been updated annually since then.

Development of the Goals

Formed in February 2002, the Sentinel Event Advisory Group (SEAG), a panel of patient safety experts including nurses, physicians, pharmacists, risk managers, and other professionals, oversees the development and improvement of the NPSG and implementation requirements. Each year, the SEAG works with the Joint Commission staff to identify potential new goals and requirements through a systematic review of the relevant literature and information from available patient safety incident databases, such as the Joint Commission's Sentinel Event Database and the U.S. Pharmacopeia's Medmarx Database. Once potential goals are identified, input is sought from practitioners, provider organizations, purchasers, consumers, and patient advocacy groups. The SEAG then determines the highest-priority goals and requirements and makes its recommendations to the Joint Commission. To maintain the focus of accredited organizations on the most salient patient safety issues, the SEAG may recommend the retirement of selected goals or requirements. Retired goals or requirements will usually continue as accreditation requirements under the relevant accreditation standards. The gaps in goal numbering indicate that a goal has been retired.

Specifically, the 2008 NPSG goals for hospitals were as follows:

Goal 1: Improve the accuracy of patient identification.

Goal 2: Improve the effectiveness of communication among caregivers.

Goal 3: Improve the safety of using medications.

Goal 7: Reduce the risk of healthcare-associated infections.

Goal 8: Accurately and completely reconcile medications across the continuum of care.

Goal 9: Reduce the risk of patient harm resulting from falls.

Goal 10: Reduce the risk of influenza and pneumococcal disease in institutionalized older adults.

Goal 11: Reduce the risk of surgical fires.

Goal 12: Implement the applicable NPSG and associated requirements by components and practitioner sites.

Goal 13: Encourage patients' active involvement in their own care as a patient safety strategy.

Goal 14: Prevent healthcare-associated pressure ulcers (decubitus ulcers).

Goal 15: Identify safety risks inherent in its patient population.

Goal 16: Improve recognition and response to changes in a patient's condition.

Last, the organization fulfills the expectations set forth in the Universal Protocol for preventing wrong-site, wrong-procedure, and wrong-person surgery, and associated implementation guidelines.

Challenges in Meeting the Goals

Depending on the goal, healthcare organizations may face various system, resource, personnel, behavioral, and/or cultural barriers to goal implementation. Some goals have been consistently criticized for the added burden they place on an already overstretched system. For example, Goal 8, the "medication reconciliation" goal, calls for healthcare organizations to obtain an accurate list of medications from patients and to define a process to ensure that information is accurately communicated from provider to provider. The intent of the goal is to prevent patient safety incidents involving adverse drug events by ensuring that healthcare providers have accurate patient medication information so that the provider can effectively care for the patient. However, inordinate attention has been paid to documentation or "obtaining the list," and therefore, the intent of the goal is sometimes lost. Organizations that have successfully implemented medication reconciliation programs are those that have integrated the practice of medication reconciliation into existing processes and then worked to refine those processes to eliminate duplication and redundancy. Organizations that struggle with implementing medication reconciliation are those that tend to add these processes on to existing systems without considering the potential implications of doing so.

Future Implications

The NPSG focus attention on problematic areas in healthcare. Successful implementation of the goals is challenging for healthcare organizations, given the complexity of organizational systems, resources, personnel, and cultures. There are no one-size-fits-all solutions, and there is only emerging research that supports the effectiveness of some of the goals. Because the goals are intended to prevent patient harm and improve safety, the Joint Commission will continue in these efforts despite the difficulties in implementation.

Gerard M. Castro

See also Adverse Drug Events; Hospitals; Institute for Healthcare Improvement (IHI); International Classification for Patient Safety (ICPS); Joint Commission; Medical Errors; Patient Safety; Quality of Healthcare

Further Readings

"2006 National Patient Safety Goals Matrix," *Joint Commission Perspectives* 25(8): 9–10, August 2005.

"Approved: Revisions to 2007 National Patient Safety Goals and Universal Protocol," *Joint Commission Perspectives* 27(3): 5–6, March 2007.

"JCAHO to Establish Annual Patient Safety Goals," *Joint Commission Perspectives* 22(5): 1–2, May 2002.

"The Joint Commission Announces the 2008 National Patient Safety Goals and Requirements," *Joint Commission Perspectives* 27(7): 1, 9–22, July 2007.

"The Joint Commission Announces the 2009 National Patient Safety Goals and Requirements," *Joint Commission Perspectives* 28(7): 11–15, July 2008.

Web Sites

Joint Commission's National Patient Safety Goals (NPSG): http://www.jointcommission.org/ PatientSafety/NationalPatientSafetyGoals

Joint Commission's Sentinel Event Advisory Group (SEAG): http://www.jointcommission.org/ SentinelEvents/AdvisoryGroup

NATIONAL PRACTITIONER DATA BANK (NPDB)

Administered by the Health Resources and Services Administration (HRSA), the National Practitioner Data Bank (NPDB) is a federal information clearinghouse responsible for receiving, storing, and disseminating information about medical malpractice payments and adverse actions taken against healthcare practitioners. Established under the Health Care Quality Improvement Act of 1986, the NPDB began collecting data on September 1, 1990. The purpose of the data bank is to improve medical-care quality and safety by restricting the ability of incompetent physicians, dentists, and other practitioners to move from state to state without the disclosure of previous medical malpractice payments and adverse actions. The NPDB is intended to be an alert system that facilitates a comprehensive review of a healthcare practitioner's professional credentials.

Types of Reports

The NPDB receives six types of reports: (1) medical malpractice payments made on behalf of a practitioner, (2) licensure actions taken by state medical and dental boards, (3) professional review actions taken by hospitals and other healthcare entities exercising significant peer review activities, (4) professional society membership actions, (5) actions taken by the U.S. Drug Enforcement Administration (DEA), and (6) Medicare and Medicaid exclusions. Medical-malpractice payments are the most common type of report received by the NPDB. Since its inception, the NPDB has received about 320,000 medical malpractice reports, which represent about 75% of all reports. State licensure actions are the next most common type of report, at 14%, followed by Medicare and Medicaid exclusion at 8.0% and clinical privileging actions at about 4%. Professional society membership and DEA actions make up less than 0.5% of all reports in the data bank.

Types of Providers Covered

While the NPDB covers a wide variety of medical practitioners, physicians are those most often reported to the data bank. Physicians make up approximately 70% of all practitioners reported to the data bank. Dentists make up the next largest group, at 13%, followed by nurses and nursing-related practitioners, who account for 9%, and chiropractors, who represent about 3% of those practitioners reported.

Types of Entities Reporting

Just as there are a variety of types of reports in the NPDB, there are also a variety of entities providing those reports. Any entity that makes a medical malpractice payment on behalf of a practitioner for full or partial settlement of a claim or judgment must submit a report to the NPDB. In general, medical malpractice reports are made by insurers or carriers; however, these reports may also be filed by other types of organizations that make such payments. Self-insured hospitals, physician groups, and managed-care organizations can also file reports. State medical and dental boards are required to report state licensure disciplinary actions related to professional competence or conduct. Other professional boards are not required to report to the data bank. Any hospital or other healthcare entity that takes a professional review action that restricts or suspends the clinical privileges of a physician or dentist for more then 30 days must report that action to the NPDB. Physicians and dentists may voluntarily surrender or restrict their clinical privileges while being investigated for possible professional incompetence or improper professional conduct in return for suspension of the investigation. In these cases, the healthcare entity must also file a report. This situation is considered a reportable clinical privileging action. Clinical privilege actions for other practitioners may also be reported, but these reports are not required. Professional societies are required to report membership actions taken for reasons related to professional competence. The DEA provides up-to-date information on revocations and voluntary surrenders of its registration numbers. Finally, Medicare and Medicaid exclusions are publicly available through the *Federal Register* and do not require a specific reporting entity.

Federal agencies are not subject to the provisions of the Health Care Quality Improvement Act of 1986. The Secretary of the U.S. Department of Health and Human Services (HHS) signed separate memoranda of understanding with various federal departments to ensure their participation in the NPDB program. The Secretary signed memoranda of understanding with the U.S. Department of Defense (DOD) in 1987, the DEA in 1988, and the U.S. Department of Veterans Affairs (VA) in 1990. Other memoranda of understanding include ones with the U.S. Public Health Service (PHS), signed in 1989 and 1990, and with the U.S. Coast Guard and the U.S. Department of Justice, Bureau of Prisons, signed in 1994. Under those memoranda of understanding, 257 medical malpractice cases were reported to the NPDB through 2005.

Access to Information

The only entities that are required to access information from the NPDB are hospitals. According to the authorizing legislation, all hospitals are required to query the data bank when a physician initially applies for employment or membership on their medical staff, and at least every 2 years thereafter. Other entities that exercise significant peer review, such as managed-care organizations and physician groups, may also query the data bank.

Healthcare practitioners may self-query the data bank about themselves at any time. A practitioner may dispute the accuracy of a report in the data bank or the fact that the report should have been filed. If the dispute between the practitioner and the report is not resolved, the practitioner may ultimately request a review of the report by the Secretary of the HHS.

Research and Impact

A great deal of research on the NPDB has focused on using the longitudinal, national data set to provide information on trends in medical malpractice claims. For example, one study compared 2001–2004 median anesthesia malpractice payments with those for a similar period a decade earlier and documented a 28% decrease in the number of anesthesia-related payments per 100,000 population but a substantial increase in the median payment amount from $69,330 to $205,222.

While studies focusing on medical malpractice payments are most common, a few studies of trends in adverse actions have also been published. These studies tend to focus on the lack of reporting in this area. For example, one research study documented that between 1991 and 1995 only 34% of hospitals reported one or more clinical privileging actions against a physician. In addition, the annual rate of reporting to the data bank for these types of actions actually fell over the period, from 12% in 1991 to 10% in 1995. Subsequent studies by the Office of the Inspector General (OIG) of the HHS found that 60% of hospitals and 84% of health maintenance organizations (HMOs) had not reported a single adverse action to the data bank in almost 10 years of data collection.

A number of studies have focused on the quality and usefulness of the data housed in the data bank. The studies determined that, in general, querying entities found the reports in the data bank useful because they confirmed information received from other sources, although they did not often change the credentialing decision of the entity. However, the studies also found a low level of completeness of data in the data bank.

Another important area of research has been the potential impact of the NPDB on medical malpractice claim settlements and adverse actions. A number of researchers and policymakers have hypothesized that in the face of the reporting requirements of the NPDB, individuals and organizations may take steps to avoid settlements or reportable adverse actions. This assumption is because a report to a federal data bank is considered onerous, notwithstanding that hospitals require physicians to submit the same information and the NPDB essentially serves as a check on physician honesty. Because of this perceived burden, some have suggested that 29-day clinical privilege suspensions, which are not reportable, are one major explanation for the limited reporting of adverse clinical privileging actions.

In the arena of medical malpractice payments, the practice of corporate shielding has become an issue of major concern to policymakers. Because medical malpractice payments on behalf of institutions are not reportable to the NPDB, some have suggested that attorneys may be working out arrangements to name institutions, such as hospitals and corporate physician groups, rather than individual physicians, in final settlements in order to avoid reportable physician payments. This practice may be responsible for the unexpectedly lower number of medical malpractice reports to the NPDB. However, a study of physician medical malpractice claim settlements before and after implementation of the NPDB found that physicians and insurers were significantly less likely to settle claims since the introduction of the NPDB, especially those less than $50,000.

Future Implications

Given the current view that quality and safety in healthcare are the responsibility of the healthcare system rather than any single individual, the approach of the NPDB may be antiquated because it focuses on incompetent practitioners. However, at this point in time, a number of factors suggest that the NPDB plays an important ongoing role in quality assurance. While hospitals are required to query the NPDB when credentialing physicians, many hospitals routinely use the data bank, asking questions that are not required, as part of their credentialing process. It is also important to note that the ideal healthcare system is not yet attainable. Fragmentation and poor communication are and will remain a reality for many years to come, and information clearinghouses that facilitate the

flow of information in the presence of those deficiencies will continue to play an important role in safeguarding the interests of both patients and providers.

Teresa M. Waters and Peter P. Budetti

See also American Medical Association (AMA); Credentialing; Health Resources and Services Administration (HRSA); Malpractice; Medical Errors; Physicians; Quality of Healthcare

Further Readings

Sandstrom, Robert. "Malpractice by Physical Therapists: Descriptive Analysis of Reports in the National Practitioners Data Bank Public Use Data File, 1991–2004," *Journal of Allied Health* 36(4): 201–208, Winter 2007.

Waters, Teresa M., Peter P. Budetti, Gary Claxton, et al. "Impact of State Tort Reforms on Physician Malpractice Payments," *Health Affairs* 26(2): 500–509, March–April 2007.

West, Rebecca W., and Charles Y. Sipe. "National Practitioners Data Bank: Information on Physicians," *Journal of the American College of Radiology* 1(10): 777–79, October 2004.

Web Sites

National Practitioner Data Bank (NPDB): http://www.npdb-hipdb.hrsa.gov

NATIONAL QUALITY FORUM (NQF)

The National Quality Forum (NQF) is charged with planning, developing, establishing, and coordinating voluntary consensus standards for healthcare quality, measurement, and reporting through a formal, structured consensus development process. Located in Washington, D.C., the NQF is a private, nonprofit organization with open membership that represents a unique consortium of over 350 public and private healthcare-related organizations including federal agencies, healthcare providers, consumers/patients, purchasers, industry, and other stakeholders. In this capacity the NQF has significant influence over healthcare policy decisions made at the federal level.

Background

In 1996, President Clinton created the U.S. Advisory Commission on Consumer Protection and Quality in the Health Care Industry. The commission was given the broad charge of investigating the changes occurring in the nation's healthcare system and recommending measures to promote and ensure healthcare quality and value and protect consumers and workers in the healthcare system. In 1998, the commission's final report recommended the creation of a public-private forum for healthcare quality measurement and reporting to focus incentives for quality improvement on national priorities while ensuring the public availability of information needed to support the marketplace and oversight efforts. By May 1999, the Quality Forum Planning Committee had put in place the structure needed to establish the National Forum for Health Care Quality Measurement and Reporting, now known as the NQF, as a voluntary consensus standard-setting body. The NQF, empowered by the federal National Technology Transfer and Advancement Act of 1995 and the Office of Management and Budget (OMB) Circular A-119, sets standards for the U.S. Department of Health and Human Services (HHS), the Centers for Medicare and Medicaid Services (CMS), and the Agency for Healthcare Research and Quality (AHRQ).

Organizational Structure

The NQF is governed by a board of directors composed of individuals from its diverse membership. The NQF members are organized into various member councils including the following: consumer council; health plan council; health professional council; provider organization council; public/community health agency council; purchase council; quality measurement, research, and improvement council; and supplier/industry council. These councils contribute expertise to the development of standards and vote on the endorsement of national consensus standards.

Functions

The NQF's primary activities fall into three categories: (1) consensus development process; (2) national healthcare priority setting and other convening functions; and (3) leadership, education, and award activities. Each of the categories is discussed below.

Consensus Development Process

The consensus development process is the formal process the NQF uses to develop and endorse voluntary national consensus standards. Projects that undergo the consensus development process may be suggested by the NQF's members, member councils, staff, and board of directors or by external entities. These projects must be consistent with NQF priorities.

Specifically, the consensus development process consists of five steps: (1) consensus standard development; (2) widespread review; (3) member voting; (4) consensus standards approval committee action and the board of directors' endorsement; (5) and evaluation. At the initiation of the consensus development process, a steering committee is formed to oversee, advise, and ensure that input is obtained from relevant parties. Steering committees reflect the diversity of the NQF membership and may also include technical advisors as needed. The measure developer (or steward) assumes responsibility for submission of candidate standards and updates to endorsed standards and provides input as requested to the deliberations of the steering committee. An NQF project officer guides this process and acts as the liaison between the committee and the NQF.

The consensus standard development procedure results in draft recommendations that are based on those of the steering committee. They are reviewed, edited, and approved by the steering committee. And the steering committee must reach a consensus before the draft recommendations can proceed for further review, with all dissenting views documented. Explicit description of the scientific base for the draft recommendations is required. Widespread review begins with NQF member and public prevoting review of the draft recommendations. Members, member councils, and the public have the opportunity to comment prior to initiation of voting. Based on the comments of members and the general public, the NQF staff may revise the draft recommendations and circulate such revisions to the steering committee for additional review prior to preparing the recommendations for voting. All comments are made available to members when voting on the draft recommendations. All members are given the opportunity to vote on the draft recommendations. Members may approve the recommendations, propose modifications and/or conditions, or vote not to approve the recommendations. All results are then forwarded to the consensus standard approval committee for consideration. That committee may approve the standard or recommend a second round of voting. The board of directors will affirm or overturn the actions of the consensus standard approval committee. Recommendations endorsed by the board of directors are designated as NQF-endorsed consensus standards. Members and the public have the opportunity to appeal an endorsement, and an appeal will be given due process review by the appropriate committees. The board of directors will then act on the appeal by responding with a rationale for maintaining or repealing the endorsement. Since its inception, the NQF has endorsed over 200 consensus standards, ranging from adult diabetes to safe practices for better healthcare.

National Healthcare Priority Setting and Other Convening Functions

The NQF is involved in numerous priority-setting activities designed to improve the quality of healthcare in the nation. One example, establishing safe healthcare practices, includes efforts in therapeutic drug management, cancer care, substance abuse, and healthcare-associated infections. The NQF is also involved in setting priorities for public reporting improvement, payment strategies, information technology, and healthcare system performance. These efforts include examination of patient safety incidence classification, pay-for-performance, electronic medical records, and healthcare equity, effectiveness, and efficiency. To obtain key stakeholder and member input as well as to inform the public, the NQF convenes high-level meetings and conferences regularly.

Leadership, Education, and Award Activities

The NQF recognizes individuals and healthcare organizations that have significantly contributed to the improvement of quality and the safety of care. The NQF and *Modern Healthcare* acknowledge the exemplary performances that have effectively used performance measurements to drive change across various settings and times, fostered a transparent and accountable culture aimed at rebuilding the social contract between healthcare and the community, and increased the expected level of a health system's performance in the areas of quality and safety with the National Quality Healthcare Award. In collaboration with the Joint Commission, the NQF presents the John M. Eisenberg Patient Safety and Quality Award annually to individuals and healthcare organizations that have made significant contributions to enhancing patient safety through performing research and providing service reflective of patients' needs and perspectives. Honorees are acknowledged for individual achievement, research, advocacy, and system innovation at the organizational, local, regional, and national levels.

Future Implications

The NQF, recognized as one of the principal organizations for quality and safety improvement in the nation, endorses consensus-driven healthcare standards, and develops national strategies for healthcare improvement. Through these major areas, the NQF will likely continue to influence the nation's future healthcare policy and promote system improvement and consumer/patient understanding.

Gerard M. Castro

See also Clinical Practice Guidelines; Hospitals; Joint Commission; Medical Errors; Patient Safety; Public Policy; Quality Indicators; Quality of Healthcare

Further Readings

Ferrell, Betty, Steven R. Connor, Anne Cordes, et al. "The National Agenda for Quality Palliative Care: The National Consensus Project and the National Quality Forum," *Journal of Pain and Symptom Management* 33(6): 737–44, June 2007.

National Quality Forum. *Safe Practices for Better Healthcare 2006 Update: A Consensus Report.* Washington, DC: National Quality Forum, 2007.

National Quality Forum. "National Quality Forum Issues Brief: Strengthening Pediatric Quality Measurement and Reporting," *Journal of Healthcare Quality* 30(3): 51–5, May–June 2008.

U.S. Advisory Commission on Consumer Protection and Quality in the Health Care Industry. *Quality First: Better Health Care for All Americans: Final Report to the President of the United States.* Washington, DC: Government Printing Office, 1998.

Wakefield, Douglas S., Marcia W. Ward, Bonnie J. Wakefield, et al. "A 10-Rights Framework for Patient Care Quality and Safety," *American Journal of Medical Quality* 22(2): 103–111, March–April 2007.

Web Sites

National Quality Forum (NQF): http://www.qualityforum.org

U.S. Advisory Commission on Consumer Protection and Quality in the Health Care Industry: http://www.hcqualitycommission.gov

NAYLOR, C. DAVID

C. David Naylor is the president of the University of Toronto. He is an internationally recognized leader in the fields of health services research, evidence-based medicine, and health policy.

Naylor received a medical degree from the University of Toronto in 1978 with scholarships in medicine, surgery, and pediatrics. As a Rhodes Scholar at Oxford University in the Faculty of Social and Administrative Studies, he earned a doctoral degree in 1983. Subsequently, he trained in general internal medicine at the University of Western Ontario and then for a year in Toronto as a Medical Research Council of Canada (MRC) fellow in clinical epidemiology.

Prior to becoming the president of the University of Toronto, Naylor was the dean of medicine and Vice Provost of Relations With Health Care Institutions at the University of Toronto. Previously, he was a senior scientist of the Medical Research Council of Canada (MRC). Naylor also developed and led a research program in clinical epidemiology at the Sunnybrook Health Science Centre in Toronto and was responsible for developing the Institute for Clinical Evaluative Sciences, where he was the inaugural chief executive officer. In addition, he was one of the founding architects of Ontario's Cardiac Care Network.

Naylor has authored or coauthored over 300 publications in diverse fields such as social history, public policy, epidemiology, biostatistics, and health economics, as well as clinical and health services research in most fields of medicine. He has been the driving force behind developing a capacity for multidisciplinary health research in Canada and was on the national task force that established the framework for the Canadian Institutes of Health Research (CIHR). In 2003, Naylor chaired the National Advisory Committee on SARS and Public Health. This Committee's report led to the creation of the Public Health Agency of Canada, to increased commitments to public health at the national level, and to the appointment of Canada's first chief public health officer.

In addition to publishing frequently cited papers, Naylor has served on several editorial boards, including the *Journal of the American Medical Association*, the *British Medical Journal*, and the *Canadian Medical Association Journal*.

Naylor's service has been recognized through major national and international awards for research and leadership in medicine, including the John Dinham Cottrell medal by the Royal Australasian College of Physicians, the Malcolm Brown award by the Royal College of Physicians and Surgeons, the Michael Smith award by the Medical Research Council, and the Research Achievement award by the Canadian Cardiovascular Society. Most recently, he was appointed a fellow of the Royal Society of Canada.

Gregory S. Finlayson

See also Academic Medical Centers; Epidemiology; Evidence-Based Medicine (EBM); Health Services Research in Canada; Infectious Diseases; Public Health; Public Policy

Further Readings

Naylor, C. David. *Private Practice, Public Payment: Canadian Medicine and the Politics of Health*

Insurance, 1911–1966. Kingston, Ontario, Canada: McGill-Queen's University Press, 1986.

Naylor, C. David, ed. *Canadian Health Care and the State: A Century of Evolution.* Kingston, Ontario, Canada: McGill-Queen's University Press, 1992.

Naylor, C. David. "Grey Zones of Clinical Practice: Some Limits to Evidence-Based Medicine," *Lancet* 345(8953): 840–42, April 1, 1995.

Naylor, C. David. "Meta-Analysis and the Meta-Epidemiology of Clinical Research," *British Medical Journal* 315: 617–19, 1997.

Naylor, C. David. "Leadership in Academic Medicine: Reflections From Administrative Exile," *Clinical Medicine* (London) 6(5): 488–92, September–October 2006.

Naylor, C. David, Cyril Chantler, and Sian Griffiths. "Learning From SARS in Hong Kong and Toronto," *Journal of the American Medical Association* 291(20): 2483–87, May 26, 2004.

Web Sites

Canadian Institutes of Health Research (CIHR): http://www.cihr.ca

Institute for Clinical Evaluative Sciences (ICES): http://www.ices.on.ca

Public Health Agency of Canada (PHAC): http://www.phac-aspc.gc.ca/new_e.html

University of Toronto: http://www.utoronto.ca

NEWHOUSE, JOSEPH P.

Joseph P. Newhouse is a preeminent health economist. He has published extensively in the fields of health economics, health policy, and health services research. He also has trained many health economists.

Born in 1942 in Waterloo, Iowa, Newhouse earned a bachelor's degree and doctoral degree in economics from Harvard University. In 1963–1964, he was a Fulbright Scholar at the Johann Wolfgang von Goethe University at Frankfurt am Main in the Federal Republic of Germany.

Since the early 1970s, Newhouse has been a leading researcher, public servant, and scholar in health economics and health policy. He conceived and carried out significant, and in some cases unique, research projects; his research spans such diverse areas as health insurance incentives, healthcare payment systems, healthcare costs, health technology, risk adjustment, medical malpractice, and the impact of poor health habits. While at the RAND Corporation (1968–1988), he markedly expanded its health research and health policy expertise. Most notable was the RAND Health Insurance Experiment (HIE), one of the largest social science experiments in U.S. history. In leading the HIE, Newhouse oversaw an unprecedented research effort for more than 15 years. HIE papers, reports, and the definitive HIE summary *Free for All?* form the canonical basis for understanding healthcare demand and the response to insurance incentives, healthcare quality, and health outcomes in America.

Newhouse left the RAND Corporation and became a faculty member at Harvard University in 1988. As of 2007, he holds the ranks of John D. MacArthur Professor of Health Policy and Management (jointly in the Faculty of Arts and Sciences, Harvard Medical School, Harvard School of Public Health, and Kennedy School of Government); Director, Division of Health Policy Research and Education; and Director, Interfaculty Initiative on Health Policy. He created a doctoral program in health policy that exemplifies productive, collegial collaboration across the major schools at Harvard and that has trained more than 100 doctoral graduates now serving on university faculties, in public health agencies, and major health foundations.

Since 1966, Newhouse has authored or coauthored 350 publications (books, reports, and peer-reviewed journal articles). In 1981, Newhouse founded the *Journal of Health Economics,* an important economics journal. He continues to lead the editorial board, having edited more than 1,000 papers in the intervening years.

Newhouse has an extensive public service record. He has served as chair of the Prospective Payment Assessment Commission (ProPAC), commissioner of the Physician Payment Review Commission (PPRC), and vice chair of the Medicare Payment Advisory Commission (MedPAC). In 1977, he was elected to the national Institute of Medicine (IOM) and served two terms on the IOM governing council.

Newhouse has been the recipient of numerous awards, including the first David N. Kershaw

Award honoring persons under 40 years of age for distinguished contributions to public policy analysis and management (1983), the Baxter Health Services Research Prize and the Administrator's Citation from the U.S. Health Care Financing Administration (HCFA) (both in 1988), and the Distinguished Investigator Award from the professional association AcademyHealth (1992). He is a past president of the Association for Health Services Research (now AcademyHealth) and the International Health Economics Association, and he was the inaugural president of the American Society of Health Economics. He was elected fellow of the American Academy of Arts and Sciences (1995) and fellow of the American Association for the Advancement of Science (2002).

Kathleen N. Lohr

See also Health Economics; RAND Corporation; RAND Health Insurance Experiment (HIE)

Further Readings

Brennan, Troyen A., Lucian L. Leape, Nan M. Laird, et al. "Incidence of Adverse Events and Negligence in Hospitalized Patients: Findings from the Harvard Medical Practice Study 1," *New England Journal of Medicine* 324(6): 370–76, February 7, 1991.

Brook, Robert H., John E. Ware, William H. Rogers, et al. "Does Free Care Improve Adults' Health? Results from a Randomized Control Trial," *New England Journal of Medicine* 309(23): 1426–34, December 8, 1983.

Cutler, David M., Mark B. McClellan, and Joseph P. Newhouse. "How Does Managed Care Do It?" *RAND Journal of Economics* 31(3): 526–48, Autumn 2000.

Cutler, David M., Mark B. McClellan, Joseph P. Newhouse, et al. "Are Medical Prices Declining?" *Quarterly Journal of Economics* 113(4): 991–1024, 1998.

Hsu, John T., Maggie Price, Jie Huang, et al. "Unintended Consequences of Medicare Drug Benefit Caps," *New England Journal of Medicine* 354(22): 2349–59, June 1, 2006.

Leape, Lucian L., Troyen A. Brennan, Nan M. Laird, et al. "The Nature of Adverse Events in Hospitalized Patients: Findings From the Harvard Medical Practice Study II," *New England Journal of Medicine* 324(6): 377–84, February 7, 1991.

Manning, Willard G., Emmett B. Keeler, Joseph P. Newhouse, et al. "The Taxes of Sin: Do Smokers and Drinkers Pay Their Way?" *Journal of the American Medical Association* 261(11): 1604–1609, March 17, 1989.

McClellan, Mark B., Barbara J. McNeil, and Joseph P. Newhouse. "Does More Intensive Treatment of Acute Myocardial Infarction Reduce Mortality?" *Journal of the American Medical Association* 272(11): 859–66, September 21, 1994.

Newhouse, Joseph P. *Pricing the Priceless: A Health Care Conundrum.* Cambridge: MIT Press, 2002.

Newhouse, Joseph P., and the Insurance Experiment Group. *Free for All? Lessons from the RAND Health Insurance Experiment.* Cambridge, MA: Harvard University Press, 1993.

Newhouse, Joseph P., Willard G. Manning, Carl N. Morris, et al. "Some Interim Results From a Controlled Trial of Cost Sharing in Health Insurance," *New England Journal of Medicine* 305(25): 1501–1507, December 17, 1981.

Web Sites

Harvard Medical School, Department of Health Care Policy: http://www.hcp.med.harvard.edu

Harvard School of Public Health, Department of Health Policy and Management: www.hsph.harvard.edu/departments/health-policy-and-management

Harvard University, John F. Kennedy School of Government: http://www.ksg.harvard.edu

NIGHTINGALE, FLORENCE

Florence Nightingale (1820–1910) was responsible for professionalizing nursing. She also was a sanitarian, a hospital administrator, and an early biostatistician. Born in Florence, Italy, in 1820, to a wealthy British couple, Nightingale grew up in England. She became well educated for a woman of those times. As a young woman, Nightingale had a calling from God asking her to do His work, though she did not discover His plan until years later. As a result of her interest in then current social issues, she began to visit the homes of the sick in villages near her home. While a woman of means would never become a nurse, on a tour in Europe, she visited a Prussian hospital and school for deaconesses in 1846. She later returned to train as a nurse, subsequently becoming, in 1853, the unpaid superintendent of a London establishment for sick gentlewomen.

The Crimean War broke out in 1854; reports criticizing the British medical facilities for the wounded resulted in her appointment to officially introduce female nurses into the military hospitals in Turkey. Although the physicians did not initially welcome her and her nurses, the women's skills were quickly appreciated. Nightingale's actions improved both the sanitary and emotional status of the wounded soldiers. Under her administration, the mortality rate of patients in the hospital decreased significantly. Her rule that she should be the only nurse in the wards at night earned her the title of the "Lady With the Lamp." Nightingale performed statistical analyses of disease and mortality. She ultimately became the general superintendent of the Female Nursing Establishment of the Military Hospitals of the Army.

Nightingale returned from the Crimean War in August 1856, soon participating in the creation of the Royal Commission on the Health of the Army. She contributed information in the form of her *Notes on Matters Affecting the Health, Efficiency, and Hospital Administration of the British Army, Founded Chiefly on the Experience of the Late War. Presented by Request to the Secretary of State for War.*

Nightingale was committed to the use of statistics, which she employed to support her ideas on healthcare and public health. She worked with the British statistician William Farr. As a result of her statistical accomplishments, she became the first woman to be elected as a fellow of the Royal Statistical Society, in 1858.

Perhaps Nightingale's greatest achievement is her elevation of the status of nursing: It became a respectable profession for women. In 1860, she established a nursing school at London's St. Thomas' Hospital. Nurses, trained in her program, worked in staff hospitals throughout Britain and abroad, establishing nursing training schools using her model.

Nightingale was an advocate of the pavilion style of hospitals: completely detached pavilions, separating medical pathologies, to prevent the spread of diseases. Her *Notes on Nursing* was first published in 1860; its latest printing was in 1992.

She campaigned to improve health standards, writing extensively on the subject. Queen Victoria awarded her the Royal Red Cross in 1883. Nightingale became the first woman to receive the Order of Merit in 1907. She died at the age of 90 in 1910.

Rosemary Walker

See also Epidemiology; Farr, William; Health Services Research, Origins; Hospitals; Nurse Practitioners (NPs) Nurses; Public Health; Quality of Healthcare

Further Readings

Dossey, Barbara Montgomery. *Florence Nightingale: Mystic, Visionary, Healer.* Philadelphia: Lippincott Williams and Wilkins, 2000.

Kudzma, Elizabeth Connelly. "Florence Nightingale and Healthcare Reform," *Nursing Science Quarterly* 19(1): 61–64, January 2006.

McDonald, Lynn, ed. *Florence Nightingale: An Introduction to Her Life and Family.* Waterloo, Ontario, Canada: Wilfred Laurier University Press, 2002.

Miracle, Vickie A. "The Life and Impact of Florence Nightingale," *Dimensions of Critical Care Nursing* 27(1): 21–23, January–February 2008.

Nightingale, Florence. *Notes on Nursing: What It Is and What It Is Not.* Philadelphia: Lippincott Williams and Wilkins, 1992.

Web Sites

Florence Nightingale International Foundation (FNIF): http://www.fnif.org/nightingale.htm

Florence Nightingale Museum: http://www.florence-nightingale.co.uk

NONPROFIT HEALTHCARE ORGANIZATIONS

A nonprofit healthcare organization is legally structured as a not-for-profit corporation and is prohibited from distributing profits to its owners, members, or other individuals with oversight for the organization. Nonprofits have a charitable mission related to the provision of healthcare services, teaching, research, and/or community service, and they are legally required to work towards the mission. These organizations are owned by their "community," which may be a religiously affiliated or unaffiliated community or other nongovernmental association. Nonprofit hospitals are the dominant type of hospital ownership in the United States. Other types of healthcare organizations may also be organized as nonprofits, including long-term care facilities and health plans. Only a small percentage of the nation's nursing homes are nonprofit, with the majority being proprietary or for-profit organizations.

Characteristics

Several characteristics conceptually differentiate nonprofit from other types of ownership, particularly for-profit healthcare organizations, including the primary stakeholders of these entities, the benefits of tax-exempt status, their sources of capital, and the provision of community benefits.

Ownership

A nonprofit healthcare organization is owned by its community, meaning that it is owned by a community or other nongovernmental association, such as a church or fraternal organization, and is governed by a voluntary, self-perpetuating board. Nonprofits may or may not be religiously affiliated. This is distinct from a for-profit healthcare organization, which is owned by its shareholders and governed by an elected board, and from a public hospital, which is owned by the federal, state, or local government and, in the case of federal and state-owned hospitals, principally serves selected populations (e.g., military) or, as in the case of local, government-owned hospitals, often serves the indigent. While for-profit organizations distribute their profits back to their shareholders, nonprofit organizations are prohibited from distributing profits to those who control the organization, although incentive-based compensation for organization leaders is common. Profits are implicitly reinvested into the organization's community—through enhanced services, new plant and equipment, or other initiatives that provide a community benefit.

Tax-Exempt Status

As tax-exempt entities, nonprofit healthcare organizations are expected to provide community benefits, commonly achieved through charity care, education and training, research, and/or community service. Tax-exempt status means that the organization is exempt from paying federal, state, and local taxes, including income, sales, and property taxes. In addition to being exempt from taxes, a nonprofit organization may use tax-exempt bond financing, which lowers its cost of capital investments. Nonprofit organizations have the advantage of being exempt from paying income taxes on interest income generated from tax-exempt bonds. Nonprofits may accept charitable donations, and donors may deduct these charitable contributions. From the federal perspective, a healthcare organization qualifies under Section 501(c)(3) of the Internal Revenue Service (IRS) tax code in the United States. Nonprofit organizations must also meet state requirements for nonprofit entities to receive a state income tax exemption as well as local requirements for local sales and property tax exemptions. These requirements vary by state and are often more stringent than federal requirements.

Sources of Capital

Nonprofit healthcare organizations rely on several primary sources for capital. These include charitable contributions, which are tax deductible by the donor, debt, retained earnings, and government grants. Having a tax-exempt status provides nonprofits with the opportunity to use tax-exempt debt as one mechanism to finance capital investments. For-profit organizations use retained earnings and debt to fund capital investments, but they also use equity capital from investors and return-on-equity payments from third-party payers.

Community Benefit

Although the provision of community benefit is the linchpin of qualifying as a nonprofit healthcare organization, there is no unambiguous definition of what community benefit entails, how it should be measured, or what qualifies as a sufficient amount in terms of measuring whether a nonprofit organization meets its community benefit obligations. Community benefit is generally considered to include services that are unprofitable but provide an important contribution to the community. Uncompensated care, Medicaid-covered services, and certain unprofitable service lines are considered to be community benefit. Uncompensated care is composed of charity care and bad debt. Charity care includes services that are provided but for which the provider does not expect a payment. Generally, the decision about whether services qualify as charity care is made prospectively or as early in the delivery of care as possible when a prospective decision is not feasible. The provider does not bill the patient or insurer, nor does the provider pursue collection of payment from an external source. Hospitals often use a sliding scale based on income to determine whether an individual is eligible for charity care and, if so, the amount of the discount. In addition, hospitals may use an asset test to determine eligibility. Bad debt, on the other hand, is care for which payment is expected to be collected by either the patient or the insurer but is ultimately not paid. Hospitals make an effort to collect these payments using internal and/or external collections processes. Some argue against the inclusion of bad debt as uncompensated care, because organizations make an active attempt to collect payment from the patient and/or insurer and, after a sufficient amount of time, elect to write off the uncollectible amount.

Medicaid-covered services are classified as a community benefit, because reimbursement from state Medicaid programs is often below the cost of providing the care. In addition, certain unprofitable services lines, such as the emergency department, high-level trauma, and labor and delivery, are considered as community benefits. Most nonprofit hospitals also provide additional community outreach programs, such as community health screenings, health education programs, immunizations, and community health assessments of unmet needs. Research that generates findings available to the community may also be included as a community benefit.

The valuation of community benefit is highly variable across organizations. No consistent guidelines exist for how to quantify or report the dollar value of these benefits. While nonprofit organizations may report a dollar amount of community benefit, cross-institution comparisons would be questionable—reports of community benefit may, for example, value charity care based on the charges for care provided to these patients, even though charges reflect neither the organization's costs nor expected payments. Organizations may or may not include bad debt and losses from services provided to Medicare and Medicaid patients.

Comparison of For-Profit and Nonprofit Organizations

The fundamental structure of nonprofits suggests that these organizations should behave in a manner that differs from for-profit entities. The charitable mission—to provide a community benefit—of a nonprofit differs from that of a for-profit, whose implicit or explicit mission is to increase the wealth of its shareholders. The difference in missions suggests that nonprofit organizations should provide more services to the community in which they reside. In addition, because of the shareholder-driven mission, for-profits conceptually have a greater incentive to provide more and more profitable services than their nonprofit counterparts, which may mean providing fewer unprofitable services and serving fewer indigent patients.

From a practical perspective, whether for-profit and nonprofit healthcare organizations are intrinsically different has long been debated. Some argue that the economic incentives inherent in the distribution of profits to shareholders are vastly different from the incentives for organizations that do not answer to shareholders. Others maintain that the ultimate motivation of both types of organizations is similar—both strive to maximize earnings over expenses (i.e., accounting profits) and must meet the needs of the patient to remain profitable and, therefore, should be expected to behave similarly. In addition, the lines between nonprofits and for-profits have blurred, due to relationships between the two.

Importance of Profit

Regardless of the type of organization, both for-profits and nonprofits must earn a profit or surplus in the long run to remain financially viable. To achieve this goal, both types of organizations must respond to their community's needs and provide high-quality care. While for-profits return a portion of their profits to shareholders, they must also make investments in their organizations to remain competitive. Likewise, nonprofits could not achieve their missions without earning profits for future investments to remain competitive.

Hybridization of Ownership Type

While some organizations are purely nonprofit or for profit, others may have elements of both within the same corporation. Examples include a nonprofit organization owning a for-profit subsidiary; a nonprofit organization contracting with a for-profit organization to provide specific services, as when a community hospital contracts with a for-profit anesthesiology group to provide anesthesiology coverage in the surgical suite; and joint ventures between nonprofit and for-profit organizations.

Efficiency

While some claim that for-profits provide less efficient care, in terms of either providing more services and more expensive care than needed or charging prices that are disproportionately higher than costs compared with nonprofits, others argue that for-profits are more efficient because of their underlying mission to generate a profit for shareholders. Systematic evidence comparing the quality of care among nonprofit and for-profit hospitals does not exist, however, to support these claims.

Quality of Care

It has been argued that for-profits provide lower quality of care than their non-profit counterparts. However, there is little consistent evidence to support this claim. While some studies have found higher quality of care in nonprofit hospitals, other studies have found no difference or higher quality in for-profits.

Uncompensated Care

Research has been mixed on whether nonprofit organizations provide more uncompensated care than their for-profit counterparts. Some studies have found that provision of uncompensated care is greater among nonprofits, while other studies

have found no significant difference. Studies of nonprofit to for-profit hospital conversions have suggested that those converting to for-profit entities do not change their level of uncompensated care provided to the community.

The Future of Nonprofit Healthcare

In recent years, nonprofit hospitals have been under increased scrutiny to explicitly quantify their benefit to the community. Two findings have led federal and state governments to investigate whether nonprofits are meeting their community benefit obligations. First, evidence has suggested that nonprofit and for-profit hospitals provide similar levels of uncompensated care, calling into question the marginal contributions that nonprofits make to the community, which are required to qualify for tax-exempt status, and whether their marginal contribution is equivalent to the tax benefits they receive from possessing tax-exempt status. Second, because insurers negotiate payment rates with hospitals that are lower than those charged by the hospitals, uninsured individuals have often been obligated to pay more for care than otherwise similar individuals with insurance. Coupled with this issue, there have been complaints about aggressive debt collection practices by nonprofit hospitals that contradict the organizations' charitable mission. Nonprofit hospitals' billing and collection processes have been questioned in light of these organizations' tax-exempt status.

States have implemented a variety of requirements for nonprofit hospitals, in particular to ensure that they are meeting their community benefit obligations. State-mandated methods of demonstrating community benefit include the requirement of a written charity care policy that is accessible to patients; mandating a minimum threshold for the value of community benefit as a percentage of net patient revenue or operating revenue; mandating that community benefit is at least equivalent to the value of the tax-exempt benefits received by the hospital; and routine documentation of the hospital's community benefit contributions. As hospital competition continues, nonprofit and for-profit hospitals will increasingly become less differentiated. The need for nonprofit hospitals to be price, quality, and outcomes competitive with for-profit hospitals will also continue. These organizations will need to justify their benefits to the community while at the same time providing care that is both of high quality and efficient.

Tricia J. Johnson

See also Charity Care; For-Profit Versus Not-For-Profit Healthcare; Hospitals; Multihospital Healthcare Systems; Nursing Homes; Regulation; Uncompensated Healthcare; Uninsured Individuals

Further Readings

Alexander, Jeffrey A., and Shoou-Yih D. Lee. "Does Governance Matter? Board Configuration and Performance in Not-for-Profit Hospitals," *Milbank Quarterly* 84(4): 733–58, December 2006.

Congressional Budget Office. *Nonprofit Hospitals and the Provision of Community Benefits.* Pub. No. 2707. Washington, DC: Congressional Budget Office, 2006.

Cutler, David M. *The Changing Hospital Industry: Comparing Not-for-Profit and For-Profit Institutions.* Chicago: University of Chicago Press, 2000.

Peregrine, Michael W. "IRS Increases Emphasis on Not-for-Profit Health Care," *Healthcare Financial Management* 61(8): 72–6, August 2007.

Potter, Sharyn J. *Can Efficiency and Community Service Be Symbiotic?: A Longitudinal Analysis of Not-for-Profit- and For-Profit Hospitals in the United States.* New York: Garland, 2000.

Salinsky, Eileen. "What Have You Done for Me Lately? Assessing Hospital Community Benefit," *Issue Brief No. 821.* Washington, DC: George Washington University, National Health Policy Forum, 2007.

Santerre, Rexford E., and John A. Vernon. "Ownership Form and Consumer Welfare: Evidence From the Nursing Home Industry," *Inquiry* 44(4): 381–99, Winter 2007–2008.

Web Sites

Alliance for Advancing Nonprofit Health Care: http://www.nonprofithealthcare.org

American Hospital Association (AHA): http://www.aha.org

Catholic Health Association of the United States (CHA): http://www.chausa.org

Internal Revenue Service (IRS): http://www.irs.gov/publications/p557/ch03.html

National Association of Community Health Centers (NACHC): http://www.nachc.com

NURSE PRACTITIONERS (NPs)

Nurse practitioners (NPs) are nonphysician clinicians who are nurses with graduate degrees in advanced-practice nursing. The primary function of nurse practitioners is to promote wellness through patient health education. Their role has expanded to include the following: taking patients' comprehensive health histories, performing physical examinations, ordering laboratory tests and procedures, and formulating and managing care regimens for acutely and chronically ill patients. Nurse practitioners work in a variety of settings, including physician offices, clinics, hospitals, and nursing home facilities. In 2008, there were about 160,000 nurse practitioners in the United States.

History

The nurse practitioner movement began in the United States in the mid-1960s, with the preparation of pediatric nurse practitioners at the University of Colorado. Initially, the profession was developed in response to a shortage of physicians, especially in rural areas where healthcare access was limited. Over time, other states also began nurse practitioner training programs, and their role in healthcare greatly expanded. Today, nurse practitioners are integral to all kinds of practices, including those located in underserved, rural, and inner-city areas and in private collaborations, independent practices, hospitals, and continuing care and nursing home facilities. Additionally, other countries such as the United Kingdom, Canada, Australia, and New Zealand have embraced nurse practitioners.

Clinical Roles

The most significant clinical role of nurse practitioners relates to their professional efficacy and autonomy in practice. They can diagnose, treat, prescribe medications, order diagnostic testing, and refer patients to other healthcare professionals. Nurse practitioners monitor and adopt evidence-based practice and bring the framework of prevention, early intervention, and patient/family health education into their work. In the United States and other countries, nurse practitioners have a specific license for practice. In the United States, most such licenses are granted and supervised by a state's board of nursing. This licensing distinguishes nurse practitioners from physicians' assistants, who typically practice under direct supervision of physicians and whose practices are authorized by a state's board of medicine.

While nurse practitioners can and often do work independently, most have collaborating physicians who review cases and provide ongoing consultation. The nursing board in a particular state may or may not require the existence of a relationship with a physician colleague. However, most advanced-practice nurses and physicians alike find the relationship stimulating and informative. The teamwork nature of such collaboration often is visible in primary-care practices or hospital specialty services, where physicians and nurse practitioners work in the same setting. Patient satisfaction and patient outcomes in these collaborative practices are similar to or better than in many traditional, physician-only practices.

Preparation

Nurse practitioners are prepared at the master's level or beyond. The educational programs are designed to make the graduate eligible for certification as a nurse practitioner in a specific area, such as care of families, children, or adults, in psychiatry, or in women's health. Certification is gained by completing the requisite educational program and passing an examination offered by specific certifying bodies. These entities are generally associated with a specific practice, such as midwifery. A significant educational requirement is actual practice under the close supervision of a licensed and certified nurse practitioner, with a minimum of 1 year of practice, or a physician. Four hundred or more hours of such practice are required. Some specialties require additional training, such as working with a minimum number of mothers in childbirth to qualify in midwifery.

Practice Standards

The American Academy of Nurse Practitioners (AANP) defines the standards of practice for nurse practitioners and updates or revises them periodically. The eight standards defining the framework for nurse practitioners are as follows: (1) the process of care, including assessment of health status, diagnosis, development of a treatment plan, implementation of the plan, and follow-up evaluation of the patient; (2) care priorities, including patient and family education, provision of competent care, facilitation of entry into the healthcare system, and a safe environment; (3) interdisciplinary and collaborative responsibilities as a member of the healthcare team; (4) accurate documentation; (5) patient advocacy; (6) quality assurance and continued competence; (7) adjunct roles, including mentor, educator, researcher, manager, and consultant; and (8) research as a basis for practice. These standards reflect an origin in the general practice of nursing. Nurse practitioners do not replace nurses in practice settings. Rather, nurses and nurse practitioners provide a broadened skill mix from which to serve patients.

Doctorate in Nursing Practice

From the comprehensive nature of these standards, nursing educators realized that the depth and extent of preparation warranted redefining the earned education credential as a practice doctorate similar to that given in other professions, such as pharmacy, medicine, and dentistry.

The American Association of Colleges of Nursing (AACN) approved a policy statement saying that the doctor of nursing practice (DNP) degree be required for entry into nursing practice as an advanced practice nurse by 2015. With this policy statement, the AACN outlined the eight essential elements of doctoral education for advanced practice nurses. These elements include (1) the scientific underpinnings for practice, (2) organizational and systems leadership for quality improvement and systems thinking, (3) clinical scholarship and analytical methods for evidence-based practice, (4) information systems/technology and patient care technology for the improvement and transformation of healthcare, (5) healthcare policy for advocacy in healthcare, (6) interprofessional collaboration for improving patient and population health outcomes, (7) clinical prevention and population health for improving the nation's health, (8) and advanced nursing practice.

Disadvantages of the requirement of the DPN degree may include the increased costs to the students due to longer programs of study. There is a nationwide shortage of faculty in nursing schools. Initially, the costs of educating DNP degree students by doctorate of philosophy (PhD)–prepared faculty may prove challenging, but the growing numbers of DNP graduates will quickly offset this shortage. Finally, the costs to the nation's healthcare system may be increased by DNPs who command higher salaries than current nurse practitioners. The additional preparation, however, should bring additional clinical leadership and skills to ensure that the latest scientific findings are readily translated into patient services.

Future Implications

While licensed independently, nurse practitioners only recently gained legal authority to bill separately from physicians. A provision in the federal Balanced Budget Act of 1997 states that nurse practitioners can receive direct Medicare Part B reimbursement, which is 85% of the physician rate. Prior to this legislation, nurse practitioners had to file under a physician's Medicare provider number. Some private insurance companies, however, did not follow the change in Medicare regulations and do not allow nurse practitioners to seek payment under their own provider number. Variations also exist among state Medicaid programs. California, for example, authorized nurse practitioners to bill its Medicaid program, Medi-Cal, directly, and be reimbursed at 100% of the physician reimbursement rate.

Many areas of the nation are expanding the role of nurse practitioners. As of 2006, all 50 states have awarded nurse practitioners prescription authority, with varying limitations. Many states also include controlled substances among the medications nurse practitioners can prescribe.

Because they possess independent licenses, nurse practitioners are viewed as challenges to healthcare quality by some groups, most notably the American Medical Association (AMA). The AMA's concern is that nurse practitioners do not have the same preparation as physicians and should, therefore, be closely supervised. State legislatures, where efforts to shape nurse practitioner practices are revisited often, can reflect this tension. An area of

typical concern is the authority of nurse practitioners to prescribe medications. While all states have authorized them to write prescriptions, this authority was approved on a state-by-state basis. Florida also has restrictions on the number and types of nurse practitioner-managed offices that physicians may supervise, and other states may choose to follow this example.

Anne R. Bavier

See also American Association of Colleges of Nursing (AACN); American Nurses Association (ANA); Hospitals; Medicare; National Institutes of Health (NIH); Nurses; Quality of Healthcare

Further Readings

American Nurses Credentialing Center. *A Role Delineation Study of Seven Nurse Practitioner Specialties*. Silver Spring, MD: American Nurses Credentialing Center, 2004.

Buppert, Carolyn. *Nurse Practitioner's Business Practice and Legal Guide*. 3d ed. Sudbury, MA: Jones and Bartlett, 2008.

Chase, Susan K. *Clinical Judgment and Communication in Nurse Practitioner Practice*. Philadelphia: F. A. Davis, 2004.

Fairman, Julie. *Making Room in the Clinic: Nurse Practitioners and the Evolution of Modern Health Care*. New Brunswick, NJ: Rutgers University Press, 2008.

Mezey, Mathy B., Diane O. McGivern, Eileen M. Sullivan-Marx, et al., eds. *Nurse Practitioners: Evolution of Advanced Practice*. 4th ed. New York: Springer, 2003.

Web Sites

American Academy of Nurse Practitioners (AANP): http://www.aanp.org

American Association of Colleges of Nursing (AACN): http://www.aacn.nche.edu

American Nursing Association (ANA): http://www.nursingworld.org

NURSES

Nurses are an integral part of the nation's healthcare system, providing treatment and care to ill or injured patients. There are currently more than 2.9 million nurses in the United States, which includes registered nurses (RNs), licensed practical nurses (LPNs), nurse practitioners (NPs), and others. While the definitions and theories about the field of nursing continue to grow and change, the role of the nurse remains vital for medical care.

History

The modern term *nurse* is derived from the Latin word *nutrire*, meaning to nourish or nurture. Florence Nightingale (1820–1910) is considered the founder of modern nursing. Recent analysis of Nightingale's letters to the Sisters of Mercy, who accompanied her to battlefields in the Crimea, reveal that she was greatly influenced by these religious women, who provided crucial skills in organizing and implementing care for the injured and wounded. On her return to England, Nightingale used this experience and knowledge to become a clear advocate for patient care, specifically the kind done by nurses. In 1859, Nightingale articulated the defining characteristic of nursing knowledge as "putting the constitution in such a state as it will have no disease," or that it can recover from disease. She provided the profession significant public respect at a time when nurses were viewed as untrained and incompetent. After the Crimean War, around 1856, the public view of nursing evolved from the negative portrayal to that of an angel of mercy, largely due to Nightingale's influence.

The image of nursing continued to form and re-form. Today, nurses are largely viewed as careerists. During the 1920s, nurses were often viewed as women whose priorities were romance, marriage, and motherhood. By the end of World War II, however, nurses were seen as heroines and professionals. This portrayal soon reverted to a "sex object" image, where nurses were seen as women who were satisfying the needs of men and male physicians. The careerist image, however, began to compete with the "sex object" image throughout the mid-1960s and into the 1980s, when it finally became predominant.

Contemporary Definition of Nursing

Virginia Henderson (1897–1996), another pioneer in nursing, was dedicated to the scientific knowledge that underpins the practice. Her view was bolstered by her singular focus to catalog relevant information from all disciplines. She and her colleagues accomplished this work long before computerized databases or nursing and allied health indexes existed. She defined nursing for practitioners worldwide as assisting individuals, sick or well, in the performance of those activities contributing to health or its recovery (or a peaceful death) that they would perform unaided if they had the necessary strength, will, or knowledge, and to do this in such a way as to help them gain independence as rapidly as possible. Henderson's definition embraces the concept that nurses meet patients wherever they are on a health, illness, and death continuum. It resonated with nurses worldwide, resulting in many translations of her work. Single-handedly, Henderson stimulated the international recognition of the common threads that join all nurses.

Struggle to Advance the Science of Nursing Practice

Continuing Henderson's work, early nursing scholars based their science on social, biological, and medical sciences. Yet they remained challenged to articulate what was specific to the practice of nursing. Beginning in the 1950s, the scholars in nursing began to develop and disseminate various nursing models. In particular, efforts were aimed at theory development so that nursing could develop specific evidence to guide its practice. Interestingly, most of the nursing research conducted into the mid-1980s focused on the individuals who were either nurses or nursing students, not on the nursing actions they performed. This approach changed dramatically after 1986, when the U.S. Congress created the National Center for Nursing Research within the National Institutes of Health (NIH). Nursing research then became part of the largest biomedical science entity in the nation. NIH funds support rigorous scientific efforts to promote the understanding of what happens to patients, without regard for the characteristics of the provider. Financial support of investigations of nursing workforce issues remained in other parts of the U.S. Department of Health and Human Services (HHS), such as the Agency for Healthcare Research and Quality

(AHRQ) and the Health Resources and Services Administration's Bureau of Health Professions (BHPr).

Nursing Theories

The nursing conceptual models describe the interrelationship of concepts and the application of theory to identify, analyze, interpret, and evaluate client-based interventions and outcomes. Four concepts appear in most nursing theories or models: the person, the environment, the nurse, and health. These theories are generally classified as middle-range or practice theories. This remains a major descriptor of nursing theories today. A thorough review of nursing theories demonstrates the continuing impact of other health disciplines, with reliance on developmental scholars, such as Helen Erikson and Abraham Maslow, and the behavioral and sociocultural sciences.

Dorothy Johnson's Behavioral System Model, established in 1959, focuses on common human needs, care and comfort, and stress and tension reduction. In 1964, Imogene King's Systems Framework, on the other hand, examined personal, interpersonal, and social systems. Myra Levine sought the need to move nursing away from the medical model and, in 1996, developed her Conservation Model, which focuses on adaptation as a means to preserve the integrity and wholeness of the person. Levine's work often is used in combination with standardized nursing nomenclatures, such as the Nursing Intervention Classification, to capture the practical benefits of this model. The Betty Neuman Systems Model, developed in 1972, also includes the concepts of adaptation, client holism, and stress in the client environment.

Dorthea Orem began developing her theory in the 1950s and formally presented her Self Care Model in 1970. The theory focused on nursing practice to move patients toward independence. That same year, Martha Rogers presented her theory of the Science of Unitary Human Being, which is not built on causality but is congruent with an action worldview. Another product of the 1970s was the Sister Callista Roy Adaptation Model, which concentrates on the adaptation processes of individuals, families, and groups.

Contemporary Nurses and Nursing

The contemporary nurse is a well-educated professional, either male or female. With more than 2.9 million nurses in the United States, RNs are the largest constituent of the nation's healthcare professions. Nursing distinguishes itself with a holistic focus on the patient and families and attention to actual or potential health problems. Nurses meet healthcare needs in virtually all settings, with more than half employed in hospitals, followed by community and public health centers, ambulatory care, nursing homes, and nursing education. Today's nurse uses assessment skills to diagnose a patient's response to illness and potential health conditions or needs and then develops an individualized plan of care. Nurses also collaborate with other healthcare professionals. A rich lexicon of nursing diagnoses and evidence supports professional nursing practice. The professional nurse continuously evaluates and modifies the patient's care plan and adjusts interventions to achieve the best possible outcomes.

Current Nursing Shortage

The United States currently faces a major crisis in nursing—the shortage of nurses presently and the increasing shortage predicted in the next 25 years. This shortage began in the late 1990s and is unlike previous shortages. Historically, classic principles of supply and demand mediated the crisis. Employers made economic and other enticements to make nursing a more desirable profession, and educational institutions increased enrollments to meet the demand. However, multiple factors make the current shortage different from those experienced in the past.

Not only is the nation's general population aging, but the nursing workforce itself is aging as well. Data from the 2004 National Sample Survey of Registered Nurses indicate that the population of nurses is aging quickly. For example, the average age of nurses in the nation is 46.8 years, with approximately 41% over 50 years of age. Only 8% are less than 30 years of age. It is anticipated that there will be more than 1 million RN vacancies by 2010. From 2000 through 2004, the average age of graduating nurses was 32.6 years, in contrast to 27.8 years in 1984. In sum, the current nursing population is aging, and those who enter the field are older than before. Clearly, there is a pressing need to expand the pipeline of those entering the nursing profession, especially at a younger age. The potential for women to enter the historically male-dominated professions, such as medicine and other fields, has changed nursing demographics and presents a challenge to increasing the number of nurses.

Nursing school leaders indicate that a national faculty shortage is the major reason that more than 32,000 qualified applicants are not enrolled annually. Nursing faculty are on average 55 years of age or older, with 20% anticipating retirement in the next 10 years. Competition for clinical placement sites and space in general science laboratory courses compounds the difficulties faced by academic administrators as they attempt to expand enrollment.

Changes in the nation's healthcare delivery system have shifted most medical care from hospitals to outpatient settings. Those patients who are admitted to hospitals today experience illness intensities comparable with those in intensive-care units less than 50 years ago. Multiple societal factors, such as major changes to how Medicare calculates reimbursements to hospitals, converged to create new strategies for cost containment and control throughout healthcare, especially in hospitals. As nurses are the largest component of most hospitals' personnel expenditures, multiple approaches were undertaken to shift from an expensive, intensive RN workforce to less expensive and less well-educated personnel.

Nurses and other healthcare workers became alarmed at the diminishing quality of care associated with the decreasing numbers of nurses directing patient care. In some states, such as California, nurses successfully lobbied for state laws that specify the ratio of nurses to patients. Other advocates, such as the national Institute of Medicine (IOM), called for systematic and systemic efforts to manage patient care and decrease medical errors. Health services researchers have examined patient outcomes in relation to the preparation of the nursing staff. These studies documented better outcomes when patient care is directed by nurses with a baccalaureate or higher degree. Seminal work supported by the American

Academy of Nursing (AAN) aimed to identify the characteristics of hospitals associated with best practices, and strong patient outcomes were identified. Now, those hospitals can become designated as Magnet Hospitals, through the American Nurses Credentialing Center. The designation is awarded by examining both qualitative and quantitative evidence of meeting 65 standards that define the highest quality of nursing practice and patient care.

Another strategy to overcome the nation's shortage of nurses is to recruit and retain nurses who were educated in other countries. The number of foreign nurses in the United States totaled approximately 90,000 in 2004, and they were most common in California, Florida, New York, Texas, New Jersey, and Illinois. In some countries, such as the Philippines, there is a deliberate effort to prepare individuals to work in their native country as well as in the United States. In general, nurses are lured from poor nations by the promise of higher wages. However, such migration patterns can deplete nations of their own healthcare workforce.

Nursing Education

Early nursing education began as informal conferences and lecture-style training by physicians to nursing students in hospital-based programs. The nation's first formal nursing school was established in 1872 at the New England Hospital for Women and Children in Boston. Using Nightingale's model of nursing preparation, other schools were soon established, including the New York Training School at Bellevue Hospital, the Connecticut Training School for Nurses, and the Boston Training School for Nurses at Massachusetts General Hospital.

Hospital-based nursing training programs used the apprenticeship model in awarding the graduate a diploma. In the middle of the 20th century, there was a shift from the diploma program to college or university preparation, with the introduction of the 2-year associate degree. Many hospital-based nursing programs were shortened from 3 to 2 years to compete, but eventually most closed or merged into academic programs. In 2006, diploma programs made up only 4% of all the basic RN education programs in the nation.

In 1952, the associate degree in nursing was developed at Teacher's College, Columbia University in New York. To alleviate the nursing shortage of that time, this degree was designed to prepare technical nurses in 2 years. Typically, associate-degree nursing programs are offered at community or technical colleges. Graduates may take the RN licensure examination, because they are taught nursing theories and have gained practical and technical experience and skills. In 2005, associate-degree programs made up 58.9% of all U.S. basic nursing education programs. The increased demand for nurses is felt keenly at the community college level, where waiting lists for admission may have more than 1,000 individuals for 60 openings.

As the demand for further professionalism grew, many programs developed to offer a baccalaureate degree in nursing. The University of Minnesota School of Nursing opened in 1909 and is considered the first university-based nursing education program in the nation. The Yale University School of Nursing opened in 1924 and offered the first program contained within an autonomous academic unit. The baccalaureate degree with a major in nursing reflects the richness of the academy's curriculum with liberal arts and science courses designed to prepare individuals as critical thinkers, both in nursing and in life. Today, the degree is earned in 4 years. However, 5-year programs existed through most of the 1960s, as nursing faculty struggled to merge clinical content into educational models of academia. In 2005, there were 573 U.S. colleges and universities offering a baccalaureate degree in nursing.

Within the nursing profession, there has been lengthy debate to define the appropriate education level for entry into practice. The American Nurses Association (ANA) and the National League for Nursing (NLN) both support the baccalaureate degree to enter general practice as an RN. Others, such as the American Association of Colleges of Nursing (AACN), support entry into general practice at the master's level and into advanced practice at the doctoral level.

It is important to note that preparation for LPNs—called licensed vocational nurses (LVNs) in some states—occurs nationwide often in the last year of a high school program or the 1st year of an associate-degree program. There were approximately 710,000 LPNs in the nation in 2005. There is a separate licensing examination for LPNs and LVNs that is overseen by the National Council of State Boards of Nursing (NCSBN). Their scope of practice is regulated by State Boards of Nursing, which typically describe LPN practice as under the direction of the RN with great emphasis on physical care and related medical procedures.

The percentage of nurses who had earned a high school diploma decreased from 63.2% in 1980 to 25.2% in 2004. During that same period, nurses graduating with an associate's degree increased from 18.6% to 42.2%, and nurses entering the profession with a baccalaureate degree or higher increased from 17.4% to 31%. With the findings that better patient outcomes are associated with nurses with a baccalaureate or higher degree directing care, there is concern that the continuing large percentage of diploma and associate-degree nurses entering the field may be a disadvantage to patients.

Licensure

To practice as RNs, all graduates must prove their competency by passing a national examination. The examination is administered by the NCSBN and called the National Council Licensure Examination for Registered Nurses (NCLEX-RN). Successful completion of the examination is necessary for licensure in all states. Individual state laws and regulations govern the practice of nursing in each state. State differences concern topics such as the requirements for continuing education, the delegation of authority to other providers, and the scope of advanced practice. A compact now exists among several states so that participating states automatically recognize and accept the nursing license of individuals from another compact state. Most states, however, accept only the test results and require an application for practice within its boundaries. With nurses increasingly using telecommunications to address patient issues across state lines, the demand for more compact state agreements will likely grow.

Future Implications

Nursing is a dynamic profession that remains focused on patient outcomes, including peaceful death. Nursing scholars continuously develop the evidence necessary to refine the practice, while healthcare leaders support and recognize the importance of nursing to the totality of healthcare in the United States.

Zepure Boyadjian Samawi,
Katie Rich, and Anne R. Bavier

See also American Association of Colleges of Nursing (AACN); American Nurses Association (ANA); Hospitals; National Institutes of Health (NIH); Nightingale, Florence; Nurse Practitioners (NPs); Quality of Healthcare

Further Readings

Buerhaus, Peter I., Douglas Staiger, and David I. Auerbach. *The Future of the Nursing Workforce in the United States: Data, Trends, and Implications.* Sudbury, MA: Jones and Bartlett, 2009.

D'Antonio, Patricia, Ellen Baer, Sylvia Rinker, et al., eds. *Nurses' Work: Issues Across Time and Place.* New York: Springer 2006.

Kalisch, Philip A., and Beatrice J. Kalisch. *American Nursing: A History.* 4th ed. Philadelphia: Lippincott Williams and Wilkins, 2003.

Katz, Janet R. *A Career in Nursing: Is It Right for Me?* St. Louis, MO: Mosby Elsevier, 2007.

Roux, Gayle M., and Judith A. Halstead. *Issues and Trends in Nursing: Essential Knowledge for Today and Tomorrow.* Sudbury, MA: Jones and Bartlett, 2009.

Ryan, Adam J., and Jack Doyle, (eds. *Trends in Nursing Research.* New York: Nova Science, 2008.

Styles, Margretta M. *Specialization and Credentialing in Nursing Revisited: Understanding the Issues, Advancing the Profession.* Silver Spring, MD: American Nurses Association, 2008.

Web Sites

American Academy of Nursing (AAN): http://www.aannet.org

American Association of Colleges of Nursing (AACN): http://www.aacn.nche.edu

American Nurses Association (ANA): http://www.nursingworld.org

Bureau of Health Professions (BHPr): http://bhpr.hrsa.gov

National Institute of Nursing Research (BHPr): http://www.ninr.nih.gov

National League for Nursing (NLN): http://www.nln.org

NURSING HOME QUALITY

Life in all its richness occurs in nursing homes. Sickness, love, caring, kindness, anger, abuse, indifference, excitement, boredom, laughter, sex, and death all transpire in nursing homes. Time-study data indicate that the average nursing home resident receives less than 1½ hours of care each day from nursing staff, indicating that treatment is a relatively small proportion of what fills the everyday life of nursing home residents. Thus, although excellent care and treatment are important, quality of care is only one aspect of quality in the nursing home. Because nursing homes are where people live, as well as receive health and rehabilitative care, discussions of nursing home quality become at the most global level deliberations about how to measure and ensure residents' well-being, in the fullest sense of the term.

While nursing homes serve a variety of populations, quality of care for long-stay residents is the focus here. This entry first provides basic information on nursing homes and their occupants. Next, it discusses how quality of care is usually measured in nursing homes. It then discusses the larger issue of quality of life. Last, it discusses the current quality assurance process in nursing homes and the future of nursing home care.

Nursing Homes and Nursing Home Residents

This discussion of nursing home quality necessarily occurs within the context of the current nursing home industry and resident population. On any given day, approximately 16,000 nursing homes in the United States provide care for roughly 1.6 million residents. Most nursing homes are for-profit, investor-owned enterprises operated by multifacility chains. The average size of nursing homes is approximately 100 beds, with an occupancy level below 90%. Over two thirds of longer-stay nursing home residents receive their care under the auspices of state Medicaid programs. Recent data indicate that state Medicaid programs pay on average about $120 per day (over $40,000 annually) for care. Private-pay residents now pay an average of about $190 per day (almost $70,000 annually). The federal Medicare program pays the bulk of costs for shorter-stay residents.

Almost all nursing homes accept Medicaid and/or Medicare funds. Receipt of these public funds requires that a nursing home be licensed by the state and certified to participate in and receive payment from these programs. Licensure and certification carry with them an elaborate array of requirements about financial reporting and resident care. The most basic of these requirements involve annual cost reports and annual on-site surveys by multimember teams who evaluate the degree to which a nursing home meets state licensure and federal certification standards.

Most admissions to nursing homes (just over 50%) come from hospitals. A large number of individuals, over the course of a year, come into nursing homes and then either die or leave within weeks. These short-stay individuals who return home are largely in the nursing home to recover from some acute disease episode such as the flu or to recover from an acute exacerbation of a chronic disease condition such as diabetes or from physical, speech, or occupational rehabilitation after a fall or stroke. On any given day, these short-stay residents constitute about 10% of a nursing home's population, but they constitute over 60% of all individuals admitted annually to nursing homes. Only about one quarter to one third of those admitted to a nursing home will be in the same nursing home 3 months after admission.

Only about 10% of long-stay nursing home residents are under 65 years of age. The average long-stay nursing home resident is a female over 75 years of age. Generally, she suffers from multiple chronic diseases and has a number of health problems, which are likely to include arthritis, hypertension, heart disease, and diabetes as well as decreased ability to see and hear. Like the majority of the residents surrounding her, she has episodes of urinary incontinence and some level of cognitive impairment. She also needs significant physical assistance with a number of activities of daily living (ADLs).

Quality of Care

Like other health services researchers, investigators conceptualize nursing home quality in terms of Avedis Donabedian's triad of structure, process, and outcome, with most researchers considering outcomes the most telling indicator of quality of care. In nursing home research, the structural quality measure with the greatest impact on process and outcome quality is nurse staffing. Turnover of direct-care staff, nursing supervisors, and administrators are also structural measures that gather considerable attention as instances where quality of care is put at risk. Some evidence indicates that for-profit ownership also tends to be associated with poorer-quality care, but part of that relationship may be attributed to the generally lower staffing levels and higher staff turnover at for-profit homes. Process quality measures that receive the most attention are the presence of urinary incontinence without a scheduled toileting plan, the use of physical restraints, psychotropic medication use, the prevalence of feeding tubes, or the use of urinary catheters.

Outcome measures of importance for measuring nursing home quality include mortality, declines in functional status or activities of daily living (e.g., ADLs), worsening cognitive status, worsening conditions (e.g., continence), accidents, falls, or hospitalizations for ambulatory-care-sensitive conditions (e.g., diabetes). Unfortunately, little research finds strong links between these outcomes and the various process quality measures noted above. For both short- and long-stay residents recovering from an acute disease episode, significant improvement is a common outcome. However, that is not the case for the average long-stay nursing home resident.

Analyses of nursing home quality are almost invariably observational studies. To enhance their validity, observational studies involving process quality or outcome quality measures usually require some type of case-mix or acuity adjustment. A major difficulty arises in studies of nursing home quality focused on outcomes. In these studies, it is difficult to determine the degree to which any undesirable outcome resulted from poor nursing home performance rather than from the natural processes of declining health beyond the nursing home's control. For example, a resident's decline in ADL function does not mean with certainty that poor care occurred. Instead, unavoidable decline in one of the resident's chronic disease or health conditions (e.g., congestive heart failure) may have adversely affected his or her ADL function. For only a few outcome quality measures is poor quality of care a truly necessary condition (e.g., medication errors).

Those researchers involved in the necessary risk adjustment process in nursing home outcome studies have two options. Either they can include variables in their models that may overadjust, giving some nursing homes undeserved credit for bad-quality care, or they can omit some variables from their models, possibly underadjusting and failing to give some nursing homes credit for good-quality care. For example, when looking at pressure ulcer rates in a nursing home, should one adjust for residents being bedfast? Being bedfast clearly raises the likelihood of a pressure ulcer. But why is a resident bedfast? The resident may be bedfast because of some natural process of declining health, such as increased respiratory distress, or he or she may be bedfast because the nursing home failed to provide an aggressive mobility program that would have kept the resident mobile. Thus, including whether a resident is bedfast in an acuity adjustment model for the presence of pressure ulcers may be overadjusting, but omitting it from the model may mean underadjusting.

Researchers can avoid confounding the impact of individual factors and nursing home performance by looking at changes over time in resident status, using only admission information as baseline data. For almost all residents, provider performance and resident characteristics are orthogonal at admission. However, using this approach, researchers must show that the early months of care that serve as the focus of most such efforts do not differ dramatically from outcomes later in a resident's nursing home stay.

Quality of Life

Quality-of-life issues for nursing homes and their residents can incorporate a long list of dimensions. These include, but are not limited to, helping preserve residents' dignity, respecting their privacy, maintaining positive relationships with staff or other residents, serving high-quality food, enhancing opportunities for resident autonomy, assuring their security, and providing a clean and pleasant physical environment.

Quality-of-life data can be gathered in two ways. Researchers can observe some of these dimensions, such as staff-resident interactions, using standardized tools. Residents can also report on their perceptions concerning all these dimensions.

Each of these approaches, however, is troublesome. Observers cannot assess all aspects of quality of life. More fundamentally, observers (even family members) are not the true recipients of care and may not share residents' perceptions of services or living arrangements. Residents are, of course, the ideal reporters. However, a large proportion of residents suffer from levels of cognitive impairment that make interviewing them difficult or impossible.

The most extensive effort aimed at developing an interviewing strategy for quality of life resulted in 10 dimensions. However, the measurement scales reflecting only a few of these dimensions demonstrated good internal consistency. Additionally, facility characteristics explained very little of the variance in quality of life. Reasonably, residents' characteristics were much stronger predictors of their quality-of-life scores. Such measures, as the developers indicate, are at this point probably best used to identify cognitively intact residents within the nursing home who might be the focus of individualized interventions. While these measures are not yet well-suited for assessing nursing homes' performance in general, they are important steps in the process of moving quality of life into the mainstream of nursing home quality measurement.

Quality Assurance

As the national Institute of Medicine (IOM), Committee on Nursing Home Regulation met over 20 years ago, the committee chair Sidney Katz described quality assurance in nursing homes as a three-legged stool requiring good assessments, good standards, and good enforcement. The IOM report from this committee provided a blueprint for a new approach to ensuring quality in nursing home care. The Nursing Home Reform Act in the Omnibus Budget Reconciliation Act of 1987 (OBRA-87) was a direct descendant of the IOM committee's report. OBRA-87 mandated a comprehensive assessment system titled the Resident Assessment Instrument or Minimum Data Set (MDS), which served as the first leg of Katz's stool. New standards in OBRA-87 that included quality-of-life issues and focused more heavily on outcomes than paper compliance formed the second leg. Then, new enforcement remedies, which included fines, temporary management, and placing a hold on Medicaid admissions to a nursing home, were added to the traditional remedies of deficiency statements from the annual certification and licensure survey conducted by the states and de-certification of the nursing home, to give the stool a truly solid base. The MDS was implemented in 1989. However, the enforcement standards and remedies were held up for many years by the nursing home industry. When finally implemented, they were watered down, and the expanded range of remedies has not been used vigorously by most states.

Current activities in quality assurance in nursing homes have begun to focus more heavily on quality indicators reporting and public information. The Centers for Medicare and Medicaid Services' (CMS) Nursing Home Compare (NH Compare) Web site allows individuals to obtain detailed information about the past performance of every Medicare- and Medicaid-certified nursing home in the nation. The reports in NH Compare include data on deficiencies cited during the annual (9–15 months apart) survey visits, quality indicators (QIs) from the MDS, and staffing data gathered during the annual survey visits. While MDS data may reflect what is in the medical records, recent research indicates that the staffing data reported to CMS by for-profit and larger nursing homes, when compared with Medicaid cost report data, may overreport staffing levels. A number of state-level reporting systems are somewhat more elaborate than NH Compare. Some state systems provide relative rankings of nursing homes (e.g., one through four stars) and include data on financial performance and expenditure patterns as well as more traditional and staffing data. Initial research findings indicate that such reports may affect nursing home activities, but there is no convincing evidence that such reports affect consumer choices.

In addition, a few researchers are now emphasizing the degree to which nursing home performance affects traditional quality indicators. Early research indicates that a relatively small percentage of the variation in ADL function over time may be attributable to nursing home performance. To the degree that this conclusion is supported by further research into other quality indicators, the quality-reporting movement in the nursing home sector may be at some risk. These reporting systems implicitly assume that nursing home performance explains a meaningful proportion of the variance in

each published indicator. That this assumption is rarely tested is, at this point, a problematic aspect of nursing home performance measurement.

Future Implications

The past few years have been marked by the nursing home industry's emphasis on quality improvement rather than quality assurance, the seeming failure of the current enforcement model, and the lack of serious enforcement activities. At the same time, a group of innovators have begun to offer alternative models of nursing home operations that focus directly on resident-centered care and enhanced quality of life. The Eden Alternative, the Pioneer Network, the Wellspring Initiative, and the Green House Movement are important examples of such alternative models of nursing home operations. All these models focus on more resident-centered care that emphasizes quality-of-life issues and better working conditions for nursing home staff. The Green House Movement takes a lesson from the group home model in community mental health and goes so far as to deconstruct the average 100-bed nursing home into a series of cottages with permanently assigned nurse aides and "circuit-riding" clinical staff.

Where these innovations have successfully been implemented and sustained, they have resulted in changes in the quality of life for residents. However, most nursing homes lack the willingness or ability to implement and sustain such innovations. With an industry dominated by for-profit, owned business entities and with high average turnover rates for senior administrative and clinical staff (ranging from 6 to 18 months), the likelihood of sustained, pervasive change in the nursing home industry seems relatively low. Some nursing homes, often not-for-profits in the least need of transformation, may change and sustain those innovations. Many nursing homes will likely focus on avoiding bad survey results and lawsuits, while maintaining the level of quality that allows them to receive an appropriate return on their investments.

A panel of distinguished experts in long-term care were recently asked what they thought would be the "one thing" that might have the greatest likelihood of enhancing quality in long-term care. The most frequent answer was additional staffing, followed closely by additional funding. But some of the less frequent answers were interesting as well. One expert said that the real problem lies in the dominance of investor-owned businesses in the nursing home industry. Another expert suggested that the greater involvement of communities in nursing homes would bring considerable benefit.

Some policy analysts, however, consider nursing quality to be something of a vestigial issue. They believe that the current "rebalancing" of long-term care reimbursement to provide more incentives for home care, combined with the growth of the assisted living industry, will sound the death knell for the nursing home industry. However, many doubt that either home care or assisted living can be the panacea that these analysts believe. They argue that home care cannot be effective without adequate staff and considerable family support; and the availability of individuals to provide either paid or informal support, both of which are largely provided by females 40 to 60 years of age, will not be increasing at the rate of increase in the number of impaired elderly 75 years old or older.

Nursing homes most likely will not be vanishing soon from the long-term care tableau. They may change in relatively unforeseen ways as the populations whom they serve change. They may, as they have in the past, go through cycles of popularity with investors on Wall Street. Much about the future of long-term care in the nation is unclear, and much about long-term care may change as policymakers begin to address the aging of society. But nursing homes and the quality of care they provide will likely not disappear from the public policy agenda.

Charles D. Phillips and Catherine Hawes

See also Activities of Daily Living (ADL); Centers for Medicare and Medicaid Services (CMS); Donabedian, Avedis; Katz, Sidney; Long-Term Care; Nursing Homes; Public Policy; Structure-Process-Outcome Quality Measures

Further Readings

Committee on Nursing Home Regulation, the Institute of Medicine. *Improving the Quality of Care in Nursing Homes.* Washington, DC: National Academies Press, 1986.

Gabriel, Celia S. "An Overview of Nursing Facilities: Data From the 1997 National Nursing Home Survey." *Advance Data From Vital and Health Statistics,* No. 311. Hyattsville, MD: National Center for Health Statistics, 2000.

National Commission on Long-Term Care Quality. *From Isolation to Integration: Recommendations to Improve Quality in Long-Term Care.* Washington, DC: National Commission on Long-Term Care Quality, 2007.

Wunderlich, Gooloo, and Peter O. Kohler, eds., Committee on Improving Quality in Long-Term Care. *Improving the Quality of Long-Term Care.* Washington, DC: National Academies Press, 2001.

Web Sites

American Association of Homes and Services for the Aged (AAHSA): http://www2.aahsa.org

American Health Care Association (AHCA): http://www.ahcancal.org

Association of Health Facility Survey Agencies (AHFSA): http://www.ahfsa.org

Centers for Medicare and Medicaid Services (CMS), Nursing Home Compare: http://www.medicare.gov

Eden Alternative: http://www.edenalt.org

Green House Project: http://www.ncbcapitalimpact.org/thegreenhouse

The National Citizens' Coalition for Nursing Home Reform, Consumer Voice for Quality Long-Term Care: http://www.nccnhr.org

Pioneer Network: http://www.pioneernetwork.net

Wellspring Initiative: http://www.wellspringis.org

NURSING HOMES

Nursing homes are licensed residential facilities with professional staff that provide continuous nursing care and health-related services for individuals who do not require hospitalization but cannot be cared for at home. These facilities provide 24-hour care for adults 18 years of age or older who are not in the acute phase of illness but who have significant functional deficiencies. Functional deficiencies are generally measured by individuals' ability to perform basic activities of daily living (ADLs), such as the ability to independently dress, eat, bathe, get around, and use the toilet themselves. Individuals may need nursing home care for a short period of time, such as for rehabilitation or recovery after an injury or illness. Other individuals may require long-term or permanent care for chronic or progressive physical or mental illness or infirmity.

Types

Nursing homes provide different levels of care designed to meet the wide range of needs of individuals. They may specialize in short-term or acute nursing care, intermediate care, or long-term, custodial nursing care. Many of the nation's nursing homes provide more than one level of care.

Skilled-Nursing Facilities

Skilled-nursing facilities (SNFs) provide relatively short-term nursing and rehabilitative care. Skilled care is generally provided to assist patients during recovery following hospitalization for acute medical conditions. These facilities are state-licensed, and registered nurses (RNs), licensed practical nurses (LPNs), and certified nurse aids (CNAs) provide care. The services of other healthcare professionals such as therapists, social workers, and dietitians are also available. Hospitals often have arrangements with skilled-nursing facilities to provide follow-up care for patients who no longer need acute hospital services. Skilled-nursing facilities provide skilled care and rehabilitation until the patient is able to return home or requires longer-term placement.

Intermediate-Care Facilities

Intermediate-care facilities provide care for individuals who are recovering from acute medical conditions but do not need continuous care or daily therapeutic services. Intermediate care is provided by skilled professionals such as RNs, LPNs, therapists, and other health professionals under the supervision of a physician.

Custodial-Care Facilities

Custodial-care facilities provide assistance to patients in activities of daily living, such as bathing, dressing, eating, and toileting. Individuals who are recovering from a disabling injury or illness may temporarily need custodial care. For other individuals who are losing their ability to function independently due to chronic or progressive disease or frailty due to advanced age, custodial care may be a long-term need. For some, ongoing professional nursing and other services may be required along with custodial care. If custodial-care residents become ill or injured, they may spend a period of time in skilled care and then return to custodial care.

Many nursing homes also provide specialized services such as hospice and respite care. Hospice care offers supportive services for terminally ill patients and their families. Nursing homes may also provide respite care for individuals who are being cared for at home to allow a family caregiver relief for short periods of time. Some nursing homes have specially equipped units for persons who are ventilator-dependent, have Alzheimer's disease, or have spinal cord injuries.

Services Provided

Nursing homes provide a wide range of services, including medical-care services; nursing-care services; other professional healthcare services; personal-care services; spiritual, social, and recreational services; and residential-care services.

Medical-Care Services

Regardless of the level of care required, all nursing home residents are under the supervision and care of a physician. Physicians certify the continuing need for nursing home care and are responsible for the resident's overall care plan. Physicians also evaluate and prescribe for the resident's medical conditions and determine the types of restorative and rehabilitative services that are required. All nursing homes must have a medical director who can address medical issues and other concerns with the resident, the resident's family, and the attending physician.

Nursing-Care Services

In the United States, all nursing homes are required to have a licensed practical or vocational nurse (LPN/LVN) on duty 24 hours a day and an RN on duty for at least one shift each day. Nursing services include the regular assessment of residents' needs, administration of medications and treatments, and coordination of care.

Other Professional Healthcare Services

Nursing homes provide rehabilitative and restorative services such as physical, occupational, respiratory, recreational, and speech therapy. In addition, dental services, dietary consultation, laboratory, X-ray, and pharmaceutical services are available.

Personal-Care Services

Nursing assistants also provide personal-care and supportive services for residents who require help with activities of daily living, such as eating, bathing, walking, and toileting.

Spiritual, Social, and Recreational Services

Nursing homes offer a wide range of services and programs to meet the spiritual and social needs of residents. Clergy and social workers are also available to support family members and friends. Most nursing homes also offer a wide variety of in-house recreational activities and organized trips.

Residential-Care Services

Nursing homes provide general supervision within a safe and secure environment along with basic housing and sustenance.

Eligibility

Each state has its own nursing home eligibility criteria. A prescreening assessment is completed for every individual being considered for nursing home admission. The assessment includes the evaluation of an individual's physical and cognitive limitations, medical conditions, the type and level of assistance required, and skilled-care needs. Although there is some variation across states, the requirements are very similar overall. For skilled-nursing facilities, a state's requirements include a need for at least one skilled service ordered by a physician, such as the administration of medications, special

catheter care, rehabilitation, or nasogastric tube for gastrostomy feedings.

Paying for Nursing Home Care

Many Americans incorrectly assume that the federal Medicare program or standard or supplemental health insurance policies will pay for nursing home care. Consequently, many people do not plan ahead financially or purchase long-term care insurance to provide for their care in the event of infirmity or an extended illness. Nationally the costs of nursing home care often exceed $50,000 annually, or more than $4,000 a month.

Medicare

The federal Medicare program is available to those nursing home residents who are eligible for the program, either through age or disability, and who require a skilled level of nursing home care. Generally, Medicare covers services after hospitalization. The number of days that Medicare will pay for skilled-nursing facility care is limited to no more than 100 days per episode of care. During the first 20 days of care, Medicare pays 100% of care. Between 21 and 100 days, Medicare requires a copayment. Many older persons have a Medicare supplement or Medigap insurance policy. This supplemental insurance pays in conjunction with Medicare, but most supplements stop paying when Medicare reimbursement ends. Medigap insurance policies are sold by private insurance companies. To buy a Medigap insurance policy, the individual must already have Medicare Part A and B insurance. Finally, each individual must buy separate Medigap insurance policies, as coverage will not be provided under a spouse or family member's insurance policy. Neither Medicare nor Medigap insurance policies will pay for custodial nursing home care.

Medicaid

If persons have exhausted their Medicare payments for nursing home care, or if they do not require skilled care, they may qualify for Medicaid coverage to pay for their nursing home care. However, Medicaid is only available to persons who have low incomes or limited resources. To qualify for Medicaid, individuals may have to spend out-of-pocket for care until their income drops to the level required for Medicaid eligibility. States vary in how they consider an individual's assets, such as the spousal home, when determining eligibility for Medicaid. Persons who stay in nursing homes for an extended period, often until death, are typically supported by Medicaid.

Long-Term Care Insurance

A relatively small number of individuals choose to purchase long-term care insurance in the event that they may need long-term care in the future. This insurance must be purchased prior to needing long-term care, and eligibility for this type of insurance is based on health status at the time of purchase. Some financial planners recommend purchasing long-term care insurance when a person is in his or her late 50s or early 60s. Premiums are based on age, health status, and type of plan purchased.

Individuals often consider three things when deciding which long-term care insurance to purchase: the daily benefit, the benefit period, and the elimination or deductible period. The daily benefit is the amount of money that the individual will receive from the insurance company for care on a daily basis. The benefit period is the length of time that benefits will be provided (options generally include 1, 2, or 3 or more years of coverage, or a lifetime plan). And the elimination or deductible period is the number of days the individual is responsible for paying for long-term care before the insurance begins to pay for the care.

Licensing and Certification

State governments are responsible for overseeing the licensing of nursing homes. Each state is contracted by the U.S. Department of Health and Human Services' Centers for Medicare and Medicaid Services (CMS) to monitor its nursing homes. Facilities that want to provide care and be reimbursed by Medicare and Medicaid must adhere to at least minimum state quality requirements. States conduct onsite inspections to determine whether a facility meets quality and performance standards. Inspections are typically yearly, but can occur more frequently, especially if

concerns are voiced or if complaints are made about the care provided. The inspection process includes observations of care processes, staff/resident interactions, and the physical environment. The inspection team also interviews a sample of nursing home residents and family members about the care in the home. Care providers and administrators are interviewed, and clinical records are reviewed based on standardized protocols. The inspection team, which includes an RN, also examines food preparation and storage, fire safety, safe construction standards, and issues related to possible resident abuse. If problems are identified, the CMS can take action against the facility. This can range from imposing a fine, to denying payment, to assigning a temporary manager or installing a state monitor. If the problems are not corrected, the CMS can terminate its agreement with the nursing home. At that point, the nursing home is no longer certified to provide care to Medicare beneficiaries and Medicaid recipients, and these residents will be transferred to other facilities. With the loss of those residents, the nursing home is very likely to close.

Selecting a Nursing Home

Although the individual requiring nursing home care should be involved as much as possible, selecting a nursing home often becomes the responsibility of a family member or friend. Fortunately, there are many resources available to assist in making the decision.

A number of steps in choosing a nursing home have been identified. Generally, the first step in choosing a nursing home is to discuss with a physician the specific types of services that are required and the level of care that is needed. Alternatives to nursing home care should also be discussed at this time. Home care services or adult day care should be considered as a possible alternative, and financial arrangements must also be taken into account.

Once it is determined that nursing home care is required, the next step is to identify local nursing homes that provide the types of services that are needed. There are a number of resources that can provide information. These include state long-term care ombudsman programs, health departments, hospital discharge planners, social workers, geriatric case managers, state or local departments of aging, the Medicare Web site and informational materials, and Web sites of individual facilities. Friends, neighbors, and clergy may also offer recommendations.

When the list has been narrowed to those local facilities that provide the needed services, family members and future residents will want to evaluate services and amenities. They should talk with administrative personnel at each facility to arrange for a tour. They should plan to visit each facility two or three times at different times of the day and arrange visits to observe meals and recreational activities. Personal observations and interactions with staff will provide the most valuable information about the quality of care provided by the nursing home.

For example, family members and individuals will need to determine if the nursing home is in a quiet, safe area that is accessible, as continued contact with family and friends is a vital aspect of a resident's well-being. They will also need to note if the building is in good repair, has adequate space, and appears clean and safe. Potential residents and families will also want to pay attention to social interactions within the facility and the availability of group activities. Residents should all have the opportunity to take part in activities that provide mental, physical, and social stimulation and decrease the likelihood of isolation. Monthly programs and activities should be posted at each nursing home.

During these initial visits and tours, families and individuals should talk to all levels of staff, including the director and nursing assistants; they should observe the staff interactions with the residents, meal presentation and preparation, and resident interactions in the dining room and other common spaces. Potential residents and family members should talk directly to the other residents, inquiring about their experience in the facility and their daily activities. Finally, they should be aware of any special services the nursing home offers to residents, such as religious services, particular diet preferences, or field trips.

It is also important to evaluate quality when selecting a nursing home. Every nursing home facility is inspected annually by its state health department. The survey results are available at the facility and the public may review the report of the facility's performance using Medicare's "Nursing Home Compare" Web site. Survey results address all aspects of care provided by the nursing home, from what might be considered minor infractions to major issues of concern. A staff representative can answer questions and provide additional information about the report and about whether identified problems have been corrected.

Often the potential nursing home resident is unable to be involved in every step of the selection process; it is essential, however, to the degree that it is possible, that he or she be involved in the final choice. Many people are reluctant to enter a nursing home, even if it is necessary. Of the options available, the facility chosen must be a place where the individual believes that he or she will be most comfortable.

Ombudsmen

In 1978, the U.S. Congress amended the Older Americans Act to include a requirement that each state develop a long-term care ombudsman program. Provisions of the act require that each state institute a program that defines the function and responsibilities of ombudsmen, addresses complaints, and advocates for improvements in the long-term care system.

The ombudsman program is administered by the federal Administration on Aging, and most state ombudsman programs are housed in their state unit on aging. There are 53 state long-term care ombudsman programs and about 600 regional programs in the nation. Over 8,400 volunteers have been certified to handle complaints. Nationally, the ombudsman program handles over 264,000 complaints annually. An individual 18 years of age or older who has the time and interest may volunteer to become an ombudsman. Although specific requirements vary from state to state, generally ombudsmen may not have a family member who is a resident in a local nursing facility, and they must not be employed by or have ownership in a long-term care facility. Volunteers must provide references, and criminal background checks are required. Once accepted into the program, ombudsman volunteers receive training and are certified.

Long-term care ombudsmen serve as advocates for nursing home residents. The ombudsmen provide a wide range of services for nursing home residents and their families, from advising in the selection of an appropriate nursing home to resolving complaints made by or for residents. They may also address a wide range of quality of care and quality-of-life concerns that can include unanswered call buttons, roommate problems, staffing issues, food concerns, and unsanitary conditions. They often visit nursing homes to reach out to residents and families, as well as receiving complaints by telephone, mail, and e-mail.

Ombudsmen conduct educational sessions for nursing home staff, family, resident councils, and others. Programs include residents' rights, restraint reduction, abuse and neglect regulations, and how to deal with difficult behaviors. They also provide general information to the public on nursing homes and other long-term care facilities and services, residents' rights, and legislative and policy issues. Nursing homes are required to clearly post information about the ombudsmen program and how residents or other concerned individuals may contact an ombudsman.

Cultural Change Movement

The cultural change movement is a grassroots effort to transform the culture of aging. This effort, led by a group called the Pioneer Network, grew out of a small group of providers and researchers who were interested in changing the culture of nursing home care into places for living and growing rather than decline and death. This group has identified 13 core values for improving the quality of long-term care in persons' homes, assisted living, nursing home, and other facilities. The Pioneer Network also acts as a liaison between long-term care researchers and nursing homes to encourage nursing homes to participate in research and to help researchers and providers to translate findings into practice.

Frances M. Weaver and Elaine C. Hickey

See also Centers for Medicare and Medicaid Services (CMS); Continuum of Care; Long-Term Care; Long-Term Care Costs in the United States; Medicaid; National Citizens' Coalition for Nursing Home Reform (NCCNHR); Nursing Home Quality; Skilled-Nursing Facilities

Further Readings

Allen, James E. *Nursing Home Administration*. 5th ed. New York: Springer, 2008.

Baker, Beth. *Old Age in a New Age: The Promise of Transformative Nursing Homes*. Nashville, TN: Vanderbilt University Press, 2008.

Cowles, C. McKeen, ed. *Nursing Home Statistical Yearbook*. McMinnville, OR: Cowles Research Group, 2006.

Grabowski, David C., Jonathan Gruber, and Joseph J. Angelelli. *Nursing Home Quality as Public Good*. NBER Working Paper No. 12361. Cambridge, MA: National Bureau of Economic Research, 2006.

Kane, Robert L. and Joan C. West. *It Shouldn't Be This Way: The Failure of Long-Term Care*. Nashville, TN: Vanderbilt University Press, 2005.

Katz, Paul R., Mathy D. Mezey, and Marshall B. Kapp, eds. *Vulnerable Populations in the Long-Term Care Continuum*. New York: Springer, 2004.

Roe, Brenda H., and Roger Beech. *Intermediate and Continuing Care: Policy and Practice*. Malden, MA: Blackwell, 2005.

Web Sites

AARP: http://www.aarp.org

Administration on Aging (AOA): http://www.aoa.gov

American Association of Homes and Services for the Aging (AAHSA): http://www.aahsa.org

American Health Care Association (AHCA): http://www.ahcancal.org

National Center for Health Statistics (NCHS): http://www.cdc.gov/nchs

National Council on Aging (NCOA): http://www.ncoa.org

Nursing Home Compare: http://www.medicare.gov/nhcompare

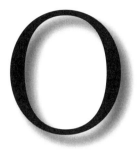

OBESITY

Obesity is a major public health problem in the United States; it has a significant impact on access, cost, and quality of healthcare. The prevalence of obesity has increased over the past 30 years to the point where many refer to it as an obesity epidemic. Today, more than 65% of adults in the nation are either overweight or obese. Additionally, 33.6% of children between 2 and 19 years of age are at risk of being overweight or are overweight. Obesity is currently the second leading cause of preventable deaths in the nation, and it may surpass smoking as the leading cause of preventable death in the future.

The link between lifestyle and obesity starts in the prenatal period. Children are exposed to parental behaviors, which they may model later in life. School lunch programs aim to meet nutritious guidelines but often do so with limited resources. An emphasis on academic standards frequently reduces time for free play and activity in school, either during recess or gym class. Computers, television, and video games are widely available to children, who often prefer these activities to physical activity after school and on weekends. Adults are bombarded with fast-food establishments, convenience foods, and demanding time constraints, which may lead to poor food selection and inactivity. Taken together, the typical American family has significant barriers to making healthy food choices and participating in physical activities.

Assessment of Risk

An important measure of weight and obesity is the body mass index, or BMI. The BMI is used to assess a person's risk of weight-related comorbidities based on his or her relative weight to height. The formula for calculating the BMI is BMI = weight (kilograms)/[height (meters)]^2. The nonmetric conversion formula is BMI = weight (pounds)/[height (inches)]^2 × 703. For example, a person who weighs 175 pounds and is 66 inches tall (or 5 foot 6 inches) has a BMI of 28: weight (175 pounds)/[height (66 inches)]^2 × 703 = 28.

A healthy BMI for adults is between 18.5 and 24.9. A BMI less than 18.5 is considered underweight and may be associated with decreased immune function, osteoporosis, decreased muscle strength, and trouble regulating body temperature. At BMIs greater than 25, a person's risk of weight-related illness or comorbidities increases. Between 25.0 and 29.9 adults are classified as overweight, and people with a BMI of 30.0 or higher are considered obese.

In children, the BMI is stratified by age and gender. This is done to control for the changes in body fat that are expected as children grow. It also allows for the differences in body fat between boys and girls. BMI-for-age tables are available from the Centers for Disease Control and Prevention (CDC) and are used to help healthcare practitioners assess adiposity (fatness) in children. A BMI-for-age that is less than the 5th percentile is considered underweight. Healthy weights include

BMI-for-age from the 5th percentile to less than the 85th percentile. A child is at risk of being overweight with a BMI-for-age from the 85th percentile to less than the 95th percentile. A BMI-for-age greater than or equal to the 95th percentile is classified as being overweight. There is no obese classification for children (2–19 years of age).

Adipose tissue (fat) that is deposited around the midsection of the body is more metabolically active than fat that is distributed in the extremities. Abdominal fat that is out of proportion to total body fat is an independent risk factor for obesity-related morbidity and mortality, even in individuals with a normal BMI. Waist circumference is used to assess the risk from abdominal obesity. Relative-risk cutoffs for waist circumference are gender specific, whereas BMI is independent of gender.

Nutrition

At the most basic level, weight gain occurs when calories taken in exceed calories expended. When a person eats more calories than he or she expends (through basal metabolism, thermic effect of food, and physical activity), he or she gains weight. If a person eats fewer calories, he or she loses weight. During the last 30 years, there have been changes in the nutrient composition of meals and portion sizes, which has contributed to the increasing calorie intakes of individuals. A public misperception regarding portion size and serving size further adds to the confusion.

Portion Size

Portion size is the amount of food or beverage that is consumed in a single eating event. Serving size is the standardized unit for measuring food that is used in dietary guidance. For example, a person might eat one bowl of pasta and consider it a serving; however, a serving size for pasta is half a cup. The bowl of pasta is the portion size that was consumed. Consider a typical breakfast from 30 years ago—coffee and a muffin. An 8-ounce cup of coffee with whole milk and sugar has approximately 45 calories. The portion size of a muffin 30 years ago was approximately 1.5 ounces (210 calories). At many restaurants today, a medium coffee (16 ounces) may have upward of 350 calories, while the muffin size has increased to

4 ounces (500 calories). This results in an increase of almost 600 calories for the same meal.

Consumers also equate size to value. When people eat in restaurants or purchase prepackaged foods, they expect a large portion for their money. Small portions are seen as cheap or insufficient, so restaurants respond by offering 12-ounce steaks and family-size bowls of pasta as single entrees. There is also an incentive to buy big at fast-food restaurants. Customers are offered the opportunity to upsize an order at minimal cost. Oversized portions are not limited to food. Beverage portions are also increasing. Soft drinks used to be served in 6- to 8-ounce portions; today consumers can choose between 12-, 20-, and 24-ounce containers. People can easily drink 150 to 180 calories per 12-ounce portion.

Breastfeeding and Infant Formula

The overconsumption of beverages starts in infancy. Formula-fed infants have their intake measured by how many ounces they consume from the bottle at each feeding. Parents often think that babies need to drink the entire bottle, even if the child shows signs that he or she is finished. When this happens, babies do not learn what satiety (fullness) feels like, and they may overeat when they are older. Breastfeeding provides an opportunity for babies to self-regulate caloric intake. Mothers are unable to measure how much milk is consumed from the breast, allowing babies to stop eating when they feel full. Some mothers may gauge consumption by monitoring how long each nursing session lasts; however, babies adjust their suck rate as hunger subsides. Nursing in response to hunger (nutritious nursing) may result in a higher milk intake than comfort nursing. The protective effects of breastfeeding on excessive weight gain in childhood may be dose dependent. The greater the opportunity children have to self-regulate intake, the more they are able to recognize hunger and satiety cues.

Parental Influence

Parental choice once children are weaned from breast milk or formula also affects the risk of excessive weight gain. When juice and juice drinks replace breast milk and formula, children consume large amounts of calories with little nutritional value. These calorie-dense beverages often take the place of nutritious foods. Children also lose out on the beneficial effects of fiber and phytochemicals that are found in fruits and vegetables. Putting infants and children to sleep with bottles of juice or milk contributes to excessive weight gain and tooth decay. For many children, their only exposure to vegetables is in the form of French fries. Children often mimic their parents and caregivers when deciding what to eat. When children see their parents eating high-fat, sugary foods, they will want to do the same. If healthy foods, including fruits and vegetables, are regularly offered, children will develop an affinity for their taste. Including children in the food-purchasing and -preparation process can also entice them to eat a variety of healthy foods. After age 2, most children can safely switch to low-fat or fat-free dairy products. Parents should avoid adding salt to food, both during the cooking process and at the table. A preference for salty foods is an acquired taste—if children do not eat salty foods when they are young, most will continue to avoid them as adults.

Dietary Guidelines

The Dietary Guidelines for Americans have been published at least every 5 years since 1980. This joint venture by the U.S. Department of Health and Human Services (HHS) and the U.S. Department of Agriculture (USDA) aims to educate Americans on healthy eating habits. There is also an emphasis on how dietary intake can help reduce the risk of several chronic diseases, including obesity. These guidelines, commonly known as the Food Guide Pyramid, received a major revision that was released in 2005. The My Pyramid food guidance system is an interactive, Web-based system that allows users to customize calorie recommendations by age and gender. It also provides recommendations for pregnant and lactating women. This system incorporates physical activity recommendations to further encourage Americans to improve their health through lifestyle modification.

Lifestyle

Technological advances, such as television, computers, and automobiles, as well as the growth of the nation's fast-food industry, have changed many individuals' lifestyles, contributing to the increase in obesity. Important elements of lifestyle are physical activity, screen time, and eating habits.

Physical Activity

The CDC and the USDA recommend at least 30 minutes of moderate-intensity activity for adults most days of the week to maintain health. To improve health and lose weight, 60 to 90 minutes of moderate-intensity activity are necessary. Children and adolescents should engage in moderate-intensity activities daily for optimal health. One way to measure daily physical activity is with a pedometer. A pedometer is a device that measures how many steps the wearer takes each day. Ten thousand steps per day correspond to approximately 60 minutes of moderate-intensity activity, or the amount recommended for healthy living and weight loss. By adjusting activities of daily living, it is possible to meet the recommended activity levels for most adults without exercising.

Individuals who are successful in maintaining their weight loss long-term have incorporated exercise into their lifestyle. Exercise enhances weight loss efforts by building muscle and bone mass and improving cardiovascular endurance. Exercise also helps control blood sugar levels, reduces blood pressure, and lessens feelings of depression and anxiety. Fifteen minutes of brisk walking or climbing the stairs for 15 to 20 (cumulative) minutes per day expends about 100 calories. The benefits of exercise are cumulative, so people can perform different activities throughout the day (in 10-minute increments) and still improve their well-being.

Screen Time

The American Academy of Pediatrics (AAP) recommends no more than 2 hours of quality screen time for children over the age of 2 each day and no screen time for children under the age of two. Screen time includes television viewing (including movies), computer usage, and playing video games. Data from the 1988 to 1994 National Health and Nutrition Examination Survey found that 26% of children watch more than 4 hours of television per day. These children had greater

BMIs than children whose television viewing was limited to less than 2 hours per day, and they were less likely to engage in vigorous physical activity. Children who engage in regular physical activity that incorporates free play and structured activities are more likely to engage in regular physical activity as adults. As opportunities for physical activity decrease during the school day, it is important that parents encourage their children to engage in active behaviors after school and on weekends. Parents can model good behaviors by designating family activity times and making healthy choices for themselves. Praising children when they accomplish new goals will further encourage them to participate in physical activities.

Eating Habits

The increase in the number of fast-food establishments, loss of family meal times, and increase in the availability of convenience foods have all contributed to obesity. Many people do not eat breakfast because of time constraints or because they think it will help them lose weight. However, skipping breakfast contributes to overeating later in the day, both at mealtimes and with snacking. It has been found that children who skip breakfast have lower test scores and more difficulty concentrating in school.

Where people eat is almost as important as what they eat. Eating a majority of meals away from home tends to result in higher caloric intakes than if the majority of meals are eaten (and prepared) at home. The loss of the family mealtime has been identified as a contributory factor in childhood obesity. Family mealtime provides an opportunity for the entire family to step back from their hectic daily schedules and focus on the family unit. It also provides an opportunity for parents to model healthy eating behaviors for their children.

Prevention

There are many national-, state-, and local-level initiatives under way to combat the obesity epidemic. Nationally, Healthy People 2010 is setting the stage for improving the health of all Americans. Among their Leading Health Indicators (a list of 10 high-priority public health issues) are physical activity and overweight and obesity. The Safe Routes to School Program is one example of a Healthy People 2010 initiative to increase physical activity and reduce overweight status in children. This $612 million program has been implemented in more than 20 states, providing support to local communities that are interested in increasing the number of children who walk or ride their bicycles to school. The Small Step campaign encourages Americans to make small efforts to improve their health and reduce their risk of weight-related medical problems.

Many states are now requiring BMI report cards; students have their BMI assessed annually at school, and the results are sent home to parents. Physicians in West Virginia will be provided with BMI wheels and training to encourage BMI assessments on all patients. And the Florida Department of Health has created the Hispanic Obesity Prevention and Education Program to help address the increasing prevalence of obesity among that ethnic group.

Nationally, Mexican American girls (under age 20) have the highest percentage of overweight; for boys, non-Hispanic Blacks have the highest percentage, followed by Mexican American boys. There is a similar trend in adult females—the age-adjusted prevalence of overweight and obesity is higher in non-Hispanic Black and Mexican American women than in non-Hispanic White women. There is little difference in prevalence among men in these three groups.

Research

Several genes are being studied to gain a better understanding of their role in regulating weight and appetite. These genes include leptin, proopiomelanocortin (POMC, a leptin receptor), prohormone covertase 1, melanocortin receptors 3 and 4, and transcription factor single-minded 1. The insulin gene is also being studied. Neurotransmitters such as serotonin, norepinephrine, and dopamine play a role in weight control and satiety and are the focus of several pharmaceutical products designed to treat obesity. The central cannabinoid (CB1) receptors are thought to play a role in the regulation of food consumption and may have a role in reducing hunger sensations.

Treatment

While many people are able to ameliorate their risk of weight-related illnesses by making healthy lifestyle choices, some are unable to achieve a healthy weight on their own. The 1998 National Institutes of Health's (NIH's) Clinical Guidelines on Managing Overweight and Obesity recommended that the U.S. Food and Drug Administration (FDA) approve weight loss drugs so that they may be used as an adjunct therapy to lifestyle modification in patients with a BMI of 30 or higher with no weight-related comorbidities or in patients with a BMI of 27 or higher with obesity-related comorbidities (or risk factors). Obesity-related comorbidities include diabetes mellitus, sleep apnea and obesity-related hypoventilation, asthma, nonalcoholic fatty liver disease, gallbladder disease, orthopedic problems, hyperinsulinemia, polycystic ovary syndrome, and metabolic syndrome (which may include hypertriglyceridemia, low-HDL cholesterol, hypertension, impaired glucose tolerance, and/or increased waist circumference).

Currently, the only FDA-approved medications for weight loss are sibutramine (Meridia) and orlistat (Xenical). Sibutramine is a norepinephrine, dopamine, and serotonin reuptake inhibitor that works by decreasing appetite. Orlistat is a gastric lipase inhibitor that reduces fat absorption in the intestines. Orlistat recently received FDA approval to be sold over the counter as Alli, although at lower doses than the prescription version.

In addition to pharmaceutical therapy, some obese individuals may benefit from bariatric (weight loss) surgery. There are four surgical procedures commonly performed in the United States for obesity: Roux-en-Y gastric bypass, adjustable gastric banding, sleeve gastrectomy, and biliopancreatic diversion (with or without duodenal switch). The adjustable gastric banding and sleeve gastrectomy work by restricting the amount of food that can be consumed at any given time by decreasing the size of the stomach pouch. The Roux-en-Y gastric bypass and biliopancreatic diversion provide restriction in addition to malabsorption. In both of these procedures, the size of the stomach pouch is reduced (restrictive component), and parts of the intestines are bypassed (malabsorptive component). Bariatric surgery should be restricted to individuals with a BMI of 40 or higher or a BMI of 35 or more with obesity-related comorbidities. Bariatric surgery programs should include education on lifestyle modification and behavioral therapy. Only the adjustable gastric banding is reversible.

Future Implications

The etiology of obesity is multifactorial and difficult to treat. There is a clear environmental impact on the increasing rates of overweight and obesity. Expansive unhealthy food selections and decreased opportunities for physical activity are significant contributory factors to America's expanding waistline. What is not fully understood is the role of genetics in the obesity epidemic. Animal studies looking at the role of various genes in appetite regulation and weight control are not easily reproduced in humans. Until scientists are able to discern the true role of genes in the obesity epidemic, it is up to families and each individual to make healthy lifestyle decisions to reduce the risk of becoming obese.

Elisa Stamm Kogan

See also Chronic Diseases; Diabetes; Disease Management; Health; Healthy People 2010; Inner-City Healthcare; Preventive Care; Public Health

Further Readings

Barrett, Deirdre. *Waistland: The(R)evolutionary Science Behind Our Weight and Fitness Crisis.* New York: W. W. Norton, 2007.

Blue Cross and Blue Shield Association, Technology Evaluation Center. *Laparoscopic Gastric Bypass Surgery for Morbid Obesity.* Chicago: Blue Cross and Blue Shield Association, 2006.

Buchwald, Henry, George S. M. Cowan, and Walter J. Pories, eds. *Surgical Management of Obesity.* Philadelphia: Saunders Elsevier, 2007.

Greer, Nancy L. *Behavioral Therapy Programs for Weight Loss in Adults.* Bloomington, MN: Institute for Clinical Systems Improvement, 2005.

Jordan, Amy B. *Overweight and Obesity in America's Children: Causes, Consequences, Solutions.* Thousand Oaks, CA: Sage, 2008.

Web Sites

American Society for Metabolic and Bariatric Surgery (ASMBS): http://www.asbs.org

Centers for Disease Control and Prevention (CDC): http://www.cdc.gov

Healthy People 2010: http://www.healthypeople.gov

My Pyramid Food Guidance System: http://www.mypyramid.gov

O'LEARY, DENNIS S.

Dennis S. O'Leary is the former long-time president of the Joint Commission, the leading healthcare accrediting body in the United States. Under his leadership, the Joint Commission's accreditation process successfully changed from being primarily focused on the structural measures of healthcare organizations to process measures and care-related outcomes. He also started cutting edge healthcare standards relating to pain management, patient safety, emergency preparedness, and the use of patient restraints. And he launched a series of public policy initiatives.

A Kansas native, O'Leary earned a bachelor's degree from Harvard University and a medical degree from Cornell University Medical College in New York. After 2 years of internal medicine training at the University of Minnesota Hospital, he completed his residency and a hematology fellowship at Strong Memorial Hospital in Rochester, New York. He is board certified in Internal Medicine and Hematology.

Prior to joining the Joint Commission, O'Leary spent 15 years at the George Washington University Medical Center in Washington, D.C. At the medical center, he was a professor of medicine, and he served as a senior manager in several positions. He was the medical director of the university's hospital for 10 years, the dean for clinical affairs at the university, and the vice president of the university's health plan, an academic health maintenance organization (HMO). In 1981, O'Leary received national attention for his role as the university hospital's spokesman for the care given to President Ronald Reagan after he was shot in a failed assassination attempt. He frequently briefed the national and international news media about the president's medical progress.

O'Leary became president of the Joint Commission in 1986. During his 21 years at the Joint Commission, he greatly expanded its scope and size. Under his leadership, the organization moved beyond its original hospital base to accredit a wide range of extended-care and ambulatory-care service organizations. It initiated an international accreditation program and a consultation services program. And the organization undertook a series of projects with the World Health Organization (WHO). Under O'Leary, the Joint Commission's budget and staff quadrupled in size.

During his career, O'Leary received many awards and honors. He is a member of the National Academy of Sciences, Institute of Medicine (IOM). He also is a master of the American College of Physicians and a fellow of the American College of Physician Executives, the American College of Healthcare Executives, and the American Dental Association. In 2000, *Modern Healthcare* magazine identified him as one of the nation's 25 most influential leaders in healthcare during the past quarter-century. In 2005, he was given the Distinguished Service Award, the highest honor from the American Medical Association (AMA), for his advancement of healthcare quality and patient safety. And in 2006, he received the Ernest Armory Codman Award from the Joint Commission for his leadership role in using performance measures to improve healthcare quality and safety.

After leaving the Joint Commission at the end of 2007, O'Leary was appointed to the board of directors of the Consumers Advancing Patient Safety (CAPS), an organization that promotes patient-centered healthcare.

Ross M. Mullner

See also Accreditation; Joint Commission; National Patient Safety Goals; ORYX Performance Measurement System; Outcomes Movement; Patient-Reported Outcomes (PRO): Quality of Healthcare; Structure-Process-Outcome Quality Measures

Further Readings

O'Leary, Dennis S. "Organizational Evaluation and a Culture of Safety and Reducing Errors in Health Care." In *Proceedings of Enhancing Patient Safety and Reducing Errors in Health Care*, edited by Adam L. Scheffler and Lori Zipperer, 34–37. Chicago: National Patient Safety Foundation, 1999.

O'Leary, Dennis S. "Accreditation's Role in Reducing Medical Errors," *British Medical Journal* 320(7237): 727–28, March 18, 2000.

O'Leary, Dennis S. "The Will to Change," *Health Affairs* 23(2): 288, 2004.

O'Leary, Dennis S. "Is 'First Do No Harm' a Lost Concept in Medical Education?" *Medscape General Medicine* 8(3): 77, September 8, 2006.

Web Sites

Consumers Advancing Patient Safety (CAPS): http://www.patientsafety.org

Joint Commission: http://www.jointcommission.org

ORYX PERFORMANCE MEASUREMENT SYSTEM

ORYX is a tool used by healthcare organizations to evaluate their ongoing performance and to inform continuous quality improvement efforts. The ORYX initiative was developed and implemented by the Joint Commission and came into use in 1997. This system for the first time included performance and outcome measures in the accreditation process that was applied to hospitals, long-term care organizations, and healthcare networks. ORYX was later expanded to also include behavioral healthcare and home care organizations.

The concept of ORYX was to be a continuous, data-driven process that evaluates a healthcare organization's standard of compliance and the outcomes of this process. Joint Commission officials note that ORYX provides purchasers and consumers of care with another level of assurance that Joint Commission–accredited organizations are evaluated on outcomes in addition to the on-site surveys that take place.

Initial policies regarding ORYX called for accredited healthcare organizations to select two of the approved measures, also known as noncore measures, and to report data on at least 20% of the patient population from a list of 60 performance measurement systems that met the Joint Commission's criteria. This information was to be collected on monthly data points and transmitted on a quarterly basis in an electronic machine-readable format via the Internet or electronic bulletin board services to an approved Performance Measurement System (PMS). The Joint Commission delayed the reporting of core measures for long-term care, home care, and behavioral-health organizations so that applicable core measures could be identified. This was in response to the lack of national consensus on appropriate performance measures for nonhospital settings of care. ORYX provides healthcare organizations with a greater degree of flexibility in selecting measures, which was identified as a problem in the past under the Indicator Measurement System (IMSystem).

In July 2002, the first ORYX measures on accredited hospitals were collected. Hospitals are required to collect and report on at least three core measures or up to nine measures if not participating in core measurement activities, to satisfy the requirements of accreditation. Nonhospitals must collect six measures to satisfy accreditation requirements. To reduce the burden of reporting requirements for hospitals and other healthcare organizations, the Joint Commission has worked closely with the Centers for Medicare and Medicaid Services (CMS), the National Quality Forum, and other entities to develop and standardize these core measures.

One criticism of the ORYX program is that healthcare organizations may focus their quality improvement efforts on only the reported measures of quality or selected measurements that they perform well on. In addition, critics cite that the measures only represent a small number of medical conditions. The Joint Commission concedes these facts; however, it is acknowledged that healthcare organizations will eventually have to report measures on a greater percentage of their population. Some professionals question how performance data will correlate with hospital accreditation and the ability of the Joint Commission, a private organization supported by the hospital industry, to objectively evaluate hospital performance.

History

The Joint Commission's history of performance measurement can be traced back to the early days of Ernest Codman, who established the concept of the data-driven "end-result" system in the 1900s. The Joint Commission's Agenda for Change had at its centerpiece the goal of incorporating performance measurement into its accreditation process. During the period leading up to this, beginning in 1986, the Joint Commission was in the process of developing, testing, and implementing standardized performance measures and also establishing the infrastructure to transmit and collect these performance measurement data. This initiative was known then as the Indicator Measurement System (IMSystem). The reason for the development of the IMSystem was that until this point compliance with standards was the basic measure of healthcare quality. This new paradigm to look at the actual results and outcome of care called for a more integrated approach to evaluation of healthcare organizations. The use of performance data by the Joint Commission would facilitate the quality improvement efforts of healthcare organizations, ensure accountability, and combine performance with standards compliance in the accreditation process.

The IMSystem was to be a national comparative measurement system comprising indicators of outcome and process measures that would reflect the appropriateness or effectiveness of performance. Outcome indicators were also to be appropriately risk adjusted to account for differences in patient-level factors. The set of performance measures under the IMSystem included perioperative care, obstetrical care, trauma care, oncology care, infection control, and medication use. The goal at the time was that hospitals would collect and start to transmit data on these measures beginning in 1995 but they would retain choice and flexibility in selecting appropriate measures to report on. The IMSystem did not take off due to the quickly changing measurement environment and because many hospitals felt that this project was not practicably feasible. Although the IMSystem never reached fruition, it served as the predecessor for the new ORYX initiative. With changing knowledge, the Joint Commission revised its original performance measures and pursued a collaborative approach in the ORYX initiative.

In 1999, the Joint Commission sought input from healthcare professionals about the initial set of hospital core measures. The Attributes of Core

Performance Measures and Associated Evaluation Criteria were used to evaluate candidate measures as potential core measures. After the core measures were developed, the Joint Commission initiated a pilot project to test the feasibility and usefulness of these measures. Out of the 11 state hospital associations that were interested in participating in this project, 5 (Connecticut, Michigan, Missouri, Georgia, and Rhode Island) were randomly selected to participate and identify a single performance measure system and participant hospitals. Through this pilot demonstration, the Joint Commission was able to receive feedback, as well as modify and assess the reliability of the core measures. After this feedback period, the Joint Commission made a series of revisions to the initial core measures prior to the full-scale implementation of this project.

During 1995, a request for PMSs to participate in the ORYX initiative was made. Candidate PMSs were evaluated against specified characteristics known as the Attributes of Conformance. The Attributes of Conformance were created by the Joint Commission to ensure that PMSs had the technical and operational infrastructure necessary to support this performance measurement initiative in the present as well as the future. The attributes of PMSs typically included appropriate performance measures that focused on organization performance, clinical processes and/or outcomes, operational database, processes that ensure data quality, risk adjustment methods, feedback to participating organizations, and usefulness and relevance to the accreditation process. The initial attributes were defined at the minimal level; however, they have been modified several times because of the growing need to maintain data quality.

After candidate PMSs passed this initial evaluation, a "request for indicators" was issued to receive PMS extant measures for review, evaluation, and approval for use in ORYX. Once they were approved, healthcare organizations could select these measures to satisfy the requirements of ORYX. The Joint Commission's database stores more than 15,000 extant performance measures.

PMSs that satisfied the selection criteria were listed for accredited healthcare organizations to select and contract with in order to meet accreditation requirements. PMSs serve as an intermediary between the Joint Commission and accredited healthcare organizations to receive and aggregate transmitted data. PMSs ensure data quality, analyze and risk adjust the data, and provide feedback to participating organizations. At present, more than 400 PMSs have been evaluated, and 98 PMSs currently participate in the ORYX initiative.

Once the Joint Commission receives the aggregated data from the PMSs, the data are passed through an automated filter process. The Joint Commission developed a software application to compare incoming data against specific statistical process control decision rules, known as the Auto-Stat process. All the data reported are run through this application, which provides comparative information and helps identify any outliers. Only data that have passed through this filtering process are then included in the Joint Commission's database. The Joint Commission conducts three types of analyses on its data: data quality assessment, intraorganizational analyses, and interorganizational analyses. These data are important in the Joint Commission's Priority Focus Process aligned with its new accreditation process, Shared Visions-New Pathways.

Data quality is assessed through the data filter process, through PMS audits, and during the on-site survey of accredited healthcare organizations. Intraorganizational analyses involve the use of control charts to assess the processes involved in the results being measured. This analysis includes evaluating the data to examine trends and patterns in organizational performance and identifying areas for improvement. The organization-specific data are also used to develop a customized on-site survey agenda and will be factored into the accreditation decision-making process. To evaluate whether an organization is performing within an acceptable range during a given period of time, the Joint Commission conducts a comparative interorganizational analysis. This analysis entails comparing an individual organization with a comparison group's data, which is then summarized in a comparison chart. The comparison chart includes an organization's observed rate, the expected rate, and the expected range or acceptance interval associated with the expected rate.

When the Joint Commission initially began to use performance measurement data, it was focused primarily on the presurvey report during the on-site visit. This presurvey report was tailored specifically for each accredited healthcare organization and included a control and comparison chart for each measure selected. The control chart examined the organization's performance over time, while the comparison chart compared the organization with other organizations collecting the same measures.

The Joint Commission also commenced to use ORYX data to detect sentinel events at facilities. If the Joint Commission learns of a sentinel event through the quarterly reporting by hospitals, this will be considered to be self-reported by the healthcare organization and would require a root-cause analysis and action plan or an evaluation of the response.

Some limitations of the ORYX initiative are that small rural hospitals do not typically have enough cases of events to draw any meaningful conclusions. Thus, hospitals with an average daily census of fewer than 10 patients and a monthly ambulatory population of fewer than 150 patients are currently exempted from submitting data on the ORYX requirements. Additionally, the issue of multiple comparisons of organizations across time and cross-sectionally may have resource implications.

As new technologies rapidly emerge and advances are made in healthcare, the Joint Commission must continue to find ways to adapt to reflect the growing sophistication of performance measurement. To meet this challenge, the Joint Commission's Performance Measurement Strategic Issues Work Group has developed areas of focus for the next 5 years. These focus areas include refining the receiving of standardized-performance measurement data from participating healthcare organizations, expanding the breadth of measure sets available that healthcare organizations may select, creating applications that will be able to use measurement data in the accreditation process as well as public reporting efforts, coordination of data demands and prioritization of measurement areas to reduce data collection burden and eliminate duplication for healthcare organizations, and continued support for the role of the National Quality Forum as the leader in setting measurement objectives.

Ongoing Activities

At present, the Joint Commission has identified five core performance measure sets for hospitals: (1) myocardial infarction, (2) heart failure,

(3) pneumonia, (4) pregnancy and related conditions, and (5) surgical infection prevention. Additionally, intensive-care unit (ICU), pain management, children's asthma care, and hospital-based psychiatric-service measures are scheduled to be implemented soon.

The process involved in creating these measures includes working with a technical expert panel, testing, and development of technical specifications. All these core measures have been reviewed and approved by the National Quality Forum.

Quality Check® was established the same year as the ORYX initiative and serves as a directory of accredited organizations and performance reports available for public use on the Joint Commission's Web site. In 2004, the debut of Quality Report became available to the general public at www.qualitycheck.org, which allowed easy access to organization-specific data that included composite scores for each set of reported measures. This result is displayed against comparative state and national data.

The use of measurement data in the accreditation process has also grown with the evolution of these measures. In addition to being used for continuous quality improvement efforts of healthcare organizations and the Joint Commission's presurvey report, performance measures are also used to focus on the on-site accreditation survey through the Priority Focus Process (PFP). The PFP compiles data from various sources and identifies one or more focus areas for the on-site survey.

Data management efforts of ORYX data have also evolved over time with newer methods. In the beginning of the ORYX initiative, data quality was focused primarily on missing data and outliers. Data integrity became even more important with public reporting and the core measures. As a result, the Joint Commission continues to monitor data quality after each quarter of data submission. Currently, the issues involved in the data management of ORYX include the aggregation of data and the reliability of data collection.

Other Health Quality Initiatives

In 1999, the National Quality Forum was formed to review and approve performance measures. The National Academy of Sciences, Institute of Medicine's report *Crossing the Quality Chasm* outlined the quality improvement objectives for the nation. With many actors now involved in health-care quality, the Joint Commission became engaged in initiatives such as the Hospital Quality Alliance.

The federal CMS heads a program similar to the Joint Commission's ORYX, known as the Hospital Quality Alliance: Improving Care Through Information. This is a public-private partnership aimed at improving care in the nation's hospitals by measuring and publicly reporting on this care. This program collects information on hospital performance measures for heart attack, congestive heart failure, pneumonia, and surgical infections, and it plans to continue to expand in the future. This initiative grew out of the collaboration between the CMS, American Hospital Association (AHA), Federation of American Hospitals, and Association of American Medical Colleges (AAMC) and is supported by the Agency for Healthcare Research and Quality (AHRQ), National Quality Forum, Joint Commission, American Medical Association (AMA), American Nurses Association (ANA), National Association of Children's Hospitals and Related Institutions, Consumer-Purchaser Disclosure Project, American Federation of Labor and Congress of Industrial Organizations (AFL-CIO), AARP, and U.S. Chamber of Commerce. A *Hospital Compare* report, which provides an easy to use interface on hospital performance, can be found at www.hospitalcompare.hhs.gov.

Future Goals

The Joint Commission envisions that performance measurement will become a seminal part of the information technology infrastructure. Some future objectives of the Joint Commission's performance measurement data include the following: the creation of a national standardized data set, continuous data monitoring and follow-up with healthcare organizations to identify areas for ongoing improvement, refining standards through the use of measure data, including measurement data in the AHRQ's National Health Care Quality and Disparities Reports, the use of measurement data to improve the quality of care through research, the use of measurement data to identify high-reliability healthcare organizations, the use of measurement data to identify evidence-based practices and establish national benchmarks, establishing processes to support increased use of measurement data by consumers, and the use of measurement data to ascertain healthcare organization reimbursements levels.

The development of new core measures will eventually replace noncore measures in nonhospital areas (long-term care, ambulatory care, home care, and behavioral health). Additionally, the Joint Commission plans to seek patient-level data, which will ensure higher levels of data quality; information regarding development; increased research related to performance measurement and quality improvement efforts; increased support for the Joint Commission's new accreditation process; and ongoing support of efforts to ensure the relevance, usefulness, reliability, and validity of the measures.

With the increasing sophistication of medical care, the Joint Commission will continue to identify measures that are no longer relevant and will find ways to randomly collect data on these "retired" measures. Additionally, the Joint Commission expects to implement patient perception of care as a core measure over the next several years through a standardized hospital patient experience-of-care tool, known as the CAHPS Hospital Survey.

As the Joint Commission continues to work with its national partners in quality improvement and performance measurement efforts, it is guided by the continued expansion and coordination of nationally standardized core measurement capabilities and increasing the use of measurement data for quality improvement efforts, benchmarking, accountability, decision making, accreditation, and research. It is anticipated that the attainment of these goals will lead to the continued improvement in patient safety and quality of healthcare organizations.

Jared Lane K. Maeda

See also Joint Commission; National Quality Forum (NQF); O'Leary, Dennis S.; Outcomes-Based Accreditation; Outcomes Movement; Quality Indicators; Quality Management; Quality of Healthcare

Further Readings

Campbell, Sandy. "Outcomes-Based Accreditation Evolves Slowly with JCAHO's ORYX Initiative," *Health Care Strategic Management* 15(4): 12–13, 1997.

Caron, Aleece, and Duncan V. Neuhauser. "Health Care Organization Improvement Reports Using Control Charts for Key Quality Characteristics: ORYX Measures as Examples," *Quality Management in Health Care* 9(3): 28–39, Spring 2001.

DeMott, Karen. "JCAHO Introduces ORYX for Outcomes-Based Accreditation," *Quality Letter for Healthcare Leaders* 9(3): 18–19, 1997.

Lee, Kwan, Jerod Loeb, and Deborah Nadzam. "Special Report: An Overview of the Joint Commission's ORYX Initiative and Statistical Methods," *Health Services & Outcomes Research Methodology* 1(1): 63–73, 2000.

Loeb, Jerod, and Alfred Buck. "Framework for Selection of Performance Measurement Systems: Attributes of Conformance," *Journal of the American Medical Association* 275(7): 508, February 21, 1996.

Morrissey, John. "Quality Measures Hit Prime Time: JCAHO's ORYX Lights Fire Under Providers," *Modern Healthcare* 27(18): 66–72, May 5, 1997.

National Academy of Sciences, Institute of Medicine. *Crossing the Quality Chasm.* Washington, DC: Institute of Medicine, 1999.

Schyve, Paul, Jerod Loeb, and Bryan Simmons. "A Collaborative Project to Study Hospital Performance Measures," *Journal of the American Medical Association* 274(19): 1497, November 15, 1995.

Web Sites

Hospital Compare: http://www.hospitalcompare.hhs.gov
Joint Commission: http://www.jointcommission.org
National Healthcare Quality Report:
    http://nhqrnet.ahrq.gov/nhqr/jsp/nhqr.jsp

OUTCOMES-BASED ACCREDITATION

Outcomes-based accreditation is an objective, data-driven process of externally evaluating providers, healthcare facilities, or health plans through the use of performance measures. Risk-adjusted outcome measures, such as mortality, quality of life, patient functional ability, and patient satisfaction, are used to compare among providers of care and healthcare organizations to make choosing a provider more meaningful to patients since patients are ultimately concerned about their health outcomes.

History

Florence Nightingale was the first to study health outcomes by measuring mortality and infection rates in British military hospitals during the Crimean War. In the early 20th century, a pioneering physician at the Massachusetts General Hospital in Boston, Ernest Codman, proposed an *end-results system* to examine patient outcomes of surgical procedures. At the time, Codman's idea was viewed as radical and against the medical establishment. Building on Codman's idea, Avedis Donabedian developed a framework for quality assessment that included structure, process, and outcomes. Structure refers to the structural characteristics of healthcare organizations, such as the number of certified staff, equipment, and medical technologies; process includes all the processes involved in providing care to the patient; and outcomes are the results of the care rendered by the provider.

Historically, accreditation reviews were primarily based on structural features since they were easy to measure; however, recently there has been a movement to further examine process and outcomes measures that give a more comprehensive view of patient care quality and enable consumers and purchasers to make informed healthcare decisions. By using the framework of Donabedian and Codman's end-result system, organizations such as the National Committee for Quality Assurance (NCQA) and the Joint Commission have started using outcomes to accredit health plans and healthcare facilities.

Accrediting Organizations

The NCQA, a private, nonprofit organization, is dedicated to improving healthcare quality by accrediting and certifying a wide range of healthcare plans through its set of performance measures known as the Health Plan Employer Data and Information Set (HEDIS). The mission of the NCQA is to provide information to purchasers and consumers on the quality of care of managed-care organizations that will allow them to make informed purchasing decisions. Beginning with HEDIS 3.0, the NCQA started to make progress by including the outcomes measures of patient function and satisfaction in its evaluation process. The major barrier to the initial implementation of outcomes measures in HEDIS was the lack of information technology infrastructure to capture these measurements. NCQA's report *A Road Map for Information Systems: Evolving Systems to Support Performance Measurements* outlined the upgrades needed to meet the demand of outcomes measurement.

The Joint Commission, an independent, private, nonprofit organization, accredits and evaluates approximately 15,000 healthcare organizations and programs in the United States. In 1997, the ORYX Performance Measurement System for the first time integrated performance measures into the Joint Commission's accreditation process. Beginning in July 2002, the first core measures on accredited hospitals were collected.

The purpose of ORYX is to link patient outcomes with accreditation to make the accreditation process more valuable while focusing on patient-centered care. ORYX is used as a supplement to the standards-based survey by continuously monitoring the performance of organizations, facilitating continuous quality improvement, and targeting the on-site survey. To meet accreditation requirements, some healthcare organizations must submit data on a specified minimum number of measures to a performance measurement system or the Joint Commission, and these data are reviewed by the surveyor(s) at the on-site survey. Using data reported from the organization's core measures, the surveyors assess the performance improvement activities of the organization during the on-site survey.

The Joint Commission intends to use ORYX to identify data trends that will enable organizations to improve the quality of care. To reduce the burden of reporting requirements for hospitals, the Joint Commission has worked closely with the Centers for Medicare and Medicaid Services (CMS) to align performance measures.

Issues of Using Outcomes

The contention surrounding the use of patient outcomes in accreditation includes the issues of risk adjustment, the case-mix of patients, and the small number of cases of individual providers. Risk adjustment is a statistical method that tries to control for the differences in patient characteristics or case-mix that may unduly affect outcomes. For example, a provider that treats a greater number of sicker patients may appear to have worse outcomes than a provider that treats relatively healthier patients. Therefore, risk adjustment statistically adjusts for these underlying differences in the case-mix of patients.

The issue of small numbers is also a problem that arises where providers may not treat a sufficient number of cases to draw statistically valid conclusions regarding a provider's performance. This may limit the comparisons that can be made among providers for a given set of conditions.

Other issues concerning the use of outcomes include the fact that a patient's outcome is shaped by many other factors outside the provider's control, even if appropriate care was given. Conversely, a patient may still have a good outcome despite the poor processes of care delivered by the provider due to the resiliency of the human body. Additionally, it may take many years before a particular health outcome is observed, and therefore, outcomes may need to be tracked longitudinally for an extended period. Furthermore, data on health outcomes can be labor intensive, costly, and difficult to collect.

The field of outcomes measurement is still young, where there are only a few available measures for specific conditions. Measuring outcomes for the purposes of accreditation relies on the collection of valid and reliable data; standardized data elements and definitions; appropriate risk adjustment methods; information technology infrastructure; and the ability to compare outcomes across providers, organizations, and health plans.

Future Implications

Outcomes measures in accreditation will continue to play an important role in evaluating healthcare providers, organizations, and health plans. The development of additional measures of outcomes will be needed to broaden the set of conditions available. With the greater availability of outcomes measures through accrediting bodies, consumers and purchasers will be able to make more informed decisions of where to seek and purchase their care and will continue to pressure healthcare providers, organizations, and health plans to continuously improve the quality of care they deliver.

Jared Lane K. Maeda

See also Accreditation; Case-Mix Adjustment; Healthcare Effectiveness Data and Information Set (HEDIS); Joint Commission; National Committee for Quality Assurance (NCQA): ORYX Performance Measurement System; Outcomes Movement; Structure-Process-Outcome Quality Measures

Further Readings

Clancy, Carolyn M., and John M. Eisenberg. "Outcomes Research: Measuring the End Results of Health Care," *Science* 282(5387): 245–46, October 9, 1998.

DeMott, K. "JCAHO Introduces ORYX for Outcomes-Based Accreditation," *Quality Letter for Healthcare Leaders* 9(3): 18–19, March 1997.

Donabedian, Avedis. "The End Results of Health Care: Ernest Codman's Contribution to Quality Assessment and Beyond," *Milbank Quarterly* 67(2): 233–56, 1989.

Harris, Marilyn D., ed. *Handbook of Home Health Care Administration.* 4th ed. Sudbury, MA: Jones and Bartlett, 2005

O'Malley, Colleen. "Quality Measurement for Health Systems: Accreditation and Report Cards," *American Journal of Health-System Pharmacy.* 54(13): 1528–35, July 1, 1997.

National Committee for Quality Assurance. *A Road Map for Information Systems: Evolving Systems to Support Performance Measurements.* Washington, DC: National Committee for Quality Assurance, 1997.

Rozovsky, Fay Adrienne, and James R. Woods Jr., eds. *The Handbook of Patient Safety Compliance: A Practical Guide for Health Care Organizations.* San Francisco: Jossey-Bass, 2005.

Web Sites

Joint Commission: http://www.jointcommission.org
National Committee for Quality Assurance (NCQA): http://www.ncqa.org

OUTCOMES MOVEMENT

The outcomes movement is an initiative designed to improve the quality of healthcare by identifying what works (and encouraging its use) and what doesn't (and discouraging the use of those treatments). It establishes links between health-care practices and procedures with specific outcomes, for the patients as well as the healthcare system. It involves evaluating in a scientific manner the consequences of medical care, diagnostic testing, and other services. This information is then pooled and analyzed and made available to the medical-practice community, healthcare administrators, and third-party payers. The goal is the development of care guidelines that improve patient outcomes and result in effective and efficient healthcare organization and delivery.

In the past, medical-care practices often developed because of anecdotal information and the experience of the individual physician and his or her colleagues. At times, this led to geographic differences in the use of a particular medical intervention. In such cases, the geographical area in which the patient would be treated served as an important predictor of the selected treatment protocol. The outcomes movement is an attempt to develop, as an alternative, a data-driven approach that makes sense across the board. This is done by systematically collecting information about patients and the medical interventions they experience. The outcomes of those interventions for the patient and the healthcare system are then documented and made available to the medical/patient community. These data are analyzed and the results used to develop best practices to improve the quality of care.

History

The value of outcomes measurement was recognized in the early 1900s, when Ernest A. Codman (1869–1940), a New England surgeon, said that treatment results and benefits should be documented. Codman created "end-result cards," which contained basic patient demographic data, the diagnosis, the treatment, the short-term outcomes, and, when possible, the outcomes after 1 year. He contended that this type of information was necessary to make sound judgments about treatment efficacy. The movement became energized in the 1960s with the work of Avedis Donabedian (1919–2000), a physician and public health academician with a strong interest in healthcare quality. Donabedian's quality model began with structure (the medical facilities and personnel), continued with process (the treatment),

and led to the outcomes (the effects of the care on patients). Donabedian stated that outcomes are crucial to judging the value of medical care and noted that mortality data alone are not sufficient. Quality-of-life indicators and patient satisfaction, though less easily measured, are also relevant and should be studied as well, in his view. At this point, the outcomes movement focused primarily on the patient rather than the healthcare delivery system as a whole.

The rapid rise in healthcare costs in the 1970s and 1980s has put the outcomes movement into an additional context. The focus now includes the financial issues and the concomitant effects on the medical system, insurance reimbursement, and federal programs. Technological innovations, the cost of new drugs and therapies, and the aging of the nation's population have thrust the issue of medical-care costs into the forefront. Insurance companies and other third-party payers as well as clinicians and hospital administrators have sought to distinguish between available therapies and those that work and matter. Researchers began to take note of the fact that different geographical areas exhibited wide variation in the use of resources and in the rates of certain medical procedures. After much investigation, however, the researchers did not find any meaningful differences in population characteristics and patient outcomes. This suggested, for example, that some surgical procedures were unnecessary, and limiting them to situations in which they would provide benefit could help contain rising costs. Other research claimed to demonstrate the lack of efficacy of some traditionally used interventions. By the 1990s, assessment and data-driven healthcare became the new mantra, and the outcomes movement came of age.

Current Usage

The outcomes movement provides an important framework for reviewing and refining medical care. Simply put, positive outcomes support the treatment or policy being studied, and negative outcomes suggest modification/elimination of that approach. At its best, outcomes research can provide information about the efficacy of the treatment and care, improve quality, save money, alter public policy in beneficial ways, and guide decision making.

As physicians and patients increasingly are able to obtain aggregated information about the harms and benefits of a medical intervention, they can make appropriately informed decisions. The medical community also uses this information to develop best practices—that is, the identification of treatment guidelines that work most effectively and with maximum benefit to the patients in specific situations. This information likewise is being used to develop and modify public policy as agencies strive to incorporate evidence in their public health initiatives. This includes disease prevention as well as the development of cost-effective and efficient disease-screening recommendations.

The trend toward shared or patient-centered decision making, likewise, has spurred interest in outcomes data. Patients increasingly are doing their own searches to ascertain the benefits and harms of specific treatment alternatives and seeking that kind of data from the medical profession. Outcomes data about survival and function probabilities are intrinsic to these efforts.

Health outcomes data are now multifaceted and include not just mortality data but also quality-of-life measures, such as the ability to function. In addition, outcome data about patient attitudes and satisfaction are becoming increasingly important to clinicians and hospital leadership, in part due to the competitive healthcare environment. Data can come from administrative and clinical databases, disease registries, clinical trial data, and census information, with an emphasis on large and more inclusive databases.

However, some critics of outcomes-based recommendations argue that solely relying on aggregated data doesn't allow for the flexibility that is necessary to adapt to the needs of the individual patient. The desire to eliminate variation can lead to treatment protocols that are too standardized, in this view. Counterarguments state that outcomes data are principally valuable when medical interventions have been carefully and thoroughly studied. Many ambiguities exist in diagnosis and treatment; so individual physician interpretation is and will continue to be crucial in complex cases. Other critics have argued that outcomes research initiatives have design limitations and are primarily cost containment strategies. Public programs such as Medicaid and Medicare require that outcomes data be designed to improve the quality of care as well as to study and monitor resource utilization.

Economic studies can be done in various ways; they can take into account cost-to-outcome data, which focus on the cost of treating a disease. Cost-effectiveness studies compare the cost of one treatment over another and the benefit of that treatment over the other in terms of a specific outcome. Cost-utility studies weight outcomes according to how they are valued. The structure-process-outcome taxonomy has been found to be useful in studying administrative and economic effects on systems. Administrative outcomes studies focus on structure, process, and personnel. Economic outcomes may include the cost of care, unnecessary or inappropriate care, length of patient stay, patient readmission, return to work, and the ability to provide self-care.

Government financial support has been an integral part of these initiatives, with research funded though organizations such as the Agency for Healthcare Research and Quality (AHRQ). Research supported by the AHRQ and other government organizations has become part of the report card for healthcare purchasers and consumers to judge healthcare quality.

The AHRQ has established evidence-based practice centers, which are designed to analyze information and develop recommendations that are relevant to decision makers. The focus areas now include the U.S. Preventive Service Task Force, which reviews evidence in clinical prevention initiatives and provides technical support; the Technology Assessment Program, which studies the clinical utility of medical interventions to help the Centers for Medicare and Medicaid Services (CMS) make outcomes-based decisions for the Medicare program; the Generalist Program, which reviews a broad spectrum of clinical, behavioral, economic, and health system delivery issues; the Effective Health Care Program, which provides comparisons of effectiveness studies for patients, clinicians, and policymakers to use in making their decisions; and the Scientific Resources Center, which provides scientific and methodological assistance to several of the above programs.

These efforts, and others that will occur in the future, are designed to provide the basis for continuous quality improvement, as medicine strives to improve patient outcomes and to do so within an efficient and effective healthcare delivery system.

Mary C. Odwazny

See also Agency for Healthcare Research and Quality (AHRQ); Centers for Medicare and Medicaid Services (CMS); Codman, Ernest Amory; Cost-Benefit and Cost-Effectiveness Analysis; Donabedian, Avedis; Health Report Cards; Quality Indicators: Quality of Healthcare

Further Readings

Bachner, Paul. "Patient Outcomes and Pathology Practice: An Introduction to the College of American Pathologists Conference XXXIV on Molecular Pathology: Role in Improving Patient Outcomes," *Archives of Pathology and Laboratory Medicine* 123: 996–99, November 1999.

Bourne, Robert B., William J. Maloney, and James G. Wright. "An AOA Critical Issue the Outcome of the Outcomes Movement." *The Journal of Bone and Joint Surgery (American)* 86(3): 633–40, March 2004.

Jeffort, Michael, Martin R. Stockler, and Martin H. Tattersall. "Outcomes Research: What Is It and Why Does It Matter?" *Internal Medicine Journal* 33(3): 110–18, March 2003.

Lee, Stephanie J., and Craig C. Earle. "Outcomes Research in Oncology: History, Conceptual Framework and Trends in the Literature." *Journal of the National Cancer Institute* 92(3): 195–204, February 2002.

MacKinnon, Joyce, David Shelledy, Cara Case, et al. "Allied Health Outcomes Research Using a Collaborative Distance Approach," *Journal of Allied Health* 29(2): 99–102, Summer 2000.

Tanenbaum, S. J. "Evidence and Expertise: The Challenge of the Outcomes Movement to Medical Professionalism," *Academic Medicine* 74(7): 757–63, July 1999.

Wilson, Ira B., and Paul D. Cleary. "Linking Clinical Variables With Health-Related Quality of Life. A Conceptual Model of Patient Outcomes." *Journal of the American Medical Association.* 273(1): 59–65, January 4, 1995.

Web Sites

AcademyHealth: http://www.academyhealth.org

Agency for Healthcare Research and Quality (AHRQ): http://www.ahrq.gov

American College of Emergency Physicians (ACEP): http://www.acep.org

Centers for Medicare and Medicaid Services (CMS): http://www.cms.hhs.gov

Health Grades: http://www.healthgrades.com

Joint Commission: http://www.jointcommission.org

OUTPATIENT CARE

See Ambulatory Care

P

PACIFIC BUSINESS GROUP ON HEALTH (PBGH)

The Pacific Business Group on Health (PBGH) is a large California healthcare business coalition. The PBGH includes more than 30 large companies as well as a subcoalition of more than 20 high-tech businesses. In total, these members represent more than 3 million employees, dependents, and retirees, accounting for about $10 billion in annual healthcare expenditures. To become a member of the PBGH, an employer must have at least 2,000 covered lives in California. Excluded from membership are healthcare consulting groups, insurance companies, health plans, hospitals, medical groups, and any other healthcare industry employers. The coalition is active in healthcare purchasing, quality improvement, and consumer engagement in health decision making.

Overview

The PBGH was founded in 1989 in San Francisco, California, with the mission of seeking to improve the quality and availability of healthcare while moderating costs. The actions taken to realize this mission have evolved from evaluating health plans to assessing other levels of healthcare delivery, such as hospitals, provider groups, and individual providers, as well as engaging the individual consumer in the process of quality assessment and cost moderation.

In the coalition's 1st years, the process of obtaining information from health plans was not in place and was not yet possible. In 1991, the PBGH introduced the Consumer Assessment Health Plan Survey, which began with a survey of the use of prevention guidelines by health plans. The survey revealed large variations. The PBGH used this information to bring together health plans to set guidelines on preventive services and to communicate these guidelines to providers. Observing the lack of data collection and reporting in California, the PBGH formed the California Cooperative Healthcare Reporting Initiative (CCHRI) in 1993. The CCHRI, which is managed by the PBGH, is a collaborative of healthcare purchasers, health plans, and many healthcare providers that produces a yearly report of performance data through a single process. Data collection and reporting has become a collaborative rather than competitive process for this group. In 2001, the CCHRI agreed on standardized diabetes treatment guidelines for the state's health plans and medical groups. The Ambulatory Quality Alliance (AQA) named the CCHRI as one of six organizations in the country to pilot physician-level performance information in 2006.

In 1996, the PBGH launched its consumer information initiative through its HealthScope. The information on the Web site is generally used by members of the PBGH to customize information for their own employees so they can make value-based decisions about their health plan. In later years, HealthScope began to include quality information on hospitals and medical groups.

Moving forward, the PBGH now also plans to assess how best to communicate physician-level choice information.

In 1997, the PBGH won a state bid to privatize a small-group purchasing pool called the Health Insurance Plan of California. The PBGH renamed the pool Pacific Health Advantage and within 4 years enrolled 147,000 members through 11,000 small employers.

The PBGH also helped form the Leapfrog Group in 2000 to communicate hospital performance measures to consumers. During this time period, the PBGH also partnered with the State of California to ask hospitals to voluntarily report performance measures related to coronary artery bypass graft (CABG) surgery. The PBGH followed in the footsteps of New York State and published risk-adjusted outcomes reports available on its HealthScope Web site. Two out of every three hospitals voluntarily participated, and, following the successful publication by the PBGH, legislation was passed in California to make the reporting mandatory starting in 2003.

That same year, the PBGH piloted a program to measure the clinical performance of individual physicians. This effort was furthered by convening a national meeting in 2004 to outline the technical and methodological issues facing the task of assessing individual physician performance. The report, *Advancing Physician Performance Measurement: Using Administrative Data to Assess Physician Quality and Efficiency*, presented significant challenges and a road map for the future. In 2005, the PBGH worked with the California Medical Association and other stakeholders to deliver unprecedented consensus on physician performance measurement. The PBGH is already providing national leadership in developing measurement and reporting systems for individual physicians, and an expanding leadership role figures largely in their plans for the future.

The PBGH's role in purchasing healthcare and controlling costs is directly manifest in The Negotiating Alliance, a mutual benefit corporation. The Negotiating Alliance promotes value-based purchasing through an annual Request for Proposals and a negotiating process on behalf of 400,000 covered lives. The alliance leverages the power of 19 large employers to obtain the best pricing as well as accountability for quality.

Future Implications

The PBGH has written and published many articles, reports, and press releases. The organization has provided testimony to many government commissions and legislatures and has offered its expertise through participation in many forums and meetings. The PBGH, through pilot programs of healthcare measurement and consumer participation, is an active participant in practical health services research. While the PBGH represents many companies with several million covered lives, its influence on healthcare delivery, both statewide and nationally, eclipses this direct service to its members. The PBGH is shaping the healthcare environment of tomorrow by providing leadership on health services measurement and the process of involving consumers in using that information.

Gregory Vachon

See also Cost of Healthcare; Health Report Cards; Leapfrog Group; Midwest Business Group on Health (MBGH); National Business Group on Health (NBGH); National Coalition on Health Care (NCHC); Outcomes Movement

Further Readings

Pacific Business Group on Health. *Advancing Physician Performance Measurement: Using Administrative Data to Assess Physician Quality and Efficiency.* San Francisco: Pacific Business Group on Health, 2005.

Pacific Business Group on Health. *Expectations for Healthcare Value: Advancing Health Plan and Providers.* San Francisco: Pacific Business Group on Health, 2006.

Pacific Business Group on Health. *Evaluation of Consumer Decision Support Tools: Helping People Make Health Care Decisions.* San Francisco: Pacific Business Group on Health, 2007.

Pacific Business Group on Health. *We Must Build Healthcare Value.* San Francisco: Pacific Business Group on Health, 2007.

Stewart, Diane. *Aligning Physician Incentives: Lessons and Perspectives from California.* San Francisco: Pacific Business Group on Health, 2005.

Thomas, J. William. *Hospital Cost Efficiency Measurement: Methodological Approaches.* San Francisco: Pacific Business Group on Health, 2006.

Web Sites

HealthScope: http://www.healthscope.org
Pacific Business Group on Health (PBGH):
    http://www.pbgh.org

PAIN

The word *pain* derives from Sanskrit and Latin roots: *pu*, meaning purification, and *poena*, meaning punishment. Pain can be physical, psychological, or sociocultural. Pain can be manifest in a variety of forms, such as back pain, bone pain, and tooth pain. Pain is a subjective and variable experience and depends on the individual, as individuals may have different thresholds. Pain is a symptom of many medical conditions, and it can have a significant impact on an individual's quality of life and daily functioning. The diagnosis and treatment of pain is based on its classification according to its duration, intensity, type, source, and location. For example, pain can be classified as either acute or chronic. Most bodily pain is able to be resolved with little or no intervention and is generally considered to be acute pain. Chronic pain, also known as persistent or intractable pain, on the other hand, is considered to be an illness and not a symptom.

Pain can be defined in many different ways. One commonly used definition defines pain as an unpleasant experience that can be sensory or emotional in nature, is generally associated with possible or actual damage to bodily tissues, and is expressed through an individual's behavior.

Importance

Pain plays an important role in health services research. Specifically, it directly affects access, cost, quality, and outcomes of healthcare. For example, the occurrence of pain is one of the most common reasons for a physician visit by individuals, resulting in about half of all Americans seeking medical care each year. In addition, pain causes visits by individuals to other ancillary healthcare providers, including physical therapists, occupational therapists, nurses, and psychologists, among others, as well as visits to complementary and alternative medical providers such as acupuncturists and massage therapists. The annual cost associated with pain exceeds $5 billion in the United States.

There are several burdens associated with pain, including costs of healthcare, disability, and lost productivity. Pain is one of the leading causes of disability and functional problems. Furthermore, back, neck, and upper extremity pain are cited as the most common reasons for being sick and taking time off from work, resulting in work and productivity losses. An estimate from a national health survey found that about 18% of U.S. workers experienced approximately 149 million days of lost work due to back pain.

Models of Pain

Historical models of pain include Descartes's mind-body model. The Cartesian model of pain held that there is a direct connection between the nerves and the brain and had a dualistic view of mind and body. Pain is the result of an injury that causes a sensation in the person's mind. The model assumed that the greater the injury, the greater the pain that is experienced by the individual. Pain was thought to result in direct tissue damage to the body. This model also held that pain is either physical or psychological in nature.

Modern models of pain integrate the biological, cognitive, emotional, behavioral, and social aspects of this phenomenon. Studies have shown that many factors may have an influence on pain perception and that this is the result of not only physiological aspects but cognitive and behavioral aspects as well. The modern models tend to view pain as a sensory and emotional experience that is not necessarily the result of tissue injury or a nerve signal.

Pain Scales

Pain has been recognized as a vital sign that should be properly monitored and alleviated. Pain management has been acknowledged to result in faster recovery, improved quality of life, and increased productivity of the individual. Healthcare providers seek to diagnose pain according to its onset, duration, character, location, and severity as well as the symptoms associated with it. The diagnosis of pain requires that the healthcare provider examine a patient's symptoms, condition, and medical history. Pain assessment generally also examines a person's pain threshold in addition to his or her pain tolerance.

A number of pain scales have been developed to assess and evaluate an individual's level of pain, using various methods. For example, the McGill Pain Questionnaire is a tool that is often used to gain a verbal assessment of an individual's pain. The Brief Pain Inventory uses an interview technique to evaluate how pain affects an individual's daily functioning. Scales have also been created to rate an individual's pain, such as the Numeric Rating Scale and the Faces Pain Scale, that assess the intensity of pain as minimal to severe as well as monitoring a person's pain over time to evaluate if the individual responds to treatment. These pain scales also enable medical researchers to compare the results between groups of patients.

Kenneth L. Vaux

See also Acute and Chronic Diseases; Complementary and Alternative Medicine; Disability; Measurement in Health Services Research; Patient-Reported Outcomes; Quality of Healthcare; Quality of Life, Health Related

Further Readings

Gelinas, Celine, Carmen G. Loiselle, Sylvie LeMay, et al. "Theoretical, Psychometric, and Pragmatic Issues in Pain Measurement," *Pain Management Nursing* 9(3): 120–30, September 2008.

Greco, Palo S., and Francesco M. Conti, eds. *Pain Management: New Research*. New York: Nova Science, 2008.

Laccetti, Margaret Saul, and Mary K. Kazanowski. *Pain Management*. 2d ed. Sudbury, MA: Jones and Bartlett, 2008.

Wittink, Harriet M., and Daniel B. Carr, eds. *Pain Management: Evidence, Outcomes, and Quality of Life: A Sourcebook*. New York: Elsevier, 2008.

Web Sites

American Academy of Pain Medicine (AAPM): http://www.painmed.org

American Chronic Pain Association (ACPA): http://www.theacpa.org

American Pain Society (APS): http://www.ampainsoc.org

NIH Pain Consortium: http://painconsortium.nih.gov

PAN AMERICAN HEALTH ORGANIZATION (PAHO)

The Pan American Health Organization (PAHO) is the world's oldest international public health agency, and it is recognized as part of the United Nations system. PAHO has over a century of experience in working to improve the health and living standards of the people in the Americas. PAHO serves as the World Health Organization's (WHO) Regional Office of the Americas as well as the health organization of the Inter-American system. The agency has scientific and technical experts located at its headquarters in Washington, D.C., at its 27 country offices, and at its 9 scientific centers that work on health issues of primary concern to countries in Latin America and the Caribbean. The mission of PAHO is to strengthen local and national health systems and to improve the health of the people of the Americas through various joint collaborative efforts.

History

PAHO was established in 1902 to work with all countries in the Americas to raise the living standards and improve the health of their peoples. PAHO comprises member states that include all 35 countries (Antigua and Barbuda, Argentina, Bahamas, Barbados, Belize, Bolivia, Brazil, Canada, Chile, Colombia, Costa Rica, Cuba, Dominica, Dominican Republic, Ecuador, El Salvador, Grenada, Guatemala, Guyana, Haiti, Honduras, Jamaica, Mexico, Nicaragua, Panama, Paraguay, Peru, Saint Lucia, St. Vincent and the Grenadines, St. Kitts and Nevis, Suriname, Trinidad and Tobago, the United States, Uruguay, and Venezuela) in the Americas, with the addition of Puerto Rico as an associate member; participating states (France, the Netherlands, and the United Kingdom and Northern Ireland); and observer states (Spain and Portugal). PAHO's policies are set through its governing bodies. To advance its organizational mission, PAHO maintains collaborative efforts with Ministries of Health, universities, nongovernmental organizations (NGOs), governmental agencies, and others.

PAHO works to promote primary healthcare strategies in communities by increasing access to care and encouraging the efficient use of limited resources. The organization has been involved in assisting countries to combat reemerging infectious diseases such as cholera, tuberculosis, and dengue as well as emerging infectious diseases such as AIDS, through technical assistance, support, and work with NGOs. In addition, PAHO works to prevent the spread of chronic diseases that have begun to afflict populations in the developing countries of the Americas. The work of PAHO is supported by the contributions of its member governments as well as outside funding that aids special programs.

The PAHO focuses its efforts to target the most vulnerable members of society, including women, children, workers, the elderly, refugees, and displaced persons as well as to address equity issues in terms of access to care. The Pan American approach of having countries cooperate and work together toward shared goals has been an essential part of PAHO's history. The agency has been pivotal in initiating multinational collaborative health ventures in Central America, the Caribbean, the Andean Region, and the Southern Cone. The height of political collaboration resulted when the American heads of state accepted the "Health Technology Linking the Americas" initiative at the Summit in Santiago.

The eradication of smallpox from the Americas in 1973, with worldwide eradication 5 years later, has been one of PAHO's great successes. Another major effort, begun in 1985, to eradicate polio, was accomplished in September, 1994, when the Americas were declared to be polio free by the International Commission. PAHO is close to its goal of eliminating measles from the Americas and continues to introduce vaccines that are available against other diseases, including the Haemophilus influenza B. vaccine to prevent meningitis and respiratory infections. PAHO continues to assist countries to secure the necessary resources to provide for the immunization and treatment of all vaccine-preventable diseases. The agency is also working to reduce morbidity and mortality from diarrheal diseases, including cholera, through case management and oral rehydration therapy, as well as to ensure the diagnosis and treatment of respiratory infections.

PAHO'S Work

PAHO distributes scientific and technical information that is made available through its publications, Web site, libraries, and documentation centers. It also provides technical assistance in the various areas of public health, in addition to organizing disaster relief coordination and emergency preparedness programs.

PAHO supports initiatives to control malaria, Chagas' disease, urban rabies, leprosy, and other diseases affecting people in the Americas. Additionally, it is collaborating with others to address nutritional deficiencies, including iodine and vitamin A deficiencies, as well as protein-energy malnutrition. The organization has also been working with countries to cope with health problems that have resulted from industrial development, including cardiovascular disease, cancer, and substance abuse. It also conducts projects on behalf of other United Nations agencies, international organizations, government agencies, and foundations.

PAHO works to enhance the health sector capacity in countries to address their priority areas. The agency is involved in training health professionals as well as increasing the capacity of national training institutions. PAHO is also working to further integrate women into society and improve the health status of women.

Priority Areas

An important priority area of PAHO is to reduce infant mortality and prevent an additional 25,000 infant deaths a year through the use of the Integrated Management of Childhood Illness strategy. The agency is also marshalling the necessary resources to train healthcare workers to evaluate the health status of children brought in to a health post or clinic as well as to diagnose, treat, and prevent disease.

Recognizing the health consequences and costs associated with tobacco use, the governing bodies of the Pan American Health Organization have directed it to curtail the use of tobacco. Additionally, with an emphasis on equity, a continued priority area of PAHO includes adequate sanitation, improvement of drinking water supplies, and increased access to healthcare for the poor. Furthermore, advocacy efforts have been directed to reduce gender inequity and address the unique health problems of women.

Jared Lane K. Maeda

See also Access to Healthcare; Emergency Preparedness; Emerging Diseases; Infectious Diseases; International Health Systems; Public Health; Tobacco Use; World Health Organization (WHO)

Further Readings

Alleyne, George A. O. "The Pan American Health Organization's First 100 Years: Reflections of the Director," *American Journal of Public Health* 92(121): 1890–94, December 2002.

Andrus, Jon Kim, and Ciro A. de Quadros. *Recent Advancements in Immunization.* 2d ed. Geneva, Switzerland: World Health Organization, 2006.

Cueto, Marcos. *The Value of Health: A History of the Pan American Health Organization.* Rochester, NY: University of Rochester Press, 2005.

Pan American Health Organization. *The Quest for a Healthy America: Celebrating 100 Years of Health.* Washington, DC: Pan American Health Organization, 2002.

Pan American Health Organization. *Health in the Americas, 2007.* Washington, DC: Pan American Health Organization, 2007.

Velzeboer, Marijke. *Violence Against Women: The Health Sector Responds.* Washington, DC: Pan American Health Organization, 2003.

Web Sites

Pan American Health Organization (PAHO): http://www.paho.org

Pan American Journal of Public Health: http://journal.paho.org

World Health Organization (WHO): http://www.who.int

PATIENT-CENTERED CARE

Patient-centered care is care that is sensitive and responsive toward the individual needs, preferences, and values of the patient. The national Institute of Medicine (IOM) named patient-centered care as one of the six domains of health-care quality. Additionally, the importance of this concept is starting to be recognized by the medical community. Studies have shown that patient-centered care results not only in increased patient satisfaction but also in improved patient medical outcomes. Licensing and regulatory bodies, as well as board certification agencies, have begun to include patient-centered criteria in their approval processes for medical professionals. Despite these various efforts, many physicians and other healthcare providers are still not currently practicing patient-centered care.

Overview

The following highlights an example of patient-centered care. A patient presents with throbbing pain in his right leg in a hospital emergency department. The nurses and physicians deal with him gently, as they seek his medical history, and discern the source of his problem. This kind of calm, tender treatment of the ill and infirm is at the core of patient-centered care.

Although patient-centered care is starting to be recognized as an important aspect in healthcare, it has been slow to be fully embraced. National surveys conducted by the Commonwealth Fund found that about 1 in 5 adults has difficulty in communicating with his or her physician. And about 1 in 10 adults has been treated disrespectfully during a healthcare visit. There have also been reports of patients who receive conflicting information from their healthcare providers or of the results of medical tests and medical records not being available at the time of the patient's visit.

As a result of these shortcomings, patients are being asked to become active partners in their healthcare. Through a patient-centered health system, there would be increased patient-provider communication and greater availability of educational materials and tools to help patients make more informed decisions. A patient-centered health system would increase access to care and include timely appointments and off-hour services. The increased use of information technology would be essential to achieve this model.

A patient-centered health system would also include greater continuity of care among primary care and specialist physicians, post-hospital-discharge follow-up, and disease management. Making sure that patients have a medical home is key to developing a patient-centered care model. Furthermore, providing patients with pertinent information on the quality of providers as well as regular feedback would contribute to an improved healthcare system.

According to a study in 2006, physicians say that they favor patient-centered care, but only 22% of physicians actually incorporate these standards into their daily practices. Some practices of patient-centered care, such as same-day appointments, have been integrated; however, other aspects related to care coordination, team-based care, and information systems have yet to be widely implemented. Some other key findings from this study were that physicians in group medical practices of 50 or more are more likely to adopt components of patient-centered care than solo practitioners and that, although 73% of primary-care physicians think that team-based care results in better care decisions, 33% think that the team process makes care cumbersome, and 21% think that it increases the likelihood of medical errors. Only 2% of primary-care physicians are paid for e-mail correspondence with patients. Additionally, 87% of primary-care physicians think that improved teamwork or communication among providers would be effective in improving the quality of patient care.

Patient Feedback

There is reported to be a significant gap between physicians' endorsement of the concept of patient-centered care and their actual adoption of practices to implement it. For example, only 36% of primary-care physicians and 20% of specialists indicated that they receive data based on patient satisfaction surveys, but more than one-quarter indicated that they were actually rewarded based on patient survey data.

Furthermore, physicians report that there is an array of barriers to their adoption of patient-centered care practices, including lack of training, knowledge, and costs. It has been suggested that different incentives might help to facilitate increased adoption of patient-centered practices. If physicians are given the correct tools and practice environment, and also develop a partnership with their patients, then a patient-centered system may be better able to take shape.

Improved Medical Outcomes

Some experts say that patient-centered care needs to be presented differently to physicians. Rather than being an abstract concept, patient-centered care should be shown as something that affects medical outcomes. Demonstrating this will increase the number of physicians who adopt the practice.

For example, health services researchers note that nearly 6% of hospital admissions are caused by patients failing to take prescribed medications (also known as *noncompliance*). The word *compliance* connotes that the patient should do exactly what the physician orders; however, physicians know that an authoritarian approach does not necessarily translate to the best medical outcomes. By being more patient-centered, physicians would treat patients as partners by involving them in planning their healthcare and encouraging them to take responsibility for their health. Experts note that a growing body of research, published during the past three decades, has shown that the nature of the physician–patient conversation has a direct bearing on compliance.

Studies have also shown that patients are more likely to take their medications, abstain from poor nutrition, and show up for appointments on time when allowed to help set their treatment plans. This ultimately promotes patient compliance and leads to better quality of care. Physicians generally underestimate the number of patients who refuse to comply with their regimens. It has been estimated that between 40% and 50% of diabetic patients do not abide by their medication regimens. Similarly, the figure for hypertensive patients is about 40%.

In addition to better medical outcomes, a patient-centered system leads to decreased costs. It has been noted that it is much less expensive to promote compliance than to hospitalize patients because they have not taken their blood pressure pills. One study found that at least half of the patients who were given a prescription did not receive the full benefit because they did not take it, they did not take the right dosage, or they stopped taking it prematurely.

Provider-Patient Communication

Communication with patients is the key to patient-centered care. There are five simple steps that physicians and other healthcare providers can take to communicate more effectively with patients.

First, the patient must determine whether he or she agrees on what the health problem actually is with the physician. A patient with a headache may believe that it is caused by a sinus infection, which should be treated with an antibiotic. However, the physician may believe that it is a migraine and needs a different medicine. If this difference is not resolved, the patient may not take the product as prescribed.

Second, once the patient and physician agree, attainable treatment goals must be set. If a hypertensive patient has a diastolic blood pressure of 120 mmHg, the physician may not want to try to bring it down below 90 mmHg immediately. Rather, the physician may suggest 110 mmHg as a short-term goal. Once this has been reached, the physician can use that to motivate the patient to reduce it even more.

Third, there is generally more than one option to treat a given condition. Physicians should review a reasonable range of alternative treatment options and discuss the benefits and possible side effects of each one in terms that the patient understands.

Fourth, the patient and physician must decide on a feasible course of treatment. They can choose the medical option that makes the most sense. For example, a patient with hypertension may have just remarried and may not want a low-cost drug that could reduce sexual drive. Therefore, he or she may opt for a high-cost product with no sexual side effects. Dosage frequency requires a similar discussion.

Last, the physician should test the patient's knowledge. He or she should ask patients to repeat what they have been told about their illness and treatment plan. It is also important for patients to demonstrate any techniques they have been taught, such as injecting insulin or using a peak flowmeter. For example, some physicians have diabetic patients practice needle sticks in their office using an orange.

There are also questions at the end of a patient visit that allow physicians to screen for likely noncompliance. An example of this is, "On a scale of 1 to 10, with 10 being the highest, how important do you think it is for you to do the things we've been talking about?" By gathering this type of information, the physician may discover that a diabetic patient is convinced that his or her disease is fatal and that any treatment would be in vain. An answer like that will inform the physician that there is a need to further discuss the disease and its management.

Additionally, a physician should probe by asking, "On a scale of 1 to 10, how confident are you that you can adhere to this treatment regimen?" A heavy smoker who is absolutely convinced that he or she needs to give up cigarettes may have a confidence level of 1 that this can be accomplished. However, by examining further, there may be signs that additional counseling and support are needed to monitor the patient closely during the withdrawal stages.

Gene J. Koprowski

See also Continuum of Care; Disease Management; Health Communication; Outcomes Movement; Primary Care; Primary-Care Physicians; Quality of Healthcare; Satisfaction Surveys

Further Readings

Audet, Anne-Marie, Karen Davis, and Stephen C. Schoenbaum. "Adoption of Patient-Centered Care Practices by Physicians," *Archives of Internal Medicine* 166(7): 754–59, 2006.

Davis, Karen, Stephen C. Schoenbaum, and Anne-Marie Audet. "A 2020 Vision of Patient-Centered Primary Care," *Journal of General Internal Medicine* 20(10): 953–57, October 2005.

Frampton, Susan B., and Patrick Charmel Planetree, eds. *Putting Patients First: Best Practices in Patient-Centered Care.* 2d ed. San Francisco: Jossey-Bass, 2009.

Mitchell, Pamela H. "Patient-Centered Care: A New Focus on a Time-Honored Concept," *Nursing Outlook* 56(5): 197–98, September–October 2008.

Sidani, Souraya. "Effects of Patient-Centered Care on Patient Outcomes: An Evaluation," *Research and Theory for Nursing Practice* 22(1): 24–37, 2008.

Wolf, Debra M., Lisa Lehman, Robert Quinlin, et al. "Effect of Patient-Centered Care on Patient Satisfaction and Quality of Care," *Journal Nursing Care Quality* 23(4): 316–21, October–December 2008.

Web Sites

American Academy of Family Physicians (AAFP): http://www.aafp.org

Commonwealth Fund: http://www.commonwealthfund.org

Institute for Healthcare Improvement (IHI):

   http://www.ihi.org

PATIENT DUMPING

Patient dumping—the denial of examination and stabilization services for persons with medical emergencies for reasons unrelated to medical need—constitutes a long-standing issue in U.S. health law and policy. It is relatively common to see the concept of patient dumping expressed strictly in relation to financial motive. In fact, financial motive is not a prerequisite to either the concept of dumping or to legal liability. Legal violation can result even without financial motive, for example, if an HIV-positive patient with a medical emergency is turned away because staff physicians refuse to treat him or her. (In such a situation, a hospital may be in violation not only of antidumping laws but also of federal and state civil rights laws that protect persons with disabilities.)

Nature and Extent

No one really knows the magnitude of patient dumping in the nation. Every so often, a headline-making incident occurs. In 2006, for example, a Los Angeles hospital was criminally charged with discharging a medically unstable homeless woman from her hospital bed—and still in her gown and slippers—to a skid-row neighborhood. But quantitative analyses do not exist, in part because there is no good way to know how many people may be turned away from hospitals with no service at all. Thus, reliable statistics are lacking regarding the number of persons who may be turned away without treatment or who may be prematurely discharged from hospitals in an unstable condition for reasons unrelated to medical need. Relatively precise standards outline the duties of hospitals where emergency care is concerned, and to estimate the dumping problem accurately, incidents would need to be aligned with an array of terms and standards that, in certain aspects, also turn on medical judgment, an added confounder. The federal government does not publicly report on the number of emergency department examinations that fail to result in a finding of an emergency

medical condition, nor are there reports on the number of persons with emergency conditions who are discharged or transferred in an unstable state.

That patient dumping is a real problem is not a matter of serious debate; indeed, the legal framework for patient antidumping standards evolved from the reports of a series of spectacular incidents. Antidumping laws are controversial, in part because of the high level of stress faced by hospital emergency departments. Between 1991 and 2003, hospital emergency department visits in the nation increased by 26%, reaching a 2003 level of about 114 million visits. Of the total number of emergency department visits, about one-third were considered to be nonurgent, meaning that about 38 million visits annually are for conditions that, on examination, may be considered nonemergent. Since antidumping duties commence with the obligation to examine, the fact that many exams reveal nonemergent conditions is actually somewhat tangential. Furthermore, emergency department statistics are predicated on individuals who become registered emergency department patients. How many individuals are actually dumped—that is, turned away without any exam or diverted away from a hospital while in an ambulance—must be factored into the equation when thinking about the true reach of antidumping laws.

The Antidumping Legal Framework

The No-Duty Principle

The starting point for understanding the consequential nature of antidumping obligation is the common law principle of "no duty." Under the common law, that is, under the long-standing principles of judicial law on which much of the U.S. legal system rests, healthcare professionals and other healthcare providers have no duty to furnish care. That is, hospitals and physicians are not considered "places of public accommodation" and thus have no legal duty to furnish care to any person they do not wish to serve. Once a provider-patient relationship is established, then, of course, healthcare providers do have a legal duty to act in a reasonable way. But this duty to behave in a reasonably professional manner does not trigger until a provider actually agrees to enter into a physician–patient relationship.

For example, a physician has no duty to come to the aid of a person suffering a medical emergency (in all jurisdictions, physicians who do provide emergency aid are covered by Good Samaritan laws that protect against all but liability for gross negligence or willful or wanton misconduct). Under common law, hospitals had no duty to treat emergencies.

Evolution of the No-Duty Principle

By the middle of the 20th century, a combination of changing emergency care technology and fundamental shifts in social values led to a fundamental legal rethinking of the no-duty principle by courts and state legislatures, at least where hospital emergency department care was concerned. (To this day, physicians have no legal duty of care.) The rise of the modern hospital, with its technologically advanced and lifesaving emergency department services, was perceived as fueling community expectations of care. The community expectation was further fueled by the considerable community support received by hospitals in the form of insurance payments, direct government support, and nonprofit tax exemptions. Indeed, the Hospital Survey and Construction Act of 1946 (more commonly known as the Hill-Burton Act) represented a national commitment to hospital construction, one that, over time, would come to be understood as creating emergency-care duties of its own.

In sum, by the middle of the 20th century, the nation's hospitals ceased to exist merely as workplaces for physicians. As complex and essential medical-care entities in their own right, hospitals were burgeoning, in great part because of a community commitment to their growth. Furthermore, this national commitment of resources took a massive leap forward with the enactment of Medicare and Medicaid in 1965.

At heart, the law is simply a highly formalized reflection of prevailing social values and beliefs. Thus, as hospitals changed as social institutions, so did their relationship to the law in many respects, including the law as it related to emergency hospital care. Similarly, as market values have come to dominate the hospital industry in recent years, the legal obligations of hospitals in response to emergency cases also have undergone a certain amount of relaxation.

The earliest patient-dumping law came from judicial decisions involving persons who died or were severely injured as a result of the denial of care. Among the principles applied to hospitals by the courts as a means of finding liability for turning people away without care under their "no duty" were the common law concepts of "detrimental reliance," "public accommodation," and "legal undertaking." A detrimental reliance claim was one in which the injured person or decedent's estate argued that the very presence of the hospital emergency department created a legal duty because the community came to rely on its presence in times of emergency; thus, the hospital could not hold itself out as the place to come for emergency care—and indeed, establish a record of furnishing such care—and then select its customers.

A public accommodation claim rested on the notion that, like innkeepers and transportation systems (which are prohibited at common law from refusing paying customers), hospitals with emergency department capacity were obligated to serve the public, even if the public could not pay at the point of service. The public accommodation theory rested on the life and death role played by inns and common carriers during the Middle Ages; thus, as hospitals came to occupy a lifesaving role in society, they came to represent a similar social good.

An undertaking claim rested on the notion that a hospital that turned someone away had actually begun to undertake care. Thus, in one celebrated court case, a hospital was found liable for essentially abandoning a patient when personnel ordered the family of a dying man to place him on an empty stretcher in the emergency department and then ignored him until he died.

In the concept of emergency care, two specific types of duties became evident from these early cases. The first was a duty to examine individuals who come to a hospital seeking care, that is, a duty to undertake care through an initial examination, regardless of factors unrelated to need. The second duty was a duty to stabilize emergency conditions in persons whose examinations revealed an emergency (typically defined as a condition that would lead to death). From the perspective of the totality of healthcare, the duty was quite narrow: Hospitals were not expected to cure or rehabilitate persons with emergencies, merely examine and stabilize them. But from the perspective of the no-duty principle, the departure was profound, particularly because it served to establish the physician–patient relationship on which professional and corporate liability rest. Furthermore, depending on the nature of the emergency, the examination and stabilization could consume considerable resources and be quite lengthy.

The Hill-Burton Act and State Anti–Patient Dumping Statutes

As judicial law shifted, so did statutory and regulatory law. By the early 1980s a number of state legislatures had enacted emergency-care statutes that conditioned licensure on not only maintenance of hospital emergency departments but also the provision of screening and stabilization services to persons with emergency medical conditions, as defined under state law.

In addition, the Hill-Burton Act became the subject of extensive litigation surrounding the meaning of its statutory "community service obligation." This obligation, a companion to the act's better-known "uncompensated care" obligation, required all federally funded hospitals to provide assurances that they would serve their communities. In revised regulations issued in 1979, the U.S. Department of Health and Human Services (HHS) had interpreted the law as requiring the provision of certain emergency-related screening and stabilization services, without regard to whether individuals could pay for the care at the point of service.

The Hill-Burton regulations reached thousands of facilities built with Hill-Burton funding. But by the end of the 1970s, funding had ceased; even during its operational period, Hill-Burton excluded for-profit facilities. Thus, hospitals built over the past generation have received no Hill-Burton funds.

The Emergency Medical Treatment and Active Labor Act

Enacted in 1986, the Emergency Medical Treatment and Active Labor Act (EMTALA) was a response to the U.S. Congress' concern over the impact of the new Medicare prospective payment system (PPS) on hospital access among indigent and uninsured patients. Its enactment followed a series of highly publicized incidents of patient dumping. In its structure and terms, EMTALA is unique in U.S. law. Indeed, EMTALA offers the only example in which U.S. law creates a legally enforceable individual right to healthcare.

EMTALA applies to all Medicare-participating hospitals that operate an emergency department, thus pushing its reach well beyond the limits of previous federal laws applicable only to hospitals built with certain forms of public financing. It obligates a covered hospital to provide an appropriate medical examination to any person who comes to the hospital's emergency department.

It is difficult to overstate the extent to which EMTALA departs from traditional U.S. health policy, given the no-duty principle described above. In short, EMTALA creates an affirmative duty of emergency care on the part of Medicare-participating hospitals with emergency departments, thereby overriding the right of covered hospitals and their staff to select the patients they will serve. This emergency duty of care principle, as noted, has evolved over decades, but EMTALA expands and clarifies the duty in ways not previously seen in law.

At the same time, EMTALA has real limits. EMTALA alone does not compel a hospital to maintain an emergency department (state licensure laws, laws governing the conditions of participation for Medicare hospitals, and accreditation standards might, of course). Nor does EMTALA mandate that hospital emergency departments meet certain staffing and equipment standards (again, accreditation, licensure, and Medicare conditions of participation standards might set performance levels). What EMTALA does require is the undertaking of emergency care in a fair and non-discriminatory fashion.

Sara Rosenbaum

See also Access to Healthcare; Emergency Medical Services (EMS); Emergency Medical Treatment and Active Labor Act (EMTALA); Hospital Emergency Departments; Hospitals; Patient Transfers; Public Policy; Uninsured Individuals

Further Readings

Taylor, Mark. "Oklahoma Hospital Settles Dumping Charges; HHS Negotiating With Other Facilities Accused of Dumping Emergency Room Patient," *Modern Healthcare* 30(33): 2, 12, August 7, 2000.

Taylor, Mark. "Patient Dumping Cases Shoot Up," *Modern Healthcare* 31(29): 6, July 16, 2001.

Taylor, Mark. "Slow Recovery: Patient Dumping Settlement Plunge; Experts Remain Mixed on Factors," *Modern Healthcare* 33(22): 8, 14, June 2, 2003.

Vesely, Rebecca. "Kaiser Probed Again: More Patient Dumping Alleged in Los Angeles Area," *Modern Healthcare* 37(29): 18–19, July 23, 2007.

Web Sites

American Hospital Association (AHA): http://www.aha.org

Centers for Medicare and Medicaid Services (CMS): http://www.cms.hhs.gov

Department of Health and Human Services, Office of Inspector General (OIG): http://www.oig.hhs.gov

PATIENT-REPORTED OUTCOMES (PRO)

In clinical and translational outcomes research, the success of a patient's medical intervention or treatment has traditionally been assessed and documented by a physician or other clinician. Direct observation of response to an intervention is limited to objective measures. An outside observer cannot always measure outcomes of illness, treatment, or health promotion that minimize physical and emotional decline or loss of independence. Interventions affecting an individual's wellness, particularly in chronic disease progression, may have benefits beyond what can be objectively studied, including the preservation of functioning, pain relief, mood enhancement, and overall improvements in quality of life and well-being. With respect to more subjective outcomes, including quality of life, functioning, and symptom reduction, tools that have been validated and deemed sensitive are required to measure the impact of disease and illness from the afflicted individual's perspective. These measures are termed *patient-reported outcomes* (PRO).

Measurement of patient-reported outcomes provides valuable insight into health and illness beyond traditional efficacy or effectiveness research. In contrast to self-evident outcomes of illness such as survival, patient-reported outcomes represent the patient's perspective on the impact of disease and its treatment on his or her everyday functioning and well-being. Instruments, typically questionnaires, can be an important measure of generic quality of life or functional status. Alternatively, they may be specific to disease, treatment, or symptom. Regardless, an instrument must be grounded in clinical and psychometric theory, be representative of domains relevant to what it attempts to measure, and have been demonstrated as valid, reliable, sensitive, and specific.

Guidance Document

Patient-reported outcomes have been defined as a measurement of any aspect of a patient's health status that comes directly from the patient (i.e., without the interpretation of the patient's responses by a physician or anyone else). Following its European counterparts, the U.S. Food and Drug Administration (FDA) released its guidance document for incorporating PRO into clinical research in 2006. This document outlines three key aspects of patient-reported outcomes that make it advantageous to include instruments in clinical and outcomes research.

1. Some Treatment Effects Are Known Only to the Patients

For some interventions, resulting success or failure can only be elucidated by querying the patient or subject. For example, level of anxiety and anxiety relief are the fundamental measures in understanding the benefit of cognitive behavioral therapy for generalized anxiety disorder. Also, pain intensity and pain relief are nearly exclusively subjective. There are little or no observable or physical measures that can be used to examine potential benefit related to treatment.

2. Patients Provide a Unique Perspective on Treatment Effectiveness

Patient-reported outcome measures can reflect what is important to a patient in terms of symptom relief, functioning, and quality of life. Thus, PRO can incorporate patient expectations related to their care. This becomes important when clinically measurable differences related to an intervention (e.g., those quantified by a laboratory test) do not always translate into a perceivable change in health or wellness status. A widely cited example is that clinically meaningful improvements in lung function as measured by forced expiratory volume (FEV1) may not correlate well with improvements in asthma-related symptoms and their impact on a patient's ability to perform daily activities. Furthermore, significant improvements in clinically observable parameters may be correlated with a significantly negative impact on a patient's subjective response to treatment, particularly if the treatment intervention is associated with bothersome or frequent untoward side effects.

3. Formal Assessment May Be More Reliable Than Informal Interview

Obtaining information from patients on symptoms and symptom relief is not new. Clinicians informally ask questions such as, "Do you get short of breath when walking up a flight of stairs?" or "Does your pain interfere with your ability to get out of bed?" However, efforts to capture and analyze subjective answers to questions such as these are prone to inconsistency and measurement error in the absence of validated instruments. There is general agreement that scientific methods for assessing subjective outcomes (e.g., psychometrics and utility measurement) are well developed and can serve as the cornerstone for patient-reported outcomes assessment. Using existing methodology to systematically and formally gather information from patients about their symptoms and the impact of those symptoms on function is the cornerstone of PRO.

Instruments completed by patients directly measure perceived treatment response. Data captured in this manner are likely to be more reliable than those obtained through indirect third-party measurements because they are not affected by inter-rater inconsistency. Use of a well-constructed instrument is also valuable in detecting change in reported outcomes over time, particularly in progressive disease. Change in functioning may be gradual, and an instrument sensitive to this change can be useful in determining longitudinal impact on decline or improvement.

Classification of PRO Measurements

Patient-reported outcomes broadly encompass several types of instruments. These include symptom scales as well as instruments that measure health-related quality of life, functional status (e.g., ability to conduct activities of daily living), satisfaction with treatment, compliance with the intervention, and medication adherence and persistence. They may be disease specific, such as the Asthma Control Test (ACT) or the Function Living Index: Cancer (FLIC); they may be treatment specific, such as the Satisfaction With Antipsychotic Medication (SWAM) scale, or they may measure the overall status of a condition such as instruments that measure the presence or absence of depression or angina.

Alternatively to these very specific applications, patient-reported outcomes instruments may also be generic and applicable across a wide variety of disease categories. Most measurements of physical functioning and activities of daily living fall into the category of generic measures. One of the earliest and perhaps the most widely known and cited generic measure was created by John E. Ware and colleagues as an outgrowth of the Medical Outcomes Study (MOS). Known as the Short Form 36 (SF-36), this instrument encompasses 36 questions representing the domains of (1) physical functioning, (2) role functioning, (3) bodily pain, (4) general health perception, (5) vitality, (6) social functioning, (7) role-emotional functioning, and (8) mental health. Item responses within these eight domains are reported as two summary measures—physical and mental health. Generic measures such as the SF-36 have been validated within numerous disease states. Depending on the disease state, the SF-36 has been used to identify both differences in overall outcome between intervention groups and also changes within intervention groups over time.

In addition to comparing patient-reported quality of life outcomes within an individual disease state, generic measures have proven valuable for comparing health perceptions across disease states. Instruments such as the SF-36 or, more commonly, the Health Utilities Index (HUI) have been validated extensively and specifically to compare quality of life across diseases. To accomplish this comparison, results from generic measures are converted to a 0 to 1 scale, with 1 representing perfect health and functioning and 0 representing the state nearest to death. To illustrate comparison of utilities, individuals with advanced metastatic medulloblastoma brain tumor may have a health utility of 0.31, as compared with 0.58 for an individual who is undergoing cardiac bypass surgery and 0.99 for someone without symptoms taking a cholesterol-lowering agent for hyperlipidemia. These "utilities" are used to calculate quality-adjusted life years (QALYs), which are used for policy decisions surrounding drug formulary placement and treatment reimbursement, particularly in Europe, Canada, and Australia.

Methodological Considerations in Developing PRO

The mechanism with which patient-reported outcome data is captured typically includes a questionnaire. Questionnaires may be self-administered, with a subject filling out a form with pen and paper or electronically via a computer. They may be clinician administered via a healthcare worker, social scientist, or other trained individual reading questions or through conducting a formal, structured interview either in person or telephonically. Methods available for questionnaire development generally are grounded in rigorous psychometric theory. The merit of patient-reported outcome questionnaires is determined based on three key properties. First, outcomes must be conceptually defined and be based on the most current understanding of domains of functioning and aspects of life quality relative to what is being assessed. Disease- or treatment-based instruments must also be framed within the context of a thorough review of the medical or psychiatric literature. Second, aspects of functioning, quality of life, or symptomatology must be suitably operationalized through the questionnaire. This includes using phraseology and terminology that can be understood and interpreted by the respondent. The time period that the subject is required to recall in order to respond to the question must be relevant to the health state studied but short enough to allow accurate reporting of experience. Scaling must be representative of the respondent's experience. Scaling typically measures intensity of the perceived health aspect (e.g., occurring none of

the time, some of the time, or all the time), as well as the intensity (e.g., mild, moderate, or severe) of the experience. The respondent burden, the time required to complete the instrument, must be minimized to promote willingness to complete the instrument and to facilitate the quality of the responses. The remaining, and perhaps most often overlooked, property of instrument development includes field testing to determine reliability, validity, and responsiveness (i.e., minimally detectable change). Creating and validating instruments typically encompasses creating a draft with input from leaders in the field of study, piloting the instrument in individuals afflicted with the condition of interest, interviewing pilot respondents to identify potential problems with the instrument, and finally, performing a full-scale validation study comparing responses to the instrument with recognized gold standards, where available (concurrent validity). Minimum requirements for validation of instruments includes demonstration of reliability, construct validity, responsiveness over time, internal consistency, and test-retest reliability. Measurements of validity and reliability typically make use of Cronbach's alpha coefficient and correlation or kappa coefficients. Agreement of .70 or greater is typically accepted for group comparisons. When investigator administered, a coefficient of .80 is typically acceptable to establish interrater reliability.

Other considerations in validation include that instruments should be able to discriminate between subgroups of individuals based on severity. Also, translation of instruments validated in one language should undergo linguistic validation during translation to alternate languages. Similarly, tools validated using one administration mode (e.g., self-administered) should be validated in an alternate mode (e.g., telephone interview administration) prior to incorporation into translational research.

In recent years, interest in incorporating patient-reported outcomes into clinical trials designed to meet regulatory requirements in the approval process for marketing of medicines has led to an explosion of instrument development. This development is geared toward developing tools sensitive and specific to changes in PRO related to specific pharmaceutical products. In response, regulators and harmonization groups have begun to adopt standards by which PRO measures are developed.

These measurement characteristics are grounded in solid theory and are now widely accepted. The ultimate objective is to develop and implement an instrument that is accurate and validated of the intended domains.

Alicia Shillington

See also Activities of Daily Living (ADL); Measurement in Health Services Research; Outcomes Movement; Quality-Adjusted Life Years (QALYs); Quality Indicators; Quality of Healthcare; Short-Form Health Surveys (SF-36, -12, -8); Structure-Process-Outcome Quality Measures

Further Readings

Atkinson, Mark J., and Richard D. Lennox. "Extending Basic Principles of Measurement Models to the Design and Validation of Patient Reported Outcomes," *Health and Quality of Life Outcomes* 4(65): 1–12, 2006.

Bergner, Marilyn. "Quality of Life, Health Status, and Clinical Research," *Medical Care* 27(3 Suppl.): S148–S156, March 1989.

Chassany, Olivier, Pierre Sagnier, Patrick Marquis, et al. "Patient-Reported Outcomes: The Example of Health-Related Quality of Life—A European Guidance Document for the Improved Integration of Health-Related Quality of Life Assessment in the Drug Regulatory Process," *Drug Information Journal* 36: 209–238, January–March 2002.

Food and Drug Administration. *Guidance for Industry. Patient-Reported Outcome Measures: Use in Medical Product Development to Support Labeling Claims.* Draft Report. Washington, DC: U.S. Department of Health and Human Services, Food and Drug Administration, 2006.

Guyatt, Gordon H., Carol E. Ferrans, Michele Y. Halyard, et al. "Exploration of the Value of Health-Related Quality-of-Life Information From Clinical Research into Clinical Practice," *Mayo Clinic Proceedings* 82(10): 1229–39, October 2007.

Kumar, Ritesh N., Duane M. Kirking, Steven L. Hass, et al. "The Association of Consumer Expectations, Experiences, and Satisfaction With Newly Prescribed Medications," *Quality of Life Research* 16(7): 1127–36, September 2007.

Lenderking, William. "Task Force Report of the Patient-Reported Outcomes (PRO) Harmonization Group: Too Much Harmony, Not Enough Melody?" *Value of Health* 6(5): 522–31, September 2003.

Lohr, K. N., N. K. Aaronson, J. Alonso, et al. "Evaluating Quality-of-Life and Health Status Instruments: Development of Scientific Review Criteria," *Clinical Therapeutics* 18(5): 979–92, September–October 1996.

Revicki, Dennis A. "Regulatory Issues and Patient-Reported Outcomes Task Force for the International Society for Quality of Life Research. FDA Draft Guidance and Health-Outcomes Research," *Lancet* 369(9561): 540–42, February 17, 2007.

Revicki, Dennis A., David Cella, Ron Hays, et al. "Responsiveness and Minimal Important Differences for Patient Reported Outcomes," *Health and Quality of Life Outcomes* 4(70): 1–5, 2006.

Sprangers, Mirjam A., Carol M. Moinpour, Timothy J. Moynihan, et al. "Assessing Meaningful Change in Quality of Life Over Time: A Users' Guide for Clinicians," *Mayo Clinic Proceedings* 77(6): 561–71, June 2002.

Ware, John E., and Barbara B. Gandek. "Overview of the SF-36 Health Survey and the International Quality of Life Assessment (IQOLA) Project," *Journal of Clinical Epidemiology* 51(11): 903–912, November 1998.

Web Sites

Cochrane Collaborative Patient-Reported Outcomes Methods Group: http://www.cochrane-hrqol-mg.org

Patient-Reported Outcomes Measurement Information System (PROMIS): http://www.nihpromis.org/default.aspx

Patient-Reported Outcome and Quality of Life Instruments Database (ProQolid): http://www.qolid.org

U.S. Food and Drug Administration (FDA): http://www.fda.gov

PATIENT SAFETY

The issue of patient safety has only gained national attention during the past decade, primarily due to the recognition that much hospital morbidity and mortality is due to medical errors. Many organizations and programs have been established to address patient safety. Most healthcare institutions have instituted patient safety measures, which are key to maintaining their accreditation and therefore to their remaining financially solvent.

Defining the Problem

Patient safety and medical errors are closely linked, and in discussing one it is often necessary to discuss the other. For this entry, patient safety is defined as freedom from accidental injury due to medical care or medical errors. *Medical error* is defined as the failure of a planned action to be completed as intended or the use of a wrong plan to achieve an aim, including problems in medical practice, products, procedures, and systems.

The term *patient safety* was first used in the name of a professional medical organization in 1984, with the establishment of the Anesthesia Patient Safety Foundation by the American Society of Anesthesiologists. Despite the recognition of patient safety issues in the field of anesthesia, the topic did not gain national attention until the late 1990s, solidified by the national Institute of Medicine (IOM) landmark report *To Err Is Human: Building a Safer Health System,* which was published in 2000. The report estimated that between 44,000 and 98,000 people die in the United States every year due to medical errors. It also estimated that the national cost of medical errors to hospitals was between $17 and $29 billion per year.

The IOM report cited commonly occurring errors, including adverse drug events and improper transfusions, surgical injuries and wrong-site surgery, suicides, restraint-related injuries or death, falls, burns, pressure ulcers, and mistaken patient identities. The report also cited an article in the *Quality Review Bulletin* (1993) that categorized medical errors broadly into diagnostic (e.g., error or delay in diagnosis, failure to employ tests, using outdated tests, and failure to act on results), treatment (error in performance or administration of treatment, avoidable delay in treatment, error in dose or method of using a drug, and inappropriate care), preventive (failure to provide prophylactic treatment and failure to monitor), or other (failure of communication and equipment failure) groups.

Following the IOM report, further studies were conducted to track medical errors and patient safety issues. A study published in the *Journal of the American Medical Association* in 2003 found that the greatest injury due to medical errors was postoperative sepsis leading to an excess length of hospital stay of 11 days, excess charges of $57,727, and excess mortality of 22%.

A HealthGrades Quality Study, which was published in 2004 and investigated hospitalized Medicare patients between 2000 and 2002, found more than 1 million adverse events resulting in up to 195,000 accidental deaths per year. Based on the Agency for Healthcare Research and Quality's (AHRQ's) 20 evidence-based patient safety indicators, the study found that the three most common errors were failure to rescue (failure to diagnose and treat in time), decubitus ulcer, and postoperative sepsis. These three errors accounted for almost 60% of all patient safety incidents among the hospitalized Medicare patients, with an estimated excess annual cost of $2.85 billion.

Addressing Medical Errors

The IOM report refuted the "bad apple" theory, which suggested that medical errors are due to specific faulty or inept practitioners; instead, it determined that errors are usually the result of faulty systems, processes, and conditions that lead people to make mistakes or fail to prevent them. Also, errors are not limited to actions but also include failure to act and avert preventable adverse outcomes.

To improve patient safety, the report recommended a four-tiered approach: (1) establish a national focus to create leadership, research, tools, and protocols to enhance the knowledge base about safety; (2) identify and learn from errors by developing a nationwide public mandatory reporting system and by encouraging healthcare organizations and practitioners to develop and participate in voluntary reporting systems; (3) raise performance standards and expectations for improvements in safety through the actions of oversight organizations, professional groups, and group purchasers of healthcare; and (4) implant safety systems in healthcare organizations to ensure safe practice at the delivery level.

Largely in response to the IOM report, the U.S. Congress allocated $50 million to the federal AHRQ in 2000 to support efforts to improve patient safety and reduce medical errors. A follow-up report from the IOM in 2001 further advocated the rapid adoption of electronic clinical records, electronic medication ordering, and computer- and Internet-based information systems to support clinical decisions to improve patient safety and reduce medical errors.

The development of evidence-based recommendations for specific medical conditions, termed *clinical practice guidelines* or *best practices,* has accelerated in the past few years. Also, the U.S. Congress passed the Patient Safety and Quality Improvement (PSQI) Act of 2005, establishing a database to improve patient safety by encouraging voluntary and confidential reporting of medical errors.

Public and Private Initiatives

Since the publication of the landmark IOM report in 2000, many government and private organizations have made patient safety a top healthcare priority. Government organizations with specific initiatives for patient safety include the AHRQ and the Centers for Medicare and Medicaid Services (CMS).

Private organizations concerned with patient safety include the American Society of Medication Safety Officers (ASMSO), Council on Graduate Medical Education (COGME), Institute for Healthcare Improvement (IHI), Institute for Safe Medication Practices (ISMP), Joint Commission, Leapfrog Group, National Academy of State Health Policy (NASHP), National Advisory Council on Nurse Education and Practice (NACNEP), National Patient Safety Foundation (NPSF), National Quality Forum (NQF), Safe Care Campaign, and the United States Pharmacopeia (USP).

Selected Patient Safety Organizations and Programs

The CMS currently has several demonstration projects underway, including a pay-for-performance program, which offers hospitals increased compensation for improvements in patient care coordination and the institution of quality measures. It also initiated a new disincentive rule in 2008, which stops hospitals from billing Medicare for any charges associated with eight serious preventable conditions. The eight conditions include (1) pressure ulcers, (2) urinary tract infections, (3) patient falls, (4) mediastinitis (an infection after heart surgery), (5) objects left in the patient's

bodies after surgery such as sponges, (6) incompatible blood transfusions, (7) air embolisms blocking blood flow, and (8) infections caused by leaving catheters in blood vessels and bladders too long.

The Joint Commission, which was established in 1951, is an independent, nonprofit organization that evaluates and accredits nearly 15,000 healthcare organizations and programs in the nation. Most healthcare organizations seek accreditation to receive federal Medicare and Medicaid funds. Many of the Joint Commission's standards for organizations directly relate to patient safety, response to adverse events, and the prevention of accidental harm. During the past decade, the Joint Commission has established a number of programs addressing patient safety, including the National Patient Safety Goals and the Speak Up initiatives, which urge patients to take an active role in preventing medical errors. In 2005, it established an International Center for Patient Safety to collaborate with international patient safety organizations.

The Leapfrog Group, which was established in 2000, is a conglomeration of large U.S. corporations that agreed to base their purchase of healthcare on principles that encouraged provider quality improvement and consumer involvement. It created the Leapfrog Hospital Rewards Program, which mandates specific quality practices such as computerized physician order entry, evidence-based hospital referral, and intensive-care unit (ICU) staffing by physicians experienced in critical-care medicine. Additionally, a Leapfrog Safe Practices Score was developed as a hospital quality ratings system to influence consumers' choices.

The NPSF is a nonprofit organization founded in 1996 by the American Medical Association (AMA), CNA HealthPro, and 3M. The foundation provides leadership training, research support, and education, and it publishes the *Journal of Patient Safety,* containing original articles and reviews on the subject.

The NQF is a nonprofit, membership organization established in 1999 to develop and implement a national strategy for healthcare quality measurement and reporting. The NQF has focused on several areas, including medical error rates, unnecessary procedures and undertreatment, and preventive care. In 2002, the NQF defined 27 events that should never occur within a healthcare facility. It grouped the "never" events into six categories (officially called Serious Reportable Events): (1) surgical events (e.g., surgery being performed on the wrong patient), (2) product or device events (e.g., using contaminated drugs), (3) patient protection events (e.g., an infant discharged to the wrong person), (4) care management events (e.g., a medication error), (5) environmental events (e.g., electric shock or burn), and (6) criminal events (e.g., sexual assault of a patient).

Important Concepts

"First, do no harm" is an often-quoted mantra attributed to Hippocrates, the father of Western medicine. The implication is that medical professionals should try to help but at a minimum should do no additional harm. Many medical errors are the direct result of inappropriate actions such as administering the wrong dose of a medication or performing surgery on the wrong limb or patient.

Prevention is a key concept as well. Inaction is considered equally as culpable as performing the wrong action. Many medical "errors" are due to not addressing foreseeable adverse events. Examples include not instituting fall precautions (e.g., raising bedrails for patients at risk of falling out of bed), not washing hands properly (leading to transmission of hospital-acquired infections), and not giving anticoagulant medicine to prevent blood clots in bed-bound patients.

Evidence-based medicine is the idea of integrating available medical research into patient care. Many clinical practice guidelines have been established in recent years, which are consensus-based recommendations for physicians to apply to care of patients. These guidelines can help create consistent care based on the most up-to-date scientific data available.

To improve patient safety, medical errors need to be identified and studied to determine possible causes. Reporting of medical errors, including near-miss events, is paramount. A near-miss event is an unplanned event that did not result in injury, illness, or damage, but had the potential to do so. Reporting of near-miss events by observers is an established error reduction technique in other industries and has recently been applied to the healthcare sector.

Future Implications

Many medical errors have been attributed to poor handwriting, manual order entry, and nonstandard abbreviations that are misinterpreted. Electronic clinical records are a new technology that has the potential to reduce some of these errors, not only by eliminating illegibility but also by having default doses for medications and alerts for potential drug interactions or allergies. Electronic clinical records could also reduce errors by improving access to information and communication among providers.

As noted above, some organizations, including the CMS, have pilot programs which use a pay-for-performance system that includes financial incentives and disincentives relating to patient safety and the occurrence of "never" events identified by the NQF. This type of reimbursement is highly controversial. Proponents suggest that financial incentives will change behavior and encourage systems improvements. Others, primarily physician groups, argue that many complications occur despite following best practice guidelines (e.g., postoperative infections), and institutions and providers will be unfairly penalized, possibly leading to compromised patient safety if healthcare organizations are denied vital resources.

Legal reform is also seen as an area for intervention. Healthcare providers are often hesitant to report errors due to the threat of legal liability. U.S. Senators Hillary Rodham Clinton (D-NY) and Barack Obama (D-IL) jointly proposed the National Medical Error Disclosure and Compensation (MEDiC) Bill of 2005, which would create an Office of Patient Safety and Health Care Quality to administer the MEDiC program. The proposed program is designed to improve disclosure of medical errors, give physicians certain protections from liability, and help facilitate appropriate compensation for affected patients, with the overall aim of improving patient safety. The bill was referred to the Senate in September 2005 and subsequently to the Committee on Health, Education, Labor, and Pensions. Neither the MEDiC Bill nor any other recent legislation addressing medical malpractice reform has been passed by both houses of Congress, but this topic will likely resurface when a new administration revisits the problems of healthcare costs and medical errors.

Stacey Chamberlain

See also Clinical Practice Guidelines; Evidence-Based Medicine (EBM); Joint Commission; Leapfrog Group; Medical Errors; National Quality Forum; Pay-for-Performance; Quality of Healthcare

Further Readings

Agency for Healthcare Research and Quality. *Patient Safety Indicators, Version 2.1, Revision 1.* Rockville, MD: Agency for Healthcare Research and Quality, March 2004.

Clinton, Hillary Rodham, and Barack Obama. "Making Patient Safety the Centerpiece of Medical Liability Reform," *New England Journal of Medicine* 354(21): 2205–2208, May 25, 2006.

Committee on Quality of Health Care in America, Institute of Medicine. *Crossing the Quality Chasm: A New Health System for the 21st Century.* Washington, DC: National Academies Press, 2001.

HealthGrades, Inc. *HealthGrades Quality Study: Patient Safety in American Hospitals.* Golden, CO: HealthGrades, 2004.

Kohn, Linda T., Janet M. Corrigan, and Molla S. Donaldson, eds., Committee on Quality of Health Care in America, Institute of Medicine. *To Err Is Human: Building a Safer Health System.* Washington, DC: National Academies Press, 2000.

Leape, Lucian L., Ann G. Lawthers, Troyen A. Brennan, et al. "Preventing Medical Injury," *Quality Review Bulletin* 19(5): 144–49, May 1993.

Zhan, Chunliu, and Marlene R. Miller. "Excess Length of Stay, Charges, and Mortality Attributable to Medical Injuries During Hospitalization," *Journal of the American Medical Association* 290(14): 1868–74, October 8, 2003.

Web Sites

Agency for Healthcare Research and Quality (AHRQ): http://www.ahrq.gov

Anesthesia Patient Safety Foundation (APSF): http://www.apsf.org

Centers for Medicare and Medicaid Services (CMS): http://www.cms.hhs.gov

Joint Commission: http://www.jointcommission.org

Leapfrog Group: http://www.leapfroggroup.org

National Quality Forum (NQF): http://www.qualityforum.org

PATIENT TRANSFERS

Patient transfers can be defined by the various methods (e.g., ground or air transport) and motives (e.g., transfer to another hospital because the patient does not have health insurance) for moving a patient from one location to another. A major classification of patient transfers is whether they are intrafacility or interfacility transfers. Intrafacility transfers are patient transfers within a given healthcare facility, either between departments or between other organizations within the healthcare facility. In contrast, interfacility transfers are patient transfers from one healthcare facility to another facility. Examples of interfacility transfers include the following: (a) hospital-to-hospital transfers, (b) clinic to hospital transfers, (c) hospital to rehabilitation facility transfers, and (d) hospital to long-term care facility transfers.

Challenges to the success of interfacility transfers include the qualifications of those delivering the care, the ability to meet the clinical needs of the patient, and the aptitude to maintain continuity of care. Due to the emergence of specialty medical systems such as cardiac centers and stroke centers, the ultimate destination of a patient is now often predicated on the patient's specific medical condition rather than the proximity of the nearest medical facility. This practice has created the need for enhanced measurement and guidelines and the evaluation of patient transfers to understand and track the different circumstances under which transfers take place.

Because of this change, the number of stakeholders involved in patient transfer protocols and instrumentations has increased and diversified over the past few years. Stakeholders include physicians at both the receiving and transferring facility, the medical staff of both institutions, the patient and the patient's family and caregivers, the third-party insurance groups, the health administration and legal staff of both facilities, and the transferring bodies such as the ambulance staff. Additional stakeholders include Emergency Medical Services (EMS) organizations and the National Highway Traffic Safety Administration (NHTSA) who enter into discussions to create EMS priority issues and establish guidelines for the EMS organization's critical-care transport. This level of transport care is provided to patients whose indication requires an expert level of provider knowledge and skills, a setting with necessary equipment, and the ability to handle the challenge of the transport.

Reasons for Patient Transfers

The rationales for transferring patients include facility capacity issues, facility or physician specialty and competency, and limitations in levels of care offered. Hospitals are often plagued with issues of overcapacity and inability to properly house and care for incoming patients. Some healthcare institutions such as clinics and nursing homes may accept only a few payment options, thereby limiting the care they provide. Additionally, many patients are transferred because the initial admitting facility is unable to support the needs of the patient. For example, some of the highest frequencies of interfacility transfers occur among obstetrics and gynecology (e.g., high-risk pregnancies) and neurology (e.g., stroke) patients, who require specialized training not available at many healthcare facilities.

Issues

Problems with interfacility patient transfers can also be unrelated to medical care. Nonclinically related issues include redundant and unnecessary transports that create financial burdens in terms of both direct and indirect costs. Direct costs may include the expenses for transport and personnel, while the indirect costs may include the expenses related to increased patient morbidity, liability issues, and overcrowding in the emergency department. Patient-related issues include the time involved, the extent of morbidity and mortality associated with wait time, lack of care continuity and poor quality of care, patient privacy issues, and patient dumping. Patient dumping occurs when unexamined or unstable patients are transferred to another facility because of nonclinical reasons, as when the patient does not have health insurance and is likely not to be able to pay for his or her care.

Public Policy

The federal Emergency Medical Treatment and Active Labor Act (EMTALA) provides broad guidelines regarding the transfer of patients after they seek care in a hospital's emergency department. EMTALA, which was passed in 1986, was designed to prevent patient dumping. It mandates that hospitals that receive Medicare and Medicaid funds provide medical screening examinations of all emergency department patients, regardless of a patient's ability to pay. If critical medical conditions are identified, EMTALA requires the hospital to stabilize the patient before transferring him or her to another facility for care. The act addresses concerns of patient safety and the ability to receive medical care regardless of demographics and socioeconomic status.

Future Implications

As the result of EMTALA, many of the nation's hospitals are changing their patient transfer protocols. They are increasingly implementing centralized transfer centers to improve overall patient flows and to control incoming patients and facility capacity. These centralized transfer centers also promise to lower costs, save time, and protect the facilities against lawsuits.

Jillian R. O'Neill

See also Access to Healthcare; Emergency Medical Services (EMS); Emergency Medical Treatment and Active Labor Act (EMTALA); For-Profit Versus Not-For-Profit Healthcare; Hospitals; Patient Dumping; Uninsured Individuals

Further Readings

Hanane, Tarik, Mark T. Keegan, Edward G. Seferian, et al. "The Association Between Nighttime Transfer From the Intensive Care Unit and Patient Outcome," *Critical Care Medicine* 36(8): 2232–37, August 2008.

Koval, Kenneth J., Chad W. Tingey, Kevin F. Spratt, et al. "Are Patients Being Transferred to Level-1 Trauma Centers for Reasons Other Than Medical Necessity?" *Journal of Bone and Joint Surgery* 88(10): 2124–32, October 2006.

Spain, David A., Michael Bellino, Andrew Kopelman, et al. "Requests for 692 Transfers to an Academic

Level 1 Trauma Center: Implications of the Emergency Medical Treatment and Active Labor Act," *Journal of Trauma: Injury, Infection, and Critical Care* 62(1): 63–8, January 2007.

Web Sites

American Academy of Emergency Medicine (AAEM): http://www.aaem.org
Centers for Medicare and Medicaid Services (CMS): http://www.cms.hhs.gov
Joint Commission: http://www.jointcommission.org

PAULY, MARK V.

Mark V. Pauly is one of America's leading health economists. Although Pauly has conducted research in many areas of health economics, he is perhaps best known for his work on moral hazard. His classic 1968 study of the economics of moral hazard was the first to point out how health insurance may affect the behavior of the insured as well as those providing healthcare services to them. His work popularized the term.

Pauly is currently the Bendheim Professor in the Department of Health Care Systems at the Wharton School of the University of Pennsylvania. He also is professor of business and public policy and insurance and risk management at the Wharton School and professor of economics in the School of Arts and Sciences at the University of Pennsylvania. Before joining the Wharton School in 1983, he taught at Northwestern University for 16 years.

Born in 1941, Pauly earned a bachelor of arts degree in classical languages from Xavier University in 1963, a master's degree in economics from the University of Delaware in 1965, and a doctorate in economics from the University of Virginia in 1967.

Over his long career, Pauly has studied the empirical and theoretical impact of health insurance coverage on preventive care, ambulatory care, and prescription drug use in managed care. He has investigated the various influences that determine the availability of health insurance coverage and, using cost-effectiveness analysis, determined the influences of medical care and health

practices on outcomes and costs. He also has studied and proposed ways to reduce the number of uninsured through the use of tax credits and ways to redesign the Medicare program.

Pauly is a prolific researcher and author. He has published many scholarly journal articles and books on various health economics topics. He is the coeditor-in-chief of the *International Journal of Health Care Finance and Economics* and the associate editor of the *Journal of Risk and Uncertainty*. He also serves on the editorial board of *Public Finance Quarterly*.

Pauly has received many awards and honors in recognition of his work. In 2007, he received the Distinguished Investigator Award from AcademyHealth and the John Eisenberg Excellence in Mentorship Award from the federal Agency for Healthcare Research and Quality (AHRQ). He is an elected member of the National Academy of Sciences, Institute of Medicine (IOM). He also is a member of the National Advisory Council for the AHRQ. He was the recipient of an investigator award in health policy research from the Robert Wood Johnson Foundation. And he previously served as a commissioner on the Physician Payment Review Commission (PPRC), which advised the U.S. Congress on Medicare physician payment.

He has consulted for national public policy and research centers such as the American Enterprise Institute for Public Policy Research (AEI), Mathematica Policy Research, and the Urban Institute; hospital associations, including the Greater New York Hospital Association; and pharmaceutical companies such as Amgen, Bayer, Glaxo, and Merck.

Pauly's current interests include the economic analysis of healthcare reform, the understanding of the conceptual foundations for cost-benefit analysis of pharmaceutical drugs, and the economic incentives in managed care. His work will continue to assist health services researchers and policymakers to better understand the economics of healthcare in America.

Pritha Dasgupta

See also Health Economics; Health Insurance; Health Insurance Coverage; Medicare; Moral Hazard; National Health Insurance; Public Policy; Uninsured Individuals

Further Readings

Pauly, Mark V. "The Economics of Moral Hazard: Comment," *American Economic Review* 58(3 pt. 1): 531–37, June 1968.

Pauly, Mark V. *Health Benefits at Work: An Economic and Political Analysis of Employment-Based Health Insurance.* Ann Arbor: University of Michigan Press, 1998.

Pauly, Mark V. "Risk and Benefits in Health Care: The View From Economics," *Health Affairs* 26(3): 653–62, May–June 2007.

Pauly, Mark V. *Markets Without Magic: How Competition Might Save Medicine.* Washington, DC: AEI Press, 2008.

Pauly, Mark V., and Bradley Herring. *Cutting Taxes for Insuring: Options and Effects of Tax Credits for Health Insurance.* Washington, DC: AEI Press, 2002.

Pauly, Mark V., and Jose A Pagan. "Spillovers and Vulnerability: The Case of Community Uninsurance," *Health Affairs* 26(5): 1304–1314, September–October 2007.

Web Site

University of Pennsylvania, Wharton School Faculty Profile: http://www.wharton.upenn.edu/faculty/pauly .html

Pay-for-Performance

The linkage of financial incentives to quality and performance is a relatively new concept in healthcare. Pay-for-performance is a way to reward healthcare providers for higher-quality healthcare. In most industries, lower costs are achieved through greater production efficiency, and financial rewards accrue to firms that produce high-quality products more efficiently. In contrast, most physicians and hospitals are paid the same regardless of the quality of the healthcare they provide, producing no financial incentives for quality and, in some cases, disincentives for quality.

In its 2001 report *Cross the Quality Chasm: A New Health System for the 21st Century,* the National Academy of Sciences, Institute of Medicine (IOM) drew attention to the poor quality of the nation's healthcare as well as factors contributing to poor quality, including the structure of the present healthcare payment system. The IOM noted that, for certain types of clinical situations, healthcare payment arrangements may actually produce disincentives for quality care. For example, in general, patients cared for under fee-for-service reimbursement systems receive more services that are under the discretion of the provider. The incentives result in overuse of services without regard to efficiency; services of high cost that are technically complex tend to be rewarded over those that are labor and time intensive, such as counseling regarding self-care of diabetes or care coordination among subspecialists. High-technology, -volume, and -cost services are preferentially rewarded over low-technology, -volume, cost preventive healthcare services.

Under fee-for-service, this imbalance in incentives for high-technology, -volume, -cost services is further compounded. When providers invest in improving outcomes of chronic diseases (such as diabetes), their income may eventually drop, as patients with excellent control of their diabetes require fewer office visits and hospital stays in the longer term, resulting in fewer opportunities to bill for services.

Other payment methods do not reimburse for services provided but pay healthcare providers prospectively. These types of payment methods may also provide disincentives for quality. For example, capitation payment methods result in lower use of healthcare services overall and may result in underuse of essential services. Furthermore, while preventive care is more likely to be rewarded under capitation than it is under fee-for-service, when patients switch healthcare plans, investments in preventive care are less likely to result in financial savings for the payer who provided and made the up-front investments in such care.

In recognition of these issues, there are increasing numbers of programs in the United Kingdom and the United States that link payment to performance. In 2004, the United Kingdom's National Health Service (NHS) began a pay-for-performance initiative. General practitioners agreed to participate in a performance program encompassing 146 quality indicators reflecting clinical care for 10 chronic diseases, organization of care, and patient experience. In return, funding for primary care was increased 20% over previous levels, permitting practices to invest in technology and staff. A startling 90% of general practitioners now use electronic prescribing, and general practitioners increased their income by $40,000 through the program.

In the United States, given the disincentives for high quality healthcare that exist in current payment methods such as fee-for-service and capitation, the objectives of pay-for-performance include rapid performance improvement to address ongoing quality deficits, innovation, structural changes in care delivery, and, ultimately, better outcomes of care. A number of issues are critical to the success of pay-for-performance programs in achieving these objectives and improving the quality of healthcare.

Measuring Quality

The methods used for defining and measuring quality are the fundamental building blocks of any pay-for-performance program and are critical to the success of a program in meeting its objectives. If measures of quality do not have a sound theoretical and methodological foundation, healthcare providers are not being rewarded for the behaviors that are desired and are even perhaps inadvertently being rewarded for behaviors that are undesirable. For example, if improving the numbers of patients who quit using tobacco is the desired outcome, but documentation of tobacco cessation advice is the rewarded measure, healthcare providers may merely document smoking cessation advice, without supplying any further tools to aid smokers in quitting.

Significant limitations exist in current clinical information systems in use by healthcare providers, which are often not designed to collect data valid for quality assessment. If the data sources for creating performance measures are not universally available, accurate, and reliable, healthcare providers become suspicious that their performance is not being accurately assessed. Furthermore, if the cohort of patients eligible for the measures does not reflect the actual panel of patients, healthcare providers participating in a pay-for-performance program may be inadvertently penalized for care provided (or not provided) by others.

Risk adjustment is also essential, where appropriate. Measures of quality that do not make appropriate risk adjustments create incentives for providers to avoid treating the sickest patients or penalize healthcare providers who care for disproportionate numbers of disadvantaged patients, who may not be able to afford their medications or comply with a treatment plan.

Chronic medical conditions are the leading cause of morbidity and mortality in the United States, and treatment of patients with these conditions consumes more than three fourths of all healthcare expenditures. Yet despite the resources devoted to the treatment of chronic conditions, chronically ill patients receive only half of the appropriate recommended care overall. Thus, many pay-for-performance programs have focused on increasing the provision of guideline-recommended care.

The effect of common, chronic, coexisting (or comorbid) conditions on measures of the quality of healthcare and patient ratings of their care is of concern to healthcare providers. Coexisting conditions complicate treatment plans and patient compliance. Some studies show that patients with chronic diseases are less likely to receive treatment for unrelated disorders or to undergo preventive healthcare services, but others show that patients with coexisting conditions are more likely to receive higher quality care. However, some studies have used a simple count of conditions as a crude marker of complexity or accessed only a limited range of conditions, possibly obscuring important relationships between types of conditions. For example, in patients with diabetes, treatment of hypertension is "concordant" with the goals of treatment for ischemic heart disease, whereas the treatment of arthritis is not, or, in other words, is "discordant." Therefore, treatment of arthritis might reduce the time available during a visit to address care for diabetes, whereas treatment of comorbid hypertension might not.

Healthcare providers are also concerned that with the increasing numbers of comorbid conditions, patient ratings of their care may suffer. This is because "high quality" care may come with a burden of large numbers of medications and healthcare use that lowers the satisfaction of patients overall. An evaluation of clinical practice guideline adherence found that a hypothetical older adult with five common comorbidities would be prescribed at least 12 medications. Also, because evidenced-based guidelines focus on single-disease processes and fail to account for patients with multiple comorbidities, the potential risks and benefits of such therapy, particularly in elderly patients, are unclear.

Process Versus Outcome Measures of Quality

In designing performance measures for incentive programs, several issues should be noted. First, the best process-of-care measures are those for which there is evidence that better performance leads to better health outcomes. Second, it is important to note that process-of-care measures may be more sensitive to quality differences than are measures of health outcomes, because a poor health outcome does not necessarily occur every time there is a quality problem.

It could be argued that, other things being equal, individual physician-level process-based incentives will create stronger incentives for improvement in processes over which the physician can exert direct control. In turn, such individual physician incentives may produce better health outcomes (assuming that the processes receiving incentives are systematically related to improved health outcomes over time). Therefore, combining outcome-based (e.g., tobacco quit rates) with process-based incentives (e.g., documentation of smoking cessation advice) may produce even greater quality improvement overall than process measures alone, by encouraging providers to balance process with attention to results. This approach may avoid the pitfalls of process-of-care measures alone that encourage gaming the system while avoiding the disadvantage of basing incentives solely on outcomes that may be relatively rare or difficult to achieve and somewhat beyond the control of the provider. Thus, a combined approach capitalizes on the advantages and complementary nature of both types of quality-of-care measures. However, the exact combination of process-based and outcome-based incentives that could be expected to produce the highest quality of healthcare is unknown.

Careful attention to quality measurement issues is important in averting healthcare provider opposition to such programs. A scientifically sound approach to quality measurement may also alleviate concerns that pay-for-performance is primarily a cost-cutting rather than a quality improvement tool.

Effectiveness

Ideally, studies of pay-for-performance would be multi-institutional, large-scale investigations of important and common medical conditions. Ideal studies include concurrent control groups to ensure that investigators can clearly infer associations between pay-for-performance and changes in performance. However, many pay-for-performance projects are implemented in an uncontrolled fashion, making it unclear whether the benefits are truly due to the financial incentives. Concurrent controls are essential to learn whether other temporal changes in the healthcare environment are resulting in improvements in the quality care, rather than a pay-for-performance program. Quality-of-care measures should be based on high-quality evidence and accepted guidelines, so as to minimize dispute over the evidence base for rewarded measures. Outcomes of care should be assessed. Unintended effects of the incentive program on performance measures that were not financially rewarded should also be assessed. To ensure face validity, clinical data should be collected consistently. However, empirical studies of the relationship between explicit financial incentives designed to improve a measure of healthcare quality and a quantitative measure of healthcare quality are rare in the literature. Rigorous research designs and methodology are necessary to determine whether performance-based payment arrangements result in meaningful quality improvements and are cost-effective. Studies meeting all the above criteria are surprisingly rare.

Despite the limitations of the literature, the available studies in general show some significant effects of pay-for-performance in improving the quality of healthcare. In studies of preventive care, with rewards to individual physicians, investigators have documented improvements in performance ranging from 8% to 19%. Rewards to provider groups generally had effect sizes of less than 10%.

Design of Financial Incentive Reward Programs

Designing financial incentives is a complex process involving decisions about whether providers should be in a "tournament" (competitive) style program, whether the recipient of the incentive should consist of an individual healthcare provider or a group of healthcare providers (including clerical support staff, nurses, and pharmacists), the amount of the reward, how frequently the reward should be given, and whether the reward should include some sort of nonfinancial component, such as audit and feedback or a public recognition program. Choices in any of these categories have advantages and disadvantages. As part of this decision-making process, policymakers should consider whether their goal is improving performance at the lower end of the spectrum versus maintaining best performance, or both.

Payment may be made according to relative performance (i.e., the participant's overall percentile ranking) or absolute performance (i.e., strictly according to performance relative to the quality standard). Payment may also be made on what is termed a "Pay as You Perform" schedule, so that each instance of the behavior is rewarded. Theoretical arguments for and against these designs from the fields of economics, social psychology, cognitive psychology, industrial/organizational psychology, and other behavioral disciplines can be made. The approach that works best in healthcare is an open question.

One could anticipate that with group- or practice-team-level incentives, individual physicians would not capture the full returns on their individual effort to improve the quality of their care. The potential for some physicians to "free-ride" on the efforts of others may lead them to reduce their individual efforts. However, the problem with rewarding individuals, but not the organization or group, is that the provision of the required institutional cooperation may not be present. Thus, theory suggests the potential for group-level incentives to support organizational and team-based efforts to improve the quality of healthcare. Some evidence regarding teams and groups exists from studies evaluating the chronic-care model. These suggest that multidisciplinary teams produce better patient outcomes. Group- or system-level incentives may provide the impetus to create infrastructure changes or to promote cooperation that is absent from traditional practice.

Attributing care to a provider or a group of providers can be challenging, particularly for patients who suffer from complex, chronic diseases, such as coexisting diabetes and chronic heart failure. Patients frequently interact with more than one provider, and treatment requires consultation with multiple subspecialists. Enhancing care coordination is essential to improving quality of care. How to identify providers who act in a coordinating role and then reward them for successfully accomplishing this role is essential to improving care for patients with chronic, complex conditions. The American College of Physicians (ACP) has proposed the concept of The Advanced Medical Home as a patient-centered, physician-guided model of healthcare to address some of these communication and coordination issues.

Most programs to date have consisted of positive rewards, rather than reduction in payments. However, this is changing. In the United States, the Centers for Medicare and Medicaid Services (CMS) has proposed eliminating payments for care that results in injury or death. As of October 2008, payments would be reduced for "never events" as defined by the National Quality Forum, such as hospital-acquired infections. And other healthcare payers are exploring similar plans.

Apart from the structure of the payment plan, the size of the bonus is almost certainly important. Possible explanations for the lack of effect or small effect in some previous studies may include the small size of the bonus. Similarly, when multiple insurers pay providers, the incentive may affect too few patients, effectively diluting the size of the incentive. On the other hand, a bonus that is perceived to be too large may produce negative feelings regarding a pay-for-performance program. Some critics have wondered whether pay-for-performance programs crowd out intrinsic motivation and negatively affect professionalism. Larger bonuses are more likely to contribute to these perceptions.

The last design issue to consider is the "end-of-year" compensation, which may not influence physician behavior as much as a concurrent fee or intermittent bonus. This is because lack of awareness of the intervention and infrequent performance feedback appear to be significant potential barriers to the effectiveness of incentives.

Regardless of the choices made, incentives require very careful design and attention to possible unintended consequences. A few studies have shown that documentation, rather than actual use of the preventive service, was significantly improved with a financial incentive. Obviously, the goal of the pay-for-performance program is to improve the quality of healthcare and not just documentation alone. Measures more likely to show evidence of unintended effects are those unrelated to reward measures, such as screening for cancer or treatment of pneumonia.

Unanswered Questions

Despite the wide adoption of pay-for-performance, research evidence of the effectiveness of pay-for-performance programs, particularly randomized trials, is very limited, and many questions remain unanswered. For example, what types of clinical conditions or healthcare services should be the target of financial incentives to improve quality—chronic diseases, acute care, and/or preventive care services? How effective (and cost-effective) are financial incentives for quality? What are the optimum magnitude, frequency, and duration of financial incentives for quality? Should insurers reward achievement of an absolute threshold of performance, improvement over baseline performance, or some combination of these? To whom should such incentives be directed—the patient, the healthcare provider, the provider group, or the hospital—or all of them? What types of quality measures should be rewarded—processes of care, health outcomes, or both? Are financial incentives for not providing inappropriate care (such as antibiotics for uncomplicated acute upper-respiratory illnesses) effective? What is the optimum "package" of nonfinancial interventions, if any, to include with financial incentives for quality—e.g., audit and feedback, recognition, clinical reminders, academic detailing, and/or information technology support? Can insurers expect that the effect of financial incentives will persist after they are stopped? Because any effective intervention will have some unanticipated effects, will important patient care activities that are not rewarded financially be neglected? Thus, despite the great enthusiasm about the potential for aligning financial incentives with high-quality healthcare, there are a number of fundamental unanswered questions about their optimal design, effectiveness, and implementation.

Rigorous research, including randomized, controlled trials and observational studies with concurrent control groups, is needed to guide implementation of explicit financial incentives for healthcare quality and to assess their cost-effectiveness. Much more research is needed to ensure that the nation's healthcare financing systems are effectively designed to encourage and promote the highest possible quality of healthcare for the nation's population.

Laura A. Petersen

See also Centers for Medicare and Medicaid Services (CMS); Medicare; National Quality Forum (NQF); Payment Mechanisms; Quality of Healthcare; United Kingdom's National Health Service (NHS)

Further Readings

American College of Physicians. *The Advanced Medical Home: A Patient-Centered, Physician-Guided Model of Health Care.* Philadelphia: American College of Physicians, 2006.

Committee on Quality of Health Care in America, Institute of Medicine. *Crossing the Quality Chasm: A New Health System for the 21st Century.* Washington, DC: National Academies Press, 2001.

McGlynn, Elizabeth, Steven M. Asch, John Adams, et al. "The Quality of Health Care Delivered to Adults in the United States," *New England Journal of Medicine* 348(26): 2635–45, June 26, 2003.

Medicare Payment Advisory Commission. *Report to the Congress: Medicare Payment Policy.* Washington, DC: Medicare Payment Advisory Commission, 2006.

National Committee for Quality Assurance. *The State of Health Care: Industry Trends and Analysis.* Washington, DC: National Committee for Quality Assurance, 2006.

Petersen, Laura A., LeChauncy D. Woodward, Tracy Urech, et al. "Does Pay-for-Performance Improve the Quality of Health Care?" *Annals of Internal Medicine* 145(4): 265–72, August 15, 2006.

Web Sites

American College of Physicians (ACP): http://www.acponline.org

Centers for Medicare and Medicaid Services (CMS): http://www.cms.hhs.gov

Joint Commission: http://www.jointcommission.org

National Academy of Sciences, Institute of Medicine (IOM): http://www.iom.edu

National Committee for Quality Assurance (NCQA):
   http://www.ncqa.org
National Quality Forum (NQF):
   http://www.qualityforum.org

PAYMENT MECHANISMS

Payment mechanisms are the methods by which healthcare providers are reimbursed for the goods and services they provide. Payment mechanisms include those made by the patient, or *first-party payments;* health insurer, or *third-party payments;* and those payments that are assumed by the healthcare provider, or *second-party payments.* Each payment mechanism has inherent economic incentives that affect utilization.

Third-Party Payment Mechanisms

Third-party payers (i.e., insurance companies, managed-care organizations, and the government) use a number of mechanisms to pay healthcare providers for the cost of services delivered to their insured patients. Both public payers (e.g., Medicare and Medicaid) and private payers (e.g., Blue Cross and Blue Shield and other insurance plans) have similar types of payment mechanisms available. These payment mechanisms include fee-for-service, fee schedule, per diem, per stay, and capitation payments. Often, a payer uses multiple payment mechanisms within a particular insurance product. For example, physician outpatient care may be reimbursed using a fee schedule and hospital inpatient care may be reimbursed on a per-stay basis.

Fee-for-Service

A fee-for-service payment mechanism reimburses healthcare providers on a per-unit basis or for each service provided. The fee may be based on the actual charges (i.e., the amount charged by the provider) or based on a schedule that lists the dollar amount to be reimbursed for each service. Under fee-for-service payment mechanisms, providers have the economic incentive to provide more services than necessary to increase revenue, since they are paid per unit. When fee-for-service payments are based on actual charges rather than a predetermined fee schedule, providers can also increase revenue by increasing their charges.

Fee Schedules

Fee schedules are a particular type of fee-for-service payment mechanism that establishes either a maximum amount or actual amount of reimbursement for a particular service. If the fee schedule were used to establish maximum fees, the provider would receive the lesser of the amount charged and the predetermined amount in the fee schedule. In practice, providers almost always charge more than the fee schedule amount to ensure receipt of the full amount established in the fee schedule. Providers have the incentive to provide more services than necessary as a means of increasing revenue, but they have no influence on the amount reimbursed per service as long as their fees are set above the fee schedule amount.

The most common fee schedule in the United States is the National Physician Fee Schedule Relative Value System, which Medicare uses to reimburse physicians for services provided to Medicare beneficiaries. The system is based on the Resource-Based Relative Value Scale (RBRVS), which was developed by William Hsiao and his associates at Harvard University. Specifically, this fee schedule establishes relative value units for each Current Procedural Terminology (CPT) and Healthcare Common Procedure Coding System (HCPCS) code, and it then converts the relative value units to a dollar amount of reimbursement using a conversion factor that is revised annually. Many third-party payers use this system as the basis for determining their physician fee schedules by modifying the conversion factor that translates relative value units to dollars of reimbursement.

Per Diem

Per diem is a payment mechanism that reimburses healthcare providers per day of stay and establishes a set fee per day. Per diem is most commonly used by third-party payers for acute, long-term, skilled nursing and psychiatric hospital stays. Providers have the incentive to keep patients in the facility longer than necessary to increase reimbursement, but they have no influence on the price paid per day.

Per Stay

Third-party payers may also use payment mechanisms that make one payment for each episode of care, such as a hospitalization stay. Per stay payments solve the incentive problem inherent in per diem payments of treating patients for longer durations of time than necessary, since a flat payment per episode is made. Providers do have an incentive, however, to increase the number of times a patient is admitted to increase reimbursement.

Medicare's prospective payment system (PPS) is a payment mechanism that reimburses services on a fixed amount per episode of care for some types of services, such as acute inpatient hospital stays and home health care, while it uses per diem payments for other services, such as skilled nursing care. Acute-care hospitals are reimbursed for each inpatient case based on the Diagnosis Related Group (DRG) assigned to the case, with one payment for each hospital stay. DRGs were developed by John D. Thompson and Robert B. Fetter at Yale University. Specifically, the total payment includes a base DRG payment component plus adjustments if the hospital has a high proportion of low-income patients or is a teaching hospital or if the case is an outlier in terms of being a high-cost case. Home health care is reimbursed based on 60-day episodes of care, with a base payment plus adjustments for factors such as case-mix (i.e., severity of illness, clinical condition, and services required).

Capitation

Capitation is a payment mechanism that reimburses a physician, medical group practice, or hospital a fixed amount per patient for a fixed period of time. Often capitation payments are paid for each insured member assigned to a provider for each month, or a per-member per-month (PMPM) capitation payment. Capitation payments cover a predetermined set of services provided within the defined time period and may include primary and specialty-care physician services, other outpatient services, diagnostic and laboratory tests, and hospital stays. The provider assumes the risk of the healthcare costs for the defined population of patients, and therefore, has the incentive to provide efficient care.

First-Party Payment Mechanisms

Healthcare providers also receive payments directly from patients. Self-pay is a first-party payment mechanism and includes situations in which the patient is the only payer and those in which the patient is responsible for a portion of the payment with a third party responsible for a balance of the payment.

Self-Pay

Self-pay is the patient's out-of-pocket payment obligation. Self-pay as a payment mechanism includes two types of patients—those with no source of health insurance coverage who are responsible for the entire fee (i.e., uninsured self-pay), and those with a third-party source of health insurance coverage who must pay a portion of the fee out of pocket (i.e., insured self-pay). Payments for uninsured self-pay patients have historically been based on hospital or provider charges with no negotiated price discounts. Many hospitals have been criticized for charging patients with the least financial means the most for care, and many are revising their policies for uninsured self-pay patients.

Payments for insured self-pay patients are based on the negotiated rates established between the third-party payer and healthcare provider. Insured self-pay payment mechanisms include three main types of demand-side cost sharing, namely deductibles, coinsurance, and copayments. A deductible is the amount that an insured individual must pay out of pocket before the insurer will start to reimburse the providers for services, and the individual usually must pay the deductible each year. From an insurance perspective, coinsurance is a general term that refers to the amount of a medical bill that the insured individual is responsible for out of pocket, which could be stated as a percentage of the total amount billed or as a flat dollar amount. In healthcare, coinsurance is commonly used to refer specifically to the proportion of the negotiated medical fees that the insured individual is responsible for (e.g., 20% coinsurance), with the insurer paying the remaining proportion of the fees. A copayment refers to the flat dollar amount of the negotiated medical fees that the insured individual must pay (e.g., $20 copayment), with the insurer paying the remaining dollar amount of the fees. The dollar amount paid out of pocket with coinsurance may vary for each visit, but the dollar amount for a copayment remains constant.

These demand-side payment mechanisms may work together in a single episode of care. For example, suppose an individual has health insurance coverage with a $500 deductible and a 20% coinsurance once the deductible is met. At the beginning of the year, the individual receives an MRI scan. This individual's out-of-pocket expenses would be $540 ($500 deductible + $40 coinsurance (20% × $200)), while the insurer's portion would be $160 ($700 – $540). Instead, if the individual has a $500 deductible with a $20 copayment, the individual's out-of-pocket expense would be $520, while the insurer would pay $180.

Provider Internal Payment Mechanisms

Hospitals, physicians, and other healthcare providers do not collect payments from all patients—either because of a decision to provide services as charity care to a patient without the financial resources to pay or because of a failure to collect payment from the patient or third-party payer. Both charity care and bad debt are classified as uncompensated care.

Charity Care

For patients without the income (or assets, in some cases) to pay for needed services, healthcare providers may render the care as charity care. Charity care includes services that are provided but for which the provider does not expect a payment. The provider does not bill the patient or insurer nor does the provider pursue collection of payment from an external source.

Bad Debt

Bad debt includes payments that are expected to be collected but are not collected from either the patient or a third-party payer. Providers attempt to collect these payments but are ultimately unsuccessful. Bad debt is an expense to providers.

Future Implications

Healthcare payment mechanisms have become increasingly diverse and complex over time. Patients undergoing the same procedure at the same hospital often use different payment mechanisms, or combination of payment mechanisms, and pay different amounts for the same services.

Even with healthcare reforms that would expand coverage to the currently uninsured population, the U.S. healthcare system is likely to continue relying on multiple sources of coverage, which will further fuel the complex web of payment mechanisms. While nations with a single-payer system have inherently simplified payment mechanisms, many nations may consider an increase in the individual's out-of-pocket responsibilities to control their own spiraling healthcare costs.

The largest change in the United States is likely to occur with respect to the balance of payments made by the individual compared with the insurer. Consumer-driven health plans are increasing the individual patient's cost-sharing obligations as a mechanism to control costs. This shift is likely to precipitate a change in how hospitals, physicians, and other healthcare providers collect first-party payments. While copayments for outpatient visits are routinely collected at the time of service, deductibles and coinsurance amounts for hospitalizations are more likely to be billed retrospectively. These payments are often collected after treatment because providers often cannot *ex ante* calculate the cost of treatment. As the size of first-party payments increases from hundreds to thousands of dollars, providers will have a greater incentive to collect them up front to guarantee payment. At face value, this change seems relatively minute; however, it could also lead to an increase in the number of potential patients denied services until they can make payment, to prevent a surge in bad debt.

Tricia J. Johnson and Michael Morgenstern

See also Capitation; Charity Care; Diagnosis Related Groups (DRGs); Fee-for-Service; Healthcare Financial Management; Prospective Payment; Resource-Based Relative Value Scale (RBRVS); Uncompensated Healthcare

Further Readings

Baron, Richard J., and Christine K. Cassel. "21st-Century Primary Care: New Physician Roles Need New Payment Models," *Journal of the American Medical Association* 299(13): 1595–97, April 2, 2008.

Davis, Karen. "Making Payment Reform in the U.S. Healthcare System Possible." *Medscape General Medicine* 9(4): 63, 2007.

Davis, Karen, and Stuart Guterman. "Rewarding Excellence and Efficiency in Medicare Payments," *Milbank Quarterly* 85(3): 449–68, September 2007.

Newhouse, Joseph P. "Medicare's Challenges in Paying Providers," *Health Care Financing Review* 27(2): 35–44, Winter 2005–2006.

Web Sites

American Hospital Association (AHA): http://www.aha.org

American Medical Association (AMA): http://www.ama-assn.org

Centers for Medicare and Medicaid Services (CMS): http://www.cms.hhs.gov

Healthcare Financial Management Association (HFMA): http://www.hfma.org

Medicare Payment Advisory Commission (MedPAC): http://www.medpac.gov

PEW CHARITABLE TRUSTS

The Pew Charitable Trusts is the single recipient of seven charitable funds initiated by the children of Joseph N. Pew, the creator of Sun Oil Company, and his wife, Mary Anderson Pew. The four founders of the Pew Charitable Trusts were Joseph N. Pew, Jr., J. Howard Pew, Mary Ethel Pew, and Mabel Pew Myrin. They established the Trusts in 1948 as a means of honoring their parents. The central aim of the Trusts is to donate to the public and add to its general health and welfare and thereby strengthen the nation's communities. Since its establishment, the Pew Charitable Trusts has stayed robust, encompassing several national organizations, while keeping its pledge to businesses and groups within the Philadelphia area.

Based in Philadelphia, with an office in Washington, D.C., the Pew Charitable Trusts provides organizations and citizens with fact-based research and practical solutions for changing issues. It investigates a large number of topics, including arts and culture, children and youth, computers and the Internet, education, environment, health, Hispanics in America, media and journalism, public opinion, and religion and public life. Specifically in the health area, it funds a number of centers and projects, including the Pennsylvania Medicaid Policy Center, the Genetics and Public Policy Center, and the Prescription Drug Project. In 2007, the Trusts spent a total of $248 million on its multitude of centers and projects.

Changing Political Views

Joseph N. Pew's political views were right of center, as were those of his heirs. In the beginning, the J. Howard Pew Freedom Trust felt that its goal was educating the American people regarding the bureaucratic morass in Washington and how important the free market was for freedom. For instance, Pew thought that Roosevelt and his New Deal were nothing more than a hoax designed to turn Americans into automatons doing exactly what Washington wanted. For many years, the Pew Charitable Trusts primarily funded conservative activities centered in Philadelphia. Initially, the recipients comprised organizations such as cancer research institutes, museums, and various universities (especially those that were historically Black). The conservative leaning of the Trusts changed when Thomas Langfitt, who was president from 1987 to 1994, and his hand-picked successor, Rebecca Rimel, shifted the Trusts' emphasis to a more liberal stance. Both Langfitt and Rimel thought that the views espoused by Pew and his heirs were outdated and that, thus, a new direction was needed.

According to Rimel, one central theme undergirding the Pew Charitable Trusts is to help politicians and policymakers in Washington make decisions that would lead to positive change for each American. As a result, the Trusts uses some of America's greatest scholars, scientists, and philosophers to envision and initiate sensible solutions to urgent public problems. Even though the Trusts now has a more international focus, great emphasis is still placed on the citizens and culture of Philadelphia.

Pew Projects

In 1999, a new era for the Trusts began when the Pew Internet and American Life Project was created. This project scrutinizes the societal and community impact of the Internet. Other projects include the Pew Research Center for the People and the Press (previously called the Times Mirror Center for the People and the Press). The center measures the changing opinions and mores of the American population. Each month, it conducts at least one major national opinion poll.

Another Trusts program is the Pew Global Attitudes Project, which conducts a series of worldwide opinion polls on a wide variety of topics. Over the years, it has conducted more than 150,000 interviews in 54 countries. In 2007, in conjunction with the Kaiser Family Foundation it conducted a global health survey that included 47 countries.

In 2001, the Trusts established the Pew Hispanic Center. Its primary goal focuses on the improvement and awareness of the diverse U.S. Hispanic populations. In addition, it seeks to record Latinos' increasing influence in the nation and to enlighten policy discussions regarding the nation's largest minority population.

The Pew Forum on Religion and Public Life sponsors an in-depth appreciation of questions at the junction of religious and public affairs. Its goal is to offer appropriate, impartial information to government leaders, journalists, analysts, and various national organizations. The forum never takes sides regarding policy and/or legislation, priding itself on being a nonpartisan entity.

Since 1999, the Pew Charitable Trusts has supported Stateline.org, an online news resource that covers state politics and policy through original reporting and by collecting news stories. Its goal is to strengthen and enrich America's political news agencies by offering data about the daily political activities taking place in each of the 50 states. Stateline.org considers itself to be an unbiased and impartial news journal; thus, the information contained therein is apolitical. Each week, approximately 20,000 viewers peruse the Web site. Stateline.org also publishes an annual *State of the States Report,* and it sponsors professional development conferences and workshops for the new media.

The Pew Charitable Trusts also funds the Pew Research Center, which operates as a self-regulating, apolitical organization. One activity of the center is to support the Pew Biomedical Scholars Program. This program provides financial assistance to talented early- and mid-career scientists who are investigating fundamental and medical areas

regarding human health. Scholars are given financial support (in the range of $240,000 for 48 months) and are encouraged to be commercial and original in their research endeavors.

Cary Stacy Smith and Li-Ching Hung

See also Access to Healthcare; Health; Kaiser Family Foundation; Medicaid; Public Health; Public Policy; State-Based Health Insurance Initiatives; Vulnerable Populations

Further Readings

Pew Charitable Trusts. *Sustaining the Legacy: A History of the Pew Charitable Trusts.* Philadelphia: Pew Charitable Trusts, 2001.
Prescription Project. *Report: Risk with No Benefit: The Marketing of Over-the-Counter Cough and Cold Medications for Children.* Philadelphia: Pew Charitable Trusts, 2007.
Stateline.org. *Report. State of the States, 2008.* Philadelphia: Pew Charitable Trusts, 2008.
Trust for America's Health and the Infectious Diseases Society of America. *Pandemic Influenza: The State of the Science.* Philadelphia: Pew Charitable Trusts, 2006.

Web Sites

Pew Charitable Trusts: http://www.pewtrusts.org
Stateline.org: http://www.stateline.org/live

PHARMACEUTICAL INDUSTRY

The pharmaceutical or drug industry historically has been one of the most innovative and profitable business sectors in the United States. Recent developments, however, portend major changes in the nation's pharmaceutical industry. Growing regulatory oversight, rising consumer distrust over advertising claims, drug safety concerns, increased cost-containment initiatives by government and private third-party payers, mandated health technology assessments to determine coverage and reimbursement policies, patent expirations of top-selling products, and the implementation of the Medicare Part D drug benefit have influenced changes in the industry's practices and strategies. This entry describes the global sales and market share of the pharmaceutical industry, the different classifications within the industry, and the future outlook for the industry in light of the recent developments.

Global Pharmaceutical Sales

Global pharmaceutical sales grew by 7% in 2006, totaling more than $643 billion (all data reported in U.S. dollars) in sales, according to industry estimates by IMS Health. This marked the third straight year of single-digit revenue growth for the pharmaceutical industry, after 5 years of double-digit increases from 1999 to 2003. The worldwide pharmaceutical market is dominated by the United States, with 44% of the world's market share, followed by Europe, with 28%, Japan, 10%, Asia Pacific, 7%, Latin America, 5%, the Middle East and Africa, 3%, and Canada, 3%. The largest European markets are France, Germany, Italy, the United Kingdom, and Spain. The Asia Pacific region includes fast-growing pharmaceutical companies, located in India and China, which mainly produce generic versions of drug products. Brazil is the largest market in Latin America.

Classification of the Pharmaceutical Industry

The pharmaceutical industry, or *pharma*, includes three primary sectors: (1) the traditional research-intensive pharmaceutical industry, (2) the research-intensive biopharmaceutical industry, and (3) the generic pharmaceutical industry. These sectors, however, are increasingly becoming blurred because of strategic company acquisitions, mergers, licensing agreements, and other business practices. For example, most traditional research-intensive pharmaceutical companies manufacture or license generic versions of their original products. The traditional research-intensive industry is attempting to gain market share and position in the biopharmaceutical industry. And the generic pharmaceutical industry is lobbying for legislation to facilitate the approval of *biogenerics* (i.e., similar versions of biotech pharmaceutical products).

Traditional Pharmaceutical Industry

The traditional research-intensive pharmaceutical industry is also known as the "brand-name" or "innovator" pharmaceutical industry. The largest companies in this sector are often referred to as "Big Pharma." They are represented by the trade association, Pharmaceutical Research and Manufactures of America (PhRMA). This sector focuses on the discovery, development, and production of new chemical entities and new biologic entities. These multibillion dollar corporations, however, are not limited solely to drug products or vaccine sales. Many of these corporations include other healthcare-related products, such as nutrition products, dietary supplements, diagnostics, medical devices, and other consumer products.

Relative rankings of the world's top pharmaceutical companies change yearly due to sales, patent expirations, mergers, acquisitions, and other practices. Based on 2007 rankings (compiled from Fortune 500 lists), 12 pharmaceutical corporations accounted for 60% of the total global pharmaceutical sales. The leading companies—based on sales, headquarters country, revenue, and profit (as a percentage of revenues)—were (1) Johnson & Johnson (U.S.), $53.3 billion, 20.7%; (2) Pfizer (U.S.), $52.4 billion, 36.9%; (3) GlaxoSmithKline (U.K.), $42.7 billion, 23.2%; (4) Novartis (Switzerland), $37 billion, 19.4%; (5) Sanofi-Aventis (France), $37 billion, 13.6%; (6) Roche Group (Switzerland), $34.7 billion, 18.1%; (7) AstraZeneca (U.K.), $26.5 billion, 22.8%; (8) Merck & Co. (U.S.), $22.6 billion, 19.6%; (9) Abbott Laboratories (U.S.), $22.5 billion, 7.6%; (10) Wyeth (U.S.), $20.4 billion, 20.6%; (11) Bristol-Myers Squibb (U.S.), $17.9 billion, 8.8%; and (12) Eli Lilly (U.S.), $15.7 billion, 17%.

Seven of the top pharmaceutical companies are American-based, and the five other top companies are headquartered in Europe. Depending on the year, other leading research-based pharmaceutical companies include Bayer (Germany), Boehringer Ingelheim (Germany), Schering-Plough (U.S.), Baxter International (U.S.), Takeda Pharmaceuticals (Japan), Procter & Gamble (U.S.), Astella Pharma (Japan), and others.

The median profit margin for the leading pharmaceutical companies was 19.5%, which is well above the median of 4% to 5% for most other industries. Median profit margins for the pharmaceutical industry have been about 17% to 18% since 2002 (with a slight dip to 14% in 2003). Industry profits increased in the United States due in part to the passage of the Medicare Part D prescription drug benefit, which the industry helped pass.

The pharmaceutical industry asserts that its profits are in line with those of other major industries in consideration of its need for a reasonable return on its investment and adequate revenue to encourage risk and innovation in the business of drug discovery. Critics counter that it is difficult to consider such a routinely profitable industry as being risky.

The research-based pharmaceutical industry strongly supports innovative drug research, swift development and approval of drug products demonstrated to be safe and effective, strong intellectual property and patent protection, and access to medicines in an open, competitive market. It also supports federal legislation that would limit liability (e.g., limits on punitive damages and on damage awards) for drug manufacturers. On the other hand, it opposes restrictive drug formularies, prior authorization policies for prescription drug coverage, limits on prescription reimbursement, price controls, and retail-level prescription drug importation from foreign sources.

The U.S. Food and Drug Administration (FDA) is the federal agency that reviews drug products for approval in America, while patents on drug products (and related chemical compounds, processes, and other intellectual property) are granted by the U.S. Patent and Trademark Office. Patents can be granted anywhere along the development lifeline of a drug compound or product. Patents are granted for a period of 20 years from the date of filing, before patent term restoration activities and court challenges. The PhRMA states that due to lost patent time during the protracted drug approval process (estimated at 11 to 12 years by the FDA and up to 15 years by the pharmaceutical industry), the effective patent life of prescription drugs in the United States is only about 11 or 12 years, as compared with more than 18 years for nondrug products. The FDA can grant exclusive marketing rights, or exclusivity, for certain time periods (ranging from 6 months to 7 years) to help promote a balance between innovation in new chemical entities and generic competition.

Biopharmaceutical Industry

The research-based biopharmaceutical industry is the newest sector and is also referred to as the "pharmaceutical biotechnology industry," or "biopharma." Its products are usually termed *biotech pharmaceuticals* or *biological medicines*. Biotech pharmaceuticals are medicines derived from living cells and proteins, the so-called large molecules. In comparison, the traditional research-based pharmaceutical industry discovers and produces drug products based primarily on small-molecule chemical substances. Examples of biopharmaceuticals include monoclonal antibodies, protein cell cultures, protein microbials, and bioengineered hormones. Biopharmaceuticals are used to treat a variety of medical conditions, though most current products are marketed as specialty medications indicated for cancers, anemia, heart disease, rheumatoid arthritis, and less prevalent diseases such as ankylosing spondylitis and Crohn's disease. A large percentage of research and development expenses (25–50% of revenue) is invested by the biopharma industry as compared with the traditional research-intensive pharmaceutical industry (which averages about 18% of revenue).

The U.S. market for biotech pharmaceuticals was $35 billion in 2006, a 17% increase in growth from 2005, which was about two times the rate of the traditional research-intensive pharmaceutical industry. Biotech pharmaceuticals accounted for 12% of total prescription sales, though the high costs for some of these products can make them prohibitively expensive. For example, treatment with Genentech's Avastin (bevacizumab)—indicated for certain types of lung cancer, advanced breast cancer, or metastatic colorectal cancer—can cost $100,000 per patient per year.

The top 10 biopharmaceutical companies, based on reported 2006 revenues, were (1) Amgen ($14.3 billion), (2) Genentech ($7.6 billion), (3) Novo Nordisk ($6.5 billion), (4) Genzyme ($3.2 billion), (5) Gilead Sciences ($3 billion), (6) UCB Group ($2.7 billion), (7) Biogen Idec ($2.7 billion), (8) Serono ($2.5 billion), (9) MedImmune ($1.2 billion), and (10) Millennium ($220 million). Eight of these companies are based in the United States. The exceptions are Novo Nordisk (Denmark) and UCB Group (Belgium).

Financial positions, relative rankings, and ownership can change quickly, especially in the more volatile biopharmaceutical sector. For example, Amgen's profits of almost $3 billion dropped by 19.7% from the levels achieved in 2005. Gilead

Sciences and Genzyme also experienced substantial profit decreases during a 1-year period. The eighth-ranked biopharmaceutical company—Serono—was acquired by Merck KGaA in 2006 and is now Merck Serono (known as EMD Serono, Inc., in the United States and Canada because Germany-based Merck KGaA is a different company from the U.S.-based Merck & Co., which has the rights to the name in North America). Similarly, AstraZeneca purchased MedImmune in 2007.

The biopharmaceutical industry has a similar product approval process to that of other pharmaceutical products. However, the approval time for a biopharmaceutical ranges between 7 and 12 years from development to approval. The development and manufacture of biologic medicines is more complex and expensive than production of small-molecule chemical entities, which is one of the reasons for their high costs. Because biologics are produced in living cells, it would be very difficult for other manufacturers to duplicate the process exactly in attempts to make generic versions of biopharmaceuticals. Thus, biosimilars may be therapeutically equivalent, rather than chemically equivalent with original products. The FDA is in the early stages of creating regulatory procedures for the review and approval of biogenerics or biosimilars, which are "generic" (or, more aptly named "similar") versions of the innovator biotech pharmaceuticals. However, it is likely to be years before that process is completed.

The major biotechnology trade association is the Biotechnology Industry Organization (BIO), and its multidisciplinary membership includes more than 1,100 biotech companies, universities, research organizations, and affiliates. In addition to biotech pharmaceutical firms, an increasing number of PhRMA companies are branching into pharmaceutical biotechnology because of the rapid growth of the industry and the lack of current processes to enable generic competition. From 2005 to 2007, Big Pharma companies spent $76 billion to acquire biotech companies. For example, Novartis, Wyeth, Abbot, and Eli Lilly have invested hundreds of millions of dollars each in the formation of in-house units for the development and manufacture of biotech pharmaceuticals and the building of new manufacturing facilities. Other Big Pharma companies have acquired smaller biotech firms to expand their pipelines.

The biopharmaceutical industry generally espouses similar position statements as the traditional research-intensive pharmaceutical companies with respect to support of market-based pricing for medicines, support of tax incentives to encourage investment in biotech-derived medicines, opposition to price controls for biotech drugs, and opposition to restrictive reimbursement programs. Similar to Big Pharma, the biotech pharmaceutical industry is using late life-cycle strategies to expand its product line and to extend the market life of its products, such as the second-generation anemia drug, EPO Aranesp (darbepoetin alfa), which is manufactured by Amgen. One area where the position of the biopharmaceutical industry differs from those of the traditional research-intensive pharmacy companies is with respect to policies on separate reimbursement mechanisms for drugs and biologicals.

Generic Pharmaceutical Industry

A generic drug product is defined as a product that is bioequivalent to a referenced innovator (brand name) drug product and is identical in active chemical ingredient, strength, dosage form, route of administration, quality, performance characteristics, safety, and treatment indication. Multisource generics are available for about three-quarters of drug products approved by the FDA. The generic pharmaceutical industry experienced a 22% growth in sales from 2005 to 2006. Nationally, 63% of prescriptions dispensed in the United States in 2006 were generic products, though generics accounted for only 20% of prescription drug sales. Over the past 20 years, the sustained growth in use of generic drug products has been promoted as a cost-saving measure by managed-care organizations, private health insurance companies, state Medicaid and other government programs, pharmacy benefit management companies, and others.

The pharmaceutical industry differentiates between unbranded generics and branded generics. Following approval of an abbreviated new drug application (ANDA) by the FDA, unbranded generics are manufactured by pharmaceutical companies unaffiliated (for that product) with the innovator company. The ANDA (and equivalent) process does not require the applicant firm to repeat the expensive preclinical and clinical research for the drug ingredients and dosage forms that were approved by the FDA for the application of the innovator company. Rather, the generic product must demonstrate bioequivalence. The median ANDA approval time in 2006 was 16.6 months. Branded generics (called "authorized generics" by the industry) are generic versions of the innovator product that are manufactured by the innovator pharmaceutical industry sponsor and/or otherwise produced and distributed by one of its licensed partners. Branded generics are not required to undergo an abbreviated FDA approval process because the innovator company is selling the same product previously approved under a brand name. In 2006, the top pharmaceutical companies for unbranded generic drug products (accounting for 54% of prescription dispensed and 10% of U.S. sales) were Teva Pharmaceuticals, Novartis (Sandoz division), Mylan Laboratories, Watson Pharmaceuticals, Pfizer (Greenstone division), Apotex Corporation, Par Pharmaceuticals, Mallinckrodt, Barr Labs, Boehringer Ingelheim, Actavis US, Qualitest Products, and Hospira, Inc.

The main generic pharmaceutical industry trade association is the Generic Pharmaceutical Association (GPhA). The association states that the generic manufacturers provide consumers with safe, effective, quality drug products at lower costs. Generic drugs are estimated to save U.S. customers $8 to $10 billion yearly at the retail level, with more savings realized when including other pharmacy distribution outlets such as hospitals and nursing homes. The generic pharmaceutical industry supports efforts to promote free market forces and supports the development of an abbreviated regulatory approval process for biogenerics or biosimilars. The generic pharmaceutical industry wants faster FDA review times for ANDAs. It is strongly opposed to brand-name (research-intensive) drug industry efforts to extend patents and other tactics to delay market introduction of generic drug products, such as patent extensions for minor changes in formulations or processes and unsubstantiated citizen petitions to block FDA approval of generic applications. The unbranded generic industry has challenged the FDA's regulatory policies in approving authorized generics. The generic pharmaceutical industry claims that by merely changing their label, the brand-name companies compete with the first generic drug company at a period in which the first generic sponsor should have exclusive marketing rights (for 180 days) without competition by any product other than the original brand label. It also opposes foreign importation of drug products at the retail level.

Future Implications

Mergers, acquisitions, and other consolidations among the major pharmaceutical companies are anticipated to continue, and the nature of the pharmaceutical industry is changing. Fewer blockbuster drug products (i.e., products with annual global sales of at least $1 billion) have been approved in recent years, with drugs in the research pipelines appearing less promising for the traditional research-based pharmaceutical industry than for the growing biotech pharmaceutical sector.

It has been estimated that Big Pharma lost $14 billion in sales as the result of patent expirations and increased generic competition in 2006. In the future, while the companies will remain profitable, revenues are likely to decline because many of their drug products are coming off patent between 2008 and 2012 (e.g., Fosamax, Valtrix, Advair, Lipitor, Plavix, and Crestor).

In light of these patent expirations, more limited pipeline resources, and declining sales, many major pharma companies are reorganizing. In recent years, many companies have attempted to have leaner operations by laying off employees and streamlining programs.

Predicted trends for the pharmaceutical industry include the increased use of outsourcing and global licensing because of reduced regulatory monitoring and decreased costs. The U.S. pharmaceutical industry (research and generic) already outsources much of its production to offshore territories (e.g., Puerto Rico) and overseas countries, especially the emerging markets of India, China, and Eastern Europe. While the FDA inspects these facilities (for drug products legitimately sold in the United States), the oversight is less stringent than the routine inspections in U.S.-based corporations.

Last, the future outlooks of the pharmaceutical industry will include increasing regulatory consideration of biosimilars. The European Commission granted Sandoz approval to market a biosimilar version of epoetin alfa, or EPO (indicated for treatment of anemia) in 2007, becoming the first biogeneric product approved in the European EPO market. While predicted to be a potential block-buster, the ultimate impact of this regulatory action is unknown. Sandoz's Omnitrope (somatropin, rDNA origin), a biosimilar version of Pfizer's human growth hormone Genotropin, was marketed under special rules in the United States and Europe in 2006. Its sales, however, represent less than 1% of the market. Perhaps its low market share was due to the drug's relatively high price and physician concerns about its bioequivalence. In 2007, legislation was introduced in the U.S. Congress (H.R. 1038 and S. 623, Access to Life-Saving Medicine Act) to provide for the licensing of therapeutically equivalent biological medicines, which would mandate the FDA to create an abbreviated approval process for biological products. However, Congress took no action.

Stephanie Y. Crawford

See also Cost of Healthcare; Direct-to-Consumer Advertising (DTCA); Medicare Part D Prescription Drug Benefit; Pharmacy; Pharmacoeconomics; Prescription and Generic Drug Use; U.S. Food and Drug Administration (FDA)

Further Readings

Angell, Marcia. *The Truth About the Drug Companies: How They Deceive Us and What to Do About It.* New York: Random House, 2004.

"By the Numbers. Top 20 Pharmaceutical Companies Ranked by U.S. Sales, October 2006 to September 2007," *Modern Healthcare* 38(1): 31, January 7, 2008.

Engelhardt, H. Tristram, and Jeremy R. Garrett, eds. *Innovation and the Pharmaceutical Industry: Critical Reflections on the Virtues of Profit.* Salem, MA: M and M Scrivener Press, 2008.

Evans, Ronald P. *Drug and Biological Development: From Molecule to Product and Beyond.* New York: Springer, 2007.

Fulda, Thomas R., and Albert I. Wertheimer, eds. *Handbook of Pharmaceutical Public Policy.* New York: Pharmaceutical Products Press, 2007.

Shayne, Gad. *Pharmaceutical Manufacturing Handbook: Production and Processes.* Hoboken, NJ: Wiley, 2008.

Sloan, Frank A., and Chee-Ruey Hsieh, eds. *Pharmaceutical Innovation: Incentives, Competition, and Cost-Benefit Analysis in International Perspective.* New York: Cambridge University Press, 2007.

U.S. Government Accountability Office. *New Drug Development: Science, Business, Regulatory, and Intellectual Property Issues Cited As Hampering Drug Development Efforts.* Report No. GAO-07-49. Washington, DC: U.S. Government Accountability Office, November 2006.

Web Sites

Biotechnology Industry Organization (BIO): http://www.bio.org

Generic Pharmaceutical Association (GphA): http://www.gphaonline.org

IMS Health: http://www.imshealth.com

Pharmaceutical Research and Manufacturers of America (PhRMA): http://www.phrma.org

U.S. Food and Drug Administration (FDA): http://www.fda.gov

PHARMACOECONOMICS

Pharmacoeconomics can be defined as the description and analysis of the costs and consequences of pharmaceutical products and services and their impact on individuals, the healthcare system, and society at large. Pharmacoeconomics as a field of research arose in the late 1970s in response to rising expenditures on prescriptions and growing concerns regarding cost containment of drug budgets. The underlying purpose of pharmacoeconomic analysis is to promote the efficient use of healthcare resources by informing treatment choices and related policy.

Background

Pharmacoeconomics has ties to both economic evaluation and health outcomes research. Many of the theoretical methods have roots in social welfare and cost-benefit analysis that are found in public finance and environmental economics. The field is also related to decision analysis and corporate finance principles often used in evaluating corporate business decisions.

Categories of Study Methods

Within pharmacoeconomics, there are four general subcategories of study methods: (1) cost-minimization analysis (CMA), (2) cost-effectiveness analysis (CEA), (3) cost-utility analysis (CUA), and (4) cost-benefit analysis (CBA). These four subcategories are differentiated according to how health outcomes are measured: CMA requires that the health effects of the alternatives in question are equal. CEA measures health outcomes in some natural unit (e.g., life years). CUA is very similar to CEA except that the unit of health is quality-adjusted life years (QALYs). These units are formed by assigning health status (e.g., mild angina) a preference-based utility score, typically between 0 and 1, where 1 represents perfect health and 0 represents death, and then multiplying life years in a particular health state by the preference score of that health state (e.g., 10 years in a health state with a utility score of 0.7 results in 7 QALYs). The scores themselves come from survey-based methods, and there are various methodologies for obtaining the utility scores. Finally, CBA measures health effects in dollars, which often involves some means of translating health gains into a dollar value. All four subcategories consider costs measured in dollars.

Data Sources

There are numerous potential sources of data for quantifying costs and outcomes for use in a pharmacoeconomics analysis, ranging from prospective data collection to analyses of administrative databases to information based on surveys of experts. In addition, information from randomized clinical trials or from pharmacoepidemiologic studies can be examined in combination with cost information. Any pharmacoeconomic study is limited by the availability of data related to what treatments it sets out to compare. In addition, data are typically available from a particular patient population, a particular time period, and a particular setting. Consequently, studies often involve the use of models to project results across patient populations, and to project costs and outcomes into time horizons beyond the research of existing data.

Determining Costs

A key aspect of pharmacoeconomics is consideration of costs beyond just the simple cost of the drug. Examples of other costs that can be included are the personnel, equipment, or facilities used in

administering treatment, the cost of treating side effects, the costs associated with healthcare utilization (e.g., physician office visits or hospitalizations), or the cost of patient time that is spent during treatment, to name a few. Finally, the costs of pain and suffering from a treatment or disease can be considered. Note, that a central element of a pharmacoeconomic analysis is the choice of the study perspective, where a societal perspective is generally felt to be the most relevant in terms of informing national policy (other perspectives include the payer perspective, the provider perspective, and the employer perspective). The study perspective fundamentally determines what costs are included in the analysis, which is a reason that studies that take a broad perspective, such as a societal perspective, are considered to be of greater importance. However, data availability and available budgets for research may limit the perspective that research can cover. More important, it is the research question (or decision to be made) that dictates the appropriate perspective.

Decision Making

In terms of how the results inform decisions, CMA identifies the lowest-cost treatment among two or more with the same effect. CEA and CUA identify treatments that cost more and provide equal or lower amounts of a health outcome, a choice that is never favorable. CEA and CUA also measure the additional spending that is required per gain in additional units of health outcome in making a treatment switch to a higher-cost, higher-effect treatment (or visa versa). By identifying the cost of increasing health in particular treatment options, CEA and CUA promote efficient treatment choices. Currently, treatment adoptions with cost-to-QALYs ratios lower than $100,000 are generally considered favorable. Cost-benefit analysis typically provides a direct calculation of the net benefit of making a treatment change, defined as the change in benefits minus the change in costs. When the change in treatment is deemed to have a positive net benefit, then that change is recommended.

Currently, CUA with a societal perspective is considered the gold standard strategy among pharmacoeconomic analysts, though this is not without controversy. While many feel that QALYs are the best available measure of general health outcomes, many also feel that the measurement techniques to acquire QALYs are flawed and that there are too many underlying assumptions that go into aggregating QALYs (e.g., that an added QALY for an elderly person is the same as for a younger person) for them to adequately inform actual policy decisions. Suffice to say that development of appropriate measures of health outcomes and notions of how to best apply aggregated results to inform policy toward health treatments is an ongoing process.

Future Implications

Pharmacoeconomics continues to grow, as measured by the number of published articles and books, the number of researchers, as well as the number of dollars spent on research in the field. Many nations require pharmacoeconomic analyses as part of the drug approval process. Although the U.S. Food and Drug Administration (FDA) does not currently require pharmacoeconomic analyses in its approval process, a growing number of healthcare organizations are including pharmacoeconomic evidence in their decision-making processes. In addition, many of the nation's pharmacy schools require pharmacoeconomics in the curriculum of their students, and there are a number of graduate programs available that include concentrations in pharmacoeconomics.

Surrey M. Walton

See also Cost-Benefit and Cost-Effectiveness Analysis; Cost of Healthcare; Health Economics; Outcomes Movement; Pharmaceutical Industry; Pharmacy; Public Policy; Quality-Adjusted Life Years (QALYs)

Further Readings

Bonk, Robert J. *Pharmacoeconomics in Perspective: A Primer on Research, Techniques, and Information.* Binghamton, NY: Haworth Press, 1999.

Drummond, Michael F., Mark J. Sculpher, George W. Torrance, et al. *Methods for the Economic Evaluation of Health Care Programmes.* 3d ed. New York: Oxford University Press, 2005.

Rascati, Karen L. *Essentials of Pharmacoeconomics.* Baltimore: Lippincott Williams and Wilkins, 2009.

Rychlik, Reinhard. *Strategies in Pharmacoeconomics and Outcomes Research.* Binghamton, NY: Haworth Press, 2002.

Schweitzer, Stuart O. *Pharmaceutical Economics and Policy.* 2d ed. New York: Oxford University Press, 2007.

Web Sites

International Society for Pharmacoeconomics and Outcome Research (ISPOR): http://www.ispor.org

Society for Medical Decision Making (SMDM): http://www.smdm.org

PHARMACY

For the general public, pharmacists are often the most accessible health professionals for patients to obtain information and advice. Currently, there are about 245,000 licensed pharmacists employed in the United States, which ranks pharmacy as the nation's third-largest health profession. There are also about 285,000 employed pharmacy technicians. Pharmacists help ensure the rational and safe use of drug therapies by working to achieve positive therapeutic outcomes, improve the quality of life for patients, reduce healthcare costs, and minimize patient risk from drug-related morbidity and mortality.

Pharmacists are increasingly expanding their roles in healthcare. Specifically, they are advising physicians, nurses, and other health professionals on medication selection, dosages, use, interactions, and side effects; dispensing medications and monitoring patients for expected outcomes and adverse effects; and educating and counseling patients on prescription and nonprescription drugs, dietary supplements, self-care, and other healthcare topics.

As recognized medication-use experts, pharmacists are well educated on the composition and characteristics of pharmaceuticals (e.g., chemical, pharmacological, and physical properties), their manufacture and/or preparation, and use. Pharmacists strive to verify the quality of drugs and related ingredients in the supply chain to help ensure drug purity, strength, and proper labeling for improved patient safety.

History of American Pharmacy

The existence of pharmacists was rare in Colonial America. Drugs and "patent medicines" (i.e., cheap and supposedly curative tonics, pills, and other concoctions, which often contained large proportions of alcohol, opium, or laxatives) were readily available and hawked for sale without a prescription at general stores and by traveling salesmen. In the late 1700s, physicians compounded drugs they prescribed (i.e., prepared specially customized medicines), or their apprentices prepared the drugs under their supervision. Apothecary shops were generally owned by physicians and were located in large cities. The local drug clerk was a shop employee whose role was more akin to a wholesaler than retailer; the drug clerk primarily compounded, stocked, and distributed medicines for physicians. The job of the drug clerk was viewed as a trade occupation, which was best learned by daily application of repetitive practices. The apprentice drug clerks eventually developed more expertise in pharmaceuticals, far beyond the knowledge of most physicians, and they enjoyed a close working relationship with physicians, since they usually operated the shops on behalf of them.

Over time, the physician-owners of the shops moved away and/or sold their businesses to their former drug clerks, which began the establishment of the independent retail drugstore trade. In the early to mid-1800s, independent apothecary shops and drugstores proliferated, and the businesses became increasingly profitable. As proprietors, the former drug clerks adopted the titled of apothecaries or druggists (and a few called themselves pharmacists). The first college of pharmacy was established in Philadelphia in 1821, and a small number of other pharmacy colleges were founded, though most druggist-practitioners lacked formal training. From the mid-1800s through the early 1900s, the country lacked laws and regulations governing foods, drugs, and healthcare practice. The sale of inefficacious, possibly poisonous, and mislabeled patent medicines were sold by self-designated apothecaries and other merchants. Some 19th-century druggists diagnosed patients and dispensed medicines, which conflicted with medical practice. Physicians widely criticized the apprentice-trained employees as unknowledgeable and unscrupulous. Many physicians continued to dispense their own medicines, and a widening rift developed between pharmacy and clinical medicine.

By the early 1900s, federal legislation and regulations helped improve safety and quality of the drug supply to some extent. Medical education, training, and practice underwent substantial change. Most physicians stopped or limited their dispensing of medicines, and druggists compromised by limiting their diagnosing to minor illnesses. During the Prohibition Era (1920–1933), drugstores were popular hangouts because druggists could dispense alcohol for medicinal purposes. Regulatory change of certain drug products to prescription-only status in the early 1900s eliminated the discretionary latitude of pharmacists in dispensing certain medications over the counter. Mass manufacturing of drug products by the pharmaceutical industry began around the same time, which greatly reduced compounding activities by pharmacists. By the 1960s, pharmacy practice started to evolve from the product-oriented distributive focus to include more patient-oriented clinical roles.

Laws and regulations, professional standards, and a professional code of ethics underpin contemporary pharmacist roles. Leaders in the profession embraced the clinical pharmacy movement in the 1970s to the 1990s, when the concept of pharmaceutical care was conceptualized. Today, pharmaceutical care is defined as assuming responsibility for providing drug therapy intended to produce outcomes that improve the patient's quality of life. The changing healthcare marketplace, societal need, shifting of some drugs from prescription to nonprescription status, advent of computerization and other automated systems, and educational reforms help shape pharmacy practice.

Education

Throughout the 20th century, inconsistent pharmacy educational requirements resulted in disjointed perceptions of pharmacists and fragmented philosophies of practice. More formalized pharmacy education programs were established by the early 1900s, including 2-year diploma programs and a few 3-year and 4-year programs. The minimum educational requirement for pharmacy increased to 3 years in 1925 and increased to a

4-year bachelor of science degree in 1932. By the 1950s, many pharmacy schools had expanded the degree program requirements to a 5-year bachelor's degree, which became the minimum standard in 1960.

Most of the nation's pharmacy degree programs in the 1960s and 1970s were heavily science based, with curriculums focused on chemistry and other physical sciences. Clinical therapeutics courses were added to the curricula at most pharmacy programs by the 1970s. A number of pharmacy schools converted their programs to a 6-year doctor of pharmacy (PharmD) degree by the 1980s, though the majority of colleges continued to offer the 5-year bachelor's degree as the entry-level degree in pharmacy. At that time, the doctor of pharmacy degree was typically available as an advanced postbaccalaureate degree.

A protracted debate ensued among members of the profession, major pharmacy providers, and the academic community as to whether there was the need for the advanced clinical degree for all pharmacists. A dual system of pharmacy education (bachelor's degree and doctor of pharmacy) persisted for decades in a contentious atmosphere of strong support for and opposition to the all-doctor of pharmacy standard for professional education. The debate ended in 1992, when the accrediting body (now the Accreditation Council for Pharmacy Education [ACPE]) announced its intent to recognize only the doctor of pharmacy as the first professional degree. Since 2004, the doctor of pharmacy has been the only professional pharmacy degree program accredited by ACPE.

The doctor of pharmacy (PharmD) is designed to take a minimum of 6 academic years, including 2 years of prepharmacy requirements and 4 years of pharmacy school. Admission to pharmacy school is highly competitive. Applicants must have high academic achievement in courses such as biology, chemistry, physics, and calculus. More pharmacy schools are also requiring students to take various liberal arts courses such as communication and economics to have a broader education. Most pharmacy schools require Pharmacy College Admission Test (PCAT) scores and interviews before applicants are considered for admission. The pharmacy school curriculum includes strong foundations in the basic pharmacy sciences (e.g., medicinal chemistry, pharmacology, pharmacognosy, or natural products, pharmaceutics, pharmacokinetics, and physiology), the social, behavioral, and administrative sciences (e.g., communications, health systems analysis and services delivery, pharmacoeconomics, and management), and pharmacotherapeutics (e.g., clinical pharmacy). Early experiential education is included throughout the curriculum, and advanced pharmacy practice experiential education (i.e., clerkships) is offered during the final year of study. Graduate programs (leading to master's and doctoral degrees) are also available in specific areas of the pharmaceutical sciences, but these research-based graduate degree programs do not generally require a background in pharmacy as a prerequisite for admission. More than 100 accredited pharmacy schools exist in the United States, and these programs graduate approximately 9,000 pharmacists annually.

Optional postgraduate training opportunities exist in pharmacy. More than 1,500 pharmacists complete a residency each year. A pharmacy residency is an organized, postgraduate training program in professional practice and management activities. Pharmacy residency programs are mainly located in the hospitals or ambulatory-care settings but also include home care and long-term care facilities, managed-care facilities, community pharmacies, and other settings. The American Society of Health-System Pharmacists (ASHP) accredits more than 800 residency programs, and the training programs cover diverse practice areas, such as ambulatory care, cardiology, critical care, informatics, psychiatric pharmacy, and transplantation. Residency programs usually last 1 year (though a few are 2 years in duration), and some pharmacists complete a second, specialized residency after 1 year of general pharmacy residency training. A pharmacy fellowship, typically lasting 2 years, is a highly individualized postgraduate training program to develop research skills for pharmacists. The pharmacy fellow is under the direction of an experienced researcher-preceptor, usually in the academic or the pharmaceutical industry sector.

Licensure and Credentialing

Graduates of accredited pharmacy programs in the United States must pass state board examinations to earn a license to practice pharmacy. Initial state licensure as a registered pharmacist is gained by passing the North American Pharmacist Licensure Examination (NAPLEX), the appropriate sections of the Multistate Pharmacy Jurisprudence Examination, both of which are administered by the National Association of Boards of Pharmacy (NABP), and/or other state requirements. Mechanisms exist to transfer NAPLEX scores (during initial licensing) and to transfer existing licenses (reciprocity) to gain licensure in more than one state or jurisdiction. A certification process is established by NABP and individual state boards to allow foreign pharmacy graduates (who pass the Foreign Pharmacy Graduate Equivalency Examination and provide documentation of sufficient foreign pharmacy education) to become eligible to take the NAPLEX. Pharmacists are expected to maintain professional competence, legal requirements, ethical standards, and continuing professional education to maintain their licensure.

At the highest recognized level of specialization, pharmacists in certain fields may become board certified through programs administered by the Board of Pharmaceutical Specialties (BPS). Board certification does not grant the recipient any legal authority. However, certification offers advantages in knowledge gained, competitive job advantages, and recognized expertise for third-party payers. BPS-specialties exist in nuclear pharmacy, nutrition support pharmacy, oncology pharmacy, pharmacotherapy (including added qualifications for subspecialists in cardiology and infectious diseases, and psychiatric pharmacy. Nearly 7,000 pharmacists (about 3% of the workforce) were board certified in 2007. In addition to BPS certification, pharmacists can develop specialized areas of practice through residency or fellowship training, certificate programs in disease state management and other areas of practice, or extensive work experience.

The role of pharmacists continues to expand, partly due to increasing numbers of pharmacists specializing in practice areas and participating in disease state management. Certain states have enacted legislation to enable collaborative practice between pharmacists and physicians based on set protocols. Through such collaborative drug therapy management agreements, qualified pharmacists may perform patient assessments, order drug-therapy-related tests, administer medications, and order and monitor drug regimens.

Pharmacy Technicians

Pharmacists often are assisted by pharmacy technicians who provide technical support. Depending on individual state practice acts and regulations, pharmacy technicians may enter medication orders, prepare medications and supplies for dispensing (e.g., counting and labeling), stock and transport medications, purchase drugs, manage narcotics inventories, answer telephone inquires, and conduct other administrative duties. Roles of pharmacy technicians are determined by their employer, and their work must be supervised under the direction of a registered pharmacist. There are no uniform qualifications for pharmacy technicians, and requirements vary across states and practice settings. Most, though not all, states require that pharmacy technicians be high school graduates or equivalent. Pharmacy technicians may be trained informally or formally on the job, in vocational programs, community colleges, or the U.S. military; training program lengths range from 1 day to 2 years. Increasingly, employers and some states are requiring that pharmacy technicians obtain certification, primarily by the Pharmacy Technician Certification Board (PTCB) or by the Institute for the Certification of Pharmacy Technicians (ICPT).

Pharmacist Associations

Hundreds of pharmacist associations exist to serve member needs, including government relations, public relations, continuing education, professional standards development, meetings, products and services, and other professional activities. The three largest pharmacist associations are (1) the American Pharmacists Association (APhA), (2) the American Society of Health-System Pharmacists (ASHP), and (3) the National Community Pharmacists Association (NCPA).

Founded in 1852, the APhA (formerly the American Pharmaceutical Association), which is located in Washington, D.C., is the oldest professional pharmacist society. The APhA has a membership of approximately 60,000 pharmacists, pharmacy students, and pharmacy technicians.

The ASHP (formerly the American Society of Hospital Pharmacists), which is located in Bethesda, Maryland, has the largest annual budget of any pharmacist association, at approximately $40 million. Its membership consists of about 30,000 pharmacists whose practice settings include hospitals, health maintenance organizations (HMOs), patients' homes, and long-term care facilities.

The NCPA, which was founded in 1898 as the National Association of Retail Druggists, is headquartered in Alexandria, Virginia. It represents approximately 23,000 members who practice in independent community pharmacies.

Other major pharmacist associations represent managed-care practitioners (Academy of Managed Care Pharmacists), clinical specialists in pharmacy practice and research (American College of Clinical Pharmacy), compounding pharmacists (International Academy of Compounding Pharmacists), and minority pharmacists (National Pharmaceutical Association).

Affiliate member status is available for pharmacy technicians in most of the major pharmacist associations, but the primary group representing them is the American Association of Pharmacy Technicians (AAPT).

Other important related associations are the National Association of Chain Drug Stores (NACDS) and the Pharmaceutical Care Management Association, which represent chain drugstores and pharmacy benefit managers, respectively.

Future Implications

Currently, about 60% of pharmacists work in community pharmacies (e.g., independently owned pharmacies, chain drugstores, mass merchandisers, and supermarket pharmacies). About 20% of pharmacists work in healthcare institutions (e.g., hospitals, nursing homes, and health clinics). The remaining pharmacists work in various areas such as the federal government, academia, the pharmaceutical industry, managed-care organizations, professional associations, and public health agencies, among others.

Although salary ranges vary widely across geographic regions and practice settings, the median annual pharmacist salaries ranged between about $83,000 and $108,000 in 2006. And because of the increasing demand for pharmacists, their salaries continue to rise each year.

The future employment outlook for pharmacists is very promising. Pharmacists are in increasing demand because of the greater use of prescription drugs, demographic trends such as the aging of the population, and the increasing incidence of chronic diseases. It is anticipated that there will be a national shortage of 112,000 to 157,000 pharmacists by 2020. It is also estimated that about 91,000 additional pharmacy technicians will be needed by 2016. Future workforce projections will be influenced by the attrition rate of older pharmacists, shifts in full-time-equivalent positions (currently 85% of practitioners) versus the growing part-time employment in pharmacy practice, the continued expansion of existing and new pharmacy school degree programs, and effective use of support personnel and automation.

Stephanie Y. Crawford and Ketsya M. Amboise

See also Direct-to-Consumer Advertising (DTCA); Medicare Part D Prescription Drug Benefit; Patient Safety; Pharmaceutical Industry; Pharmacoeconomics; Prescription and Generic Drug Use; U.S. Food and Drug Administration (FDA)

Further Readings

Chisolm, Stephanie. *The Health Professions: Trends and Opportunities in U.S. Health Care.* Sudbury, MA: Jones and Bartlett, 2007.

Kelly, William N. *Pharmacy: What It Is and How It Works.* 2d ed. Boca Raton, FL: CRC Press, 2007.

Knapp, Katherine K., and James M. Cultice. "New Pharmacist Supply Projections: Lower Separation Rates and Increased Graduates Boost Supply Estimates," *Journal of the American Pharmacists Association* 47(4): 463–70, July–August 2007.

Manasse, Henri R., and Marilyn K. Speedie. "Pharmacists, Pharmaceuticals, and Policy Issues Shaping the Work Force in Pharmacy," *American Journal of Pharmaceutical Education* 71(5): 82–3, October 15, 2007.

McCarthy, Robert L., and Kenneth W. Schafermeyer, eds. *Introduction to Health Care Delivery: A Primer for Pharmacists.* 4th ed. Sudbury, MA: Jones and Bartlett, 2007.

Poirier, Therese. "A New Vision for Pharmacy Education: It Is Time to Shift the Old Paradigm and

Move Forward," *American Journal of Pharmaceutical Education* 71(5): 103–104, October 15, 2007.

Smith, Michael I., Albert I. Wertheimer, and Jack E. Fincham, eds. *Pharmacy and the U.S. Health Care System*. 3d ed. New York: Pharmaceutical Products Press, 2005.

Web Sites

Accreditation Council for Pharmacy Education (ACPE):
  http://www.acpe-accredit.org

American Association of Pharmacy Technicians (AAPT):
  http://www.pharmacytechnician.com

American Pharmacists Association (APhA):
  http://www.pharmacist.com

American Society of Health-System Pharmacists (ASHP):
  http://www.ashp.org

National Association of Boards of Pharmacy (NABP):
  http://www.nabp.net

National Association of Chain Drug Stores (NACDS):
  http://www.nacds.org

National Community Pharmacists Association (NCPA):
  http://www.ncpanet.org

Pharmaceutical Care Management Association (PCMA):
  http://www.pcmanet.org

Pharmacy Technician Certification Board (PTCB):
  http://www.ptcb.org

PHYSICIAN ASSISTANTS

Physician assistants play an important role in America's healthcare system, working in areas often not directly served by physicians. In 2008, there were about 68,000 physician assistants delivering healthcare in the nation. Physician assistants are trained to diagnose health conditions and administer therapy under the direction of a supervising physician. They are an integral part of healthcare teams. They often take patients' medical histories, examine and treat patients within their respective range of knowledge, and order and interpret laboratory tests and X rays, as well as make specific diagnoses. They may perform simple medical procedures such as stitching cuts and splinting and casting broken limbs. Physician assistants are allowed to prescribe medications in 48 states and the District of Columbia; they may also be responsible for managerial duties, such as ordering supplies and equipment and supervising others.

Background

During the 1960s, the United States had a shortage of physicians. During the Vietnam War, many medical corpsmen returned from their tour of duty looking for suitable employment in which to apply the skills they learned while in military service. The physician assistant vocation was viewed as a measure to aid the delivery of primary care, while extending the practice of physicians.

The first program in the nation to train physician assistants was established at Duke University in 1967. The program's goal was to make healthcare available to all people, especially those living in underserved areas. Federal grants allowed the expansion of physician assistant programs, and between 1970 and 1980 the number of programs grew from 12 to 56.

Education Programs

Today, about 12,000 students are enrolled in 141 accredited physician assistant educational programs in the nation. Most programs (121) offer students the opportunity of earning a master's degree. The other programs allow students to earn either a bachelor's degree or an associate degree. Each program has its own admission requirements, but all require at least 4 years of college and some healthcare experience prior to admission.

Like medical students, physician assistant students take a variety of science courses, such as biology, chemistry, and mathematics. They also take courses in various subspecialties, including pharmacology, human growth and development, and human physiology. The students receive their clinical training in various medical specialties, such as obstetrics-gynecology, general surgery, and otolaryngology. Depending on the program, some students have the option of serving on more than one clinical rotation.

Physician assistants are not bound to one specialty. That is, if a physician assistant wants additional education to gain new skills, he or she has the option of doing so. For example, it is common for physician assistants to receive additional instruction in specialties such as pediatrics or emergency medicine. To meet common healthcare challenges found in underserved areas, many physician assistants enroll in postgraduate educational programs that emphasize disciplines critical to rural and/or inner-city communities.

Licensure

To gain licensure, each state requires a physician assistant to complete an accredited, recognized curriculum of study as well as pass a qualifying examination. Physician assistant programs typically last 2 years and require full-time attendance. Some courses in the curricula are given in university health clinics, medical schools, and traditional colleges and universities, while others are given at community colleges, in military establishments, or in hospitals.

Each state and the District of Columbia have laws specifying the requirements and qualifications needed to become a physician assistant. All require physician assistants to successfully pass the Physician Assistant National Certifying Examination (PANCE), which is given by the National Commission on Certification of Physician Assistants (NCCPA). The examination is available only to graduates of accredited physician assistant education programs. To retain certification, physician assistants need to take 100 hours of continuing medical education every 24 months. Every 72 months, they must take a recertification examination.

Scope of Work

All professional medical services provided by physician assistants are under the guidance of a physician. However, in many rural areas where there are few physicians, the physician assistants are often the primary medical-care providers. In scenarios such as this, the physician assistants discuss each case with the overseeing physician, as mandated by statutory law. Unlike many physicians, physician assistants visit patients in their home, travel to various hospitals and nursing homes to see how patients are progressing, and then report everything back to the physician.

Like physicians, physician assistants often specialize in areas such as general practice, cardiology, and psychiatry. Other specialty areas include neurology, internal medicine, and surgery. Physician assistants with specialties in surgery provide both preoperative and postoperative treatment and are often the physician's primary assistants if major surgery is required. The physician assistant's work setting depends on his or her supervising physician. For example, some work mainly in an office, whereas others assist with surgeries. Physician assistants working in hospitals usually have a variety of schedules and are often on call. On the other hand, physician assistants employed in physicians' clinics usually work 40 hours per week.

Future Implications

The demand for physician assistants is expected to continue to grow in the future much faster than the average job growth for all occupations in the nation. The U.S. Bureau of Labor Statistics projects rapid job growth for physician assistants because of the general expansion of healthcare and an emphasis on cost containment, which will result in the increasing use of physician assistants by healthcare organizations. Job opportunities will likely be in rural and inner-city clinics because these settings have difficulty attracting physicians.

Cary Stacy Smith and Li-Ching Hung

See also Access to Healthcare; Nurse Practitioners (NPs); Nurses; Physicians; Physician Workforce Issues; Primary Care; Public Health

Further Readings

Ballweg, Ruth, Sherry Stolber, and Edward M. Sullivan, eds. *Physician Assistant: A Guide to Clinical Practice.* 4th ed. Philadelphia: Saunders-Elsevier, 2008.

Cassidy, Barry A., and J. Dennis Blessing, eds. *Ethics and Professionalism: A Guide for the Physician Assistant.* Philadelphia: F. A. Davis, 2008.

Hooker, Roderick S., and James F. Cawley. *Physician Assistants in American Medicine.* 2d ed. St. Louis, MO: Churchill Livingstone, 2003.

Keir, Lucille, Barbara A. Wise, and Connie Krebs. *Medical Assisting: Administrative and Clinical Competencies.* 6th ed. Clifton Park, NY: Thomson Delmar Learning, 2008.

Web Sites

American Academy of Physician Assistants (AAPA)
    http://www.aapa.org
Bureau of Health Professions (BHPr): http://bhpr.hrsa.gov
Bureau of Labor Statistics (BLS): http://www.bls.gov
Duke University, Physician Assistant History Center
    (PAHx): http://www.pahx.org

PHYSICIANS

Physicians are medical practitioners who focus on improving human health through the study, diagnosis, and treatment of disease and injury. Physicians are able to apply their knowledge and the science of medicine after much training and specialized studies. Physicians play a vital role in the nation's healthcare system, and they may work directly with patients in a clinical setting or conduct medical research. Although physicians make up less than 10% of the nation's total medical workforce, they command enormous resources, and the entire healthcare industry is usually subordinate to their professional authority in clinical matters and research.

Overview

Modern medicine in the United States dates back to the latter half of the 18th century when the first medical school was founded at the University of Pennsylvania. Quickly thereafter, there was a push to standardize the practice of medicine. In 1847, the American Medical Association (AMA) was established; with this came the initiation of licensing laws and accreditation standards for medical schools. The strength of the AMA was illustrated with the publication of the landmark report *Medical Education in the United States and Canada,* more commonly known as the Flexner Report, in 1910, which subsequently led to the closure of a number of medical schools that did not meet the AMA's criteria. Another consequence of the Flexner Report was the curtailment of the supply of physicians. Standardization of medicine continued in many ways, including the establishment of the National Board of Medical Examiners (NBME) in 1915, whose function was to administer a standardized licensing examination to physicians, the United States Medical Licensing Examination (USMLE).

Entrance Into Medical School

Motivations to enter the field of medicine, while unique to the individual who pursues this path, generally include factors such as the desire to help others in a healing capacity, service in the context of science, technology, and research, and preference for an autonomous profession. Medical school admission requirements include successful completion of the Medical College Admissions Test (MCAT), a standardized test comprising three sections of physical sciences, biological sciences, and verbal reasoning, scored from 1 to 15 points, as well as two writing samples. An application is typically submitted through the American Medical College Application Service (AMCAS), which processes applications for the majority of allopathic medical schools, or through the American Association of Osteopathic Medicine (AACOM) for osteopathic medical schools.

This highly selective and competitive process draws serious and motivated students. Applicant data are collected annually and shows that most accepted applicants earned an average of 10 to 15 points on each section of the MCAT. Moreover, they have an undergraduate cumulative grade point average in science of 3.75 on a 4.0 scale. Recently, there have been an increasing number of female applicants to medical schools, and approximately 60% of students are female. Most applicants are White. Blacks, Native Americans, Mexican Americans, and mainland Puerto Ricans comprise about 12% of all medical students, while these groups together comprise about 20% of the nation's overall population.

On graduating from medical school, physicians enter medical residency programs to continue their training. These programs run from 3 to 8 years in length, and, generally, osteopathic physicians must complete a 12-month rotation prior to entry. After residency, physicians obtain a state license to practice medicine. Licensing laws are set by state boards of medicine that require graduation from an accredited medical school and passing the three steps of the USMLE to obtain a license. Furthermore, these boards set certain standards for physicians, such as qualifications for a license and standards of practice, and they have authority over disciplinary action.

Allopathic and Osteopathic Physicians and International Medical Graduates

All physicians, including allopathic physicians (MDs) and osteopathic physicians (DOs) have the role of evaluating, diagnosing, and treating patients. However, these medical providers accomplish their goals in distinct roles, as most MDs are specialists whereas most DOs are primarily general practitioners.

Allopathic medicine is generally regarded as the traditional (Western) practice of medicine and its study leads to the doctor of medicine degree (MD) in any of the 126 accredited schools of medicine in the nation. These schools are accredited by the AAMC and graduate about 14,500 students per year.

Osteopathic medicine, however, has a history distinct from the allopathic school of thought. In 1892, Andrew T. Still, the father of osteopathic medicine, founded the American School of Osteopathy, which has since changed it name to the Kirksville College of Osteopathic Medicine, in Kirksville, Missouri. The school was founded on the core beliefs of osteopathy that stress holistic medicine, manipulative therapies, and the importance of the neuromusculoskeletal system. These beliefs still prevail today and are taught in conjunction with academic courses similar to those offered in allopathic schools of medicine. At the completion of their four-year education in one of the 19 U.S. osteopathic schools of medicine, osteopathic students earn a DO (or doctor of osteopathy or doctor of osteopathic medicine) degree, and they can then enter into either osteopathic or allopathic residency programs. About 2,500 students graduate from osteopathic schools of medicine annually, and about two thirds of DOs go through allopathic medical residencies. Ultimately, most DOs are in general practice, and they account for about 6% of all active physicians in the nation.

International Medical Graduates (IMGs) comprise about 25% of all residency positions and account for about a quarter of all active physicians in the nation. These individuals have graduated from medical schools in countries outside the United States, including Puerto Rico and Canada. The Educational Commission for Foreign Medical Graduates (ECFMG) must certify IMGs prior to their entrance into U.S. graduate medical education programs. To receive certification, IMGs must pass both the Test of English as a Foreign Language (TOEFL) and the USMLE. In addition, as of 1988, IMGs must also pass the Clinical Skills Assessment (CSA) examination. Many influential organizations, including the AMA, the national Institute of Medicine (IOM), and the Pew Health Professions Commission have called for a reduction in the number of IMGs in residency programs citing the fact that they are not helping the problem of the maldistribution of physicians in the nation. Despite the fact that most IMGs train in underserved areas, most practice in nonunderserved areas.

Need for Physicians

The federal government plays an important but indirect role in the number of physicians in the United States by funding both medical school education and medical residency programs. Moreover, the government also influences the number of physicians practicing in specialties or primary care by regulating the amount of funds for training in these areas. Importantly, some believe that access to healthcare itself can be managed by exercising control over the supply of physicians.

Supply of Physicians

In the early 1960s, the ratio of physicians to the population was 140 physicians per 100,000 people in the nation. Many felt this ratio was too low and that there was a national physician shortage. To overcome the shortage, the U.S. Congress enacted the Higher Education Facilities Act (PL 88–204) in 1963, and efforts were made to both increase the enrollment of students in existing medical schools and create new schools across the nation. Eventually, 40 new medical schools were created, and many more physicians graduated from medical school. By 1980, the ratio of physicians to the population rose to 202 physicians per 100,000 people. The federal Civil Rights Act of 1964 (PL 88–352) also increased the national supply of physicians, particularly of Blacks and women. In fact, between 1965 and 1999, the number of women graduates from the nation's medical schools increased from 7% to 43%. Similarly, there was an increase in the total number of women physicians in active practice from 7% in 1970 to 21% in 1999.

The Graduate Medical Education National Advisory Committee (GMENAC), which consisted of a panel of prominent experts, was established in 1976 to assess the success of the effort to overcome the national physician shortage problem. Commissioned by the U.S. Department of Health and Human Services (HHS), GMENAC was given the task of determining the following: (a) the number of physicians required to meet the healthcare needs of the nation, (b) the most appropriate specialty distribution of these physicians, (c) the most favorable geographic distribution of physicians, (d) appropriate ways to finance the graduate medical education of physicians, and (e) the strategies that can achieve the recommendations formulated by the committee. GMENAC published its findings in 1980 and concluded that there was no longer a national shortage of physicians. Rather, it predicted, there would be an excess number of physicians by the 1990s. Also, the committee noted concerns related to geographic and primary-care shortages, specifically in the areas of general medicine and child psychiatry, and failure to meet its suggested ratio of between 145 and 185 physicians per 100,000 people. The trend of training more physicians continued, with the number of physicians in the nation increasing by 173% between 1950 and 1990. Consequently, the Pew Commission published data in the mid-1990s predicting that there would be a surplus of physicians and called for the closing of 20% of medical schools and for a 25% reduction in the number of medical residency positions. Along with the increasing number of physicians there were also rising costs associated with their training. To curtail this, the federal Balanced Budget Act of 1997 capped the total number of medical residents funded by the Medicare program and also reduced payments to residency programs.

Demand for Physicians

The demand for physicians is a function of access to healthcare. The total number of physicians and the physician to population ratio do not present an entirely accurate picture of access to care, as there are significant problems with the maldistribution of providers. In particular, physicians are not evenly distributed across geography or by specialty, which has resulted in shortages in rural areas and in primary care. The geographic maldistribution of physicians generally means that some areas lack adequate numbers of physicians whereas others have a sufficient number or even an oversupply. There are severe shortages of healthcare services in many rural areas, particularly in areas with populations of less than 5,000 individuals. People who reside in these areas must rely on only 5 physicians per 10,000 residents. Approximately 20% of the nation's population lives in these areas, which only have about 9% of the nation's physicians. Furthermore, although cities generally report an adequate number of practicing physicians, in many instances, they are not distributed equally within the cities. As a result, there are local communities that need more physicians. In fact, some urban areas have physician to population ratios as low as 10 physicians per 100,000 people.

Some steps have been taken to compensate for these shortages of physicians. In 1970, the federal National Health Service Corps (NHSC) was established with the mission of recruiting and retaining physicians and other health professionals in shortage areas. To entice people to join the NHSC, scholarships and loan repayments are offered, providing that the minimum 2 years of service are completed. This program has placed more than 20,000 health professionals since its inception. Additionally, guidelines were developed for the designation of Medically Underserved Areas (MUAs) in 1973. MUA status was determined by using a four part Index of Medical Underservice that looked at the percentage of the population below the federal poverty level, the percentage of the population 65 years of age or older, the infant mortality rate, and the physician to population ratio. In 1976, similar guidelines were set for the designation of Health Manpower Shortage Areas (HMSAs) under the Health Professionals Education Assistance Act. These guidelines outlined three different types of primary-care HMSAs: (1) geographic areas, (2) population groups, and (3) medical facilities. Another effort to combat the geographic shortage of physicians was the development of Community and Migrant Health Centers

(C/MHCs), which have been important in providing services to patients in rural areas. For example, in 2000, about 53% of all C/MHCs were located in rural areas and served more than 9 million people. The enactment of the federal Rural Health Clinics Act in 1977 instituted a successful reimbursement strategy to help deal with the lack of physicians in rural areas. This legislation allowed physician assistants, nurse practitioners, and certified nurse midwives associated with rural clinics to practice without the supervision of a physician. Also, this act gave rural health clinics eligibility for reimbursement from Medicaid at a higher rate, matching that provided by Medicare.

Medical schools have also taken steps toward overcoming the physician shortages in rural areas. Schools such as Philadelphia's Thomas Jefferson School of Medicine and the University of Illinois College of Medicine have implemented programs to deal with geographic shortages. A 2001 study of the Physician Shortage Area Program of the Thomas Jefferson School of Medicine found that it was successful in contributing to the supply of physicians practicing in rural and underserved areas. The study noted that the program's selection criteria, which almost exclusively favor admission for students from rural areas, coupled with its emphasis on primary care during training were the key reasons for its success.

The imbalance between specialists and primary-care physicians is another obstacle limiting access to healthcare. Reasons for specialty maldistribution include medical technology, reimbursement methods, and specialty-oriented medical education. Medical technology is expanding at a rapid pace, and it may appeal to medical students who are further attracted into specialties because their training is organized around it. Moreover, reimbursement and remuneration of specialists is higher compared to primary-care physicians, which may deflect interest in pursing a career in primary care. These factors have been linked to fluctuations in the number of medical students who match residencies in internal medicine, pediatrics, and family care. These fields were most popular in 1998 and had a match rate of 53%, but interest has dropped, and in 2002 only 44% of students matched in these areas of practice. Specifically, rates between 1998 and 2002 decreased from 24% to 22% in internal medicine, 16% to 10% in family medicine, and 13% to 12% in pediatrics. However, it is difficult to predict the numbers of medical residents who will actually practice in primary care, since many of them enter fellowship programs and subspecialize. This dichotomy has grown larger over time, such that two thirds of physicians are specialists.

Impact of Managed Care

Managed care has greatly influenced the practice of medicine. Managed-care organizations such as health maintenance organizations (HMOs) and preferred provider organizations (PPOs) were the preferred choice of employers and the government in the 1980s as a means to contain the costs of healthcare. Managed-care organizations either contract with physicians or directly employ them. They use three principal types of payments: (1) payments to preferred providers with discounted fee schedules, (2) capitation payments, and (3) salaries. The consequence is that these organizations exercise control over physicians by way of constraints on payments, and they tend to use a capitation or discounted rate payment scheme. This approach results in disincentives for physicians to refer patients to specialists and to limit inpatient hospital stays. The use of primary-care physicians as gatekeepers to specialty care has also jeopardized patient care by imposing barriers to specialty care. On the other hand, the managed-care organizations offer incentives to physicians depending on their productivity. Despite this, the objective of cost containment has not been realized since the wide-scale implementation of managed care. And healthcare costs continue to rise.

Future Implications

In 2009, there will be about 890,000 active physicians in the United States, or approximately 295 per 100,000 people. Future projections, however, indicate that there will be a growing national shortage of physicians. According to several reports, although the total number of physicians will increase, the demand for their services will outpace supply. Factors such as the accelerating rate of retirements of older physicians, the aging of the nation's population, with associated chronic medical conditions, and restrictions on the number of hours medical residents work will contribute to the physician shortages. To prevent the shortage, there is a push to increase the enrollment of students in medical schools across the nation. While this is a feasible solution, its effects will not be realized in the short term, because it takes 12 to 15 years to train a physician. Also, financial factors complicate this issue and influence the number of students who apply to medical school. It is problematic that the costs of education have consistently risen against a background of decreasing physician reimbursement. With an average of about $200,000 in educational costs incurred postgraduation, coupled with less return on the investment today as compared with the past, interest in medicine has declined and so have the number of applicants to medical schools. A more immediate solution to the shortage of physicians may be achieved by having a greater number of IMGs enter residency programs. Another possibility is the greater use of nonphysician practitioners (NPPs), who represent a large portion of healthcare providers. Specifically, nurse practitioners (NPs) and physician assistants (PAs) are popular medical careers that can be helpful in combating the need for care in underserved areas at a lower cost, typically 40% less than the cost of a physician. NPs, who complete registered nursing degrees in addition to extended study, are able to write prescriptions in most states. PAs practice under the supervision of a physician and also tend to practice in primary-care fields. Pooling resources from multiple areas, including more domestic medical graduates and IMGs, along with the greater use of NPPs, will help to equilibrate the imbalance between physician supply and demand and also promises to help with the problem of geographic and specialty maldistribution.

Kristen Friscia

See also American Medical Association (AMA); American Osteopathic Association (AOA); General Practice; Managed Care; Medical Group Practice; Physicians, Osteopathic; Physician Workforce Issues; Primary Care Physicians

Further Readings

American Medical Association. *Physician Characteristics and Distribution in the U.S.* Chicago: American Medical Association, 2008.

Blumenthal, David. "New Steam From an Old Cauldron: Physician-Supply Debate," *New England Journal of Medicine* 350(17): 1780–87, April 22, 2004.

Bujak, Joseph S. *Inside the Physician Mind: Finding Common Ground with Doctors.* Chicago: Health Administration Press, 2008.

Cooper, Richard A., "Weighing the Evidence for Expanding Physician Supply," *Annals of Internal Medicine* 141(9): 705–714, November 2, 2004.

Ginzberg, Eli, and Panos Minogiannis. *U.S. Health Care and the Future Supply of Physicians.* New Brunswick, NJ: Transaction Publishers, 2004.

Mitka, Mike. "Looming Shortage of Physicians Raises Concern about Access to Care," *Journal of the American Medical Association* 297(10): 1045–1046, March 14, 2007.

More, Ellen S., Elizabeth Fee, and Manon Parry, eds. *Women Physicians and the Culture of Medicine.* Baltimore: Johns Hopkins University Press, 2008.

Rabinowitz, Howard K., James J. Diamond, Fred W. Markham, et al. "Critical Factors for Designing Programs to Increase the Supply and Retention of Rural Primary Care Physicians," *Journal of the American Medical Association* 286(9): 1041–1048, September 5, 2001.

Whelan, Gerald P., Nancy E. Gary, John Kostis, et al., "The Changing Pool of International Medical Graduates Seeking Certification Training in U.S. Graduate Medical Education Programs, " *Journal of the American Medical Association* 288(9): 1079–1084, September 4, 2007.

Web Sites

American Association of Colleges of Osteopathic Medicine (AACOM): http://www.aacom.org
American Medical Association (AMA): http://www.ama-assn.org
Association of American Medical Colleges (AAMC): http://www.aamc.org
Bureau of Health Professions (BHPr): http://bhpr.hrsa.gov

PHYSICIANS, OSTEOPATHIC

There are currently about 61,000 osteopathic physicians in the United States; they constitute about 7% of the nation's practicing physician workforce. But osteopathic physicians are responsible for

16% of patient visits in small communities with populations of fewer than 2,500 individuals. In addition, 22% of all osteopathic physicians practice in rural and medically underserved areas.

The osteopathic medical philosophy emphasizes preventive care and focuses on the unity of all body parts. Instead of just treating specific symptoms or illnesses, osteopathic physicians regard the body as an integrated whole, and they help patients develop attitudes and lifestyles that help prevent illness. Like allopathic physicians, osteopathic physicians are fully licensed to prescribe medications and practice in all medical specialty areas, including surgery.

Osteopathic physicians also receive extra medical training in the musculoskeletal system, the body's interconnected system of nerves, muscles, and bones that make up two thirds of its body mass. This training provides osteopathic physicians with a better understanding of the ways that an injury or illness in one part of the body can affect another.

Furthermore, osteopathic physicians incorporate osteopathic manipulative treatment into their medical care. With this treatment, osteopathic physicians use their hands to diagnose injury and illness and to encourage the body's natural tendency toward good health.

Background

Andrew Taylor Still (1828–1917) was the father of osteopathic medicine as well as the founder of the first college of osteopathic medicine. Born in a log cabin in Jonesville, Virginia, Still decided at an early age to follow in his father's footsteps and become a physician. As an apprentice physician to his father, he learned both from being at his father's side as well as from the course of study. Still later served in the Civil War as a surgeon in the Union Army.

It was not until the early 1870s that Still separated himself from his allopathic counterparts by his pervasive criticism of the misuse of drugs common in that day. Believing that medicine should offer the patient more, he supported a philosophy of medicine different from the practice of his day, and in its place he advocated the use of osteopathic manipulative treatment.

Still identified the musculoskeletal system as a key element of health and recognized the body's ability to heal itself. He stressed preventive care, eating properly, and keeping fit. In 1892, Still founded the American School of Osteopathy, now known as the Kirksville College of Osteopathic Medicine of the A. T. Still University of Health Sciences, in Kirksville, Missouri.

Osteopathic Medical Education

Currently, there are 26 osteopathic medical schools in the United States. Students in these programs take courses in anatomy, physiology, microbiology, histology, osteopathic principles and practices, including osteopathic manipulative medicine, pharmacology, clinical skills, physician–patient communications, and systems courses that focus on each major system of the body, such as the cardiac and respiratory systems.

Many osteopathic medical schools have students assigned to work with physicians beginning early in their 1st year of study. This process continues throughout the 2nd year in conjunction with the necessary science courses. In the 3rd and 4th years, osteopathic medical students spend time learning about and exploring the major specialties in medicine through clinical rotations.

One unique aspect of the osteopathic medical student's education is how these rotations are conducted in community hospitals and physicians' offices across the nation. Because few osteopathic medical colleges have their own hospitals, the schools partner with community hospitals to deliver the final years of curriculum as well as internship and residency training. This model of medical education developed by the osteopathic medical profession has been touted as the new model for all medical education. Current pilot studies are being developed on a national level to evaluate this model of medical education.

Medical Licensure

Licensing boards in each state provide osteopathic physicians with licensure to practice medicine. Requirements vary by state, but there are generally three ways an osteopathic physician can become licensed. First, osteopathic physicians must successfully complete a medical licensing examination administered by the state licensing board. State boards may prepare their own examination or administer an examination that has been prepared and purchased from a specialized agency. Today, the United States Medical Licensing Examination (USMLE) and the Comprehensive Osteopathic Medical Licensing Examination (COMLEX-USA) are the most widely used tests. The osteopathic physician can also accept the certificate issued by the National Board of Osteopathic Medical Examiners (NBOME), awarded after an applicant has satisfied the requirements, including the successful passage of a rigorous series of tests. Finally, licensure can be granted through reciprocity or endorsement of a license previously received from another state. This typically has to be issued on the basis of a written examination.

Future Implications

Osteopathic physicians are one of the fastest growing segments of healthcare professionals in the nation. By the year 2020, an estimated 100,000 osteopathic physicians will be in active medical practice. Approximately 60% of all practicing osteopathic physicians specialize in the primary-care areas of family practice, internal medicine, obstetrics and gynecology, and pediatrics. Many of these physicians will continue to fill a critical need by practicing in rural and medically underserved areas of the nation.

American Osteopathic Association

See also Access to Healthcare; American Osteopathic Association (AOA); Health Professional Shortage Areas (HPSAs); Health Workforce; Physician Workforce Issues; Physicians; Preventive Care; Primary Care

Further Readings

Gevitz, Norman. *The DOs: Osteopathic Medicine in America.* 2d ed. Baltimore: Johns Hopkins University Press, 2004.
Still, Andrew T. *Autobiography of Andrew T. Still: With a History of the Discovery and Development of the Science of Osteopathy.* Whitefish, MT: Kessinger, 2007.
Still, Andrew T. *Philosophy of Osteopathy.* New York: Ams Press, 2008.
Stone, Caroline. *Science in the Art of Osteopathy: Osteopathic Principles and Models.* Cheltenham, UK: Nelson Thornes, 2000.

Web Sites

American Association of Colleges of Osteopathic Medicine (AACOM): http://www.aacom.org
American Osteopathic Association (AOA): http://www.osteopathic.org
Bureau of Health Professions (BHPr): http://bhpr.hrsa.gov
Bureau of Labor Statistics (BLS): http://www.bls.gov

PHYSICIAN WORKFORCE ISSUES

The rate of change throughout the healthcare industry has had profound effects on the composition of the physician workforce. Yet while many health services researchers study issues involving the physician, including healthcare insurance and managed care, quality of care and outcomes, and malpractice and tort reform, direct evidence of changes in the physician workforce is relatively scant. Researchers, however, are able to use information from the studies that do exist to help develop efficient and effective healthcare management and policy.

Nature and Function of the Physician Workforce

More than 15 centuries ago, the Greek physician Hippocrates advocated that all physicians pay attention to the individual patient. In this rebellion against the Cnidian convention that favored diagnosis and classification of diseases, Hippocrates modernized the practice of medicine. While the physician has historically trained as an apprentice and basic responsibilities have remained the same over time, the physician is no longer simply someone who is a skilled healer. Today's physician is a healer who is formally trained—and legally qualified—to practice medicine. More stringent standards have existed only since the early 20th century, when Abraham Flexner's report on the status of medical education in North America largely resulted in the advent of scientifically based university medical schools and teaching hospitals similar to those that had been established in Europe.

The physician workforce is presently composed of individuals educated and trained in primary care and various specialties. A primary-care physician is a Medical Doctor (MD) or Doctor of Osteopathic Medicine (DO) who, as a generalist, serves as the patient's first entry point into the healthcare system; a specialist physician is one who is qualified to diagnose and care for specific ailments or injuries. Physicians also may choose to practice in surgical specialties, which include the branches of medicine that treat injury or disease by operative procedures, or medical specialties, which include the branches of medicine that deal with nonsurgical techniques.

Various specialty boards, recognized by the American Board of Medical Specialties (ABMS) and the American Medical Association (AMA), individually certify physicians as specialists based on specific requirements, such as training, examination, and continuing education. Recognized specialties include the following: Allergy and Immunology, Anesthesiology, Colon and Rectal Surgery, Dermatology, Emergency Medicine, Family Practice, Internal Medicine, Medical Genetics, Neurological Surgery, Nuclear Medicine, Obstetrics and Gynecology, Ophthalmology, Orthopedic Surgery, Otolaryngology, Pathology, Pediatrics, Physical Medicine and Rehabilitation, Plastic Surgery, Preventive Medicine, Psychiatry and Neurology, Radiology, Surgery, Thoracic Surgery, and Urology. A majority of the specialties also acknowledge various subspecialties.

Many factors influence the choice of specialization as well as the choice to pursue a career in medicine. These factors become more defined as the individual's career, status, and function change over time. Among these factors are career opportunities; academic opportunities; practical experience during medical school; role models or mentors in the specialty; length of training required; lifestyle and work hours, especially during residency; likelihood of obtaining a residency position; concern about loans and debt; call schedules; post-training lifestyle, work hours, and financial rewards; intellectual challenges; interactions with patients; potential patient demographics; and within-specialty gender distribution. Medical students also have expressed that receiving early exposure to positive role models and opportunities in a certain specialty is likely to influence their career pursuits in that specialty.

At the same time, lifestyle issues are increasingly and conclusively central to career choice decisions of medical school students. Measuring the determinants of specialty choice and overall satisfaction among generalists and specialists in different types of workplaces and organizations also requires the consideration of various factors, including possible postponement of family plans. And as the physician workforce experiences the introduction of younger professionals and the development of new opportunities for older ones, there is an increased need to consider the availability of role models and mentors, gender demographics, assurance in expressing emotions at work, development of personal relationships, parenthood during residency, family plans, and geographic location—all of which act as important factors in choices made by physicians throughout their careers. That is, the manner in which physicians view quality of life, both at work and at home, is of increasing importance when considering issues in and of the physician workforce.

Work Conditions

Although the majority of physicians continue to work in private offices or clinics, typically assisted by a small staff of nurses and administrative personnel, the professional lives of American physicians are increasingly—and almost entirely—being defined by group practice relationships and health maintenance organizations (HMOs). The HMO model, originated by Kaiser Permanente, is vertically integrated to link financial concerns with healthcare delivery and horizontally integrated to connect healthcare services, with the intent of providing continuity of care to patients who are members. This healthcare delivery structure is also designed to reduce scheduling and administrative by using a team approach to coordinating patient care. The model does, by definition, however, decrease the amount of independence solo practitioners experience by increasingly centralizing power within the organizational hierarchy.

Such organizational structures have had a significant impact on physician working conditions. Where excessive workloads, professional- and personal-time demands, and interpersonal communication hassles have long contributed to physician dissatisfaction at work, there are strong indications that HMO and other managed-care physicians base work satisfaction on a combination of professional expectations and characteristics of the workplace as well as whether they are working for one managed-care organization or more. As with physicians in other practice types, these physicians' satisfaction is based on the extent of autonomy, administrative issues, resources, work-related relationships, and the amount of time allotted to visit with patients. In keeping with Max Weber's early-20th-century analyses of bureaucratic organizations as fundamentally impersonal and constraining of individuals' behaviors, managed-care physicians increasingly report less job satisfaction as compared with nonmanaged-care physicians. The enjoyment that they individually sense in their daily work or career, however, is contingent on whether the physicians can accept the differences between work in the context of managed care and prior to its arrival.

Adaptation to the Work Milieu

Federal and state governments have taken interest in regulating the number of medical resident work hours, in response to growing public concerns over medical errors and the national Institute of Medicine's (IOM) seminal report, *To Err Is Human*. Although there is no conclusive evidence of a significant relationship between medical errors and the number of hours worked, the reduction in medical resident work hours has affected educational, practical, and patient care experiences. There is also a focus in government institutions and public and private organizations on modernizing information technology systems used by healthcare providers in ways that align with the implementation of service-outcome and quality improvement programs.

To further understand physicians' motivation to act on issues in the work environment, there must be an account of concerns over capitation-based income, negotiability of other work incentives, and whether physicians have autonomy when arranging work schedules and the like. But physicians have also cited decreased control over medical decisions, decreased control over referral processes, the proliferation of malpractice lawsuits, ethical concerns due to managed-care arrangements, federal Health Insurance Portability and Accountability Act (HIPAA) compliance requirements, and reduced income as reasons for diminished satisfaction at work. Where these effects of managed care may be interpreted or overinterpreted by any human being as an affront to personal self-image, they may have a consequent effect on how physicians view their work environments and how they perform in them.

Time and Money

Irrespective of the type of organization or environment in which a physician practices medicine, the amount of time a physician spends at work may exceed an average of 60 hours per week, especially during medical residency. Physicians who are on call also have to contend with patients' concerns over the telephone and have to prepare to make emergency hospital visits; the emergence of e-mail as a physician–patient communication channel has also had an impact on physicians' time considerations. These considerations have emerged on top of the expansion of managed care, which has arguably had an adverse effect on the quantity and quality of time physicians can dedicate to patient care.

The requisite time commitments provide challenges in scheduling individually desired work shifts. In instances where physicians negotiate new and more flexible schedules, coworker resentment can emerge. Thus, physicians and the organizations for which they work are discovering that they have to amicably determine some form of compensation when desired schedules cannot be realized.

One potential trade-off to the amount of time spent in professional activities is the income generated by most physicians. The latest reports on physician distribution from the American Medical Association (AMA) and the U.S. Department of Labor (DOL) indicate that almost 900,000 active physicians in the United States practice professional activities in hospital-based, office-based, and academic medical settings. The number of physicians spread across these diverse practice settings, combined with an increasingly consumerist healthcare system, are a cursory signal of the market forces that facilitate physician income streams. With incomes generally holding across the six-figure range, medicine remains one of the highest paid professions in the nation.

Yet physicians report that their service commitment is disproportionate to the financial reward. Physicians are seeing more patients, or have simply had to increase the price of their services, in an effort to keep pace with rising operational costs and the rate of inflation. This development runs in line with a public perception that physicians seek a "target income" that is accomplished through their increasing the volume of services. Plus, the relative disparity in income between specialists and primary-care physicians and the variability of income across the profession, combined with the implications of managed care, government reform, and the economy in general, have conceivably led many physicians to seek alternative sources of remuneration.

Malpractice and Tort Reform

Among the healthcare issues that further affect physician income is the current condition of medical malpractice litigation in the nation. The original intent of medical malpractice litigation, which first materialized in the nation during the 19th century, was to safeguard patients against sham or hazardous medical practices and to equitably compensate patients injured by such practices. Over time, and despite the medical profession having become more regulated, the per-person cost of malpractice litigation in the United States is proportionately more than that in any other country in the world. The considerable number of plaintiffs in medical malpractice cases who have received multimillion-dollar monetary awards has led to a widespread assertion that there is a national malpractice crisis. This crisis has in turn caused a great number of professionals in the healthcare field to share the belief that malpractice litigation has surpassed reasonable levels and that some correction is overdue. The concomitant fallout has profoundly affected the medical profession.

Physicians have recently experienced enormous changes with regard to professional liability insurance. These circumstances have been attributed to a systemwide failure to adopt tort reform that includes caps on noneconomic damages. This view

has been contrarily refuted by scores of plaintiff attorneys and like-minded advocacy groups. Increases in malpractice insurance premiums have nevertheless reached a point where many physicians have considered practicing without malpractice insurance coverage, while others have difficulty obtaining insurance—in some cases despite having never faced a claim. Coverage from many insurers has now become cost-prohibitive. The existing malpractice conundrum has thrown professional practices into a state of confusion.

Physicians generally function on the basis that a majority of the litigious claims are erroneous allegations made by patients whose medical cases resulted in negative outcomes. To whatever extent this belief is true, malpractice claims seem to be in large part contingent on the physician–patient relationship and how actively engaged the patient judges the physician to be when communicating during office, clinic, or hospital visits. Although effective communication between the physician and the patient is an obvious means toward reducing liability, the sheer number, financial and reputation costs, and jury awards associated with malpractice suits brought against physicians have also significantly contributed to a shift in the way physicians practice medicine.

In an attempt to avoid litigation, some physicians are said to be practicing defensive medicine, whereby patient care decisions are predicated more on reducing the physician's liability risk than by what treatments may be considered accurately in the best interest of the patient. For example, physicians may feel compelled to order excessive tests, treatments, and services and may even avoid certain high-risk procedures and entire specializations altogether for fear of being sued for malpractice. As physicians increasingly diminish the types of procedures they are willing to perform and find their incomes being reduced by rising malpractice fees, a palpable cascade effect affects the delivery of care to patients. The decrease in income and decision-making opportunities may further help explain why physicians have been seeking out and clinging onto the vestiges of their autonomy and self-esteem.

Also striking is the finding that younger physicians are likely to seek a job as opposed to wanting to establish a practice. This trend may be due to a movement away from the less-satisfying, productivity-based compensation of private practice, which has long been a risky but lucrative system for medical professionals. Even though production-based compensation leads to increased productivity among physicians, physicians have reported being satisfied when an emphasis is placed on quality of care and dissatisfied when productivity is emphasized in their work. This finding echoes earlier conclusions that time pressure may lead to suboptimal work performance and overall satisfaction levels, which lead to potential compromises in patient care. In today's healthcare system, the amount of time a physician spends with a patient or on a given task is regulated to an extent by the size and structure of the organization in which the physician works.

Demographic Changes

A number of economic factors have clearly influenced change throughout healthcare. Yet the central management concern in healthcare lies in two significant social transformations that have occurred with a minimum of attention: The older generation of physicians assert different expectations about their work as compared with the younger generation; and the physician workforce in the United States, which before the last quarter or third of the 20th century had been male dominated, is now becoming female dominated.

Many of the age-based changes may be seen in the contrasts between baby boomers, born between 1946 and 1964, and Generation X-ers, born between 1965 and 1981. Within the medical profession, baby boomers and the first half of Generation X comprise upward of 60% of the physician workforce, while the latter half of Generation X accounts for slightly less than 20% of the total. Physicians of the baby boomer generation experienced enormous practice management changes throughout their careers. They most likely began and spent most of their careers in private practice as solo practitioners or in small groups but are now likely to be employed by or associated with a large healthcare organization. Yet they may assert a sense of confidence about their work and are often accused of caring more about their work than their lives outside work. They convey satisfaction in their jobs because they are often at a point in their careers where they are given opportunities

to voice their opinions and make high-level decisions. And practicing medicine has provided a respectable level of affluence for most of them because of less-stringent economic constraints on medicine during the early and middle years of their careers. But younger physicians have entered the field during a time when medical-practice management has been increasingly enveloped by the bureaucratic systems of managed care.

Another change is that women now account for about half of all medical school applicants; 35 years ago, they comprised less than 1/10 of the applicant pool. While this shift may well alter the physical image of the physician in the popular imagination, the increasing number of women in the workforce has already changed things. Chief among the changes has been the growth in the number of women who join the physician workforce and who also continue to involve themselves in traditional roles at home, which has been the motive behind flexible work schedules. Female physicians born between the early 1960s and as late as 1980 were among the first physicians to demand flexibility and variety in their schedules. When these requests were accommodated by administrators, male physicians of the same generation requested similar elasticity in their schedules, and then so, too, did more senior physicians.

Information about physicians' attitudes toward work and home life is becoming more focused on illuminating physician-specific healthcare-related trends and could be integrated into plans to improve individual and organizational performance abilities and functions.

Physician Supply

There are now indications that the United States will face a shortage of physicians in the coming decades. Reasons for this supply shortage include the following: (a) the overall growth of the nation's population, (b) an increased demand for physicians' services due to economic expansion, (c) an increased demand for more medical care by aging baby boomers, (d) an increase in performance of physicians' services by nonphysician clinicians who will need to be supervised, (e) an increase in malpractice insurance premiums and concomitant legal issues, (f) insurance carriers that dictate practice methods and income, (g) salaries that lag behind the rising rate of inflation, (h) the retirement of practicing physicians, (i) a decline in physician work effort, (j) the suddenly low number of applications to medical schools, and (k) geographically dependent lifestyle effects. As the composition of the physician workforce continues to change, and with it ideas about the length and meaning of work, questions abound as to how positions will be filled throughout the workplace.

Future Implications

Contemporary healthcare facility and medical school administrators must contend with challenges related to physician recruitment and retention, especially as the U.S. population consumes more healthcare as it moves through midlife and into old age. But complex social, economic, political, organizational, and individual factors have influenced the creation of new institutions throughout healthcare. To understand and capably manage the new aims, physicians and their employers, patients and their advocates, politicians, and the press will have to examine all facets of the physician at work. It is physicians who on a daily basis participate in healthcare more than any other stakeholder, which means that they are a valid point from which to assess the thoughts and behaviors of the people, organizations, and systems that have an impact on healthcare.

Lee H. Igel

See also American Medical Association (AMA); Association of American Medical Colleges (AAMC); General Practice; Malpractice; Medical Group Practice; Physicians; Primary-Care Physicians

Further Readings

American Medical Association. *Physician Characteristics and Distribution in the U.S.* Chicago: American Medical Association, 2008.

Arnold, Mark W., Anna F. Patterson, and A. S. Li Tang. "Has Implementation of the 80-Hour Work Week Made a Career in Surgery More Appealing to Medical Students?" *American Journal of Surgery* 189(2): 129–33, February 2005.

Bureau of Labor Statistics. *Occupational Outlook Handbook, 2008–09 Edition.* Washington, DC: Bureau of Labor Statistics, 2008.

Cooper, Richard A., Thomas E. Getzen, Heather J. McKee, et al. "Economic and Demographic Trends Signal an Impending Physician Shortage," *Health Affairs* 21(1): 140–54, January–February 2002.

Linzer, Mark, Thomas R. Konrad, Jeffrey Douglas, et al. "Managed Care, Time Pressure, and Physician Job Satisfaction: Results From the Physician Worklife Study," *Journal of General Internal Medicine* 15(7): 441–50, July 2000.

Murray, Alison, Jana E. Montgomery, Hong Chang, et al. "Doctor Discontent: A Comparison of Physician Satisfaction in Different Delivery System Settings, 1986 and 1997," *Journal of General Internal Medicine* 16(7): 452–59, July 2001.

Williams, Eric S., Mark Linzer, Donald E. Pathman, et al. "What Do Physicians Want in Their Ideal Job?" *Journal of Medical Practice Management* 18(4): 179–83, January–February 2003.

Web Sites

American Board of Medical Specialties (ABMS): http://www.abms.org

American Medical Association (AMA): http://www.ama-assn.org

Association of American Medical Colleges (AAMC): http://www.aamc.org

Council on Graduate Medical Education (COGME): http://www.cogme.gov

PREFERRED PROVIDER ORGANIZATIONS (PPOs)

A preferred provider organization (PPO) is a healthcare delivery system where providers contract with the PPO at various reimbursement levels in return for patient steerage into their practices and/or timely payment. PPOs differ from other healthcare delivery systems in the way they are financed as well as by providing more choice, benefit flexibility, and enrollee access to providers and medical services both in and out of network.

History

While PPOs have been in existence in some form or another for decades, the development of modern

PPOs was the result of key legislative actions at the state and national level. In the 1970s and 1980s, many states passed enabling legislation to specifically allow for the development of PPOs. In 1974, the U.S. Congress enacted the Employee Retirement Income Security Act (ERISA). A very small portion of this law gave Taft-Harley Funds and other organizations the right to self-insure their healthcare benefits. Under the new law, organizations that self-insured would not be subject to various state coverage mandates or to state premium taxes; instead, they were now free to develop employee healthcare benefit programs. Recognizing the unique opportunity, third-party administrators began providing some or all of the services required by the self-insuring companies.

As a rule, however, these third-party administrators did not develop their own delivery networks and instead looked to another fledgling group of companies—preferred provider organizations—to credential and supply networks of physicians and healthcare institutions. Insured products grew and employers and other purchasers came to see PPOs as the middle ground between health maintenance organizations (HMOs) (traditionally lower cost but more restrictive) and indemnity insurance plans (permissive but more expensive). This fueled the development of local PPO organizations in the 1970s and 1980s and—beginning in the 1990s—encouraged the expansion of a limited number of national PPOs. The growth in PPO plan enrollment at the expense of traditional indemnity insurance and point of service plans is shown in Figure 1.

Today PPOs are tremendously popular. Over the past few years, there has been a consolidation of the PPOs marketplace resulting in fewer regional PPOs and larger national plans as regional plans merge or are bought by larger national plans.

In 2007, more than 158 million individuals were enrolled in a PPO program, which represents 64% of all Americans with healthcare coverage. One reason for this strong market share is that PPOs have delivered what the public has called for: choice, flexibility, and a balance between delivery of appropriate care and cost control.

Characteristics and Types of PPOs

There are two basic types of PPOs: a nonrisk PPO and a risk PPO. A nonrisk PPO's primary focus is to contract with providers in a geographical area to form an interconnected network of providers and services. The nonrisk PPO network leases and/or "rents" its network for a fee to insurance companies, self-insured employers, union trusts, third-party administrators, business coalitions, and associations. In contrast, a risk PPO assumes the financial risk for an enrollee's healthcare costs.

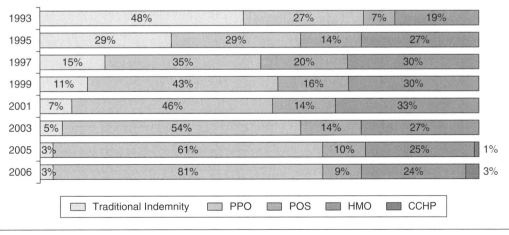

Figure I   A Comparison of Medical Plan Enrollment, 1993 to 2006

Source: Association of Preferred Provider Organizations (2007).

Traditionally, insurance companies offer a risk PPO that includes a benefit plan and network services either provided by the risk PPO or leased from a nonrisk PPO.

Insurance companies own most PPOs. They are also owned by hospitals, hospital consortiums, individual entrepreneurs, and private equity groups.

Enrollees in PPOs typically have benefit plans that provide both in-network and out-of-network coverage. Enrollees who seek care from providers within the PPO network receive in-network coverage, generally at a greater benefit level or lower coinsurance or copayment. Enrollees may still seek care outside the PPO network, but the benefit level is usually lower, and the enrollee may incur additional costs due to balance billing from the nonnetwork provider. Enrollees can choose, each time they seek care, to use an in-network or out-of-network provider. PPOs benefit enrollees by supporting their need to take a more active role in their healthcare.

PPOs also benefit providers. The financial considerations of the PPO healthcare delivery model do not override patient care decisions but rather work in conjunction with PPO providers in delivering patient care.

Claims from providers are usually handled in several ways. The PPO can give access to its fee schedule to the claims-paying entity. This is often done by providing a computerized record of the payment amount. If the PPO does not share its fee schedule with the payer, the PPO usually reprices the claims and then sends them to the payer, which pays the bill. Claims from hospitals and professional providers are sent to the PPO. The PPO adds information to each claim about the fees that should be used to process the claim. The fee information includes the PPO's negotiated and contractual rate. The claims are then sent to the paying entity (HMO, insurance company, third-party administrator) for processing. Of course, some PPOs pay claims for all providers as well.

In addition to comprehensive network PPOs, some PPOs are dedicated to specialty networks. Specialty network PPOs facilitate and support the delivery of specialized healthcare services, such as dental, vision, chiropractic, radiology, behavioral health, and other areas. Often, these types of providers have unique reimbursement and benefit issues.

Lynn Huls

See also American Association of Preferred Provider Organizations (AAPPO); Employee Retirement Income Security Act (ERISA); Healthcare Financial Management; Health Insurance; Hospitals; Managed Care; Physicians

Further Readings

Association of Preferred Provider Organizations. *PPO Outlook: 2007 Market and Industry Trend Report.* Louisville, KY: Association of Preferred Provider Organizations, 2007.
Greenrose, Karen, J. Stephen Ashley, American Association of Preferred Provider Organizations, American Accreditation HealthCare Commission/ URAC. *Rise to Prominence: The PPO Story.* Arlington, VA: American Association of Preferred Provider Organizations; Washington, DC: URAC, 2000.
Joint Commission. *Accreditation Manual for Preferred Provider Organizations.* 3d ed. Oakbrook Terrace, IL: Joint Commission, 2004.
National Committee for Quality Assurance. *Standards and Guidelines for the Accreditation of PPO Plans.* Washington, DC: National Committee for Quality Assurance, 2004.
U.S. Congressional Budget Office. *CBO's Analysis of Regional Preferred Provider Organizations Under the Medicare Modernization Act.* Washington, DC: U.S. Congressional Budget Office, 2004.

Web Sites

American Association of Preferred Provider Organizations (AAPPO): http://www.aappo.org
America's Health Insurance Plans (AHIP): http://www.ahip.org
Joint Commission: http://www.jointcommission.org
National Committee on Quality Assurance (NCQA): http://www.ncqa.org

PRESCRIPTION AND GENERIC DRUG USE

The pharmaceutical industry in the United States represents a multibillion dollar a year enterprise that has helped fuel increasing healthcare costs. In 2006, America's spending alone on drugs increased to over $250 billion, accounting for more than

41% of worldwide expenditures. New foreign markets, primarily in Asia, have seen more drastic annual expenditure increases than the United States, however. Reasons cited for the increase in drug expenditures include the introduction of new, more expensive drugs to the marketplace, a population that is aging and requiring more pharmaceuticals for disease management, increasing prices on the manufacture of existing drugs, and the use of drugs as a substitute for other forms of healthcare services.

Historically, the pharmaceutical industry has grown with the development of new drugs, new drug therapies, and the expansion of medical knowledge and practice. This expansion has required an increased focus on new drug efficacy and safety. Tighter government scrutiny and control have been realized through the Prescription Drug Marketing Act of 1987 and the U.S. Federal Drug Administration (FDA) approval process. Many, especially within the pharmaceutical industry, view the FDA's approval process as prohibitive; others view it as necessary to ensure public safety. The length of the approval process delays a drug's entry into the marketplace and quite possibly drives the developmental costs upward. It is estimated that the total development costs for a new drug in the United States, including losses to nonapproval of previous drugs, is around $1 billion each year. The accepted estimate is around $860 million per new medication developed, although some recent estimates put development costs at somewhere between $500 million and $2 billion per new drug. Companies try to recoup these costs as quickly as possible, which leads to higher prices when the drugs arrive on the marketplace for use by the public.

Although pharmaceutical companies typically receive a 20-year patent on the new drugs they develop, the FDA approval process may take as long as 12 years in and of itself. This lengthy period considerably reduces the effective income-producing potential of any new drug produced. Because of the shortened brand name shelf life for a drug, the companies must make profits within a relatively short amount of time. When the patent expires, other companies may produce the drug in its generic form. Generic drugs represent a cheaper alternative to the branded versions of the drug when released by the companies.

This entry presents an overview of the 12-step FDA approval process and discusses orphan and generic drugs. Then, this entry discusses the factors associated with those who use prescription drugs. Next, the prescription drugs' cost dilemma is addressed; and last, future implications are considered.

The FDA Approval Process

Once a pharmaceutical company has developed a new drug, the company must apply to the FDA for approval to market and sell the drug. The FDA process involves 12 steps, beginning with animal testing. This is designed to increase the size of clinical studies until the drug has been proven to have the desired effect while being safe.

Animal testing, referred to as preclinical testing, involves establishing the efficacy of the drug before it is given to humans. Many new drugs are stopped at Stage 1 because the FDA has not deemed the drugs reasonably safe for human usage because of their side effects or their lack of desired effect on the animals tested.

If the drug shows promise and is considered safe for further testing, a protocol for human testing is developed and must be approved by a local institutional review board (IRB) and the FDA in Stage 2. The IRB is composed of scientists and researchers who must determine whether human subjects are adequately protected from possible negative outcomes. It also determines whether the study is scientifically acceptable. This stage represents the company's proposal for clinical trials, involving human subjects, of the new drug.

Once the protocol is established and approved by the IRB, the company may move on to Stage 3 of the process. Stage 3 includes what is generally referred to as Phase 1 clinical trials. Phase 1 studies involve testing the drug on a small group of human subjects. The size of the group is generally between 20 and 80 healthy volunteers. The observance and notation of negative or frequent side effects of the drug is particularly important during Phase 1. If significant side effects are not detected, Phase 2 clinical trials may begin. Occasionally, alternative uses for a drug may be uncovered at this stage. That is, it is possible that a side effect may have a significant impact on another medical condition. An example of such unintended uses of a drug is the case of AZT. AZT was originally developed as an anticancer drug in the 1960s, but its trial results were disappointing. Twenty years later, AZT was discovered to be a viable treatment for HIV/AIDS.

Phase 2 studies, Stage 4 in the FDA approval process, increase the size of the subject panels from several dozen to a few hundred participants. The focus of Phase 2 clinical trials shifts from the safety focus of Phase 1 trials to a focus on effectiveness. Safety is continually monitored, though. Rather than testing on healthy individuals, Phase 2 trials use volunteers with the condition that the drug attempts to alleviate. These studies often involve the use of cohorts comparing the effectiveness of the drug to a placebo. A cohort study represents a type of epidemiological approach to investigating the incidence and prevalence of disease across a fixed population group over time. Investigators compare outcomes between a group of individuals who have a risk factor believed to be associated with the outcome to a group without that factor. Cohort studies can be conducted prospectively or retrospectively, but the concept of control is extremely important to determining a drug's efficacy.

Should the evidence from the Phase 2 clinical trials point to the drug's safety and effectiveness, the pharmaceutical company moves its application to Stage 5 of the approval process. In Stage 5, Phase 3 clinical trials include a larger number of participants, usually up to a few thousand subjects, and they continue to scrutinize the safety and effectiveness of the drug. On successful completion of these drug trials, the process moves to Stage 6.

Stage 6 is sometimes referred to as the pre–New Drug Application, or pre-NDA, stage. At this point in the approval process, drug company representatives meet with FDA representatives to review the proposed product. If it is determined safe and effective, the pharmaceutical company moves to the next stage of the process.

Stage 7 involves the submission of the New Drug Application (NDA) to the FDA. The NDA represents a formal request from the pharmaceutical company for the FDA's approval of the drug. The FDA has 60 days to decide whether to consider approval. The agency's decision itself is considered Stage 8 of the overall process. A positive decision leads the FDA to file the application as Stage 9. It also assigns a team to evaluate the evidence collected from the three phases of the clinical trials.

In Stage 10 of the FDA approval process, the focus is on the review of the proposed labeling of the drug. The FDA ensures that the patient instructions are clear and understandable. Its review team also visits the pharmaceutical company's production facilities and evaluates its processes to ensure quality control in Stage 11.

Finally, in Stage 12 of the process, the FDA reviews all submitted evidence and documentation. The agency arrives at a final decision of "approvable" or "not approvable." Assuming that the data indicate an acceptable risk and demonstrable benefit, the drug is ready for manufacture and sale.

The length of time between drug development and sale is obviously long. For drugs that can potentially save patients with immediate and life-threatening conditions where no drug currently exists, the FDA may allow the company to engage in an accelerated approval process. This more expedient process involves using "surrogate endpoints" or alternative data to establish the drug's efficacy. In some cases, the larger Phase 3 clinical trials may be waived based on the promise of data from the smaller Phase 2 trials. Accelerated approval, however, is relatively rare. It tends to be used on drugs developed to treat diseases with very poor projected outcomes where other treatments have been shown to be ineffective. Most recently, drugs used to treat HIV/AIDS have been approved through an accelerated process because the benefits of the drug to patients are deemed to outweigh the risks when the disease is terminal.

The entire FDA drug approval process is designed to ensure the public's safety and its confidence that these drugs achieve the results that the pharmaceutical companies maintain. It is long, arduous, and expensive to the developers of new pharmaceuticals. Even then, however, it is still possible that long-term negative effects may surface at a later date, necessitating a change in the FDA's initial ruling. Therefore, even after a drug has obtained FDA approval, it is continuously monitored for safety. This postapproval safety monitoring may cost the pharmaceutical industry an additional $50 million annually.

Orphan Drugs

Although the FDA approval process is clearly intended to protect the public's interest and guarantee their safety, it can become cost-prohibitive for pharmaceutical companies to use their resources to develop drugs for conditions that affect a relatively small number of patients. Relatively rare diseases are sometimes referred to as orphan diseases. Similarly, drugs developed to treat such diseases are called orphan drugs. Orphan drugs have received special federal regulations that allow for a 7-year monopoly on the production of the drugs as well as tax reductions. The orphan drug rules are in effect for diseases that affect fewer than 200,000 people in the United States.

Generic Drugs

A generic drug is a prescription drug that is produced and sold without a brand name. Once the patent for a drug expires, companies may make generic versions for sale to the public. Generic drugs are generally less expensive than their branded counterparts, primarily because they are not advertised and because of increased competition among pharmaceutical companies. Many health insurance companies encourage their beneficiaries to use generic equivalents whenever possible because they provide significant cost savings. The Congressional Budget Office (CBO) estimates that generic drugs save consumers between $8 and $10 billion annually.

If a pharmaceutical company wishes to sell a drug as a generic, it must file an abbreviated new drug application with the FDA prior to introducing it in the marketplace. The company must demonstrate that the generic version of the drug is identical to the brand version in order to obtain FDA approval to sell the drug. Not only must the generic version be chemically identical, but the same strict manufacturing procedures previously adhered to for the brand version must also be used to make the generic version of the drug.

Some health insurance companies require the substitution of a generic equivalent to be covered. Patients who request not to receive a generic drug may have to pay the additional cost out of pocket. Not all drugs have generic counterparts, however. Presently, only around 50% of brand name drugs have generic equivalents. Patients desiring a generic equivalent may ask their physician if an equivalent exists and whether a substitution is appropriate.

Prescription Drugs Users

As previously mentioned, age is an important factor in who uses prescription drugs. The National Center for Health Statistics (NCHS) reports that nearly 85% of all Americans over the age of 65 had at least one prescription in the previous month and nearly 52% had three or more prescriptions. The percentage of those using prescription drugs increases steadily with age.

Gender also plays a significant role in prescription drug use. The data reported by NCHS indicate that a higher percentage of women use prescription drugs than do men across every age group except those under 18. Women are more likely than men to use prescription drugs across racial/ethnic groups as well.

Whites, for both men and women, are the most likely to use prescription drugs, followed by African Americans and Hispanics, respectively. Because access to prescription drugs is restricted, disparities in their use are similar to disparities in healthcare resulting from different levels of access to physician services and medical care.

Prescription Drug Cost Dilemma

The widespread use of generic drugs represents one way in which consumer costs can be reduced. Generic drugs are lower in price because they do not incur a number of the high costs associated with brand name drugs. First, there are no new research and development costs. Once a patent expires on a brand name drug, pharmaceutical companies can make generic equivalents through a reverse engineering process. Second, they do not have marketing costs. Generic equivalents tend to benefit from previously marketed brand drugs. In addition, companies tend not to provide free samples of generic drugs to physicians. Third, generic drugs do not have the costs associated with the 12-stage FDA approval process; rather, they only have to demonstrate the biochemical equivalence of the brand version. Finally, because multiple drug companies can sell generic equivalents after the patent expires, there is greater competition, which results in lower costs to the consumer.

The elderly have been especially affected by spiraling drug costs because they often live on a lower, fixed income than younger cohorts, and older adults use prescription drugs more frequently. In 2003, the federal government enacted the Medicare Prescription Drug, Improvement, and Modernization Act, which is generally referred to as Medicare Part D, to assist the elderly in accessing necessary prescription drugs in a more cost-effective manner. Medicare Part D was implemented in 2006 and allowed eligible elderly and disabled Medicare patients to select enrollment into one of a set of government-approved private prescription plans.

Different approved prescription drug plans tend to cover different drugs. An early complaint from Medicare recipients about the selection process was that it was too complicated. The enrollee is expected to make a plan choice by matching a list of the prescriptions they receive against the lists of approved drugs and their prices to arrive at the most cost-effective choice given their personal situation. After initial problems, however, the process has gone considerably more smoothly. Revenues from Medicare Part D premiums are expected to be nearly $750 million by the year 2015.

Future Implications

The use, and the expense associated with that use, of prescription drugs has spiraled upward in the past and is likely to increase even more in the future. As this happens, efforts to make drugs more accessible will escalate. In some cases, this may mean that some prescription drugs may be made available over the counter if they have demonstrated very long-term efficacy and safety. This practice allows greater exposure and availability of the drug to a wider public consumer audience. It also typically reduces the unit cost because of higher expected sales.

The percentage of the population, adjusted for age, that has received at least one prescription has increased from 38% in the early 1990s to over 45% in the early 21st century. For the elderly, the increase is even more dramatic. Pharmaceutical companies strive to bring more and better drugs to the marketplace as part of their financial strategic plans. The net effect on the consumer and the physician is a wider selection of drugs that can be used to treat a wider array of conditions.

Ralph Bell

See also Cost of Healthcare; Inflation in Healthcare; Medicare Part D; Pharmaceutical Industry; Pharmacoeconomics; Pharmacy; Randomized Controlled Trials (RCT); U.S. Food and Drug Administration (FDA)

Further Readings

Adams, Christopher P., and Van V. Brantner. "Estimating the Cost of New Drug Development: Is It Really $802 Million?" *Health Affairs* 25(2): 420–28, March–April 2006.

Gooi, Malcolm, and Chaim M. Bell. "Differences in Generic Drug Prices Between the U.S. and Canada," *Applied Health Economics and Health Policy* 6(1): 19–26, 2008.

Grabowski, Henry G., and Y. Richard Wang. "The Quantity and Quality of Worldwide New Drug Introductions, 1982–2003," *Health Affairs* 25(2): 452–60, March–April 2006.

Griffith, H. Winter, and Stephen Moore. *Complete Guide to Prescription and Nonprescription Drugs.* New York: Perigee Group, 2007.

Sloan, Frank A., and Chee-Ruey Hsieh, eds. *Pharmaceutical Innovation: Incentives, Competition, and Cost-Benefit Analysis in International Perspective.* New York: Cambridge University Press, 2007.

Stagnitti, Marie N. *Trends in Brand Name and Generic Prescribed Medicine Utilization and Expenditures, 1999 and 2003.* Statistical Brief No. 144. Rockville, MD: Agency for Healthcare Research and Quality, October 2005.

Voet, Martin A. *The Generic Challenge: Understanding Patents, FDA, and Pharmaceutical Life-Cycle Management.* 2d ed. Boca Raton, FL: Brown Walker Press, 2008.

Web Sites

AARP: http://www.aarp.org

Agency for Healthcare Research and Quality (AHRQ): http://www.ahrq.gov

Henry J. Kaiser Family Foundation (KFF): http://www.kff.org

National Center for Health Statistics (NCHS): http://www.cdc.gov/nchs

Pharmaceutical Research and Manufacturers of America (PhRMA): http://www.phrma.org

U.S. Food and Drug Administration (FDA): http://www.fda.gov

PREVENTIVE CARE

Preventive care is a set of measures taken before symptoms begin to prevent illness or injury. While the number of preventive services has expanded in recent years, particularly in the areas of cancer and ischemic heart disease, preventive care is still best exemplified by routine physical examinations and immunizations. The emphasis remains to prevent disease before it occurs. Physicians, nurses, and public health officials perform preventive services in various settings, including physicians' offices, clinics, health departments, and hospitals. Public and private health insurance plans generally pay for preventive services, and the literature and expert consensus agree that healthcare systems focused on preventive care are more cost-effective. A number of barriers to preventive care exist, and medicine, public health, and policymakers must work to eliminate them.

Background

While traditional preventive strategies of medicine and public health, such as routine physical examinations and immunizations, have been around for many years, the science of preventive care was first formalized with the establishment of the U.S. Preventive Services Task Force (USPSTF) in 1984. The task force, first convened by the U.S. Public Health Service (PHS) and since 1998 sponsored by the Agency for Healthcare Research and Quality (AHRQ), is the leading independent panel of private-sector experts in prevention and primary care. The task force ensures that the clinical guidelines for providing preventive care are evidence based. Specifically, the task force conducts rigorous, impartial assessments of the scientific evidence for the effectiveness of clinical preventive services, including health screening, counseling, and preventive medications. Its recommendations are considered the gold standard for clinical preventive services. The task force is made up of primary-care clinicians along with nurses. The task force evaluates the benefits of individual services based on age, gender, and risk factors for disease and offers recommendations that have formed the basis of the clinical standards for many professional societies, health organizations, and medical

quality review groups. Its work has established the importance of including prevention in primary care and prompted insurance coverage for effective preventive services.

Types of Prevention

Preventive care can be categorized into three levels: (1) primary, (2) secondary, and (3) tertiary prevention. Primary prevention services avert disease development and include population-based health promotion activities such as vaccination and safe water supplies. Secondary prevention services target early detection of asymptomatic disease with the goal of preventing the progression of disease (exemplified by the pap smear to detect precancerous cervical changes). Secondary prevention services may also include prophylaxis to reduce the chance of disease recurrence (e.g., aspirin, blood pressure control, and lipid-lowering medications for the secondary prevention of ischemic heart disease following an initial myocardial infarction, or heart attack). Tertiary prevention services reduce the impact of already established disease. Preventive care encompasses both therapeutic interventions, such as immunizations or antibody prophylaxis and diagnostic examinations that screen for early asymptomatic disease. Screening examinations often detect early disease at a point where interventions improve health outcomes.

Preventive-Care Services

The historical foundation of preventive care rests on routine medical history taking, physical examination, and healthy lifestyle counseling, but rapid advances in medical technology provide new devices and laboratory tests to screen for disease. Amid the rapid growth of preventive-care services, clinicians must decipher the evidence of each service. The USPSTF offers the most rigorous evaluation of preventive services and provides guidance for clinicians to make evidence-based decisions. The task force's *Guide to Clinical Preventive Services, 2007* provides recommendations on 58 services made from 2001 to 2006. These services are grouped into clinical categories, including cancer; heart and vascular diseases; infectious diseases; injury and violence; mental health conditions and substance abuse; metabolic, nutritional, and endocrine conditions; musculoskeletal disorders; obstetric and gynecological conditions; pediatric disorders; and vision and hearing disorders.

The task force recommends that clinicians discuss the 58 preventive services, based on their strength of evidence, with their eligible patients. The services include the following: abdominal aortic aneurysm screening (one-time screening by ultrasonography in men 65 to 75 years of age who have ever smoked); alcohol misuse and behavioral counseling interventions (for men, women, and especially pregnant women); aspirin for the primary prevention of cardiovascular events (for men and women at increased risk for coronary artery disease); asymptomatic bacteriuria screening (for pregnant women); breast cancer (mammography every 1–2 years for women 40 years of age and older and discussion of chemoprevention in high-risk populations); breast and ovarian cancer susceptibility (genetic testing and counseling); promotion of breastfeeding (structured education and behavior counseling for pregnant women); cervical cancer screening (for women over 18 who are sexually active); chlamydial infection screening (for women 25 and younger and other asymptomatic women at risk of infection); colorectal cancer screening (for men and women 50 years of age and older); dental caries prevention (oral fluoride supplementation to preschool children in areas where water sources are deficient in fluoride); depression screening (for men and women within established clinical systems); diabetes mellitus (Type 2) screening in adults (for men and women with hypertension or hyperlipidemia); diet counseling (for adult men and women with hyperlipidemia and other known risk factors for cardiovascular and diet-related chronic disease); gonorrhea screening (for all sexually active women at increased risk for infection, including pregnant women); prophylactic gonorrhea treatment (including ocular topical medications for all newborns); hepatitis B virus infection screening (for pregnant women at first prenatal visit); high blood pressure screening (for adult men and women at all visits); HIV screening (for all adolescents and adults at risk for HIV infection and all pregnant women); iron deficiency anemia prevention (including routine iron supplementation for asymptomatic children 6–12 months of age who are at risk for iron deficiency); iron deficiency anemia screening (for asymptomatic pregnant women);

lipid disorder screening (for men 35 years of age or older and women 45 years of age or older, and for younger adults with other risk factors for coronary disease); obesity screening (including intensive counseling and behavioral interventions to promote sustained weight loss for obese adults); osteoporosis screening (for women 65 years of age and older and women 60 years of age or older who are at increased risk for osteoporotic fractures); Rh(D) incompatibility screening (including blood typing and antibody testing at the first pregnancy-related visit); syphilis infection screening (for persons at risk and all pregnant women); tobacco use and tobacco-caused disease counseling (including cessation interventions for those who use tobacco); and visual impairment screening (for children younger than 5 years of age to detect amblyopia, strabismus, and defects in visual acuity).

It should be noted that the task force did not make recommendations for newborn screening, which aims to identify treatable genetic, endocrinologic, metabolic, and hematologic diseases. It also did not address immunizations.

Immunizations

Immunization is the process in which the body develops a defense against foreign agents (e.g., bacteria, viruses, and fungi). Exposure to these foreign molecules prompts the immune response to protect the body. A hallmark of the immune system is its memory. After first exposure to most agents, the human body develops immunological memory, such that later exposure to the same agent will result in quick, efficient, and successful protection from the agent. A common example is the lifetime protection conferred to most people after infection with Varicella (chickenpox). It is this feature of the immune system that provides the basis for successful vaccines, which have become a cornerstone of public health and preventive care. Under typical conditions, immunizations expose the body to nonvirulent doses of foreign agents, enabling it to develop immunological memory, which confers lifetime protection to the specific agent. Since the original work of Edward Jenner in the early 19th century, biomedical research has developed many successful vaccines, of which many are given routinely to children and are considered compulsory for attending school.

Immunizations have led to worldwide eradication of smallpox and the dramatic decline in mortality and morbidity from diseases such as polio, measles, diphtheria, whooping cough, hepatitis B, and bacterial meningitis.

The Advisory Committee on Immunization Practices (ACIP), a branch of the Centers for Disease Control and Prevention (CDC), provides evaluation of the literature and offers evidence-based recommendations for immunization schedules for adults, infants, and toddlers, preteens and adolescents, college students and young adults, parents, pregnant women, healthcare workers, people with specific diseases/conditions, racial and ethnic populations, and travelers. The ACIP is composed of 15 experts who are selected by the Secretary of the U.S. Department of Health and Human Services (HHS). This committee provides advice and guidance to the Secretary, the Assistant Secretary for Health, and the CDC on the control of vaccine-preventable diseases. The committee develops written recommendations for routine administration of vaccines with the goal of reducing the incidence of vaccine-preventable diseases in the nation and ensuring safe use of vaccines. Under this guidance, immunizations remain one of the most valuable services of preventive care.

Providers

Primary-care physicians (i.e., internal medicine, pediatrics, family medicine, and obstetrics and gynecology), nurses, physician assistants, and nurse practitioners represent the majority of the clinicians who provide preventive-care services on a daily basis. They provide these services in various settings, including physicians' offices, outpatient clinics, public health departments, and hospitals. Importantly, these professions have incorporated preventive care into their missions of providing care and ensuring health among their patients.

While primary-care physicians provide the bulk of preventive services, as recommended by the USPSTF, the profession of medicine further formalizes and emphasizes preventive care through designated training in the specialty of preventive medicine. Preventive medicine is one of 24 medical specialties recognized by the American Board of Medical Specialties (ABMS). The specialty encompasses multiple population-based and clinical approaches

to healthcare and draws on several core competencies, including biostatistics and epidemiology, management and administration, clinical preventive medicine, and occupational and environmental health. Board-certified physicians in preventive medicine can hold many positions within a variety of healthcare settings, yet a common undercurrent of their work in all venues involves an approach to health that seeks systemic and population-based interventions to improve the health of individuals.

Preventive medicine residencies are offered at more than 75 institutions in the nation and include a general medicine internship, a year of classwork to attain a master of public health (MPH) degree, and a year of practicum work, which is often tailored to an individual's career interests and aspirations. The three specialty areas within preventive medicine residencies are (1) public health/general preventive medicine, (2) occupational medicine, and (3) aerospace medicine.

Another venue for potential preventive care that has received much attention is the school—more specifically, the role of school nurses in obesity prevention. Schools present a critical setting for addressing the significant and increasing public health problem of childhood obesity. School nurses are uniquely positioned to address obesity and offer preventive services such as height, weight, and body mass index (BMI) measurements along with healthy diet and lifestyle counseling.

Reimbursement

The USPSTF's rigorous evaluation of the literature offers authority to clinicians' utilization of many preventive services. The consensus among clinicians, researchers, and public health officials regarding the value of routine preventive services, as recommended by the USPSTF and described above, has prompted their reimbursement by both public and private health insurance plans.

The nation's Medicare program, for example, offers its beneficiaries many preventive services, including screening tests for heart disease; mammograms, pap smears, and pelvic examinations; bone mass measurements; colon cancer screening; prostrate screening; diabetes testing; diabetes self-management training; foot care and supplies; flu shots; pneumonia vaccine; hepatitis B vaccine; and glaucoma screening. Despite these services, however, Medicare falls short of providing comprehensive preventive care for its beneficiaries. One deficiency is that Medicare only covers one routine preventive physical examination that must be received within 6 months of initial enrollment in the program.

All the nation's state Medicaid programs provide inclusive preventive care for eligible recipients, who are mostly children and pregnant women, groups that benefit significantly from preventive services. The Early and Periodic Screening, Diagnostic, and Treatment (EPSDT) service is Medicaid's comprehensive and preventive child health program for individuals under 21 years of age. Defined by law in 1989, the EPSDT includes periodic screening, vision, dental, and hearing services. EPSDT guarantees that physicians will provide initial and periodic evaluations of children and assures that health problems are diagnosed and treated early, preventing complications, and improving health outcomes.

Although private health insurance coverage varies with respect to the preventive services covered, most private insurance policies provide comprehensive preventive care, especially for children and pregnant women.

Cost-Effectiveness

Intuitively, it is easy to accept the notion that prevention is more cost-effective than treatment. However, with respect to medicine and public health, this notion needs to be verified with evidence. While an emerging body of literature supports specific preventive-care interventions, no studies of the overall cost-effectiveness of preventive services have been conducted.

Recent literature tends to show that the cost-effectiveness of specific preventive services depends greatly on the particular intervention and its target population. For instance, a recent systematic review of the cost-effectiveness of preventive interventions for Type 2 diabetes mellitus suggests that primary prevention of that disease is highly cost-effective. Other interventions, such as strict blood pressure control, have also been shown to be overwhelmingly cost-effective. However, other individual interventions aimed at lowering weight, average blood glucose, and cholesterol levels varied significantly in their cost-effectiveness.

Although much more research is needed, it appears that the potential impact of preventive care both economically and with respect to improved health outcomes may be highly significant. For example, it has been estimated that about 800,000 deaths in the nation (40% of the total annual mortality) in 2000 were from preventable causes, such as tobacco use, poor diet, physical inactivity, and alcohol misuse. It also has been shown that preventive measures, such as tobacco cessation programs and screening for colorectal cancer, can reduce mortality at low cost or even at cost savings. It seems logical that if preventive services were more widely used they would lower mortality and likely lower the total cost of healthcare.

Barriers

Individuals face a number of barriers to receiving preventive care. One important barrier is lack of health insurance coverage. It is clear that individuals without health insurance often delay needed healthcare and many times entirely forgo preventive care. However, even individuals with health insurance coverage face significant barriers to receiving preventive care. Many characteristics of the physician–patient interaction have been found to hinder the delivery of preventive care, including the following: the physician's attitudes toward prevention, unfamiliarity with the USPSTF's recommendations, belief that some healthcare services do not fall under the physician's scope of care; hurried office visits and lack of time to address prevention; lack of financial incentives to provide preventive care; and patients' attitude toward preventive care. Another important dynamic of the physician–patient relationship that affects preventive services is continuity of care. Several studies confirm that identifying a regular site of care is associated with increased access to preventive services, particularly for women and children. The medical literature supports the value of both site and provider continuity in preventive care. Despite the growing rhetoric among policymakers and politicians about the importance of preventive care, the day-to-day infrastructure of healthcare delivery does not support this ideal. And a concerted effort must be made to overcome the many barriers to preventive care.

Benedict S. Dillon

See also Child Care; Diabetes; Disease; Health; Obesity; Primary Care; Public Health; Tobacco Use

Further Readings

Cohen, Joshua T., Peter J. Neumann, and Milton C. Weinstein. "Does Preventive Care Save Money? Health Economics and the Presidential Candidates," *New England Journal of Medicine* 358(7): 661–63, February 14, 2008.

Institute for Clinical Systems Improvement. *Health Care Guideline: Preventive Services for Adults.* 13th ed. Bloomington, MN: Institute for Clinical Systems Improvement, 2007.

Institute for Clinical Systems Improvement. *Health Care Guideline: Preventive Services for Children and Adolescents.* 13th ed. Bloomington, MN: Institute for Clinical Systems Improvement, 2007.

Ross, Joseph S., Susannah M. Bernheim, Elizabeth H. Bradley, et al. "Use of Preventive Care by the Working Poor in the United States," *Preventive Medicine* 44(3): 254–59, March 2007.

Starfield, Barbara. "U.S. Child Health: What's Amiss, and What Should Be Done About It?" *Health Affairs* 23(5): 165–70, September–October 2004.

Woolf, Steven H., Steven Jonas, and Evonne Kaplan-Liss, eds. *Health Promotion and Disease Prevention in Clinical Practice.* 2d ed. Philadelphia: Wolters Kluwer/Lippincott Williams and Wilkins, 2008.

Web Sites

Advisory Committee on Immunization Practices (ACIP): http://www.cdc.gov/vaccines/recs/ACIP/default.htm
American College of Preventive Medicine (ACPM): http://www.acpm.org
Institute for Clinical Systems Improvement (ICSI): http://www.icsi.org
Office of Disease Prevention and Health Promotion (ODPHP): http://odphp.osophs.dhhs.gov
U.S. Preventive Services Task Force (USPSTF): http://www.ahrq.gov/clinic/uspstfix.htm

PRIMARY CARE

Primary health care, as defined by the World Health Organization (WHO), is "essential health-care" that is delivered in a "practical, scientifically sound and socially acceptable" way; it is "universally accessible" to all in the community who seek it; it is affordable; and it is geared toward "self-reliance and self-determination." Primary care includes basic, routine, and preventive care that is often provided in an office or clinic by a provider who coordinates all aspects of a patient's health-care needs. It is often the patient's first contact with the healthcare system for a given health problem. Physicians, nurses, or other healthcare professionals can provide primary care. Primary-care physicians are generally considered to include those trained in family medicine or general practice, general pediatrics, and general internal medicine. Sometimes physicians in obstetrics and gynecology are also considered primary-care physicians. After briefly discussing problems with the U.S. health services system, this entry summarizes primary care's role in health services and how health policies can foster the provision of quality primary care to patients.

Background

Every complex organization, whether biological or social, requires a framework to support and coordinate its different functions. Healthcare systems rank among the various social systems that require a unified framework for appropriate functioning. Among industrialized nations, the United States is an anomaly because it lacks such a unified framework. A highly developed nation with well-developed and long-standing systems in many areas, such as education, it lacks any semblance of a health services delivery system with a structural framework. Historically, health services developed without any planning or regulation of their supporting structures and rules of conduct.

As a result, the United States stands alone among industrialized nations in its inability to respond to new imperatives and new challenges to public health. At the mercy of unaccountable market forces, the healthcare system reacts unpredictably, or sometimes not at all, to changing needs of the population for services of various kinds. Market-oriented organizations, including private universities and hospitals, medical-device manufacturers, pharmaceutical companies, professional organizations, and disease-oriented consumer advocacy groups, can set agendas for the operation of health services according to the likelihood of these services furthering the interests of the group in particular ways of defining health needs. They can create unwarranted health demands, particularly among population groups whose care contributes to high rates of profit for the industry. Some in the health services research field believe that the federal and state governments have abdicated responsibility or accountability. This current system has resulted in continuing escalation of costs, proliferation of unnecessary and potentially harmful technology, and declining population health as measured by the United States' relative position in the world.

Importance of Primary Care

Numerous research studies in the United States have found that a greater primary-care physician supply is associated with a variety of positive health outcomes, including fewer instances of all-cause mortality; cancer, heart disease, stroke, and infant mortality; low birth weight; increased life expectancy; and higher self-rated health. These results were consistent across study years and geographic areas. Pooled results for all-cause mortality indicate that an increase of one primary-care physician per 10,000 people is associated with an average mortality reduction of 5.3%, or 49 fewer deaths per 100,000 deaths per year. Mortality rate reductions for the Black population were higher than those for the White population, indicating improved equity and effectiveness. At a national level, a 5.3% reduction in all-cause mortality in the year 2000 would have translated into about 130,000 averted deaths. In comparison, a decline in the number of deaths of about 2,000 is considered sufficient to justify a national focus on screening the entire adult population for colorectal cancer. An increase of one primary-care physician per 10,000 people would require a 12.6% overall increase in the primary-care physician supply, or an absolute one-time increase of 28,726 primary-care physicians, based on the supply in the year 2000.

These results are consistent with international comparisons of nations differing in the strength of primary care. Nations with strong primary-care infrastructures have lower mortality rates, with the greatest reductions for causes particularly sensitive to primary-care interventions, such as asthma, heart and cerebrovascular diseases, and pneumonia. These results remain consistent after controlling for other important influences on health, including differences in age structure of the population, income per capita, gross domestic product (GDP) per capita, and behavioral factors such as smoking and alcohol consumption.

The evidence of the benefits of primary care is not limited to studies of the supply of primary-care physicians. There are demonstrated benefits from improving access to and use of primary-care practitioners as people's regular source of care, as well as from better experiences with the four cardinal features of primary care, which are detailed below. The greater the reported use of primary-care physicians as the regular source of care, the better the 5-year survival rates of patients, even after controlling for a variety of sociodemographic characteristics and initial health status: the better the experiences with the receipt of primary-care services, the better the self-reported health.

Beneficial Impact on Health and Costs

Primary-care services are the supporting spine of healthcare systems by virtue of four cardinal features: (1) They are generally the first contact point of access and use, (2) they are person-focused care over time instead of being disease focused, (3) they are comprehensive in the sense of taking care of all health-related needs except those too uncommon to maintain competence, and (4) they coordinate and integrate care that is more appropriately provided elsewhere.

In combination, these four functions constitute primary care. Their achievement makes it possible for care to be patient focused, family oriented, and relevant to the needs of the community in which people live and work. Primary care, when organized to carry out these functions, makes it possible to achieve more appropriate, safer, and less costly care. It helps people navigate the healthcare system so that they avoid the unnecessary or duplicated interventions that increase the risk of adverse effects and that are becoming common in the experiences of people.

Evidence for the beneficial impact of each of the four cardinal features of primary care is strong. That is, the filtering of patients by primary care, the first-contact feature, is effective in reducing unnecessary visits to specialists that both increase costs and increase the risk of overuse and adverse effects. Moreover, the person focus of primary-care practitioners leads to better overall improvement in health. The third feature of primary care, comprehensiveness, is an important contributor to the beneficial impact of primary care. The breadth of problems that are dealt with in primary care as opposed to being provided by specialists is the most consistent distinction between nations that have strong primary care and nations with weak primary care. Both national studies and international comparisons show that the greater the number of physicians involved in caring for an individual patient, the worse the outcome. And last, the coordinating feature of primary care is responsible for reducing duplication of medical tests and adverse effects of interventions. These four features, which in combination may be referred to as "primary-care practice," are associated with increased access to care for relatively deprived population groups, improved quality of care overall, better preventive services overall, better early interventions for health problems, fewer hospitalizations, and reductions in referrals to specialists, with resulting better population health at considerably lower costs.

A focus on achieving the combination of these four features explains why studies of people's experiences with primary care are even more consistent in showing benefits than are studies that seek to correlate the supply of primary-care physicians to health outcomes. The mere presence of such clinicians does not assure that good primary care is being provided; some population subgroups may lack access to existing primary-care resources, and some purported primary-care practices may not be adequate in their provision of first-contact, person-focused, comprehensive, and coordinated care. Moreover, an excess of directly accessible specialists may detract from the benefits of existing primary-care resources by discouraging coordination and person-focused care, as well as by leading to unnecessary and excessive interventions in the context of the patient's needs. Studies in the United States have shown that a greater supply of specialists available to the population does not improve the outcomes of care and, in fact, often worsens it. In 35 research studies dealing with differences between various geographic areas and rates of

mortality (total deaths, deaths from heart disease, cancer, and stroke, and infant deaths), 28 of the studies found that the greater the primary-care physician supply, the lower the mortality. And in 25 of the studies, it was found that the higher the specialist to population ratio was, the higher the mortality.

Primary Care's Growing Importance

Four major challenges to health services delivery in the nation will make the role of primary care increasingly important in the future. First, the morbidity burden of the population will increase as a result of increased survival from individual diseases. Most people, particularly as they age, accumulate a higher burden of morbidity—that is, comorbidity. Coexisting illnesses cause the focus of medical attention and quality assessments on particular diseases to be inadequate. Clinical practice guidelines are based, at best, on randomized controlled trials (RCTs) that attempt to exclude individuals with coexisting disease, even though they may constitute the majority of people otherwise eligible to participate in the trial. Consequently, the results of the trial are not applicable to most people with the disease for which the guidelines are implemented. A major, largely unrecognized defect in the application of results of the trials is the assumption that their findings apply to all populations even though it is known that the properties of tests and interventions differ according to the characteristics of the target population: general communities, patients in primary-care settings, or patients in specialty settings. When applied in a general community, in the example of fecal blood screening for colon cancer, the proportion of false-positive tests is much greater than would be the case if the intervention were applied in primary-care settings or specialty-care settings; intervention applied to the whole population will lead to many more unnecessary interventions, with a much greater likelihood of adverse effects and greatly decreased cost-effectiveness. For most medical interventions directed at individuals in the population, it is much more effective and efficient to focus on their application to patients in primary-care settings than in community-based settings, with referral to specialists from primary care as needed.

Second, an increase in the morbidity burden of the population exists because of growing rates of diagnosis of existing and new health problems. In the past two decades, the prevalence of diagnosed disease has increased markedly, largely due to lowered thresholds for diagnosis of individual diseases or inclusion of one or more risk factors as a proxy for a diagnosed disease. The increase has greatly expanded the market for use of medications, many of which have subsequently been shown to be dangerous. Primary care bears the burden, from increasing workloads to the challenges of dealing with adverse effects.

A third challenge is presented by an increase in the frequency of occurrence of adverse effects in medical interventions. These negative effects are estimated to precipitate more than 200,000 deaths annually in the nation. Between 4% and 18% of patient visits are also associated with adverse effects.

The rate of withdrawal of drugs from the market due to lack of safety has greatly increased since 1992, when the Food and Drug Administration (FDA) drug approval process was relaxed. Rates of nonindicated prescriptions have also increased. For example, the rate of prescribing medications for the common cold is 50% higher than the national desirable target, and the percentage of the elderly receiving a prescription for 1 of the 11 always-contraindicated drugs remains unchanged at about 3% per year. Deaths associated with medication errors increased markedly, by more than 65% in the nation just between 1990 and 1993. Only 40% of coronary angiographies are done competently; one fourth of those are erroneously read as showing severe disease; 6% of patients are informed that the test was normal although it was not; and one third of those individuals with misread tests have had surgery that was of uncertain benefit. The more physicians a patient sees, the greater the likelihood of adverse effects. Primary-care physicians, as the locus of responsibility for the ongoing care of patients, are in the best position to identify and deal with these adverse effects. Electronic health records, portable across a variety of settings, provide a way to facilitate identification of adverse effects and conduct research to establish more effective ways of dealing with these effects. However, to do this, a system of coding patients' problems, in the form of symptoms and signs, will have to become routine. Such a system exists but is not widely used in the

United States. To have it incorporated into medical practice will require considerable leadership from professional and policy-making bodies.

Finally, the imperative to reduce disparities in health resulting from avoidable differences in outcomes across different population subgroups remains a challenge to the healthcare system. In contrast to specialty services, which are distributed inequitably in most nations, primary-care services are generally equitably distributed. The exception is in the United States, however. The equity-facilitating influence of primary care is well documented, both from studies in the nation and elsewhere. The benefits of a greater supply of primary-care physicians are even greater for the Black population in this nation than for the majority White population and are greater in socially deprived areas than in more advantaged areas. Populations receiving their care from Federally Qualified Health Centers (FQHCs), which are required to maintain standards for primary-care practice, have fewer disparities in health outcomes between Black and White populations; studies in other industrialized nations such as the United Kingdom and in developing nations have had similar results. Thus, the move toward primary care can be considered a move toward equity in health.

Public Policy Directions

The supply of primary-care physicians in the nation is declining at a rapid rate, as is evident from the 45% reduction from 1997 to 2003 in the number of medical school students intending to enter a primary-care specialty. Chronic underfunding of primary-care services as compared with specialists has contributed to this decline in the attractiveness of primary-care practice, as the level of reimbursement for fee-for-services payment is set by reference to historical levels of relative reimbursement rather than to the difficulty and time requirements of practice. As a result of media focus on the technologic and pharmacologic aspects of health services, the public has come to believe that specialty care is superior to primary care; hence, population groups with rich insurance coverage and the ability to pay out of pocket have set the standard of seeking out specialty care directly. Research on the quality of care, however, is consistent in showing that primary care is superior to specialty care when the outcomes are broad rather than focused on diseases. Recent literature reviews indicate that even outcomes for specific common diseases are at least as good if not better when care is provided by primary-care physicians, appropriately buttressed by care from specialists. Early studies purporting to demonstrate the superiority of care from specialists were fraught with methodological inadequacies, especially with regard to controlling for overall morbidity burden. Even the extensive focus on evidence-based quality of care fails to give sufficient attention to the special benefits of primary care in relation to person- and population-focused outcomes rather than disease outcomes. This failure is due to the inappropriateness of guidelines for "all-or-nothing" performance measures.

The health services research community has not been in the forefront of primary care, most of which is carried out by primary-care physicians. In view of the evidence that some health system structures and processes have a major impact on outcomes, this seems to be a notable oversight concerning an important aspect of investigations into the role and impact of health services.

Preliminary evidence indicates that at least three features of health systems and two features of practice have a notable influence on health indicators at national levels. The systemic features include (1) national efforts to distribute health service resources according to need, (2) nonuse of copayments for primary-care services, and (3) tax-based health or regulated financing systems ensuring universal benefits. The practice characteristics most consistently associated with strong primary care are (1) comprehensiveness of services within primary care and (2) family orientation of health services. None of these characteristics are covered by U.S. health policy—and practically none by health services research in the nation.

Future Implications

The way that specialists and primary-care physicians provide healthcare differs. Their roles are different and need to be separately identifiable. There are almost certainly large differences in costs and activities, and high national health services costs and poor health outcomes result at least in part from an underuse of primary care and an overuse and misuse of specialty care. Both primary care and specialty care have important roles to play in the care of the population, and researchers can help policymakers make rational, evidence-based decisions about the relative functions and appropriate contributions of each.

Barbara Starfield

See also Equity, Efficiency, and Effectiveness in Healthcare; Physician Workforce Issues; Physicians; Preventive Care; Primary Care Case Management (PCCM); Primary Care Physicians; Public Health; Public Policy.

Further Readings

American College of Physicians. *How Is A Shortage of Primary Care Physicians Affecting the Quality and Cost of Medical Care? A Comprehensive Evidence Review.* Philadelphia: American College of Physicians, 2008.

Bodenheimer, Thomas, and Kevin Grumbach. *Improving Primary Care: Strategies and Tools for a Better Practice.* New York: McGraw-Hill, 2007.

Buttaro, Terry Mahan, JoAnn Trybulski, Patricia Polgar Bailey, et al. *Primary Care: A Collaborative Practice.* 3d ed. St. Louis, MO: Mosby, 2007.

Showstack, Jonathan, Arlyss Anderson Rothman, and Susan B. Hassmiller, eds. *The Future of Primary Care.* San Francisco: Jossey-Bass, 2004.

Starfield, Barbara. "Access, Primary Care and the Medical Home: Rights of Passage," *Medical Care* 46(10): 1015–1016, October 2008.

Starfield, Barbara. "An Evidence Base for Primary Care," *Managed Care* 17(6): 33–6, 39, June 2008.

Starfield, Barbara. "Refocusing the System," *New England Journal of Medicine* 359(20): 2087–2091, November 13, 2008.

Steinwald, A. Bruce. *Primary Care Professionals: Recent Supply Trends, Projections, and Valuation of Services.* Report No. GAO-08–472T. Washington, DC: U.S. Government Accountability Office, 2008.

Stenger, Joseph, Suzanne B. Cashman, and Judith A. Savageau, "The Primary Care Physician Workforce in Massachusetts: Implications for the Workforce in Rural, Small Town America," *Journal of Rural Health* 24(4): 375–83, Fall 2008.

Web Sites

American Academy of Family Physicians (AAFP)
http://www.aafp.org

American Academy of Pediatrics (AAP)
   http://www.aap.org
American College of Physicians (ACP)
   http://www.acponline.org
American Osteopathic Association (AOA)
   http://www.osteopathic.org

PRIMARY CARE CASE MANAGEMENT (PCCM)

The Centers for Medicare and Medicaid Services (CMS) defines Primary Care Case Management (PCCM) as case management–related services, including the locating, coordinating, and monitoring of healthcare services provided by a physician, a physician group practice, or an entity employing or having other arrangements with physicians under a PCCM contract with a state. These contracts can also be with nurse practitioners, certified nurse midwives, and physician assistants. State Medicaid agencies administer PCCM programs in which primary-care providers are responsible for managing the care of Medicaid recipients, including routine primary and preventive services, coordination of care, and arrangements for specialty services, usually without network restrictions. The primary-care providers receive reimbursement on a fee-for-service basis for the services they provide as well as a flat per-member-per-month fee or an increase in their preventive service fees to compensate for care management.

History

PCCM as an approach to Medicaid was enabled by an amendment to Title XIX of the Social Security Act in the Omnibus Budget Reconciliation Act of 1981. The addition of Section 1915(b) authorized the waiver of statutory requirements that Medicaid programs offer comparable benefits statewide and offer recipients freedom of choice in obtaining services. The amendment also specified that PCCM services would be Medicaid-covered and that qualifying PCCM programs must make provisions for 24-hour emergency treatment and reasonable geographic availability delivery sites as well as have a sufficient number of physicians to

serve the Medicaid population promptly and without compromise to the quality of care.

The Balanced Budget Act of 1997 further amended the Social Security Act to include a new Section 1932 state plan option as an alternative to seeking waivers under Section 1915(b) and research and demonstration projects under Section 1115. The new authority permitted states to implement mandatory managed care without waivers and without the cost-neutrality requirements associated with Section 1115. Approval could be obtained through a state plan amendment, and there was no time limit on the approval. The managed-care state plan was also required to offer enrollees in urban areas a choice between at least two managed-care organizations or between a PCCM system and a managed-care organization. In rural areas, there could be one managed-care organization or PCCM as long as there was a choice of physicians or case managers.

Growth of PCCM Programs

By the mid-1980s, states interested in increasing access to healthcare while holding providers accountable and controlling costs began enrolling Medicare recipients in PCCM programs. These programs attempted to reduce inappropriate hospital emergency department use and other types of high-cost care. In many instances, states developed PCCM programs as a stepping stone to risk-based managed care, and these programs grew steadily during the 1990s. When commercial managed-care organizations began declining to serve Medicaid populations in many markets, even those states that originally intended to move all their Medicaid recipients to risk-based managed care began considering PCCM as a viable method for maintaining Medicaid managed-care delivery systems.

Presently, 30 states in the nation use PCCM, and it is the model of choice for rural areas, where a relative scarcity of providers and a scattered population have resulted in weaker managed-care penetration. Due to its flexibility, PCCM is also used in urban areas. It is frequently the default enrollment for Medicaid recipients who fail to make a choice of a plan. Furthermore, PCCM may be used only in specific markets and also statewide, under either voluntary or mandatory conditions. In markets where feasible, states commonly offer both PCCM programs and risk models. The resulting competition increases recipient choice and motivates both managed-care organizations and PCCM programs to improve quality and service. However, states must be careful to apply access, quality, and reporting standards evenly to avoid encouraging managed-care-organizations' withdrawal.

In addition to the benefits associated with PCCM's flexibility from the perspective of states, it has enjoyed popularity with both patients and primary-care providers. Medicaid recipients entering PCCM programs report finding stable relationships with their physician and appreciating the lack of restrictions usually associated with managed care. And primary-care providers are pleased not to have to assume the financial risk for the care of their patients and find that they have greater control over medical decision making as well as less administrative burden. They also recognize that states are willing to take their concerns seriously and to find better ways to support them.

Comparison of PCCM Programs and Managed-Care Organizations

PCCM programs, which are legally recognized as managed-care plans, are similar to managed-care organizations in several ways. Notably, the structure of PCCM programs includes a panel of physicians, and one primary-care provider is charged with the primary responsibility for each recipient. PCCM also structures incentives for both physicians and recipients to encourage appropriate use of healthcare services. Additionally, PCCM programs typically conduct utilization reviews, patient education programs, and quality-monitoring activities.

An important difference is that states themselves are in charge of PCCM programs rather than a managed-care organization contractor, which means that state Medicaid agencies either directly administer PCCM or manage a contractor to handle administrative functions. Although such responsibilities are demanding for Medicaid agencies, this aspect of PCCM programs offers states an important opportunity to tailor programs to their policy goals in terms of populations, culture, and public health priorities. Furthermore, PCCM provides an assurance of continuity; unlike a for-profit managed-care organization, a state agency cannot consider leaving when a market turns unprofitable.

Another major difference between PCCM programs and managed-care organizations is the sharing of financial risk. PCCM physicians, with fee-for-service reimbursement supplemented by a management fee, do not take on additional risk. Therefore, PCCM programs are attractive to physicians because they are not disadvantaged when they have a sicker-than-average group of patients.

Trends in PCCM Practices

State PCCM programs differ because each state has taken a different approach that depended on its particular managed-care environment, and policy goals of states also vary. Nevertheless, several trends in the structure and operation of PCCM are apparent and reflect the significant evolution of PCCM over time.

Expanded Eligibility

In addition to enrolling a core population of individuals receiving Temporary Assistance for Needy Families (TANF), PCCM is also frequently being used to extend health insurance coverage to hard-to-serve populations, such as Supplemental Security Income (SSI) disabled children and adults, the aged, and children in foster care. Since the advent of the State Children's Health Insurance Program (SCHIP), most states have incorporated SCHIP members into their PCCM programs as well. Many states have also targeted individuals with chronic medical conditions and have integrated disease management into their PCCM programs.

Provider Recruitment and Retention

States are focusing on improving provider recruitment and retention by supporting participating providers through specially designated outreach staff, operating provider hotlines, implementing feedback mechanisms such as provider profiling, and devising strategies to gain providers' input and suggestions. Rather than second-guessing the decisions of physicians, states frequently provide tools to allow providers to police themselves and, when necessary, dedicate resources for working with outliers to improve their practices. States also have found that providing educational outreach, as by disseminating best practices and making available online instructional models, to be an effective support for providers. Taken together, these activities may produce strong state-provider relations and ultimately result in increased commitment from a wide variety of providers.

Quality Activities

Increasingly, states are applying many of the principles commonly used in network management to ensure that Medicaid recipients receive quality care from PCCM programs. For example, states are putting tighter language into their provider contracts and dedicating staff to monitor compliance with the stricter standards. In some cases, PCCM programs also are including strict provider credentialing, member surveys, care coordinated across multiple providers and conditions, 24-hour member services and nurse advice lines, community-based preventive health campaigns, Healthcare Effectiveness Data and Information Set (HEDIS) reporting to gauge the primary-care provider's performance, member education and health needs assessment, disciplined utilization management, disease management programs, complaint log reviews, and provider profiles.

Enrollment Process

Informing prospective members about Medicaid managed care and its requirements in a manner that ensures a full understanding of the PCCM program and how to access services remains a critical challenge. To overcome the intrinsic issues associated with enrollment, private enrollment vendors or brokers are increasingly being used to conduct enrollment and other functions. A variety of enrollment strategies is used, including providing informational materials and instructions about how to enroll, holding group educational sessions, operating toll-free help lines, and offering individual face-to-face counseling.

The mobility of Medicaid recipients also presents a significant challenge, creating discontinuity between the time individuals are enrolled in Medicaid and the time they enroll in PCCM. To address this issue, states are conducting telephone outreach at the time of the initial Medicaid eligibility determination. Additionally, some state agencies responsible for Medicaid eligibility determination

are educating recipients about PCCM and encouraging timely enrollment.

Increasing PCCM Active-Care Coordination

Some states are including an active care coordination component in their PCCM programs, recognizing that the referral process is the key to managing services, and they are making significant efforts to streamline prior authorization for providers. Additionally, care coordinators who are familiar with available resources and the community are often employed to more effectively respond to questions and concerns from both members and providers. These care coordinators may also be expected to collaborate with existing services, such as the Women, Infants, and Children (WIC) program, as well as empower local communities to change their service delivery system. Care coordinators may also be deployed to work with community service agencies and other providers to coordinate resources and services on the behalf of members with special needs.

Provider Reimbursement

States with incentive payment systems have found that these systems can be very effective in reinforcing primary program goals, and some state Medicaid agencies have gone beyond the basic fee approach. To encourage the provision of certain primary-care services, some states are reimbursing primary-care providers at enhanced rates rather than reimbursing them at the standard per-member-per-month fee. Other states have adopted partial capitation for primary care, paying a capitated amount for basic office visits and an enhanced payment for targeted services. Still other states allow primary-care providers to receive a per-member-per-month payment and also participate in a bonus pool that is distributed annually based on a composite measure of the physician's Medicaid caseload, hospital emergency department use, and defined prevention and quality goals.

Future Implications

The primary goals of PCCM programs are to reduce costs while improving patient outcomes.

Few evaluations of these programs have been conducted, and those that have been conduced are dated. They tended to focus on cost saving and service utilization, but they did not address patient outcomes except to suggest that PCCM programs improved access, especially to primary care.

In general, existing evaluations of PCCM programs have recorded initial savings in the range of 5% to 15% as compared with a similar fee-for-service population. This level of savings is considered comparable to the savings achieved by managed-care organizations. Savings from PCCM programs have been reported to result from changes in utilization patterns. Costs typically increase for primary-care services and prescription drugs, but the increases are offset by decreases in the costs of hospital emergency department use and inpatient services. In addition to the positive evaluations, a few of the early evaluations were negative, and as a result some state PCCM programs were abandoned in favor of full-risk or managed-care-organization-only models. Given the millions of Medicaid recipients enrolled in state PCCM programs, much more research needs to be conducted to evaluate the long-term benefits and problems of these programs.

Deann Muehlbauer

See also Access to Healthcare; Case Management; Cost of Healthcare; Managed Care; Medicaid; Primary Care; Quality of Healthcare; State Children's Health Insurance Program (SCHIP)

Further Readings

Adams, E. Kathleen, Janet M. Bronstein, and Curtis S. Florence, "Effects of Primary Care Case Management (PCCM) on Medicaid Children in Alabama and Georgia: Provider Availability and Race/Ethnicity," *Medical Care Research and Review* 63(1): 58–87, February 2006.

Garrett, Bowen, Amy Davidoff, and Alshadye Yemane. *Effects of Medicaid Managed Care Programs on Health Services Access and Use.* Discussion Paper Assessing the New Federalism 02–01. Washington, DC: Urban Institute, 2002.

Momany, Elizabeth T., Stephen D. Flach, Forrest D. Nelson, et al. "A Cost Analysis of the Iowa Medicaid Primary Care Case Management Program," *Health Services Research* 41(4 pt. 1): 1357–71, August 2006.

Rawlings-Sekunda, Joanne, Deborah Curtis, and Neva Kaye. *Emerging Practices in Medicaid: Primary Care Case Management.* NASHP Pub. No. MMC61. Portland, ME: National Academy for State Health Policy, 2001.

Smith, Vernon K., Terrisca Des Jardins, and Karin A. Peterson. *Exemplary Practices in Primary Care Case Management: A Review of State Medicaid PCCM Programs.* Princeton, NJ: Center for Health Care Strategies, 2000.

Walsh, Edith G., Deborah S. Osber, C. Ariel Nason, et al., "Quality Improvement in a Primary Care Case Management Program," *Health Care Financing Review* 23(4): 71–85, Summer 2002.

Web Sites

American Case Management Association (ACMA): http://www.acmaweb.org

Case Management Society of America (CMSA): http://www.cmsa.org

National Association of State Medicaid Directors (NASMD): http://www.nasmd.org

PRIMARY-CARE PHYSICIANS

Primary-care physicians generally serve as the first point of contact to the healthcare system for nearly all of a patient's medical and healthcare needs, including the treatment and diagnosis of health conditions and the provision of preventive and continuing care. Under the managed-care model, the primary-care physician also acts as a gatekeeper who controls access to specialists or costly procedures as a mechanism to control healthcare costs. Primary-care physicians may follow patients in a variety of healthcare settings, including outpatient clinics, offices, hospitals, long-term care facilities, and the patient's home.

Physicians trained in family medicine, general internal medicine, and general pediatrics typically are considered to be primary-care physicians. Additionally, health insurance plans may differ in regard to whether pediatricians and obstetricians/gynecologists, who specialize in the care of women, are considered primary-care physicians. Family physicians generally provide comprehensive care to patients from infancy till the end of life. Pediatricians are considered primary-care physicians for children, adolescents, teenagers, and young adults, while internists, who are practitioners of general internal medicine, provide care to adults.

Because of the aging of the nation's population, greater focus on prevention efforts and lifestyle changes, and the prevalence of acute and chronic diseases, the need for primary-care physicians has grown substantially. In recent years however, the number of primary-care physicians in the United States and other developed nations has been declining, as most physicians tend to specialize in an area of practice. A survey conducted by the University of Missouri-Columbia and the U.S. Department of Health and Human Services (HHS) predicts that by the year 2025, there will be a national shortage of 35,000 to 44,000 primary-care physicians. As a result, the current and future shortage of primary-care physicians is of concern among policymakers and healthcare planners.

Overview

Early practitioners of the science and art of medicine were primarily generalists. The breadth of their practice included diagnosing and treating a variety of illnesses, using apothecaries, and performing surgery. The concept of primary care, however, began to be formalized in the 1960s when the term appeared in the medical literature attempting to define its content and the scope and the role of the primary-care physician. Prior to this time in the United States, a movement toward specialization beginning in the early 1900s resulted in the first medical/physician specialty board being formed in 1916. The American Board of Medical Specialties (ABMS) was established in 1933 to ensure that physicians had a certifiable body of knowledge. ABMS's mission was to establish and maintain high standards for the delivery of safe, quality medical care by certified physician specialists. The American Board of Pediatrics (ABP) and the American Board of Internal Medicine (ABIM) were later established in 1935 and 1936, respectively. Today, ABMS member boards certify physicians in more than 130 different specialties and subspecialties.

After World War II, the rise of specialized care and provider specialization continued. This growth was supported by economic and professional incentives. And the decline in the number of general practitioners that had already begun before the war accelerated. The percentage of primary-care physicians in the nation declined from more than 80% in the early 1900s to less than 20% by 1960.

In response to the growing public concern over the reduced number of general practitioners, the American Academy of General Practitioners (now the American Academy of Family Physicians) was founded in 1947 to assist these practitioners in preserving and advancing the specialty. The American Academy of Family Physicians later joined with the American College of Physicians, representing internal medicine, and the American Academy of Pediatrics to become one of the largest organizations representing the primary-care specialty of family medicine. Eventually, in 1969, family medicine was established as the 20th primary medical specialty recognized by the American Board of Medical Specialties, and as a result of these efforts, general medicine was reborn.

Primary-Care Practice

The scope of primary-care physicians' practice generally includes the basic diagnosis of common health conditions and nonsurgical treatment and interventions. During the clinical encounter, primary-care physicians gather information about the patient's condition, symptoms, and medical history through interviewing. Primary-care physicians are also trained to order and interpret medical tests such as routine labs, electrocardiograms, and X rays. For more complicated diagnoses, however, they may refer the patient to a specialist with further specialized training or experience. After obtaining medical test results, primary-care physicians will make a diagnosis and may send the patient for further testing, referral to specialized care, therapy, diet or lifestyle changes, treatment, and/or follow-up. Primary-care physicians may also perform routine screenings and immunizations as well as counsel patients on health behaviors and self-care.

With more than 130 physician specialties and subspecialties, there inevitably exist overlapping boundaries in care. Yet the decision-making of primary-care physicians does differ from other specialized physicians who include some primary-care services in their practices.

The structure of the primary-care practice may include a team of physicians and nonphysician health professionals charged with establishing and sustaining a long-term, personal relationship and partnership with individuals and their families. Primary-care physicians and members of the healthcare team serve as advocates for the patient in coordinating the use of the entire healthcare system to benefit the patient. Additionally, primary-care physicians assist with helping patients navigate the system. For example, they may coordinate a full array of services that are essential for maintaining and improving the individuals' health status while providing nonepisodic interventions early in the disease process.

Future Implications

The ultimate goal of a healthcare system is to provide the highest quality of care, at the lowest possible cost, to the greatest number of people. Possible strategies to help accomplish this include increased financing to support primary-care practices, revitalizing primary-care education, and promoting the value of care that is accessible, comprehensive, coordinated, continuous, and accountable, provided by primary-care physicians and other nonphysician primary-care clinicians.

Javette C. Orgain

See also Acute and Chronic Diseases; American Academy of Family Physicians (AAFP); American Academy of Pediatrics (AAP); General Practice; Physicians; Preventive Care; Primary Care; Primary Care Case Management (PCCM)

Further Readings

Pathman, Donald E., Thomas R. Konrad, Rebekkah Dann, et al. "Retention of Primary Care Physicians in Rural Health Professional Shortage Areas," *American Journal of Public Health* 94(10): 1723–29, October 2004.

Pham, Hoangmai H., Deborah Schrag, J. Lee Hargraves, et al. "Delivery of Preventive Services to Older Adults by Primary Care Physicians," *Journal of the American Medical Association* 294(4): 473–81, July 27, 2005.

Sandy, Lewis G., and Steven A. Schroeder. "Primary Care in a New Era: Disillusion and Dissolution?" *Annals of Internal Medicine* 138(3): 262–67, February 4, 2003.

Schoen, Cathy, Robin Osborn, Phuong Trang Huynh, et al. "On the Front Lines of Care: Primary Care Doctors' Office Systems, Experiences, and Views in Seven Countries," *Health Affairs* 25(6): w555–w571, November–December 2006.

Yarnall, Kimberly S. H., Kathryn I. Pollack, Truls Ostbye, et al. "Primary Care: Is There Enough Time for Prevention," *American Journal of Public Health* 93(4): 635–41, April 2003.

Web Sites

American Academy of Family Physicians (AAFP): http://www.aafp.org

American Academy of Pediatrics (AAP): http://www.aap.org

American Board of Medical Specialties (ABMS): http://www.abms.org

American College of Physicians (ACP): http://www.acponline.org

PROJECT HOPE

Project HOPE (Health Opportunities for People Everywhere) is a nonprofit, international organization that is dedicated to improving the quality of life of the most vulnerable members of society, with a particular emphasis on women and children. Project HOPE's mission is to attain sustainable advances in healthcare globally by implementing health education programs and humanitarian assistance. Project HOPE is well-known in the field of health services research for its health policy journal *Health Affairs*.

Background

Celebrating its 50th anniversary in 2008, Project HOPE was founded as a floating hospital by William B. Walsh. After witnessing poor health conditions, particularly of young children, in the South Pacific while serving as a medical officer during World War II, Walsh persuaded President Eisenhower in 1958 to donate a naval ship to provide charity healthcare. The ship was later transformed into the S.S. HOPE and Project HOPE was formed. In September, 1960, the *S.S. HOPE* set sail from San Francisco to Indonesia. Although the *S.S. HOPE* was eventually retired in 1974, it made a total of 11 voyages to various countries around the world. Today, Project HOPE continues to operate land-based programs, including medical training and health education in more than 30 countries across 5 continents.

Project HOPE is dedicated to providing sustainable solutions to health problems by helping people assist themselves. The organization improves the local capacity to sustain improvements in health and improve access to healthcare. It has programs across the globe, in locations including Africa, the Americas and the Caribbean, Asia and the Middle East, Central and Eastern Europe, and Russia/Eurasia. Project HOPE's current programs in Africa are fighting to combat HIV/AIDS, malaria, and other diseases; poverty and hunger; infant mortality; and maternal mortality. Its programs in South American countries target access to healthcare services for women and children. And in Asia its programs are focused on addressing infectious diseases and women's health issues.

Project HOPE also provides humanitarian and emergency assistance in areas that are affected by disasters. Additionally, the organization strives to provide long-term access to essential medicines and medical supplies to underserved areas. Since 1987, Project HOPE has shipped nearly $1 billion in humanitarian assistance globally.

The organization also maintains expertise in various health and medical disciplines and provides health professionals education through various programs, ranging from the training of rural health promoters in primary care to the establishment of specialized tertiary-care medical programs. Project HOPE's implementation of train-the-trainer methodologies has resulted in millions of healthcare professionals being better equipped worldwide. Project HOPE has also laid the foundation for a healthier future by building, and training the staff needed to operate, hospitals and clinics, especially those targeting the special needs of children. The facilities serve as national training centers for healthcare providers in addition to being an invaluable resource to improve the health of children in developing countries.

Project HOPE is a registered organization of the U.S. Agency for International Development (USAID) and is a member of the Partnership for Quality Medical Donations. The organization maintains close collaborations with local partners to ensure that efforts are not duplicated in meeting the needs of those it serves.

Health Affairs

Project HOPE has published the leading peer-reviewed health policy journal, *Health Affairs*, since 1981. The journal consistently ranks at the top of its categories in the *Journal Citation Report*. Its founding editor, John K. Iglehart, is a member of the National Academy of Sciences, Institute of Medicine (IOM) and national correspondent for the *New England Journal of Medicine*. The idea for *Health Affairs* was spawned in the 1970s when Walsh, Project HOPE's founder, concluded that it should expand its reach by publishing a journal to focus on the U.S. healthcare system.

Health Affairs is a multidisciplinary journal that covers topics such as access, costs, and quality of healthcare; Medicare; Medicaid; healthcare reform; and prescription drug coverage. The journal is nonpartisan and publishes a wide range of timely health articles, which focus on research and commentary that are of concern both domestically and abroad.

Health Affairs is published six times a year with additional supplements and is also available online. The authors that contribute to the journal include acclaimed scholars, policymakers, and leaders in the healthcare industry. The journal averages about 33,000 readers per printed issue, and the readership includes legislators, healthcare leaders and professionals, academics and researchers, health policy analysts, and advocates. *Health Affairs* is widely cited in the national media and press, including *The Washington Post, The New York Times, The Wall Street Journal*, and CNN, and it has been referred to as the "bible of health policy." Between January and July, 2006, alone, the journal was cited 18 times in U.S. congressional testimony, which is illustrative of its policy influence.

The journal is divided into the sections of Feature Articles, Commentary, Interviews, Narrative Matters, Health Tracking, DataWatch, GrantWatch, UpDate, Book Reviews, and Letters to the Editor. *Health Affairs* also publishes thematic issues each year that explore a topic in depth as well as on "variety issues."

Future Implications

Project HOPE continues its work to improve the lives of people throughout the world, particularly among low- and middle-income countries, by educating healthcare professionals and volunteers, training community workers, providing essential supplies and medicines, and combating infectious diseases. Additionally, *Health Affairs* remains an influential force in informing the public policy debate on issues that are of particular concern in healthcare.

Jared Lane K. Maeda

See also Access to Healthcare; Healthcare Reform; Health Services Research Journals; International Health Systems; Medicaid; Medicare; Quality of Healthcare; Vulnerable Populations

Further Readings

Hebert, Paul L., Jane E. Sisk, and Elizabeth A. Howell. "When Does a Difference Become a Disparity? Conceptualizing Racial and Ethnic Disparities in Health," *Health Affairs* 27(2): 374–82, March–April 2008.

Igelhart, John K. "Forging a New Path Down a Very Challenging Road," *Health Affairs* 25(2): 310–311, March–April 2006.

Project Hope. 2007 *Project Hope Annual Report*. Millwood, VA: Project Hope, 2007.

Ridley, David B., Henry G. Grabowski, and Jeffrey L. Moe. "Developing Drugs for Developing Countries," *Health Affairs* 25(2): 313–24, March–April 2006.

Smedley, Brian D. "Moving Beyond Access: Achieving Equity in State Health Care Reform," *Health Affairs* 27(2): 447–55, March–April 2008.

Web Sites

Health Affairs: http://www.healthaffairs.org
Project HOPE: http://www.projecthope.org
Project HOPE: Forty Years of American Medicine Abroad: http://americanhistory.si.edu/hope

PROSPECTIVE PAYMENT

The manner in which healthcare organizations are paid for the services they provide can influence their organizational behavior. Healthcare organizations are generally paid in three ways: (1) on a cost-based basis, (2) on a capitation basis, or (3) on a case-based basis. On a cost-based basis, such as fee-for-service, the organization is paid for all the services it provides, which is a powerful incentive for high levels of effort and service. Payment on a capitation basis consists of a flat payment to the organization per person cared for, with the organization assuming the risk that the payment will cover the cost of the patient's care. On a case-based basis, the organization is paid a single payment for an episode of care, and the payment does not change if fewer or more services are provided. The various payment types may be either retrospective or prospective.

Medicare's Prospective Payment System

The best-known example of case-based payment in healthcare is Medicare's prospective payment system (PPS), which was mandated by the U.S. Congress to control community hospital inpatient costs in 1983. Under this system, the Medicare program changed its mode of payment for hospital inpatient care from a retrospective cost-based system to a prospective case-based system.

After the Medicare program was established in 1965 the costs of hospital care soared. One of the major factors that led to rising costs was the retrospective cost-based payment system. Under this system, hospitals submitted their bills to Medicare after the care had been given and the costs to the hospital were known. Hospitals were then paid for the care they provided, as allowed by Medicare rules, regardless of whether the costs were high or low, excessive or appropriate. Consequently, there was little incentive for hospitals to be cost-effective.

On the other hand, the prospective case-based payment system set payment rules prior to when the care was given. By setting a fixed reimbursement level per case based on diagnosis, the PPS provided economic incentives to conserve the use of resources. Hospitals that used more resources than covered by the flat rate lost the difference. Those with costs below the rate retained the difference.

Diagnosis Related Groups

Under Medicare's PPS, the amount paid to hospitals is based on their patients' Diagnosis

Related Groups (DRGs). Specifically, each patient is assigned into one of more than 500 DRGs, based on principal diagnosis, age, and medical complications. The DRGs aggregate patients with similar resource-consumption and hospital length-of-stay patterns. Medicare then pays the hospitals a set amount for each DRG. The government calculates the payment for each DRG based on national averages. It also modifies that amount somewhat based on local wage rates, geographic location (e.g., rural versus urban area), and whether the hospital is a teaching hospital.

Effects of Medicare's Prospective Payment System

Extensive research has been conducted to examine the impact of Medicare's PPS on hospitals and patients. This research has focused on the system's impact on average hospital length of stay, access to and quality of care, financial condition of hospitals, overall effects on costs, and hospital management.

Average Hospital Length of Stay

Since Medicare's PPS pays hospitals a fixed amount based on the patient's DRG, there is an incentive for hospitals to discharge their patients as soon as possible. Given that revenue is fixed, the time a patient spends in the hospital will determine the profit or loss. As a result, one of the ways to increase profits is to reduce the number of days of care taken to treat a patient. Many studies have reported that hospital average length of stay did drop after the introduction of the system.

Access to and Quality of Care

With the introduction of Medicare's PPS, many policymakers and the general public were concerned that it would induce hospitals to save on costs by cutting corners—reducing access to care and the quality of care—by refusing to treat costly patients or by closing treatment units. Researchers have addressed these issues to some extent; however, the results have been mixed so far.

Financial Conditions of Hospitals

Because Medicare's PPS puts a degree of financial stress on hospitals, particularly on those that have higher than usual costs, there was a concern about their financial viability. When PPS was first established, its fixed payment rates proved sufficiently generous, and average hospital operating margins increased. However, over time, the rates were lowered. By the late 1980s and through the early 1990s, average operating margins for the Medicare segment of hospital patients tended to be negative.

Overall Effects on Costs

The main objective of the Medicare PPS was to control hospital costs. With regard to the effect of PPS on reducing hospital expenditures, one study found that for a sample of California hospitals, those under the strongest pressure from PPS responded by reducing expenditures. Another study found that PPS reduced Medicare's hospital costs substantially. In terms of Medicare's overall budget, the PPS appears to have been effective in slowing down expenditures. The PPS reduced the historic rates of growth in total Medicare spending. However, the reduced growth in inpatient spending was partially offset by increases in spending on hospital outpatient care, skilled nursing care, home health care, and physician payment increases.

Hospital Management

The Medicare PPS was designed to create incentives for the balancing of costs and benefits in treating patients. It led hospitals to begin to explore mechanisms for more accurate product costing. Under cost-based payment, when healthcare providers were directly reimbursed for whatever costs they incurred, accurate cost measurement was of little concern. However, under PPS, the revenue per patient is not merely a reflection of reported cost but is instead a fixed amount. If the true underlying cost is substantially more than the revenue for a certain type of patient, the hospital must be aware of it. Similarly, hospitals must also be aware if the cost is much less than the revenue. Medicare's PPS encouraged the use of product-line costing, which led to more efficient hospital financial management.

Future Implications

After applying PPS to community hospitals, the federal government developed and applied similar systems in other healthcare settings. Medicare now uses PPSs for hospital outpatient services, inpatient psychiatric hospital care, inpatient rehabilitation hospital care, inpatient long-term hospital care, skilled-nursing facility care, home health care, and hospice care. It seems likely that these systems will remain in use for many years to come.

Tae Hyun Kim

See also Centers for Medicare and Medicaid Services (CMS); Cost Containment Strategies; Cost of Healthcare; Diagnosis Related Groups (DRGs); Healthcare Financial Management; Hospitals; Medicare; Medicare Payment Advisory Commission (MedPAC)

Further Readings

Kulesher, Robert R. "Impact of Medicare's Prospective Payment System on Hospitals, Skilled Nursing Facilities, and Home Health Agencies: How the Balanced Budget Act of 1997 May Have Altered Service Patterns for Medicare Providers," *Health Care Managers* 25(3): 198–205, July–September 2006.

Mayes, Rick, and Robert A. Berenson. *Medicare Prospective Payment and the Shaping of U.S. Health Care.* Baltimore: Johns Hopkins University Press, 2006.

Sood, Neeraj, Melinda Beeuwkes Buntin, and Jose J. Escarce. "Does How Much and How You Pay Matter? Evidence From the Inpatient Rehabilitation Care Prospective Payment System," *Journal of Health Economics* 27(4): 1046–1059, July 2008.

White, Chapin, "Why Did Medicare Spending Growth Slow Down?" *Health Affairs* 27(3): 793–802, May–June 2008.

Web Sites

Centers for Medicare and Medicaid Services (CMS): http://www.cms.hhs.gov

Healthcare Financial Management Association (HFMA): http://www.hfma.org

Medicare Payment Advisory Commission (MedPAC): http://www.medpac.gov

PROVIDER-BASED RESEARCH NETWORKS (PBRNs)

Provider-based research networks (PBRNs) are collaborative partnerships between academically based investigators and community-based physicians who share an ongoing commitment to developing and conducting health-related research. PBRNs provide the infrastructure and support necessary to conduct community-based clinical research studies on an ongoing basis, thus providing stability and continuity that transcends individual studies. PBRNs address many shortcomings of academic medical centers–only research and present several distinct advantages to it; most notably, these entities provide access to a much larger population of prospective clinical research trial participants.

Clinical research trials are the means by which medical researchers explore and answer specific questions about health. Clinical trials, translational research, epidemiological research, health services research, and several other categories are included in the broader definition of clinical research.

Academic medical centers (AMCs) have long been the centers of clinical research, the development of new knowledge, and the transfer of that knowledge to the next generation of researchers and care providers. There, teams of investigators develop research questions and methods for examining them and also carry out the research through voluntary enrollment of study subjects who are often patients at the centers. Having AMCs as the center of the clinical research universe has many advantages, including the presence of both clinical and research infrastructure and the synergy that can be developed among academics, researchers, and clinicians; but it also has several limitations.

In 1961, one of the founders of health services research in the United States, Kerr L. White, presented a statistical estimate with far-reaching implications for both medical education and population-based clinical research: For every 1,000 adults at risk of being ill or using health services in a given month, only one will be referred to an AMC. While the precision of this estimate has been debated and patterns of care may have shifted since 1961, the implications remain relevant today. If this estimate is accurate, although the overwhelming majority of clinical research is conducted in AMCs, less than 1% of the relevant population is being seen at AMCs, and only a small subset of these individuals is enrolling in clinical research trials. A tremendous risk of selection bias exists then, jeopardizing the external validity of the majority of clinical research. Furthermore, limiting clinical research access to only AMCs induces a bottleneck in completing clinical research studies, consequently slowing the pace of medical progress.

In 2006, a contract research organization, Westat, completed and published the *Inventory and Evaluation of Clinical Research Networks: A Complete Project Report,* a comprehensive worldwide study of clinical research networks. This report identified 262 PBRNs with a variety of funding sources and organizational structures, and spanning multiple types of research and subject populations. The majority of these networks are less than 10 years old; however, others have been in existence for 50 years. Currently, 62% of these networks are funded by the federal government. Another 10% are funded by nonprofit organizations, 9% are funded by a government outside the United States, and 8% are funded by academia. Approximately 60% receive funding from more than one source; 52% report operations in the United States only, while 32% report operations in the United States and internationally, and 16% report exclusively international operations. Universities and AMCs continue to play a dominant role in many networks, while other network members span the healthcare spectrum and include the following: state and federal government healthcare facilities, community hospitals, individual or group physician practices, clinical laboratories, pharmaceutical companies, foundations, contract research organizations, and health maintenance organizations (HMOs).

The research areas vary widely, and include epidemiology, behavior modification, health communication, patient care, medical practice, clinical quality improvement, research-centered surveillance, and clinical process improvement, among others. Approximately 60% of the studies conducted through PBRNs are clinical trials, 24% are epidemiology and other observational studies, 6% are other interventional research, and 2% are outcome oriented. As far as the populations being studied are concerned, these research network projects are variously organized by demographic characteristics (e.g., age group, gender, and race), disease type (e.g., AIDS, cancer, and heart disease), practice type (i.e., primary care and specialty services), and point on the care continuum (i.e., prevention, early detection, treatment, or disease survivorship).

Research Generalizability and Medical Progress

Among its many benefits, PBRNs broaden the access points between clinical research studies and the total potential participant population, helping ensure better research with more generalizable findings. PBRNs broaden clinical research's reach to include more members of the more than 99% of the population described by White as being "at risk" but not seen at AMCs, thus offering inclusion of people who would not seek care at the centers for any number of reasons, including their geographic relation to them, insurance coverage, perceived nonnecessity of AMC-based care, or other factors. By including members of this larger, more diverse population, the research is more likely to result in findings that are more broadly representative of it and therefore generalizable. More comprehensive population representation is of increasing importance with, for example, the current growth of genetics research. With striking limitations on the geographic reach of AMCs, PBRNs help give such genetics-based studies a broader reach, which may prevent the exclusion of potentially geographically clustered and genetically distinctive populations. These efforts help medical researchers improve the understanding of genetic pathways of disease and extend the applicability of research findings to these populations.

By opening the access points to a larger population, PBRNs also serve to expedite the pace of medical discovery. Simply put, patient enrollment is one of the most time-consuming components of most clinical trials. Individual studies can spend many years enrolling a sample of individuals sufficient to allow the statistical power to demonstrate an intervention's effectiveness. With PBRNs' access to a broader population, there is an increased probability of an individual with the right trial-specified clinical characteristics seeking care at a location that offers access to the trial. This greater rate of patient-to-trial exposure can translate into more rapid overall trial enrollment and, consequently, more rapid trial completion. A prime example of this is cancer prevention research, which is often conducted among healthy populations.

Because cancer prevention trials often require a very large participant sample size to allow for statistically powerful analysis, this type of project may be impractical at an AMC. Beyond potentially limited trial access to the less than 1% of individuals at risk who seek care at AMCs, a large proportion of patients have considerable health concerns that would preclude their enrollment in the trial. PBRNs open the door to a dramatically larger, generally healthier population that sees their geographically more accessible practitioners for everything ranging from annual checkups and flu shots to symptom-induced visits for transient health issues to ongoing care needs that are not severe enough to either warrant referral to the AMC or preclude the patient from a prevention trial. Most recently, this benefit of PBRNs has perhaps been visible as a significant component of the National Institutes of Health's (NIH's) Roadmap, which is the federal plan for medical research in the 21st century.

Translating Research Into Practice

As part of NIH's Roadmap, the importance of developing new partnerships among patient communities, community-based physicians, and academic researchers is recognized. Indeed, several institutions and federal agencies are developing PBRNs or have them already in place. To this end, the NIH and other federal agencies are aware of the role PBRNs can play in both translating research results into better care and closing the gap between discovery and delivery.

For many medical-care innovations, providers often remain unconvinced that sufficient evidence exists to support the implementation of research-tested clinical services in real-world practice settings. The national Institute of Medicine's (IOM) 1998 report, *Bridging the Gap Between Practice and Research: Forging Partnerships With Community-Based Drug and Alcohol Treatment*, describes how the clinical-care community perceives an excess of "efficacy" research and a simultaneous dearth of "effectiveness" research. Many have noted that most research on clinical services takes place in AMCs, yet

most care is delivered in community settings. Consequently, for many community-based providers, evidence-based practice awaits more practice-based evidence. These observations suggest that the acceptance and implementation of evidence-based clinical services in community-based practice settings depends less on dissemination, which connotes a one-way flow of knowledge from researchers to providers, than on knowledge exchange, which involves two-way communication between researchers and providers. In PBRNs, this exchange is structurally facilitated, as community-based providers assume primary responsibility for seeing patients and for collecting research data and participating in other aspects of the research process. On the discovery-to-delivery continuum, the process of seeing patients represents the critical process of implementation, which remains a daunting challenge no matter how strong or credible the evidence.

For all but the simplest clinical services, successful implementation depends on administrative support, adequate financial and human resources, and organizational culture that values scientifically based practice. Indeed, systematic reviews indicate that multifaceted interventions that target organizational staffing, office workflow, and information systems are more effective in changing provider behavior than interventions that increase provider awareness and knowledge, such as continuing education and academic detailing. These findings suggest that the implementation of evidence-based clinical services necessitates systemic organizational changes, including the development of a supportive infrastructure and culture for both academic settings and, perhaps more important, community-based practice settings.

These systemic organizational changes are of growing importance because the recent healthcare market trends emphasize efficiency and may serve to erode the professional values and norms that emphasize scientifically based practice and the conduct of historically inefficient clinical research.

PBRNs involve both knowledge exchange and systemic organizational changes. As such, they are a promising model for both disseminating and implementing evidence-based clinical services and, ultimately, improving the quality of care. Knowledge exchange occurs through community-based participatory research (CBPR). By engaging providers in the research process, researchers gain insight into the clinical issues and needs of community-based practice settings, obtain provider input on study design and the feasibility of implementation, and discover the tacit practice-based knowledge that exists in community-based practice settings and the acceptability of the intervention. CBPR promotes a sense of trust and ownership that enhances providers' acceptance of clinical research results and strengthens their commitment to acting on research findings. However, CBPR does not occur spontaneously or effortlessly.

Keys to Success

Substantial federal commitment exists to develop and support PBRNs as a means for improving and advancing the nation's research agenda as well as disseminating and implementing evidence-based clinical services in community settings. Yet reports indicate that PBRNs themselves are encountering challenges to implementation and sustainability. Several studies have elucidated characteristics that are associated with successful performance of PBRNs and the challenges they face, including developing a research agenda, obtaining member buy-in and sustaining member interest, consistently obtaining sufficient funding, creating a clinical research infrastructure, and coping with regulatory compliance issues.

Perhaps the most fundamental characteristics associated with PBRN success is the commitment of both the lead- and coinvestigators and their continuous active involvement in the PBRN. These individuals must establish a clear vision for the organization, typically in the form of scientific focus, goals, and priorities. They must also keep a close watch on the environment and remain open to new ideas and ways of remaining energized and at the forefront of research, including through continually developing new relationships with new investigators. They must also develop the relationship both inside and outside the PBRN, including those partners with the relevant patient populations, the prospective partners who would interact with those populations, and the funding groups or agencies that support the ongoing infrastructure necessary to conduct the research. Indeed, the sustainability of PBRNs has been strongly and directly tied to the ability to acquire ongoing sponsorship of research, which can be a very costly endeavor.

For all practical purposes, PBRNs cannot function without independent funding. Traditionally, clinical practice has cross-subsidized concomitant clinical research; however, this is no longer sustainable because the healthcare environment increasingly emphasizes efficiency as well as increasingly complex, burdensome, and resource-intensive research and regulatory requirements. Lack of such resources has had a negative impact on PBRNs' abilities to pursue specific lines of research and on some PBRNs' abilities to complete already initiated studies. The pressures and uncertainty of obtaining new and ongoing funding are ever present, and the time spent seeking funding displaces the time that could be spent performing the research. Restrictions placed on some funding sources can further limit how and where PBRN efforts are directed. Some PBRNs receive stable funding through federal support, which mitigates some of this pressure and uncertainty, and enables more consistent operations, while some PBRNs take as much of a business perspective as a research perspective when determining research agendas and carrying out research, as they constantly focus on costs and efficiency of operations.

In addition to being costly, clinical research is time-consuming. Investigators in PBRNs often experience exceptional time pressure because they are often also responsible for maintaining a viable clinical practice. These investigators often have little or no directly supported time to develop or conduct research, let alone analyze study data or develop and publish the findings. As such, their success is often tied to their ability to create an organizational infrastructure to support the many time-consuming aspects of clinical research. PBRN member provider organizations often must implement systemic changes in organizational staffing, office workflow, information systems, and reward structures to appropriately encourage staff support and participation and operational success. Some PBRNs have a more centralized model, where the research staff is funded in dedicated support of research, operate out of a central nonclinical office setting, and only interact with clinical staff to identify and enroll patients and carry out the strictly research-related aspects of study participants' otherwise usual course of care. Some PBRNs, on the other hand, employ a more decentralized model in which the same staff members support both patient care and the requirements of the clinical research protocol. In either case, two infrastructure elements, good staffing and strong information technology (IT), remain key components to success.

Successful PBRNs consistently extol the value of a well-trained staff to carry out the many specialized functions within the PBRN. These roles include data managers and statistical support staff who assist in the development of research protocols and also help manage and analyze data, research nurses who interact with study participants, administrative staff who help ensure that all sorts of regulatory requirements, including interactions with local institutional review boards (IRBs) and government agencies such as the Food and Drug Administration (FDA), are met, and study coordinators and managers who oversee and coordinate all these roles. To fulfill these roles, PBRN staff efficiency, effectiveness, and general productivity are often influenced by having IT systems.

As it pertains both to internal PBRN operations as well as PBRN interaction with sponsors and other agencies, many recent advances in IT have been facilitators of PBRN success. With many PBRNs spread across multiple states and even multiple countries, the utility of an IT resource for communication and operations support is obvious. New government-sponsored IT resources such as the Clinical Trials Support Unit (CTSU), cancer Biomedical Information Grid (caBIG), Network for Effective Collaboration Technologies through Advanced Research (NECTAR), and other resources have facilitated access to information on clinical trial availability, contributed to relieving the regulatory burden of trial participation for practitioners, and allowed much greater consistency and efficiency in participant enrollment and ongoing trial management. Some other, more forward-looking research programs have begun to develop patient-centric IT systems in which patients enter responses to trial-relevant questions on checking in for a clinic visit. With implications for practice at both AMCs and community-based practices, these data are stored for trial analysis with other patients' responses. Additionally, they are analyzed in real time to inform and improve practice immediately by both providing useful educational information to participants or patients and also informing the care provider regarding the most pertinent matters to address during the concomitant clinic visit.

Future Implications

PBRNs have broadly demonstrated their success in allowing access to new populations and enhancing enrollment in clinical trials. To cite just one example, a National Cancer Institute (NCI) PBRN, the Community Clinical Oncology Program, has allowed a successful expansion from cancer treatment trials into cancer prevention and control trials. In addition to effectively opening the door to prevention trials, it currently accounts for 30% of all enrollments to treatment trials sponsored by the NCI.

Although many PBRNs have shown that they can complete studies and advance medical knowledge, the extent to which PBRNs actually promote the use of evidence-based clinical services in community-based practice settings remains largely unknown. The few studies that have been done have demonstrated a benefit of enhanced utilization of new therapies for nontrial patients compared with patients in practices that do not do clinical research. The scope, details, and generalizability of these relationships largely remain to be proved, since many PBRNs are too new, too small, or lack reliable outcome data to measure their impact as a model for dissemination. With the NIH Roadmap's recent emphasis on PBRNs, a growing opportunity exists to conduct empirical evaluations of the benefits of PBRNs in terms of their ability to directly influence clinical practice and facilitate the translation of research into practice.

William R. Carpenter and Bryan J. Weiner

See also Academic Medical Centers; Clinical Practice Guidelines; Community-Based Participatory Research (CBPR); Evidence-Based Medicine (EBM); Quality Indicators; Quality of Healthcare; Randomized Controlled Trials (RCT); White, Kerr L.

Further Readings

Kuo, Grace M., Jeffrey R. Steinbauer, and Stephen J. Spann. "Conducting Medication Safety Research Projects in a Primary Care Physician Practice-Based Research Network," *Journal of the American Pharmacists Association* 48(2): 163–70, March–April 2008.
Lamb, Sara J., Merwyn R. Greenlick, and Dennis McCarty, eds. *Bridging the Gap Between Practice and*

Research: Forging Partnerships With Community-Based Drug and Alcohol Treatment. Washington, DC: National Academy Press, 1998.

Lindbloom, Erik J., Bernard G. Ewigman, and John Hickner. "Practice-Based Research Networks: The Laboratories of Primary Care Research," *Medical Care* 42(4 Suppl.): III45–III49, 2004.

Tierney, William M., Caitlin C. Oppenheimer, Brenda L. Hudson, et al. "A National Survey of Primary Care Practice-Based Research Networks," *Annals of Family Medicine* 5(3): 242–50, May–June 2007.

Zerhouni, Elias A. "Medicine: The NIH Roadmap," *Science* 302(5642): 63–72, October 3, 2003.

Web Sites

Agency for Healthcare Research and Quality (AHRQ): http://www.ahrq.gov

Center for Participatory Research (CPR): http://hsc.unm.ed/som/fcm/cpr

National Institutes of Health (NIH): http://www.nih.gov

Networks for Clinical Research: http://www.clinicalresearchnetworks.org

PUBLIC HEALTH

Public health involves promoting health and preventing disease for all people in a community. The mission of public health is to promote health and mental health and prevent disease, injury, and disability for all the inhabitants of a community or other jurisdiction. Society has an interest in protecting its population and making assurances to that population that the society will endeavor to create conditions for all people to be healthy. Public health practitioners carry out the mission of public health through assessment, policy development, and the application of the essential public health services. The vision of public health is to promote a healthy people in healthy communities agenda. At a scientific level, this means that research and practice will be oriented to preventing disease before it occurs (primary prevention), finding ways to prolong life, encouraging healthy lifestyles with individual responsibility for maintaining these lifestyles, and developing a public health system that promotes health for all its population through organized community efforts and collaboration. This latter point is tied to a major concern about health equity for all. At a practice level, this agenda would also be pursued by preventing epidemics and the spread of disease, protecting people from environmental hazards, prevention of injuries, responding to disasters and helping people and communities in the recovery period, and assuring accessibility of health services for everyone. Public health is thus population based and not generally a provider of clinical services. Public health agencies work with other community health partners to carry out the mission of public health and a vision for a healthier future.

Major Functions and Essential Services

Public health has 3 major functions and 10 essential services that will successfully impact a local public health system. The first function is *assessment*, which involves the identification of health problems in a community and a determination of all quantitative and qualitative considerations of that problem. The function of *policy development* involves the creation of solutions and action steps with appropriate rules, regulations, statutes, and laws, and protocols related to these solutions. The final function involves *assurance*, which relates to the implementation of the solutions in the area of action.

A clarification of these core functions involves the public health system carrying out the 10 essential public health services:

1. Monitor health status to identify community problems.

2. Diagnose and investigate health problems and health hazards in the community.

3. Inform and educate people about health issues and empower them to deal with the issues.

4. Mobilize community partnerships to identify and solve health problems.

5. Develop policies and plans that support individual and community health efforts.

6. Enforce laws and regulations that protect health and ensure safety.

7. Link people to needed personal health services and ensure the provision of healthcare when otherwise unavailable.

8. Ensure a competent public health and personal healthcare work force.

9. Evaluate effectiveness, accessibility, and quality of personal and population-based services.

10. Conduct research for new insights and innovative solutions to health problems.

Structure of the American Public Health Service System

Most public health agencies in the United States are found at the state and local levels. Although the American public health system tends to be decentralized, with different structures between states and localities, it is possible to see a public health presence at the national level. The U.S. Public Health Service includes the Office of Public Health and Science (OPHS) and eight operating agencies. These agencies are (1) the Health Resources and Services Administration (HRSA), (2) Indian Health Service (IHS), (3) Centers for Disease Control and Prevention (CDC), (4) National Institutes of Health (NIH), (5) Food and Drug Administration (FDA), (6) Substance Abuse and Mental Health Services Administration (SAMHSA), (7) Agency for Toxic Substances and Disease Registry (ATSDR), and (8) the Agency for Healthcare Research and Quality (AHRQ).

There are also 10 Regional Health Administrators for the federal regions of the country. Under Section 330 of the Public Health Service Act, there are also a number of Community Health Centers (CHC) around the country that provide ambulatory healthcare in areas where there are few health services for a population or a special needs population. These centers coordinate federal, state, and local resources to deliver health and social services to a designated population. The federal government also provides funds to the states for designated program development, such as HIV/AIDS programs. In fact, the federal government is the largest purchaser of health-related services.

All 50 states have a public health presence within some state agency. State public health agencies are either freestanding or units of a multipurpose health and human services agency. These agencies are responsible for identifying and meeting the health needs of the residents of the states. They are often responsible for monitoring federal funding in the state. However, the subdivisions within state agencies are not common among all states. For example, environmental public health programs may be in a different agency than population-based programs. In Illinois, for example, family health programs are in the Illinois Department of Human Services and not in the Illinois Department of Public Health. State health agencies are involved in a range of activities from drinking water regulation; vital statistics and epidemiologic surveillance; food safety; tobacco prevention and control; Women, Infants, and Children (WIC) programs; health professions licensing; health facility regulation; medical and forensic examination; public health laboratories; mental health; drug and alcohol abuse prevention; environmental health and regulation; and Medicaid.

On a day-to-day basis, most of the work of public health professionals is carried out at the local level. It is estimated that there are about 3,200 local health departments in the United States at the regional, district, county, or municipal level. About 60% of these local health departments are county based. The remainder are city-county agencies, multicounty agencies, or some other hybrid. In terms of governance, these entities are either a freestanding part of the local government, a local agency where all staff are part of the state agency, a mixed model with both state and local shared responsibility, a mixed pattern, or, in a few instances, a not-for-profit agency such as a hospital contracting with the local government to manage the public health programs of the jurisdiction. Most local health departments are small organizations. About 70% serve a population of 50,000 or less. More than 80% of these agencies are associated with a local board of health.

In recent years, there has been an initiative to develop an operational definition of a functional local health department. In concert with this activity, there has been an initiative to develop a voluntary national accreditation process for local health departments. Some experts believe that an operational definition may lead to a reduction in the number of local health departments as some smaller programs consolidate with other local agencies or other small agencies into some regionally based model. Regardless of structure or pattern of governance, a functional health department would need to meet certain standards, such as the following:

- Understand the specific health issues confronting the community.
- Investigate health problems and health threats.
- Prevent, minimize, and contain adverse health effects from communicable diseases, disease outbreaks from unsafe food and water, chronic diseases, environmental hazards, injuries, and risky health behaviors.
- Lead planning and response activities for public health emergencies.
- Collaborate with other local responders and with state and federal agencies to intervene in other emergencies with public health significance.
- Implement health promotion programs.
- Engage the community to address public health issues.
- Develop partnerships with public and private healthcare providers and institutions, community-based organizations, and other governmental agencies engaged in services that affect health to collectively identify, alleviate, and act on the sources of public health problems.
- Coordinate the public health system's efforts in an intentionally noncompetitive and nonduplicative manner.
- Address health disparities.
- Serve as an essential resource for local governing bodies and policymakers on up-to-date public health laws and policies.
- Provide science-based, timely, and culturally competent health information and health alerts to the media and the community.
- Provide its expertise to others who treat or address issues of public health significance.
- Ensure compliance with public health laws and ordinances using enforcement authority when appropriate.
- Employ well-trained staff members who have the necessary resources to implement best practices and evidence-based programs and interventions.
- Facilitate research efforts, when approached by researchers, that benefit the community.

- Use and contribute to the evidence base of public health.
- Strategically plan its services and activities, evaluate performance and outcomes, and make adjustments as needed to continually improve its effectiveness, enhance the community's health status, and meet the community's expectations.

These standards are closely allied to the core functions and essential public health services discussed above. These standards can serve as guidelines for the fundamental responsibilities of the local health department. They also will be critical in any agency accreditation process.

Public Health Workforce

The public health workforce is composed of individuals from diverse backgrounds, education, and training in fields including medicine, nursing, psychology, social work, epidemiology, biostatistics, laboratory science, law, public administration, business, economics, pharmacy, veterinary medicine, social sciences, education, and public health. This diversity serves both as strength and a weakness in the definition of public health and in the dimensions of how to carry out the work of public health. The U.S. census reports about 250,000 full-time equivalent health workers employed by local governments. In 2004, there were about 550,000 full-time equivalent workers in the governmental sector at the federal, state, and local levels. In a more recent survey of the public health workforce in local public health departments, it was estimated that there were 160,000 in 2005. Managers and administrators constitute about 6%, nurses 24%, environmental specialists/scientists 10%, clerical staff 27%, health educators 3%, nutritionists 3%, and other designated health professionals such as physicians constitute about 4%; the remaining 23% are uncategorized workers. With regard to physicians, it is estimated that there will be a need for 10,000 more public health physicians in the coming decades than we have now. Currently, there are about 10,000 public health physicians.

It is also estimated that there will be critical shortages of public health nurses, environmental health specialists, health educators, epidemiologists, and information technology (IT) specialists in the future. Since September 11, 2001, there has been an increase in the number of public health workers involved in emergency preparedness and response. As federal funding for these activities declines, it is predicted that there will be some decline in the governmental public health workforce.

Public Health Education Programs

Although there are many individuals in the public health workforce, many have not been specifically trained in public health. Schools of public health and public health programs that are accredited by the Council on Education for Public Health (CEPH) provide academic training in public health. Currently, there are 39 accredited Schools of Public Health and 67 accredited graduate public health programs in the United States. All the schools have curricula that are competency based. A credentialing process has been developed to credential master's of public health (MPH) graduates of the schools and other accredited public health programs. The first credentialing examination was held in the summer of 2008.

There are a number of core competencies that have been developed to demonstrate the skills that are needed for successful public health practice. These competencies include analytic/assessment skills; policy development/program planning skills; community dimensions of practice skills; basic public health sciences skills; communication skills; cultural competency skills; financial planning and management skills; and leadership and systems thinking.

Prior to 2002, five major curriculum content areas were designated as important for public health practice: (1) biostatistics, (2) epidemiology, (3) environmental health sciences, (4) health services administration, and (5) social and behavioral sciences. A number of educational programs also included content on community health and laboratory sciences.

During this first decade of the 21st century, the national Institute of Medicine (IOM) has strongly advocated the addition of a number of other content areas that are critical for public health practice in the new century. They have identified 11 additional content areas: (1) informatics, (2) genomics, (3) communication, (4) cultural competence, (5) community-based participatory research, (6) global health, (7) policy and law, (8) ethics, (9) leadership, (10) public health emergency preparedness, and (11) clinical and community preventive services.

Public Health Emergency Preparedness

Since the terrorist attacks of September 11, 2001, emergency preparedness and response have become major activities for local public health departments. These local entities have significantly increased their ability to address public health emergencies with federal funding from the Centers for Disease Control and Prevention (CDC). Whereas only 20% of local health departments had comprehensive emergency response plans in 2001, more than 90% have such a plan in late 2007. Funding is beginning to be cut, with concern about the ability to maintain this emergency preparedness momentum in the future. About 20% of local health departments hold that they are fully prepared now, and 77% hold that improvements have been made since 2001. Since 2005, funding has declined by almost 30%. With these funding cuts, local public health agencies have had to cut or lay off staff. Workforce training programs have been curtailed as a result. More than 55% of local public health agencies do not think that they can achieve their deliverables within the designated time frames. In addition, local public health agencies are finding it difficult to find and hire emergency preparedness planners, epidemiologists, and nurses. The only positive element has been an increase in funding for pandemic influenza planning. Staff have been redeployed to address this new health priority.

Louis Rowitz

See also American Public Health Association (APHA); Centers for Disease Control and Prevention (CDC); Community-Based Participatory Research (CBPR); Community Health; Community Health Centers (CHCs); Emergency and Disaster Preparedness; Epidemiology; Preventive Care

Further Readings

Aday, Lu Ann, ed. *Reinventing Public Health: Policies and Practices for a Healthy Nation.* San Francisco: Jossey-Bass, 2005.

Institute of Medicine. *The Future of the Public's Health in the 21st Century.* Washington, DC: National Academies Press, 2003.

Institute of Medicine. *Training Physicians for Public Health Careers.* Washington, DC: National Academies Press, 2007.

National Association of County and City Health Officials. *Operational Definition of a Functional Local Health Department.* Washington, DC: National Association of County and City Health Officials, 2005.

National Association of County and City Health Officials. *Federal Funding for Public Health Emergency Preparedness.* Washington, DC: National Association of County and City Health Officials, 2007.

National Association of County and City Health Officials. *Informatics at Local Health Departments.* Washington, DC: National Association of County and City Health Officials, 2007.

National Association of County and City Health Officials. *The Local Health Department Workforce.* Washington, DC: National Association of County and City Health Officials, 2007.

Rowitz, Louis. *Public Health for the 21st Century: The Prepared Leader.* Sudbury, MA: Jones and Bartlett, 2006.

Turnock, Bernard J. *Public Health: What It Is and How It Works.* 3d ed. Sudbury, MA: Jones and Bartlett, 2004.

Web Sites

American Public Health Association (APHA): http://www.apha.org

Association of Schools of Public Health (ASPH): http://www.asph.org

Association of State and Territorial Health Officials (ASTHO): http://www.astho.org

Council on Education for Public Health (CEPH): http://www.ceph.org

National Association of County and City Health Officials (NACCHO): http://www.naccho.org

Trust for America's Health (TFAH): http://www.healthyamericans.org

PUBLIC HEALTH POLICY ADVOCACY

Almost every decision made by policymakers influences public health. Whether a given policy is directly related to healthcare, or whether it indirectly affects human health or the environment, public health advocates must be cognizant of the policy-making process and how to influence that process. Examples of issues affecting public health range from environmental regulation to education policy and from transportation projects to consumer protection. And, of course, key to public health policy analysis are issues involving access, costs, and quality of healthcare.

Developing a Policy Action Plan

To advocate for a public health policy, a policy action plan should be developed. The basic issues for developing such a plan are discussed below.

The "Commodity" of Information

For each issue, information must be collected, analyzed, assimilated, and delivered. A Policy Action Plan should be developed to clearly and concisely provide a strategy for consensus building. Types of information to be collected include data from research-based studies, epidemiological studies, and cost-benefit analyses as well as information about previous policy approaches to addressing the issue from other jurisdictions, and adopted policies. Information about policymakers should also be collected. Who cares most about this issue? Why? Can they assist in advocacy efforts? Advocacy channels are also a key consideration. Is the issue best addressed by legislators, or should relief be sought through administrative routes?

Legislative Branch

Most policy-making venues have both legislative and executive branches. Understanding how to navigate through the policy-making infrastructure is key to effective policy advocacy. On the legislative side, advocates need to familiarize themselves with the bill-making process, committee structures, and individual legislators and their staff. Each jurisdiction has slightly different rules for how a bill becomes law. Key legislative committees will include those relating to healthcare, public health, health disparities, education, justice reform, environment, and transportation, to name a few. Appropriations committees often operate under a different set of rules that may significantly influence how programs are funded and administered.

Executive Branch

On the executive side, policy advocates need to understand the agency structure, the rule-making process, and key administrators. Executive branches at the local, regional, state, and federal level often mirror each other. For instance, at the federal level, the U.S. Department of Health and Human Services (HHS) houses most of the key public health and healthcare agencies, including the Centers for Disease Control and Prevention (CDC) and the National Institutes of Health (NIH). At the same time, most federal funding flows through state departments of health and human services, which have subagencies for each relevant funding stream.

The administrative rulemaking process determines how funds flow to various agencies and the rules under which those funds will be distributed. At the federal level, information on the rulemaking process is found in the *Federal Register*. Typically, each state's administrative code can be accessed through the state's official Web site. While many localities also house their ordinances and local rules online, advocates may be required to make the trip to city hall to obtain a copy of relevant regulations.

Identifying Stakeholders

Effective public health policy advocacy must include an analysis of the various stakeholders. The inquiry should begin by identifying the proper venue for advocacy. Is the issue best addressed at the local, state, country, or international level? For example, if the issue concerns children's health in

school, it may be best to seek out solutions at the local school level. If the issue concerns county health departments, it may be most effective to advocate the issue with the proper county policymakers. An effective advocate will determine which local or regional policymakers chair the relevant committees, which ones are passionate about the topic, which ones have direct experience with the topic, and so on. The same analysis holds true with issues at the state, federal, and international levels.

Identifying external stakeholders is another important exercise that policy advocates must undertake. What constituency and interest groups will support or oppose the initiative? Which organizations will take a lead role in assisting in advocacy efforts? Other external stakeholders, including private-sector organizations such as hospitals, healthcare systems, insurance companies, and pharmaceutical companies, should also be catalogued as potential advocacy channels. Which organizations' Web pages, newsletters, or events can be used for advocacy? Advocates should also research private funders, including nonprofit foundations and corporate foundations, to determine opportunities to leverage funding.

Delivering Information/Direct Advocacy Channels

Often, advocates have opportunities to discuss their issue directly with policymakers. A single meeting, if handled correctly, can have a tremendous impact on the policy-making process. Direct advocacy channels range from formal meetings to happenstance encounters at, say, the pharmacy. Most often, formal meetings can occur in an elected policymaker's capital or district office. Careful consideration should be given to where the meeting occurs and who attends. Elected policymakers are often passionate about public health issues and can easily be approached to discuss a specific issue. Most direct advocacy opportunities, however, will occur in a short meeting; advocates must be well prepared to maximize the contact.

Formal and informal meetings with administrative policymakers are an often overlooked opportunity for effective issue advocacy. Regulators are generally well informed about the intricacies of the policy-making process as well as the complexities of implementing policies on particular issues. Establishing relationships with regulators can provide unmatched advocacy opportunities, particularly when the individual has a direct interest in the issue or where the affected agency has the issue as a core competency.

Advocacy Tools

In addition to direct contact with policymakers, advocates deliver information in various written formats. The most widely used written document is a fact sheet—a one-page summary of the issue, recommended action, and rationale for the proposed action. Fact sheets should also include a messaging component as well as a clearly articulated summary of the request. Other written advocacy tools include issue papers, correspondence, letters to the editor, brochures, and Web pages, to name a few. Policymakers pay significant attention to handwritten letters from their constituents. Other types of letters include form letters signed by individuals and those listing supporting organizations. In addition to written communications, advocates sometimes use messaging tools such as pins and bumper stickers.

Future Implications

To be most effective, public health policy advocates should carefully map out a policy action plan for each issue. Methods for collecting, analyzing, assimilating, and delivering relevant information to policymakers at the local, regional, state, national, and international levels should be carefully considered. Tools for advocacy should include face-to-face meetings as well as written communication. Meetings should be short, and written documents should be clear and concise. Without question, public health policy advocates can influence the policy-making process on significant issues relating to healthcare, health disparities, and the environment, among others.

William C. Kling

See also Equity, Efficiency, and Effectiveness in Healthcare; Forces Changing Healthcare; Healthcare Reform; Health Disparities; Public Health; Public Policy; Regulation

Further Readings

Bodenheimer, Thomas S., and Kevin Grumbach. *Understanding Health Policy: A Clinical Approach.* 3d ed. New York: McGraw-Hill, 2002.

Dye, Thomas R. *Understanding Public Policy.* 12th ed. New York: Prentice Hall, 2007.

Longest, Jr., Beaufort B. *Health Policymaking in the United States.* 4th ed. Chicago: Health Administration Press, 2006.

Teitelbaum, Joel B., and Sara E. Wilensky. *Essentials of Public Health Law and Policy.* Sudbury, MA: Jones and Bartlett, 2007.

Web Sites

American Public Health Association (APHA): http://www.apha.org

Henry J. Kaiser Family Foundation (KFF): http://www.kff.org

National Association for Public Health Policy (NAPHP): http://www.naphp.org

PUBLIC POLICY

Public policy represents the codification of mainstream values. Policy comes in the form of legislation, regulation, executive decisions, budget allocations, and court decisions. Public policy represents the official direction or pronouncement of governmental institutions (the legislature, executive, or judicial branches) on a particular subject or issue. In the United States, public policy is promulgated at the federal, state, and local levels of government by elected and appointed officials. As mainstream values change over time, so does public policy. This change may be the result of elections, interpretations of the courts concerning legislation, lobbying, or public opinion. Policy represents the product of a priority-setting process. Public policy in the area of healthcare, therefore, represents the official decisions of government on access, allocation of resources, delivery, financing, and organization of healthcare services.

Basic Premises

In the United States, the basic value at the foundation of public policy concerning healthcare is that healthcare is not a legal right of citizenship. Instead, healthcare is considered to be a privilege usually associated with a benefit of employment. Only for those 65 years of age or older and those with very low incomes has the nation created a legal entitlement to health insurance coverage, thus establishing a right to healthcare for these citizens.

The basic model is that healthcare is an individual, private responsibility for all those in the age range of 18 to 65 whose incomes do not fall below the poverty line and who are not disabled, veterans, American Indians, or Alaska Natives.

The U.S. healthcare system stands out in two other ways, which also reflect mainstream values. The first is that it devotes the largest share of its gross domestic product (GDP) to healthcare in contrast to other developed nations. In the middle of the 20th century, less than 5% of its GDP was devoted to healthcare. That percentage rose to nearly 14% by the end of the century. Yet the system does not necessarily produce superior health outcomes (e.g., low infant morality or greater life expectancy). The second unique feature of the U.S. healthcare system is that it is not based on some form of universal healthcare. The system relies, for the most part, on private healthcare providers with a mix of private and public insurance as well as extensive government regulatory intervention.

Policy-Making Process

Policy is the product of a process consisting of the following stages: (a) problem definition; (b) formulating options for consideration; (c) debate and deliberation over the available options; (d) adoption of a particular option; (e) implementation of the selected option, including appropriation of resources to support the option; and (f) assessment or evaluation. This process may vary depending on which political institution or level of government is involved.

Legal and Regulatory Foundations

Much of public policy since World War II in the healthcare area can be traced to changes in laws and regulations related to healthcare. These policies relate to access, financing, organization, and service delivery. Taken together, these laws and regulations represent public policy in American healthcare.

Hospital Expansion

After World War II, President Truman assigned a high priority to health insurance. He built on the proposals developed in 1938 and included the following components: expansion of hospitals, increased support for public health, support for maternal and child health services, increased federal support for medical research and education, and, most significantly, a single health insurance program to provide coverage for all segments of society. These reforms were defeated for the same reasons and by the same coalition that had defeated these kinds of proposals in the past.

It was, however, during the Truman Administration that part of his vision was realized: the expansion of hospitals. The U.S. Congress passed the Hospital Survey and Construction Act, also known as the Hill-Burton Act of 1946, which provided for $1 dollar of federal funds for every $2 spent by states in the construction of community-based hospitals.

With the defeat of the various proposals for universal health insurance coverage between 1915 and 1946, the post–World War II era in healthcare was characterized by an expansion of Blue Cross and Blue Shield and other commercial insurance products as well as an increase in prepaid, direct service plans, such as the one developed by Henry Kaiser.

Medicare and Medicaid

With the passage of the Title XVIII (Medicare) and Title XIX (Medicaid) amendments to the Social Security Act in 1965, the role of the federal government was fundamentally changed. These programs represented a major change in the government's approach to the design, financing, and delivery of healthcare. As part of the New Frontier, President Kennedy had flirted with the reintroduction of a national health insurance proposal. President Johnson, subsequently, succeeded in the enactment of Medicare, which provided an entitlement to every citizen who reached the age of 65. Part A of the Medicare program (i.e., reimbursement for inpatient, hospital-based treatment) was mandated, and Part B (i.e., outpatient care and reimbursement for physicians) was to be voluntary. Between 1965 and 1985, Medicare helped restructure financing and reimbursement policies for all the American healthcare system and not just for this particular program, because private insurance companies adopted reimbursement policies that were indexed to Medicare.

Medicaid represented a federal-state partnership to provide medical services to low-income individuals who meet the eligibility criteria. The theory behind Medicaid was that eligible individuals should be given the buying power in the healthcare marketplace that would provide free choice of providers and open-ended reimbursement, based on reasonable costs and fee-for-service, for noninstitutional providers. The statute also provided nonhospital providers with the choice to accept or reject Medicaid patients. The program provided for a core minimum set of services that all states must provide and a second set of services that states had the option to provide.

Health Maintenance Organization Act

Subsequent to Medicare and Medicaid, the U.S. Congress enacted the Health Maintenance Organization (HMO) Act of 1973. This statute represented a new approach in federal healthcare policy: It was an attempt to gain control over healthcare pricing by encouraging the development of fully integrated healthcare organizations that imposed vertical controls on the cost of services furnished to their member providers. Congress envisioned that 1,700 HMOs would be developed by 1976, but only a fraction of that number was ultimately developed. This innovative legislation, proposed by the Nixon Administration, foresaw a trend in American healthcare that would ultimately become quite popular in the 1990s. In 1988, for example only 25% of those with employer-based insurance were enrolled in managed-care plans; by 1997, the number increased to 80%.

Emergency Medical Treatment and Active Labor Act

Federal involvement in healthcare was augmented in 1986 with the enactment of the Emergency Medical Treatment and Active Labor Act (EMTALA). This statute was a response to the growing problem of access to healthcare in the United States. This law was also in response to what appeared to be a grow-

ing trend of hospitals not providing treatment to those who could not afford to pay for the services they were receiving. EMTALA requires hospitals that are receiving any Medicare revenues (which includes almost all the hospitals in the nation) to provide treatment to all patients seeking care for emergency medical conditions regardless of the ability to pay and regardless of their eligibility for Medicare. The statute requires hospitals to provide patients with "appropriate medical screening," and patients must also be stabilized, before they can be transferred to another facility.

At approximately the same time, there was increasing concern in the public and private sector alike over the rising costs of healthcare and more intensive skepticism over the effectiveness of the traditional fee-for-service system. This system was considered to be user-friendly, allowing for flexibility and discretion for providers and patients alike. However, it did not seem that it could control costs. Health insurance premium increases, for example, of 15% to 20% per year were commonplace in the mid- to late 1980s. In 1990, when employer-sponsored group insurance premiums increased "by only 14%," this was considered to be good news, because they had risen by 24% in the previous year. This inability to control cost increases was considered to be the fatal flaw of the fee-for-service system.

This indictment led to the increased popularity of managed-care arrangements. The term *managed care* encompasses a broad range of healthcare organizational arrangements that are intended to eliminate unnecessary and inappropriate care and to reduce costs. The basic theory of managed care is to control costs by restricting access and services while maintaining quality. The basic features of managed care include contractual arrangements with selected providers to furnish a comprehensive set of healthcare services to its members, significant financial incentives to steer patients toward providers and treatments/medical procedures within the plan, and ongoing accountability of providers for their clinical and financial performance through formal quality assurance and utilization review. A central feature of managed care is the use of a limited number of providers who are selected on the basis of their clinical-practice patterns and specialty and their acceptance of financial incentives for cost conscious utilization of resources.

These managed-care arrangements allow for the provision and financing of healthcare in a structure substantially different from the accepted fee-for-service arrangement, and they enable managed-care organizations to take an active role in monitoring and controlling the amount and type of services provided to patients by physicians and other caregivers. They differ in the amount of financial risk that the managed-care organizations assume, the way they share risk with providers, the restrictiveness of the provider policies, and the level of out-of-pocket costs that the beneficiaries bear.

Health Security Act

With the growing concern over costs, the critique of the fee-for-service system, and the growing popularity of managed care, healthcare became a campaign issue in the 1992 presidential race. Following his election, President Clinton introduced a comprehensive proposal (Health Security Act [HSA] of 1993) to reform the American healthcare system. The proposed legislation began with the premise that healthcare was a legal right for all citizens. This act envisioned universal access to healthcare for all citizens. It used principles of managed competition to increase access and quality of healthcare at the same time. The plan was to restructure the financing and delivery of services through providing incentives to private insurance companies, enabling the formation of small groups and purchasing cooperatives, and by increasing the role of government in providing access and services, as required. During this same time period, at least 10 alternative proposals to reform the nation's healthcare system were introduced by members of the U.S. Congress. None of these proposals, including the HSA, were adopted.

Health Insurance Portability and Accountability Act

The debate over Clinton's proposed health plan, did, however, highlight some of the problems of the nation's healthcare system. This recognition led to the adoption of the Health Insurance Portability and Accountability Act (HIPAA) of 1996. HIPAA provides for continued health insurance coverage for individuals who might otherwise lose their coverage as part of a group plan (e.g., for leaving one job to accept another). It also bars exclusionary practices of insurance companies that are designed to deny coverage to individuals who are bad risks because of preexisting medical conditions.

Employee Retirement Income Security Act

State government has traditionally held the right to regulate the insurance industry. Insurance law, certification, and licensing requirements have provided states with a measure of control over the healthcare industry. However, in 1974, the U.S. Congress passed the Employee Retirement Income Security Act (ERISA), a comprehensive, uniform national system for employee benefit plans, which mandated inclusion of healthcare benefits. ERISA provisions have resulted in preemption of state initiatives, especially those oriented at universal coverage provided through employer mandates. In addition, ERISA has often been interpreted by the federal courts to preempt virtually all of the vast body of state insurance, contracts, and other laws or regulations applicable to healthcare plans.

As already indicated, the focus of healthcare policy and law since 1930 has been containment of healthcare expenditures. Cost containment efforts have led to a transformation in the organization and financing of the American healthcare system, with the government-financed Medicare program serving as a standard for reimbursement. However, neither the cost-containment initiatives nor the new programmatic statutes such as EMTALA or HIPAA have addressed what many employers, consumers, and third-party payers consider to be the major flaws with the traditional fee-for-service system. This has led to the growing acceptance of managed care.

National data suggest that managed-care organizations are substantially more efficient than indemnity plans in controlling costs. The average premiums paid for by employers for health benefits decreased substantially between 1989 and 1999. Health insurance premiums began to increase again over the past several years. It could be argued that these rate increases are linked to the negative impact of regulation on managed care. In 1989, the average premium increase per year was 18%, and by 1996 it was only 1%. The sweeping changes in the organization and financing of the healthcare system can be attributed to the spread of managed care.

However, the growing reliance on managed care in the private marketplace and in Medicaid programs was also accompanied by consumer and provider dissatisfaction with these new financing, administrative, and organizational arrangements. Providers and consumers have advocated for a larger panel of providers in managed-care networks and less restrictiveness on stepping outside the network to obtain reimbursable medical services from nonnetwork providers. Consumers are looking for less restricted access to providers than they have in many managed-care plans. Providers, being shut out of selective contracting and fearing loss of income from the closed panels of managed-care organizations, are advocating for unrestricted access for patients. Providers are also demanding that the administrators of these organizations remove themselves from, in effect, making therapeutic decisions that result from financing decisions. For example, providers and consumers alike strongly object to so-called gag clauses, which prevent providers from informing patients about treatment options that the managed-care plan does not cover; to policies that limit hospital stays for childbirth; and to restrictions on patients' rights to sue managed-care organizations for denial of needed care.

In response to the growing criticisms of managed care by providers and consumers and the increasingly adverse coverage of managed care by the popular press, state legislatures and the U.S. Congress began to respond with a regulatory strategy. Since the defeat of the Clinton healthcare reform proposal, states have taken the lead in enacting a set of laws limiting the flexibility of managed-care organizations in their contracting for and delivery of services.

The specific features of managed-care regulation vary from state to state, but the types of regulation can be divided into two categories: (1) laws that regulate the relationship between managed-care organizations and healthcare providers and (2) laws that regulate the relationship between managed-care organizations and healthcare consumers.

Laws that regulate the relationship between managed-care organizations and healthcare providers affect how the organizations select, deselect, compensate, and control the physicians whom they employ directly or contract with to provide healthcare. These include laws that limit the ability of managed-care plans to direct the flow of patients to specific providers, prohibit contracts between managed-care plans and provisions that establish exclusive relationships (contracts that do not permit providers to sign contracts with other managed-care plans), and mandate that any provider willing to meet the price terms of the health plan must be accepted into the network—the so-called Any Willing Provider legislation (statutes that stipulate that any provider who meets the criteria for inclusion in a managed-care organization's network must be given the opportunity to join the managed-care organization); at least 14 states have enacted comprehensive Any Willing Provider laws, and another 14 states have enacted more limited versions of these laws.

Proposed laws that regulate the relationship between managed-care organizations and healthcare consumers include legislation that would allow patients direct access to specialists without a referral (the so-called direct access laws), which mandates a minimum stay in hospitals for births and other procedures, and that allows enrollees to sue managed-care organizations for refusing necessary treatment.

The commonality between these various forms of managed-care regulation is that they all focus on issues of cost and access. A central feature of managed care's ability to restrain the rapid rise of healthcare costs is its restriction on access and choice. Managed care restricts access through the use of a limited number of providers who are selected to be part of the plan and through the use of financial incentives to steer patients to providers who are part of this plan. Elimination or restraint of either of these features significantly affects the ability of the managed-care organization to control costs. Issues of increased access to a broad set of providers and, hence, increased choice and cost control appear to be mutually exclusive if one is trying to adhere to principles of managed care.

The plethora of anti-managed-care regulations put forward appears to be a disjointed attempt by state legislators to satisfy disgruntled constituencies by violating the fundamental principles of managed care that can make it successful. The continued pressure on state legislatures to respond to constituent pressure for relief from managed-care restrictions is not the only issue healthcare reformers will face in the future. Insurance premium costs are increasing after several years of slow or flat growth. It could be argued that these rate increases are linked to the negative impact of regulation on managed care. While managed-care penetration into the healthcare market increased in the 1990s, will rising costs cause employers to discontinue healthcare coverage for their employees or shift ever-larger portions of healthcare costs onto them? Growing numbers of healthcare purchasers are opting to move into self-insured plans; this is done, in part, to avoid state regulation. Self-insurance plans "protect" employers from state regulation because of the ERISA preemption.

State Policy

Public policy in the arena of healthcare has not only been formulated at the national level, but there also have been policies promulgated in the states. In the past decade or so, the majority of states have passed legislation regulating the issuance, content, and pricing of private group health insurance plans. The purpose of this legislation is to increase the number of insured persons by expanding and securing coverage and to ensure that those who are sick receive the appropriate care. A variety of factors have motivated these laws. One prominent reason for states' aggressive regulation of the private health insurance market was the large number of uninsured individuals who were employed. In 1987, prior to the implementation of many of the regulations, there were 23 million uninsured individuals between the ages of 18 and 64, many of whom were employed. Moreover, there was a significant increase in the number of uninsured workers in small firms during the latter half of the 1980s. Many believe that insurance industry practices such as experience rating and redlining (i.e., refusing to sell insurance to firms deemed high risk) were major reasons that workers in small firms accounted for one out of every two uninsured workers. In response, many states limited these practices through legislation collectively referred to as small group reform.

The other major type of state (and federal) regulation is mandated health insurance benefits, regulation that requires that all group insurance plans pay for certain medical procedures and/or providers. These reforms have a longer history than small group insurance reform. They initially arose as a

response to lobbying pressures by provider groups and as a way to address possible market failures, but recent mandates have been primarily motivated by the rise of managed-care organizations. Regulation of the content of insurance plans is an attempt to counter managed-care organizations' efforts to limit utilization. To ensure that people still receive appropriate care, states have specified the types of treatments and kinds of providers an insurance plan must cover. An example of such a mandate is minimum maternity hospital stays. The popularity of mandated benefits has grown dramatically over time. In the first 6 months of 1997 alone, more than 600 new state health insurance benefit mandates were introduced across the nation.

Future Implications

There have been debates over healthcare reform in the United States since the Progressive Era. However, large-scale reform has not been achieved. Future policy deliberations will need to address some fundamental tensions, such as balancing the need for cost containment while providing access to the growing number of uninsured individuals. They will also need to address many questions, such as the following: Can increased access be achieved without introducing mandates for employers or individuals? With increasing life expectancy, how can the costs of Medicare be brought under control? Will the United States ever commit itself to providing healthcare as a right of citizenship?

Robert F. Rich

See also Access to Healthcare; Cost of Healthcare; Healthcare Reform; Health Insurance; Medicaid; Medicare; National Health Insurance; Regulation

Further Readings

Barr, Donald A. *Introduction to U.S. Health Policy: The Organization, Financing, and Delivery of Health Care in America.* 2d ed. Baltimore: Johns Hopkins University Press, 2007.

Feldstein, Paul J. *Health Policy Issues: An Economic Perspective.* 4th ed. Chicago: Health Administration Press, 2007.

Longest, Beaufort B. *Health Policymaking in the United States.* 4th ed. Chicago: Health Administration Press, 2006.

Luft, Harold S. *Total Care: The Antidote to the Health Care Crisis*. Cambridge, MA: Harvard University Press, 2008.

Schoeni, Robert F., ed. *Making Americans Healthier: Social and Economic Policy as Health Policy*. New York: Russell Sage Foundation, 2008.

Teitelbaum, Joel B., and Sara E. Wilensky, eds. *Essential Readings in Health Policy and Law*. Sudbury, MA: Jones and Bartlett, 2009.

Web Sites

AARP: http://www.aarp.org

Brookings Institution: http://www.brookings.edu

Commonwealth Fund: http://www.commonwealthfund.org

Congressional Budget Office (CBO): http://www.cbo.gov

Henry J. Kaiser Family Foundation (KFF): http://www.kff.org

RAND Corporation: http://www.rand.org

Urban Institute: http://www.urban.org

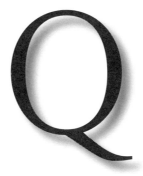

QUALITY-ADJUSTED LIFE YEARS (QALYS)

A quality-adjusted life year (QALY) is an outcome measurement of health over time related to a disease or condition under study. The quality of life can be determined by using various tools to measure the preference toward a health state of the general public or of a specific individual or group in a certain state of disease or wellness. This measure of the quality of life in each health state is multiplied by the time spent in each health state to obtain the QALY. The QALY is not just a measure of life years but also a measure of the quality of health in each of those years, therefore a measurement of both morbidity and mortality. A QALY will be equal to or less than the total number of life years studied.

Calculation Methods

A QALY can be calculated in several ways using various methods. The quality of life can be measured using preference scales to implicitly rate the quality of health experienced by either individuals or the public in general. These tools can be either based on general attitudes or disease specific. Preference scales commonly used are the Visual Analog Scales (VASs), or feeling thermometers, the Standard Gamble (SG), and the Time Trade Off (TTO) preferences. The use of preference scales allows for the measurement of the quality of health from the perspective of the individuals toward whom the health system is directed.

The VASs use number or category rating scales, marked or unmarked line scales, or combinations of either. While the scales vary, the final measure is transformed into a scale of 0 to 1, where 0 is *dead* and 1 is *perfect health*. The individual is presented with two choices: One is treatment, which may result in a chronic health state leading to either a better state or immediate death; the other is no treatment, therefore remaining in a chronic health state leading to death. The assumption is that the life years are longer in the treatment state. This tool could also be used with temporary health states that do not lead to death. One such scale is the Health Related Quality of Life Scale (HQRL). The HQRL uses a vertical scale, analogous to a thermometer, from 0 to 1, 10 divisions between each integer, with 0 being *dead* and 1 being *perfect health*. The subjects are asked to indicate where on the scale they feel the quality of their health lies. Another published scale using preference scores is the Quality of Well-Being Scale (QWB). The preference scores can be plotted on the vertical axis of a graph against the time spent in each score or health state with time on the horizontal axis. Integrating the area under the plotted curve is a measure of the total QALY.

The SG method measures preferences for chronic states by presenting the subject with a choice between treatment, leading to either a healthy state or death, and no treatment, resulting in a continued chronic state until death, much like the VASs. However, the time in each state, if listed as a probability, can be altered to determine the subject's preference. SG techniques are offered by direct interview, paper, or computerized questionnaires. Any of these can be enhanced with visual aides. Variations for temporary health states can accommodate conditions not having a fatal outcome. Examples of tools incorporating SG are the Short-Form-6D and the Health Utility Index (HUI), both of which were generated from general public preferences.

The TTO method is used by the EuroQoL Group (an organization initiated in Europe to develop a common instrument for describing and assessing health and quality of life) and is similar to the SG. In this method, subjects choose between living in a certain chronic state until death and a healthy state of shorter duration until death. Or for temporary states, the subject can choose between a poor health state or one that is worse but with treatment leading to a better state. The time spent in each state can be adjusted until the subject feels about the same toward each.

Other methods include the Rosser Index and the Person Trade-Off (PTO), which is basically a TTO with the trade-off considered for others rather than oneself.

QALY measures do not look at the monetary cost of arriving at a particular state of health quality but are used in cost-effectiveness and cost-utility analyses to determine the ratio of cost to outcome or cost per QALY. In these analyses, the cost per unit of health can be measured in several ways, one of which is the cost per life year gained. When choosing an instrument to measure QALY, consideration must be given to the population used in developing the tool. Attempting a pilot test prior to choosing, or using several tools may be advisable. The resulting cost-effectiveness or cost-utility analysis may vary greatly depending on the method used to evaluate the quality of life. A thorough analysis using several methods could yield results better suited for economic evaluations. The use of QALYs is also recommended to facilitate comparisons across studies for various medical and healthcare interventions. On the individual scale, a small improvement in health over many years may yield the same QALYs as a large benefit over only a few years. Similarly on the societal level, a small improvement for many people may equal a large benefit for a few individuals.

When calculating QALYs into the future, discounting of future benefits or health states can be done to gain the relative weight in the current year. With escalating healthcare costs, increasing emphasis is placed on government and private control measures, individual contributions, and universal coverage. Developing decision models using cost per QALY comparisons could assist in public and private policy-making decisions on the allocation of resources. A limitation is the long-term observation period required for the analysis of newer treatments. The ongoing collection of data sets and league tables listing costs per QALY, available in public registries, lends convenient access for such purposes.

Ann L. Viernes

See also Cost-Benefit and Cost-Effectiveness Analyses; Health Economics; Measurement in Health Services Research; Mortality; Quality of Healthcare; Rationing Healthcare; Short-Form Health Surveys (SF-36, -12, -8); Williams, Alan H.

Further Readings

Bell, Chaim M., Richard H. Chapman, Patricia W. Stone, et al. "A Comprehensive Catalog of Preference Scores from Published Cost-Utility Analyses," *Medical Decision Making* 21(4): 208–215, 2001.

Bowling, Ann. *Measuring Health: A Review of Quality of Life Measurement Scales.* 2d ed. Philadelphia: Open University, 1997.

Drummond, M. F., M. J. Sculpher, G. W. Torrance, et al. *Methods for the Economic Evaluation of Health Care Programmes.* 3d ed. Oxford, UK: Oxford University Press, 2005.

McDowell, Ian. *Measuring Health: A Guide to Rating Scales and Questionnaires.* 3d ed. New York: Oxford University Press, 2006.

Raisch, D. W. "Understanding Quality-Adjusted Life Years and Their Application to Pharmacoeconomic Research," *Annals of Pharmacotherapy* 34(7): 906–914, 2000.

Web Sites

Cost-Effectiveness Registry: https://research.tufts-nemc.org/cear/default.aspx
EuroQoL Group: http://www.euroqol.org

QUALITY ENHANCEMENT RESEARCH INITIATIVE (QUERI) OF THE VETERANS HEALTH ADMINISTRATION (VHA)

The Quality Enhancement Research Initiative (QUERI) of the Veterans Health Administration (VHA) is a multidisciplinary, data-driven, quality improvement program designed to ensure excellence in all places where VHA provides healthcare services, including inpatient, outpatient, and long-term care settings. QUERI aims to identify best practices, systematize their use, and provide the feedback necessary to maintain ongoing improvement. The National Academy of Sciences, Institute of Medicine's (IOM) seminal report *Crossing the Quality Chasm* (2001) identified QUERI as one of the nation's best examples of synthesizing the medical evidence base and applying it to clinical care.

The VHA is the healthcare delivery system for the U.S. Department of Veterans Affairs. It runs many hospitals, outpatient clinics, and long-term care facilities. One of the main offices of the VHA is the Office of Research and Development (ORD). QUERI is based within the Health Service Research and Development Service of ORD. From its onset in 1998, QUERI has been fully integrated into the VHA's strategic framework for quality management. Being within the VHA, with its central management and centralized database that is used by all its facilities, the clinicians and researchers associated with QUERI have the unique opportunity of putting their research findings into practice.

Organization

QUERI is organized into three parts: QUERI centers, a Research and Methodology Committee, and a National Advisory Council (NAC).

QUERI brings together VHA's Health Services Research and Development researchers and VHA's clinicians and administrators and provides them the unique opportunity to transfer research findings into patientwide and systemwide improvements. QUERI centers currently focus on nine conditions that are prevalent and high risk among veterans: chronic heart failure, diabetes, HIV/hepatitis, ischemic health disease, mental health, polytrauma and blast-related injuries, spinal cord injury, stroke, and substance use disorders. Each QUERI center consists of a research and clinical coordinator and a 15-member executive committee that includes researchers and clinicians with expertise in specific areas for each center from around the country.

The Research and Methodology Committee serves as the oversight committee for the entire QUERI process. It is composed of VHA senior researchers, clinicians, and policymakers. It meets semiannually to evaluate the performance of each QUERI center by reviewing their research methods, plans, and projects. It approves requests for solicitations, and it ensures that the QUERI process is being followed by each center.

The NAC is composed of senior VHA policy leaders from the U.S. Department of Veterans Affairs' (VAs') central office in Washington, D.C. It provides general policy guidance and direction, and it ensures that QUERI is integrated into the VHA's operational policies and structure.

Process

The specific activities of the QUERI centers follow a standard process or sequence of activities that were specified at the time the centers were established. Through literature reviews and experience, six steps were identified as necessary to systematizing quality improvement in the VHA. The six steps are discussed below.

Step 1: Identify conditions associated with high risk of disease and/or disability and/or burden of illness for veterans. The QUERI leadership chose the conditions. Most of the conditions chosen were high volume and among the most common discharge diagnoses in the VHA. For two of the conditions, spinal cord injury and HIV/AIDS, the VHA is the nation's largest provider of care. The individual QUERI executive committees could choose to concentrate on specific high-priority subtopics within their condition. This was done with the approval of the QUERI leadership.

Step 2: Identify best practices. Following the identification of the disease or condition, each QUERI group identified evidence-based best-practice recommendations and processes. For many of the QUERI conditions, a range of systematic reviews, evidence-based clinical practice guidelines, and other clinical recommendations were already available for review, refinement, and implementation. In some areas, evidence-based clinical practice guidelines were unavailable. In these cases, each QUERI center was expected to do literature reviews, evaluate care models, and use other best-practice programs. If necessary, the QUERI centers were to initiate their own research to close existing gaps in knowledge and practice. They were also encouraged to work with VHA's National Clinical Practice Guideline Council to facilitate the development of new evidence-based guidelines.

Step 3: Define existing practice patterns and outcomes across VHA and current variation from best practice. Following the identification of evidence-based best practices, each QUERI center conducted research to document and assess current VHA practice patterns and identify gaps and shortcomings in VHA policies, clinical practices, and outcomes. The VHA's national database greatly expedited this process. This process identified opportunities for improvement. Where VHA databases did not allow the collection of such data, the QUERI centers worked with VHA to refine and develop such data or tools.

Step 4: Identify and implement interventions to promote best practices. Following completion of Step 3 (which included data collection and analysis activities and the identification of important performance variations and gaps), each QUERI center worked to diagnose the cause of documented performance problems and to identify and implement programs and strategies to improve healthcare quality and outcomes. In areas where published literature provided evidence regarding promising strategies, the QUERI centers worked to adapt and implement the established strategies. In areas where such guidance was not available, the QUERI researchers designed new strategies. The specific interventions and projects conducted in Step 4 included (1) efforts to translate clinical research findings and recommendations into routine clinical practice through refinements and reorganization of clinical-practice systems and processes and (2) efforts to translate successful facility-level programs into systemwide policies and practices.

Since the field of translation research is relatively new, several coordinated efforts were launched to support and encourage the investigators associated with the QUERI centers. These included special funding and solicitations, a separate scientific review board with experience to review grant proposals from the QUERI centers, annual conferences to examine methods and processes of quality improvement and strategies for organizational behavioral change in healthcare delivery, translation consultants identified and made available to the QUERI centers, and supplemental funding made available to each QUERI center to hire dedicated translation experts (with formal training and experience in individual and organizational behavior change and quality improvement). Each QUERI center was responsible for having a plan outlining where in the six steps it was for each condition or subtopic and a separate translation plan. These plans were updated annually and reviewed by the Research and Methodology Committee.

Step 5: Document that best practices improve outcomes. An important feature of the QUERI process and a critical element in its success is its focus on measurement and improvement in patient and system outcomes. If QUERI was to promote sustained quality improvement and attain support from VHA patients, staff, managers, and external stakeholders (e.g., the U.S. Congress), it must demonstrate continued improvement in patient care and systems outcomes. Although process and structure data were also needed, outcome measurement was prioritized. Outcomes were generally measured in QUERI through a diverse set of tools and sources, including VHA's computerized data and surveys of patients, their caregivers, and VHA clinicians. Together, these sources provided a comprehensive assessment of relevant patient and system outcomes, ensuring value and helping to further refine the QUERI quality enhancement programs and other interventions implemented in Step 4. Outcomes of interest typically included mortality, morbidity, functional status, health-related quality of life (HRQOL), access, utilization, costs, and patient satisfaction. In circumstances where valid outcome measures did not exist, studies were proposed in the strategic plan, which was then reviewed, by the Research and Methodology Committee. Where appropriate, risk-adjusted models were also developed and tested. Finally, the development of relevant feedback mechanisms was encouraged.

Step 6: Document that outcomes are associated with improved HRQOL. The final QUERI step was to link practices with improved HRQOL, functional status, and patient satisfaction. Although patient outcomes were addressed in Step 5 of the QUERI process, HRQOL measures are so important and so often neglected that they were emphasized separately in the QUERI process. Separating HRQOL in Step 6 ensured that QUERI projects emphasize this critical outcome and that adequate attention be given to its measurement and improvement.

Progress and Results

Several of the QUERI centers have already demonstrated improved patient outcomes. For example, the chronic health failure QUERI implemented a multifaceted intervention to improve the patient's outcomes and to reduce the length of stay and readmission rates, by using coordinated case management, patient education, and related tools. They have shown a significant decrease in 14-day readmission rates (from 14.2% to 4.8%) and increased patient stability on discharge and at the first outpatient visit.

The diabetes QUERI designed interventions to increase clinician awareness of diabetic-patient risk factors and to increase use of aggressive appropriate therapy. Impacts include increased provider awareness of the importance of blood pressure control and significant improvements in controlled blood pressure, lipids, and glycosylated hemoglobin (HA1c). This has led to decreasing cardiovascular events and death.

The spinal cord injury QUERI has targeted influenza vaccination of its patients. This led to a VHA-wide policy to identify and target spinal cord injury patients as a high-risk, high-priority group for flu vaccination. As a result of the policy, vaccination rates improved from 26% in the late 1990s to 74% for influenza and 89% for pneumonia in 2007.

The mental health QUERI has facilitated the spread of collaborative care for depression in VA primary-care settings.

The ischemic heart disease QUERI has implemented computerized decision support for treatment of hypertension.

In addition to the accomplishments of each QUERI center, the leadership of QUERI recognized the need to advance the field of implementation by promoting the sharing of insights and results among scientific peers. To accomplish this, it recently participated in the establishment of an online reviewed journal focused on implementation science.

John G. Demakis

See also Clinical Practice Guidelines; Evidence-Based Medicine(EBM); Health Services Research at the Veterans Health Administration (VHA); Quality of Healthcare; Quality of Life, Health-Related; Satisfaction Surveys; Structure-Process-Outcome Quality Measures; U.S. Department of Veterans Affairs (VA)

Further Readings

Asch, Steven M., Elizabeth A. McGlynn, Mary M. Hogan, et al. "Comparison of Quality of Care for Patients in the Veterans Health Administration and Patients in a National Sample," *Annals of Internal Medicine* 14(12): 938–45, December 2004.

Committee on Quality of Health Care in America, Institute of Medicine. *Crossing the Quality Chasm: A New Health System for the 21st Century.* Washington, DC: National Academy Press, 2001.

Demakis, John G., Lynn McQueen, Kenneth W. Kizer, et al. "Quality Enhancement Research Initiative (QUERI): Collaboration Between Research and Clinical Practice," *Medical Care* 38(6 Suppl. 1): 117–25, June 2000

Francis, Joseph, and Jonathan B. Perlin. "Improving Performance Through Knowledge Translation in the Veterans Health Administration," *Journal of Continuing Education in the Health Profession* 26(1): 63–71, 2006.

Hagedorn, Hildi, Mary Hogan, Jeffery Smith, et al. "Lessons Learned about Implementing Research Evidence Into Clinical Practice: Experiences from the VA QUERI," *Journal of General Internal Medicine* 21(Suppl. 2): S21–S24, February 2006.

McQueen, Lynn, Brian S. Mittman, and John G. Demakis. "Overview of the Veterans Health Administration (VHA) Quality Enhancement Research Initiative (QUERI)," *Journal of the American Informatics Association* 11(5): 339–43, September–October 2004.

Web Sites

Implementation Science:
    http://www.implementationscience.com
Quality Enhancement Research Initiative (QUERI):
    http://www.hsrd.research.va.gov/queri
U.S. Department of Veterans Affairs (VA):
    http://www.va.gov

Quality Improvement Organizations (QIOs)

Quality Improvement Organizations (QIOs) are nonprofit organizations whose statutory missions are to improve and protect the quality of Medicare services while safeguarding the integrity of the Medicare Trust Fund. QIOs accomplish their mandates by working with physicians, hospitals, and other healthcare providers to ensure that Medicare beneficiaries receive care consistent with professionally recognized standards of practice, mediating complaints about quality of care, and performing utilization review to ensure that services are medically necessary and appropriate. QIOs stem from a federally mandated program aimed at improving quality through national oversight and the monitoring of Medicare services. These organizations are relevant to health services research because they investigate why costs of care are increasing and how they can be contained without jeopardizing quality.

Background

The concept of QIOs emerged soon after the passage of the Medicare program (Title XVIII of the Social Security Act) in 1965, at a time when national priorities were directed on efforts to contain rising healthcare costs. Prior to that time, hospital and medical peer groups had set the precedent in establishing quality assessment criteria and in the creation of a hospital-accrediting organization (today, the Joint Commission) to enforce quality standards. These efforts not only laid the groundwork for the standards for hospitals participating in the Medicare program, they also propelled the U.S. Congress to authorize a pilot program in 1971 for an experimental medical care review organization (EMCRO) to assess and monitor utilization of inpatient and ambulatory services, which served as the initial model for a national quality review program. A year later, the professional standards review organizations (PSROs) were established as the first national quality assurance program to focus on utilization review of hospitals and physician outliers as a way to control costs. Physician groups, however, opposed the PSROs, because they were unable to demonstrate that results from such approaches affected cost containment. A decade later, the passing of the federal Peer Review Improvement Act of 1982 (as part of the Tax Equity and Fiscal Responsibility Act of 1982) led Medicare to replace the PSROs with peer review organizations (PROs). The PROs refocused their efforts on monitoring utilization and outcomes for specific Diagnosis Related Group (DRG) assignment, readmissions, hospital operations, complications, and mortality rates. The success of the PROs led to expanding reviews in nursing facilities, home health agencies, hospital outpatient services, physician offices, and managed-care organizations. By the end of the 20th century, Medicare shifted away from a quality assurance focus on case review to quality improvement approaches that influenced patterns in clinical-care processes and outcomes. Hence, by 2002, the PROs were renamed quality improvement organizations (QIOs) to reflect the changing definitions of quality and national priorities toward measurement and population-based improvement effects.

Evolution and Current Status

QIOs constitute the nation's foremost infrastructure for quality improvement that is administered by the Centers for Medicare and Medicaid Services (CMS) as part of a larger program financed mainly through monies from the Medicare Trust Fund. CMS contracts with QIOs to provide services in all 50 states, the Virgin Islands, the District of Columbia, and Puerto Rico, plus several QIO support centers that operate solely as national resource clearinghouses. Moreover, CMS has developed and oversees a complex communication and information systems technology service for the QIO program comprising a standard data-processing system (SDPS) that serves as a centralized repository of clinical data information interfacing with two clinical data abstraction centers (CDAC) and all QIOs. In addition, this service operates a centralized case review information system (CRIS) to track and report on case review activities as well as a protected intranet Web site used by the QIO community to share measurement tools and resources for the SDPS used in the national measures reporting activities.

As of 1984, QIOs have operated from a statement-of-work contract, in 3-year cycles, which has transformed over the decades in three distinctive phases. In the first phase, under the first and third statement-of-work contract cycles, the PROs emphasized the utilization and case review, which was gradually extended to other provider settings. During the second phase, under the fourth and fifth statement-of-work cycles, the PROs focused on transitioning healthcare providers into measurement-based quality improvement project activity rooted in systematic data collection methods using case review to validate measurements. The second phase continued under the sixth and seventh statement of work, with the PROs transitioning into the QIOs, with quality improvement projects aimed at high-cost, high-volume medical conditions (e.g., cardiac care, pneumonia, diabetes), technical assistance to providers in building performance measurement systems, and focusing cost containment on reducing the number of payment errors in hospital settings. The third phase, under the eighth statement-of-work cycle, shifted the QIOs' role to building capacity in performance-based measurement and reporting systems, adapting health information technology, redesigning processes of care, and transforming organizational culture across all provider settings.

Future Implications

The U.S. Congress completes an independent evaluation of the QIOs' program prior to the end of each 3-year statement-of-work contract cycle to determine its effectiveness in meeting quality goals and to define future directions. Current trends indicate that under the ninth statement-of-work contract cycle, slated to begin in 2009, emphasis will remain on supporting the expansion of national systems for quality measurement and reporting to sustain performance improvement activity and on supporting emerging changes in payment systems aimed at pay-for-performance of healthcare.

Iris Garcia-Caban

See also Centers for Medicare and Medicaid Services (CMS); Joint Commission; Medical Errors; Medicare; Outcomes Movement; Patient Safety; Pay-for-Performance; Quality of Healthcare

Further Readings

Bradley, Elizabeth H., Melissa D. Carlson, William T. Gallo, et al. "From Adversary to Partner: Have Quality Improvement Organizations Made the Transition?" *Health Services Research* 40(2): 459–76, April 2005.

Committee on Redesigning Health Insurance Performance Measures, Payment, and Performance Improvement. *Medicare's Quality Improvement Organization Program: Maximizing Potential.* Washington, DC: National Academies Press, 2006.

Rollow, William, Terry R. Lied, Paul McGann, et al. "Assessment of the Medicare Quality Improvement Organization Program," *Annals of Internal Medicine* 145(5): 342–53, September 5, 2006.

Snyder, Claire, and Gerard Anderson. "Do Quality Improvement Organizations Improve the Quality of Hospital Care for Medicare Beneficiaries?" *Journal of the American Medical Association* 293(23): 2900–2907, June 15, 2005.

Web Sites

American Health Quality Association (AHQA): http://www.ahqa.org
Centers for Medicare and Medicaid Services (CMS): http://www.cms.hhs.gov
Medicare Quality Improvement Community: http://www.qualitynet.org

QUALITY INDICATORS

Healthcare quality indicators are tools to measure and monitor the quality of care. Quality indicators are used to determine how well a healthcare system is performing and how it can be further improved. Because poor healthcare quality can adversely affect people's lives and lead to unnecessary healthcare expenditures, quality measurement is important.

Definition

Healthcare quality indicators are the instruments and methods for quantitatively assessing clinical processes and/or patient outcomes. They are used to document the quality of care delivered by providers, evaluate patient outcomes and institutional performance, make comparisons over time and between providers, inform and help purchasers and patients make wise decisions in selecting providers, support accountability and quality improvement efforts, and create transparency in the healthcare system.

Based on the published literature, some of the key characteristics of healthcare quality indicators are as follows: They are based on agreed definitions, described exhaustively, are highly specific and sensitive, are valid and reliable, discriminate well, are relevant, permit useful comparisons, and are evidence based. Quality indicators should be explicit statements of structure, process, or outcome dimensions.

Quality indicators should be developed in the planning and development phase. The planning phase should consist of choosing the clinical area for evaluation and organizing the measurement team. The development phase should comprise providing an overview of existing evidence and practice, selecting clinical indicators and standards, designing the measure specification, and performing pilot tests. The development of quality indicators should be closely tied to both the definition and efforts to improve the quality of care.

Quality indicators can be categorized based on the type of healthcare provided (preventive, chronic, or acute); function (screening, diagnosis, treatment, or follow-up); modality (history, physical examination, laboratory/radiological study, medication); whether they are generic or disease specific, and whether they are rate based or sentinel.

Overview

Recent reports have highlighted the major deficiencies in the U.S. healthcare system. The National Academy of Sciences, Institute of Medicine's 2000 report, *To Err Is Human,* estimated that between 48,000 and 98,000 people die each year in American hospitals from preventable medical errors. And another study (Barbara Starfield's) estimated that 225,000 deaths occur each year in the nation as the result of iatrogenic causes—unnecessary surgeries, medication errors, other hospital errors, hospital-acquired infections, and adverse effects of medications.

Studies have also shown that healthcare quality in the United States varies greatly among providers and across geographic regions. Healthcare often does not meet professional standards, with most adults in the nation only receiving about half of the recommended care for common acute and chronic conditions as well as preventive services. Additionally, studies have shown that the quality of care varies according to where an individual lives in the country. As a result, there remains significant room for quality improvement across all states.

Variation in healthcare quality is not unique to the United States. Many national and international studies on the quality of care have found that the care provided in most countries is substandard. Furthermore, many countries lack performance evaluation systems to measure the quality of care. Extensive research demonstrates that quality of care does not depend on the payment system. Even countries with single-payer systems have problems with quality. Additionally, the level of quality does not appear to depend on the level of healthcare expenditures. For example, the United States has the highest healthcare expenditures per capita, but it still does not have the best measurable outcomes. Overall, there remains a general lack of investment in measuring the quality of care.

The growing concern that healthcare provides poor value relative to the amount of resources spent have led many industrialized countries to develop and implement quality indicators to better manage health production and increase the quality of care. As a result, numerous quality improvement initiatives have been implemented in the healthcare system of nations, since Florence Nightingale first measured infection rates at the Crimean barracks hospital in the 1860s.

Early efforts in the development of quality indicators were focused on disease-specific criteria for process-based evaluations of individual physicians. With the development of clinical practice guidelines and pay-for-performance initiatives, the focus of quality indicators has been expanded to cover organizational performance.

International Quality Indicators

The development of quality indicators by the United States has resulted in the international community adopting similar practices to address the low levels of healthcare quality. Following the lead of the U.S. Agency for Healthcare Research and Quality (AHRQ), a number of other organizations are developing healthcare quality indicators, including the World Health Organization (WHO), the Canadian Association for Health Services and Policy Research (CAHSPR), and the Organization for Economic Cooperation and Development (OECD). Through these efforts, many quality indicators have been developed and are being increasingly used to evaluate the performance of individual practitioners, hospitals, and other institutional providers. Consequently, a number of countries, including Canada, England, the Netherlands, and Denmark, have launched quality indicator programs.

In particular, the OECD countries have advanced the development of quality indicators and extended these methodologies. The OECD's Health Care Quality Indicators (HCQI) project developed a conceptual framework and a set of indicators to allow for the comparison of healthcare quality across its member countries. The HCQI integrates proven concepts and methods into a health performance framework.

The OECD's framework of health determinants consists of a comprehensive multistage hierarchical model that includes four major components: health, nonhealthcare determinants of health, healthcare system performance, and health system design and context. The OECD's healthcare quality indicators focus on the healthcare system's performance, which consists of healthcare needs and specific dimensions of healthcare performance.

Healthcare needs consist of staying healthy, getting better, living with illness or disability, and coping with end-of-life problems. The dimensions of healthcare performance consist of quality (effectiveness, safety, and responsiveness/patient centeredness), access, and costs.

The Dutch healthcare system's performance evaluation is an example of a quality indicators framework that has been implemented at the national level. The Dutch model, which is based on the Canadian Lalonde model, has the dual goals of constructing a conceptual framework for national healthcare performance and selecting quality indicators for measurement. The performance system combines population health and management information into the quality indicators. The system is based on a balanced scorecard, which provides information from the consumer, financial, internal business processes, and innovation perspectives.

The Commonwealth Fund in the United States also recently developed a scorecard method and applied it to healthcare quality indicators to allow for state, national, and international comparisons. These quality indicators consist of 37 indicators of performance. This initiative is the first comprehensive means of measuring and monitoring health outcomes, quality, access, efficiency, and equity of care.

Limitations

Many of the quality indicators currently in use have conceptual and measurement issues, as they do not provide a complete assessment of a provider's performance. Furthermore, the use of quality indicators in the practice setting requires a sophisticated infrastructure that generally includes information technology, which is lacking in many clinical environments. Some of the shortcomings of quality indicators and quality-monitoring initiatives are as follows: Many healthcare systems do not have adequate documentation of the quality of care for many diseases; there are no appropriate benchmarks; there is limited evaluation of quality management efforts; and there is a lack of outcomes assessment. As a result, quality indicators have had limited success in comparing the performance between providers and organizations.

Future Implications

In the future, the quality indicators will increasingly be developed and used to monitor the performance of healthcare systems at the regional, national, and international levels. However, many conceptual and methodological issues need to be addressed. Issues such as the differences in cultural context, healthcare delivery systems, data specifications, and data availability make comparisons of healthcare performance among organizations and countries challenging. These differences must be considered if an acceptable model is to be developed. It is hoped that as healthcare quality indicators continue to be developed, evolve, and be refined to better measure, monitor, and compare against universal standards of care, the quality chasm will be crossed.

Sang-O Rhee

See also Agency for Healthcare Research and Quality (AHRQ); Codman, Ernest Amory; Donabedian, Avedis; Joint Commission; Medical Errors; Nightingale, Florence; Quality of Healthcare; Structure-Process-Outcome Quality Measures

Further Readings

Brook, Robert H., Elizabeth A. McGlynn, and Paul G. Shekelle. "Defining and Measuring Quality of Care: A Perspective of U.S. Researchers," *International Journal for Quality in Health Care* 12(4): 281–95, August 2000.

Committee on Quality of Health Care in America, Institute of Medicine. *To Err Is Human: Building a Safer Health System*. Washington, DC: National Academies Press, 2000.

Committee on Quality of Health Care in America, Institute of Medicine. *Crossing the Quality Chasm: A New Health System for the 21st Century*. Washington, DC: National Academies Press, 2001.

Hussey, Peter S., Gerard F. Anderson, Robin Osborn, et al. "How Does Quality of Care Compare in Five Countries?" *Health Affairs* 23(3): 89–99, May–June 2004.

Mainz, Jan. "Defining and Classifying Clinical Indicators for Quality Improvement," *International Journal for Quality in Health Care* 15(6): 523–30, December 2003.

Mainz, Jan, and Paul D. Bartels. "Nationwide Quality Improvement: How Are We Doing and What Can We Do?" *International Journal for Quality in Health Care* 18(2): 79–80, April 2006.

Mattke, Soeren, Arnold M. Epstein, and Sheila Leatherman. "The OECD Health Care Quality Indicators Project: History and Background," *International Journal for Quality in Health Care* 18(Suppl. 1): 1–4, 2006.

Schuster, Mark A., Elizabeth A. McGlynn, and Robert H. Brook. "How Good is the Quality of Health Care in the United States?" *Milbank Quarterly* 76(4): 517–63, December 1998.

Starfield, Barbara. "Is U.S. Health Really the Best in the World?" *Journal of the American Medical Association* 284(4): 483–85, July 26, 2000.

Thompson, Richard, Sally Taber, Joanne Lally, et al. "UK Quality Indicator Project (UK QIP) and the UK Independent Health Care Sector: A New Development," *International Journal for Quality in Health Care* 16(Suppl. 1): i51–i56, 2004.

Web Sites

Agency for Healthcare Research and Quality (AHRQ): http://www.ahrq.gov

Canadian Association for Health Services and Policy Research (CAHSPR): http://www.cahspr.ca

Commonwealth Fund: http://www.commonwealthfund.org

Joint Commission: http://www.jointcommission.org

National Quality Forum (NQF): http://www.qualityforum.org

National Quality Measures Clearinghouse: http://www.qualitymeasures.ahrq.gov

Organization for Economic Cooperation and Development (OECD): http://www.oecd.org

World Health Organization (WHO): http://www.who.int

QUALITY MANAGEMENT

Quality management can be described as a method that is used to make sure that all the aspects pertaining to the design, development, and implementation of a service or product are handled in an efficient and effective manner. Quality management is critical to ensuring that certain standards are met when there is a high production volume. In healthcare, quality management has gained significant attention because of the number of deaths and injuries reported due to medical errors. In 2000, the national Institute of Medicine (IOM) published a highly influential report, *To Err Is Human: Building a Safer Health System,* which highlighted the large number of medical-error-related deaths that occur each year in the nation's hospitals. Although the nation's manufacturing industry has been using for many years quality management techniques that encourage teamwork and communication, the healthcare industry has only recently adopted these practices.

Overview

There is no singular widely accepted definition of quality management as there are various forms of this concept, including total quality management (TQM), continuous quality improvement (CQI), and statistical control processes. The definition of quality is relevant only to the extent that it provides value to the customer. However, the main components of quality management include quality control, assurance, and improvement.

The concept of quality management evolved from the work of several important figures in the field, including W. Edwards Deming (1900–1993), Joseph M. Juran (1904–2008), Walter A. Shewhart (1891–1967), and Frederick Winslow Taylor (1856–1915). Taylor, the father of scientific management, was one of the first to lay the foundation for quality management through standardization and to advocate improved organizational practices. Continuing to advance the field, Shewhart, the father of statistical quality control, introduced the concept of the control chart. Shewhart developed his concepts at Bell Laboratories, later describing the principles of statistical quality control in his book *Economic Control of the Quality of Manufactured Products* (1931). Statistical quality control is the discipline that involves applying statistical methods to process-related data that identify the critical variables or root causes that result in reduced variation of processes or the elimination of problems.

Following in Shewhart's footsteps, Deming shared his knowledge of statistical methods to achieve quality control during World War II as well as his 14 points that served as a basis for quality management principles. Because of Deming's extensive knowledge, he consulted with post–World War II Japan to help that nation improve the quality of its products. Japan would recognize Deming by establishing a prize for quality achievement in his honor. Deming popularized the Plan-Do-Check-Act (PDCA) cycle developed by Shewhart, also known as Deming's Cycle, or Shewhart's Cycle, which is a four-step process in quality control. In this cycle, the Plan step consists of determining goals and targets as well as the methods of reaching these goals, Do involves implementing the processes, Check assesses the results of the implementation, and Act entails taking appropriate action to improve the processes.

Juran is regarded as one of the eminent quality experts, and he was one of the first to deal with the broad management concept of quality. Juran introduced the cost of quality concept in *The Quality Control Handbook* (1951). He advocated structured improvement initiatives, a sense of urgency, extensive training, and strong upper-level management commitment.

Quality Management Strategies

Six Sigma is a quality management technique based on statistical process control to emphasize the continuous decrease in process variation. Developed at the Motorola Corporation in 1986, Six Sigma strives to reduce and eliminate sources of errors in the manufacturing process. This concept eventually led to the concept of TQM, which is a strategy that aims to improve quality among all organizational levels and processes. Another quality management strategy that arose in corporate environments and has been implemented in healthcare is CQI. This concept focuses on a team approach to quality improvement as opposed to having a culture of blame.

One of the difficulties with quality management is how to define and ensure quality. The consumer, or payer, ultimately decides what the attributes of quality are. Additionally, quality can be used as a differentiating factor between an organization's products or services.

Quality Management in Healthcare

Quality management in healthcare only began to flourish in the mid-1980s when the healthcare industry moved toward a more outcomes-based approach. The Hospital Corporation of America (HCA) was one of the leaders in adopting Deming's PDCA cycle as FOCUS-PDCA. FOCUS stands for F—find a process that can be improved, O—organize to improve that process, C—clarify what is currently known, U—understand why there is variation, and S—select a process improvement strategy.

Research on quality management initiatives to improve patient safety and reduce medical errors has been undertaken by many national organizations and agencies such as the Joint Commission, American College of Surgeons, Agency for Healthcare Research and Quality (AHRQ), and Centers for Medicare and Medicaid Services (CMS). Computerized physician order entry, flagging alert systems, and various provider-patient communication tools are just some of the quality management techniques that have been implemented in healthcare systems in recent years.

Baldrige Award

There are several national awards given out to recognize quality; however, in the United States, the Baldrige award is the most prestigious. To recognize achievements in quality, the Malcolm Baldrige National Quality Award is given out annually by the U.S. National Institutes of Standards and Technology (NIST). Established by the U.S. Congress in 1987 and named after former U.S. Secretary of Commerce Malcolm Baldrige, this award program, inspired by total quality management practices, highlights businesses and healthcare, educational, and nonprofit organizations that deliver quality services. The original intended purpose of the Baldrige award was to increase quality awareness, acknowledge the quality achievements of companies, and highlight successful quality strategies. Recent winners of the Baldrige award in healthcare include Mercy Health System of Janesville, Wisconsin (2007); Sharp Healthcare of San Diego, California (2007); and North Mississippi Medical Center of Tupelo, Mississippi (2006).

Future Implications

Because of the wide recognition of the significant gaps in the U.S. healthcare system, quality management will remain at the forefront of the healthcare agenda as a way to reduce medical errors and adverse events while improving patient safety, outcomes, and overall quality. The increasing use of technology, improved communication strategies, and performance assessment will be integral to implementing quality management practices in healthcare. Quality management initiatives will continue to play an important role in ensuring the consistent delivery of high-quality care for all.

Jared Lane K. Maeda

See also Agency for Healthcare Research and Quality (AHRQ); Institute for Healthcare Improvement (IHI); Joint Commission; National Committee for Quality Assurance (NCQA); National Quality Forum (NQF); Quality Improvement Organizations (QIOs); Quality of Healthcare; Outcomes Movement

Further Readings

Committee on Quality of Health Care in America, Institute of Medicine. *To Err Is Human: Building a Safer Health System.* Washington, DC: National Academies Press, 2000.

Ferlie, Ewan B., and Stephen M. Shortell, "Improving the Quality of Health Care in the United Kingdom and the United States: A Framework for Change," *Milbank Quarterly* 79(2): 281–315, June 2001.

Jha, Ashish K., Jonathan B. Perlin, Kenneth W. Kizer, et al. "The Effect of the Transformation of the Veterans Affairs Health Care System on the Quality of Care," *New England Journal of Medicine* 348(22): 2218–27, May 29, 2003.

Juran, Joseph, M. *The Quality Control Handbook.* New York: McGraw-Hill, 1951.

McLaughlin, Curtis P., and Arnold D. Kaluzny. *Continuous Quality Improvement in Health Care: Theory, Implementation, and Applications.* 3d ed. Sudbury, MA: Jones and Bartlett, 2006.

Ortendahl, Monica. "Different Time Perspectives of the Doctor and the Patient Reduce Quality in Health Care," *Quality Management in Health Care* 17(2): 136–39, April–June 2008.

Shewhart, Walter A. *Economic Control of the Quality of Manufactured Products.* New York: D. Van Nostrand, 1931.

Shortell, Stephen M., Robert H. Jones, Alfred W. Rademaker, et al. "Assessing the Impact of Total

Quality Management and Organizational Culture on Multiple Outcomes of Care for Coronary Artery Bypass Graft Surgical Patients," *Medical Care* 38(2): 207–217, February 2000.

Web Sites

Agency for Healthcare Research and Quality (AHRQ):
    http://www.ahrq.gov
Baldrige National Quality Program, Health Care Criteria
    for Performance Excellence: http://www.quality.nist
    .gov/HealthCare_Criteria.htm
Institute for Healthcare Improvement (IHI):
    http://www.ihi.org
Joint Commission: http://www.jointcommission.org
National Committee for Quality Assurance (NCQA):
    http://www.ncqa.org
National Quality Forum (NQF):
    http://www.qualityforum.org

QUALITY OF HEALTHCARE

Quality of healthcare refers to the degree to which healthcare services for individuals and populations increase the likelihood of desired health outcomes that are consistent with current professional knowledge. To improve the quality of healthcare, many evaluation and standardization practices have been developed. This entry discusses several aspects of healthcare quality, including the history of healthcare quality evaluation, the major organizations and programs created to increase the quality of healthcare, the role of academe in the quality of healthcare, evaluation phases, and incentives for improving quality.

History

During the first quarter of the 20th century, a confluence of events served as a strong impetus to the institutionalized, systematic evaluation of hospital quality. Abraham Flexner's report on medical education in the United States and Canada, published in 1912, called attention to the serious deficiencies in the training of American physicians. Ernest A. Codman successfully persuaded his fellow surgeons that the development of hospital standards, along with complete, accurate records

of care and outcomes and the development of clinical databases for the study of end results, was necessary for the improvement of medical care.

In 1917, the new American College of Surgeons (ACS), created in 1913, established its Hospital Standardization Program, fundamentally embodying Codman's proposal. The ACS formulated a one-page "Minimum Standard" on the basis of which its volunteer member-surveyors began surveying hospitals that wished to obtain ACS accreditation, the badge of excellence. Early hospital surveys revealed that medical records were for the most part utterly inadequate as documentation. The entire medical community was alerted to the need for the formulation of standards for medical and surgical care and to the need for a system of medical records that would thoroughly and accurately document patient care.

Foundation Organizations and Programs

For 35 years the ACS conducted its Hospital Standardization Program, using as surveyors its own members who volunteered their services. Over the years, it became obvious that the logistical and financial burdens of a single-organization volunteer program had become too great for the ACS to support on its own. In 1952, the ACS was joined by the American College of Physicians (ACP), American Hospital Association (AHA), American Medical Association (AMA), and Canadian Medical Association (CMA) in forming the Joint Commission on Accreditation of Hospitals (JCAH). A few years later, the CMA withdrew to become a founding member of the new Canadian Council on Hospital Accreditation (CCHA).

With the passage of the federal Medicare program in 1965, the U.S. Congress conferred "deemed status" on JCAH-accredited hospitals in the nation, granting accredited hospitals automatic eligibility for Medicare reimbursement. In view of this delegation of federal authority, as it was perceived by many critics, it became imperative to develop objective standards for the evaluation of hospital performance. The JCAH responded by completely overhauling its research and standards development programs from 1967 to 1970 and publishing updated, more objective standards with which compliance could be measured.

In 1988, in recognition of its expansion to include mental health, long-term care, home-care, and ambulatory-care providers, the JCAH changed its name to the Joint Commission on Accreditation of Healthcare Organizations (JCAHO). Since then, it has expanded its reach to include non-hospital-based clinical laboratories and office surgery practices. As a result, it has recently changed its name to simply the Joint Commission.

The growth of health maintenance organizations (HMOs) during the 1980s spurred the development of managed-care organizations and large multispecialty group practices. In 1990, the National Committee for Quality Assurance (NCQA) was established. The mission of the NCQA was to develop performance standards and conduct accreditation surveys of managed-care organizations. Since 1992, NCQA has used the Healthcare Effectiveness Data and Information Set (HEDIS), a set of standards of organizational performance with a significant emphasis on the use of screening procedures in covered populations, as its principal tool in evaluating the performance of managed-care organizations. Over the years, HEDIS has been systematically updated and expanded.

The Role of Academe

Medical schools came to system-oriented quality management slowly. Their interpretation of the concept of quality focused on the efficacy of the individual physician's clinical performance and traditionally tended to ignore the physician's role as a member of a system for providing care. While, beginning in the 1960s, small groups of inquisitive scholars on the faculties of medical schools and colleges of nursing were beginning to study ways to measure and improve the quality of hospital care, very little information about their findings and recommendations appeared in course content. In 1987, in response to an informal questionnaire survey sent to the members of the Association of American Medical Colleges (AAMC), 20% of the responders replied that they did include some material on quality assessment in the curriculum. However, the most common offering cited, typical of the affirmative responses, was a 2-hour elective lecture in the 1st or 2nd year of medical school. When the survey was repeated in 1993, the results were essentially the same.

Some respondents commented that the curriculum was so crowded with mandatory courses that no room was left for the study of organizational quality management. In another study, researchers found that 54% of the study sample of medical residents indicated that their training had not included content on medical errors.

Phases in Evaluation

In the United States, hospital-wide patient-care evaluation has gone through three recognizable phases in its evolution. The first phase was implicit review. This, the traditional method, involved assessing care on the basis of process norms or criteria derived from the assessor's personal experiences, values, and professional opinions. The criteria used were not formulated or published in advance and often varied from one expert assessor to another.

Accreditation-driven evaluation by the JCAH prior to the early 1980s focused primarily on a hospital's organizational structure and its presumed ability to provide good care, without explicitly incorporating the outcomes of care in the evaluation equation. The Joint Commission's criteria were essentially structural, although during the 1970s, research and development were moving in the direction of process-oriented surveys. Evaluation criteria focused on the organizational structure; the presence of an organized medical staff; credentials of the medical staff members; the presence of adequate numbers of qualified nurses; and the presence of acceptable plant, equipment, and instruments.

Process-oriented patient-care audits represented the second phase in institutional healthcare evaluation. During the late 1970s and 1980s, quality assurance audits performed periodically by hospitals involved the application of preestablished hospital-generated process criteria. However, the audit system had some basic flaws that weakened its potential for stimulating improvements in patient-care outcomes. When a conventional audit was performed, it was easy to pounce on a few episodes of care that failed to meet the criteria, to conclude that the observed care was acceptable, or to dismiss the whole exercise with the notation "Audit completed." The obligation had been fulfilled. Those care episodes that failed to meet the criteria had been identified. Although it served to identify performance flaws, this approach did nothing to help professionals understand the reasons for poor performance or to point the way toward improvement. The major contribution of this approach was the fact that the criteria were established in advance of the audit and an attempt was made to quantify the evaluation findings.

Meanwhile, the Joint Commission was laying the groundwork for new techniques focusing on assessing patient clinical outcomes. Improving outcomes entails improving the systems of care. In this third, or system-oriented, phase, the healthcare industry began applying the principles of continuous quality improvement (CQI) and total quality management (TQM) to its organizational behavior. One popular approach, the "Plan, Do, Check, Act" (PDCA) cycle, gained wide acceptance. Diagnosis-specific clinical measures came into use as criteria of good care and then gave rise to the use of end-results data in developing treatment benchmarks, related "best-practices" guidelines, and evidence-based medicine. Although they were being formulated by highly credentialed groups, such as teams formed by medical specialty societies, the concepts of best practices and benchmarks met with some early resistance on the part of traditionalists, who decried their use as "cookbook medicine." Over time, benchmarking and best practices have become generally accepted as parts of the quality management armamentarium. Reminiscent of Codman's emphasis on end results was the development, during this time, of the concept of evidence-based medicine as a guide to practice.

Access to Care and Patient Satisfaction

Along with the reduction of medical errors and the improvement in clinical outcomes, two additional components of healthcare quality are access to good care and patient satisfaction. Access to care is a process that usually is addressed through strategies such as insurance programs, nondiscrimination policies and laws, architectural and environmental modifications, adequate public transportation, and community health education programs. Achieving widespread access to good quality care depends on legislative and public financial support at the municipal, state, and federal levels.

Over the past quarter-century, patient satisfaction has come to be recognized as an important factor in the quality of care, subject to measurement and improvement. An active consulting industry has developed around the need for objective analysis of the needs, desires, and reactions of patients and their families with regard to many elements in their care, such as the quality of hospital food, pain control, staff courtesy and responsiveness, and environmental features. Patients routinely respond to lengthy, detailed survey instruments designed to elicit their reactions to each element in the hospital experience. On the basis of analytical study of the responses, hospital managements evaluate patient satisfaction levels and institute indicated changes.

Development of New Tools

It was not enough to formulate and publish standards of performance, such as benchmarks and practice guidelines. New sets of tools for quantifying assessment and behavioral change were necessary. The need for new tools was answered in large part by the introduction of statistical process control (SPC) to healthcare quality management during the 1980s and 1990s. Derived from the work of Walter Shewhart, W. Edward Deming, and Joseph Juran and long established in industry, SPC in all its manifestations has become solidly established in healthcare.

SPC involves the use of control charts to show the degree to which a group's performance varies from a preestablished optimal or normative range. Investigators sought to differentiate between the special causes of variation, stemming from factors peculiar to the specific case under study, and the common causes of variation, related to factors inherent in the system of care itself. During the same period, the healthcare industry came to recognize that problems of quality and safety were system problems and that their resolution was an organizational responsibility.

The use of SPC in the healthcare industry received valuable support from the publication of two seminal reports by the national Institute of Medicine's (IOM) Committee on Quality of Health Care in America. In the first report, *To Err Is Human: Building a Safer Health System*, published in 2000, the committee explored issues of patient safety ranging from staff training to falls and medication errors. This report sparked universal support, on the part of both consumers and the healthcare community, for methods of ensuring the safety of patients from medication and treatment errors. In the second report, *Crossing the Quality Chasm: A New Health System in the 21st Century,* published in 2001, the committee set forth broad strategic plans for redesigning the nation's healthcare delivery system with an emphasis on patient safety, accountability, and evaluation based on objective evidence.

Another widely used transplant from industry is Six Sigma, a method for bringing about quantifiable improvement in group performance, again as measured against a charted normative level. The objective of following the Six Sigma process is to reduce errors to a rate of 3.4 errors per 1 million opportunities. Following the example set by the rest of the corporate world, healthcare organizations increasingly have retained consultants to teach executives and clinical personnel how to plan and run their own Six Sigma programs in order to attain excellence in organizational performance. An important feature of Six Sigma is "Poko-yoke, or "mistake-proofing," the designing of systems that make it easy for personnel to perform their tasks correctly without error. The mistake-proofing approach has a long history in Japanese industry. While Six Sigma can be superficially described as a quantitative method of reducing errors in patient care, applying it across a healthcare organization is a complex task. It requires problem detection (often through the use of process control charting); causal analysis; problem solving, including mistake proofing and the revision of procedures; and retraining personnel.

Evidence-Based Medicine and Electronic Tools

Nine decades after Codman's call for improving end results, the same theme—the need for concrete evidence to support assessment and guideline development—continues to shape the healthcare industry's efforts to improve the quality of care. In the late 20th and early 21st centuries, the concept was called evidence-based medicine. Researchers rely on this concept to guide studies and identify optimal diagnostic and therapeutic strategies for

dissemination to clinicians. Without the nearly universal use of electronic ordering and database building in hospitals, physicians' offices, and other sites of care, it would have been impossible to reach Codman's goal of documenting and analyzing the end results of medical care.

The development and expansion of electronic ordering and medical record systems in hospitals and other care centers, which began in the 1980s and continues today, is making it possible to build and maintain the patient databases needed for SPC and the Six Sigma approach. Using the clinical-pathway model based on critical-path analysis, tracing every phase of the patient's treatment from admission to discharge, quality investigators can determine whether the treatment of individuals or of groups was consistent with best practices. Database development on a national scale made it possible for the Joint Commission, the NCQA, and the federal Centers for Medicare and Medicaid Services (CMS) to publish national performance data.

Widespread media dissemination of the information derived from these programs, along with the development of readily accessible Internet reference sources, is providing consumers with improved access to healthcare information and stoking their interest in finding and supporting improved therapies. The existence of a critical mass of well-informed consumers, theoretically, will play a role in the widespread improvement of the quality of healthcare. However, the risks of spreading misinformation also arise from uncritical, often sensationalized media presentation of clinical breakthroughs (e.g., untested "miracle cures") and ongoing developments in patient care. In the long run, the spread of information facilitates competition, which historically results in improvements in the quality of the product or service.

Creating Incentives

Leapfrog Group

The revelations contained in the IOM's 2000 report, *To Err Is Human,* resonated with the large American corporations that provide healthcare benefits to their employees. The report focused on the prevalence of hospital-related preventable medical errors, leading to an estimated 44,000 to

98,000 deaths per year. The issue was one of simple economics: The evidence indicated that employers were not getting what they were paying for—good healthcare in return for their premiums. In 2000, a group of these large corporate employers founded an association that they named the Leapfrog Group. The name reflected the need to leap forward in developing strategies to correct the existing conditions.

A principal Leapfrog Group objective is to promote high-quality healthcare by providing incentives and rewards, through their health benefits plans, to providers that use computerized physician order entry systems; base hospital referrals on evidence-based medicine; require specialized training for physicians working in intensive-care units; and adopt the 30 Safe Practices, addressing processes across a range of areas, formulated by the National Quality Forum (NQF).

Pay-for-Performance

The CMS has conducted several incentive-based monitoring and evaluation programs under the umbrella title pay-for-performance, or as they are commonly known, P4P. The general objective of pay-for-performance is to try to ensure that providers of services to Medicare beneficiaries and Medicaid recipients meet certain standards of care consistent with those of the NQF, Joint Commission, NCQA, Agency for Healthcare Research and Quality (AHRQ), AMA, and other nationally recognized bodies involved in setting quality standards. Demonstrated, documented compliance with quality measures endorsed by pay-for-performance is rewarded through an incentive system. Managed-care groups, in particular, have been quick to recognize the value of the pay-for-performance approach and have begun to develop formal mechanisms to participate in it.

PEPPER, MACS, and the False Claims Act

Many clues to the quality and effectiveness of clinical care can be found by tracing a patient's billing record. Complications and misdiagnoses are often reflected in unusually long hospital inpatient stays and very early hospital inpatient readmissions. Another resource at the disposal of the CMS, in its efforts to improve quality and efficiency, is

the Program for Evaluating Payment Patterns (PEPPER). A PEPPER is an electronic data report containing hospital-specific billing data for 13 targeted Diagnosis Related Groups (DRGs) and discharges that have been identified as carrying a high risk of payment errors. Using a PEPPER and the associated database, the CMS and hospital reviewers can home in on admissions that resulted in extended hospital stays or early readmissions for the same diagnosis. This process can point to the occurrence of clinical complications and inadequacies—poor quality—in patient care and alert hospitals to the need for change.

One factor making it difficult to follow up on patients after discharge to assess the end results of hospital care has been the strong possibility that a Medicare patient who received poor care, resulting in a complication, may not return to the same provider and hospital but may go to another physician and another hospital. Thus, the patient's postdischarge history lacks continuity and is lost to quality evaluation research. This would not happen in the presence of a single national database of Medicare patients. Beginning in 2007, and expected to be operational by 2012, a new plan called the Medicare Administrative Contractor System (MACS) will be functioning. Under the MACS plan, data from Medicare Part A and Part B plans will be combined into a single database for each Medicare region, with the entries identified by patient. Thus, all the Medicare patient's care, whether office, ambulatory, or inpatient, will be traceable in one database, facilitating long-term study.

As purveyors of services to Medicare patients, healthcare providers are subject to the terms of the federal False Claims Act. Therefore, they can be prosecuted for defrauding the federal government if their services are shown to have been other than appropriate and of good quality. A growing body of case law reflects the successful prosecution of healthcare providers found guilty of such fraud. The severe financial and operational sanctions provided for in the amendments to the act can be a strong deterrent to clinical behavior that fails to meet established norms and standards.

Future Implications

The quality of healthcare will remain an important issue in the future. With the greater availability of information and quality measurement tools, insurers and individual consumers will, it is hoped, be able to more wisely choose healthcare organizations and individual practitioners who provide high-quality care.

Jean Gayton Carroll

See also Agency for Healthcare Research and Quality (AHRQ); Clinical Practice Guidelines; Evidence-Based Medicine (EBM); Joint Commission; Leapfrog Group; National Committee for Quality Assurance (NCQA); Pay-for-Performance; Quality Management

Further Readings

Agency for Healthcare Research and Quality. *National Healthcare Quality Report, 2007*. Rockville, MD: Agency for Healthcare Research and Quality, 2008.

Committee on Quality of Health Care in America, Institute of Medicine. *To Err Is Human: Building a Safer Health System*. Washington, DC: National Academies Press, 2000.

Committee on Quality of Health Care in America, Institute of Medicine. *Crossing the Quality Chasm: A New Health System for the 21st Century*. Washington, DC: National Academy Press, 2001.

Dhillon, B. S. *Reliability Technology, Human Error, and Quality in Health Care*. Boca Raton, FL: CRC Press, 2008.

Earp, Jo Anne L., Elizabeth A. French, and Melissa B. Gilkey, eds. *Patient Advocacy for Health Care Quality: Strategies for Achieving Patient-Centered Care*. Sudbury, MA: Jones and Bartlett, 2008.

Hagland, Mark. *Transformative Quality: The Emerging Revolution in Health Care*. New York: Productivity Press, 2009.

Ransom, Elizabeth R., Maulik S. Joshi, David B. Nash, et al., eds. *The Healthcare Quality Book: Vision, Strategy, and Tools*. 2d ed. Chicago: Health Administration Press, 2008.

Trusko, Brett E., Carolyn Pexton, H. James Harrington, et al. *Improving Healthcare Quality and Cost With Six Sigma*. Upper Saddle River, NJ: FT Press, 2007.

Web Sites

Agency for Healthcare Research and Quality (AHRQ): http://www.ahrq.gov

Centers for Medicare and Medicaid Services (CMS): http://www.cms.hhs.gov

Joint Commission: http://www.jointcommission.org

Leapfrog Group: http://www.leapfroggroup.org

National Committee for Quality Assurance (NCQA): http://www.ncqa.org

National Quality Forum (NQF): http://www.qualityforum.org

QUALITY OF LIFE, HEALTH-RELATED (HRQOL)

Health-related quality of life (HRQOL) refers to an individual's or a group's physical and mental well-being over time. Healthcare providers and health services researchers use HRQOL tools to measure patients' chronic illness and to see how these conditions affect a person's daily life. Additionally, public health professionals use HRQOL to measure disorders, disabilities, and diseases in various populations. By tracking HRQOL, groups with poor physical and mental health can be properly identified. Policies to improve the health of these groups can then be appropriately developed.

Overview

The following highlights an example of the use of HRQOL for one individual. A 5-year old girl presents at a hospital with acute lymphoblastic leukemia, the most common type of childhood cancer. For the physicians, as well as the parents, the child's current quality of life is a key concern. How much pain is the child in now? What is her emotional condition? How did she respond to earlier therapies?

Examining the HRQOL in patients is of increasing concern in the medical community, and these concerns are affecting the way new therapies are administered and randomized controlled trials (RCTs) are planned. HRQOL provides important information on the improvements that new therapies offer as well as an outcome measure for economic evaluations.

Recently developed HRQOL measures and applications are important contributions to this emerging field. Information from these tools is used to adjust therapy or improve treatment for the patient. The quality-of-life information is also used to prevent and control disease, injury, and disability in others.

According to researchers, the domains of quality of life refer to areas of behavior that are measured. The subjective domains of quality-of-life include the following: physical functioning, occupational functioning, psychological functioning, social functioning, and perceptions about health status. Some researchers have also defined "social health" as the dimension of an individual's well-being that concerns how he or she gets along with others, how other people react to the individual, and how the person interacts with social institutions and norms.

From an objective standpoint, health status can be measured by laboratory or diagnostic tests, psychology tests, measures of socioeconomic status, and the degree of social support. Experts note that the so-called objective measures of quality of life often bear little relationship to life satisfaction. Thus, patients' subjective satisfaction should always be considered in routine assessment and clinical interventions as it is a useful source of information.

Clinicians have for many years had to substitute physiological or laboratory tests for the direct measurement of people's health. During the past 20 years, however, clinicians have recognized the importance of direct measurement of how people are feeling and how they are able to function in daily activities. Investigators have now developed sophisticated methods of measuring quality of life.

Healthy Day Measures

The Centers for Disease Control and Prevention (CDC) employs what it calls Healthy Day Measures to monitor the quality of life of individuals. This measure is a survey which can be administered to any population and from which data about the individual's state of health can be determined. These questions include the following:

1. Would you say that in general your health is excellent, very good, good, fair, or poor?

2. Now thinking about your physical health, which includes physical illness and injury, for how many days during the past 30 days was your physical health not good?

3. Now thinking about your mental health, which includes depression, stress, and problems with emotions, for how many days during the past 30 days was your mental health not good?

4. During the past 30 days, for how many days did poor physical or mental health keep you from doing your usual daily activities, such as self-care, work, or recreation?

The CDC indicates that "unhealthy days" are an estimate of the overall number of days during the preceding 30 days when the respondent felt that his or her physical or mental health was "not good." To obtain this estimate, responses to Questions 2 and 3 are combined to calculate a summary index of overall unhealthy days, with a maximum of 30 unhealthy days. For instance, a person who reports 4 "physically unhealthy days" and "2 mentally unhealthy days" is assigned a value of 6 unhealthy days, while someone who reports 30 physically unhealthy days and 30 mentally unhealthy days is assigned a maximum of 30 unhealthy days.

The CDC reports that the majority of individuals report "substantially different" numbers of physically unhealthy days versus mentally unhealthy days. For example, according to the 1998 Behavioral Risk Factor Surveillance System (BRFSS), 68% of the 68,600 adults who reported any unhealthy days indicated only physically unhealthy days or mentally unhealthy days, while 4% indicated "equal numbers" for each measure. Additionally, evidence demonstrates that the reported days do not overlap. Just 10% of the 250 persons who reported both 15 physically unhealthy days and 15 mentally unhealthy days also reported more than 15 days of recent activity limitation due to poor physical or mental health.

History

The World Health Organization (WHO) broadly defines health as a state of complete physical, mental, and social well-being and not just the absence of disease. For two decades, the four core Healthy Days Measures have been part of the CDC's state-based BRFSS's sample. Beginning in 2000, the Healthy Days Measures were also incorporated by CDC's National Center for Health

Statistics (NCHS) into the examination part of its National Health and Nutrition Examination Survey (NHANES).

The measures and data have also been used for research and program planning by CDC's Cardiovascular Health and HIV/AIDS programs. Other users have included the Public Health Foundation, the Foundation for Accountability, and numerous other academic and government programs.

Recently, several organizations have found these Healthy Days Measures useful at the national level for determining health disparities, following population trends, and creating broad coalitions around a measure of population health compatible with the WHO's definition of health.

The Healthy Days Measures and data have been employed by state and local public health departments for tracking the overall progress in achieving the two major goals of the federal government's Healthy People 2010 initiative, increasing the quality and years of healthy life and eliminating health disparities.

Major National Research Findings

The CDC has reported a number of key findings related to the nation's adult HRQOL, including the following: Americans on average report that they felt "healthy and full of energy" for only about 19 days per month; they said that they felt unhealthy—physically or mentally—for about 6 days per month; nearly one third of Americans said that they suffer from some mental or emotional problems every month—including 10% who reported that their mental health was not good for 14 or more days per month; younger American adults, between 18 and 24 years of age, said that they suffered mental health distress the most; older American adults suffered the most from poor physical health and activity limitation; Alaska Natives and other Native Americans reported the highest levels of unhealthy days among American race/ethnicity groups; those Americans with the lowest income and education reported more unhealthy days than did those with higher income or education; and Americans with chronic diseases and disabilities reported high levels of unhealthy days.

The CDC also reported on HRQOL for individuals suffering from specific diseases, including chronic arthritis, breast cancer, heart disease, and diabetes mellitus. They found the following: Adults with chronic arthritis reported 4.6 more unhealthy days per month compared with adults without arthritis; among adults with arthritis, the largest number of unhealthy days was experienced by women, younger persons, and persons without a college education; women with breast cancer reported experiencing 8.5 unhealthy days per month compared with 6.1 unhealthy days per month for women without breast cancer; individuals who had a heart attack, coronary heart disease, or a stroke reported an average of 10 unhealthy days for the previous month compared with 5 unhealthy days reported among persons not having one of these conditions; and individuals with diabetes reported experiencing 9.9 unhealthy days per month compared with 5.1 unhealthy days per month for adults without diabetes.

Controversy

Researchers typically measure HRQOL by using survey questionnaires that include questions about how individuals are feeling or what they are experiencing associated with response options such as "yes" or "no" or point scales. As discussed earlier, researchers then aggregate the responses to these questions into domains or dimensions—such as physical or emotional function—that yield an overall quality-of-life score. However, controversy exists over the extent to which individual values must be included in its measurement. Increasingly, researchers are asking if it is sufficient to know that individuals with chronic obstructive lung disease in general value being able to climb stairs without getting short of breath? Or does medical science need to establish that the individual values climbing stairs with dypsnea (difficulty in breathing)?

Additional controversy exists about the value of the scoring systems developed by the CDC and other health research organizations. Researchers are wondering whether it is enough to simply know that both dypsnea and fatigue are important to people with lung disease. Or does medicine need to establish their relative importance? Furthermore, if establishing their relative importance is necessary, which of the many available approaches should be used?

An emerging consensus indicates that medicine is ready to accept an individual's own statements about what he or she values without a very precise determination of ranking of that information on a scale. However, experts note that not all treatment and therapies lead to an improvement in HRQOL for patients. Many life-prolonging treatments have a negligible impact on the quality of life that individuals experience. This may lead them and their families to be concerned with the very small gains in life span that come at a great price. Some examples of this include chemotherapy for cancer and treating HIV disease. Although life may be prolonged, the individual may worry about how his or her quality of life may be affected.

When the physician's goal for treatment is to improve how patients are feeling rather than to merely prolong their lives, HRQOL measurement is vital. Difficult decisions occur, however, when the relationship between laboratory measures and HRQOL outcomes is uncertain. In the past, physicians have relied on substitute outcomes, not because they were not interested in making patients feel better but because they assumed a strong link between physiologic measurements and the well-being of the patient.

A recent RCT of patients with symptomatic postmenopausal osteoporosis studied the effect of sodium fluoride on bone density and vertebral fractures. The researchers reasoned that increased bone mass and fewer vertebral fractures would most definitely lead to decreased pain and increased functionality. The question to be asked, however, is does the failure of the researchers to measure the effect of treatment in areas of unequivocal importance to patients, including pain, physical function, and household and leisure activities, affect the clinical message of the results? Based on research related to HRQOL, the answer would be yes.

Fear of Recurrent Disease

The relationship between physiological and clinical measures and patients' symptoms is usually somewhat modest. Each clinician must therefore rely on his or her own threshold. However, increasing consultation with the patient is becoming the norm.

Studies of cancer survivors reveal that many of them fear the recurrence of the disease. Studies show that HRQOL measures can also be successfully used with former as well as current cancer patients.

Future Implications

As HRQOL measures continue to be developed and expand in their use, they will likely have a growing impact on improving the health of populations. HRQOL tools hold much potential in facilitating a more effective healthcare system and enhancing patient outcomes.

Gene J. Koprowski

See also Activities of Daily Living (ADL); Acute and Chronic Diseases; Cancer Care; Disability; Measurement in Health Services Research; Mental Health; Quality of Well-Being Scale; Short-Form Health Surveys (SF-36, -12, -8)

Further Readings

Cantrell, Mary Ann, and Paul Lupinacci. "Investigating the Determinants of Health-Related Quality of Life Among Childhood Cancer Survivors," *Journal of Advanced Nursing* 64(1): 73–83, October 2008.

Centers for Disease Control and Prevention. *Measuring Healthy Days: Population Assessment of Health-Related Quality of Life.* Atlanta, GA: Centers for Disease Control and Prevention, November 2000.

Krouse, Robert S., M. Jane Mohler, Christopher S. Wendel, et al. "The VA Ostomy Health-Related Quality of Life Study: Objectives, Methods, and Patient Sample," *Current Medical Research and Opinion* 22(4): 781–91, April 2006.

Lis, Christopher G., Digant Gupta, and James F. Grutsch, "Patient Satisfaction With Health-Related Quality of Life: Implications for Prognosis in Prostate Cancer," *Clinical Genitourinary Cancer* 6(2): 91–96, September 2008.

Strandberg, Arto Y., Timo E. Strandberg, Kaisu Pitkala, et al., "The Effect of Smoking in Midlife on Health-Related Quality of Life in Old Age: A 26-Year Prospective Study," *Archives of Internal Medicine* 168(18): 1968–74, October 13, 2008.

Web Sites

Centers for Disease Control and Prevention (CDC), Health-Related Quality of Life: http://www.cdc.gov/hrqol

Centre for Health Evidence (CHE): http://www.cche.net/usersguides/life.asp

Quality of Well-Being Scale (QWB)

The Quality of Well-Being Scale (QWB) is a widely used general health index that summarizes an individual's current symptoms and disabilities in a single number. It represents a judgment of the health problems of an individual or population, and it can be expressed in terms of quality-adjusted life years (QALY). The QWB can be used as an outcome measure to estimate present and future healthcare needs, and it can be used with any type of acute or chronic disease.

Overview

The first version of the QWB was developed in the 1970s by J. W. Bush and his colleagues at the University of California at San Diego. It was later refined to its current forms in the late 1990s by Robert M. Kaplan. The QWB is a general health-related questionnaire that measures quality of life as defined by four major domains—symptoms, mobility, physical activity, and social activity. Scores from the questionnaire are often translated into an economic assessment for studies of cost-effectiveness of treatment and also to approximate an individual's QALY. The QWB exists in two formats—self-administered (QWB-SA) or given by a trained interviewer, often a healthcare provider. Each type of QWB takes about 20 minutes to complete. The QWB has been translated into Spanish, German, Chinese, and many other languages.

Scoring

In terms of finding a person's place on the scale, the QWB combines weighted values for symptoms and functioning. Functioning is evaluated by questions that gather information about limitations over the previous 3 days, within three areas—mobility, physical activity, and social activity. In addition, symptoms are evaluated by asking simple questions about how the individual feels with regard to the presence or absence of common symptom complexes (e.g., sore throat, joint pain). The scores (which are arranged in a roughly normal distribution) from these four areas are tallied to provide a numerical evaluation of an individual's well-being at a given point in time, somewhere on the continuum between the extremes of *death* (0.00) to *complete health* (1.00). In addition to using morbidity descriptors, the QWB also uses mortality data from life tables, clinical experience, and direct measurement to help determine quality-adjusted life expectancy (current life expectancy corrected for decreased quality of life associated with disabilities and disease states).

Validity and Reliability

Many research studies have shown the QWB to be very reliable (consistency of measurement) in the short term, especially when it is given on back-to-back days, with a 96% reliability rate in the general adult population and ranging from 83% reliability in burn patients to 98% reliability in chronic obstructive pulmonary disease (COPD) patients, when considering the population with morbidities. Many studies have also shown the QWB to be highly valid (correctness of measurement) in repeated randomized controlled trials (RCTs). One study, for example, found that individuals with Alzheimer's disease scored significantly lower on the QWB, while the degree of cognitive impairment was also found to be related in a systematic way, leading to lower QWB scores. Another study found that the QWB scores were highly correlated with performance and physiological findings relevant to the health status of those with COPD. At the same time, the QWB was capable of being translated into well-year units for studies of cost-effectiveness and also served as an outcome predictor and measure for the disease.

Criticisms

Criticisms of the QWB include the fact that there is no mental health component, which some would argue makes evaluating psychiatric patients very difficult (although Kaplan disagrees with this notion). Another difficulty with the QWB is assessing the potential impact of the interviewer on the responses of the individual. The QWB has also been criticized as being long, complex, expensive, and difficult to administer. To some extent the self-administered

QWB alleviates many of these problems. It has been shown that the self-administered version of the QWB is highly correlated with the interviewer-administered QWB and that it retains the same validity and reliability.

Future Implications

The QWB has been used in numerous RCTs and research studies to evaluate medical and surgical treatments for conditions such as arthritis, atrial fibrillation, COPD, cystic fibrosis, diabetes mellitus, and lung transplantation. In addition, the QWB was used to prioritize medical procedures and ration health resources by Oregon's Medicaid program in the late 1980s and early 1990s. The innovative, and highly controversial, Oregon Plan attempted to extend Medicaid cost-effective health services such as prenatal care but eliminated costly, ineffective services such as organ transplants. After the deaths of several individuals who required transplants, the plan was suspended. With the increase in the nation's aging population and growing concerns over the cost-effectiveness of healthcare, it seems likely that quality-of-life measures such as the QWB will be more widely used by healthcare organizations, practitioners, and researchers to measure various treatments and allocate resources.

Sumul Gandhi

See also Cost-Benefit and Cost-Effectiveness Analyses; Health; Quality-Adjusted Life Years (QALYs); Quality Indicators; Quality of Healthcare; Quality of Life, Health-Related; Short-Form Health Surveys (SF-36, -12, -8)

Further Readings

Frosch, Dominick L., Robert M. Kaplan, Theodore G. Ganiats, et al. "Validity of Self-Administered Quality of Well-Being Scale in Musculoskeletal Disease," *Arthritis Care and Research* 51(1): 28–33, February 15, 2004.

Kaplan, Robert M., Theodore G. Ganiats, William J. Sieber, et al. "The Quality of Well-Being Scale: Critical Similarities and Differences With SF-36," *International Journal for Quality in Health Care* 10(6): 509–520, December 1998.

McDowell, Ian. *Measuring Health: A Guide to Rating Scales and Questionnaires.* 3d ed. New York: Oxford University Press, 2006.

Smith, Michael T., Timothy P. Carmody, and Michelle S. Smith. "Quality of Well-Being Scale and Chronic Low Back Pain," *Journal of Clinical Psychology in Medical Settings* 7(3): 175–84, September 2000.

Web Sites

Medical Outcome Trust: http://www.outcomes-trust.org
University of California, San Diego, Health Outcomes Assessment Program (HOAP): http://famprevmed.ucsd.edu/hoap

R

RAND Corporation

The RAND Corporation is the largest policy analysis think tank in the United States. The RAND (a contraction of "research and development") Corporation is an independent, nonprofit institution that conducts research and analysis for the U.S. and foreign governments, international organizations, industry, foundations, universities, professional associations, and other organizations. Headquartered in Santa Monica, California, with branch offices in Washington, D.C., and Pittsburgh, Pennsylvania, the RAND Corporation employs about 1,600 people. It annually receives over $200 million in contracts and grants, and at any given time its staff is working on about 500 projects. Of its nine research divisions, the RAND Health division consists of over 170 employees. Each year, it produces many reports concerning various aspects of health services research.

Background

During the various military campaigns of World War II, the U.S. War Department, the Office of Scientific Research and Development, and industry identified the need for a private organization to link military planning with research and development. To establish such an organization, the U.S. Army Air Forces (USAAF) in the fall of 1945 issued a special contract to the Douglas Aircraft Company in Santa Monica, California, to create Project RAND, which would eventually become the RAND Corporation.

A number of people participated in the creation of Project RAND, including H. H. "Hap" Arnold, U.S. Secretary of War and Commanding General of the USAAF; Edward Bowles, a professor of electrical engineering at the Massachusetts Institute of Technology (MIT) and a consultant to the Secretary of War; General Lauris Norstad, Assistant Chief of Air Staff for Plans, USAAF; Major General Curtis LeMay of the USAAF, who was in charge of the strategic bombing of Japan; Donald Douglas, President of Douglas Aircraft Company; Arthur Raymond, Chief Engineer at Douglas; and Franklin Collbohm, Raymond's assistant.

The first report of Project RAND, which was published in 1946, was years ahead of its time. It addressed the design and possible use of an experimental, world-circling spaceship.

In 1948, with the approval of the U.S. Air Force (which was established in 1947), RAND became an independent, nonprofit corporation. And Project RAND was transferred to the new corporation. During much of the Cold War era, the RAND Corporation worked closely with the defense industry, the military, and the federal government, helping to develop policies and strategies and to improve decision making. In the 1960s, RAND expanded its scope to also include national, social, economic, political, and healthcare delivery and financing issues.

Organizational Structure

The RAND Corporation's mission is to help improve policy and decision making through research and analysis. Its core values are quality and objectivity. To accomplish its mission, RAND is governed by a 23-member Board of Trustees, which is composed of leaders from the business, academic, and nonprofit sectors. The corporation is also guided by 16 advisory boards, composed of experts in various areas. It has nine research divisions, including the following: RAND Army Resource Division; RAND Education; RAND Europe; RAND Health; RAND Infrastructure, Safety, and Environment; RAND Institute for Civil Justice; RAND Labor and Population; RAND National Security Research Division; and the RAND Project AIR FORCE.

RAND Health Division

Originating in the 1960s, the RAND Health division currently consists of three programs: Economics, Finance, and Organization; Quality Assessment and Quality Improvement; and Health Promotion and Disease Prevention. The division also includes four strategic initiatives: Compare; Global Health; Public Health Preparedness; and Military Health. The division's research agenda is very broad, including areas such as aging and health; complementary and alternative medicine; diversity and health; end-of-life care; global health; health economics; health security; HIV, sexually transmitted diseases, and sexual behavior; informatics and technology; maternal, child, and adolescent health; mental health; military health; neighborhood influences on health; overweight and obesity; public health; quality of care; substance abuse: alcohol, drugs, and tobacco; and violence and health.

Past and Present Healthcare Research

Over the decades, the RAND Corporation has conducted a number of innovative and influential health services research studies. For example, in the early 1970s to the mid-1980s, it conducted the RAND Health Insurance Experiment (HIE). The HIE was one of the largest and most important social experiments in U.S. history. It randomly assigned several thousand families in various regions of the nation to insurance plans with various levels of cost-sharing arrangements and then followed them for up to 5 years to evaluate the effects on healthcare expenditures and health status. The study helped shape health services research in the nation and greatly influences policies for healthcare financing.

In the late 1980s and early 1990s, RAND conducted the Medical Outcome Study (MOS), the first large-scale study attempting to measure medical outcomes in terms of how individuals feel, function, and perform. As part of the study, a brief, health-screening survey instrument was developed: the Short Form 36-Item Health Survey, or SF-36. Today, the SF-36 and other versions of it are widely used throughout the world.

In late 1990, RAND conducted the HIV Cost and Services Utilization Study (HCSUS), the first comprehensive national survey on healthcare use of persons in care for HIV. The study provided information on the barriers to access, the costs of HIV care, and the effects of HIV on quality of life.

In the 2005, RAND released the first comprehensive study of the costs and quality effects of computerizing clinical records. The study found that computerizing records dramatically increased efficiency, greatly increased safety, and led to various health benefits.

Currently, the RAND Health division is conducting research in health economics, public health, and quality of care. For example, in 2007, its researchers provided technical assistance to the U.S. Department of Health and Human Services (HHS) on how to improve the readiness of state and local health departments to respond to emergencies. They conducted research to determine what percentage of children in the United States are receiving recommended care for acute and chronic medical problems. And they helped global health officials address the threat of an influenza pandemic in Southeast Asia.

Frederick S. Pardee RAND Graduate School

The RAND Corporation established a graduate school in public policy analysis in 1970. The school, originally the RAND Graduate Institute, changed its name to the RAND Graduate School in 1987, and in 2004, its name was again changed to honor Frederick S. Pardee, a former RAND researcher and philanthropist. The graduate school, which is part of RAND and an autonomous entity within it, primarily awards the Doctor of Philosophy (PhD) degree. It also awards a Master of Philosophy (MPhil) degree. About 25 new students are accepted each year, and currently there are about 100 students enrolled in the school. Doctoral students (called fellows) are required to take course work and qualifying examinations and to write a dissertation. They also are required to take a practicum by working on various RAND projects. To date, the school has awarded about 200 doctoral degrees, making it the world's leading producer of doctorates in public policy analysis. Graduates from the school are employed in research and public service, as well as in the private sector.

Ross M. Mullner and Cherie Weinewuth

See also Brook, Robert H.; Health Economics; Newhouse, Joseph P.; Public Policy; RAND Health Insurance Experiment; Short-Form Health Surveys (SF-36, -12, -8); Ware, John E.

Further Readings

Abella, Alex. *Soldiers of Reason: The RAND Corporation and the Rise of the American Empire.* Orlando, FL: Harcourt, 2008.

Collins, Martin J. *Cold War Laboratory: RAND, the Air Force, and the American State.* Washington, DC: Smithsonian Institute Press, 2002.

Kaplan, Fred M. *The Wizards of Armageddon.* New York: Simon and Schuster, 1983.

RAND Corporation. *Project AIR FORCE 50 Years: 1946–1996.* Washington, DC: RAND Corporation, 1996.

Web Sites

Frederick S. Pardee RAND Graduate School: http://www.prgs.edu

RAND Corporation: http://rand.org

RAND Health: http://rand.org/health

RAND HEALTH INSURANCE EXPERIMENT

The RAND Health Insurance Experiment (HIE) was one of the largest and most important social experiments in U.S. history. The HIE randomly assigned several thousand families in various geographic areas of the nation to insurance plans with various levels of copayments and then followed up for 5 years to evaluate the effects on healthcare expenditures and health status. The experiment ran from approximately 1974 to 1982. At the time, there was limited information on the impact of cost sharing or of prepaid care on health expenditures, and there was almost no information on the impact of health insurance on health status. The experiment's results encouraged the restructuring of the nation's private health insurance, and they are still widely cited today.

Background

To assess the potential economic and health impacts of decisions on what insurance coverage to provide, how generous the cost sharing should be, and how services should be delivered (traditional fee-for-service-based insurance plans versus prepaid, health maintenance organization [HMO]–style managed care), there are two research strategies. The first is to collect more and better observational data, including information on insurance structure, health status, and other confounders that could lead to biased assessment of the effect of health insurance on either expenditures or subsequent health status. The second is to design and conduct a randomized trial that would experimentally assign coverage to remove the potential bias from residual confounding or to avoid adverse selection effects. Both strategies were followed from the 1970s through the end of the century. Major observational data sets were collected under the auspices of the National Center for Health Services Research (NCHSR), the Agency for Health Care Policy and Research (AHCPR), the Agency for Healthcare Research and Quality (AHRQ), and the National Center for Health Statistics (NCHS). The RAND Corporation designed and conducted the randomized trial known as the HIE with financial support from the Office of the Assistant Secretary for Planning and Evaluation (ASPE). The health economist Joseph Newhouse was the principal investigator for the project throughout its length.

Study Design and Sample

The HIE enrolled families in six sites—Dayton, Ohio; Seattle, Washington; Fitchburg, Massachusetts; Franklin County, Massachusetts; Charleston, South Carolina; and Georgetown County, South Carolina—starting in 1974. The last of the enrollees exited the study in 1982. The sites were selected to represent the four geographic census regions, to represent the range of city sizes to reflect the complexity of the medical delivery system, to cover a range of waiting times to appointment and physician per capita ratios (in order to test for the sensitivity of demand to non-price rationing), and to include both urban and rural sites in the North and the South.

Health Insurance Plans

Families participating in the experiment were randomly assigned to 1 of 14 different fee-for-service or 2 prepaid group practice health insurance plans. The fee-for-service plans had different levels of cost sharing that varied over two dimensions: the coinsurance rate and an upper limit on out-of-pocket expenses. The coinsurance rates (percentage paid out of pocket) were 0%, 25%, 50%, or 95% for all health services. Each plan had a stop-loss or upper limit on out-of-pocket expenses of 5%, 10%, or 15% of family income up to a maximum of $1,000. Beyond the maximum out-of-pocket dollar expenditure amounts, the insurance plan reimbursed all expenses in full. One plan had different coinsurance rates for inpatients and ambulatory medical services (25%) than for dental and ambulatory mental health services (50%). Finally, on one plan, the families faced a 95% coinsurance rate for outpatient services, subject to a $150 annual limit on out-of-pocket expenses per person ($450 per family). In this plan, all inpatient services were free; in effect, this plan had an outpatient individual deductible. The coinsurance rate for this plan was changed to 95% after the 1st year of the study in the first site (Dayton, Ohio).

To illustrate how one of the plans worked, we consider a plan with a family coinsurance rate of 25% up to a stop-loss of $1,000 in 1970s dollars (or $3,400 in 2007 dollars, corrected by the all-item consumer price index). For the first $4,000 of

expenditures on any health service (dental, medical, or mental health), the family pays 25% of the bill, and the insurance company pays 75%. Beyond that point (the stop-loss), the family pays nothing more out of pocket for the remainder of that year. The following year, the family again will incur out-of-pocket expenses of 25% of the bill until it reaches its stop-loss or upper limit on out-of-pocket expenses.

In addition to the fee-for-service-based health insurance plans, the HIE had two groups enrolled in a prepaid staff model HMO, Group Health Cooperative of Puget Sound (GHC). The scope of benefits was comparable with that of all the fee-for-service plans. Like the free plan, there was no out-of-pocket cost as long as enrolled individuals stayed within the plan.

All plans covered the same wide variety of services, including inpatient and outpatient medical care, mental healthcare, dental services, drugs and supplies. However, there were some benefit exclusions: nonpreventive orthodontia, cosmetic surgery, and outpatient psychotherapy services in excess of 52 visits per year per person.

The families were enrolled on their experimental health insurance plans as a group, subject to the same coinsurance rate(s) and stop-loss, with the exception of the Individual Deductible Plan with its separate individual deductible for outpatient care. Only individuals eligible for the experiment could participate. Families were either offered one experimental plan or were allowed to continue with their existing coverage. To prevent refusals, families were given a lump-sum payment greater than the worst-case outcome in their experimental plans relative to their previous plan; thus, families were always better off financially for accepting the enrollment offer. Moreover, because of a bonus for completion, they were always better off completing the study. Hence, there is a theoretical presumption of no bias from refusal or attrition. In fact, study researchers have detected negligible effects from refusal and attrition.

Families were assigned to treatments using the finite selection model. This model is designed to achieve as much balance across plans as possible while retaining randomization; that is, it reduces the correlation of the experimental treatment with health, demographic, and economic covariates.

Refusal and Attrition

There are two potential threats to the balance of health and other characteristics across insurance plans: (1) nonrandom refusal of the offer to participate and (2) nonrandom attrition from the study. Refusals of the plan offer varied across plans. However, analysis of these refusals to participate indicates that the only significant difference between those who accepted and those who rejected the offer was that the latter had lower education and income. Income is controlled for in the analysis of experimental data, and education had no detectable (partial) effect on use. There is no evidence that those who rejected the offer to participate were sicker or that there was an interaction between plan, sickness, and refusal of the offer.

Individuals on the cost-sharing plans were more likely to leave the study early than were individuals on the free plan. These early departures were also sicker on average than those who stayed. Thus, people on the cost-sharing plans at the end of the study were healthier on average than those on the free plan. This could lead to an overestimate of the response to the cost-sharing insurance plans. To correct for such a potential bias, baseline health status measures were included as covariates.

Population Sampled

The individuals enrolled in the experiment were drawn from a random sample of each site's noninstitutionalized civilian population, excluding those 62 years of age and older at the time of enrollment, those with incomes in excess of $25,000 in 1973 (or $115,000 in 2007 dollars—this excluded 3% of the families contacted), those eligible for the Medicare disability program, and veterans with service-connected disabilities. The HIE also included a group in GHC. A group of nonelderly individuals already enrolled in GHC were randomly selected and invited to participate as a control group. Another group of nonelderly, noninstitutionalized civilians in the fee-for-service system were randomized to be an experimental group at GHC from the same pool as those enrolled in the fee-for-service plans.

Estimation Samples

Estimation samples varied from the study groups being examined—the whole population, adults, children, fee-for-service plans, or comparisons between fee-for-service and prepaid group plans (in Seattle only). Interim results were reported in the first two fifths of the data and final results on the full sample of those enrolled for the 3- to 5-year duration.

Outcomes (Dependent) Variables

The analysis of the economic effects of cost sharing focused on medical care utilization (inpatient hospital stays, outpatient visits, episodes of treatment) and related healthcare expenditures (including drugs and supplies), based on information collected on health insurance claims. All expenditures, including out-of-pocket payments and payments by the insurance carrier, were relevant. For the prepaid plans, medical records were abstracted in the form of claims data and assigned prevailing fee-for-service prices; these were augmented with information on out-of-plan use.

The effects of cost sharing focused on a number of health status measures developed as a part of the HIE. These included scales based on self-reported health status in a number of health domains (general health, mental and social health, physical and role limitations, pain, etc.), the presence and severity of health conditions, as well as assessments based on physical examinations that were given to a random percentage of families at enrollment and to all families at normal completion. Nearly 77% of all noncompletion cases (85% of the survivors) were located and had their health assessed.

Independent Variables

Most analyses of the HIE report simple averages by health insurance plan or by groups of plans. However, any analysis must rely on results that already control for demographic, health status, and socioeconomic measures in addition to fixed effects for study sites and the health insurance plan.

Unit of Analysis

The unit of analysis is a person-year for the analysis of utilization and expenditures, because the stop-loss is an annual limit. The researchers used the person as the unit of observation because the major determinants of the use of services are individual (e.g., age, gender, and health status) rather than family (e.g., insurance coverage and family income).

The unit of analysis for the health status studies is the person, again because the major determinants of health are individual. Children (under age 13) were separated from adults because the instrumentation of health status was different.

Results

Healthcare Utilization and Expenditures

The results from the HIE indicate that increases in out-of-pocket cost sharing reduced healthcare use and costs. Since all these plans had a stop-loss on the financial risk incurred by the family, this is the effect of first-dollar cost sharing, not the effect of a change in out-of-pocket price throughout the year. Thus, each response is a response to price for part of the year and having free care (beyond the stop-loss or deductible) for the remainder of the year. Specifically, higher coinsurance rates reduce expenditures by about 20% for moderate levels of cost sharing and nearly 30% for high levels of cost sharing. This response corresponds to a price elasticity of approximately −0.2 once the effect of the stop-loss has been eliminated. Though less dramatic, the same response is observed for the probability of any care and for any admission during the year. Most of the response to cost sharing can be traced to the reduction in the likelihood of having any healthcare during the year.

Although children and adults exhibited similar responses to insurance plans for outpatient care, they had different responses to cost sharing for inpatient hospital care. There was little response for children but a significant response for adults. The experiment did not detect any differential response to cost sharing by income group, gender, health status, or site.

Other healthcare goods and services exhibited different or more complicated responses. The expenditures for outpatient prescriptions followed the same pattern as that for outpatient care. The response of emergency department use to cost sharing was very similar to that for general medical care, but this masked a major difference in response depending on the urgency of the diagnosis. Urgent emergency department demand had half the response to cost sharing that less urgent care did. Dental-care demand surged on the free plan by 46% during the 1st year of the experiment. After that, plans with out-of-pocket cost sharing were about a quarter less expensive than the free plan. Outpatient mental healthcare was almost twice as responsive to cost sharing as outpatient care.

In an attempt to understand whether cost sharing had a greater effect on the appropriateness of care, the study examined the appropriateness of inpatient care for conditions other than maternity, pediatric, or psychiatric, using a methodology that indicated whether the care had to be done in a hospital or could have been done as an outpatient service. The free and cost-sharing plans had very similar and statistically insignificantly different fractions of hospitalizations that were inappropriate. Thus it appears that cost sharing is a blunt instrument for reducing inappropriate care because it reduced both appropriate and inappropriate care by approximately the same amount.

The HMO experimental group had 28% lower annual expenditures than the free fee-for-service plan. Both had the same benefits and the same out-of-pocket costs. This lower expenditure rate was achieved largely by a 39% lower admission rate at the HMO. Outpatient visit rates were comparable for both the HMO experimental group and the free fee-for-service plans. Other fee-for-service plans also had higher expenditure rates than the HMO, except for the 95% plan, which acts like a large deductible plan. That plan had significantly lower visit rates and insignificantly higher admission rates than the HMO experimental group. The individual deductible plans followed a similar pattern.

One of the concerns motivating this experiment group was that HMOs were experiencing favorable selection that would help explain the difference in utilization and costs. The experimental comparisons suggest that such an explanation did not account for the differences observed in this mature HMO. A further comparison of those HMO enrollees who self-selected into the HMO versus those who were randomized in indicates only modest differences. If anything, the controls were slightly older and sicker than the experimental group, which partially accounts for the difference in visit rates.

Health Status

Despite the substantial reduction in healthcare utilization and expenditures, there was little evidence that cost sharing had an adverse effect on the overall health status of the HIE's enrollees. There was no statistically significant effect on average for adults on general health or separately for physical, mental, or social health or on an index of the risk of dying. Nor was there an effect on the economically poorest part of the adult population. However, there was some evidence that those individuals who were both poor and sick at the beginning of the experiment had better health status at the end of the experiment if they were on the free plan rather than on the cost-sharing plans. This group constituted about 6% of the HIE population.

There were some areas of health that were better with the free plan than with cost sharing. These included hypertension control and vision; there was also a reduction in the number of decayed teeth among young adults.

There was no statistically significant effect of cost sharing on children's health status relative to the free plan. Nor was there evidence of an effect for at-risk or poor children.

For both children and adults, there was no evidence of an overall effect of the prepaid, staff model HMO compared with the free fee-for-service plan.

Policy Implications

The HIE found that health insurance plans with first-dollar cost sharing and moderate deductibles could have a major impact on total healthcare utilization and healthcare costs without having an adverse effect on the health status of nonelderly individuals. Although there were healthcare reductions, the cost sharing appeared to be a blunt policy instrument in that it reduced both medically appropriate and medically inappropriate hospitalization nearly equally. However, it is important to recognize that the word *inappropriate* has a more limited use in this and other studies of the period. Here, an inappropriate hospital stay means that the treatment could have been given in an outpatient setting, while an inappropriate inpatient stay means that the stay was inappropriate

or that the patient had unnecessary days at either the beginning or the end of the stay.

If cost sharing reduced both inpatient and outpatient care, why were the changes in health status so modest—largely limited to blood pressure control, corrected vision, and decreases in dental decay? Why weren't there more substantial changes in overall health status or mortality? Several explanations have been offered: The nonelderly population as a whole is healthy relative to the elderly or the disabled, and thus there is less room for improvement; the similar effect on appropriate versus inappropriate care may mean that there are offsetting effects of cost sharing; the data are from the 1970s and early 1980s, before the major drops in inpatient utilization in the nation, and thus there may have been more discretionary care in the healthcare system than has been the case in the past decade; and the presence of a stop-loss on the plans means that cost sharing was never large enough to deter any major or important utilization (none of the health plans involved unlimited cost sharing or left the family completely uninsured). Finally, it is worth remembering that one of the major benefits of health insurance is to protect risk-averse individuals against the uncertainty involved with large healthcare bills, especially ones that may be sufficiently large to impoverish the individuals. All these explanations are plausible to some degree. A single study, even one as well designed and executed as the HIE, is not sufficient to answer these questions.

There were some findings from the HIE that raise concerns. There was some evidence that cost sharing could have an adverse effect on the health of those who were *both* sick and poor—not sick *or* poor, but having both characteristics. This could provide an argument for differentially lower cost sharing or the elimination of cost sharing for this group.

The prepaid versus fee-for-service findings suggest that large drops in inpatient use can be achieved without major adverse effects on the overall populations. This was consistent with the major drops in inpatient use during the 1990s and the spread of managed care and managed indemnity plans. However small the differences in health status, there were major differences in patient satisfaction, which is consistent with the widespread reaction to the spread of managed care.

If cost sharing coupled with stop-losses can reduce healthcare costs without much risk to the health of the general nonelderly population, then is the long-term decrease in cost sharing responsible for a large part of medical care inflation? The answer is "Probably not." It is true historically that more generously covered services have experienced more rapid inflation than less generously covered ones. But the magnitude of the post-HIE changes in healthcare utilization (visits and stays) is not enough to account for medical care inflation; it is not the demand response to cost sharing per se that increased healthcare expenditures. That part is too small. It appears that the relation of costsharing to the rapid growth in healthcare expenditure is more complex and involves linkages to more rapid rates of technological progress and adoption of more generously covered service plans by institutions.

Willard G. Manning

See also Coinsurance, Copays, and Deductibles; Cost of Healthcare; Health Economics; Health Insurance; Health Surveys; Newhouse, Joseph P.; RAND Corporation

Further Readings

Brook, Robert H., John E. Ware Jr., Allyson Davies-Avery, et al. "Overview of Adult Measures Fielded in RAND's Health Insurance Study," *Medical Care* 17(7 Suppl.): iii–x, 1–131, 1979.

Gruber, Jonathan. *The Role of Consumer Copayments for Health Care: Lessons From the RAND Health Insurance Experiment and Beyond.* Publication No. 7566. Menlo Park, CA: Henry J. Kaiser Family Foundation, 2006.

Manning, Willard G., Joseph P. Newhouse, Naihua Duan, et al. "Health Insurance and the Demand for Medical Care: Evidence From a Randomized Experiment," *American Economic Review* 77(3): 251–77, June 1987.

Newhouse, Joseph P. "Consumer-Directed Health Plans and the RAND Health Insurance Experiment," *Health Affairs* 23(6): 107–113, November–December 2004.

Newhouse, Joseph P., Robert H. Brook, Naihua Duan, et al. "Attrition in the RAND Health Insurance Experiment: A Response to Nyman," *Journal of Health Politics, Policy and Law* 33(2) 295–308, April 2008.

Newhouse, Joseph P., and the Insurance Experiment Group. *Free For All? Lessons From the RAND Health Insurance Experiment.* Cambridge, MA: Harvard University Press, 1993.

RAND Corporation. "The Health Insurance Experiment: A Classic RAND Study Speaks to the Current Health Care Reform Debate," *RAND Research Highlights,* 2006.

Web Sites

America's Health Insurance Plans (AHIP): http://www.ahip.org

American Economic Association (AEA): http://www.vanderbilt.edu/AEA

American Society of Health Economists (ASHE): http://healtheconomics.us

Henry J. Kaiser Family Foundation (KFF): http://www.kff.org

RAND Health Insurance Experiment (HIE): http://rand.org/health/projects/hie

RANDOMIZED CONTROLLED TRIALS (RCTs)

In medicine, a clinical trial is an experimental study conducted on human subjects to answer or confirm a research question. Clinical trials can be designed at the discretion of the researcher and must meet certain ethical criteria to ensure the protection of human subjects. Of the many research design options for clinical trials, the randomized controlled trial (RCT) has evolved as the gold standard in the investigation of several types of treatments, including (but not limited to) new therapies, community interventions, and diagnostic techniques. The RCT is often referred to as a randomized clinical trial, and the terms are used interchangeably throughout the literature.

Historical Beginnings

The earliest reference to research that meets the definition of a controlled trial dates back to 605–562 BC, when King Nebuchadnezzar II carried out the first controlled trial by ordering that a strict diet of meat and wine be followed by a small group of children for 3 years while four children of royal blood were allowed to exchange bread and water for the required meal. After only 10 days, those who had switched to bread and water appeared healthier than those who ate only wine and meat.

In 1537, the French Renaissance surgeon Ambroise Parè (1510–1590) blended a mixture of oil of rose, turpentine, and egg yolk as a replacement for the accepted regimen for treating open wounds. One day after the unintentional trial, Parè observed that the wounds treated with the traditional formula were swollen and extremely painful, while the wounds treated with the experimental mixture were not painful, indicating that the new balm was more favorable than the oil usually applied.

Active Controls

The Scottish naval surgeon James Lind (1716–1794) is often credited with originating controlled trials, since he was the first to introduce a control group into his experiments in approximately 1747. A control is when the investigator, or the individual conducting the study, controls the treatment or stimulus to be received by the subject. In this context, one can study the treatment or stimulus, defined as the experimental group, by comparison with (or as a supplement to) the standard of care, defined as the control group. Lind studied the great sea plague, scurvy, of the time. On long naval voyages, it was not uncommon for scurvy to kill two thirds of a ship's crew. To prevent scurvy, Lind conducted the first planned, controlled trial, supplementing the diet of a small number of sailors with fresh citrus fruit and lemon juice (the experimental group). He then compared the incidence of scurvy among those men with that among other sailors on the same ship who ate the normal vitamin-poor naval diet (the control group). Finding that citrus fruit prevented the disease, Lind recommended dietary changes for all sailors, which ultimately resulted in the eradication of scurvy from the British navy. Hence, British sailors are still referred to as "limeys."

Blinding and Placebo Control

By 1863, controlled trials began to evolve with more rigorous study designs, including the use of placebo treatments. A placebo can be considered a type of control in which no active treatment or stimulus is introduced, but rather subjects assigned to a placebo receive an inactive or sugar pill if the treatment is a pill medication or an injection of salt water if the treatment is a fluid injection, or they go through the routine of having an X ray without the instrument being activated. The placebo has the broadest indication in medicine, as it is effective to a greater or lesser extent in almost all medical settings, necessitating additional design enhancements to minimize bias addressing this phenomenon, known as the placebo effect.

The introduction of a matching placebo allows for the blinding or masking of what treatment, if any, the subject is receiving. In controlled (clinical) trials, treatments are often compared to assess the experimental treatment's effect as compared with what should be the noneffective treatment of the placebo. Participants in the control group receive a placebo instead of an active treatment, and the results from the placebo group are then compared with the results from the experimental group, which received the treatment. Blinding can also be used when comparing different active treatments. The process of blinding, with or without the use of a placebo, helps control for bias that is introduced if the subject or the researcher (or both) is aware of the treatment group to which the subject has been assigned. In a single-blind design, the subjects do not know what treatment they are receiving. In a double-blind design, neither the person delivering nor the one receiving the therapy knows which treatment has been assigned.

Randomization

In 1912, the U.S. Congress passed the Sherley Amendment to the 1906 U.S. Food and Drugs Act, prohibiting labeling medicines with false treatment claims. This amendment ultimately raised experimental standards to the level of requiring the conduct of controlled trials for new treatments. This stimulated the growth of the RCT and further added to the design rigor expected to prove the effectiveness and safety of drugs approved for marketing in the United States.

Generally, a researcher uses randomization to indiscriminately allocate subjects between or among the different treatments or stimuli, thus performing a "randomized" controlled trial. The major strength of this approach, known as random assignment, is a theoretical equal distribution of potential confounding factors that are known, unknown, or not measurable. Without this, the treatment groups may be different and not comparable. Because biases are minimized by randomization and the treatment groups are directly comparable as a result, associations demonstrated in RCTs are more likely to be causal associations than those demonstrated using other research study designs. If the study is powered sufficiently (i.e., is sufficiently large to detect true differences), the assigned treatment is the most likely explanation of any observed differences in the outcomes, whether an improvement or a worsening of the disease state, between the treatment groups.

The English statistician Sir Ronald Aylmer Fisher (1890–1962) first introduced randomization in the 1920s in the science of agriculture. In Fisher's experiment the assignment of a plant strain to a plot of land was made randomly. In a controlled (clinical) trial, the same principle results in the assignment of a treatment to subjects by chance, by placing the subjects randomly into three treatment groups (i.e., subjects are assigned to the active treatment group, to the nonactive treatment group, or to the placebo group). In this example, effective randomization would give a subject a 50% chance of being in any one treatment group or arm. This technique deliberately introduces noise into the study such that, over all RCTs that could have been conducted with the experimental treatment, each subject has an equal chance to be in any one treatment group or arm. Therefore, Fisher's technique, adding the noise of randomization to a controlled trial, allows for a fair comparison to be made between treatments.

In 1879, while at Johns Hopkins University, the American mathematician Charles Peirce (1839–1914) may have been the first to use randomization in a research study, to see if blindfolded people could notice the difference between a 1- and a 2-kilogram weight. Peirce would add or remove weight based on a specially designed deck of cards so as to remove the bias from the researcher making the weight adjustments.

Among the earliest randomized trials was one by the American physician James Burns Amberson Jr. (1890–1979). Amberson, an international authority on chest disease and tuberculosis, conducted a controlled (clinical) trail from 1926 to 1927 (published in 1931) of sanocrysin, a gold preparation, in pulmonary tuberculosis. The study used a flip of a coin to assign treatment to groups receiving either sanocrysin (active group) or distilled water (control group). Subjects were not aware of which treatment was administered.

A subsequent study, often referenced as the first documented trial to correctly use randomization to assign subjects to treatment and control groups, was carried out by the British Medical Research Council (MRC) in 1948 and involved the use of streptomycin to treat pulmonary tuberculosis. The British statistician Sir Austin Bradford Hill (1897–1991) played a major role in designing the trial, which featured a double-blind assignment to treatment groups, where neither the researchers nor the subjects knew which treatment group each subject was in during the conduct of the study, enabling unbiased analysis of the results.

Randomizations are usually balanced to ensure that, overall, the same quantity, or number, of subjects receives each of the available treatments; this is referred to as a simple or nonstratified randomization. A stratified randomization can be used to minimize the risk of imbalance or bias occurring because of the preponderance of a particular factor relative to the disease or its treatment in one of the treatment groups. To do this, the subjects are separated into groups (or the groups are predefined if the subjects have yet to be identified) according to the factors that are important, such as age, duration of illness, laboratory value, etc. A separate randomization plan or schedule is then prepared for each predefined group.

Multicenter Trials

Multicenter RCTs were first used in the 1940s. Multicenter studies are conducted at several different sites or locations, but all use the same research protocol. When numerous subjects are necessary to detect a meaningful difference in treatment, multicenter studies are typically conducted, making the studies large in scale. Data collected from subjects treated at each site can be pooled so that the greater numbers give increased statistical "power" to the overall results found. Multicenter RCTs are most commonly conducted by government and industry researchers and in some instances also by not-for-profit health organizations.

Trial Design

When comparing different treatments in an RCT, subjects may be given only one of the treatments prospectively as part of a parallel group design, or all treatments, each on different occasions, as part of a crossover design (also called within-subject comparison).

In the parallel-group study of treatments, each subject would be randomized to receive only one treatment. In the crossover study of treatments, each subject would receive each treatment one after the other. With the crossover design, the order in which the treatments are given is random to avoid the best or worst treatment always being taken first, thereby minimizing any bias in the results obtained from the alternative treatment. Depending on the type of treatment, there may also be a washout period (e.g., a period when the drug is shed from the body until there is no trace of the drug) between crossover design treatments such as placebo, no treatment, or an alternative noncompeting treatment (e.g., one that satisfies the needs of the subject in minimizing discomfort). The crossover study design typically requires fewer subjects than the parallel-group design, but the disease itself may have changed over the time of the treatment period, confounding the results, and the studies typically take longer to conduct, making the crossover study less favored and the parallel-group design the most commonly used.

Human-Subject Protection

RCTs should be carried out adhering to accepted standards of safety, subject welfare, and data interpretation. However, history shows that subject welfare was not always a high priority. To prevent atrocities such as those that occurred in World War II, the Nuremberg Code was developed in 1947. With it, the mid 20th century witnessed a period of protectionism for human subjects. The protection of human subjects has had an impact on the conduct of RCTs, as represented in the World Medical Association's development of the Declaration of Helsinki (first released in 1964, and subsequently amended in 1975, 1983, 1989, 1996, 2000, and 2001).

Most recently in 2001, the Declaration of Helsinki was revised to reaffirm its position that extreme care must be taken in conducting a placebo-controlled trial and that in general this methodology should only be used in the absence of existing proven therapy. However, a placebo-controlled trial may be ethically acceptable, even if proven therapy is available, if there are compelling and scientifically sound methodological reasons for its use—for example, if it is necessary to determine the efficacy or safety of a prophylactic, diagnostic, or therapeutic method or if a prophylactic, diagnostic, or therapeutic method is being investigated for a minor condition and the subjects who receive the placebo will not be subject to any additional risk of serious or irreversible harm. An investigator must propose and defend such research to an institutional review board (IRB)/institutional ethics committee for review to gain conduct approval.

Problems

RCTs are not without their problems. Conducting an RCT often has potential problems inherent in the study design and can be ethically and logistically challenging to perform. Examples of ethically problematic RCT designs include the use of a placebo when an alternate therapy is available, the use of a surrogate end point when the target end point is not reasonably attainable, or the establishment of a short-term follow-up period when the treatment may be intended for long-term application. In addition, randomized controlled (clinical) trials are expensive and artificial. The RCT results are applicable to efficacy (the effect of the treatment or stimulus in a controlled environment) but may not demonstrate effectiveness (the effect of the treatment or stimulus in an uncontrolled environment). This can be further explained by assuming that the severity of a disease is normally distributed, whereas an RCT is designed to include eligible subjects typically represented at the extremes from the mean, median, or mode to demonstrate a pronounced effect of the treatment or stimulus as compared with the control. Thus, the RCT does not represent a typical response expected from the majority of subjects that lie within a few standard deviations of a disease state distribution. However, when an RCT is robustly designed and of sufficient size, the results of the trial can be applied to the general population.

Future Implications

RCTs continue to be the gold standard for demonstrating safety and efficacy and will continue to be the model by which other experimental designs are judged, but they likely will continue to be critiqued. In the future, there will be continued scrutiny of the controlled (clinical) trial and its inherent design efficacy as opposed to effectiveness, especially considering public concerns over pharmaceutical treatment risks not fully elucidated until after FDA approval for use among the general population, leading to product withdrawals and black-box warnings. Additionally, U.S. policymakers have not fully endorsed the 2001 amendment to the Declaration of Helsinki and its limits on the use of placebos, in terms of the conduct of RCTs for novel treatments. It is important to note that regulatory agencies are beginning to make changes in their standards for approval of new drugs for the good of public health, but further discussions and development of policies are needed. There will be continued examination of the increasing expenditures for the development of novel treatments and of the development costs of conducting the RCTs necessary for approval, estimated at more than $1 billion for every new treatment in the United States. While there should always be a balance between medical progress and public health, the regulation and policy analysis of controlled (clinical) trials must ensure that this balance is acceptable and reasonable.

Daniel J. O'Brien

See also Association for the Accreditation of Human Research Protection Programs (AAHRPP); Epidemiology; Ethics; Evidence-Based Medicine (EBM); Pharmaceutical Industry; Public Health; Quality of Healthcare; U.S. Food and Drug Administration (FDA)

Further Readings

Biswas, Atanu. *Statistical Advances in the Biomedical Sciences: Clinical Trials, Epidemiology, Survival Analysis, and Bioinformatics.* Hoboken, NJ: Wiley, 2008.

Cook, Thomas D., and David L. DeMets. *Introduction to Statistical Methods for Clinical Trials.* Boca Raton, FL: Taylor and Francis, 2007.

Devereaux, P. J., and S. Yusuf. "The Evolution of the Randomized Controlled Trial and Its Role in Evidence-Based Decision," *Journal of Internal Medicine* 254(2): 105–13, August 2003.

Friedman, Lawrence M., Curt D. Furberg, and David L. DeMets. *Fundamentals of Clinical Trials.* 3d ed. New York: Springer Science+Business Media, 1998.

Furberg, Bengt, and Curt Furberg. *Evaluating Clinical Research: All That Glitters Is Not Gold.* New York: Springer Verlag, 2007.

Hulley, Stephen B., Steven R. Cummings, Warren S. Browner, et al. *Designing Clinical Research.* Philadelphia: Lippincott Williams and Wilkins, 2001.

Meinert, Curtic L. *Clinical Trials: Design, Conduct, and Analysis.* New York: Oxford University Press, 1986.

Rozovsky, Fay A., and Rodney K. Adams. *Clinical Trials and Human Research: A Practical Guide to Regulatory Compliance.* San Francisco: Jossey-Bass, 2003.

Spilker, Bert. *Guide to Clinical Trials.* Philadelphia: Lippincott Williams and Wilkins, 2000.

Torgerson, David J., and Carole Torgerson. *Designing and Running Randomized Trials in Health, Education, and the Social Sciences.* New York: Palgrave Macmillan, 2008.

Web Sites

Clinical Trials: http://clinicaltrials.gov
National Cancer Institute (NCI): http://www.cancer.gov
National Institute of Mental Health (NIMH): http://www.nimh.nih.gov/health/trials/index.shtml
U.S. Food and Drug Administration (FDA): http://www.fda.gov/oashi/clinicaltrials/default.htm
World Health Organization (WHO), International Clinical Trials Registry Platform (ICTRP): http://www.who.int/ictrp/en

RATIONING HEALTHCARE

Rationing typically refers to the distribution of some good or service insufficient in supply to meet the available demand for it. Most people think of rationing as a situation when scarce commodities such as fuel during wartime are not sufficiently available. The fuel available could be rationed by price and given to the highest bidder, but such price rationing is seen as unfair. Thus, a system of allocation is designed that seeks to incorporate broader values such as equity, need, potential benefit, fair share, positioning in the queue, and so on.

The situation best exemplifying such scarcity in contemporary America is the lack of available hearts, kidneys, livers, and lungs for transplantation, where need in many cases far exceeds supply. Almost everyone regards price rationing for such available organs as unfair, so an alternative distribution system must be designed. Such distributions have been called "tragic choices" because there is no correct answer on how to do this.

Some analysts note that many of the instances in medicine referred to as rationing do not involve scarcity in that the needed supply is available but consumers are unwilling or unable to pay the price demanded. However, most instances of scarcity are imposed by policy choices reflecting culture and ethical values. There are numerous ways to increase the availability of scarce organs were we not bound by our values and norms. These include allowing people to buy and sell them, paying relatives to agree to the use of organs of their loved ones who no longer have brain function, or appropriating the organs of people who are brain dead by fiat regardless of family wishes. Or we can do what occasionally has been done in China—take the organs of prisoners following execution or solders killed in war. We can even imagine societies where people are bred for spare organs. Most societies view all the above solutions to scarcity as unethical.

Price Rationing

It is commonly asserted that healthcare is not rationed in America. This might be substantially true if price rationing is excluded. Our healthcare system has the capacity to provide an adequate level of care to all who need it. But many lack access because they are uninsured or have little of the disposable income needed to purchase care. Thus, many people forgo needed care because of cost and as a consequence have poorer health. To most economists, allocation by price is simply an instance of supply and demand. Most people would not think that luxury cars are rationed simply

because many persons cannot afford to buy them. But societies think differently about some necessities such as healthcare than about ordinary commodities. The special claims for healthcare stem from the belief that adequate health is a precondition for fair competition.

Levels of Rationing

Most nations seek to control the resources devoted to healthcare relative to other societal needs. The United Kingdom, for example, establishes a central health budget each year and seeks to live within it, while other nations use a variety of price controls and other regulations to hold healthcare expenditures in check. Since no nation provides all the care the population would wish, all must have some rationing rules to determine the distribution of available health resources.

The rationing context is established in most countries by macro decisions that shape the amounts and types of care available: decisions concerning the number and types of health professionals trained; the distribution of funds among varying types of technologies, services, and specialists; the numbers and locations of hospitals and clinics built; the definition of reimbursable providers; the amounts of payment for varying kinds of services; the distribution between primary-care physicians and specialists and among different types of health professions; and the distribution of funding among types of providers and geographic locations. These decisions may be more or less centralized and involve fierce politics and interest-group advocacy. The history and culture of each country shapes the design of benefits and the extent to which patients are expected to share in the costs. Definitions of care services will vary among nations. In some, respite care in spas is covered under the basic health plan.

Some planning decisions may remain highly centralized, such as decisions about overall budgets, new hospital buildings, or acquisition of new, expensive technologies, while others may be delegated to regions or local entities and provider organizations, such as insurance plans, hospitals, clinics, and provider groups. Managers in these more decentralized settings make many intermediate decisions, such as how to distribute their available funding, the numbers and types of reimbursable facilities and providers, the balance between general practice and specialty care, the numbers of specialists in each type of service, and the like. These decisions will make care more or less available in varying categories, such as cardiac care or mental health, and make rationing more or less needed, depending on the resources allocated to each function.

Many rationing decisions are predetermined by benefit design and coverage decisions by the purchaser (government) of the healthcare plan. Important services may or may not be covered or may be restricted in various ways, such as dental care, prescription drugs, long-term care, certain preventive services, specified surgical interventions, some appliances and devices, and so on. All healthcare systems exclude some services seen as less important or too expensive, such as various cosmetic surgical interventions, some reproductive services, "lifestyle" drugs, psychoanalysis, and the like. These decisions may be controversial and politically contested, but they are part of the overall design process. Decisions made at the point of service are much more difficult, because people cannot access care or are denied services they believe they need at the point where they believe their health is at stake.

Explicit and Implicit Rationing

A central issue is the extent to which rationing should be allowed at the point of service delivery and whether it should be explicit or implicit. One advantage of implicit rationing, where clinicians make discretionary judgments about what services to provide, is that it more readily takes account of differences in medical and social circumstances, patient preferences, and situations that cannot be known beforehand, given the iterative nature of patient care and decision making. Thus, it is flexible and readily adaptable to different and changing situations. Its strengths are also its weaknesses, in that it makes decision making less transparent and opens greater opportunities for personal bias and discrimination under the guise of clinical decisions. Physicians sometimes make care decisions on the basis of age, gender, race, and other prejudices and may respond differently if they like or dislike particular patients.

Critics of implicit rationing seek more transparent decision making and clear, explicit rules about who should have access to varying interventions. They also see this as a way to ensure professional accountability. They commonly advocate having such rules established through public participation so that decisions reflect the dominant values of the community. The most publicized effort to develop rules for explicit rationing was the Oregon Health Plan, which sought to provide healthcare coverage to more people by rationing the services available. Efforts were made to distinguish between more and less useful interventions in order of priority as a way of defining the services available within that state's Medicaid program. Oregon began with a series of public meetings and meetings of various advisory committees, to develop consensus on priorities. Through this exercise, medical services were classified into a number of condition-treatment pairs that were ranked and prioritized through judgments of medical efficacy and community values. Initially, 700 categories were established, but it was determined that the state budget could only support the first 588.

When the rankings were examined, there were a variety of seemingly bizarre outcomes. Tooth capping, for example, ranked higher than surgery for ectopic pregnancy or appendectomy, interventions that save lives. Thus, the rankings were criticized for failure to give the "rule of rescue" sufficient priority and for other reasons. The list was then reordered to give more influence to clinical understanding. The public was involved, but most participants in the various meetings and committees were health professionals. Observers viewed the process as a rational and fair way to make difficult decisions about allocations of limited budgets. The system was never really implemented as expected, and relatively little rationing actually took place. All such efforts function in a broader political, organizational, economic, and social context, and implementation depends on factors that may have little to do with the approach itself.

The psychometric techniques used are uncertain because of the difficulty of rating needs and experiences one has not personally encountered. The general public makes different assessments from those who actually have the illnesses in question. Moreover, explicit rationing has many problems beyond the technicalities of developing rational and evidence-based priorities. Given the complexities of people's lives and their medical histories and varying social situations, it is impossible to anticipate all the issues that may arise in caregiving. Explicit decisions can be inflexible and misdirected. It is also difficult to modify them in a timely way as new knowledge and understanding evolves.

In the United States, rationing has largely involved excluding many services in the benefit design, requiring cost sharing when using services, and requiring waits to get appointments to see the physician. Most denials do not occur at the point of service, and patients commonly do not think of these access limitations as rationing. Managed care changed this a great deal in the 1990s by explicitly denying care at the point of service. The rationing approaches used by managed-care organizations included utilization review (precertification for and concurrent review of inpatient care and other expensive interventions), requiring clients to enroll with a primary-care physician from a predetermined list, and requiring formal referrals for specialty care. Prescription plans similarly developed drug formularies and required substitution of generic for brand-name medications. They sometimes limited the number of prescriptions a patient could fill in a month (as in some state Medicaid programs) and limited the number of pills a patient could receive per month (as in coverage for lifestyle drugs such as Viagra). This was the first major experience American patients and physicians had with explicit rationing at the point of service, and they disliked it, resulting in a major backlash. Many of these controls were then relaxed, contributing to a new cost spiral.

Explicit rationing at the point of service is "rationing in your face" and is less acceptable than more impersonal types of explicit rationing, as in benefit design. The most successful types of rationing are often those that people don't perceive as rationing at all. When people and their loved ones are seriously ill, most will use every means to get the services they believe they need. Thus, rational efforts under managed care to limit some types of care resulted in public attacks and litigation, leading managers to back down in order to avoid bad publicity. One example was bone marrow transplants in patients with advanced breast cancer, a treatment ultimately proven to have no value in such instances. But explicit rationing is inherently political, and the transparency of decision making encourages confrontation and public acrimony. Although implicit rationing is less fair and more easily open to favoritism, it allows people's preferences to be met when some feel more strongly than others. But it also gives advantages to those who are more educated and sophisticated and who know better how to manipulate bureaucratic systems. Nevertheless, explicit rationing at the point of service is extraordinarily difficult to sustain politically. Few successful examples exist beyond organ transplantation.

Types of Rationing

The easiest types of rationing are often those where the public fails to perceive it. Rudolf Klein and his associates have described seven types of rationing. The most apparent is denial of service because individuals lack health insurance or cannot pay the required cost or because the managed-care reviewers do not believe that the service is justified. Rationing by selection refers to the choice of individuals among competing patients because of assessments of likelihood of benefit, place on a queue, or some rule about what is fair. Rationing by deflection refers to sending patients elsewhere because of heavy load, as often occurs in ambulance deflection from emergency departments or "turfing" what are seen as undesirable patients (because of age, chronicity, or social characteristics) to some other service. Rationing by deterrence involves making it difficult to receive a service by unresponsive telephone systems, inaccessible locations, dismissive receptionists, dismal surroundings, and making people feel unwelcome. A related type of rationing is by delay, making it difficult to obtain an appointment or very long waiting times in the clinic or office. A particularly serious form of deterrence involves marketing efforts by health plans that avoid enrolling people with serious illness by making program enrollment less accessible to them. Rationing also occurs by dilution, involving short consultations with little content and the need to make repeated visits for basic services that could be provided in fewer visits. Finally, some patients face rationing by termination when they seek services but are told that nothing more can be done for them and health personnel withdraw. Such rationing commonly occurs at the end of life.

Setting Limits Fairly

It is inevitable that more rigorous rationing will be needed as new technologies and rapidly developing biomedical science provide new and expensive possibilities for treating disease. Some believe that given the large amount of waste in the U.S. healthcare system, it will be possible to improve access and quality without rationing care by introducing new organizational rationalities, restructuring physician and hospital payment and other incentives, and emphasizing evidence-based treatment. However, this may be wishful thinking. Healthcare in America has always been rationed in the ways described and likely will be rationed even more as new possibilities pose enormous cost demands. The hope is that we can ration in constructive and health-promoting ways rather than simply allocating care to those with the greatest ability to pay. Rational allocation schemes require significant changes in healthcare practice organization and broad implementation of information technology, but American medicine has been slow to make these changes. The experience of large practice systems such as the Veteran's Affairs (VA) healthcare system and large health maintenance organizations (HMOs) such as Kaiser-Permanente suggests that change is feasible.

One major challenge is to have the capacity to make evidence-based assessments credible to the public and insulated from everyday political pressures and influences. One example is the United Kingdom's National Institute for Health and Clinical Excellence (known as NICE), which makes such judgments and gives advice to the National Health Service (NHS). A number of models have been proposed for such a function in the United States, including one fashioned like the U.S. Federal Reserve System, which makes monetary policy significantly insulated from everyday political pressures. Some large organizations such as the VA and Kaiser-Permanente have their own processes to make such judgments, building on evidence from sophisticated databases such as those maintained by the Cochrane Collaboration, a large effort to bring together and assess the findings from randomized controlled trials and other research from all over the world.

Knowing the evidence, however, does not ensure a fair and credible allocation process. Norman Daniels and James Sabin have developed a rationing approach to achieve legitimacy with patients. They call their approach "accountability for reasonableness" and define four necessary elements. First, they argue, decisions and their underlying rationales must be public and easily accessible. Here they endorse, as do many ethicists, explicit rationing. Second, the decisions must be based on evidence, principles, and justifications that all participants see as relevant to decisions about how best to allocate resources that are too few to give everyone whatever they might demand. Third, they recognize the uncertainties in medical care and do not demand certainty but maintain that the evidence and decision making should be plausibly consistent. Fourth, any decisions should be open to challenge and revisable when new information becomes available. In short, there must be clear organizational mechanisms in place to appeal against and revise decisions. Finally, there must be organizational mechanisms in place to ensure that the aforementioned conditions are met. No system has implemented this approach in full, although some of the elements have been used in particular kinds of decisions in some organizations. It is not clear, however, if this explicit rationing approach can be implemented to its full extent for the reasons discussed earlier. However, such thoughtful theory is helpful as we go forward.

Rationing remains an unbroachable topic in discussions of American healthcare, and professionals and patients commonly believe the myth that healthcare is not rationed. If we are to make thoughtful and prudent decisions, the public must understand rationing realities. The question is not whether to ration but how to ration more thoughtfully and effectively. This will be a continuing challenge.

David Mechanic

See also Access to Healthcare; Cost of Healthcare; Economic Barriers to Healthcare; Health Economics; Medical Sociology; Public Policy; United Kingdom's National Institute for Health and Clinical Excellence (NICE); U.S. Department of Veterans Affairs (VA)

Further Readings

Aaron, Henry J., William B. Schwartz, and Melissa Cox. *Can We Say No?: The Challenge of Rationing Health Care.* Washington, DC: Brookings Institution Press, 2005.

Daniels, Norman, and James E. Sabin. *Setting Limits Fairly: Can We Learn to Share Medical Resources?* New York: Oxford University Press, 2002.

Jacobs, Lawrence, Theodore Marmor, and Jonathan Oberlander. "The Oregon Health Plan and the Political Paradox of Rationing: What Advocates and Critics Have Claimed and What Oregon Did," *Journal of Health, Politics, and Law* 24(1): 161–80, February 1999.

Klein, Rudolf, Patricia Day, and Sharon Redmayne. *Managing Scarcity: Priority Setting and Rationing in the National Health Service.* Philadelphia: Open University Press, 1996.

Mechanic, David. "Muddling Through Elegantly: Finding the Proper Balance in Rationing," *Health Affairs* 16(5): 83–92, September–October 1997.

Mechanic, David. "The Rise and Fall of Managed Care," *Journal of Health and Social Behavior* 45(Suppl.): 76–86, 2004.

Mechanic, David. *The Truth About Health Care: Why Reform Is Not Working in America.* New Brunswick, NJ: Rutgers University Press, 2006.

Mechanic, David, Lynn B. Rogut, David C. Colby, et al., eds. *Policy Challenges in Modern Health Care.* New Brunswick, NJ: Rutgers University Press, 2005.

Web Sites

American Public Health Association (APHA): http://www.apha.org

American Society of Health Economists (ASHE): http://healtheconomics.us

American Sociological Association, Medical Sociology Section: http://dept.kent.edu/sociology/asamedsoc

Brookings Institution: http://www.brookings.edu

National Center for Policy Analysis (NCPA): http://www.ncpa.org

REGULATION

Regulation is the formal process through which health policy governs behavior. It takes the form of rules, procedures, adjudications, and administrative actions implemented by a regulatory authority. Such an authority can function at the federal, state, or local governmental level or through numerous private organizations. Because of the breadth of the healthcare industry, the regulatory framework is particularly complex.

Health services researchers study the effects of regulation as a tool for achieving policy goals. Such investigations are often referred to as program evaluations, as they evaluate the effectiveness of regulatory programs. The outcomes of health services research may also influence the development of regulations and of legislation that forms its legal basis. Research findings are often cited by members of the U.S. Congress, state legislators, members of private bodies, and courts in the development and evaluation of regulatory policy.

Health services research is itself subject to regulation. The National Research Act of 1974 requires that all federally funded research involving the use of human subjects be approved and supervised by an institutional review board (IRB) at the sponsoring institution. IRBs are composed of professional peers of the investigators and members of the community at large, and their role is to ensure that subjects are adequately protected, in particular through procedures for obtaining informed consent concerning possible research risks. The federal Health Insurance Portability and Accountability Act of 1996 (HIPAA) limits the use and distribution of medical information that can identify individual patients. Health services researchers who rely on clinical data must either use information from which patients cannot be identified or obtain the consent of the patients involved.

Purpose and Functions

The primary purpose of government regulation is to develop and enforce the detailed rules that effectuate statutes. When the U.S. Congress or a state legislature enacts a law, it cannot account for all the technical aspects of implementation, as legislators do not have the time or the expertise to do so. Statutes typically set overall policy guidance in a field and direct an agency to bring it to fruition. For example, the U.S. Congress mandated that the Food and Drug Administration (FDA) ensure the safety and efficacy of all new drugs and devices but left it to the agency to determine the manner in which clinical testing will be conducted. The legislature in every state has required that physicians be licensed by a medical board to practice and directed these boards to set the actual qualifications for licensure.

In a private context, regulation implements policy decisions of professional and industry organizations. For example, the hospital members of the Joint Commission seek to have all institutions function at a uniform level of quality. Committees within the organization devise the actual standards that must be met to exhibit quality and the procedures for enforcing them. Similarly, the physician members of medical specialty societies seek to ensure that practitioners display minimum levels of skill and competence. Committees of these bodies develop examinations and practice guidelines to assess these attributes.

Government regulators serve four main functions. First, they promulgate rules and standards that fill in the details of legislation, as when the FDA specifies the procedures for testing a new drug. This activity is known as rulemaking. Second, they conduct adjudications that enforce those rules and that grant rights and privileges under them, such as the right to practice medicine. Third, they administer government functions, such as hospital operations in the Veterans Administration (VA). Fourth, they disperse funding for targeting purposes—for example, support for biomedical research by the National Institutes of Health (NIH).

In performing these tasks, regulators take on the roles of each branch of government. Rulemaking extends the reach of the legislative branch by adding detailed directives to the general guidance contained in laws. Adjudication mimics the activity of the judicial branch by resolving disputes over regulatory enforcement. Administration of government operations and of funding programs carries out functions of the executive branch by directly managing government activities.

Regulatory authority may be vested in bodies known as boards, commissions, agencies, or departments. They are headed by officials who are appointed by the president or, for state-level programs, the governor, and who are generally subject to confirmation by the Senate or the state legislature. When there is a single agency head, leadership changes with each new administration. Members of boards and commissions are often appointed for fixed terms that are staggered to extend beyond election cycles in order to provide for continuity of leadership across administrations. Senior agency officials just below the top leadership also tend to be political appointees. Their role is to provide overall policy guidance. Most of the day-to-day work of regulatory agencies is conducted by a permanent professional staff.

In cutting across the traditional divisions of responsibility between branches of government, regulators play an anomalous role. They derive their authority from legislative enactments, yet they are directly accountable to the executive that appoints their leadership, and all their actions are subject to review by the courts for consistency with the underlying statutes and with the federal or state constitution. The mixing of governmental roles has at times proved controversial, in that it can be seen to blur the conventional separation of powers.

Process

Under the constitution, basic legal powers are vested in the states unless one of several enumerated national concerns is involved. Therefore, most regulation of routine aspects of healthcare, such as medical practice, hospital operations, and sanitation, fall under the jurisdiction of state agencies. States may delegate some of these functions to municipal and county governments, as is the case, for example, for restaurant inspections. Most federal regulation of healthcare falls under the constitutional authority to regulate interstate commerce, as seen in the regulation of drugs by the FDA, or under the power to spend funds to address national needs, as is done in the Medicare program.

Private regulators are usually sponsored by the regulated industry or the profession itself, as in the examples of the Joint Commission and medical specialty boards. They do not exercise actual legal authority to govern behavior and cannot impose legal sanctions for violations of their rules. Their power derives from their ability to influence reputations and professional recognition. The Joint Commission does not determine whether or not a hospital may legally operate, but accreditation by the Joint Commission adds essential credibility to an institution's claim to quality, and it is required for reimbursement by virtually all governmental and private payers. Board certification does not control the legal right to practice medicine, but it exerts similar effects on credibility and reimbursement eligibility.

Government regulators are subject to the restrictions on authority contained in the federal constitution. In particular, they may not violate the rights of those whom they oversee to due process when life, liberty, or property are at stake. Healthcare regulation affects property interests in many ways—for example, by controlling a physician's ability to earn a living, determining when a drug company can sell a new product, or deciding when a hospital can construct a new facility. Due process requires that such actions be taken only after full consideration of all relevant factors and after all affected parties have had a chance to be heard. As a guide to ensure that these steps are taken, the U.S. Congress in 1946 enacted the Administrative Procedures Act (APA), which imposes standards that federal regulators must follow. Most states have similar laws.

To meet the Administrative Procedures Act's requirements, regulatory actions must be preceded by a series of prescribed steps. The agency involved must conduct a thorough fact-finding effort that builds a record to support the action. Adequate notice must be provided to the general public of pending activities, which is generally accomplished through publication in a regular journal of the federal government known as the *Federal Register*. Particular care must be given to notifying parties who may be directly affected by an adjudication. Those with a direct interest in the outcome must also be afforded the opportunity for input through written comments or at a hearing, and after an initial decision is made, they must be able to bring an appeal. At the end of the process, a regulatory action is considered final, but appeal to the courts is still possible. They can review regulatory actions for consistency with the APA, the underlying statute that authorized the action, and the Constitution.

Private regulators are not components of the government, so they are not subject to the Administrative Procedure Act. However, there are several legal rules that circumscribe their actions. They may not discriminate based on impermissible factors such as race, religion, or national origin. In many states, they are subject to a requirement of "fundamental fairness" in their actions. They may also be held accountable for complying with their own internal rules and bylaws. Some private organizations that exercise regulatory powers, such as hospitals that grant staff privileges to physicians, are considered by the courts to be "quasi-governmental" actors because of their tax-exempt status and receipt of government funding. This brings with it a requirement to provide due process for parties affected by their actions. Beyond these legal dictates, private regulators also have a strong interest in safeguarding their own reputations for fairness, if they are to remain credible as arbiters of professional competence and quality.

History

Over the course of the past 150 years, the focus of healthcare regulation has expanded, so that it now covers almost every aspect of the field. For the most part, each regulatory program addresses one of three key policy concerns—enhancing quality, ensuring access, or controlling costs. As the focus of policy has shifted over the years, new programs have been added by a range of different authorities, and in many instances sets of regulatory requirements are layered, one upon another.

The earliest regulation of healthcare in America addressed public health concerns. As science first revealed the role of germs in causing disease and as the means of contagion, state and local governments responded with preventive measures. These included sanitation, clean drinking water, food inspections, mandatory vaccinations, and quarantine in the face of epidemics. At the start of the 20th century, the quality of healthcare services and products became the focus as states imposed licensure requirements for physicians and private bodies affiliated with the umbrella professional organization for the medical profession, the American Medical Association (AMA), instituted procedures for accrediting the medical schools at which their members trained. In 1906, the U.S. Congress passed the first national drug safety law and established the FDA. The law was overhauled and strengthened in 1938 and again in 1962. In overall effect, these actions improved the level of quality in American healthcare and to a sufficient extent that by the 1920s the country could claim a credible system.

During the mid 20th century, the focus of regulatory activity turned largely to enhancing access. State laws passed in the 1930s facilitated the first Blue Cross and Blue Shield plans that provided insurance on a nonprofit basis. A federal ruling in

1943 helped link insurance to employment. The War Labor Board exempted employer-paid insurance premiums from a freeze on wage and price increases during World War II and permitted firms to add health coverage as a fringe benefit without restriction. Further encouragement for this benefit came after the war, when the Internal Revenue Service (IRS) ruled its value to be exempt from the calculation of income for purposes of taxation. In 1946, the U.S. Congress passed the first major federal healthcare spending initiative in the form of the Hill-Burton Act, which allocated billions of dollars for hospital construction, especially in rural areas.

The most significant regulatory expansion of access occurred in 1965 with the enactment of Medicare and Medicaid. These programs offered insurance to millions of citizens who lacked eligibility for employer-sponsored coverage—Medicare to the elderly who were no longer working and Medicaid to several categories of the poor who lacked employment. The programs were supplemented in 1997 by the state Children's Health Insurance Program (SCHIP), which permits states to extend coverage to children of families with incomes that are low but not low enough to qualify for Medicaid. In exercising its spending power through these programs, the U.S. Congress has added various regulatory restrictions over the years. For example, to receive reimbursement, institutions and practitioners must meet quality criteria embodied in the conditions of participation. Hospitals that operate emergency rooms, a category that includes almost all, must provide open access regardless of ability to pay. All providers must structure their financial dealings to avoid the exchange of remuneration in return for the referral of patients.

Not surprisingly—to many healthcare analysts—the expansion of access that Medicare and Medicaid achieved imposed tremendous pressure on costs, and healthcare spending in the United States began to accelerate rapidly in the late 1960s. In response, many regulatory programs enacted over the next 30 years focused on different kinds of cost control strategies. In 1973, the U.S. Congress passed the Health Maintenance Organization Act to encourage the use of managed care. The next year, it passed the Employee Retirement Income Security Act (ERISA) to assist large, multistate employers in self-insuring for employee healthcare expenses. During the 1970s, all states passed, with federal encouragement, certificate-of-need (CON) programs to limit the expansion of healthcare services and facilities that were deemed superfluous. In 1983, the U.S. Congress changed the mechanism for reimbursing hospitals under Medicare to a prospective payment system based on Diagnosis Related Groups (DRGs) to eliminate incentives for overtreatment.

The actual effectiveness of these programs in stemming the rise in healthcare spending has been a matter of debate among health policy analysts and health services researchers. Costs for healthcare services continue to rise relentlessly and represent more than 16% of the gross domestic product (GDP), more than the proportion in any other country. However, from a research perspective, cost control programs have provided considerable fuel for studying the effects of economic incentives on the behavior of institutions, practitioners, and patients.

More recent regulatory programs address a range of concerns. Various federal and state reporting laws require that government authorities be informed of medical errors, which have been found to represent a major threat to quality, especially in hospitals. The U.S. Congress has empowered the FDA to take more assertive action when safety hazards are discovered in approved drugs. Access to prescription medications was expanded for the elderly with the enactment of Part D of Medicare. HIPAA restricts the ability of insurers to refuse coverage based on preexisting conditions to members of employer-sponsored groups.

In separate provisions, HIPAA also protects the privacy of patient medical information. This last regulatory thrust may be a harbinger of much future health policy. Healthcare has been slower than many other industries to adopt information technology, but substantial efforts are under way to accelerate the computerization of many aspects of the industry. This trend will raise new kinds of concerns, particularly regarding threats to patient privacy, that regulatory policy will have to address. Other applications of information technology, such as electronic medical records, telemedicine, and Internet-based services, will undoubtedly also command the attention of policymakers to an increasing extent as inevitable issues and conflicts arise.

Current Regulatory Structures

With a history of over 100 years of expansion, regulation today affects almost every aspect of American healthcare. In most cases, a variety of regulators, rather than a single authority, is involved. Each sphere of the industry is subject to its own complex structure, characterized in most cases by a dynamic interplay between oversight bodies and programs that have arisen at different times.

Physicians and other healthcare professionals are subject to licensure at the state level. Many healthcare professions also maintain a certification process through which expertise in a specialty is recognized. To achieve a financially viable practice, most kinds of practitioners must also meet the conditions for participation in Medicare and Medicaid and abide by the requirements for participation in the provider networks of private managed-care organizations should they wish to qualify for reimbursement. Physicians who seek to practice at or admit patients to a hospital are also subject to review and supervision by that institution's credentials committee.

Hospitals and other healthcare institutions are similarly subject to licensure by the states. Most also seek accreditation by the Joint Commission. About two thirds of all states maintain CON laws, which restrict the ability of hospitals to add new services or facilities without state approval based on a demonstration of community need. Hospitals must also abide by the numerous requirements that go with receipt of Hill-Burton funding, including nondiscrimination, indigent care, and maintenance of emergency rooms, and by additional rules that accompany participation in Medicare.

Healthcare finance in America has substantial components at both the private and the governmental level, both of which function within a complex regulatory framework. The business of insurance is regulated by the states, but ERISA preempts state authority over some aspects of employer-sponsored coverage, which represents over 90% of the market. In its place, this law provides for minimal oversight of health plan finances by the U.S. Department of Labor. The premiums paid for employment-based health insurance receive favorable tax treatment, which effectively creates a large government subsidy for this kind of coverage.

The federal government finances healthcare directly for the elderly, the totally disabled, and those suffering from end-stage renal disease through Medicare. Government financing is shared jointly between the federal and state governments for those categories of the extremely poor who are covered by Medicaid and for SCHIP. All these programs rely on regulatory mechanisms to operate.

Drugs and other healthcare products are regulated primarily by the FDA. This agency administers a regulatory structure that oversees all aspects of drug and device testing and determines whether test results indicate sufficient safety and efficacy to justify approval for marketing. Once a drug is on the market, the FDA oversees the advertising and promotion of approved products and evaluates postmarket safety data. Manufacturers must also obtain patents from the federal Patent and Trademark Office to protect new discoveries from competition. The federal Drug Price Competition and Patent Term Restoration Act of 1984 determines when generic copies of patented drugs and devices may be manufactured, tested, and sold.

Public health in America, the oldest subject of governmental regulation, is today one of the most disjointed. Most basic public health regulatory functions, such as oversight of sanitation, restaurant inspections, and epidemic investigations, are handled at the state or local level. The federal government takes the lead with regard to food safety. It also coordinates state efforts, monitors national disease trends, and develops recommendations through the Centers for Disease Control and Prevention (CDC). Environmental pollution is addressed by the federal Environmental Protection Agency (EPA) and by similar bodies in many states. Occupational safety and health is primarily a federal concern, subject to oversight by the Occupational Safety and Health Administration (OSHA).

Business relationships between healthcare entities are regulated in distinctive ways that do not apply to other industries. Antitrust laws are enforced by the federal U.S. Department of Justice, the Federal Trade Commission, and many state attorneys general. Federal guidance has been issued to advise healthcare providers that compete with one another on permissible forms of collaboration. Payments that providers exchange to encourage the referral of patients are strictly prohibited by federal law, and the boundaries of legitimate financial relationships are defined in regulations issued by the Office of Inspector General of the Medicare program. Tax exempt hospitals must abide by the rules of the IRS regarding charitable activities. All healthcare providers are subject to regulations issued under HIPAA concerning the privacy of patient data.

Biomedical and other health-related research is regulated by various government agencies that provide funding and also by the FDA when results are used to support applications for approval of new drugs or devices. The National Institutes of Health (NIH), the largest single research-funding source in the world, reviews proposals of private investigators, as do the National Science Foundation (NSF), the Agency for Healthcare Research and Quality (AHRQ), and other agencies. Scientists who receive support must abide by IRB oversight concerning the use of human subjects and by numerous accounting rules.

Future Implications

Regulation is the force that translates health policy into action. Its scope is broader with regard to healthcare than with regard to most other industries. Healthcare regulators operate at all levels of government and in private settings, and they address, in one form or another, each of the three key policy concerns of enhancing quality, controlling costs, and ensuring access.

To those within the industry, regulation represents a complex and often bewildering array of restrictions. However, it has also helped foster the industry's growth over the past century. Regulatory programs have channeled much of the country's healthcare activity, for example, through the National Institutes of Health (NIH) support for basic biomedical research; enhanced the public's respect for the field, for example, through the licensure of healthcare professionals; and served as the conduit for injecting huge amounts of federal money into the system, for example, through the Medicare program. As a result, regulation serves as both a fertile ground for health services research and an outlet for implementing research findings. Because of the importance of healthcare to the nation's well-being and to its economy, regulation will always play a central role in determining the industry's shape and in guiding its functioning.

Robert I. Field

See also Accreditation; Antitrust Law; Certificate of Need (CON); Employee Retirement Income Security Act (ERISA); Health Insurance; Health Insurance Portability and Accountability Act of 1996 (HIPAA); Joint Commission; Public Policy; U.S. Food and Drug Administration (FDA)

Further Readings

Brown, Lawrence D. "Political Evolution of Federal Health Care Regulation." *Health Affairs* 11(4): 17–37, Winter 1992.
Committee on Assessing the System for Protecting Human Research Subjects, Institute of Medicine. *Responsible Research: A Systems Approach to Protecting Research Participants*. Washington, DC: National Academies Press, 2002.
Committee to Study the Role of Allied Health Personnel, Institute of Medicine. *Allied Health Services: Avoiding a Crisis*. Washington, DC: National Academies Press, 1989.
Department of Health and Human Services, Office of Inspector General. *The External Review of Hospital Quality: The Role of Medicare Certification*. Report No. OEI-01–97–00052. Washington, DC: Department of Health and Human Services, 1999.
Field, Robert I. *Health Care Regulation in America: Complexity, Confrontation, and Compromise*. New York: Oxford University Press, 2006.
Hilts, Philip J. *Protecting America's Health: The FDA, Business, and One Hundred Years of Regulation*. New York: Knopf, 2003.
Kurian, George T., ed. *A Historical Guide to the U.S. Government*. New York: Oxford University Press, 1998.
Longest, Beauford B. *Health Policymaking in the United States*. Chicago: Health Administration Press, 1998.
Lubbers, Jeffery S. *A Guide to Federal Agency Rulemaking*. 3d ed. Chicago: ABA Books, 1998.
Weissert, Carol S., and William G. Weissert. *Governing Health: The Politics of Health Policy*. Baltimore: Johns Hopkins University Press, 2002.

Web Sites

Centers for Medicare & Medicaid Services (CMS): http://www.cms.hhs.gov

Federal Trade Commission (FTC): http://www.ftc.gov

Joint Commission: http://www.jointcommission.org

National Academy for State Health Policy (NASHP): http://nashp.org

Occupational Health and Safety Administration (OHSA): http://www.osha.gov

U.S. Department of Health and Human Services (HHS): http://www.hhs.gov

U.S. Department of Labor (DOL): http://www.dol.gov

U.S. Food and Drug Administration (FDA): http://www.fda.gov

U.S. Government Accountability Office (GAO): http://www.gao.gov

Reinhardt, Uwe E.

Uwe E. Reinhardt is a well-known and highly respected health economist and health services researcher. Reinhardt is an insightful, and often humorous, commentator on economic, political, and public policy issues in healthcare. He frequently writes on the uninsured and compares healthcare in the United States with that in other countries.

Born in 1937 in Germany, Reinhardt immigrated to Canada. He earned a bachelor's degree in commerce and economics from the University of Saskatchewan, Canada, in 1964 and was awarded the Governor General's Medal as the Most Distinguished Graduate of his class. He did his graduate work at Yale University, earning a master's degree and a doctorate in economics in 1970.

Reinhardt has taught at Princeton University since 1968, rising through the academic ranks from assistant professor of economics to his current position of James Madison Professor of Political Economy and professor of economics and public affairs. At the university, he has taught courses in micro- and macroeconomics, accounting, financial management, and health economics and policy.

Reinhardt has served on a number of government committees and commissions. He served on the National Council on Health Care Technology of the U.S. Department of Health and Welfare from 1979 to 1982. He was a member of the Special Medical Advisory Group of the Veterans Administration (VA) from 1981 to 1985. He also

served as a commissioner on the Physician Payment Review Commission (PPRC), which advised the U.S. Congress on reforms of Medicare policies for paying physicians, from 1986 to 1995.

He has also served as a member of many private-sector organizations, including the Council on the Economic Impact of Health Reform, the National Leadership Coalition on Health Care, and the National Institute for Health Care Management. He is currently on the board of trustees of Duke University Health System and the Teachers Insurance and Annuity Association. And he is the chairman of the Coordinating Committee of the International Program in Health Policy of the Commonwealth Fund.

Reinhardt is a prolific researcher and writer who has authored or coauthored over 200 journal articles, books, and editorials. He also has served on the editorial boards of many prestigious medical and health services research journals, including *Health Affairs, Journal of the American Medical Association, Journal of Health Economics, Milbank Quarterly,* and the *New England Journal of Medicine.*

In recognition of his work, Reinhardt has received many awards and honors. For example, he was elected to the National Academy of Sciences, Institute of Medicine (IOM), in which he has been a member since 1978. He is a past president of the Association of Health Services Research and the Foundation for Health Services Research. In 2004, he received the Distinguished Investigator Award from AcademyHealth.

Reinhardt has been a consultant to many organizations, including the World Bank, as well as to various federal legislators. He frequently is called to testify before the U.S. Congress.

Erin R. Page

See also Commonwealth Fund; Healthcare Financial Management; Healthcare Reform; Health Economics; Health Insurance; International Health Systems; Public Policy; Uninsured Individuals

Further Readings

Reinhardt, Uwe E. "Does the Aging of the Population Really Drive the Demand for Health Care?" *Health Affairs* 22(6): 27–39, November–December 2003.

Reinhardt, Uwe E. "The Swiss Health System: Regulated Competition Without Managed Care," *Journal of the American Medical Association* 292(10): 1227–31, September 8, 2004.

Reinhardt, Uwe E. "The Pricing of U.S. Hospital Services: Chaos Behind a Veil of Secrecy," *Health Affairs* 25(1): 57–69, January–February 2006.

Reinhardt, Uwe E. "Assessing U.S. Health Insurance Coverage," *Journal of the American Medical Association* 297(10): 1049, March 14, 2007.

Reinhardt, Uwe E. "U.S. Health Care Stands Adam Smith on His Head," *British Medical Journal* 335(7628): 1020, November 17, 2007.

Reinhardt, Uwe E., Peter S. Hussey, and Gerard F. Anderson. "U.S. Health Care Spending in an International Context: Why is U.S. Spending so High, and Can We Afford It?" *Health Affairs* 23(3): 10–25, May–June 2004.

Web Sites

Princeton University, Woodrow Wilson School of Public and International Affairs: http://wws.princeton.edu

RELMAN, ARNOLD S.

Arnold S. Relman is Professor Emeritus of Medicine and of Social Medicine at Harvard Medical School. He has been a medical research scientist, a clinical practitioner and consultant, a medical-school teacher and department head, a university and medical-school trustee, the editor of two influential medical journals, a writer on medical and healthcare policy issues, and a member of a state board of licensure and discipline.

Born in New York City in 1923, Relman graduated from Cornell University in 1943 and received his medical degree from Columbia University in 1946. After residency training at Yale-New Haven Hospital, he moved to Boston in 1949 to be a National Research Council Fellow in the Medical Sciences at Boston University School of Medicine. He remained on the Boston University faculty, rising to the position of Conrad Wesselhoeft Professor of Medicine and Director of the Boston University Medical Services at the Boston City Hospital. From 1962 to 1967, he served as the editor of the *Journal of Clinical Investigation*. In 1968, he

moved to Philadelphia to become the Frank Wister Thomas Professor of Medicine and chair of the Department of Medicine at the University of Pennsylvania School of Medicine and Physician-in-Chief at the Hospital of the University of Pennsylvania. In 1975–1976, he was a Macy Foundation Faculty Scholar at Oxford University, England, and a visiting scientist in biochemistry at Merton College, Oxford. In 1977, he returned to Boston to become the editor of the *New England Journal of Medicine,* professor of medicine at Harvard Medical School, and senior physician at the Brigham and Women's Hospital. In 1991, he became Editor Emeritus of the *New England Journal of Medicine* and professor of medicine and of social medicine at Harvard University. In 1994, he became Professor Emeritus. From 1995 to 2001, he was a member of the Massachusetts State Board of Registration in Medicine and chair of its committee on quality.

Relman began his career as a medical research scientist and clinical practitioner and teacher. His research focused on renal disease and physiology and on fluid and electrolyte metabolism. He published many original studies that contributed to the understanding of the regulation of acid-base balance by the kidney, the renal effects of potassium depletion, and the diagnosis and treatment of kidney disease. He became a leader in academic medicine, serving as president of major national organizations such as the American Federation for Clinical Research, the American Society of Clinical Investigation, and the Association of American Physicians (the only person to hold all three positions) and as a member of the Council of the National Academy of Sciences, Institute of Medicine (IOM).

When Relman assumed the editorship of the *New England Journal of Medicine* in 1977, his primary interest shifted to healthcare policy and issues of medical professionalism. Since then, he has written widely on the economic, ethical, legal, and social aspects of healthcare and the practice of medicine. In 1980, he published a seminal article, "The New Medical-Industrial Complex," which first called attention to the growing commercialization of medical care in the United States and its consequences. In many articles since then in professional journals and in the lay media, he has continued to explore this theme. Relman has also been interested in the ethical and professional principles that govern the writing, editing, and publishing of medical research reports. He was a cofounder, in 1978, of the International Committee of Medical Journal Editors, which has promulgated influential guidelines in this area.

In 1966 and 1974, Relman was a coeditor of two volumes of *Controversy in Internal Medicine*. In 2007, he published *A Second Opinion: Rescuing America's Health Care*, which summarizes his assessment of the problems of healthcare in the United States and proposes major reforms in both the insurance and the delivery systems. In this book, he says that the uniquely high costs of the nation's healthcare are due primarily to the investor-owned businesses that own most of the private insurance system, most of the ambulatory services and facilities, and a large fraction of the short- and long-term inpatient facilities. He argues that investor ownership demands continued growth of income and this has changed all of the system into an expanding commercial market that has become unaffordable. As a solution, he proposes a publicly regulated single-payer insurance system and a not-for-profit delivery system based on prepaid multispecialty medical groups with salaried physicians.

Marcia Angell

See also For-Profit Versus Not-For-Profit Care; Health Services Research Journals; National Health Insurance; Physicians; Physician Workforce Issues; Politics of Healthcare Reform; Public Policy.

Further Readings

Relman, Arnold S. "The New Medical-Industrial Complex," *New England Journal of Medicine* 303(17): 363–70, October 23, 1980.

Relman, Arnold S. "A Proposal for Universal Coverage," *New England Journal of Medicine* 353(1): 96–7, July 7, 2005.

Relman, Arnold S. *A Second Opinion: Rescuing America's Health Care: A Plan for Universal Coverage Serving Patients Over Profit*. New York: Public Affairs, 2007.

Relman, Arnold S. "Medical Professionalism in a Commercialized Health Care Market," *Journal of the American Medical Association* 298(22): 2668–70, December 12, 2007.

Relman, Arnold S. "The Problem of Commercialism in Medicine," *Cambridge Quarterly of Healthcare Ethics* 16(4): 375–76, Fall 2007.

Relman, Arnold S., Franz J. Ingelfinger, and Maxwell Finland, eds. *Controversy in Internal Medicine*. 2 vols. Philadelphia: W. B. Saunders, 1974.

Web Sites

Harvard Medical School: http://www.hms.harvard.edu

RESOURCE-BASED RELATIVE VALUE SCALE (RBRVS)

The Resource-Based Relative Value Scale (RBRVS) is the method used to construct Medicare's physician payment schedule for ambulatory services. The RBRVS transformed the way physicians were reimbursed by establishing a method of standardization of payment. Other nations have also used the method to reimburse their physicians.

Background

The method and rate of physician payment constitute powerful incentives under which physicians make clinical decisions, such as how much time to spend with patients and hours of work supplied. Fee-for-service is the dominant payment method for physician services in most countries, including the United States, Germany, Canada, Japan, Australia, and Singapore. Their fees are largely based on what physicians have charged in the market place. In a market economy, prices are determined by supply and demand and by competition. However, nations have learned from experience that the market for physician services does not satisfy the conditions that define a reasonably competitive market. These imperfections in the market often distort the payment rates for different services.

First, widespread health insurance coverage reduces patients' sensitivity to fees. Physicians can overcharge patients, particularly for the diagnosis and treatment of urgent and life-threatening medical conditions. Moreover, there is an asymmetry of information between physicians and patients.

While in a few specialties, such as family medicine and pediatrics, patients may be able to make reasonably informed choices, in others, such as oncology and neurosurgery, patients have to rely primarily on physicians' decisions. Consequently, physicians can induce demand and raise their fees. Finally, legal restrictions specify who can provide medical services, admit patients to hospitals, and prescribe drugs. Although such restrictions protect patients from unqualified providers, they also tend to grant monopoly power to the medical profession. Physicians can use this monopolistic power to raise their fees.

These market distortions result in the fees for some specialties being higher than those for other specialties. A distorted fee schedule can cause an under- or oversupply of physicians by specialty and therefore also a lack of medical services in areas where there is an undersupply, excess service provision (which can be harmful to patients) in areas where there is an oversupply, and higher health expenditures when unnecessary services are rendered. To avoid distorted fees, policymakers in the United States and several other advanced economies have sought a systematic and rational foundation for determining physician fees.

Once a nation decides to move away from paying physicians according to their charges, the question becomes, "What rational foundation and methodology can be used to develop a relative value scale and set the conversion factor?" Equally important is the question of whether the medical profession will accept a new approach to administering their fees. The RBRVS was developed when the United States was grappling with these questions.

Theoretical Foundation

In 1979, William C. Hsiao and William B. Stason published an article that outlined a rational foundation for setting a physician fee schedule. It was to be based on the theory of competitive markets, whereby the price of a service would be equal to the cost of the input resources required to produce it efficiently. A fee schedule based on the price that a perfectly competitive market would yield has the advantage that the fees will allocate resources efficiently and services will be produced efficiently.

In 1986, the U.S. Congress requested and appropriated funds for developing a new method to set physician fees for the nation's Medicare program on a more rational basis. A Harvard University research group, headed by Hsiao, was selected from several competing organizations to conduct the study. Hsiao proposed to develop the new fees based on the principles of his earlier work. A year later, the U.S. Physician Payment Review Commission (PPRC), an advisory body to the U.S. Congress, also endorsed the method based on input resource costs. The commission reasoned that a resource-cost basis would reflect estimates of what relative values would be in a hypothetical market that functions perfectly and that in such a market, competition drives relative prices to reflect the relative costs of efficient producers.

Method and Data

The Harvard research group identified three main resource inputs required to produce physician services: (1) the total work input by the physician (TW); (2) the relative practice costs, including professional liability insurance premium (RPC); and (3) the amortized value of the opportunity costs of postgraduate specialty training (AST). These three components are combined to produce the RBRVS. Specifically, RBRVS = (TW)(1 + RPC)(1 + AST). The TW, RPC, and AST are each expressed as an index. The total work is divided into pre-, intra-, and postservice work. The intraservice period is the time when a physician sees the patient or performs a procedure, while the preservice and postservice periods represent the time spent on the patient before and after the intraservice period.

To investigate the work and other costs, the RBRVS study relied on the Physician's Current Procedural Terminology (CPT-4), a coding system designed by physicians, to identify more than 7,000 distinct services, visits, and procedures.

In their study, the Harvard research group found that physician work consists of two key components: time and intensity of time. The intensity has four dimensions: mental effort and clinical judgment, technical skill, physical effort, and stress due to risk. The study employed the magnitude estimation method to measure work inputs for a given service. Magnitude estimation method is a way of measuring subjective perceptions and judgments;

its usefulness in obtaining reliable, reproducible, and valid results for work input has been repeatedly demonstrated.

The Harvard research group randomly selected 6,841 physicians from the American Medical Association's Physician Masterfile and surveyed them by telephone. They were asked to estimate the time and intensity of the work of selected services performed by that specialty. The survey covered 33 specialties. The overall response rate was 69%, ranging from a high of 84% for nuclear medicine to a low of 56% for obstetrics and gynecology. The responses were tested for reliability, consistency, and validity with different statistical methods such as the intraclass correlation method and regression analysis. The study found the results from the surveys to be reliable, consistent, and reproducible. A panel of more than 200 practicing physicians who served as consultants to the study, representing the 33 specialties, then reviewed the results. The research group found that the results had face validity.

In the national survey, physicians in each specialty used a different service as a standard against which to rate the work of other services. To create a common scale for all specialties, the research group had to link the separate scales. They developed a method whereby their physician consultant panels identified pairs of services from different specialties that required approximately equal amounts of intraservice work. They connected each specialty to others by at least four of the pairs, creating a set of linkages. They then used a weighted-least-squares method to find the best-fit location for each link. A jackknife analysis of the residual sum of squares suggested that the choice of links was appropriate.

Practice costs can vary widely between different specialties and different services. Such costs would include compensation for supporting staff, office space, equipment, and supplies. The RBRVS study divided practice costs into direct and indirect costs. The identification of direct costs is straightforward—these are the resources used to render a service. In contrast, indirect costs consist of all the remaining costs; they are allocated based on commonly accepted allocation methods used in cost accounting, such as time or space occupied.

Physicians master their clinical judgment and skills through post–medical school residency training, which can range from 3 to 7 years depending on specialty. To undertake residency training, the physicians forgo the compensation they could have earned as medical school graduates. This loss in earnings constitutes the opportunity cost of residency training. The RBRVS study developed an index of the opportunity costs for different specialties by calculating the opportunity costs for each specialty and amortizing these costs over their working lifetime.

Last, the three components of the RBRVS are combined into one index.

Epilogue

The RBRVS study was completed for all specialties in late 1991. On its completion, the U.S. Congress immediately passed a law to adopt its use for the nation's Medicare program by January 1, 1992. Many private insurance plans in the nation adopted it as well. Responsibility for updating the RBRVS was given to the American Medical Association (AMA). Subsequently, several other nations, including Australia and France, and private insurance plans in England also adopted the RBRVS method to set their physician fees.

William C. Hsiao

See also American Medical Association (AMA); Centers for Medicare and Medicaid Services (CMS); Healthcare Financial Management; Health Economics; Medicare; Pay-for-Performance; Payment Mechanisms; Supplier-Induced Demand

Further Readings

American Medical Association. *Medicare RBRVS 2008: The Physician's Guide.* Chicago: American Medical Association, 2008.

Hsiao, William C., and William B. Stason. "Toward Developing a Relative Value Scale for Medical and Surgical Services," *Health Care Financing Review* 1(2): 23–38, Fall 1979.

Jan Bergman, Martin. "Resource-Based Relative Value Scale (RBRVS): A Useful Tool for Practice Analysis," *Journal of Clinical Rheumatology* 9(5): 325–27, October 2003.

Johnson, Sarah E., and Warren P. Newton. "Resource-Based Relative Value Units: A Primer for Academic Family Physicians," *Family Medicine* 34(3): 172–76, March 2002.

Rotarius, Timothy, and Arron Liberman. "An RBRVS Approach to Financial Analysis in Health Care Organizations," *The Health Care Manager* 19(3): 17–23, March 2001.

Williams, Tim R. "A Geologic Survey of the Medicare RBRVS System," *Journal of the American College of Radiology* 1(3): 192–98, March 2004.

Web Sites

American Medical Association (AMA):
    http://www.ama-assn.org
Centers for Medicare and Medicaid Services (CMS):
    http://www.cms.hhs.gov
Healthcare Financial Management Association (HFMA):
    http://www.hfma.org

RICE, DOROTHY P.

Dorothy P. Rice is a noted health economist and statistician who developed and applied methodologies for estimating the cost of illness and directed the federal National Center for Health Statistics (NCHS).

Rice was born Dorothy Rebecca Pechman in Brooklyn, New York, in 1922. Her parents had immigrated from Poland about a decade before. She attended Brooklyn College for 2 years and then transferred to the University of Wisconsin, where she earned a bachelor's degree in economics in 1941.

Immediately after college, she began her career as a federal civil servant—as an assistant statistical clerk for the Railroad Retirement Board, and in 1942, she moved to the War Production Board. There, she met her future husband, John D. (Jim) Rice, whom she married in 1943 and remained married to until his death 62 years later. In 1946, she worked as a health economist for the U.S. Public Health Service on the Hill-Burton Act, which supported the post–World War II growth of hospitals. Thereafter, she had three children, Kenneth, Donald, and Thomas and was out of the labor force, raising them and volunteering for various nonprofit organizations, from 1949 to 1960.

Rice reentered the labor force in 1960 and joined the U.S. Public Health Service. There, she helped develop, refine, and apply a methodology for estimating the cost of a human life. Called the "human capital method," it approximates the economic value of life by calculating the discounted value of future earnings. One of her innovations was developing and refining methods for imputing values for those not in the labor force, such as housewives. One purpose of calculating the value of a life was to estimate the aggregate cost of disease. Rice estimated the costs of cardiovascular disease and cancer (1965) and then the overall cost of illness in the United States (1966).

She became Chief of the Health Insurance Research Branch of the Social Security Administration (SSA) in 1965 and then Deputy Assistant Commissioner for Research and Statistics at SSA in 1972. During the early 1960s, much attention was being devoted to national health insurance. She analyzed data from a comprehensive survey of the aged and found that more than half of the citizens aged 65 and older did not have adequate health insurance. These data were used in developing proposals that resulted in the Medicare program.

In 1976, Rice was appointed the director of the National Center for Health Statistics (NCHS). NCHS is the leading national agency that oversees the collection, analysis, and dissemination of health data. Her stewardship lasted until 1982, when she retired from the federal government and moved to California.

In 1982, Rice was appointed as a professor in the Department of Social and Behavior Sciences in the School of Nursing and at the Institute for Health and Aging at the University of California, San Francisco (UCSF). At UCSF she revisited her work on estimating the cost of illnesses, applying it to injuries, aging, mental illness, and AIDS. She devoted considerable attention to the cost of smoking and contributed to the Tobacco Settlement of $246 billion between the state attorneys general and the tobacco companies.

Rice's honors include election to the national Institute of Medicine (IOM); the American Public Health Association's Sedgwick Memorial Medal for Distinguished Service in Public Health; the Presidential Award for Leadership and Contributions to Health Services Research from the Association for Health Services Research (now AcademyHealth); and the Jack C. Massey Award for Achievement in Health and Related Sciences. She also holds an honorary doctorate of science from the College of Medicine and Dentistry at New Jersey. Rice is the author of more than 250 articles, chapters, books, and monographs. In 1999, the University of California, San Francisco, established the Dorothy Pechman Rice Center for Health Economics.

Thomas Rice

See also Acute and Chronic Diseases; Cost of Healthcare; Health Economics; Hospitals; Medicare; National Center for Health Statistics (NCHS); Tobacco Use, Women's Health Issues

Further Readings

Hoffman, Catherine, Dorothy P. Rice, and Hai-Yen Sung. "Persons With Chronic Conditions: Their Prevalence and Costs," *Journal of the American Medical Association* 276(18): 1473–79, November 1996.

Rice, Dorothy P., Peter J. Fox, Wendy Max, et al. "The Economic Burden of Alzheimer's Disease Care," *Health Affairs* 12(21): 164–76, Summer 1993.

Rice, Dorothy P., Thomas A. Hodgson, Peter Sinsheimer, et al. "The Economic Costs of the Health Effects of Smoking, 1984," *Milbank Quarterly* 64(4): 489–547, 1986.

Rice, Dorothy P., Wendy Max, Jacqueline Golding, et al. *The Cost of Domestic Violence to the Health Care System: Final Report.* Report prepared for the Office of the Assistant Secretary for Planning and Evaluation. Washington, DC: U.S. Department of Health and Human Services, 1997.

Rice, Dorothy P., L. Paringer, and E. Wittenberg. *Development of AIDS Studies Protocols: Comparing the Cost of AIDS to the Cost of Other Illnesses.* San Francisco: University of California, Institute for Health and Aging, 1988.

Web Sites

University of California, San Francisco, Institute for Health and Aging, Faculty Profile: http://nurseweb.ucsf.edu/iha/faculty/rice.htm

RISK

Risk refers to the potential negative impact of some event or exposure. It can refer to the probability of a particular (typically negative) event or, more generally, to a magnitude that is a combination of the probability of a negative event and the magnitude of loss associated with the given event. The more likely the event is to occur and the more harsh and costly the results if the event occurs, the greater the overall risk.

Risk in Epidemiology and Biostatistics

In the context of epidemiology, the term *risk* refers to the probability that some event will occur within a particular time period. Typical events are death (mortality) or disease (morbidity) incidence. The fixed time period is essential for defining the probability. Related measures of risk per unit time are instead referred to as *rates*. In the area of biostatistics, risk also refers specifically to the probability of the occurrence of a particular event during a defined time period. Biostatistical analyses along with epidemiologic study designs have been used extensively to analyze risk in this sense. Estimation of risk can be done based on a random sample of the population for whom the status of the given event is defined during the given time period; the estimate is then simply the number who experience the event divided by the total. It is essential that the entire sample be at risk of the outcome event. For example, if the event is the incidence of some disease, the population at risk is the subset of the population that has been diagnosed with the disease. It is also essential that each individual in the population can be properly classified as either having the event or not having the event during the given time period. Statistical theory addressing estimation of probabilities of risk is based on the binomial distribution. Confidence intervals can be computed that reflect the variation in the estimate due to sampling, based on the sample size and the assumption of a random sample.

An area within biostatistics known as survival analysis addresses the problem of incomplete information, or censoring, in the estimation of risk. Right censoring occurs when an individual known to be at risk of the event for some time period is then lost to follow-up or when the individual's subsequent status is unknown for some reason. The latest time the individual is known to still be at risk, or has still had the event, is his or her right-censored time. Such persons are said to be at risk of the event until they are right-censored. Given a sample of right-censored observations at any time point, the subset that is still known to be a risk is called the risk set. The product-limit estimate, or Kaplan-Meier estimate, is a method of estimating the cumulative risk of an event at any time point, based on conditional probabilities within the risk set. The entire set of risk estimates for different time points is the estimated survival curve.

Often risk is studied in terms of an instantaneous rate per unit time, which is then applied to a time interval to compute a risk or probability. Specifically, the rate is the potential for change in a numerator quantity—in this case, event occurrence, or change from no event to an event—relative to change in a denominator quantity—in this case, time. Under the assumption of a constant rate across time, the rate can be estimated easily from a sample of observations with varying amounts of time at risk. For example, a study of disease incidence might record disease status across time for a sample of persons initially free of the disease, and the observed time at risk might vary. If time is measured in months, the total person-time for the study is the sum of the number of months observed at risk across all individuals in the study. The average rate is then the number of events divided by the total person time and will be the event rate per month. This estimate is also known as the average incidence density.

Risk Factors and Risk Markers

A factor demonstrated to be associated with the risk of a particular outcome is called a risk factor. Examples of risk factors include environmental exposure, personal behaviors or lifestyles, or inborn or inherited characteristics. A risk marker is something shown to be associated with a particular health outcome but not necessarily as a causal factor. A factor that does seem to cause the given health outcome is referred to as a determinant of the health outcome. A determinant that can potentially be altered with intervention is a modifiable risk factor.

Risk Ratio, Odds Ratio, and the Risk Difference

There are three statistical measures used to summarize the association between a binary exposure or other factor and risk of a given outcome; these are the risk ratio, the odds ratio, and the risk difference. The risk ratio is the risk of the outcome in those who are exposed divided by the risk of the outcome in those who are not exposed. A risk ratio of 2.0, for example, suggests that the exposure doubles the probability of the outcome. Similarly, the odds ratio is the ratio of the odds of the outcome in those who are exposed relative to those who are not exposed, where *the odds* is defined as the risk probability divided by 1 minus the risk probability. The odds ratio has become popular with researchers because, unlike the risk ratio, it is not altered when the proportion with exposure or disease is fixed in the sample by design. Considering a two-by-two table that is a cross-tabulation of exposure by disease outcome, another way of stating this property is that the odds ratio remains constant if the marginals of the table are altered. In case-control studies of disease outcomes that are rare in the population, the estimated odds ratio from the sample provides a reasonable estimate of the risk ratio in the population.

The risk difference is the risk of the outcome in those who are exposed minus the risk of the outcome in those who are not exposed. This measure of association is preferred by some researchers because its interpretation is directly tied to the number in the population affected by the exposure. There are several more variations on the risk difference. The rate difference is a difference in rates, rather than risks tied to a particular time period, between the exposed and unexposed. The population risk difference is the risk in the entire population minus the risk in the unexposed population, which corresponds to the theoretical improvement in the population risk if the exposure were entirely eliminated. The attributable risk is the population risk difference divided by the risk of disease in the population, or the proportion of risk that could theoretically be eliminated if exposure in the population were eliminated. The attributable risk among the exposed is the risk difference divided by the risk of disease given exposure, or the proportion of risk within the exposed population that could theoretically be eliminated.

Use of Statistical Regression

Epidemiological study designs along with statistical regression modeling have been used extensively to identify factors related to risk. Logistic regression and Poisson regression are both used to model risk of disease, or any other binary variable, as the outcome measure. Logistic regression assumes linear effects on the logarithm of the odds of the outcome and produces a simple estimate of the odds ratio, whereas Poisson regression assumes linear effects on the logarithm of the risk of the outcome and produces a simple estimate of the risk ratio. Multiple regression, either logistic or Poisson, is used to adjust for confounders as additional independent variables and obtain a more accurate estimate of association of a given factor with disease risk. Inclusion of interactions as independent variables can allow for the magnitude of association between a factor and the outcome to vary with other characteristics. Factors or exposures under study are concluded to be risk factors for the outcome if the model coefficients representing their effects are statistically significantly different from zero, typically using the criterion of Type I error rate equal to .05. A statistically significant association in this case means that there is less than a 5% probability that the observed association arises only due to the particular random sample and that there is really no association in the population.

The epidemiologic literature refers to the following criteria for deciding that something is a risk factor: strength of the association, as elaborated above; dose-response effect (more exposure is associated with higher risk); lack of temporal ambiguity (the risk factor precedes the outcome); consistency of findings across different studies; biological plausibility; coherence of evidence; and specificity of the association.

Risk Assessment

Risk assessment is the estimation of risk of adverse effects resulting from negative exposures to health hazards or from absence of beneficial or positive exposures. Specifically, the amount of risk is estimated in terms of a probability and in terms of different magnitudes or doses of exposure. In the context of negative environmental exposures, or ecological risk assessment, the process typically consists of four steps. The hazardous negative exposure, conditions of exposure, and the potential target population must be identified (hazard

identification), and the resulting adverse events to be investigated must be described (risk characterization). The exposure to the relevant population must then be quantified and measured (exposure assessment); this could be done based on measures of emissions or environmental levels of the toxic substance, reflecting potential exposure in a particular area, or directly from biological monitoring of subjects from a representative sample. The final step (risk estimation) consists of combining information to make a statement about expected health effects in the target population.

Health risk appraisal is a form of risk assessment that addresses individual behaviors or lifestyles that play the role of exposure. In this case, the purpose of the risk assessment would be to identify high-risk people and motivate them to change their negative exposures or behaviors. Promoting awareness of negative effects would hopefully create a tension in high-risk individuals. There is a vast literature addressing numerous intervention programs designed to motivate change in high-risk behaviors.

The process of taking steps to reduce levels of risk is called risk management. Typically, this refers to an active hazard and control process to deal with environmental agents of disease such as toxic substances. There are three steps involved in risk management: risk evaluation, exposure control, and risk monitoring. Specifically, *risk evaluation* refers to the determination of acceptable versus unacceptable risk by comparing risk estimates with some standard for level of acceptable risk. *Exposure control* refers to actions taken to keep exposure below the acceptable maximum level. *Risk monitoring* is the process of measuring reduction in the risk as a result of exposure control.

Risk-benefit analysis refers to the process of analyzing and comparing the benefits, or expected positive outcomes, with the costs, or expected negative outcomes, of a particular action. When this is done on a single scale, results can be summarized as a risk-benefit ratio, defined as the ratio of risks to benefits. For example, the single measurement scale could be dollars.

In the context of economics, financial risk is often defined as the unexpected variability of returns, including both worse than expected and better than expected outcomes. In this case, the process of assessing risk involves predicting the range or variability of possible outcomes of a given action.

Sally A. Freels

See also Disease; Epidemiology; Infectious Diseases; Mental Health Epidemiology; Morbidity; Mortality; Mortality, Major Causes in the United States; Public Health

Further Readings

Gordis, Leon. *Epidemiology.* 4th ed. Philadelphia: Elsevier/Saunders, 2008.

Kleinbaum, David G., and Mitchel Klein. *Logistic Regression: A Self-Learning Text.* 2d ed. New York: Springer, 2002.

Kleinbaum, David G., and Mitchel Klein. *Survival Analysis: A Self-Learning Text.* 2d ed. New York: Springer, 2005.

Vose, David. *Risk Analysis: A Quantitative Guide.* 3d ed. Hoboken, NJ: Wiley, 2008.

White, Emily, Bruce K. Armstrong, and Rodolfo Saracci. *Principles of Exposure Measurement in Epidemiology: Collecting, Evaluating and Improving Measures of Disease Risk Factors.* New York: Oxford University Press, 2001.

Web Sites

American Society for Healthcare Risk Management (ASHRM): http://www.ashrm.org

Mayo Clinic, Genetic Epidemiology and Risk Assessment Program: http://cancercenter.mayo.edu/mayo/research/genetic_epidemiology_program

National Institute of Mental Health (NIMH): http://www.nimh.nih.gov

Risk World: http://www.riskworld.com

Toxicology Excellence for Risk Assessment (TERA): http://www.tera.org

ROBERT WOOD JOHNSON FOUNDATION (RWJF)

Located in Princeton, New Jersey, the Robert Wood Johnson Foundation (RWJF) is the largest U.S. foundation exclusively funding health-related activities and research. It played a major role in creating the new field of health services research, and because of its large size and the number of projects it funds, the foundation continues to have an important impact on the field.

Robert Wood Johnson II (1893–1968), who built the family firm of Johnson & Johnson into one of the world's largest health and personal-care products entities, established the foundation in 1936. On his death, he left the vast majority of his personal fortune to the foundation. Since that time, the RWJF has funded research, education, and services in a wide variety of areas but with the priorities of access to affordable primary care, medical and nursing education, and quality-of-care initiatives. The foundation does not fund direct care or biomedical research. Hospitals, universities, public schools, professional associations, research organizations, community groups, and state and local governments are eligible for funding.

In 2006, the RWJF awarded over 900 grants and contracts totaling $403 million. Grants from the foundation average $300,000 for a project period of 3 years. Many types of organizations have been funded; priority is given to public agencies, public charities, and organizations deemed tax-exempt under Section 501(c)(3) of the U.S. Internal Revenue Code. Only projects located in the United States are funded; no international projects are supported. Many types of projects are funded, including service demonstrations, surveillance, data collection and analysis, secondary data analysis, public education (including health professions training programs), policy development and analysis, health services and public health services research, technical assistance, communication activities, and evaluation projects.

Background

In 1952, the foundation, which was originally located in New Brunswick, New Jersey, and called the Johnson New Brunswick Foundation, moved to Princeton, New Jersey, and changed its name to the Robert Wood Johnson Foundation. At this time, it also expanded its scope and began funding projects throughout New Jersey; previously it only funded local projects in New Brunswick.

In its early decades, the Johnson Foundation developed a set of priorities that still guide its funding: hospitals and healthcare; scholarship support, primarily in the health professions; and community service programs focusing on vulnerable and underserved populations. In its early years, over half of all its grant funds went to support hospitals and healthcare, primarily in New Brunswick. It also established a large number of educational scholarships for medical, dental, nursing, and pharmaceutical students from low-income backgrounds; approximately 25% of its funds were spent in this area. The remainder of the foundation's spending was directed to community agencies serving indigent people, particularly youth. This included secular organizations such as the Boy Scouts and Girl Scouts as well as religion-affiliated organizations such as the Hillel Foundation and the Christ Church of New Brunswick.

In 1968, when Robert Wood Johnson II died, the foundation had a net worth of over $53 million. In his will, he bequeathed $300 million in Johnson & Johnson stock to the foundation. In the 3 years it took to probate his estate, the value of the stock increased to more than $1 billion. This radically changed the foundation, making it the largest health-focused philanthropy in the nation. In 1971, the foundation's policy committee decided that the foundation's grants would have a national focus and that its primary purpose would be to contribute to the advancement of healthcare in the United States. Three specific objectives were adopted: expand access to medical care services for underserved populations through large-scale testing of promising approaches; improve the quality of medical care through measures including funding health professions training programs, especially those designed to increase minority representation in the primary-care disciplines; and develop approaches designed to allow the objective analysis of health-related public policies. Broadly speaking, the RWJF has kept this focus while continuing to maintain a more diverse giving strategy in the New Brunswick, New Jersey, area.

In 1971, the foundation had $1.2 billion in assets, and in the next funding year, it dispersed $45 million; this compares with a total of $4.4 million in giving during the previous 34 years. Faced with the responsibility of managing this large grant program, the foundation leadership set several priorities for giving. They decided that the foundation would provide seed money to test new programs and ideas, especially in the areas of access to care for underserved populations, improving the quality of health and medical care, and developing methodologies that would lead to objective analysis of policy interventions. They also decided to fund outcomes over process, positioning the foundation to be an early leader in the area of program evaluation. Finally, they committed the foundation to devoting significant resources to communication, thereby ensuring that their findings would be well-known and available to researchers, academic leaders, elected officials, and government policymakers.

Many of these basic approaches and areas of interest have stood the test of time. The RWJF continues to fund communications and evaluations, health professions training, and testing of new ideas through large demonstration projects. Specific issues and strategies have changed over time and will continue to evolve as the health-related needs of the nation change and develop.

Current Priorities

Specific information regarding the foundation's current funding priorities is available on its Web site. Funding is available through specific calls for proposals (CFPs); unsolicited proposals are rarely accepted except in three program areas: human capital, vulnerable populations, and pioneer projects. Proposals can include funding for service demonstrations, gathering and monitoring of health statistics, public education, health professions training and fellowship programs, policy analysis, health services and public health services research, technical assistance, communications activities, and evaluation activities. The foundation does not fund general operating expenses, existing deficits, endowment or capital campaigns, biomedical research, research on drug therapies or devices, direct support of individuals, or any kind of lobbying activities. As of 2008, the foundation no longer accepts proposals related to long-term care, end-of-life care, physical activity for adults over 50, and specific chronic conditions not otherwise covered in their priority areas.

Affordable Primary Care, Access to Care, and Health Professions Education

The giving practices of the RWJF show that it views these three issues as intertwined. From its earliest days, the foundation sponsored programs to expand health insurance and access to care, to explore the efficacy of prepaid group plans, and to promote primary care. Between 1972 and 1975, the foundation provided over $50 million to academic medical centers to improve the delivery of primary care and to train health professionals in the primary-care disciplines. The Clinical Scholars Program was also initiated during this time. During the mid-1970s, the foundation funded a demonstration project to improve dental care for disabled persons, a project that permanently changed the standard-of-care and service delivery approach for this population. In the late 1990s, the foundation targeted efforts toward health insurance coverage for children. In 1997, it launched Covering Kids and Families at a cost of $13 million. A month later, the U.S. Congress passed the $20 billion State Children's Health Insurance Program (SCHIP). The foundation added $34 million to help states enroll children in the program.

This area of grant making is driven by CFPs issued by the foundation; unsolicited proposals are not accepted. In 2006, a wide variety of projects received funding, including 47 proposals totaling $19.6 million designed to address affordable healthcare coverage through the development of policies and programs to expand healthcare coverage and maximize enrollment in existing coverage programs.

Quality Initiatives

During the 1970s, the foundation funded Georgetown University to develop a methodological tool to measure the quality of diagnostic services and follow-up care. Since that time, the foundation's interest in this area has broadened. In 2006, 133 grants totaling $43.1 million were awarded. Many projects are designed to assist communities—especially communities facing lower standards of care—to improve the quality of healthcare in ways that matter to their residents. These efforts take a variety of approaches, including coalition building, developing performance measures, and encouraging public disclosure of healthcare quality measures and quality improvement projects. Program and policy evaluation are also funded under the foundation's quality initiative. The foundation also uses its national resources to ensure that results are effectively communicated to all stakeholders.

Health Services Research and Public Policy

Historically, the foundation's commitment to health services research has been embedded in its commitment to evidence-based public policy. In the 1990s, the foundation became interested in understanding and accessing the changes wrought by managed care in terms of access, cost, and quality. To facilitate this interest, the foundation established a new organization, the Center for Studying Health System Change. This organization, located in Washington, D.C., continues to design and conduct research on the nation's healthcare system to inform policymakers in government and private industry.

During the 2001 decade, the RWJF increased its efforts in this area, coming forward and espousing a need to refocus the national health services research agenda to include public health services and systems research. It is the intent of the foundation to direct more private and public dollars towards building a strong public health research infrastructure, one that continues to generate epidemiological data as well as address the social and community conditions that promote physical and mental health in the population. In announcing its increased interest in this area of research, the foundation expressed concern over the fragility of the nation's public health system and stated that, in its estimation, the best remedy is to increase the science base and ensure that recommendations are based on findings, not political expediency. While in terms of grant-making dollars this is a new initiative, it is consistent with the foundation's long-standing interests and builds on its activities to support the 1988 National Academy of Sciences, Institute of Medicine (IOM) report, *The Future of Public Health*, participation in the Turning Point Initiative, and the goals and objectives of Healthy People 2010.

Funding under this giving area is in response to specific CFPs issued by the foundation. In 2006, 137 projects were funded, totaling $43 million. Most of these projects were designed to improve the performance of public health agencies, increase advocacy for public health resources and policy changes, and, to these ends, build an evidence base for public health policy and practice. Funding to build the evidence base included assessing the potential of a public health accreditation system and other quality improvement efforts; projects that actively engage public health research partners; support for survey research concerning public health activities; and research to assess the potential health impacts of a variety of projects and policies.

Of note, the National Association of City and County Health Officials (NACCHO) and the Association of State and Territorial Health Officials (ASTHO) were among the public health organizations funded to create a national public health accreditation system to serve as the basis for ongoing quality assessment, greater transparency, and increased accountability.

A variety of advocacy initiatives were also funded in 2006. They included tobacco control measures, including smoke-free-air laws and tobacco taxes.

Healthy Communities and Lifestyles

Beginning in the 1990s, the RWJF became interested in the nonmedical factors that influence health. Since that time, it has funded many approaches to ensuring healthy communities and to encouraging healthy lifestyle choices. Projects have been funded on a broad array of topics, including smoking, diet, sexual behavior, substance abuse, and environmental exposures. Beginning in 2006, the foundation specifically directed efforts toward the childhood obesity epidemic in the belief that the long-term consequences of childhood obesity will negatively affect the health status of an entire generation and will further stress systems of primary care and limit resources. In that year, 128 grants totaling $41.8 million were funded to support the priority of reversing the epidemic by 2015 by improving access to affordable healthy foods and increasing opportunities for physical activity in schools and communities across the nation. Three integrated strategies guide this area of grant making. The foundation prioritized funding projects that will build an evidence base to ensure that the most promising efforts are replicated throughout the nation. It also funds action strategies for schools and communities, including coalition building to disseminate promising approaches at the local level. Advocacy efforts also receive funding under this initiative.

The foundation funds the Leadership for Healthy Communication initiative, which works with national organizations that represent elected and appointed officials—such as the National Conference of State Legislatures and the U.S. Conference of Mayors—to educate their members about successful approaches to increasing physical activity and healthy eating among children and young adults.

In 2008, the foundation announced a new initiative in this area, the Commission to Build a Healthier America. This commission, funded for 2 years, is charged with identifying proven interventions capable of successful replication, especially those interventions that take into account economic, social, and physical environment factors. This program area accepts unsolicited proposals.

Vulnerable Populations

This area of giving is designed to support promising ideas and strategies to overcome health disparities. Unsolicited proposals are accepted. In 2006, 154 grants totaling $83.7 million were approved. This area of giving supports promising new ideas to help overcome long-standing health challenges for groups that bear an excess of the burden of disease. Projects often address poor health status in the context of other factors such as housing, education, and poverty. Changes in healthcare service delivery and organization are funded, as are initiatives to improve policy, financing, and service integration among local service providers and state and federal agencies. The Community Oriented Correctional Health Services project funds continuity-of-care approaches to connect the healthcare provided in local correctional centers with healthcare providers in the community.

This giving area also funds projects that bring together nontraditional partners and multiple-service systems to address health disparities and care for vulnerable populations. As an example, the Green House Project is taking a new approach to skilled-nursing homes and assisted living facilities by creating residences for small groups of individuals who require skilled nursing care in a homelike setting.

The foundation also funds projects to address rapid demographic changes occurring in the nation, including the Community Partnership for Older Adults and the New Routes to Community Health projects.

Human Capital

This giving area funds a wide variety of training programs and leadership development programs. In 2006, 195 grants totaling $115.1 million were awarded. Unsolicited proposals are accepted. This area includes some of the foundation's most long-standing programs, such as the Clinical Scholars Program. It also funds programs to increase the racial and ethnic diversity of the health professions, train people in specific subdisciplines such as quality improvement, ameliorate the nursing shortage, and involve scholars from a variety of fields (e.g., business, engineering, and law) in research studies on the policy issues in health and healthcare. Diversity training and cultural-competence projects are also funded. The foundation maintains many midcareer awards, including its Health Policy Fellowship Program, Community Health Leaders Program, and the Executive Nurse Fellows Program.

Pioneering Projects

This area of giving allows the foundation to be an early participant in new approaches to important problems, approaches deemed capable of developing breakthrough improvements in health, healthcare, and public health. The foundation tends to fund projects that it feels have the potential to become long-term foundation initiatives. Unsolicited proposals are accepted. In 2006, 29 grants totaling $8.3 million were made in this area. This included funding for new approaches to fighting drug-resistant diseases; improving the public health system's ability to predict influenza outbreaks; a national program to reform medical liability by developing a system of specialized health courts; the Myelin Repair Foundation, to develop a fast-track process for "bench to bedside" translational research; and Project Health Design, which is designing strategies to expand the use of personal health records and develop a "smart" system capable of helping individuals comply with treatment guidelines and engage in preventive measures.

Science Evaluation

Beginning in the 1970s, the foundation became committed to program evaluation. It has consistently funded evaluation components for its projects. Over the years, the foundation has remained interested in program evaluation, outcome evaluation, and the evaluation of specific policy initiatives. Funding for evaluation is embedded in all successful grant proposals. However, specific evaluation projects are also funded.

Impact on Health Services Research

The RWJF's commitment to health services research has been consistent throughout its history. It has supported research, evaluation, and the dissemination of results toward the end of supporting an evidence-based approach to the development and evaluation of public policy. Health services research is a major focus of the foundation; this is clearly evident in its rhetoric, its requests for proposals, and the allocation of its grant funds. In many ways, its support of other issues such as building healthy communities, supporting health professions education, and addressing discrete issues such as childhood obesity is toward the end of evidence-based public policy. The foundation will likely continue to play a dominant role in the funding of the field of health services research in the future.

Judith V. Sayad

See also Access to Healthcare; Center for Studying Health System Change; Health Insurance; Primary Care; Public Policy; Quality of Healthcare; State Children's Health Insurance Program (SCHIP); Vulnerable Populations

Further Readings

Colby, David C. "Health Services Research." In *To Improve Health and Health Care*, vol. 11: *The Robert Wood Johnson Foundation Anthology*, edited by Stephen L. Isaacs and David C. Colby, 35–57. San Francisco: Jossey-Bass, 2007.

Foster, Lawrence G. *Robert Wood Johnson: The Gentleman Rebel*. State College, PA: Lillian Press, 1999.

Institute of Medicine. *The Future of Public Health*. Washington, DC: National Academy of Sciences, Institute of Medicine, 1988.

Issacs, Stephen L., James R. Knickman, and David J. Morse. "Health, Health Care, and the Robert Wood Johnson Foundation: A Ten-Year Retrospective, 1996–2006." In *To Improve Health and Health Care*, vol. 10: *The Robert Wood Johnson Foundation Anthology*, edited by Stephen L. Isaacs and David C. Colby, 3–21. San Francisco: Jossey-Bass, 2006.

Lavizzo-Mourey, Risa. "Childhood Obesity: What It Means for Physicians," *Journal of the American Medical Association* 298(8): 920–22, August 22, 2007.

Showstack, Jonathan, Arlyss Anderson Rothman, and Susan B. Hassmiller, eds. *The Future of Primary Care*. Public Health/Robert Wood Johnson Foundation. San Francisco: Jossey-Bass, 2004.

Voelker, Rebecca. "Robert Wood Johnson Clinical Scholars Mark 35 Years of Health Services Research," *Journal of the American Medical Association* 297(23): 2571–73, June 20, 2007.

Warner, Kenneth E., ed. *Tobacco Control Policy*. Robert Wood Johnson Foundation Series on Health Policy. San Francisco: Jossey-Bass, 2006.

Web Sites

Robert Wood Johnson Foundation (RWJF): http://www.rwjf.org

ROEMER, MILTON I.

Milton I. Roemer (1916–2001) was a pioneer in health services research, a health administrator, and a teacher. Roemer was a scholar in the areas of international health, primary care, rural health, and healthcare organization. He was the first to identify, in the early 1960s, the phenomenon of supplier-induced demand. Specifically, he found that when health insurance is widespread in a community, increased utilization of services results in an increase in the supply of hospital beds, or, in short, a hospital bed built is a bed filled. This finding became known as the *Roemer effect* or *Roemer's law*. It would contribute in the 1970s to the enactment of federal certificate-of-need (CON) legislation and comprehensive health planning.

Born in Paterson, New Jersey, in 1916, Roemer earned a master's degree in sociology from Cornell University in 1939, a medical degree from New York University in 1940, and a master's degree in public health from the University of Michigan in 1943.

In the early 1940s, Roemer was a county health officer for Monongalia County, West Virginia. Later, he was a medical officer for the New Jersey State Health Department. During World War II, he joined the U.S. Public Health Service, where he served as a medical officer for the War Food Administration and the Medical Care Administration of the States Relations Division. In 1951, Roemer began his international work when he was appointed Chief of Social and Occupational Health at the newly formed World Health Organization (WHO). At the WHO, he was responsible for a wide range of services, including hospital administration, occupational health, and the organization of medical care, among others. However, he was forced out of his position when the U.S. government withdrew its approval of his appointment under pressure of McCarthyism. In 1953, Roemer moved to Canada, where he worked for the Saskatchewan Department of Public Health as the Director of Medical and Hospital Services. He eventually returned to the United States and taught at Yale and Cornell universities. In 1962, Roemer joined the faculty of the School of Public Health at the University of California, Los Angeles (UCLA). He taught courses in comparative national health systems, hospital administration, medical care, and public health. And he served as the chairman of the Department of Health Services for 8 years. While at the university, he undertook extensive work in Asia and Latin America. In 1986, Roemer retired from the university and became Professor Emeritus.

During his 60-year career, Roemer conducted a wide range of research projects in international health, and he was a prolific writer. He worked in 71 countries and authored or coauthored 32 books and 430 scholarly articles. One of his best-known publications is *National Health Systems of the World*, a monumental two-volume comparative analysis of international healthcare systems.

Roemer received many awards and honors in recognition of his work. He was a member of the National Academy of Sciences, Institute of Medicine (IOM). He received the International Award for Excellence in Promoting and Protecting the Health of People in 1977, the Sedgwick Memorial Medal for distinguished service in public health in 1983, and the Lifetime Achievement Award in 1997 from the American Public Health Association (APHA). He also received the Joseph W. Mountain award from the Centers for Disease Control and Prevention (CDC) in 1992 and the Distinguished Career Award from the Association for Health Services Research in 1997. Roemer died in 2001 at the age of 84.

Ross M. Mullner

See also Certificate of Need (CON); Comparing Health Systems; Health Planning; International Health Systems; National Health Insurance; Public Health; Public Policy; Supplier-Induced Demand

Further Readings

Jonas, Steven, and Milton I. Roemer. *An Introduction to the U.S. Health Care System.* 3d ed. New York: Springer, 1992.

Kaplan, Diane. *Preliminary Guide to the Milton Irwin Roemer Papers.* Manuscript Group 1786. New Haven CT: Yale University Library, 2003.

Mott, Frederick Dodge, and Milton I. Roemer. *Rural Health and Medical Care.* New York: McGraw-Hill, 1948.

Roemer, Milton I. *Health Policy.* New York: Marcel Dekker, 1981.

Roemer, Milton I. *National Health Systems of the World.* Vol. 1, *The Countries.* New York: Oxford University Press, 1991.

Roemer, Milton. *National Health Systems of the World.* Vol. 2, *Issues.* New York: Oxford University Press, 1993.

Roemer, Milton I. *National Strategies for Health Care Organization: A World Overview.* Ann Arbor, MI: Health Administration Press, 1985.

Web Sites

University of California, Los Angeles (UCLA), School of Public Health: http://www.ph.ucla.edu

ROOS, LESLIE L.

Leslie L. Roos is a Distinguished Professor at the University of Manitoba (Canada), the founding director of the Population Health Research Data Repository, and Senior Researcher at the Manitoba Centre for Health Policy. Roos is a recognized expert in the use of administrative databases in conducting health services research.

Roos received a bachelor's degree with honors in psychology and biology from Stanford University in 1962. With awards from the National Science Foundation and Social Science Research Council, he earned a doctoral degree in political science from the Massachusetts Institute of Technology (MIT) in 1966. He then completed a postdoctoral fellowship in political science at MIT. Following academic appointments at Brandeis and Northwestern Universities, in 1973, Roos joined the University of Manitoba as an associate and was subsequently full professor in the Faculty of Administrative Studies (now the Asper School of Business). His early research resulted in three books and numerous papers on social science methods and organizational behavior. Roos moved to the University of Manitoba's Department of Community Health Sciences, Faculty of Medicine in 1990.

Roos's substantive work includes a number of papers comparing health and healthcare in Canada and the United States, looking at primary and secondary prevention among socioeconomic groups over time, and analyzing alternative approaches to funding Canadian Medicare. Roos's studies have helped transform research approaches in health services, health policy, and population health. Recent papers are expanding the applicability of his work in epidemiology, economics, and sociology. Current research has been examining the effects of family and place on well-being.

Roos has received over $20 million in research support (several grants have been in collaboration with researchers based across Canada as well as at several U.S. universities), and he has been invited to venues as diverse as Australia and Spain to give short courses on his work.

Roos's contributions in health services research have been recognized nationally and internationally and through the ongoing success of the Manitoba Centre for Health Policy. He has published approximately 186 peer-reviewed papers and book chapters with collaborators from leading universities. Roos has been honored as a "Highly Cited Investigator" by the Institute of Scientific Information. His citations recently tallied almost

2,800, the highest number of citations by any Canadian social scientist. Journals in which he has published include *Health Affairs, Health Services Research, Journal of Clinical Epidemiology, Journal of the American Medical Association, Medical Care, Milbank Quarterly, New England Journal of Medicine,* and *Social Science and Medicine.*

Roos received career funding from the National Health Research and Development Program for over 20 years. He is a fellow of AcademyHealth and an associate of the Canadian Institute for Advanced Research. His work contributed substantially to the Manitoba Centre for Health Policy's receipt of the 2001 Health Services Research Advancement Award from the Canadian Health Services Research Foundation (CHSRF) and the 2005 regional Knowledge Translation award from the Canadian Institutes for Health Research.

Roos has received awards from the University of Manitoba for research excellence, outreach, and graduate student mentorship.

Gregory S. Finlayson

See also Canadian Association for Health Services and Policy Research (CAHSPR); Canadian Health Services Research Foundation (CHSRF); Data Sources in Conducting Health Services Research; Health Services Research in Canada; Roos, Noralou P.

Further Readings

Carriere, Keumhee C., Leslie L. Roos, and Douglas C. Dover. "Across Time and Space: Variations in Hospital Use During Canadian Health Reform," *Health Services Research* 35(2): 467–487, June 2000.

Roos, Leslie L., Marni Brownell, Lisa Lix, et al. "From Health Research to Social Research: Privacy, Methods, Approaches," *Social Science and Medicine* 66(1): 117–29, January 2008.

Roos, Leslie L., Jennifer Magoon, Sumit Gupta, et al. "Socioeconomic Determinants of Mortality in Two Canadian Provinces: Multilevel Modelling and Neighborhood Context," *Social Science and Medicine* 59(7): 1435–47, October 2004.

Roos, Leslie L., Leonie Stranc, Robert C. James, et al. "Complications, Comorbidities, and Mortality: Improving Classification and Prediction," *Health Services Research* 32(2): 229–38, June 1997.

Roos, Leslie L., Randy Walld, Julia Uhanova, et al. "Physician Visits, Hospitalizations, and Socioeconomic Status: Ambulatory Care Sensitive Conditions in a Canadian Setting," *Health Services Research* 40(4): 1167–85, August 2005.

Web Sites

Manitoba Centre for Health Policy: http://www.umanitoba.ca/centres/mchp

National Bureau of Economic Research Working Papers: http://www.nber.org/cgi-bin/author_papers .pl?author=leslie_roos

Providing Information to Regional Health Care Planners: A Manitoba Case Study: http://www.pitt.edu/~super1/ lecture/lec2881/index.htm

Studying Health and Health Care: http://www.pitt.edu/~super1/lecture/lec1011/index.htm

Studying Health Care: Some ICD-10 Tools: http://www.pitt.edu/~super1/lecture/lec22371/index.htm

Working More Productively: Tools for Information-Rich Environments: http://www.pitt.edu/~super1/lecture/ lec11441/index.htm

ROOS, NORALOU P.

Noralou P. Roos is a professor at the University of Manitoba (Canada) and the founding director of the Manitoba Centre for Health Policy, where she is a senior researcher, having stepped down from the directorship in 2004. Her research interests include the use of administrative data for managing the healthcare system; the relationship between healthcare use and population health; and, most recently, the impact of early childhood experiences, education, community environment, and healthcare interventions on the health of children.

Roos received a bachelor's degree with distinction and departmental honors in political science from Stanford University in 1963. As a Woodrow Wilson Fellow and a Woodrow Wilson Dissertation Fellow, she earned a doctoral degree in political science from the Massachusetts Institute of Technology (MIT) in 1968. Her first academic appointment was in political science at MIT. She then moved to a faculty position in the Graduate School of Management at Northwestern University, followed by a year as a medical program specialist and Sears-Roebuck Foundation Federal Faculty Fellow at the National Center for Health Services Research Development. In 1973, Roos joined the University of Manitoba as an associate and subsequently full professor in the Faculty of Administrative Studies (now the Asper School of Business) (1973–1988) and the Faculty of Medicine (1973 to present).

As founder of the Manitoba Centre for Health Policy and Evaluation (later called the Manitoba Centre for Health Policy), Roos established a prototype for successfully conducting research using administrative data. The Centre holds anonymized and linkable health administrative data for all health services provided within the province of Manitoba. Using these data, Roos and her colleagues have addressed many important questions about the health and healthcare of Manitobans, and their findings have been valuable not only in Manitoba but in other healthcare systems in Canada and elsewhere around the world.

Roos is an Institute for Scientific Information Highly Cited Researcher, placed in the top half of 1% of published scientists with over 2,800 citations. Her early work built on her doctoral research and focused on public administration in Turkey. Subsequently, she shifted her scholarship to evaluation and to evaluating health programs in particular. She has published over 200 scholarly articles and academic reports and has collaborated extensively with authors throughout North America and elsewhere in the world. She has published in journals such as *American Journal of Public Health, Health Affairs, Health Services Research, Medical Care, Milbank Quarterly,* the *New England Journal of Medicine,* and *Social Science and Medicine.*

Over the course of her career, Roos has received over $45 million in research support, including being continuously funded as a National Health Research Scientist from 1973 to 1998, an associate with the Canadian Institute for Advanced Research from 1988 to 2002, and a Tier 1 Canada Research Chair in Population Health Research from 2001 to the present. She was a member of the Prime Minister's National Health Forum from 1994 to 1997 and a member of the Medical Research Council from 1997 to 2000.

Her work and collaborations were recognized in 2001 through the Canadian Health Services Research Foundation (CHSRF) awarding the Manitoba Centre for Health Policy the Health Services Research Achievement Award. In 2005, Roos was the recipient of the Order of Canada in recognition of her lifetime of outstanding achievement, dedication to the community, and service to the nation.

Gregory S. Finlayson

See also Canadian Association for Health Services and Policy Research (CAHSPR); Canadian Health Services Research Foundation (CHSRF); Data Sources in Conducting Health Services Research; Health Services Research in Canada; Roos, Leslie L.

Further Readings

Mitchell, Lori, Noralou P. Roos, and Evelyn Shapiro. "Patterns in Home Care Use in Manitoba," *Canadian Journal on Aging* 24(Suppl. 1): 59–68, Spring 2005.

Reid, Robert J., Noralou P. Roos, Leonard MacWilliam, et al. "Assessing Population Health Care Need Using a Claims-Based ACG Morbidity Measure: A Validation Analysis in the Province of Manitoba," *Health Services Research* 37(5): 1345–64, October 2002.

Roos, Noralou P., Charles Burchill, and Keumhee Carriere. "Who Are the High Hospital Users? A Canadian Case Study," *Journal of Health Services Research and Policy* 8(1): 5–10, January 2003.

Roos, Noralou P., Evelyn Forget, Randy Walld, et al. "Does Universal Comprehensive Insurance Encourage Unnecessary Use? Evidence From Manitoba Says 'No.'" *Canadian Medical Association Journal* 170(2): 209–214, January 2004.

Roos, Noralou P., Kip Sullivan, Randy Walld, et al. "Potential Savings From Reducing Inequalities in Health," *Canadian Journal of Public Health* 95(6): 460–64, November–December 2004.

Web Sites

Canada Research Chairs: http://www.chairs.gc.ca/web/home_e.asp

Manitoba Centre for Health Policy (MCHP), http://umanitoba.ca/medicine/units/mchp

ROREM, C. RUFUS

The field of health economics was still in its infancy when C. Rufus Rorem (1894–1988) was asked to join the landmark Committee on the Costs of Medical Care (CCMC) in 1929. From that time onward, Rorem's groundbreaking work established his reputation as a pioneer in this new field. Along the way, Rorem proved to be an innovative and influential advocate for group medical practice, hospital prepayment, uniform hospital accounting, and areawide health planning.

Born in Radcliffe, Iowa, in 1894, Rorem was the son of Norwegian immigrant parents who were members of the Religious Society of Friends, or Quakers. Rorem attended Oberlin College, majoring in political science. After graduation, he accepted a position with the Goodyear Tire and Rubber Company. But he soon left to join the U.S. Army for service in World War I. After the war, Rorem decided to pursue a career in education, and he took a position teaching accounting and business courses at Earlham College, a small Quaker college in Richmond, Indiana. To establish his credentials in accounting, he passed the Indiana Certified Public Account (CPA) examination. At that time, Rorem saw where his future lay, for he enrolled in graduate studies at the University of Chicago. He received an instructorship in accounting, and he completed a master's and a doctoral degree in economics. Soon Rorem was promoted to assistant professor at the university, and in 1928 was appointed assistant dean of its School of Commerce and Administration. And in 1929, he became an associate professor.

While at the University of Chicago, Rorem developed a friendship with a colleague who had a lasting influence on his life. In 1928, he met Michael M. Davis. Davis was a major figure in the nation's medical-care circles; he was the director of medical services at the Julius Rosenwald Fund and an executive committee member of the CCMC. The CCMC was organized in 1927 and supported by a number of large foundations to conduct a 5-year study of the financing and delivery of medical care in the nation.

In 1929, Davis asked Rorem to become the associate director of medical services at the Rosenwald Fund. He also asked Rorem to lead a study of hospital capital investment for the CCMC, which had not been studied previously. The project appealed to Rorem because of his background and his interest in public finance and nonprofit corporations. It was not long before Rorem was a full-time staff economist for the CCMC. In 1930, he moved to Washington, D.C., where he assisted in preparing a number of CCMC reports, including the landmark *Final Report of the Committee on the Costs of Medical Care*, which was published in 1932.

While at the University of Chicago, Rorem also met Isidore S. Falk. Falk would become widely recognized in medical-care circles for his work on health and Social Security issues. Eventually, Falk became the associate director of the CCMC research staff, linking him professionally with both Rorem and Davis.

Rorem's work at CCMC led to his interest in the prepayment of healthcare. He became associate secretary of the American Hospital Association (AHA) and later, executive secretary of the Committee on Hospital Service, where he assisted in the approval of prepaid group hospitalization in 1934. It has been said that Rorem more than anyone else shaped the movement of prepaid healthcare. Ultimately, Rorem's activities at the AHA helped enormously in laying the foundation for the formation of Blue Cross and Blue Shield plans around the nation. In his work, Rorem was influenced by E. A. Filene's emphasis on applying the principles of scientific management to the healthcare field and by his advocacy for group prepayment and regional health planning.

In 1946, Rorem testified before the U.S. Senate Committee on Education and Labor, describing the rapid growth of Blue Cross plans in America as having "enrolled more participants in less time than any voluntary movement in the history of the world."

Among the principles Rorem supported were not-for-profit operation in healthcare, appointing physicians and community leaders to hospital governing boards, patients' choice of physician and hospital, financial integrity, and "dignified promotion." He believed strongly that health is wealth and access to health services is a basic right, essential to the effective pursuit of happiness. He also held the opinion that while healthcare is an economic commodity, it differs sharply from other commodities.

Rorem was a prolific writer. His first publication on medical care costs was *The Public's Investment in Hospitals* (1930). In the book, he underscored the fact that most hospital capital came from public rather than from private sources. He also published *Private Group Clinics* (1931). Rorem contributed to 5 of the 28 reports issued by the CCMC, and he was the author of numerous other publications.

Rorem remained at the American Hospital Association for 10 years, leaving in 1947 to take the position of executive director of the Hospital Council of Greater Philadelphia. He remained there until 1960, when he took a post in Pittsburgh as the director of the Hospital Planning Association of Alleghany County.

During his long career, C. Rufus Rorem received many honors, including membership in the Health Care Hall of Fame. He was admired for his soft-spoken and self-effacing manner and respected for his view of healthcare as more than just a business. He had no sympathy for the view of many hospital spokesmen and physicians who described their activities as an "industry." He was a gentle and wise man who made an indelible mark on American health economics and medical care.

Samuel Levey and James Hill

See also American Hospital Association (AHA); Blue Cross and Blue Shield; Committee on the Costs of Medical Care (CCMC); Davis, Michael M. ; Health Economics; Hospitals; Medical Group Practice

Further Readings

Committee on the Costs of Medical Care. *Medical Care for the American People. Final Report of the Committee on the Costs of Medical Care.* Publication No. 28. Chicago: University of Chicago Press, 1932.
Goldsmith, S. B. "C. Rufus Rorem: A Profile," *Journal of Ambulatory Care Management* 6(2): 75–78, May 1983.
Rorem, C. Rufus. *The Public's Investment in Hospitals.* Chicago: University of Chicago Press, 1930.
Rorem, C. Rufus. "The Hospitals of America: The Same Roots as Churches and Schools," *Vital Speeches of the Day* 5(4): 118–20, December 1938.
Rorem, C. Rufus. *Private Group Clinics.* New York: Milbank Memorial Fund, 1971. (Reprint of the Committee on the Costs of Medical Care Publication No. 8. Chicago: University of Chicago Press, 1931)
Rorem, C. Rufus. *A Quest for Certainty.* Ann Arbor, MI: Health Administration Press, 1982.
Sigmond, Robert M. "C. Rufus Rorem, PhD, CPA: Obituary," *Journal of the American Medical Association* 260(19): 2845, November 1988.
Weeks, Lewis E. "C. Rufus Rorem: A First-Person Profile," *Health Services Research* 18(2 pt. 2): 325–41, Summer, 1983.

Web Sites

American Hospital Association (AHA), Center for Hospital and Health Administration History: http://www.aha.org

ROSENBAUM, SARA

Sara Rosenbaum is a leading health policy expert whose professional accomplishments have transformed the lives of ordinary Americans by advocating for more equitable and effective policies to increase access to healthcare for low-income, minority, and medically underserved populations. Rosenbaum has been pivotally involved in designing national and state legislative and regulatory health policies in a variety of areas, including Medicaid, private health insurance, employee health benefits, health services for medically underserved populations, maternal and child health, civil rights, and public health.

Sara Rosenbaum is the Harold and Jane Hirsh Professor of Health Law and Policy and is the founding chair of the Department of Health Policy at the George Washington University School of Public Health and Health Services in Washington, D.C. She is also the director of the Hirsh Health Law and Policy Program and the Center for Health Services Research and Policy at the university.

Rosenbaum received her bachelor's degree from Wesleyan University in 1973 and her Juris Doctorate degree from the Boston University School of Law in 1976. She began her career as a community legal services attorney in Vermont and California and also worked at the Children's Defense Fund in Washington, D.C.

Rosenbaum's research interest focuses on the ways in which the law intersects with the nation's healthcare and public health systems, with a particular interest in quality of care, managed care, insurance coverage, and civil rights. She has published extensively and is coauthor of the widely used health law textbook *Law and the American Health Care System.*

Rosenbaum serves on many boards and committees, including AcademyHealth, the National Board of Medical Examiners, and the Committee on Child Health Research of the American Academy of Pediatrics and on study committees of the national Institute of Medicine (IOM), and she serves in an advisory role to the March of Dimes and the Centers for Disease Control and Prevention's (CDC) National Center on Birth Defects and Disabilities. During the Clinton administration, from 1993 to 1994, Rosenbaum worked for the White House Domestic Policy Council, where she directed the drafting of the Health Security Act and oversaw the development of the Vaccines for Children program.

Rosenbaum has received numerous accolades for her work, including the Investigator Award in Health Policy from the Robert Wood Johnson Foundation, and has been recognized by the U.S. Department of Health and Human Services for distinguished national service on behalf of Medicaid beneficiaries. In addition, she has been named one of the nation's 500 most influential health policymakers by McGraw-Hill.

Rosenbaum has advised the U.S. District Court for the Middle District of Tennessee in *John B. v. Groetz,* a class action suit that challenges the adequacy of health services for children in that state. She also continues to champion the needs of the most marginalized members of our society and mentors students interested in improving healthcare for the poor.

Jared Lane K. Maeda

See also Access to Healthcare; Medicaid; Public Health; Public Policy; Regulation; State Children's Health Insurance Program (SCHIP); Uninsured Individuals; Vulnerable Populations

Further Readings

Rosenbaum, Sara. "New Directions for Health Insurance Design: Implications for Public Health Policy and Practice," *Journal of Law, Medicine and Ethics* 31(4 Suppl.): 94–103, Winter 2003.

Rosenbaum, Sara. "A Dose of Reality: Assessing the Federal Trade Commission/Department of Justice Report in an Uninsured, Underserved, and Vulnerable Population Context," *Journal of Health Politics, Policy and Law* 31(3): 657–70, June 2006.

Rosenbaum, Sara "U.S. Health Policy in the Aftermath of Hurricane Katrina," *Journal of the American Medical Association* 295(4): 437–40, January, 2006.

Rosenbaum, Sara. "Medicaid and Documentation of Legal Status: Implications for Public Health Practice and Policy," *Public Health Reports* 122(2): 264–67, March–April 2007.

Rosenbaum, Sara. "SCHIP Reconsidered," *Health Affairs* 26(5): 608–17, September–October 2007.

Rosenblatt, Rand E., Sylvia A. Law, and Sara Rosenbaum. *Law and the American Health Care System.* New York: Foundation Press, 1997.

Web Sites

George Washington University Department of Health Policy, http://www.gwumc.edu/sphhs/healthpolicy

RTI International

RTI International is an independent, nonprofit research organization dedicated to improving the human condition by turning knowledge into practice through cutting-edge study and analysis in health and pharmaceuticals, education and training, surveys and statistics, advanced technology, democratic governance, economic and social development, energy, and the environment. Founded in 1958 by three universities (Duke University, North Carolina State University, and the University of North Carolina) in North Carolina's Research Triangle Park, RTI was the initial research organization and focal point for research in the Park; its first projects included applied statistics and environmental research. Today, with a staff of more than 2,600 individuals, RTI conducts research in 40 countries. Headquartered in North Carolina, RTI has seven U.S. regional offices and eight international offices. Its clients include most federal cabinet departments (particularly the U.S. Department of Health and Human Services), numerous state and public health agencies, and a variety of private foundations.

Health Services Research

Health services research encompasses investigations into healthcare delivery and interventions from prevention and screening through diagnosis and treatment to rehabilitation; a broad set of health policy issues concerning access to care, costs of care, and quality of care; health insurance; effectiveness and efficiency of care processes; patient outcomes, including quality of life and satisfaction; workforce issues; and a wide array of social problems with health implications, including domestic violence and criminal justice, substance use and abuse, and environmental toxicities. Health services research at RTI concerns individuals, families, organizations and institutions, communities, and populations.

RTI's research portfolio is highly multidisciplinary and applies sophisticated quantitative and qualitative methods from many fields, including social sciences such as sociology, psychology, anthropology; statistical, economic, and mathematical sciences including advanced modeling techniques; epidemiologic and public health fields that employ community-based methods; and biological and life sciences, particularly medicine, nursing, and pharmacy. RTI projects employ advanced survey techniques based on both traditional and modern measurement theory, all possible administration modes, and program evaluation and policy analysis.

Exceptionally strong survey and computer processing capabilities support health services research at RTI. Healthcare surveys may be small area, national, or international in scope, and they may be either cross-sectional or longitudinal in nature. RTI specializes in recruiting and following hard-to-reach populations, such as children in the foster care system, the low-income elderly, and homeless persons. RTI has an outstanding capacity for using administrative data, with programmers able to link claims and enrollment data from multiple sources to create episodes of care or to follow cohorts of patients over time.

Principal Areas of Research

RTI research is heavily oriented toward improving the health and well-being of individuals and populations (both domestically and internationally), enhancing healthcare and social programs, and strengthening public policy through an extensive health services research and policy analysis portfolio. Particular emphasis is placed on applying multiple disciplines, methods, and theoretical frameworks to healthcare financing and payment; healthcare quality; aging and persons with disabilities; child, adolescent, and family well-being; early childhood development; women's and reproductive health; and health and social organizations. RTI conducts research on substance abuse, mental health, and criminal justice issues using a wide range of multidisciplinary social science methods on broad topics of behavioral health and related policy issues. Research foci include substance abuse prevention and treatment; HIV/AIDS; problems of the urban poor; risk behaviors and family research; and transdisciplinary research that links genetic, neurobiological, and behavioral factors in the study of substance abuse, crime, and violence.

RTI also conducts a broad range of applied research and evaluation in health promotion, disease prevention, health and environmental economics, and technology transfer, with special emphasis on individual, social, and environmental factors that affect modifiable health behaviors and human welfare. A growing collection of research focuses on health communications, including literacy and health literacy. Among social and environmental factors of interest are public policies and regulation, media and communications, communities, schools and workplace, and interpersonal and individual psychology.

Special Areas of Focus and Strength

Economic research covers healthcare costs and cost-effectiveness, behavioral health economics (especially substance abuse and mental health), prevention effectiveness economics, and payment and reimbursement issues. Particular emphasis is placed on healthcare financing, insurance, payment, and reimbursement issues, especially those affecting Medicare and State Children's Health Insurance Programs (SCHIPs). RTI conducts extensive evaluation and research for the Centers for Medicare and Medicaid Services (CMS). RTI's Medicare payment research includes developing risk adjustment algorithms for managed care and Medicare Part D (prescription drug) plans, implementing and evaluating competitive bidding and pay-for-performance demonstrations, redesigning provider payment systems (e.g., for post-acute-care providers and for psychiatric hospitals and units), and making technical refinements of prospective payment systems and physician fee schedules. Medicaid and SCHIP research has focused on enrollment and retention, managed care, long-term care, and evaluations of 1,115 waiver demonstrations, including the Oregon Health Plan. Many of these studies are mandated by the U.S. Congress and are used to support new federal policies and regulations.

RTI performs cost-of-illness studies and cost-effectiveness analysis. This work includes designing and evaluating interventions to prevent obesity, diabetes, coronary heart disease, cancer, infectious diseases, injuries, and other preventable causes of disability and death. Related research evaluates strategies to boost positive health behavior and reduce risky behaviors such as smoking, substance abuse, and domestic violence.

Research on access to healthcare, apart from the wide variety of projects concerned with public and private insurance schemes, focuses on vulnerable populations such as minority or low-income populations; on patient populations defined by substance use and abuse, tobacco use, mental illness, and HIV/AIDS; and on incarcerated persons. Many studies focus on subsets of these vulnerable populations, such as low-income children and elderly persons belonging to racial and ethnic minority groups. Health and healthcare delivery for active-duty military populations and dependents are expanding targets of RTI research. Numerous projects concern the elderly and disabled, especially with respect to long-term care and rehabilitation. Health and healthcare disparities represent a growing portion of the health services research portfolio, with particular emphasis on access to cancer screening and treatment, family planning services, preventive and primary care, high-tech surgery, and prescription drugs. Geospatial analysis (e.g., for breast cancer) and complex modeling techniques are increasingly being applied.

RTI addresses quality of healthcare through several broad programs, including an Evidence-Based Practice Center (EPC) for conducting systematic and comparative effectiveness, a Developing Evidence to Inform Decisions About Effectiveness Center (DEcIDE) for projects related to the comparative effectiveness of therapies and delivery systems, and an Accelerating Change and Transformation in Organizations and Networks (ACTION) to study change within healthcare organizations; all are supported by the U.S. Agency for Healthcare Research and Quality (AHRQ). RTI researchers develop and evaluate quality measures and indicators of patient safety such as injury detection triggers, refine and apply methods for detecting adverse drug events, develop and test methods for public reporting of quality performance, and analyze the effect of payment policy on quality of healthcare. Applying methods to assess quality of life and patient-reported outcomes is a growing feature of RTI research. Research involving clinical measures of quality, processes of care, and outcomes addresses issues for the U.S. Department of Health and Human Services, the Department of Defense, and international pharmaceutical clients and foundations.

Virtually all health technologies and interventions fall within the purview of RTI health services research: counseling and behavioral interventions, diagnostic and screening tests, prevention activities such as immunization or chemoprevention, all forms of therapeutics (especially pharmaceuticals), and rehabilitation services. Similarly, virtually all types of chronic diseases (e.g., cancer, cardiovascular diseases, depression, and obesity), many prevalent and emerging infectious diseases (e.g., HIV/AIDS, avian influenza), genetic conditions (e.g., Fragile X), and various lifestyle behaviors (e.g., smoking, poor nutrition, physical inactivity, obesity, smoking, and the use of alcohol and licit or illicit drugs) figure prominently in the RTI research portfolio.

Kathleen N. Lohr and Janet B. Mitchell

See also Agency for Healthcare Research and Quality (AHRQ); Centers for Medicare and Medicaid Services (CMS); Healthcare Financial Management; Medicaid; National Center for Health Statistics (NCHS); Public Health; Public Policy; Women's Health Issues

Further Readings

Bray, Jeremy W., Gary A. Zarkin, Keith L. Davis, et al. "The Effect of Screening and Brief Intervention for Risky Drinking on Health Care Utilization in Managed Care Organizations," *Medical Care* 45(2): 177–82, February 2007.

Drozd, Edward M., Jerry Cromwell, Barbara Gage, et al. "Patient Casemix Classification for Medicare Psychiatric Prospective Payment," *American Journal of Psychiatry* 163(4): 724–32, April 2006.

Finkelstein, Eric A., Christopher J. Ruhm, and Katherine M. Kosa. "Economic Causes and Consequences of Obesity," *Annual Review of Public Health* 26: 239–57, 2005.

Gavin, Norma I., E. Kathleen Adam, Willard G. Manning, et al. "The Impact of Welfare Reform on Insurance Coverage Before Pregnancy and the Timing of Prenatal Care Initiation," *Health Services Research* 42(4): 1564–88, August 2007.

Gibbs, Deborah A., Sandra L. Martin, Lawrence L. Kupper, et al. "Child Maltreatment in Enlisted Soldiers' Families During Combat-Related Deployments," *Journal of the American Medical Association* 298(5): 528–35, August 1, 2007.

Greenwald, Leslie, Jerry Cromwell, Walter Adamache, et al. "Specialty Versus Community Hospitals: Referrals, Quality, and Community Benefits," *Health Affairs* 25(1): 106–118, January–February 2006.

Lohr, Kathleen N. "Rating the Strength of Scientific Evidence: Relevance for Quality Improvement Programs," *International Journal of Quality in Health Care* 16(1): 9–18, February 2004.

McCormack, Lauren A. and Jennifer D. Uhrig. "How Does Beneficiary Knowledge of the Medicare Program Vary by Type of Insurance?" *Medical Care* 41(8): 972–78, August 2003.

Mitchell, Janet B., Susan G. Haber, Galina Khatutsky, et al. "Impact of the Oregon Health Plan on Access and Satisfaction of Adults With Low Income," *Health Services Research* 37(1): 19–31, February 2002.

O'Keeffe, Janet, and Joshua M. Wiener. "Public Funding for Long-Term Care Services for Older People in Residential Care Settings," *Journal of Housing for the Elderly* 18(3–4): 51–79, 2004.

Trisolini, Michael G., Kevin W. Smith, Nancy T. McCall, et al. "Evaluating the Performance of Medicare Fee-For-Service Providers Using the Health Outcomes Survey: A Comparison of Two Methods," *Medical Care* 43(7): 699–704, July 2005.

Wechsberg, Wendee M., Wendy K. K. Lam, William A. Zule, et al. "Efficacy of a Women-Focused Intervention to Reduce HIV Risk and Increase Self-Sufficiency Among African American Crack Abusers," *American Journal of Public Health* 94(71): 1165–73, July 2004.

Web Sites

RTI International: http://www.rti.org

RTI's Developing Evidence to Inform Decisions About Effectiveness (DEcIDE): http://www.rti.org/decide

RTI's Evidence-Based Practice Center (EPC): http://www.rti.org/epc

RURAL HEALTH

What constitutes rural in healthcare depends on the definition being used for rurality, and that is sometimes dependent on the type of healthcare being delivered. There currently is no consensus definition of what rural is in the United States, either for health or for other policy domains. Since 1910, the U.S. Census Bureau has used a threshold of 2,500 people living in an incorporated place as its definition of rural; that definition remains in place today, but it is seldom used except for classification purposes in the census. A more widely used and recognized definition is the "metropolitan" designation process developed by the U.S. Office of Management and Budget (OMB), the White House office responsible for devising and submitting the president's annual budget proposal to Congress. The OMB classifies counties as metropolitan if they include a central city of at least 50,000 people or contain an urban cluster of that size or if they are closely tied to central metropolitan counties by commuting or economic trade patterns. The OMB originally identified only metropolitan counties but later designated core and other metro counties. In 2000, the nonmetropolitan counties with small urban centers were classified as "micropolitan." The U.S. Department of Agriculture (USDA) has created several different classifications of nonmetropolitan counties (non–Core Based Statistical Areas, functional regions based around an urban center of at least 10,000 people) that are often used to scale the degree of rurality of counties. These include the Rural Continuum Code and the Urban Influence Codes. An alternative, fine-grained classification system based largely on commuting patterns, the Rural Urban Commuting Areas (RUCA) codes, is based on clusters of census blocks or block groups; it has been adapted to apply to U.S. Postal Service ZIP code areas. Federal and state policies that apply to health programs and regulations often specify one or more of these classification systems to guide the allocation of funds or application of rules to rural communities and populations.

The Rural Population in the United States

The United States was, for most of its history, a rural, agricultural nation. It was not until the 1920 census that the urban population of the nation exceeded the rural for the first time. In that year, the rural population was 50,866,899, or 48.1% of the total U.S. population. Since that time, the nation's rural population has remained relatively stable, growing to 59,274,456 in 2000. However, the rural proportion dropped to just over 20% of the total population of the nation. Alternatively, since the 1950s, the OMB chose to develop the metropolitan statistical areas designation to separate urbanized or city-oriented from other counties. In 2005, a total of 1,090 counties in the nation were metropolitan and constituted 83.2% of the U.S. population; 693 counties were micropolitan, 10.3% of the nation's population; and 1,358 counties were non–Core Based Statistical Areas, 6.6% of the total population. In 2005, the estimated total U.S. population living in nonmetropolitan counties was 54,566,948.

Rural Health Services Research

Rural health services research grew out of social and policy concerns with access to medical care and the health consequences of poverty that are closely associated with many rural areas. The problem of the relative deprivation of rural areas and its effects on health was noted in the 1920s, with structural assessments completed by the Farm Security Administration (FSA), a product of the New Deal. The FSA promoted prepaid medical group practice cooperatives as one way to meet the healthcare access needs of rural areas. This laid the foundation for the development of the staff model managed-care systems and health maintenance organizations (HMOs). The FSA also supported analysis of these programs and their outcomes and impacts, and this work was an early forerunner of health services research.

Plans for regionalization of healthcare services were proposed early in the 20th century as one way to ensure that rural places would receive the necessary care. In Great Britain, the work of Lord Dawson of Penn in his plans for a hierarchical system of clinics and hospitals stimulated future American healthcare planners associated with the Committee on the Costs of Medical Care (CCMC), which met from 1927 to 1932. The committee began work to estimate the necessary minimum population that could support what were termed "primary" medical centers that would provide medical services in the smaller towns and villages. The idea of a hierarchical structuring of regionalized medical services became part of the federal Hospital Survey and Construction Act, also known as the Hill-Burton Act, which supported the construction of hospitals in many rural communities from 1946 through the 1960s. The basic planning methodologies developed in the process of implementing the Hill-Burton Act formed the structure for later analytic work attempting to balance place-based needs with services. The subsequent federal planning legislation of the 1970s supported the development of methods to allocate resources, project supply, and anticipate demand. This work formed the underpinnings for determination of appropriate levels of utilization of services, a theme that later emphasized the ability of populations to gain access to healthcare.

The relative supply of physicians between rural and urban places was a concern of Milton I. Roemer and Frank G. Dickenson of the American Medical Association. Their work in the 1950s was centered on the development of appropriate geographic service areas to properly assess and guarantee distribution of care. This assessment of geographic distribution and variations in supply anticipated the later work of John E. Wennberg at Dartmouth Medical School.

In the 1950s and early 1960s, the problems of overall physician supply were apparent, and rural-focused research emphasized the analysis of health manpower needs as well as the development and assessment of alternatives to resolve that problem. The economics of physician workforce distribution with a specific emphasis on rural places developed in the emerging field of health services research with the work of health economists including Rashi Fein, Uwe E. Reinhardt, and Frank A. Sloan. The primary-care needs of rural places became one of the principal reasons for the development of the new professions of nurse practitioner and physician assistants, and evidence supporting their efficacy was collected in many rural communities. These same economists tackled the issues of substitution and complementarity of clinical roles as these "new health professionals" found political acceptance.

The late 1960s and 1970s saw the emergence of subsidized primary care programs and clinics in the form of comprehensive community health centers, hospital-based clinics, nurse practitioner–staffed clinics, outreach programs, and physician leadership programs. Given the relative shortage of resources, many of the clinics were established in rural places, and a number of programs stimulated their development. The variety of organizational structures of rural primary-care systems stimulated a series of studies that compared the relative efficiency and effectiveness of these organizational forms via work led by Stephen M. Shortell and Cecil G. Sheps with funding from various foundations and the federal government.

The Medicare program based its payments for hospitals and physician services partly on the location of the provider during this period. The system recognized wide geographic differences in costs and charges in the "usual, customary, and reasonable" payment system that was eventually modified into a system that differentiated between cities and the rural parts of states and regions. Medicare structured its payments to hospitals using a geographic modifier to account for past payment patterns and underlying labor costs. This created a pattern of inexplicably and dramatically different payment levels between seemingly similar adjacent counties but a relatively consistent gradient between urban and rural areas, with providers in metropolitan areas receiving higher payments than those outside those places. This differential was especially apparent with the release of payment indexes for managed-care organizations after the passage of the federal Tax Equity and Fiscal Responsibility Act (TEFRA) of 1982. The system created an average adjusted per capita cost (AAPCC) mechanism to guide managed-care payments; these created very large gaps between urban and rural payment levels. This formalized system generated an organized political response that, in turn, unified the several differing advocacy organizations representing rural interests into the National Rural Health Association (NRHA), which, in turn, pressed for a lead federal agency to promote the cause of rural healthcare in the federal government. Legislation creating the federal Office of Rural Health Policy (ORHP) was passed in 1987 and was organized in the following year. The authorizing legislation for the ORPH called for a research agenda, which led to the funding of a group of rural research centers in 1988.

One of the first issues the rural research centers investigated was the viability of small, rural hospitals. In the 1980s there was concern that these institutions would not be able to weather the effects of a rural economic downturn. The Inspector General's Office in the U.S. Department of Health and Human Services noted that there was an alarming trend toward closure of small rural hospitals, which could be attributed to aggressive competition from urban hospitals and the demands of rapidly developing technologies that required significant economies of scale. The problems of rural hospitals were identified in various research studies as lack of technology and gaps in management and leadership as well as a fundamentally skewed payment system in Medicare. A demonstration of a new form of provider, the Medical Assistance Facility (MAF), was fielded in Montana in 1987. The MAFs were scaled-down hospitals that restricted their size and range of services but maintained emergency and limited inpatient facilities in remote, frontier communities. The Health Care Financing Administration (now the Centers for Medicare and Medicaid Services [CMS]) granted a waiver allowing Medicare payments to these institutions. That was followed by a seven-state demonstration of the Essential Access/Rural Primary Care Hospital provider type authorized under the federal Omnibus Budget and Reconciliation Act of 1989, which was replaced in the Balanced Budget Act of 1997 by the Medicare Rural Hospital Flexibility Program, which created critical-access hospitals (CAH). These demonstrations were accompanied by evaluation and research that showed the viability of the concept of a limited-service rural hospital. By 2007, there were over 1,250 CAHs dispersed through all but two states in the nation.

Rural healthcare systems have used several options to guide their structure, with networks and consortia being the primary organizational tool. Early rural hospital cooperatives and consortia were created in the upper Midwest, which allowed many smaller hospitals to share resources and promoted their survival. Networks are promoted by federal legislation, including the Medicare Rural Hospital Flexibility Program, which requires the CAHs to link with a larger, more complex hospital as well as emergency services and policy development partners. The trend toward networking and collaboration was given a boost by the Institute of Medicine (IOM) in a 2005 report that found that cooperation among providers allowed for better access and quality of care.

Health Services and Vulnerability

Data from the National Health Interview Survey (NHIS) and the Medical Expenditure Panel Survey (MEPS) indicate that self-reported health status is generally worse among rural residents than among urban residents and that this situation has persisted over the past two decades. After adjusting for differences in age, NHIS respondents living in nonmetropolitan counties were more likely than metropolitan residents to rate their health as only fair or poor. Similar patterns in self-reported health status were also found among MEPS respondents. Likewise, most chronic diseases have been, and continue to be, more prevalent in rural areas. Data from the NHIS also confirm these patterns for chronic conditions such as various types of joint pain, low back and neck pain, and vision and hearing problems. In addition, data from the U.S. Centers for Disease Control and Prevention (CDC) show higher rates of obesity, cigarette smoking, and total tooth loss in nonmetropolitan counties.

During the past decade, rural areas have seen a steep decline in manufacturing jobs (which tended to offer higher rates of employer-sponsored health insurance coverage than other jobs), accompanied by a rise in service-sector employment, where access to health insurance has been much lower. This has resulted in a greater percentage of rural residents being uninsured than urban residents. In 2001–2002 nearly 4 million rural families (30%) had at least one uninsured member. And many rural residents with private health insurance may face large out-of-pocket costs for care as a result of being underinsured.

Some of the earliest research on rural healthcare focused on the geographic distribution of physicians. That has continued in studies of the distribution of primary-care practitioners as part of policies intended to identify the places with the fewest health professional resources, either as health professional shortage areas (HPSAs) or as medically underserved areas (MUAs). These designations are used by the federal government to qualify localities for a multiplicity of programs that allow them to seek grants for clinics, placement of practitioners, and special payment regimes under Medicare and Medicaid. Underserved areas are defined and designated by the Shortage Designation Branch of the Health Resources and Services Administration's (HRSA) Bureau of Health Professions. Both geographic areas and population groups can be classified as either shortage or underserved areas. The percentage of both metropolitan and nonmetropolitan counties with either a single-county or a part-county primary-care HPSA designation increased from 1987 to 2004. Over 75% of nonmetropolitan counties were designated as HPSAs by 2004.

Other Health Professions and Services

The geographic distribution of health professionals in rural areas has long been identified as a problem; more than half of all the nation's counties have no licensed psychiatrist or psychologist, and virtually all these counties are rural. As of 2004, 79% of nonmetropolitan counties and 55% of metropolitan counties were identified as being either single- or part-county mental health HPSAs. Counties with mental health HPSA designations have a shortage of psychiatrists and/or other core mental health professionals such as clinical psychologists and clinical social workers.

Rural communities have proportionately fewer dentists than urban places. In 2004, there were 3.8 general practice dentists per 10,000 urban residents but only 2.3 per 10,000 rural residents. The geographic distribution of registered nurses in nonmetropolitan counties is proportional to the general population distribution, but in the least populous and most isolated rural counties, the numbers are below the general population share. Public health agencies in rural places also tend to have smaller staffs, lower budgets, and less technical capacity than in urban areas.

Persistent Problems

The nature of rural places makes them less attractive to many professionals and less able to invest in high-technology, high-cost healthcare services. This economic reality presents a challenge to public policies that attempt to equalize access to services in government programs such as Medicare and Medicaid and for the regulation of private health insurance. A constant challenge to researchers and policymakers is to identify optimal minimums of healthcare services that should be provided to small and isolated populations. The same problems of scale affect the diffusion of clinical as well as organizational innovations. Rural communities often have less access to newer medical technologies and specialized treatments. Health reform programs that depend on market forces, such as managed-care programs or group practices, often do not work well in rural places.

Rural communities and rural health policies remain an important part of national healthcare policy due to the structure of the U.S. Congress, which gives proportionately greater power in the U.S. Senate to the residents of the more sparsely populated states of the West and Midwest. This political reality has provided a balancing force to even out the market forces that often leave rural communities at a disadvantage.

Thomas C. Ricketts

See also Access to Healthcare; Geographic Barriers to Healthcare; Health Planning; Health Professional Shortage Areas (HPSAs); Health Resources and Services Administration (HRSA); Medicaid; Medicare; Primary Care

Further Readings

Committee on the Future of Rural Health Care, Institute of Medicine. *Quality Through Collaboration: The Future of Rural Health Care.* Washington, DC: National Academies Press, 2005.

Geyman, John, ed. *The Handbook of Rural Medicine.* New York: Wiley, 2000.

Glasgow, Nina, Lois Wright Morton, and Nan E. Johnson, eds. *Critical Issues in Rural Health.* Ames, IA: Blackwell, 2004.

Ricketts, Thomas C., ed. *Rural Health in the United States.* New York: Oxford University Press, 1999.

Web Sites

Health Resources and Services Administration (HRSA), Office of Rural Health Policy: http://ruralhealth.hrsa.gov

National Organization of State Offices of Rural Health (NOSORH): http://www.nosorh.org

National Rural Health Association (NRHA): http://www.RuralHealthWeb.org

Rural Assistance Center (RAC): http://www.raconline.org

Rural Policy Research Institute (RUPRI): http://www.rupri.org

U.S. Department of Agriculture (USDA), Economic Research Service, Rural Definitions: http://www.ers.usda.gov/Data/RuralDefinitions

S

SACKETT, DAVID L.

David L. Sackett is widely regarded as one of the originators of evidence-based medicine (EBM), which is the integration of the best research evidence and clinical expertise in the care of individual patients. Evidence-based medicine has revolutionized the thinking of many clinical practitioners.

Over the years, Sackett has developed and mentored a cadre of applied clinician-scientists who have disseminated the practice of evidence-based medicine throughout the world. These research teams have been at the forefront of medicine. They were the first to validate the efficacy of aspirin and carotid endarterectomy for patients with threatened stroke. They developed strategies for hypertensive patients to comply with their drug regimes. And they found compelling evidence for the effectiveness of nurse practitioners.

Sackett was the founding chair of the Department of Clinical Epidemiology and Biostatistics at McMaster University in Hamilton, Ontario. He rose through the academic ranks at the university and became professor and chair of the Division of Internal Medicine. After nearly 27 years at McMaster University, Sackett moved to Oxford University in 1994 to become founding director of the Centre for Evidence-Based Medicine and professor of Epidemiology in the Nuffield Department of Clinical Medicine. He also was founding chair of the Cochrane Collaboration Steering Group, which is an organization dedicated to the dissemination of systematic reviews of the effects of healthcare interventions.

Sackett has authored many books in the field of epidemiology, including *Clinical Epidemiology: A Basic Science for Clinical Medicine* and *Evidence-Based Medicine: How to Practice and Teach EBM*. He has also authored or coauthored over 300 journal articles. Sackett has been involved in hundreds of randomized controlled trials (RCTs) as a principal investigator, consultant, or member or chair of a data safety monitoring board.

Sackett has received numerous honors and awards, including the Trillium Clinical Scientist Award, the Zinkoff Honor Award, the J. Allyn Taylor International Prize in Medicine, and the Health Services Research Prize from the Baxter International Foundation, and he was elected to the Canada Medical Hall of Fame. He is a fellow of the Royal College of Physicians of London and Edinburgh. He is also an elected member of many learned societies, including the Royal Society of Canada, the American and Canadian Societies for Clinical Investigation, the Association of American Physicians, the Canadian Society for Internal Medicine, and the Pan American Health Association.

Born in Chicago, Sackett earned a bachelor's degree from Lawrence College in 1956. He earned a second bachelor's degree from the University of Illinois in 1958. He then went on to earn his medical degree from the University of Illinois College of Medicine, followed by a medical residency at the University of Illinois Research and Educational Hospital. Sackett then completed a postdoctoral fellowship in nephrology and earned a master of science degree in epidemiology from the Harvard School of Public Health. He also was awarded a doctor of science degree from the University of Bern.

Currently, Sackett resides in Canada, where he continues to write and teach. He is the founder and director of the Kilgore S. Trout Research and Education Centre in Hamilton, Ontario, an organization dedicated to training young researchers.

Jared Lane K. Maeda

See also Clinical Practice Guidelines; Cochrane, Archibald L.; Epidemiology; Evidence-Based Medicine (EBM); Outcomes Movement; Public Health; Quality of Healthcare; Randomized Controlled Trials (RCTs)

Further Readings

Daly, Jeanne. *Evidence Based Medicine and the Search for Science of Clinical Care.* Berkeley: University of California Press and Milbank Memorial Fund, 2005.

Hayes, R. Brian, David Sackett, Gordon Guyatt, et al. *Clinical Epidemiology: How to Do Clinical Practice Research.* 3d ed. Philadelphia: Lippincott Williams and Wilkins, 2006.

Sackett, David. *Evidence-Based Medicine: How to Practice and Teach EBM.* New York: Churchill Livingstone, 1997.

Sackett, David. "Clinical Epidemiology: What, Who, and Whither," *Journal of Clinical Epidemiology* 55(12): 1161–66, December 2002.

Sackett, David, Brian R. Haynes, and Peter Tugwell. *Clinical Epidemiology: A Basic Science for Clinical Medicine.* 1st ed. Boston: Little, Brown, 1985.

Sackett, David, William Rosenberg, Ja Muir Gray, et al. "Evidence Based Medicine: What It Is and What It Isn't," *British Medical Journal* 312(7023): 71–72, January 13, 1996.

Web Sites

Trout Research and Education Centre at Irish Lake: http://users.sitewaves.com/index.cfm?member=sackett

SAFETY NET

The nation's healthcare safety net is a patchwork of responses to the health needs of underserved populations. Some responses reflect governmental mandates, while others represent institutional missions or charitable initiatives to offer free or reduced-fee care. In its 2000 report, *America's Health Care Safety Net: Intact But Endangered,* the national Institute of Medicine (IOM), arrived at a two-tiered definition of safety net providers. Most broadly, it defines the safety net as including those organizations that provide healthcare services to the uninsured, Medicaid recipients, and other vulnerable populations. In addition, it singled out a subset of core safety net providers with two distinguishing characteristics: (1) by legal mandate or explicitly adopted mission, they maintain an "open door," offering access to services to patients regardless of their ability to pay, and (2) a substantial share of their patient mix is composed of uninsured, Medicaid recipients, and other vulnerable patients. Taken together, these providers and the resources that support them constitute a distinct system of care for the nation's most vulnerable individuals.

This entry provides an overview of how the safety net emerged as the nation's healthcare system evolved. Subsequent sections describe components, sources of financing, threats to stability, and resources for monitoring the safety net. Health services researchers and policymakers have become increasingly interested in and concerned about the nation's safety net as healthcare costs rise and the number of uninsured persons continues to grow.

History

At the beginning of the 20th century, medical care was neither particularly costly nor effective for most conditions. Middle- and upper-middle-income families typically received medical care in their home. The major economic concern associated with illness was lost wages. Hospitals were most often charitable institutions supported by local government appropriations predominantly serving as respites for the poor. Private donations and fees supported a smaller number of religious or ethnically affiliated institutions. However, as services became more sophisticated and costs rose—with the advent of modern anesthetic techniques, antiseptics, and antimicrobial agents—medical care became a valuable and costly commodity. Health insurance began to emerge during the Great Depression as prepaid hospital plans. During World War II, at a time when the U.S. Congress had instituted wage and price controls, employers competed for scarce labor by offering health insurance benefit packages. In addition, the federal government waived payroll taxes for employer contributions to employee health insurance plans. These incentives established the linkage between employment status and access to private health insurance that characterizes the United States today.

Government support of private approaches to insuring healthcare coverage evolved in the context of several failed attempts to institute a universal health coverage program dating back to the early years of the 20th century, again during the Great Depression, and following the election of President Harry S. Truman in 1948. The continued rise in healthcare costs accompanied by incremental rather than universal expansion of health insurance created serious gaps as more Americans found themselves in need of services they could not afford. In 1946, the U.S. Congress passed a law called the Hill-Burton Act, which gave health facilities grants and loans for construction and modernization. In return, the facilities agreed to provide a reasonable volume of services to persons unable to pay for care. The 1960s saw the emergence of Medicare to improve access for the elderly and disabled and Medicaid to improve access to those most impoverished and ill.

Despite governmental incentives and subsidized programs, there existed no guarantee of basic care to those without coverage for an emergency condition. It was not until 1986 that the U.S. Congress passed the Emergency Medical Treatment and Active Labor Act (EMTALA) to prevent hospitals that have entered into provider agreements under the Medicare program from denying medical services to patients with emergency medical needs because of their inability to pay. The essential provisions of the statute are that every patient must receive a medical screening examination and obtain appropriate stabilizing treatment or be transferred to another facility, if clinically indicated, for an emergency condition. The law applies to any hospital-based provider, including off-site clinics and primary-care centers that operate under the name, ownership, and financial and administrative control of the institutions that contract with Medicare.

An important difference between EMTALA and other incremental reforms to improve access, however, is that EMTALA is an unfunded mandate. In other words, the law provides no financial support for the required services. As a result, it places an enormous burden on patients who are shouldered with bills they cannot pay and on the hospitals that serve them and accrue the resulting bad debt.

In sum, over the past century incremental reforms to broaden access to healthcare have followed failed attempts to establish any system of universal healthcare coverage, resulting in federal and state programs, incentives, and statutes that benefit some individuals but not others. The emergence of a safety net system of providers has been an outgrowth of this process.

Components

As noted above, the IOM has distinguished between core providers and other providers in the healthcare safety net system. Core providers include two groups. First, there are "essential community providers," defined by the U.S. Congress in 1993 as those located in federally designated Medically Underserved Areas (MUAs); these include Community Health Centers/Federally Qualified Health Centers (FQHCs), FQHC Look-Alikes (FQHC-LA), and many public hospitals and local public health departments. These facilities are typically eligible for various federal and state grants or subsidies. Second, there are mission-driven organizations that may not meet the criteria for essential community provider but nevertheless serve a disproportionately poor and uninsured population. Although the care of the uninsured is concentrated among core providers, the absolute volume of uncompensated care is larger across the many, primarily not-for-profit community hospitals and academic medical centers, private practitioners, and school-based health centers that make up what has been called the hidden safety net. Finally, although considered distinct from the safety net system because they serve two narrowly circumscribed populations, the Veterans Health Administration (VHA) and the Indian Health Service (IHS) provide care to two large groups that include many otherwise uninsured Americans.

Geographic regions of the nation vary greatly in their dependence on core versus noncore healthcare safety net providers. New York, Los Angeles, Chicago, and Atlanta all have major public hospitals or healthcare systems that cater primarily to the indigent and underserved. At the other end of the continuum are regions that rely on mainstream private institutions. Instead of directing low-income patients to a public hospital system, indigent patients are dispersed across a subset of private hospitals and clinics with a mission that includes them. Philadelphia, for instance, has not had a public hospital since 1978, and inpatient services for the uninsured are distributed across the 25% of mostly private hospitals in Pennsylvania that provide more than half of all services to the state's Medical Assistance Program. Proponents of the former emphasize the specialized services (e.g., assisting patients with language and cultural barriers) and focus of core providers. Proponents of the latter emphasize that mainstreaming safety net care avoids a potentially two-tiered healthcare system.

In differentiating core from noncore safety net providers, it is also useful to distinguish between the two types of uncompensated care: charity care and bad debt. Whereas the former refers to free or discounted health-related services to individuals deemed unable to pay, the latter relates to charges that hospitals or other providers have not collected from patients who are expected to pay. While both core and other safety net providers deliver unusually high amounts of uncompensated care, core providers typically stand out for their willingness not to bill many of their patients and to employ generous sliding-fee scales, thereby providing much charity care. Unfortunately, there has been a lack of available data about the proportion of uncompensated care that is due to bad debt versus charity care at many institutions—mainly due to inconsistent hospital bookkeeping and reporting practices, but core safety net providers are clearly the major source of the latter. Whereas the distinction has not, historically, been so significant to providers since both represent unreimbursed costs, for patients the inability to pay medical bills or even the fear of accruing such debt can significantly affect access to needed care. Health services–related bad debt is now the leading cause of personal bankruptcy in America.

In recent years, there has been a public outcry over the aggressive collection practices of many hospitals attempting to reduce bad debt while at the same time reporting high levels of uncompensated care. In the case of not-for-profit hospitals, the issue is that these entities receive considerable tax benefits with the expectation that they will "give back to their communities" an amount that is at least commensurate with those benefits. The concern is that hospitals that claim high uncompensated care costs but are primarily accruing those losses because of bad debt are not really serving a safety net function. An alternative argument, however, is that the willingness of some of these hospitals to provide certain services—such as trauma care—at a predictable loss in poor communities, to care for many publicly insured or uninsured patients despite their inability to pay at cost, and to write off losses from the latter without using overly aggressive collection practices constitutes an essential safety net function even if there is little documented charity care.

Financing

To care for some patients at a loss while still remaining in business, healthcare providers must be able to offset those losses from the revenues generated by other payers—a process known as cost shifting, from private donations, or from government funds or government-mandated charity-care pools. Alternatively, they must cut their expenses. Historically, prior to World War II, most charity care was financed by private donations. Then, with rising healthcare costs and the growth of indemnity health insurance, cost shifting became an important presumed mechanism to finance the care of the poor. More recently, however, economists have questioned the role of cost shifting. Empirical analysis of hospital charges to private insurers provides little evidence that markups have correlated with or offset rising uncompensated care costs, even during the pre-managed-care era, when hospitals were thought to have the capacity to raise prices. Instead, in the absence of other sources of revenue, such as federal subsidies, providers with a high indigent care burden cut costs by reducing personnel, limiting charity care, eliminating service lines that are loss leaders, and putting off pay increases for staff.

Because of the limited capacity of providers to shift costs, they depend on a variety of funding sources at the federal, state, and county levels. One important source has been Medicaid disproportionate-share (DSH) hospital payments. Established in 1981 by the U.S. Congress, the Medicaid DSH program requires state matching funds. Initially this dampened its appeal, until states adopted a number of ways to count various state expenses from other agencies to justify federal dollars in the 1990s, through a process known as Inter-Governmental Transfers (IGT). Unfortunately, some states misdirected the funds obtained toward ineligible healthcare or even non-healthcare-related expenses. Another problem was that since DSH payments were linked to Medicaid volume rather than to the volume of uninsured, an increasingly poor correlation between these two payer groups (as more and more upscale providers competed for Medicaid dollars but not for the uninsured) diluted the program's benefit to the safety net. As a result, the U.S. Congress passed laws limiting DSH payments to states (state DSH allotments) and to hospitals (hospital-specific DSH caps), the latter linked to the hospital's overall uncompensated-care costs. States and their hospitals must also currently comply with new auditing requirements that demonstrate that DSH payments are in fact offsetting the costs of care of indigent patients receiving medical services.

Although Medicaid DSH payments were originally established to fund hospitals, a number of states have found innovative and legitimate strategies to direct the funds toward primary- and preventive-care services, often with hospitals' support. In Maine, unused state DSH funds contributed to a Medicaid expansion for uninsured adults without dependent children called Access Health. In Georgia, DSH hospitals contribute funds to extend primary-care services through a program called the Georgia Indigent Care Trust Fund, which includes case management for the uninsured chronically ill and for pharmaceutical support. In Massachusetts, an uncompensated-care pool that supports both inpatient and community-based care is financed with DSH funds in addition to assessments on hospitals and health plans. In sum, Medicaid DSH funds are being successfully stretched across the safety net in many locales to cover a broader range of services than was originally intended.

Medicare DSH payments have also been an important source of additional revenue for safety net providers. Also dating to the 1980s, this adjustment was originally intended to compensate those hospitals serving a disproportionate number of low-income Medicare patients, who tend to be sicker and therefore more costly to serve than others with the same diagnosis. Specifically, the DSH payment is an add-on to the Diagnosis Related Group (DRG) payment, established 2 years after Medicare's prospective payment system (PPS) began in 1983. Although Medicare's PPS was established with no new money—by lowering the basic DRG rate and decreasing indirect medical education (IME) payments to teaching hospitals (which benefit from the DSH payments)—the program grew in the 1990s as the U.S. Congress added money for various categories of hospitals, particularly safety net providers. More than 95% of Medicare DSH payments goes to urban hospitals. Hence, while the original intention of the Medicare DSH payment was to offset the higher costs of caring for poor Medicare patients, it has come to serve the broader purpose of financially assisting hospitals serving low-income populations in order to preserve access to care.

DSH payments represent just one mechanism of many for funding safety net providers that rely on a patchwork of support from federal, state, county, and other sources. These include, at the federal level, funding from the Ryan White Care Act, which supports the unmet healthcare needs of individuals living with HIV; the Public Health Service Act, which provides Section 330 grants to eligible community and migrant health centers, homeless programs, and public housing primary-care programs; the Rural Health Clinics program, which allows enhanced Medicare and Medicaid reimbursement to encourage nurse practitioners, physicians, and physician assistants to work together in provider shortage areas; and the Critical Access Hospitals program, which provides cost-based reimbursement in an effort to reduce hospital closures in medically underserved areas.

Although states support the safety net primarily with federal matching programs, the presence of state-only programs can broaden access by extending coverage to residents who would otherwise fall through the cracks. For instance, MediKan in Kansas covers individuals trying to get Social Security disability benefits but who are not yet approved; Wisconsin's General Assistance Medical Program (GAMP) covers indigent Milwaukee County residents who are not eligible for Medicaid or the State's Children's Health Insurance Program (SCHIP); and Minnesota Care and Basic Health (in Washington state) both provide subsidized insurance to Medicaid-ineligible residents not covered by other programs. Such state-only programs are relatively few and far between because of the challenge of enacting adequate financing mechanisms, usually through new taxes or cuts in other services.

In some states, counties contribute substantial funds and services to safety net care, while in others they do not. In Texas, for instance, counties are legally responsible for funding indigent care. Uninsured individuals receive services through county hospitals or local public health departments. In regions of the state without public hospitals or health systems, counties are required to administer an indigent healthcare program for eligible residents by funding services in the private sector. Counties receive state subsidies or matching funds depending on the cost and volume of the indigent care services they provide. As in Texas, the 58 counties in California play a crucial and state-mandated role in financing and delivering safety net services. Within these states, counties have substantial discretion in how they interpret requirements, so services vary widely. In contrast, in Alabama and Mississippi, few county programs exist for indigent care beyond those funded by Medicaid.

Finally, in addition to the federal, state, and county support, the safety net receives some support and resources from foundation grants, managed-care companies, and manufacturer's indigent drug programs. For instance, the Virginia Health Care Foundation was initiated in 1992 as a public-private partnership to raise private funds to supplement public indigent care services.

Challenges

The challenges affecting the nation's healthcare safety net include the rising numbers of uninsured individuals needing care and the changing structure and environment of the healthcare marketplace. The impact of these challenges and the resilience of the safety net vary regionally, based on local support and structural factors that affect the safety net providers. Structural factors include the degree to which safety net services are concentrated among providers, such as a few public hospitals versus a wider network; the extent to which the burden is shared by both public and private entities; and the overall price competitiveness of the marketplace.

Equally important is the purposefulness with which healthcare administrators and policymakers have responded to local challenges to develop or maintain robust safety net systems. In some cases, adaptation has led to mergers, as in the joining of publicly owned Boston City Hospital and the private Boston University Hospital to establish Boston Medical Center. There have also been conversions of public hospitals to not-for-profit private status to facilitate joint ventures or improve efficiencies, as in the creation of the non-profit Cambridge Hospital, previously an agent of city government. And there have been restructured relationships within the public system resulting in administratively independent entities such as Denver Health, which consists of an extensive horizontally integrated system that includes a medical center with Level 1 trauma services, nine family health centers in underserved communities, 11 school-based clinics, and a wide range of detoxification, correctional-care facilities and behavioral health services that have provided over $100 million in charity-care services annually. In addition, Denver Health established the vertical integration of insurance, hospitals, and clinicians to create a large and financially viable Medicaid HMO called Colorado Access.

Other geographic regions of the nation have been less successful in building viable safety net systems or are greatly struggling to meet the growing needs of a large indigent population. Such locales typically lack strong core providers or mainstream health systems that are able and willing to provide substantial inpatient and outpatient safety net capacity. Little Rock, for instance, has struggled with inadequate safety net infrastructure and growing poverty, individuals without health insurance, and an influx of undocumented immigrants. A generous public insurance program for children has helped, as well as the engagement of faith-based charities and the participation of the city's academic medical center, where waits for specialist appointments for uninsured patients average 6 to 9 months. Even the most evolved safety net systems, however, remain vulnerable to the vicissitudes of public revenue streams, particularly Medicaid funding. For example, although it has been successful for over a decade, Colorado Access was forced to drop its physical health Medicaid contract in 2006 because of a 15% drop in the state's reimbursement rate. It has adapted by focusing on providing access for low-income children and for those needing behavioral health services and on Medicare Part D products; but 65,000 individuals lost their Medicaid coverage. In sum, success depends on adopting good business models that improve productivity, collections, economies of scale, and technical expertise and diversifying revenue streams—but with a mission to providing care for the poor.

Monitoring

Given the precarious nature of the healthcare safety net, with its wide variation across geographic regions of the nation, the IOM recommended a monitoring system for tracking its stability and performance in meeting the needs of vulnerable populations. Beginning in 2000, the federal Agency for Healthcare Research and Quality (AHRQ) and the Health Resources and Services Administration (HRSA) embarked on a joint safety net monitoring initiative with three strategies: to provide baseline information on hundreds of local safety nets throughout the nation, to establish and disseminate a standardized methodology for regional analysts to monitor the ongoing status of their safety nets, and to provide specific tools for assessing local capacity and performance. Initially, two data books were produced that described the status of safety nets in over 1,800 U.S. counties, with information on demand for safety net services (based on measures of poverty, individuals without health insurance, and illness), financial support for indigent care (including funding for Medicaid, DSH payments, and community health centers), descriptions of safety net structure, and measures of outcome of safety net performance (such as preventable hospitalizations and barriers to accessing care). A subsequent publication detailed how to estimate local demand for uncompensated care, assess safety net provider financial status, and measure performance

and outcomes, among other strategies to aid regional analysts. Finally, the project generated Web-based tools, including a worksheet for evaluating an entity's financial risk relative to a distribution of other safety net providers.

Future Implications

America's healthcare safety net is a complex patchwork of institutions, providers, and funding streams that offer medical services to individuals who lack the financial resources to pay for the care they need. Although various federal initiatives fund safety net programs, there are wide regional differences that reflect local variations in funding, political priorities, and demand for uncompensated care. Recently, a growing number of states have been leading innovators in identifying ways to reduce the burden on the safety net by expanding health insurance coverage. For the foreseeable future, however, the safety net will remain a vast but limited resource for many in America who must try to access it when they need healthcare.

Saul J. Weiner

See also Access to Healthcare; Community Health Centers (CHCs); Federally Qualified Health Centers (FQHCs); Health Insurance; Medicaid; Rationing Healthcare; Uninsured Individuals; Vulnerable Populations

Further Readings

Geyman, John P. *Falling Through the Safety Net: Americans Without Health Insurance.* Monroe, ME: Common Courage Press, 2005.

Hadley, Jack, and Peter Cunningham. "Availability of Safety Net Providers and Access to Care of Uninsured Persons," *Health Services Research* 39(5): 1527–46, October 2004.

Lewin, Marion Ein, and Stuart Altman, eds., Committee on the Changing Market, Managed Care, and the Future Viability of Safety Net Providers, Institute of Medicine. *America's Health Care Safety Net: Intact but Endangered.* Washington, DC: National Academy Press, 2000.

Lurie, Nicole. "Strengthening the U.S. Health Care Safety Net," *Journal of the American Medical Association* 284(16): 2112–14, October 25, 2000.

Waitzkin, Howard. "The History and Contradictions of the Health Care Safety Net," *Health Services Research* 40(3): 941–52, June 2005.

Werner, Rachel M., L. Elizabeth Goldman, and R. Adams Dudley. "Comparison of Change in Quality of Care Between Safety-Net and Non-Safety-Net Hospitals," *Journal of the American Medical Association* 299(18): 2180–87, May 14, 2008.

Web Sites

Agency for Healthcare Research and Quality (AHRQ), Safety Net Monitoring: http://www.ahrq.gov/data/safetynet

Center for Studying Health System Change (HSC): http://www.hschange.com

National Association of Public Hospitals and Health Systems (NAPH): http://www.naph.org

Urban Institute: http://www.urban.org

SATISFACTION SURVEYS

Obtaining information on how patients rate a healthcare facility and its providers and how satisfied they are with the care they receive has become a major focus of healthcare organizations. Although healthcare providers have been collecting such information for decades, in the past, it was viewed as a routine function with little practical utility. Patients were plentiful, and a consumerist approach was not in vogue. Patient satisfaction was not seriously considered as a method to improve quality and reduce costs.

Today, healthcare organizations are increasingly aware of the importance of keeping their patients satisfied as a way of preventing their shifting to other providers for their healthcare needs. As revenues become scarcer and competition more acute, many healthcare organizations are using patient satisfaction data to improve their services, increase revenue, and attain a superior market position.

Many healthcare providers view the delivery of care differently from their patients. They often view care as "fragmented," or being provided in "silos." Patients, on the other hand, tend to evaluate their total care experience as an integrated whole. Thus, the way patients view and evaluate their experiences may be completely different from the isolated view of providers and healthcare organizations. The implication, of course, is that low satisfaction levels for one or two aspects of care may result in significantly lower subjective assessments of the quality of the entire organization. And one or two positive experiences, on the other hand, may not be generalized to the whole experience.

Background

In the past, many healthcare organizations viewed patients as an unlimited resource. If patients became dissatisfied with their health care, and chose to switch their source of care, most healthcare facilities firmly held the attitude that there were "plenty more where they came from." Patient satisfaction therefore was of neither practical nor theoretical interest. However, in the 1970s, patient satisfaction became a phenomenon of theoretical interest to health services researchers. Patient satisfaction was used as a subjective measure of realized access to care. As such, satisfaction with care became a dependent variable of research interest as well as a predictor of other healthcare outcomes, including compliance with medical advice and return visits for care.

Today, there is an unprecedented revolution in healthcare. The informed consumer, who through an information explosion propelled by scientific and technological advances, mass media coverage, and the Internet better understands treatment options, is not afraid to challenge healthcare providers if the care does not meet his or her standards. Since patients can no longer be viewed as an unlimited resource, consumers have taken control and, in some cases, have more information regarding their specific diagnosis than some of their healthcare providers. Information flow helps set the standards for individual health behavior and for patient involvement in the diagnostic, treatment, and curative processes. Properly analyzed, patient satisfaction data can point to areas of patient concern, which when corrected will improve quality, reduce costs, and bring the patient back into the process of care.

Importance of Patient Perceptions

There are many reasons why all healthcare organizations should be concerned about patient perceptions of quality and their level of satisfaction. First, satisfied patients are more compliant, which results in better medical outcomes. That is, they will follow treatment protocols, such as completing drug regimens. Second, satisfied patients are more likely to return for follow-up visits. Third, patient satisfaction data provide managers with useful information regarding the outcomes of care themselves. Since satisfaction can be viewed as a proxy measure for the outcome of care, patient perceptions can point out process areas needing improvement. Fourth, patient satisfaction is a subjective measure of access to care. Fifth, patients who are satisfied tend not to file lawsuits. Sixth, satisfied patients, even if the medical outcome is not positive, tend to view the healthcare they were provided as a quality experience if they were satisfied with the level of care provided. Finally, patients, like all consumers, want and deserve to be satisfied with the products and services they purchase.

The Joint Commission recognizes patient satisfaction as part of its ORYX performance measurement system requirements. In addition, the National Committee for Quality Assurance's (NCQA) Healthcare Effectiveness Data and Information Set (HEDIS), ISO 9000, many state agencies, and the Malcolm Baldrige National Quality Award competition all consider patient satisfaction to be of very high importance. All contain regulations and guidelines for the measurement and reporting of specific satisfaction indicators. Many hospitals, health systems, and business cooperatives are publishing report cards with the same patient satisfaction indicators.

Data Collection Methods

The main way to collect data on patients' perceptions of the care they receive is to ask them. Doing so requires the use of a questionnaire and a survey process. Healthcare organizations use different survey techniques to collect their data. They must decide whether to interview their patients retrospectively at some time after they received care or to use a more prospective, point-of-service approach to capture patient perceptions as close to the time when they received care as possible. They also must decide the specific data collection strategy they will use. In general, there are three choices: a self-administered questionnaire, a personal interview, or a telephone survey. Each approach has its own set of advantages and disadvantages that affect cost, response rates, and ease of follow up. Personal interviews of past patients tend not be used because they are very costly to conduct.

Using mail surveys can be the most cost-effective and reliable method to collect patient satisfaction information. Response rates should generally be in the 50% range. Major costs in conducting a mail survey include the printing of the survey and cover letter; postage, including survey return postage; follow-up reminder letters or postcards after the first mailing; and a second mailing letter and survey for a portion of the original sample. Staff time is needed for the process as well. Time must be allocated for assembling the cover letter and survey, addressing the envelope package, mailing the package, compiling return surveys, and preparing the responses for analysis. Information-system time is also required to generate a random sample of patients to be surveyed and to produce their addresses and mailing labels. In terms of time, as many as 40 hours per survey may be required to successfully complete the process. If a healthcare organization uses a third party vendor to conduct the survey, it should compile and distribute regular reports within the organization. If the survey is being conducted in-house, resources necessary to generate reports should also be considered.

Advantages of conducting mail patient satisfaction surveys include the following: the healthcare organization maintains control of the process; costs are limited to printing, postage, and staff time to administer the surveys; the result of the surveys are likely to be reliable; ongoing investment in the process of conducting the surveys can be constant and predicable for budgeting purposes; the surveys can be customized without much effort; the results from the surveys can produce data for benchmark comparisons; the surveys may provide actionable results within acceptable statistical variance; and they may be less expensive to conduct than using an outside company.

Disadvantages of conducting mail satisfaction surveys include the following: intensive internal staff effort is required to prepare the surveys for distribution; there is loss of control over individual questionnaires once they are mailed; the functional illiteracy rate in the United States is high, and patients may not understand the language used in the survey; it may be difficult to locate patients such as those who are homeless; foreign-language-speaking patients may not be able to respond; return rates may vary greatly given the population being sampled; the lag time of results reporting can be from 30 to 60 days post survey mailing; if the survey is changed, it must be reprinted, thus increasing the costs; increases in postal rates can negatively affect the survey's budget; and staff departments involved in the survey process may stop or delay the timing of the survey.

The main difference between a mail survey and a telephone survey approach is the use of an interviewer. Using a telephone as the delivery mechanism, rather than the mail, means that an interviewer is necessary to ask the questions once a respondent is contacted. Interviewers are useful because they can circumvent the illiteracy problem, they can establish a sense of personal relationship, and they can assist the respondent if the questions are unclear.

Advantages of telephone patient satisfaction surveys include the following: there is immediate response and feedback, as it is a relatively fast process; callbacks are easy and inexpensive; it generally produces a greater response rate; no staff time is involved in data collection; standard questions are available; sample size and response by demographic group are more controllable; they produce reliable statistical results; they can produce large comparative benchmark databases; and they produce actionable reports and results.

Disadvantages of telephone patient satisfaction surveys include the following: they are more costly than mail surveys; customized questions may be available but at a premium price; patients receiving the telephone calls may view them as intrusive; individuals conducting the calls may be inconsistent in their presentations; some patients may not have a telephone; patients with multiple telephone numbers may be called several times; there may be multiple callbacks to obtain a response; the results of the survey may be difficult to compare with other survey methods if change is implemented; and comparative databases are generally unavailable for customized questions.

Point-of-service strategies include exit or discharge surveys, bedside surveys, or surveys of patients at any time during their visit or hospital stay. These data collection approaches are relatively simple for organizations to implement in-house, but if done on a large scale, they can become complicated.

The advantages of point-of-service patient satisfaction surveys include the following: there is immediate feedback; the patient can enter information via a kiosk or a computer terminal; any problems or concerns presented can be immediately addressed; they are cost-effective in that the patient does the work with little direct staff involvement; reports can be computer generated from the database; it is easy to change or add questions; the surveys can be used as an ongoing method to acquire information; computer software to conduct the surveys is easily updated; and data from the surveys can be continuously collected.

Disadvantages of point-of-service patient satisfaction surveys include the following: responses to the survey's questions may be biased due to the patient's medical condition; patients may perceive a lack of confidentiality and/or anonymity; the data collection method usually involves nonprobability samples, making any generalizations difficult; the initial costs of point-of-service systems are generally high; no comparative database may be available; there is no method to control respondents, which may result in oversampling of population groups; patients may respond more than once during their stay; the results may not be statistically reliable; patients may be fearful of computers; and there is the potential problem of safeguarding electronic information.

The method by which an organization chooses to measure patient satisfaction will be based on issues such as cost, philosophy toward satisfaction, and how the results will be used. Perhaps the most frequently used strategy is a self-administered questionnaire approach. Usually, healthcare organizations rely on a mail survey approach because of its low cost and low pressure on patients to respond. Another approach, growing in popularity, is to use kiosks located around the healthcare facility. This allows patients to stop at their convenience to assess the level and quality of care received. The problem with this approach is that the resulting sample of patients is not random and may not include all patients in the population base. Should the sample not be indicative of the total population of patients, the results may be biased and not nearly as useful to administrators.

No matter what data-gathering approach is used, the heart of the process is the questionnaire itself. Those using patient satisfaction surveys should be concerned about their validity and reliability. Making meaningful quality and cost improvements requires high-quality, valid, and reliable data. *Validity* refers to whether a survey's question actually measures what it is intended to measure. *Reliability* refers to whether a survey's question measures the same thing each time it is used. Validity ensures reliability, but a reliable question is not necessarily valid. That is, a survey's question may be measuring the same thing each time it is used, but it is not measuring what it is intended to measure. Obviously, when it comes to using patient satisfaction data for improving the quality of care an organization provides, both issues are key. In addition, issues such as sample size, response rate, generalizability, and statistical significance must also be recognized to generate usable results.

To make quality decisions regarding improvement strategies, it is important that the data used to make such decisions is of high quality. The old data processing adage of "garbage in-garbage out" (GIGO) is relevant and applicable to using patient satisfaction data for quality and performance improvement.

Many healthcare organizations currently outsource patient satisfaction data collection to proprietary companies. The reasons for outsourcing the data collection are usually related to cost, convenience, and organizational competence. That is, some healthcare organizations feel that it is less expensive to outsource the work than to maintain a qualified staff of survey and statistical experts. Others organizations may feel that receiving satisfaction data from a proprietary company on a regular basis is convenient and reduces the non-clinical functions within the organization. Still others may feel that they do not have the necessary level of competence within the organization to carry out the tasks associated with collecting their own patient satisfaction data.

Even if a healthcare organization outsources its patient satisfaction data collection process, it would be unwise to haphazardly select a company without considering several key factors. The fact that a company is in the business of collecting data for hospitals and other healthcare organizations does not automatically ensure that it provides a quality product. Before selecting any data collection company, issues surrounding two key questions must be satisfactorily addressed. First, is the data collection instrument valid and reliable? Second, what specific questions are asked?

Measuring Patient Satisfaction

There are two general approaches to measuring patient assessment of care. The first is to ask questions directly related to satisfaction levels. For example, "How satisfied were you with the overall quality of care at your last visit?" The respondent selects a response from a list of possible answers, such as very satisfied, somewhat satisfied, somewhat dissatisfied, and very dissatisfied.

An alternative approach is to use a patient rating system. An example of this strategy is to ask, "How would you rate the overall quality of the care you received at your last visit?"—with the possible responses of "excellent," "good," "fair," and "poor." Although it could be argued that these two strategies tap into different perceptions, they tend to be viewed within the healthcare industry as interchangeable.

A strategy that is used to accumulate data on the patient's experience with care is to divide the visit into its component parts. For example, questions pertaining to waiting time, appointment time, staff and physician communications, and so on are presented as separate items. This allows an analysis of the various parts that make up the whole visit or hospital stay. Usually, the last question asks about the overall satisfaction with the visit or stay. This approach permits the relative importance of each item to be measured against the patient's overall perception of the care, and it will identify where problem areas exist. The approach allows healthcare managers to focus intervention strategies for quality improvement where they are most needed. It also can be used to highlight areas where the providers do an especially good job, which allows the opportunity to establish best-practices protocols that can be used across the organization.

Future Implications

Querying patients about all dimensions of the care they receive across the health system provides the opportunity to identify areas where the process of care fails to provide an encompassing, satisfying experience. Satisfaction is a valuable weapon that provides an organization an edge in a highly competitive marketplace. If a hospital or other healthcare organization is not using available tools to understand and interpret patient satisfaction data, it is missing a valuable opportunity for improvement. Patient satisfaction data reflect the voice of the customer. That voice provides a very personal view of the process of care within the organization.

It is important that the patient's input be taken seriously when attempting any improvement strategies. Early on, patient satisfaction surveys were conducted primarily to show the patient that the healthcare organization "cared," with little practical use for the results. With the move by healthcare-accrediting organizations, insurance companies, and government agencies to obtain and use more patient outcome measures, healthcare organizations are now being required to demonstrate how patient satisfaction survey results are used to improve care.

Ralph Bell

See also Healthcare Effectiveness Data and Information Set (HEDIS); Health Report Cards; Health Surveys; Hospitals; ORYX Performance Measurement System; Patient-Centered Care; Pay-for-Performance; Quality of Healthcare

Further Readings

Applebaum, Robert, Jane K. Straker, and Scott Geron. *Assessing Satisfaction in Health and Long-Term Care: Practical Approaches to Hearing the Voices of Consumers.* New York: Springer, 2000.

Bell, Ralph, and Michael J. Krivich. *How to Use Patient Satisfaction Data to Improve Healthcare Quality.* Milwaukee, WI: ASQ Quality Press, 2000.

Morales, Leo S., Juan Antonio Puyol, and Ron D. Hays. *Improving Patient Satisfaction Surveys to Assess Cultural Competence in Health Care.* Oakland, CA: California Healthcare Foundation, 2003.

Press, Irwin. *Patient Satisfaction: Understanding and Managing the Experience of Care.* 2d ed. Chicago: Health Administration Press, 2005.

Shelton, Patrick J. *Measuring and Improving Patient Satisfaction.* Gaithersburg, MD: Aspen, 2000.

Web Sites

American Academy of Family Physicians (AAFP): http://www.aafp.org

Consumer Assessment of Healthcare Providers and Systems (CAHPS): http://www.cahps.ahrq.gov

Council of American Survey Research Organizations (CASRO): http://www.casro.org

Health Resources and Services Administration (HRSA) Health Center Patient Satisfaction Survey: http://bphc.hrsa.gov/patientsurvey

SCOTT, W. RICHARD

W. Richard (Dick) Scott has made significant contributions to the field of organizational theory and the application of this theory to healthcare organizations. He has conducted extensive research on professional organizations, with particular emphasis on social welfare, educational, and medical organizations. Scott is Professor Emeritus of Sociology, with appointments in the Graduate School of Business, the School of Education, and the School of Medicine at Stanford University.

Scott has spent his entire academic career at Stanford University, where he was the founding director of the Stanford Center for Organizations Research. Scott's early research focused on the sociological study of authority and control relations in organizations. Along with his colleagues John W. Meyer and James G. March at Stanford, Scott soon became a key theorist of organizational analysis within the school of neoinstitutionalism. This school examines how organizations operate in institutional and societal environments that govern behavior beyond market forces.

Scott is well-known for his historical study examining changes in the healthcare delivery system of the San Francisco Bay Area over a 50-year period. The study, which is published in *Institutional Change and Healthcare Organizations: From Professional Dominance to Managed Care* (2000), examines the profound transformation of healthcare organizations in the Bay Area. It charts changes since World War II in the number and types of organizations delivering healthcare services as these have been affected by changes in the resource environment—for example, demography, financing, supply of health professionals—and in the institutional environment—for example, changes in institutional logics and governance systems.

Scott has authored or coauthored many books and has published over 150 scholarly articles. Specifically, he has authored three widely used textbooks on organizations, *Formal Organizations: A Comparative Approach* (1962), *Organizations and Organizing: Rational, Natural and Open Systems* (2007), and *Institutions and Organizations: Ideas and Interests* (2008).

Scott has received many awards and accolades throughout his distinguished career. He is an elected member of the National Academy of Sciences, Institute of Medicine (IOM), and was a fellow of the Center for Advanced Study in the Behavioral Sciences. Scott also received the Distinguished Scholar Award from the Management and Organization Theory Division of the Academy of Management as well as the Richard D. Irwin Award for a career of distinguished scholarly contributions to management. In 2000, the American Sociological Association, Section on Organizations, Occupations, and Work created an award in Scott's name to recognize his contributions to the field of organizational sociology. The award is given annually to honor the most outstanding article contributing to the advancement of the field.

Scott was born in 1932 in Parsons, Kansas. He graduated from Parsons Junior College with an associate degree in 1952. He went on to receive a bachelor's and a master's degree from the University of Kansas and later completed his doctoral degree in sociology at the University of Chicago in 1961. While at the University of Chicago, he studied under Peter M. Blau, one of the founders of the field of organizational sociology. Scott has received honorary doctorates from the Copenhagen School of Business (2000) and the Helsinki School of Economics (2001).

Scott continues to teach doctoral-level seminars and conduct scholarly work at Stanford. He is currently engaged in the theoretical work of combining institutional theory in organizations with social movement theory as well as conducting research on institutional change at the community and the transnational level.

Jared Lane K. Maeda

See also Healthcare Organization Theory; Hospitals; Managed Care; Medical Sociology; Mental Health

Further Readings

Blau, Peter M., and W. Richard Scott. *Formal Organizations: A Comparative Approach*. San Francisco, CA: Chandler, 1962.

Meyer, John W., and W. Richard Scott. *Organizational Environments: Ritual and Rationality*. Beverly Hills, CA: Sage, 1983.

Scott, W. Richard. *Institutions and Organizations: Ideas and Interests*. 3d ed. Thousand Oaks, CA: Sage, 2008.

Scott, W. Richard, and Bruce L. Black, eds. *The Organization of Mental Health Services: Societal and Community Systems*. Beverly Hills, CA: Sage, 1986.

Scott, W. Richard, and F. Gerald Davis. *Organizations and Organizing: Rational, Natural and Open Systems*. Upper Saddle River, NJ: Pearson Prentice Hall, 2007.

Scott, W. Richard, Martin Ruef, Peter J. Mendel, et al. *Institutional Change and Healthcare Organizations: From Professional Dominance to Managed Care*. Chicago: University of Chicago Press, 2000.

Web Sites

Stanford Center for Health Policy/Center for Primary Care and Outcomes Research: http://healthpolicy.stanford.edu/people/wrichardscott

Stanford University Department of Sociology: http://sociology.stanford.edu

SELECTIVE CONTRACTING

Selective contracting is when an insurer, usually a managed-care plan, contracts with some but not all healthcare providers in a market. In essence, the insurer trades patient volume in return for lower provider prices. Selective contracting has been the comparative advantage that managed-care plans have used to enter and eventually dominate the nation's private health insurance market during the past 20 years. The selective contracting process was successful in introducing price competition into healthcare markets in the 1990s. The rapid increase in health insurance premiums in the past several years can be attributed, at least in part, to the erosion of selective contracting.

Overview

The basic idea surrounding selective contracting is that insurers contract with hospitals, physicians, pharmacies, and other healthcare providers based on factors such as services, quality, amenities, location, and, potentially, price. In the 1970s and 1980s, competition in healthcare was characterized as a medical arms race. More competitors in a market, measured as more hospitals in a geographic area, were associated with higher, not lower, prices as simple economic theory would predict. In as much as consumers were reasonably well insured and insurers entered into contracts with all local providers, there was little reason for a provider to offer a lower price. A lower price would garner little additional patient volume. Instead, more services, greater quality, and additional amenities attracted physicians and their patients. Thus, costs were higher in areas with greater nonprice competition.

Empirical Evidence

Efforts largely beginning in California began to change the medical arms race. California's state legislature passed laws that made it clear that insurers did not have to contract with all licensed providers in a market. Prior to the laws, hospital costs were higher in highly competitive markets in California. However, after enactment of the laws, cost increases were much smaller in the more competitive hospital market areas—the opposite of the medical arms race scenario.

Even more compelling evidence was found in an analysis of the hospital prices that were negotiated by the Blue Shield of California preferred provider organization (PPO). An analysis of the medical-surgical price per day that the PPO negotiated with 190 California hospitals showed that the PPO was able to obtain a lower price when there were fewer hospitals in the market; when the PPO had a larger share of a hospital's admissions; when a hospital had only a small share of the PPO's local book of business; and when there was idle capacity in the hospital or, indeed, in the local hospital market. These findings were strong evidence that the standard economic model was functioning in the hospital market. A number of other recent studies have generalized these findings beyond California.

Managed Care

The success of managed care in reducing health-care costs is attributed to selective contracting and the reduction of expensive services on the part of managed-care plans. There is substantial evidence that managed-care plans, particularly health maintenance organizations (HMOs), have attracted lower utilizers of healthcare. It is less clear, however, whether this reduction comes about as a result of actions that the health plans take to enroll lower utilizers and shun high users or whether their enrollment reflects individuals who disproportionately like the concept of health maintenance and who dislike interacting with the healthcare system. The evidence that managed-care plans discourage the use of expensive services is scarce.

There is some evidence that sorts out the relative impacts of selective contracting, favorable selection, and treatment intensity on the lower use of healthcare in the case of managed care relative to conventional plans. Researchers examining the per-enrollee expenditures for eight medical conditions (acute myocardial infarction, live birth, four types of cancer, and Types 1 and 2 diabetes) among Massachusetts state employees in the mid-1990s found that the HMOs offered by the state had per-person claims costs that were $107 lower for these conditions than the analogous claims costs for the same conditions in the conventional plan offered. Fifty-one percent of the difference was attributable to favorable selection. The HMOs attracted younger enrollees and people with a lower incidence of the medical conditions. An additional 5% was attributable to lower treatment intensity. Selective contracting accounted for 45% of the lower claims costs. As an example, the HMOs on average paid $20,302 for an angioplasty procedure, while the conventional plan paid $37,330.

Increase in Insurance Premiums

Selective contracting also provides a potential explanation for the more rapid increase in health insurance premiums that the country has observed during the past decade. Two explanations are typically advanced for this increase. One is a backlash against managed care. The other is a consolidation among providers. Both suggest an undermining of the comparative advantage that was offered by selective contracting.

The managed-care backlash is said to consist of physician and patient complaints about the nature of the restrictions that managed-care plans imposed on access to healthcare. These include restrictions on self-referral and the use of various utilization management techniques. In addition, patients seem to be concerned about the quality of the providers potentially available to them in their managed-care panel. As a consequence, there has been growth in the preferred provider organization (PPO) model of managed care at the expense of HMOs. PPOs allow subscribers to use a wider set of healthcare providers if they are willing to pay higher copays to use non-panel providers. Whatever the merits of this shift, it has the consequence of undermining selective contracting. By expanding their networks and allowing subscribers to step outside the established network of providers, managed-care plans are unable to trade patient volume for lower prices. As a result, health insurance premiums continue to increase.

The consolidation explanation for higher health insurance premiums holds that hospitals have combined through mergers and acquisitions and physician groups have entered into larger groups and formed marketing networks to negotiate with managed-care plans. These activities also have the potential to undermine selective contracting. Consolidations and marketing networks reduce the number of competitors, remove idle capacity from the market, and increase the share of the insurer's subscribers using the new entities. All these actions have the potential to raise the prices that managed-care firms could negotiate through selective contracting.

Michael A. Morrisey

See also Competition in Healthcare; Healthcare Markets; Health Economics; Health Insurance; Health Maintenance Organizations (HMOs); Hospitals; Managed Care; Preferred Provider Organizations (PPOs)

Further Readings

Dranove, David. *The Economic Evolution of American Health Care: From Marcus Welby to Managed Care.* Princeton, NJ: Princeton University Press, 2000.

Morrisey, Michael A. *Health Insurance.* Chicago: Health Administration Press, 2007.

Zwanziger, Jack, Glenn A. Melnick, and Anil Bamezai. "The Effects of Selective Contracting on Health Cost and Revenues," *Health Services Research* 35(4): 849–67, October 2000.

Web Sites

America's Health Insurance Plans (AHIP): http://www.hiaa.org

National Conference of State Legislatures (NCSL): http://www.ncsl.org

SEVERITY ADJUSTMENT

A common problem with comparing performance among healthcare providers is how to adjust for differences in the disease severity of patients. For example, the mortality rate of patients in Hospital A may be higher than in Hospital B, but unfair and misleading conclusions may be drawn if patient characteristics in the two hospitals are not taken into consideration. Perhaps Hospital A is more likely to serve a large number of indigent patients, who lack health insurance coverage and tend to delay care until later stages of the disease, while Hospital B serves a large number of upper-middle-class patients, who have access to routine and preventive care. When assessing the relative performance of these two hospitals, these patient differences must be accounted for in some way, a process referred to as severity adjustment.

Although severity adjustment might initially appear to be straightforward, the process may be very complex. Methods of severity adjustment depend on the availability of data, the accuracy of the data, and the costs of data collection. A large number of factors may affect the outcomes of care, including the patient's age, gender, race and ethnicity, coexisting diseases, and psychosocial and socioeconomic characteristics. There are also a number of different severity adjustment methods and models available that often do not lead to similar conclusions.

History

The first attempts to measure patient severity took place in the 1970s. Later, particular attention was paid to severity adjustment in 1983, when the nation's Medicare program adopted a Diagnosis Related Group (DRG)–based prospective payment system (PPS) for hospitals. Hospitals were concerned that the new system would not pay for the provision of care to "sicker" patients. There was also concern about the accuracy of the DRG concept, since it assigns patients based mainly on principal diagnosis codes. Since compensation levels were at stake, critics argued that diagnosis severity could be exaggerated by hospitals in an attempt to improve their "bottom lines." These issues prompted debate over the use of code-based versus medical record surveys to assess patient complexity; thus, there were considerable efforts by developers of severity measures to explore and test a number of systems, such as disease staging, severity scores of Patient Management Categories (PMCs), and All Patient Refined Diagnosis Related Groups (APR-DRGs).

Selection of Performance Outcome

In the process of severity adjustment, healthcare managers and researchers must decide on a performance outcome of interest. Outcome measures that could be attributable to healthcare quality include morbidity, mortality, readmission rates, complication rates, functional status, and patient satisfaction. By far, mortality has been the most frequently used generic measure of hospital performance. Advantages of using mortality include the wide availability of this information, its clearly definable end point, and its importance. Further decisions about the mortality outcome measure may include whether to use in-hospital mortality, 10-day mortality, 30-day mortality, or 1-year mortality.

While a generic measure of hospital performance such as all-cause mortality may be used, it may be of greater interest to evaluate a disease- or procedure-specific mortality (e.g., in-hospital mortality among patients with congestive heart failure or in-house mortality after abdominal aortic aneurysm repair). Instead of mortality, healthcare managers and researchers may be interested in performance indicators such as the number of cesarean deliveries among high-risk women,

urinary-catheter-associated infections, or postoperative sepsis. Sometimes, selection of performance indicators may be hampered by small sample size, leaving inadequate statistical power to properly assess priority outcomes.

Selection of Severity Indicators

Fundamental to risk adjustment strategies is the selection of specific indicator variables that will help healthcare managers and researchers arrive at an adequate disease severity measure. If disease severity is poorly represented, then differences in healthcare performance outcome may be inaccurately estimated.

The selection of risk adjustment variables may be made on an individual level, the hospital or organization level, or both. For example, common variables to control for at the patient level include demographic factors such as age, gender, and race. Obviously, a hospital that treats more elderly patients will likely have a high mortality rate. Examples of health status variables at the patient level include the presence of coexisting diseases such as congestive heart failure, cancer, or chronic renal failure. An example of a health status indicator at the hospital level is the all-payer, DRG-based case mix index. Socioeconomic indicators at the county level, which could help adjust for case-mix differences among organizations, may also be incorporated into adjustment models. Variables might include per capita income, unemployment rate, or college graduation rate.

Data Sources

Decisions regarding the manner in which data are collected for severity adjustment may vary. For example, it may be less costly and less time-consuming to use routinely collected data already present in a hospital's computer system. However, this type of data may be very limited in nature and have questionable accuracy, depending on the habits of individual healthcare providers within the settings of interest. For these reasons, some experts have advocated going directly to medical records to extract relevant information. However, data extraction alone for a single hospital can cost tens of thousands of dollars and may therefore be prohibitive and not worth the net gain in added precision.

Severity Adjustment Methods

There have been numerous attempts to design the most ideal disease severity adjustment method, which have resulted in a variety of commercial products that are compared and contrasted in the literature. Due to the complexities of severity adjustment, practical limitations, and the evolving nature of the field, selection of an appropriate severity measure can be difficult. Different adjustment models require different inputs. Some models use clinical information that may only be extracted from the medical record, while others may require coding data that are already available in an electronic format.

Examples of severity measurement models include Acute Physiology and Chronic Health Evaluation (APACHE III—APS), MedisGroups Score, Severity Scores on Patient Management Category Severity Scales (PMCs), Disease Staging, Charlson Severity Score, and the All Patient Refined Diagnosis Related Groups (APR-DRGs).

Daniel K. Roberts

See also Case-Mix Adjustment; Diagnosis Related Groups (DRGs); Disease; Epidemiology; Health Report Cards; Outcomes Movement; Quality of Healthcare; Risk

Further Readings

Arca, Massimo, Danilo Fusco, Anna P. Barone, et al. "Risk Adjustment and Outcome Research: Part I," *Journal of Cardiovascular Medicine* 7(9): 682–90, September 2006.

Fleming, Steven T. *Managerial Epidemiology: Concepts and Cases.* 2d ed. Chicago: Health Administration Press, 2008.

Iezzoni, Lisa I., ed. *Risk Adjustment for Measuring Health Care Outcomes.* 3d ed. Chicago: Health Administration Press, 2003.

Kominski, Gerald F. *Medicare's Use of Risk Adjustment.* Washington, DC: National Health Policy Forum, 2007.

Web Sites

Agency for Healthcare Research and Quality (AHRQ), Healthcare Cost and Utilization Project (HCUP): http://www.hcup-us.ahrq.gov

American Health Information Management Association (AHIMA): http://www.ahima.org

Leapfrog Group: http://www.leapfroggroup.org

SHAPIRO, SAM

Sam Shapiro (1914–1999) was both a founder and an exemplar of health services research as a recognized field of inquiry in public health and medical care. He was an innovative researcher, a dedicated teacher of a generation of health services researchers, a generous mentor to younger researchers, and a valued partner in research to colleagues.

Shapiro is widely recognized for research begun in the 1960s with Drs. Philip Strax and Louis Venet that demonstrated the effectiveness of screening mammography, combined with a clinical examination, in reducing breast cancer mortality. At the time, Shapiro was director of Research for the Health Insurance Plan of Greater New York. He, Strax, and Venet initiated a clinical trial that, between 1963 and 1968, enrolled 62,000 women aged 40 to 64 who were randomly assigned screening mammography and clinical examination versus regular care. Ten years later, cumulative mortality among women randomized to screening was about 30% lower than in the regular care group. In recognition of the importance of this work, Shapiro and Strax were awarded the Charles E. Kettering Prize for outstanding contributions to cancer diagnosis or treatment in 1988. Shapiro was the first public health researcher to receive this prize.

Shapiro was born and raised in Brooklyn, New York, and attended Brooklyn College, where he earned a bachelor's degree in mathematics in 1933. In the 1934–1935 academic year, he did graduate work in mathematics and statistics at Columbia University but left to work in Home Relief, a Depression-era program in New York City. In early 1943, he went to Washington, D.C., where he worked for the Selective Service System. In 1944–1946, he served in the U.S. Navy.

After being discharged from the Navy in 1946, he joined the National Office of Vital Statistics (now the National Center for Health Statistics), a component of the Public Health Service. It was there he began his work in public health, with responsibility for birth and infant death statistics. Among his earliest published papers are several concerned with the development and completeness of birth registration data and applications of these statistical data to answer public health questions.

He spent a year (1954–1955) as senior study director at the National Opinion Research Center (NORC) in Chicago, developing research designs and questionnaires for national and local studies on health services use. He joined the Health Insurance Plan (HIP) of Greater New York in 1955 as associate director of Research and Statistics and was promoted to vice president and director of Research and Statistics in 1959.

His research at HIP focused initially on the effects of prepaid group practice on health outcomes. With Paul Densen and others, he authored two research papers in 1958 and 1960 comparing prematurity and perinatal mortality among HIP members and the general population; he reported that women in the HMO began prenatal care earlier and had lower prematurity and perinatal mortality rates and that this occurred for both White and non-White groups. Differences were also observed between women seeing private physicians and those seeing "general-service" physicians.

Concurrently with the perinatal-care work, he and Densen examined patterns of ambulatory services utilization and hospitalizations. They designed and implemented one of the very early, if not the first, routine collections of encounter data in a prepaid group practice plan to support research on patterns of service utilization. His work in mental health began with analyses of prescriptions for psychotropic medications and patterns of medical care related to mental illness. Shapiro also conducted research showing that encounters for elderly patients took more time than for adults under age 65. This provided the basis for higher capitation payments by Medicare for elderly enrollees.

Under Shapiro's direction, HIP launched a longitudinal study of the course of newly diagnosed coronary heart disease among its members in the early 1960s, taking advantage of the plan's enrolled population, ready access to medical records, and extensive information on procedures and treatments available from the encounter data system. Over the next 10 years or so, a number of research papers were published describing, for instance, analyses of factors associated with the incidence of myocardial infarction and angina, lifestyle changes after a diagnosis of myocardial infarction or angina, and the disease course for women as compared with men.

In March 1973, Shapiro accepted the position of director of the Health Services Research and Development Center (HSRDC) at Johns Hopkins University. During the next 9 years, he developed an interdisciplinary team of health services researchers that competed successfully for a 5-year core support grant for the HSRDC from the National Center for Health Services Research and Development and for project grants from foundations and several of the National Institutes of Health (NIH).

His own research during this period addressed several disparate topics, including surveys of defined populations in Baltimore concerning utilization of health services for chronic and preventive care; the development of statistical procedures for measuring health status in geographic areas using vital statistics and hospital discharge data; evaluation of a Maryland statewide initiative to improve blood pressure control; and, with Ellen Mackenzie, reliability testing of the Injury Severity Scale (ISS) and its underlying Abbreviated Injury Scale (AIS) for evaluating trauma injuries.

In 1974–1976, with support from the National Center for Health Statistics (NCHS), Shapiro and Richard Yaffe conducted a pilot study to assess the costs and effectiveness of alternative methodologies for obtaining survey data on medical expenditures. The results of that work influenced the design of the 1977–1978 National Medical Care Expenditure Survey (now the Medical Expenditure Panel Survey).

Continuing his interest in perinatal care issues, he undertook between 1975 and 1981, with Marie McCormick and Barbara Starfield, an evaluation of the effects of Robert Wood Johnson Foundation (RWJF)–supported regionalized networks for high-risk pregnancy care. They found that while the program's regions did not show better outcomes than nonprogram regions, its implementation coincided with increased centralization of high-risk pregnancy care nationally so that the decrease in neonatal mortality was accompanied by a decrease in selected morbidity overall.

In 1979, Shapiro joined with Morton Kramer and Ernest Gruenberg to lead the Eastern Baltimore Mental Health Survey, one of five sites for National Institute of Mental Health's Epidemiologic Catchment Area Survey, which developed population-based estimates for the incidence and prevalence of mental disorders in the United States and for met and unmet needs for mental health care among people with mental disorders.

Shapiro stepped down as HSRDC director in 1982, at the age of 68, but continued his active research career, publishing more than 55 research papers and two books over the next 15 years. In 1992, at the age of 78, he began his last major investigation, with Dr. Janet Hardy. The study traced the biological and social conditions experienced by a cohort of children born at Johns Hopkins Hospital between 1960 and 1965 and assessed their status at ages 27 to 33 years with regard to their health, educational attainment, employment experience, and family formation.

In the course of his long career at Johns Hopkins University, Shapiro was advisor to a large number of students, many of whom have gone on to make major contributions in health services research. He was also a mentor to many young faculty members who are now leaders in the field in their own right.

Shapiro received many awards in recognition of his unique contributions. The American Public Health Association gave him its Award for Excellence in Promoting and Protecting the Health of People in the Domestic Field in 1977, citing the breadth and groundbreaking nature of his contributions to our knowledge of health services and their contribution to the public's health. He was elected to the national Institute of Medicine (IOM) (1974); received the Distinguished Achievement Award of the American Society of Preventive Oncology (1985); was selected to give the American Public Health Association Lowell Reed Lecture (1989); was chosen to present the 14th Wendell G. Scott Memorial Lecture of the American College of Radiology (1992); and was made an honorary fellow of the American College of Radiology (1993). Shapiro was a key participant in the formation of the Association for Health Services Research (now AcademyHealth) in 1981, in recognition of which he was given the first Distinguished Investigator Award in 1985.

Shapiro's research defined standards for preventive services and provided new epidemiologic information on major risk factors for coronary heart disease. His research on organization and finance demonstrated that HMOs could provide care of equal or better quality than the alternatives.

He developed one of the first information systems to capture utilization and diagnostic information on each physician visit and demonstrated its potential value. Today, we rely on administrative data systems that are built on this experience, including Medicare and Medicaid. One of their uses is to analyze variations in medical-practice patterns and their relationship to patient outcomes and costs as a way to identify opportunities to improve the effectiveness and efficiency of health care. His work spanned pregnancy to old age, included physical and mental health problems, focused on prevention of disease and disability, and examined alterative approaches to the organization and payment of services to ensure that those who need care receive it. His contributions to the development of this new field of knowledge, health services research, were recognized by the Johns Hopkins University in 1998 with an honorary doctorate in humane letters, "for changing the face of American health care in this half-century." Shapiro died in Baltimore in 1999 at the age of 85.

Elizabeth A. Skinner

See also Health Services Research, Origins; Mental Health Epidemiology; National Center for Health Statistics (NCHS); Preventive Care; Public Health; Robert Wood Johnson Foundation (RWJF); Starfield, Barbara; Women's Health Issues

Further Readings

Shapiro, Sam. "End Result Measurements of Quality of Medical Care," *The Milbank Memorial Fund Quarterly* 45(2 pt. 1): 7–30, 1967.

Shapiro, Sam. "Measuring the Effectiveness of Prevention: II," *Milbank Memorial Fund Quarterly/ Health and Society* 55(2): 291–306, 1977.

Shapiro, Sam. "Determining the Efficacy of Breast Cancer Screening," *Cancer* 63(10): 1873–80, May 15, 1989.

Shapiro, Sam. "Epidemiology and Public Policy," *American Journal of Epidemiology* 134(10): 1057–1061, November 15, 1991.

Shapiro, Sam, Harold Jacobziner, Paul M. Densen, et al. "Further Observations on Prematurity and Perinatal Mortality in a General Population and in the Population of a Prepaid Group Practice Medical Care Plan," *American Journal of Public Health* 50(9): 1307–1317, September 1960.

Shapiro, Sam, Wanda Venet, Philip Strax, et al. "Ten- to
    Fourteen-Year Effect of Screening on Breast Cancer
    Mortality," *Journal of the National Cancer Institute*
    69(2): 349–55, August 1982.
Shapiro, Sam, Eve Weinblatt, Charles W. Frank, et al.
    "The HIP Study of Incidence and Prognosis of
    Coronary Heart Disease: Preliminary Findings on
    Incidence of Myocardial Infarction and Angina,"
    Journal of Chronic Diseases 18: 527–58, June 1965.

Web Sites

Johns Hopkins University, Health Services Research and
    Development Center (HSRDC):
    http://www.jhsph.edu/HSR

SHEPS, CECIL G.

Cecil G. Sheps (1913–2004), one of the founders of the field now known as health services research, was the Taylor Grandy Distinguished Professor of Social Medicine and Epidemiology at the University of North Carolina at Chapel Hill (UNC-CH), the university's former Vice Chancellor for Health Affairs, and founding director of UNC-CH's Health Services Research Center (renamed in 1991 as the Cecil G. Sheps Center for Health Services Research), where he maintained an active presence until his death in 2004.

Sheps spent two different periods of his long career as a member of the UNC-CH faculty. He first came to Chapel Hill in 1947, shortly after having completed his public health training at Yale University. He was born and had grown up in Winnepeg, Canada, and he took his medical degree at the University of Manitoba. At UNC, he was first employed in the Office of Planning for the newly created Division of Health Affairs, and he was on the campus as the School of Medicine expanded to become a 4-year curriculum and the School of Public Health was made a distinct academic unit. He taught basic courses in public health administration, biostatistics, and epidemiology in the latter school until he departed for Boston in 1953 to become director of the Beth Israel Hospital, one of the principal teaching hospitals affiliated with the Harvard Medical School, where he held a faculty position.

In 1958, he left Boston to become professor of Public Health and head of the graduate program in medical care administration at the Graduate School of Public Health at the University of Pittsburgh. After only 5 years in that position, he was lured back into an administrative position as director of the Beth Israel Hospital in New York and as a professor at the Mount Sinai School of Medicine.

In 1968, the University of North Carolina at Chapel Hill received one of five major grants from the U.S. Public Health Service to begin a multidisciplinary center for health services research. A search for an initial director of this new center began, and several faculty members suggested that an approach be made to Sheps to return to Chapel Hill to launch this new multidisciplinary center. Sheps and his wife decided to accept separate offers to return to North Carolina, he as director of the Health Services Research Center and as professor of family medicine and she as professor of Biostatistics in the UNC School of Public Health.

Sheps had developed a keen interest in multidisciplinary problem-focused research, especially research focused on the issues of concern to the field of healthcare. He had formed a multidisciplinary unit to carry out this sort of research at Beth Israel in Boston, one of the first hospital-based research institutes of its kind. Several of the investigators he attracted to work in that unit later became the leading figures in the emerging field of health services research, a field he helped to create and name. He was the first chairperson of the initial study section of the U.S. Public Health Service, giving grants to support the work of scholars in what was then called healthcare studies.

Sheps believed that the problems in assuring access to quality medical care for everyone were surmountable. He believed that one of the challenges of health services was to discover ways of converting an array of disconnected healthcare services into coherent and consumer/patient-centered programs of healthcare serving defined populations by offering clearly defined and needed care.

Throughout his career, Sheps had a strong interest in international healthcare issues and in the development of both research and educational programs addressing healthcare issues. He traveled and was actively involved in health services research in the United Kingdom, and he was one of the consultants involved over a number of years in the development of a new community-oriented medical school at Ben Gurion University of the Negev in Israel.

Sheps published over 140 articles in scientific journals and wrote or edited nine books, including *Needed Research in Health and Medical Care: A Biosocial Approach* with Eugene E. Taylor and *The Sick Citadel: The American Academic Medical Center and the Public Interest* with Irving J. Lewis. Sheps passed away on February 7, 2004.

Gordon H. DeFriese

See also Academic Medical Centers; Access to Healthcare; Comparing Health Systems; Epidemiology; Health Planning; Health Services Research, Origins; International Health Systems; Public Health

Further Readings

Lewis, Irving J., and Cecil G. Sheps. *The Sick Citadel: The American Academic Medical Center and the Public Interest.* Cambridge, MA: Oelgeschlager, Gunn and Hain, 1983.
Madison, Donald L. "Remembering Cecil," *North Carolina Medical Journal* 65(5): 301–6, September–October 2004.
Sheps, Cecil G. *Medical Schools and Hospitals: Interdependence for Education and Service.* Evanston, IL: Association of American Medical Colleges, 1965.
Sheps, Cecil G. *Higher Education for Public Health: A Report of the Milbank Memorial Fund Commission.* New York: Milbank Memorial Fund, 1976.
Sheps, Cecil G., and Eugene E. Taylor. *Needed Research in Health and Medical Care: A Bio-Social Approach.* Chapel Hill: University of North Carolina Press, 1954.

Web Sites

University of North Carolina at Chapel Hill, Cecil G. Sheps Center for Health Services Research: http://www.shepscenter.unc.edu

SHORTELL, STEPHEN M.

A highly distinguished scholar and well-respected leader in health services delivery systems in the United States, Stephen M. Shortell has had a very productive and influential career. His groundbreaking, interdisciplinary research projects have sought to identify and understand the interactions among business strategies, organizational structures, quality improvement processes, and performance of healthcare systems. One important outcome of Shortell's research has been a typology of healthcare systems alliances. His research also has focused on organizational attributes of physician group practices, with an ongoing interest in quality, outcomes of care, and strategic alliances between physicians and other healthcare entities. Woven throughout his ongoing program of research are questions about the effectiveness of total quality management (TQM), strategic change in the healthcare sector, and ways to enhance community-based initiatives to improve health. At the heart of his scholarly and intricate studies is a concern for improving the organization of health services as a means to improve the health of populations.

After receiving his bachelor's degree in business from the University of Notre Dame, Shortell completed a master of public health degree from the University of California at Los Angeles. Next, he received a master of business administration and a doctoral degree in behavioral science from the University of Chicago. In 1998, Shortell became dean of the University of California, Berkeley, School of Public Health; Blue Cross of California Distinguished Professor of Health Policy and Management; and a professor of Organization Behavior at the Haas School of Business. He concurrently holds appointments in the Department of Sociology at Berkeley and the Institute for Health Policy Research at the University of California, San Francisco. For the 16 years prior to arriving at Berkeley, Shortell was A. C. Buehler Distinguished Professor of Health Services Management in the Kellogg Graduate School of Management at Northwestern University.

Over his long career, Shortell has received numerous distinguished awards for his various contributions. He received the Baxter-Allegiance Prize for innovative research and the Gold Medal from the American College of Healthcare Executives (ACHE). He was elected to the National Academy of Sciences, Institute of Medicine (IOM), in 1986 and served two terms on the Governing Council. He has served as editor-in-chief of *Health Services*

Research, president of the Association for Health Services Research, and chair of the Accrediting Commission for Graduate Education in Health Services Administration. More recently, Shortell was a fellow at the Center for Advanced Study in the Behavioral Sciences at Stanford University. He has received three "Book of the Year" awards from professional associations ranging from the American Nurses Association to the Academy of Management. The textbook Shortell wrote with Arnold D. Kaluzny is now in its fifth edition. It was one of the first textbooks written specifically for health services managers and researchers.

The extent of Shortell's accomplishments is a testament to both his keen intellect and his ready willingness to engage with others in the pursuit of knowledge.

L. Michele Issel

See also Healthcare Organization Theory; Health Services Research Journals; Hospitals; Medical Sociology; Multihospital Healthcare Systems; Physicians; Public Health; Public Policy

Further Readings

Casalino, Lawrence, Robin R. Gillies, Stephen M. Shortell, et al. "External Incentives, Information Technology, and Organized Processes to Improve Health Care Quality for Patients With Chronic Diseases," *Journal of the American Medical Association* 289(4): 434–41, January 22, 2003.

Dukerich, Janet M., Brian R. Golden, and Stephen M. Shortell. "Beauty Is in the Eye of the Beholder: The Impact of Organizational Identification, Identity, and Image on the Cooperative Behaviors of Physicians," *Administrative Science Quarterly* 47(3–4): 507–33, September 2002.

Shortell, Stephen M., Robin R. Gillies, David A. Anderson, et al. *Remaking Health Care in America: The Evolution of Organized Delivery Systems.* San Francisco: Jossey-Bass, 2000.

Shortell, Stephen M., and Arnold D. Kaluzny, eds. *Health Care Management: Organization Design and Behavior.* 5th ed. Clifton Park, NY: Thomson Delmar Learning, 2006.

Shortell, Stephen M., Jill A. Marsteller, Michael Lin, et al. "The Role of Perceived Team Effectiveness in Improving Chronic Illness Care," *Medical Care* 42(11): 1040–1048, November 2004.

Shortell, Stephen M., Julie Schmittdiel, Margaret C. Wang, et al. "An Empirical Assessment of High Performing Physician Organizations: Results From a National Study," *Medical Care Research and Review* 62(4): 407–34, August 2005.

Web Sites

University of California, Berkeley Hass School of Business Faculty Profile: http://www.haas.berkeley.edu/faculty/shortell.html
University of California, Berkeley School of Public Health Faculty Profile: http://sph.berkeley.edu/faculty/shortell.html

SHORT-FORM HEALTH SURVEYS (SF-36, -12, -8)

The Short-Form Health Survey (SF-36) is a generic, multipurpose, 36-item survey that is widely used to measure the health status of general and specific populations for a variety of purposes. Specifically, the SF-36 survey instrument measures eight health domains, including the following: general health, physical functioning, role limitations due to physical health problems, role limitations due to emotional problems, social functioning, bodily pain, vitality, and mental health. The survey is usually self-administered and takes only 5 to 10 minutes to complete. Shorter versions of the SF-36 are available. The SF-36 has been translated into dozens of languages, and its use has been documented in thousands of published studies. Applications of SF-36 include comparing and evaluating health outcomes related to specific medical treatments, estimating and/or comparing the burden of different disease states, and comparing health status over time.

Survey Development

Most of the items used in the SF-36 have evolved from other survey instruments applied over several decades, but its immediate roots can be traced to the development of a 149-item Functioning and Well-Being Profile (FWBP) developed by researchers involved in the RAND Corporation's Health Insurance Experiment (HIE) and Medical Outcomes Study (MOS). The 149 items used in the FWBP were taken and modified from a variety of other survey instruments, including the General Psychological Well-Being Inventory and the Health Perceptions Questionnaire. An initial version of the SF-36, the SF-20, was published in 1988 but received criticism for being too short and lacking sensitivity to health status changes. The SF-20 was therefore transformed into the SF-36, which has withstood considerable evaluation and scrutiny since then.

The SF-36 is currently published and coordinated by QualityMetric, Inc., a company that develops and markets patient-reported outcome instruments that measure health-related quality of life. The company publishes several manuals that contain detailed information pertaining to the survey's administration and scoring, as well as comparisons with other tools.

Due to time and cost constraints on the amount of data that can be collected for many studies, even shorter versions of the SF-36 have been developed that provide acceptable degrees of information for certain applications. The SF-12, a 12-item survey that fits on a single page, consists of a subset of the SF-36. Although it improves efficiency and lowers research costs, the shorter survey has limitations. Similarly, the 8-item SF-8 also has limitations, and it may be used in lieu of the SF-36 and SF-12.

Description and Content

The SF-36 contains 11 numbered sections, some of which have multiple items (Table 1). Each "item" is essentially a specific question; therefore, as the survey's name implies, there are 36 total questions or items that address eight health domains. Depending on needs and preferences, some variation may be applied to the scoring and analysis of the SF-36. The fundamental information provided, though, consists of two sets of scores, including eight individual domain scores and two summary scores. One summary score is calculated for the "physical health component" function and the other for the "mental health component." The physical health component summary score is derived from the physical-functioning domain, the role limitation due to

physical health domain, the bodily pain domain, and the general health domain. The mental health component summary score is derived from the general mental health domain, the vitality domain, the role limitation due to emotional problems domain, and the social-functioning domain.

All the items in the current version of the survey instrument (SF-36 Health Survey Version 2.0) have three or more Likert Scale responses (i.e., data that are categorical in nature yet have a hierarchical sequence). For example, for the question that asks how much pain the individual has experienced during the past 4 weeks, the possible ordered responses are "none," "very mild," "mild," "moderate," "severe," and "very severe." This type of question format provides more data than the older version of SF-36, which used simple "yes" and "no" responses. And the greater number of response categories in lieu of the dichotomous response options has resulted in greater measurement precision as well as a reduction in "floor" and "ceiling" effects whereby the survey instrument may fail to differentiate responses at the margins.

Although the SF-36 contains eight of the health domains most frequently used in other popular surveys, symptoms and problems connected to a specific medical condition are not included among the questions. Thus, it does not encompass content areas such as self-esteem, sleep adequacy, and cognitive functioning.

Survey Administration

The overall purpose of the SF-36 is to measure aspects of a person's health for those 14 years of age or older in a manner that is relatively comprehensive and from the individual's perspective. It is also intended to be brief. The survey instrument is designed to be self-administered, but it may also be administered through face-to-face or telephone interview. Computerized administration is also possible. When the survey is administered, individuals are not "coached," or provided with advice relative to its interpretation. Rather, instructions are limited to those printed on the survey. If any assistance is required, due to poor visual acuity, for example, it is limited to reading the survey verbatim.

Table 1   Short-Form 36 Health Survey

Your Health and Well-Being

This survey asks for your views about your health. This information will help keep track of how you feel and how well you are able to do your usual activities. *Thank you for completing this survey!*

For each of the following questions, please mark an X in the one box that best describes your answer.

1. In general, would you say your health is:

Excellent	Very good	Good	Fair	Poor
▼	▼	▼	▼	▼
☐₁	☐₂	☐₃	☐₄	☐₅

2. <u>Compared to one year ago</u>, how would you rate your health in general <u>now</u>?

Much better now than one year ago	Somewhat better now than one year ago	About the same as one year ago	Somewhat worse now than one year ago	Much worse now than one year ago
▼	▼	▼	▼	▼
☐₁	☐₂	☐₃	☐₄	☐₅

3. The following questions are about activities you might do during a typical day. Does <u>your health now limit you</u> in these activities? If so, how much?

	Yes, limited a lot	Yes, limited a little	No, not limited at all
	▼	▼	▼
a. <u>Vigorous activities</u>, such as running, lifting heavy objects, participating in strenuous sports	☐₁	☐₂	☐₃
b. <u>Moderate activities</u>, such as moving a table, pushing a vacuum cleaner, bowling, or playing golf	☐₁	☐₂	☐₃
c. Lifting or carrying groceries	☐₁	☐₂	☐₃
d. Climbing <u>several</u> flights of stairs	☐₁	☐₂	☐₃
e. Climbing <u>one</u> flight of stairs	☐₁	☐₂	☐₃
f. Bending, kneeling, or stooping	☐₁	☐₂	☐₃
g. Walking <u>more than a mile</u>	☐₁	☐₂	☐₃
h. Walking <u>several hundred yards</u>	☐₁	☐₂	☐₃
i. Walking <u>one hundred yards</u>	☐₁	☐₂	☐₃
j. Bathing or dressing yourself	☐₁	☐₂	☐₃

4. During the past 4 weeks, how much of the time have you had any of the following problems with your work or other regular daily activities as a result of your physical health?

	All of the time	Most of the time	Some of the time	A little of the time	None of the time
a. Cut down on the amount of time you spent on work or other activities	☐1	☐2	☐3	☐4	☐5
b. Accomplished less than you would like	☐1	☐2	☐3	☐4	☐5
c. Were limited in the kind of work or other activities	☐1	☐2	☐3	☐4	☐5
d. Had difficulty performing the work or other activities (for example, it took extra effort)	☐1	☐2	☐3	☐4	☐5

5. During the past 4 weeks, how much of the time have you had any of the following problems with your work or other regular daily activities as a result of any emotional problems (such as feeling depressed or anxious)?

	All of the time	Most of the time	Some of the time	A little of the time	None of the time
a. Cut down on the amount of time you spent on work or other activities	☐1	☐2	☐3	☐4	☐5
b. Accomplished less than you would like	☐1	☐2	☐3	☐4	☐5
c. Did work or other activities less carefully than usual	☐1	☐2	☐3	☐4	☐5

6. During the past 4 weeks, to what extent has your physical health or emotional problems interfered with your normal social activities with family, friends, neighbors, or groups?

Not at all	Slightly	Moderately	Quite a bit	Extremely
☐1	☐2	☐3	☐4	☐5

7. How much bodily pain have you had during the past 4 weeks?

None	Very mild	Mild	Moderate	Severe	Very Severe
☐1	☐2	☐3	☐4	☐5	☐6

8. During the past 4 weeks, how much did pain interfere with your normal work (including both work outside the home and housework)?

Not at all	A little bit	Moderately	Quite a bit	Extremely
☐1	☐2	☐3	☐4	☐5

Table 1 (Continued)

9.   These questions are about how you feel and how things have been with you <u>during the past 4 weeks</u>. For each question, please give the one answer that comes closest to the way you have been feeling. How much of the time during the <u>past 4 weeks</u>...

	All of the time	Most of the time	Some of the time	A little of the time	None of the time
	▼	▼	▼	▼	▼
a. Did you feel full of life?	☐1	☐2	☐3	☐4	☐5
b. Have you been very nervous?	☐1	☐2	☐3	☐4	☐5
c. Have you felt so down in the dumps that nothing could cheer you up?	☐1	☐2	☐3	☐4	☐5
d. Have you felt calm and peaceful?	☐1	☐2	☐3	☐4	☐5
e. Did you have a lot of energy?	☐1	☐2	☐3	☐4	☐5
f. Have you felt downhearted and depressed?	☐1	☐2	☐3	☐4	☐5
g. Did you feel worn out?	☐1	☐2	☐3	☐4	☐5
h. Have you been happy?	☐1	☐2	☐3	☐4	☐5
i. Did you feel tired?	☐1	☐2	☐3	☐4	☐5

10.   During the <u>past 4 weeks</u>, how much of the time has your <u>physical health</u> or <u>emotional problems</u> interfered with your social activities (like visiting friends, relatives, etc.)?

All of the time	Most of the time	Some of the time	A little of the time	None of the time
▼	▼	▼	▼	▼
☐1	☐2	☐3	☐4	☐5

11.   How TRUE or FALSE is <u>each</u> of the following statements for you?

	Definitely true	Mostly true	Don't know	Mostly false	Definitely false
	▼	▼	▼	▼	▼
a. I seem to get sick a little easier than other people	☐1	☐2	☐3	☐4	☐5
b. I am as healthy as anybody I know	☐1	☐2	☐3	☐4	☐5
c. I expect my health to get worse	☐1	☐2	☐3	☐4	☐5
d. My health is excellent	☐1	☐2	☐3	☐4	☐5

THANK YOU FOR COMPLETING THESE QUESTIONS!

QualityMetric, Inc., the Medical Outcomes Trust (MOT), and the Health Assessment Laboratory (HAL) are co-copyright and trademark holders of the SF-36, -12, and -8 surveys. Use of them requires a commercial license or permission for use in scholarly research.

When using the SF-36 to measure health status repeatedly over time, the standard form is designed for a 4-week recall. An acute (1 week) recall version is also available when it is desirable to measure health status weekly or biweekly. The 1-week recall version is more sensitive to recent changes in health status than the standard 4-week recall version. The 1-week recall form was created by changing the words "in the past four weeks" to "in the past week" in the health domain questions for which this is applicable.

Scoring the Survey

As with many other survey instruments, although the raw recorded data may appear straightforward initially, there are important considerations, and choice of analysis method may depend on the specific applications. There are many considerations, including whether health status is being compared among different populations or within the same population over time. Detailed manuals are best consulted for in-depth explanations and scoring options. Computer software is also available to assist with scoring, but expertise is required nonetheless.

Fundamental to the SF-36 is that it yields eight scale scores, one for each health domain, and two summary scores, one being a physical component score (PCS) and the other a mental component score (MCS). An initial step in the process of scoring requires some transformation of the data such that "better health" is represented by consistently higher values (on the original survey form, the numeral 1 may correspond to the "best" health response or the "worst" health response). Each item is then scored on a 0 to 100 scale such that the score 0 represents the poorest health option and 100 represents the best health option. Thus, an item's answer represents the percentage of the maximum achievable score. Because the intervals in a Likert Scale are not typically proportional, an item that has five possible responses cannot simply be assigned 0, 25%, 50%, 75%, and 100%.

Instead, special weights that have been determined from Likert analyses must be used.

Domain scores are calculated by using averaging methods of the scores from each domain's relevant items. Similarly, the summary scores (i.e., the PCS and the MCS) are derived using averaging methods applied to the relevant domain scores. During the scoring process, unanswered items may simply be ignored altogether while averaging a domain's remaining items, but this can be handled in several different ways. Commercial software designed specifically for the survey instrument can be used to create imputed values to replace "missing" data if desired.

To make it easier to compare the eight domain scores, different populations, and survey results acquired using the SF-36, Version 2.0, with published results using the SF-36, Version 1.0, norm-based scoring algorithms were developed that yield standardized scores (with a mean score of 50 and a standard deviation of 10). This type of standardization allows an interpretation such that scores 0 to 49 are below average and scores 51 to 100 are above average.

Reliability and Validity

Developing an in-depth understanding of the reliability and validity of the SF-36 is complex, and assistance from someone familiar with the voluminous SF-36 literature and with expertise in survey research is desirable. Although the appropriateness of the short-form surveys must be considered in relation to specific applications, the survey instruments are generally both reliable (yield consistent results) and valid (accurately measure what is being tested). Numerous studies, using both internal consistency and test-retest methods, support the reliability of the eight health domain scores as well as the two summary measures. In particular, the physical and mental summary scores usually have exceeded median reliability coefficients. Reliability trends have been found to span many different sociodemographic groups and medical diagnoses.

Systematic comparisons of the SF-36 content validity with that of other widely used surveys show that the health domains addressed are some of the most frequently used for similar purposes. There are many different health domains, or content areas, that are used in other surveys, but the SF-36 is designed to be a nonspecific, generic health survey. Thus, it will not indicate condition-specific problems, nor should it be expected to do so, because of its general nature.

Shorter Versions of the Survey

Both the SF-12 and SF-8 were developed as shorter alternatives to the SF-36. Having these shorter survey instruments to measure health status in a manner that is reasonably as accurate as the SF-36 is frequently necessary when there is a need to also collect other information that adds to cumulative testing time.

The initial version of the SF-12 was published in 1995, and it has been widely used. It contains only 12 items extracted from the SF-36, it fits on one page, and it takes only about 2 minutes to complete. Each of the eight health domains is addressed with only one or two items. Similar to the SF-36, the SF-12 has evolved so that all items have more than just a "yes" or "no" response, and this has improved the possible conclusions from the survey. Version 1.0 of the SF-12 was developed so that two summary scores, the PCS and the MCS, could be calculated with about 90% of the accuracy of the SF-36.

The SF-8, the shortest questionnaire, has only one item for each of the eight health domains. Unlike the SF-12, the SF-8 has only one item that has the same language as the SF-36. Scores from the SF-8 can be compared directly with scores from other SF surveys. Similar to the SF-36, the SF-8 is available in 1-week and 4-week recall formats. The SF-8 has also been modified into a 24-hour recall format.

Daniel K. Roberts

See also Disability; Disease; Health; Health Indicators, Leading; Health Surveys; Measurement in Health Services Research; Quality of Life, Health Related; Ware, John E.

Further Readings

Frank-Stromborg, Marilyn, and Sharon J. Olsen, eds. *Instruments for Clinical Health-Care Research*. 3d ed. Sudbury, MA: Jones and Bartlett, 2004.
McDowell, Ian. *Measuring Health: A Guide to Rating Scales and Questionnaires*. 3d ed. New York: Oxford University Press, 2006.
Ware, John E. "Improvements in Short-Form Measures of Health Status: Introduction to a Series," *Journal of Clinical Epidemiology* 61(1): 17–33, January 2008.
Ware, John E. *SF-36 Health Survey: Manual and Interpretation Guide*. Lincoln, RI: Quality Metric, Inc., 2003.

Web Sites

Agency for Healthcare Research and Quality (AHRQ): http://www.ahrq.gov
QualityMetric, Inc.: http://www.qualitymetric.com
RAND Corporation: http://www.rand.org

SINGLE-PAYER SYSTEM

The term *single-payer system* refers to any healthcare scheme in which a sole source of funding provides payments to physicians, hospitals, laboratories, and other providers for services rendered to patients. While healthcare reform advocates often propose single-payer systems as a means to achieve universal healthcare, the terms should not be considered synonymous. Single-payer systems may serve patients grouped by government constituency (e.g., national citizens or state citizens) or by patient community. By this standard, the U.S. government currently manages several single-payer systems, including Medicare, for individuals 65 years of age and older, and the Veterans Health Administration (VHA), for eligible armed services veterans.

The payer in such a system may be a government entity or other designated insurance organization. But typically, when policy analysts refer to the United States moving to a single-payer-based healthcare system, they envision a system of national health insurance, implemented similarly to the system currently employed in Canada. Canada's national health insurance scheme works according to a federal model, with mandates and guidelines set by the national government; it is implemented and provided by the individual provincial governments. Just as in the United States, Canada's healthcare providers exist as a mix of public, private not-for-profit, and for-profit, investor-owned organizations. Approximately 70% of Canada's healthcare expenditures run through its national health insurance plan, with the remaining expenditures made up of out-of-pocket costs and supplementary private insurance payments.

Canada's system originated with provincial-level programs, starting with Saskatchewan in 1946, and some advocates have proposed a similar approach to instituting single-payer systems in the United States. To date, state legislatures have evaluated proposals for state-level single-payer systems in California, Oregon, Massachusetts, and Illinois. Of these, only one bill, the 2006 Health Care for all Californians Act, passed the state legislature, but it went down to veto by California's Governor Arnold Schwarzenegger.

Advantages

Advocates of a single-payer approach to reforming the U.S. healthcare system point to several assumed advantages, chiefly cost reductions through administrative efficiency and bargaining power; increased access to insurance and healthcare; and improved healthcare quality and outcomes.

Approximately 31% of U.S. healthcare spending goes to overhead costs and profits. In contrast, Canada's national health insurance program spends a little more than 1% of its budget on overhead, and in the United States, the federal government keeps Medicare's administrative costs to less than 4% of the total spending. U.S. hospitals devote roughly one quarter of their budgets to administration and billing, while Canadian hospitals only spend about half as much for the same functions. In theory, a single-payer system would enable these savings on a nationwide basis. Policy analysts speculate that further cost reductions would come from the bargaining power a national-sized insurance plan would have to negotiate prices with service providers, drug companies, medical-device makers, and other suppliers.

While single-payer systems need not require individual coverage, most proposals for implementing national health insurance in the United States include either mandates or strong economic incentives to include as many persons in the pool as possible. Advocates of this approach point to lower costs of entry for individuals, as

well as reduced costs for those people currently insured, by virtue of enlarging the risk pool. The resulting equality of coverage should break down many of the current barriers to care experienced in the United States, particularly by persons of lower socioeconomic status, persons at high risk for disease or injury, and other populations that have trouble securing insurance, such as the self-employed.

With the massive spending outlays on billing and administration by hospitals and other healthcare providers comes a great drain on human resources. Advocates of the single-payer approach highlight the amount of time spent by U.S. physicians dealing with insurance paperwork and bureaucracy and suggest that moving to a simplified national insurance program would free providers to spend more time with their patients, improving quality of care.

Disadvantages

Even some advocates of single-payer systems criticize the Canadian model as preserving what both they and some critics see as a problematic fee-for-service delivery model. By itself, implementing the single-payer system in the United States would do nothing to address the broader quality-of-care issues that many analysts link to fee-for-service delivery.

More specifically, opponents of single-payer systems often argue against them on broad economic or philosophical grounds that sometimes have more to do with the means than the ends of such reform proposals. But in terms of the specifics of implementing a single-payer system in the United States, critics identify some potential pitfalls: healthcare rationing, insufficient redress of healthcare inequality, illusionary cost savings, and the general repercussions of reducing competition in healthcare.

Many single-payer system plans operate on a global budget, specifying a maximum government outlay for healthcare during a given year. To remain within those budgets, countries such as Canada enforce limitations on resources, such as the number of appointments available, and on implementation of expensive technology, such as magnetic resonance imaging scanners. Opponents note that for the covered population, these limitations can result in increased waiting times for nonemergency services and noncoverage of some services readily available in third-party-payer systems.

Despite assertions that a single-payer model would address health disparities, critics point out that even in nations with single-payer-based universal coverage, serious health disparities remain. One study, for example, found that Canada's system increased access to psychiatric services for persons in higher socioeconomic groups with lower morbidity while failing to address the needs of persons in lower socioeconomic groups with greater need for care.

Opponents of single-payer models argue that the cost savings seen in existing systems do not represent true savings but actually cost-shifting from patients and payers to caregivers and vendors. In other words, if a single-payer entity negotiates the fee for a service from $1000 down to $750, the payer may "save" $250, but this transaction "charges" the provider $250, leaving the social cost the same.

Finally, critics of single-payer systems suggest that reducing competitive payment from the U.S. healthcare system will ultimately harm patients by eliminating incentives for providers to compete through lower fees, increased convenience, and innovations in products and services. These policy analysts offer examples such as Lasik surgery and fee-based telephone physician consultation as the types of services that would not emerge and thrive under a monopolistic single-payer model.

Future Implications

With growing healthcare costs, swelling ranks of the uninsured, and increased global competition, few policy analysts would argue that the U.S. healthcare system does not require some kind of intervention and reform. But like so many issues of national policy, the question of whether or not to implement a single-payer system hinges on political and philosophical questions at least as much as questions concerning its potential economic and social impact. Most opponents of a single-payer system favor market-based solutions that minimize government's role in healthcare. In many ways, single-payer versus market reforms perfectly represents the broader fault lines in American politics.

For decades, policymakers have tried to sidestep the broader questions embedded in the healthcare debate by implementing incremental changes that both expand government's role as single payer for some populations (e.g., as in Medicare Part D) and use incentives to make healthcare more like traditional markets (e.g., as in health savings accounts). But while few analysts seriously propose eliminating government's role as a payer entirely, advocates on both sides of the debate increasingly acknowledge that these incremental, balanced approaches do not yield satisfactory results. At the same time, despite a growing sense of crisis about U.S. healthcare, observers find scant evidence that the political will exists to fully embrace either approach.

Despite the growing size and power of its national government, the United States remains a federalist nation. Just as Canada's national health insurance system originated in a single province, one or more U.S. states may pass single-payer legislation and thus serve as laboratories for a single-payer experiment. Success on the state level could well lead to a national tipping point for the single-payer system or, in the event of failure, a backlash favoring market-based solutions.

Jason Rothstein

See also Cost of Healthcare; Equity, Efficiency, and Effectiveness in Healthcare; Healthcare Financial Management; Health Insurance; Health Services Research in Canada; International Health Systems; National Health Insurance; State-Based Health Insurance Initiatives

Further Readings

DeGrazia, David. "Single Payer Meets Managed Competition: The Case for Public Funding and Private Delivery," *The Hastings Center Report* 38(1): 23–33, January–February 2008.

Emanuel, Ezekiel J. "The Problem With Single-Payer Plans," *The Hastings Center Report* 38(1): 38–41, January–February 2008.

Himmelstein, David U., Steffie Woolhandler, John C. Goodman, et al. "Our Health Care System at the Crossroads: Single Payer or Market Reform?" *Annals of Thoracic Surgery* 84(5): 1435–46, November 2007.

McCormick, Danny, David U. Himmelstein, Steffie Woolhandler, et al. "Single-Payer National Health

Insurance: Physicians' View," *Archives of Internal Medicine* 164(3): 300–4, February 9, 2004.

Reinhardt, Uwe E. "Why Single-Payer Health Systems Spark Endless Debate," *British Medical Journal* 334(7599): 881, April 28, 2007.

Sharfstein, Steven S. "Some Interesting Lessons From Canada," *Psychiatric Services* 57(3): 297, March 2006.

Web Sites

American Medical Student Association (AMSA): http://www.amsa.org

National Association of Health Underwriters (NAHU): http://www.nahu.org

Physicians for a National Health Program (PNHP): http://www.pnhp.org

Single Payer Now: http://www.singlepayernow.net

SKILLED-NURSING FACILITIES

Skilled-nursing facilities play a vital role in the continuum of healthcare services, providing care in one of the most intensive healthcare settings outside hospitals. Skilled-nursing facilities meet the short-term care needs of individuals with intensive medical and rehabilitation needs or needs for hospice or respite services, and they provide more continuous long-term care for persons with disabilities, chronic conditions, and custodial care needs. For individuals with short-term care needs, skilled-nursing facilities play a transitional role in facilitating care that is less intensive than that provided in acute care settings and more intensive than care provided at home. For individuals with long-term care needs, skilled-nursing facilities provide services that may be rendered until the end of their lives.

The Nature of These Facilities

A skilled-nursing facility is a specific category of nursing home. A nursing home is defined as an establishment of three or more beds that provides individual care and services to the aged, infirm, and chronically ill. Nursing homes are licensed institutions that have the option to pursue additional certification as skilled-nursing facilities. Nursing homes without skilled-nursing facility certification provide a less intensive, custodial level of care. Skilled-nursing facilities may be either independent, freestanding facilities or distinct units within a larger nursing home, hospital, continuing-care retirement community, or long-term care hospital.

There are approximately 15,000 skilled-nursing facilities throughout the United States. The majority of these facilities are proprietary (for-profit), followed by not-for-profit facilities, with the smallest number of facilities being government owned. Regardless of ownership, most skilled-nursing facilities are affiliated with a chain, while a smaller number are independent facilities. The majority of skilled-nursing facilities in the nation are located in the Midwest and South. And most facilities are located in metropolitan areas. The average size of these facilities is about 100 beds. Most skilled-nursing facilities are certified by both Medicare and Medicaid, although a small number of them are certified by only Medicare. Smaller facilities and those certified by only Medicare are often designated distinct units within larger institutions such as hospitals.

Problems

While the number of skilled-nursing facilities in the nation has been on the rise, the overall occupancy rate of these facilities has been declining. The decline in occupancy rate is the result of shorter lengths of stay and alternative options for care. Shorter lengths of stay are spurred by many factors, including changes in financing mechanisms and advances in medical treatment. Consumer interests, changes in financing mechanisms, and the development of various technologies are creating alternative options of care. Alternative settings to nursing facilities include the patient's home (in-home care), assisted living and supportive living facilities, and continuing care retirement communities.

Criteria for Care

Most individuals who are admitted to skilled-nursing facilities for short-term transitional needs must meet the criteria established by Medicare, private health insurance companies, and/or the states. The criteria individuals must meet under Medicare and insurance companies typically include medically necessary nursing and therapy services provided by a licensed practitioner such as a physical, occupational, respiratory, or speech therapist or a licensed, vocational, or registered nurse. These services must be ordered by a physician and initiated and executed within specific time frames. With the qualifying criteria met, Medicare will pay for services rendered in a certified skilled-nursing facility; however, this benefit is limited to 100 days and may be discontinued prior to 100 days if the individual no longer meets the qualifying criteria. Financial coverage through private health insurance companies follows similar guidelines; however, the full extent of the coverage is specific to each individual insurance policy.

Individuals may be admitted to a skilled-nursing facility and not meet the qualifying criteria for coverage through Medicare or private health insurance. They may continue to live in a skilled-nursing facility after they no longer meet the qualifying criteria for financial coverage under Medicare or private insurance. They may also no longer meet qualifying coverage because they have exhausted their coverage benefit or because they no longer demonstrate a need that qualifies them for coverage.

Qualifying criteria associated with long-term care in a skilled-nursing facility vary from state to state. The criteria may correlate to payment for skilled-nursing facility care under the individual state's Medicaid payment program. This criterion often uses two variables associated with an individual's capacity in the areas of cognition and independence. An individual is scored to have a qualifying level of cognitive impairment through the administration of various tests, such as the Folstein Mini-Mental State Examination (FMSE). Criteria that measure an individual's independence are typically scored through the Activities of Daily Living (ADL) or the Instrumental Activity of Daily Living (IADL). These tests measure an individual's level of independence in a number of categories, including bathing, grooming, ambulation, shopping, and housekeeping.

Services Provided

Skilled-nursing facilities may provide a wide range of services. These services may be organized into dedicated units within the facility or offered as standard levels of care throughout the facility. These services may include intensive nursing care associated with ventilator care; intensive rehabilitation associated with postacute, postsurgical, or neurological needs; and complex medical care emphasizing the intensive combination of both nursing and rehabilitation. These varieties of highly skilled care may be referred to as subacute care. Skilled-nursing facilities may also offer specialized services for persons with Alzheimer disease, those in need of hospice care, or persons with respite-care needs. Other services provided include education of the individual patient and family, meals, medications, social services, activities, and dietary consultation.

As skilled-nursing facilities become more competitive and occupancy rates continue to decline, they are increasingly looking toward specialization in one or more of these services, to maintain or develop a position in the marketplace.

Future Implications

Skilled-nursing facilities play an important role in the delivery of healthcare services in the nation. They provide some of the most intensive settings for medical care outside hospitals. Providing both short-term and long-term care, skilled-nursing facilities meet the transitional needs of individuals who require care between the hospital and their home. They also play an important role in the provision of long-term care for individuals who are cognitively impaired or are dependent in a significant number of activities of daily living. A number of financing mechanisms pay for care in a skilled-nursing facility; however, individuals must often meet qualifying criteria to be admitted to the facility. As the need for skilled-nursing facilities evolves, more of them are developing specialized services or units focusing on specific conditions, treatments, and services.

Kimberly R. Clawson

See also AARP; Access to Healthcare; Long-Term Care; Health Insurance; Medicaid; Medicare; Nursing Home Quality; Nursing Homes

Further Readings

Allen, James E. *Nursing Home Administration.* 5th ed. New York: Springer, 2008.

Baker, Beth. *Old Age in a New Age: The Promise of Transformative Nursing Homes.* Nashville, TN: Vanderbilt University Press, 2007.

Cowles, C. McKeen, ed. *Nursing Home Statistical Yearbook.* McMinnville, OR: Cowles Research Group, 2006.

Golant, Stephen M., and Joan Hyde, eds. *The Assisted Living Resident: A Vision for the Future.* Baltimore, MD: Johns Hopkins University Press, 2008.

Web Sites

AARP: http://www.aarp American Association of Homes and Services for the Aging (AAHSA): http://www.aahsa.org

American Health Care Association (AHCA): http://www.ahcancal.org

Centers for Medicare and Medicaid Services (CMS): http://www.cms.hhs.gov/center/snf.asp

STARFIELD, BARBARA

Barbara Starfield is an internationally recognized health services researcher who is known for her work in primary care. She has devoted much of her career to studying the role and impact of primary care on health systems and the health of populations. She is also a strong advocate for the greater use of primary care as a way to improve quality and lower healthcare costs. Many of her publications are seminal works in the field. Two of her best-known publications are *Primary Care: Concepts, Evaluation, and Policy* and *Primary Care: Balancing Health Needs, Services, and Technology.*

Born and raised in New York City, Starfield earned her bachelor's degree from Swarthmore College in 1954, her medical degree from the State University of New York (through the Health Sciences Center in Brooklyn) in 1959, and her master of public health degree from Johns Hopkins University in 1963.

Starfield has been at Johns Hopkins University for most of her career. From 1959 to 1963, she was a fellow in the pediatrics department at the university's medical school. From 1963 to 1966, she was an instructor in the pediatrics department and medical director of the pediatric medical care clinic. From 1966 to 1975, she was a professor in the department of medical care and hospitals at the university's School of Public Health. From 1975 to 1994, she was the head of the Division of Health Policy in the Department of Health Policy and Management. She is now University Distinguished Service Professor in the Department of Health Policy and Management and director of the Primary Care Policy Center at Johns Hopkins University.

Starfield is a prolific researcher and writer. She has authored or coauthored over 200 journal articles, 15 books and monographs, and 57 book chapters.

In recognition of her work, Starfield has received numerous awards and honors. She has been a member of the National Academy of Sciences, Institute of Medicine (IOM) since 1977. She received the Distinguished Investigator Award from the Association of Health Services Research in 1996 and the Baxter International Foundation Prize for Health Services Research from the Association of University Programs in Health Administration (AUPHA) in 2004. She was awarded the John G. Walsh Award for Lifetime Contributions to Family Medicine by the American Academy of Family Physicians (AAFP), and she received an honorary doctoral degree from the University of Montreal in 2005. She received the Annual Award for Excellence and Innovation and Value Purchasing from the National Business Group on Health and the Avedis Donabedian Award for Quality Improvement from the American Public Health Association in 2007.

Starfield was the cofounder and first president of the International Society for Equity in Health, a scientific society devoted to equity in the distribution of health care services.

Ross M. Mullner

See also Community Health; Equity, Efficiency, and Effectiveness in Healthcare; Physicians; Primary Care; Primary Care Physicians; Public Health; Public Policy

Further Readings

Starfield, Barbara. "Health Services Research: A Working Model," *New England Journal of Medicine* 289(3): 132–36, July 19, 1973.

Starfield, Barbara. *Primary Care: Concepts, Evaluation, and Policy.* New York: Oxford University Press, 1992.

Starfield, Barbara. *Primary Care: Balancing Health Needs, Services, and Technology.* New York: Oxford University Press, 1998.

Starfield, Barbara. "Is U.S. Health Really the Best in the World?" *Journal of the American Medical Association* 284(4): 483–85, July 2000.

Starfield, Barbara, and Leiyu Shi. "Primary Care and Health Outcomes: A Health Services Research Challenge," *Health Services Research* 42(6 pt. 1): 2252–56, December 2007.

Starfield, Barbara, Leiyu Shi, and James Macinko. "Contributions of Primary Care to Health Systems and Health," *Milbank Quarterly* 83(3): 457–502, September 2005.

Web Sites

Johns Hopkins Bloomberg School of Public Health: http://www.jhsph.edu

STARR, PAUL

Paul Starr is a noted professor of sociology and public affairs at Princeton University, where he holds the Stuart Chair in Communications and Public Affairs at the Woodrow Wilson School of Public and International Affairs. Starr was awarded the Pulitzer Prize for Nonfiction and the Bancroft Prize in American History in 1984 for his book *The Social Transformation of American Medicine.* This seminal work details the history of the nation's healthcare system over the past centuries. The book stimulated many scholars and students in history, political science, and public health to take stock of medicine's historical and future directions.

The Social Transformation of American Medicine documents the transformation of the nation's healthcare from a household service to one that has become dominated by market forces and the emergence of private medical practice. In the book, Starr details the institutionalization and professionalization of American medicine and the rise in influence of the medical profession and its authority over healthcare. He elaborates how physicians have been able to exert their control over almost every aspect of the healthcare system and how hospitals have served as the medical workshops of physicians, subsidized by various government programs. As a result of the dominance of physician control, healthcare costs have risen dramatically, and the public has become increasingly frustrated. This also has led to corporate conglomerates exerting greater influence over the burgeoning healthcare system.

Starr also authored the book *The Logic of Health Care Reform,* which advocated a national health insurance system and managed competition based on President Clinton's healthcare reform proposal. During 1993, Starr served as a senior advisor to the White House and was the chief architect of the Clinton administration's proposed healthcare reform plan. Starr laid out a variation of a managed-competition scheme to cover all Americans, regardless of employment status or pre-existing conditions, which was to be funded through employer contributions and government subsidies.

Starr has published extensively on issues in politics, American society, and domestic and foreign policy. His most recent book, *Freedom's Power: The True Force of Liberalism,* argues that modern democratic liberalism is the only viable solution to the challenges confronting our modern society. Starr also is the coeditor of *The American Prospect,* a liberal monthly magazine about politics, policies, and ideas that he cofounded in 1990 along with Robert Kuttner and Robert Reich.

Starr previously served as the project director for the Center for the Study of Responsive Law from 1971 to 1972, and he was the director of the Century Institute from 1999 to 2003. Starr was assistant professor of sociology from 1978 to 1983 and associate professor of sociology from 1983 to 1985 at Harvard University. He received his bachelor's degree in 1970 from Columbia University and a doctoral degree in sociology from Harvard University in 1978. Starr also received in 1986 an honorary Doctor of Humane Letters from the State University of New York.

Jared Lane K. Maeda

See also American Hospital Association (AHA); American Medical Association (AMA); Hospitals; Medical Sociology; National Health Insurance; Nurses; Physicians; Public Policy

Further Readings

Starr, Paul. *The Social Transformation of American Medicine: The Rise of a Sovereign Profession and the Making of a Vast Industry.* New York: Basic Books, 1982.

Starr, Paul. *The Logic of Health Care Reform.* Knoxville, TN: Grand Rounds Press, 1994.

Starr, Paul. "What Happened to Health Care Reform?" *The American Prospect* 20: 20–31, Winter 1995.

Starr, Paul. *Freedom's Power: The True Force of Liberalism.* New York: Basic Books, 2007.

Wailoo, Keith, Timothy Stoltzfus Jost, and Mark Schlesinger. "Professional Sovereignty in a Changing Health Care System: Reflections on Paul Starr's *The Social Transformation of American Medicine,*" *Journal of Health Politics, Policy, and Law* 29(4/5): 557–68, August–October 2004.

Web Sites

Princeton University Faculty Profile: http://www.princeton.edu/~starr

STATE-BASED HEALTH INSURANCE INITIATIVES

Many states in the nation, including Illinois, Maine, and Massachusetts, have created state-based health insurance initiatives to expand coverage. These state-based initiatives have incrementally expanded existing health insurance programs as well as created new programs. Their varied attempts have resulted in equally varied results and outcomes. These varied outcomes mirror the states' diverse populations and situations. Their successes have been limited by federal laws, financial constraints, and political wills.

In 2006, approximately 47 million Americans, or about one in six residents, did not any have health insurance coverage. Nationally, 15.8% of the population were uninsured, but the variation across states ranged from a low of 8.5% for Minnesota to a high of 24.1% for Texas. Individuals without health insurance receive no care, inadequate care, or care paid for by a third party such as the government, a charity, or involuntary subsidy. Inadequate healthcare often means more expensive care. Healthcare for the uninsured is often delivered after a disease has progressed, when the disease is more difficult and expensive to treat. Preventive healthcare is likely to be the first type of care that uninsured people do without. When uninsured Americans finally do receive healthcare, other citizens and businesses ultimately pay for the cost of that care.

Individuals, businesses, and governments all have incentives to create an efficient and equitable health insurance coverage system. The federal government addresses this problem through several insurance entitlements and funding mechanisms. However, the federal government programs have not been able to provide all Americans with guaranteed health insurance. The unmet cost of healthcare for these uninsured Americans then falls to local charities and governments, and these entities have tried to meet this demand.

Many states are attempting to expand healthcare coverage in spite of the continued rise in the cost of health insurance and the decline in employer-sponsored health insurance coverage. The health insurance landscape creates many challenges. The states themselves, faced with budgetary constraints, political interest groups, and federal regulations, find their attempts to provide health insurance difficult. No state has been able to provide universal health coverage. In addition to the financial and political hurdles the states must face, they must also conform to federal laws. And federal law prevents them from mandating businesses to provide health insurance benefits.

Health Services Research Issues

State-based health insurance initiatives must address three health services research issues: access, cost, and quality of care. However, access issues have been their primary focus. State-based initiatives have mainly attempted to expand health insurance coverage through improved financing (increasing state funds) and lowering the cost of health insurance premiums. Funds for these goals can come from state taxes or from federal government programs and grants.

Access

State governments can increase access to healthcare by expanding eligibility to state-sponsored health insurance (largely Medicaid and State Children's Health Insurance Programs, or SCHIP). They can encourage employee-sponsored insurance by providing subsidies to businesses that offer it or by providing premium assistance to employees who elect to take the insurance. The states can modify eligibility rules, and they also can attempt to increase access by lowering the costs of health insurance premiums. Lower health insurance premiums may increase the number of people who opt to purchase insurance.

Cost

Many states have attempted to lower the cost of health insurance by creating high-risk pools that organize high-risk individuals (individuals with preexisting medical conditions, individuals employed in small businesses, and others) into larger groups, thereby spreading the risk of insurance across the larger group of people. These high-risk pools do require higher premiums, but they provide insurance access that would otherwise not exist. The states have also provided liability protection to insurance companies (reinsurance) to limit the insurance companies' exposure from high-risk individuals' insurance claims. The states also have lowered health insurance costs by allowing decreased benefits (however, this can decrease quality). However, states have limited means to actually decrease the costs of healthcare.

Quality

Many states have attempted to increase the quality of care via expanded coverage within the state-sponsored entitlement programs or through rules mandating specific coverage benefits that insurance products must offer. Some states have set up commissions to address the quality of healthcare.

Types of State Initiatives

The individual states have taken several specific initiatives to increase health insurance coverage. These initiatives include the following: expanding eligibility for Medicaid and other federal programs, offering reinsurance, creating high-risk pools, establishing mandated and limited-benefit plans,

imposing individual mandates, allowing group purchasing arrangements, adding dependent coverage, and providing administrative assistance.

Medicaid and Other Federal Programs

Medicaid is the nation's largest health insurance program for the poor, covering over 40 million Americans. Medicaid is a joint federal-state government program. It is financed by both the federal government and the individual states. The federal government matches state spending on qualified Medicaid recipients.

Both the federal government and the states set the rules for Medicaid eligibility. The Medicaid program was created by the federal government to provide health insurance to needy members of society—impoverished families with children, the disabled, and elderly individuals. As a federal program, Medicaid is not a purely state-based coverage initiative; but the states define eligibility (within limits) and administer their own Medicaid programs. The federal government establishes some minimum and maximum eligibility criteria, but the states have some flexibility in determining who qualifies for Medicaid. Additionally, multiple waivers are available to allow the states to expand coverage beyond their historical limits. As a result, state control of the Medicaid program is the most important means for a state to provide coverage for its uninsured residents.

The states may expand Medicaid eligibility beyond the federal criteria, but matching federal funds will not be provided unless the state has a waiver for the expanded coverage. Certain groups are eligible for Medicaid, including children living under a specific federal poverty level, parents of children living under a specific federal poverty level (which differs from state to state), pregnant women below the poverty level, elderly and disabled social security insurance beneficiaries with incomes less than the poverty level, some working disabled, and Medicare buy-in groups. Other groups, if designated by the state, are allowed to be covered without special waivers. These optional Medicaid-eligible groups include some subsets of the same groups (children, parents of children, disabled, and elderly) that exceed the specific federal poverty limits—for example, children over the age of 6 who live over 100% of the federal poverty level but are still impoverished by state-set standards. Other groups, such as the medically needy, may be permissible. The federal government sets specific guidelines for these groups, but multiple avenues exist for states to try to expand coverage and still receive matching funds. The flexibility of coverage criteria results in a wide range of eligibility standards from state to state. This range of eligibility variability will likely continue to expand.

The federal Personal Responsibility and Work Opportunity Reconciliation Act of 1996, better known as the Welfare Reform Act, created options for the states to expand Medicaid. The provisions in Section 1931 of the act require states to continue to cover families with incomes below the 1996 Aid to Families With Dependent Children (AFDC) income limits regardless of whether they receive cash assistance. More important, Section 1931 gives states greater flexibility to extend eligibility to more low-income families. The states are allowed to disregard some of an individual's income or assets. By ignoring some income or assets, many additional individuals meet the federal criteria for poverty.

Federal SCHIP allows states to provide health insurance coverage to uninsured children in low-income families that are not otherwise eligible for Medicaid. The states are allowed to include children from families with higher income levels than otherwise allowable. Additional funds were designated for this program, and additional rules for copayments and benefits are allowed. The federal matching rate is higher for this program than for traditional Medicaid, but the total SCHIP funds available to all the states, in aggregate, are capped, and new funds will determine the future of this program.

The federal Ticket to Work and Work Incentives Improvement Act of 1999 provides another way to increase Medicaid eligibility. Under this law, states may permit working individuals with disabilities to maintain their Medicaid eligibility.

Another major initiative of the federal government to encourage the states to explore novel ways to expand coverage is Section 1115 of the Social Security Act. This law allows the federal government to waive certain Medicaid requirements in order to conduct pilot, experimental, or demonstration projects that expand or improve health insurance coverage.

In 2001, the Health Insurance Flexibility and Accountability Act expanded Section 1115. It encourages new comprehensive state approaches to increase the number of individuals with health insurance coverage with current-level Medicaid and SCHIP resources. However, these new initiatives cannot increase a state's federal matching funds.

Reinsurance

Reinsurance, insurance for insurance companies, provides an avenue for insurance carriers to lower their risk and therefore lower the premiums they charge. The state is likely to be the source of the reinsurance, but reinsurance can be a private enterprise that is encouraged by the state. The reinsurance is specifically created to cap the risk exposure from high-risk health insurance policies. The reinsurance premium is paid by the insurance carriers in exchange for limiting their risk. For example, maximum 1-year claims may be capped at a predetermined figure. Any claims higher than the capped amount would be covered by the state reinsurance fund. Limiting the insurance carriers' liability should entice the carriers to offer policies to higher-risk individuals, groups, or small businesses. Only a few states currently have reinsurance plans.

High-Risk Pools

High-risk pools create a source of health insurance to high-risk individuals who could otherwise not access it. The high-risk pools attempt to create an option for individuals who are the most difficult to insure—those who do not qualify for entitlement programs, have preexisting medical conditions, and do not have access to group insurance policies. The high-risk pools are state associations specifically created as a last option for health insurance. Most states have created high-risk pools. The federal Health Insurance Portability and Accountability Act of 1996 (HIPAA) requires that people leaving a group health insurance policy be able to access an individual policy. Each state sets its own premium rates (usually significantly higher than group insurance rates) and then uses specific insurance carriers to administer the health insurance. High-risk pools usually require additional funds to cover the claims expenses, as many of the covered individuals have costly healthcare needs. Most states view high-risk pools as a last resort and establish strict guidelines on accessing them to encourage individuals to seek other options first.

Mandated and Limited-Benefit Plans

State legislatures require health insurance policies to offer specific benefits. Each state has its own list of mandated benefits. Most of these mandated benefits are essential and needed safeguards, while a few of the mandates emerged as reactions to isolated public events. These mandates generally increase the quality of healthcare, but they also increase overall healthcare expenses. In an attempt to make health insurance more affordable, and thereby increase coverage, many states have allowed (and/or encouraged) insurance carriers to offer bare-bones policies. These policies usually suspend the state mandates and frequently offer a reduced set of healthcare benefits, such as catastrophic coverage only.

Several states have limited-benefit plans, but their effectiveness in expanding coverage has been small. The limited-benefit plans tend to be only slightly less expensive than comprehensive plans; they do not sell well, and insurance companies do not like to market them. Additionally, when individuals who previously had a comprehensive plan purchase limited-benefit plans, many of them actually reduce their health coverage, creating an unintended effect.

Individual Mandates

Individual mandates require individuals to obtain health insurance coverage. Presumably a financial penalty (added to an individual's state tax obligation) would ensue for those failing to obtain health insurance. Individual mandates have been passed by a few state legislatures, but they have not been effective. Impoverished or low-income individuals, those most likely to be uninsured, do not generally pay state income taxes.

Group Purchasing Arrangements

Group purchasing arrangements are small groups or individuals who join together to purchase health insurance. The goal is to create a large group that can qualify for lower health insurance premiums. Group purchasing arrangements can be formed outside state governments, but many states have organized these groups to facilitate individual purchase of health insurance. Little evidence exists, however, that these groups actually have access to less expensive health insurance.

Dependent Coverage

Dependent coverage allows minors to receive health insurance through their parent or guardian. Young people older than 18 years often go without health insurance. Several states have changed laws to allow these individuals to continue qualifying for dependent coverage past age 18 and school enrollment. These arrangements are quite effective as the dependent coverage can be reasonably priced and involves no expense for the states.

Administrative Assistance

Some states encourage their residents to access health insurance by providing various kinds of administrative assistance. For some states, this means offices to enroll residents in Medicaid, but for other states the assistance can be quite extensive. Some states attempt to find private insurance or offer additional state financial benefits for individuals who use local government medical services.

Federal Limits on State Power

The federal Employee Retirement Income Security Act (ERISA) of 1974 created employer mandates for health insurance coverage. This federal law sets guidelines for companies offering health insurance coverage. The states may not pass laws with additional health benefit rules for specific companies. As a result, no state can expand health insurance coverage by placing the burden on business enterprises. However, the states are allowed to raise revenues from businesses and individuals to pay for state health insurance coverage schemes. Several states have implemented "play or pay" laws that force businesses to pay additional taxes if they do not provide additional state-mandated coverage. These laws seem to be allowable by the courts if the businesses are given a real option between the tax and employer-sponsored insurance. If the tax poses a choice that is not much better than providing employer-sponsored insurance, it is unlikely to be considered legal under ERISA.

Future Implications

Increased globalization and the competitive economy are pushing many companies to decrease employer-sponsored health insurance. Without a national health insurance program, the states are being forced to develop expanded coverage systems. The states have implemented and proposed a wide variety of health coverage initiatives. State-based coverage initiatives have explored a range of proposals, but no state has successfully eliminated the problem of the uninsured. Many proposals are being tested, and many remain to be explored. As some states are finding ways to expand coverage, other states may follow their lead.

Richard A. Guthmann

See also Access to Healthcare; Economic Barriers to Healthcare; Employee Retirement Income Security Act (ERISA); Health Insurance; Health Insurance Coverage; Medicaid; Public Policy; Uninsured Individuals

Further Readings

Coughlin, Teresa A., and Stephen Zucherman. "State Responses to New Flexibility in Medicaid," *Milbank Quarterly* 86(2): 209–40, June 2008.

Hackey, Robert B., and David A. Rochefort, eds. *The New Politics of State Health Policy.* Lawrence: University Press of Kansas, 2001.

Isaacs, Stephen L., and Steven A. Schroeder. "California Dreamin': State Health Care Reform and the Prospect for National Change," *New England Journal of Medicine* 358(15): 1537–40, April 10, 2008.

Monheit, Alan C., and Joel C. Cantor, eds. *State Health Insurance Market Reform: Toward Inclusive and Sustainable Health Insurance Markets.* New York: Routledge, 2004.

Riley, Trish, and Barbara Yondorf. *Access for the Uninsured: Lessons From 25 Years of State Initiatives.* Portland, ME: National Academy for State Health Policy, 2000.

Steinbrook, Robert. "Health Care Reform in Massachusetts: Expanding Coverage, Escalating Costs," *New England Journal of Medicine* 358(26): 2757–60, June 26, 2008.

Weil, Alan. "How Far Can States Take Health Reform?" *Health Affairs* 27(3): 736–47, May–June 2008.

Web Sites

Alliance for Health Reform: http://www.allhealth.org

Commonwealth Fund: http://www.commonwealthfund.org

Families USA: http://www.familiesusa.org

Henry J. Kaiser Family Foundation (KFF): http://www.kff.org

National Academy for State Health Policy (NASHP): http://www.nashp.org

State Coverage Initiatives (SCI): http://www.statecoverage.net

STATE CHILDREN'S HEALTH INSURANCE PROGRAM (SCHIP)

The federal Balanced Budget Act of 1997 created the State Children's Health Insurance Program (SCHIP) as part of Title XXI of the Social Security Act. SCHIP is the single largest expansion in health insurance coverage since the enactment of Medicaid in 1965. The goal of SCHIP is to increase the medical coverage of low-income, uninsured children up to the age of 19 by extending eligibility for public insurance to children in families earning too much to qualify for Medicaid yet earning too little to afford private health insurance, which generally includes families earning between 100% and 200% of the federal poverty level. The SCHIP legislation apportioned more than $40 billion in federal matching funds over 10 years beginning in FY1998. States are allowed to use these funds to expand Medicaid eligibility, develop new insurance programs, and increase outreach for children already eligible for public coverage.

Program Design

Like Medicaid, SCHIP is a joint federal-state program, though SCHIP offers states more flexibility with respect to eligibility criteria, program design, and benefits. States had three broad options for implementing SCHIP. They could expand their Medicaid programs by either increasing income eligibility thresholds or extending coverage to age groups that were not eligible for Medicaid previously, create a new separate health insurance program for children, or do both. At the time of implementation, a key argument for expanding Medicaid was that states could build on existing infrastructure for administration, enrollment, and processing of claims. The main disadvantages of this approach were the requirement of conforming to existing federal rules that some states considered burdensome as well as the effect of any negative reputation associated with Medicaid. The main argument for creating a new insurance program for children was that it would allow greater flexibility in designing a program that better met the needs of children in a particular state. However, a separate program must contend with the potentially higher costs associated with start-up and outreach.

Unlike Medicaid, the law creating SCHIP included specific provisions that mandated states to include outreach efforts as a part of their expansion. As part of this effort, states created television, radio, and print advertising campaigns to increase awareness about the programs. Toll-free information lines and Web sites were also established. In California, for example, the outreach campaign included two main components, (1) the use of community-based "application assistants" to reduce the process and outcome costs of enrolling and (2) a media campaign to increase awareness of the program and reduce the information costs of enrolling, with roughly $7 million devoted to each component in the 1st year. Nearly every state also instituted a number of administrative reforms, such as simplifying application forms and eliminating face-to-face interviews, which had previously been required of Medicaid applicants.

Another innovative aspect of SCHIP is the explicit attempt to limit the degree of substitution from private insurance in favor of public insurance, or crowd-out. The most common strategy taken by states to reduce crowd-out was the requirement that children be without health insurance coverage for some period of time (typically 3–6 months) prior to enrolling in the program. In addition, a few states used sliding-scale premium contributions for families with incomes above 150% of the federal poverty level and subsidies to encourage parents to take up employer-based health insurance coverage when it was available.

Like Medicaid, SCHIP financing features a federal matching rate for state dollars contributed to the program. The federal medical assistance percentage (FMAP) is the rate at which the federal government shares the expenditures associated with each state's Medicaid program. The FMAP formula is calculated annually and is a function of the average per capita income of the state relative to the national average. States with lower average per capita incomes receive a higher FMAP, while states with higher per capita incomes receive a lower FMAP. To encourage state participation in SCHIP, states receive an enhanced FMAP for their SCHIP expenditures. While the Medicaid FMAP ranges from 50% to 76% in FY2006, the enhanced SCHIP FMAP ranged from 65% to 83% across states.

Title XXI of the Social Security Act specifically states that children with insurance, including children with Medicaid coverage, are not eligible to enroll in SCHIP. To prevent states from shifting enrollees from Medicaid to SCHIP to take advantage of the more generous federal matching rates, the legislation requires that children who apply for SCHIP be screened for Medicaid eligibility and those found to be eligible only be enrolled in Medicaid. Because of this rule, it is possible that SCHIP "marketing" may have indirectly increased the Medicaid enrollment of children who were already eligible for but not covered by that program.

The benefit package for SCHIP enrollees was mandated to contain at least the benefits required for Medicaid recipients, though additional benefits could be added by states if they chose.

Implementation

States implemented SCHIP at various times and in various ways. Thirty-four states enacted their programs in 1998. Eleven states did so in 1997, and the remaining six states began in 1999 or 2000. Nineteen states have expanded their Medicaid programs to include SCHIP, 15 states created a separate new program, and 17 states implemented a combination of expanded Medicaid and the new program. States that implemented both Medicaid expansions and a separate SCHIP expansion were able to start these components at different times, usually expanding Medicaid eligibility first.

States differed in their initial preprogram eligibility criteria, and within states, rules tended to be more generous for younger children. Prior to SCHIP, states were required to cover children 6 years of age and under up to 133% of the federal poverty level and were allowed to expand coverage up to 185% and still receive federal matching dollars. As of 1996, several states had used their own funds to expand eligibility beyond 185% of the poverty level. Since eligibility increases were larger in states that previously had lower eligibility limits for Medicaid, the SCHIP expansions have reduced the cross-state variation in public insurance eligibility standards. Likewise, in many states, prior to SCHIP, income eligibility limits were substantially higher for younger children than for older children. By increasing income limits more for older than for younger children, the SCHIP expansions largely eliminated this within-state variation in eligibility.

Effects on Insurance Coverage

The early experience with SCHIP was fraught with some degree of anxiety that enrollment was not meeting expectations. Some of this concern might have been rooted in the ambitious nature of many state expansion plans. A large number of studies have examined the impact of SCHIP on children's health insurance coverage. Fewer studies have examined the effect of SCHIP on children's health.

The best available evidence points to a modest effect of SCHIP on the health insurance coverage of children. Studies have found that about 8% to 10% of children meeting eligibility standards for SCHIP enrolled in the new program.

Recent Developments

In 2007, SCHIP came up for reauthorization. Considerable disagreements were apparent between those who wanted to expand the income eligibility limits for the program and those who wanted to maintain the status quo with respect to the program. Several expansion bills were passed by the U.S. Congress but were vetoed by the President. Ultimately, the program was not expanded.

In December 2007, the U.S. Congress passed—and the President signed—the Medicare, Medicaid,

and SCHIP Extension Act to continue SCHIP coverage through March 2009. This legislation maintains the current federal SCHIP funding level at $5 billion a year. The bill also includes additional funds for states with projected shortfalls.

The ongoing reauthorization debate over SCHIP has created uncertainty among states regarding their programs. Several states, anticipating a lack of federal funding, are operating on contingency plans. Others have established enrollment caps and implemented more cost-sharing measures, including increasing premiums.

Anthony T. LoSasso

See also Access to Healthcare; Child Care; Crowd-Out; Health Insurance; Medicaid; Public Policy; State-Based Health Insurance Initiatives; Uninsured Individuals

Further Readings

Cousineau, Michael R., Gregory D. Stevens, and Trevor A. Pickering. "Preventable Hospitalization Among Children in California Counties After Child Health Insurance Expansion Initiatives," *Medical Care* 46(2): 142–47, February 2008.

Ewing, Mary T., ed. *State Children's Health Insurance Program (SCHIP)*. New York: Nova Sciences, 2008.

Kenney, Genevieve. "The Impacts of the State Children's Health Insurance Program on Children Who Enroll: Findings From Ten States," *Health Services Research* 42(4): 1520–43, August 2007.

Rosenbaum, Sara. "The Proxy War-SCHIP and the Government's Role in Health Care Reform," *New England Journal of Medicine* 358(9): 869–72, February 28,2008.

William, Susan R., and Margo L. Rosenbach. "Evolution of State Outreach Efforts Under SCHIP," *Health Care Financing Review* 28(4): 95–107, Summer 2007.

Web Sites

American Academy of Pediatrics (AAP): http://www.aap.org

Centers for Medicare and Medicaid Services (CMS): http://www.cms.hhs.gov

Henry J. Kaiser Family Foundation (KFF): http://www.kff.org

National Academy for State Health Policy (AASHP): http://www.aashp.org

National Conference of State Legislatures (NCSL): http://www.ncsl.org

STEVENS, ROSEMARY A.

Rosemary A. Stevens is a well-known and highly respected social medical historian. She began her career as a National Health Service (NHS) hospital administrator in Great Britain, and much of her subsequent academic work describes comparatively the orientation of healthcare in the United Kingdom and the United States. In her various scholarly works, Stevens has described how American hospitals are unique: a combination of public and private institutions that are at once charities and businesses, social welfare institutions and icons of American science, wealth, and technical achievements. This rare combination of public and private is different from hospitals in other advanced nations, especially her native United Kingdom. American hospitals have little concern with improving public health. Also, many professional healthcare organizations function largely as interest groups, jostling with others for political favors. Stevens' work is an alternative vision—one in which professionals, healthcare institutions, and government serve the public interest. She describes the American healthcare system without bitterness or anger. According to Stevens, this is how it is; it is not all bad, but it could be better.

Born in Lincolnshire, England, in 1935, Stevens attended Oxford University as an undergraduate, majoring in English literature. Later, she pursued graduate studies at Yale University, earning a master of public health degree in hospital administration and medical care in 1963 and a doctoral degree in epidemiology in 1968. After graduation, she taught at Yale University for 8 years, followed by a 2-year appointment at Tulane University. In 1979, she joined the University of Pennsylvania, where she has spent most of her career. Stevens served as chair of the department of history and sociology of science from 1980 to 1983 and again from 1986 to 1991, when she was appointed the first woman dean of the University of Pennsylvania's School of Arts and Sciences. In 2002, she moved to Cornell University. Currently, she is the DeWitt Wallace Distinguished Scholar at the Weill Cornell Medical College in New York City.

Stevens's scholarly works include *Medical Practice in Modern England: The Impact of Specialization and State Medicine* (1966) and *American Medicine and the Public Interest* (1971). In 1974, in conjunction with Robert B. Stevens, she published *Welfare Medicine in America: A Case Study of Medicaid*. This was followed by *In Sickness and in Wealth: American Hospitals in the Twentieth Century*—arguably her best-known work. Stevens organized and coedited *History and Health Policy in the United States: Putting the Past Back In*. Her most recent book, *The Public-Private Health Care State: Essays on the History of American Health Policy*, includes 17 of her essays, spanning a 40-year period, from 1961 to 2001.

Stevens has received many awards and honors. For example, she received the Robert Wood Johnson Foundation Investigator Award in Health Policy Research for the years 1998–2003. In 2003, she received the Lifetime Achievement Award from the American Association for the History of Medicine. She also has been given four honorary doctoral degrees.

Stevens has served on numerous boards and committees, including the American Board of Medical Specialties, the Educational Commission for Foreign Medical Graduates, and the Milbank Memorial Fund. She has been a member of the National Academy of Sciences, Institute of Medicine (IOM), since 1973.

Blair D. Gifford

See also Comparing Health Systems; Hospitals; International Health Systems; Physicians; Public Policy; United Kingdom's National Health Service (NHS)

Further Readings

Stevens, Rosemary A. *In Sickness and in Wealth: American Hospitals in the Twentieth Century.* New York: Basic Books, 1983.

Stevens, Rosemary A. *The Public-Private Health Care State: Essays on the History of American Health Policy.* New Brunswick, NJ: Transaction, 2007.

Stevens, Rosemary A., Charles E. Rosenberg, and Lawton R. Burns, eds. *History and Health Policy in the United States: Putting the Past Back In.* New Brunswick, NJ: Rutgers University Press, 2006.

Web Sites

University of Pennsylvania, University Archives and Records Center, Rosemary Stevens' Papers: http://www.archives.upenn.edu/faids/upt/upt50/stevensr.html

STRUCTURE-PROCESS-OUTCOME QUALITY MEASURES

Avedis Donabedian (1919–2000), a physician and professor of public health at the University of Michigan, first proposed the conceptual model of assessing the quality of healthcare using structure-process-outcome measures in the 1960s. Donabedian's model continues to be widely used for evaluating quality within healthcare. Structure measures in the model include the characteristics and traits of the healthcare providers, their tools and resources, and their physical and organizational work settings. Process measures include the set of activities that occur with and between the providers and patients. Outcome measures include the change in a patient's current and future health status due to the care he or she received. Each of these measures is discussed in more detail below, along with the methods used to obtain information, research studies using this model, and future implications.

Structure Measures

Structure measures refers to the conditions under which care is provided, with the notion that if the structure is appropriate, good-quality medical care will follow. Material resources such as adequacy of facilities and equipment are taken into consideration, as are professional and organizational resources that support and direct provision of care (e.g., staff credentials, facility-operating capacities, performance review, and fiscal organization). Donabedian's concept of structure is especially relevant for organizational learning, in terms of encompassing the more stable characteristics of the care delivery system: staffing, equipment, facilities, and the way these are organized to deliver care. It also includes formalized organizational routines, such as the process of passing patient information across shifts.

Using structure to measure the quality of care leads to relatively concrete and accessible information. Structure data are essential to system-level organizational learning and improvement. The primary limitation in using structure is that the relationship between structure and process or structure and outcomes is rarely well established.

Process Measures

Process measures of quality refer to things done to or for the patient by practitioners in the course of treatment, including clinical history taking, the appropriateness and thoroughness of physical examinations, the number and type of diagnostic tests given, and technical competence in diagnostic and therapeutic procedures such as surgery. Other process measures include preventive management, coordination and continuity of care, referral criteria, and patient education. Estimates of quality obtained through process measures are not as stable or final as those obtained from outcome measures. Many times, process measures are used to identify whether medicine was practiced properly or not. Process-of-care evaluation has several advantages. It is directly related to the practice of medicine and is relatively easy to conduct. Many diseases have established, peer-reviewed models on which to base evaluations. In addition, data can be analyzed for population studies or health delivery systems where computerized data networks are available. Such measurements provide direct indicators to the areas needing quality improvement.

Two methods are used to measure process quality: explicit and implicit review. Explicit review is based on analyzing medical care from medical records. Under ideal circumstances, the analysis should be based on a set of concrete values formulated by experts or recognized professional organizations such as the American Heart Association. The measurement criteria are developed after careful evaluation of clinical trials, cohort studies, and established practice protocols to produce evidence-based quality indicators. Explicit reviews suffer some drawbacks in that the complexity and variety of medical care makes congruency in formulating such indicators difficult, and each organization can have different criteria. Also, they can be incomplete and fail to reflect the totality of care offered to a patient, as not only physicians are involved in care. To make explicit reviews more meaningful, there is a need to identify the processes that truly improve outcomes and correlate them with clinical judgments individually and not collectively, as each person can have unique factors that can influence outcomes.

In contrast, implicit review involves a personalized, critical appraisal of the quality of care received and has no set protocols as yet. It is particularly relevant to physicians, as it takes into consideration the exigencies and limitations of the situation while administering care. Medical errors are commonly subjected to implicit reviews, which can be expensive and time-consuming. There can be significant differences in assessments between reviewers due to divergence of views in the absence of set protocols. Attempts to improve the quality of implicit reviews include the creation of standard review forms and coding criteria, aggregating scores, and making statistical adjustments for bias. Other changes include the process of simplifying the clinical factors under review to eliminate reviewer bias and the tendency to give credence to outcomes over process.

Quality improvement research suggests that process measures are more sensitive than outcome measures to differences in quality across providers and/or time. Process measures are easier to interpret, partly because accountability is clearer.

Outcome Measures

Outcome measures are the desired states resulting from care processes. Outcome measures such as recovery, restoration of function, and survival have been frequently used as indicators of the quality of medical care. Technical outcomes encompass the physical and functional aspects of care, such as the absence of postsurgical complications and the successful management of chronic conditions, while interpersonal outcomes encompass dimensions of the "art" of medicine, such as patient satisfaction with care and the influence of care on the patient's quality of life as perceived by the patient.

Outcome measures can also be divided into five broad categories: death (mortality), disease (morbidity), disability (days of disability, work loss), discomfort (pain), and dissatisfaction (patient dissatisfaction, compliance with treatment regimens, provider retention). Excessive focus on the worst outcomes, such as death and severe disability, could lead to insufficient attention to prevention of minor disabilities, discomfort, and dissatisfaction.

Theoretically, lower mortality and morbidity rates, fewer readmissions or hospitalizations, and higher quality-of-life measures are equated with better quality of care. However, blind acceptance of these statistics is not justified, as these numbers may not adequately reflect the case-mix differences in various categories of hospitals. For example, a large inner-city public hospital may treat patients with more complications, due to delays in seeking care because patients lack health insurance coverage, as compared with a suburban private hospital. To compare outcomes without accounting for these differences may lead to biased and false conclusions. Such measures act as disincentives to offering treatment to disadvantaged and more severe patients, to preserve rankings, and they also perpetuate disparities in care. There are few case-mix computerized data models available on which a fair evaluation of surgical and medical outcomes can be made. To improve quality-of-care outcomes research, it is imperative to create and use such assessment tools. In the absence of such tools, limited case-mix models are being used to judge whether quality of care was optimal at all levels: emergency department, inpatient, outpatient, and follow up.

Outcome measures can be viewed from several different perspectives, depending on the objectives of a study. Long-term, intermediate, and short-term outcomes need to be judged on different criteria. Consider, for example, patients suffering from heart attacks; for these patients, prevention of death soon after the attack is a short-term outcome involving different levels of care, while the long-term morbidity, quality-of-life, and mortality outcomes are viewed differently. Health outcomes are governed considerably by many factors outside the clinical domain, including social, psychological, environmental, socioeconomic, and personal factors, which need to be accounted for when studying health outcomes. Patients' preferences for treatment and adherence to it, their will to recover, and their assessment of quality of service are difficult to quantify, though these may significantly influence health outcomes.

Outcome measures tend to have more face validity than process measures and are more meaningful in the discussion of patient safety. Outcomes tend to be concrete, and the use of outcome measures lends itself to precise measurement where validity is rarely questioned.

The advantages of outcome measurement include the ease of measuring concrete factors such as death or functional recovery from strokes or injuries. They can be used as screening tools to indicate the areas that need process measurement to improve the quality of outcomes. The disadvantages of outcome measurement are that they tend to be focused on aggregate data rather than on individual cases. They are therefore not equipped to change individual behaviors. Second, they are retrospective, so that on-the-spot treatment decisions cannot be analyzed and changed for the better. Third, outcome measures have scant correlation to process measures in many areas, thus limiting reliance on outcome measures exclusively. Last, most patients receive care from several different physicians and facilities over their lifetimes, thus blurring the clear delineation of entry to and exit from care and the fixing of responsibility. The high costs of conducting such evaluations also act as barriers.

Several limitations exist in using outcome as a quality-of-care measure. Sometimes a particular outcome measure is irrelevant, or the outcome measure is not the most relevant measure. Factors outside medical care, such as genetic factors and personal history, can influence the outcome. Some outcomes are not clearly defined or can be difficult to measure: patient attitudes and satisfactions, social restoration, physical disability, and rehabilitation. The limitations of outcome measures do not mean that they are inappropriate indicators of quality; they just simply must be used carefully.

Sources and Methods of Obtaining Information

Patient medical records are often used for assessing the quality of healthcare. However, questions arise about how thorough or appropriate these records are as a source of information. For example, are the records complete, is the record or the care provided being rated, and should the entire record or only the abstracted information be used for evaluation purposes?

Patient medical records are often not adequate to serve as a basis for evaluation in general practice. Observation of a physician by a qualified colleague is the best alternative, though some dimensions of care are not observable and would not be included in the evaluation. The major limitation of direct observation is the change of usual practice by those who know that they are being observed.

Studying behaviors and opinions is an indirect method of obtaining information about quality. For instance, in seeking care for themselves and their families, physicians exhibit critical and valid judgments concerning the capacity of their colleagues to provide a high quality of care. An *autoreputational* approach is one in which hospital personnel (managerial, profession, and technical) and knowledgeable community members rank and rate the hospital's quality of medical care.

Patient evaluation constitutes the consumer's perspective of the quality of care. Healthcare organizations and practices exist to serve patients, and their objective is to satisfy consumer needs and aspirations to the best of their ability. Collecting patient feedback provides valuable insights into perceived shortfalls in treatment and care and is gaining increasing acceptance as a way to evaluate quality of care. Patient evaluations are also able to provide feedback on organizational shortcomings in structure and process measures, such as long waiting times, unsatisfactory clinical care, or wrong billing. Constant review of patient evaluations is helpful in initiating changes to improve the overall quality of care.

Research Studies Using the Model

Most research studies using the structure-process-outcome model examining ambulatory care have focused on structure and the process of care rather than the outcomes of care. Physician characteristics that were found to be associated with greater conformity to standards of care are length of training, primary-care specialization, practicing area of specialty training, and continuing education.

In terms of inpatient hospital care, evidence supports a volume-quality relationship; that is, mortality rates are lower in high-volume facilities. A variety of structural measures have not been conclusively associated with outcomes, including: public versus private institutions, teaching hospitals and patient satisfaction, physician capabilities (board certification, years of experience), and nurse to patient staffing ratios. Higher registered nurse staffing and years of nursing experience have been found to be associated with better postsurgical outcomes but not with mortality rates.

Studies of the association between nursing home structure and resident-care outcomes focus on capacity and capability measures. Outcome-centered studies demonstrate the lack of a consistent relationship between bed size and measures of mortality, discharge status, patient functioning, patient satisfaction, and quality of life. Registered nurse to resident ratios have been found to be associated with better physical functioning, lower mortality rates, higher likelihood of discharge back to the resident's home, and less unnecessary hospitalization.

A serious lack of information exists concerning whether structural characteristics make a difference in outcomes of home health care services.

The structure-process-outcome model is frequently used for assessing internal quality-of-care measures, which do not need to be very stringent. There is a lack of computerized systems that provide data on the continuum of care, so essential in managing chronic diseases, which now form the bulk of medical care. The use of integrated health systems that have community outreach is necessary to really assess quality outcomes in healthcare. This is now the focus of many health services researchers who are implementing such models.

Future Implications

Health services research using structure-process-outcome quality measures focuses on organizational capacity and capability. Concepts of structure and outcome are evolving as perspectives on what constitutes meaningful measures have changed.

The accrediting organizations, the government, and the general public are increasingly demanding quality and patient safety data from healthcare organizations. Clinical practice guidelines designed to capture the essence of state-of-the-art and evidence-based care have become more prevalent. And efforts to measure patient satisfaction have grown.

However, many challenges remain in identifying excellent quality of healthcare. Clinical knowledge is constantly changing; therefore, the definition of quality healthcare must evolve. Furthermore, individual patients tend to value different aspects of care. Researchers suggest broadening the current quality measurement lens, specifically incorporating patient preferences, and adding a focus on the organization. Encouraging the development and use of integrated, computerized systems that can provide data on parameters of quality of care in its continuum will likely help improve the quality of healthcare at all levels.

Karen E. Peters, Benjamin C. Mueller, Nicole E. Stoller, and Sunanda Gupta

See also Case-Mix Adjustment; Donabedian, Avedis; Evidence-Based Medicine (EBM); Joint Commission; Quality Indicators; Quality of Healthcare; Outcomes Movement; Volume-Outcome Relationship

Further Readings

Dlugacz, Yosef D. *Measuring Health Care: Using Quality Data for Operational, Financial, and Clinical Improvement*. San Francisco: Jossey-Bass, 2006.

Donabedian, Avedis. "Evaluating the Quality of Medical Care," *Milbank Memorial Fund Quarterly: Health and Society* 44(3 pt. 2): 166–203, 1966. (Reprinted in *Milbank Quarterly* 83(4): 691–729, 2005)

Glickman, Seth W., Kelvin A. Baggett, Christopher G. Krubert, et al. "Promoting Quality: The Health-Care Organization From a Management Perspective," *International Journal for Quality in Health Care* 19(6): 341–48, December 2007.

Lighter, Donald E., and Douglas C. Fair. *Quality Management in Health Care: Principles and Methods*. 2d ed. Sudbury, MA: Jones and Bartlett, 2004.

Lloyd, Robert. *Quality Health Care: A Guide to Developing and Using Indicators*. Sudbury, MA: Jones and Bartlett, 2004.

Wan, Thomas T. H., and Alastair M. Connell. *Monitoring the Quality of Health Care: Issues and Scientific Approach*. New York: Springer, 2002.

Web Sites

Agency for Healthcare Research and Quality (AHRQ): http://www.ahrq.gov

American Society for Quality (ASQ): http://www.asq.org

Institute for Healthcare Improvement (IHI): http://www.ihi.org

Joint Commission: http://www.jointcommission.org

National Quality Forum (NQF): http://www.qualityforum.org

SUBSTANCE ABUSE AND MENTAL HEALTH SERVICES ADMINISTRATION (SAMHSA)

The Substance Abuse and Mental Health Services Administration (SAMHSA) is a unit of the U.S. Department of Health and Human Services (HHS). Established in October 1992 as a result of Public Law 102–321, SAMHSA has as its statutory mission the provision of prevention and treatment services for people at risk of or suffering from mental or substance abuse disorders. SAMHSA works in partnership with states, communities, and private organizations to address the needs of people with substance abuse and mental illnesses as well as the community risk factors that contribute to these illnesses. SAMHSA's most recent strategic plan describes its vision as providing a life in the community for everyone and its operating mission as the building of resilience and facilitating recovery. A matrix of priorities based on cross-cutting principles and programs and issues delineates the overall scope of its services and program expectations.

Background

Prior to the creation of SAMHSA in 1992, the Alcohol, Drug Abuse, and Mental Health Administration (ADAMHA) was charged with both drug and alcohol research and the provision of treatment services. A study in early 1992 led to the decision to separate the research function from the treatment function to more efficiently and effectively use resources. As a result of this study, SAMHSA was created to provide treatment and mental health services, and research funding was moved to the National Institutes of Health (NIH), where two institutes—the National Institute for Drug Abuse (NIDA) and the National Institute on Alcohol Abuse and Alcoholism (NIAAA)—serve as the repositories for research into alcohol and drug abuse. A third NIH institute, the National Institute of Mental Health (NIMH), conducts and supports research on mental health and mental illnesses.

In the decade leading to the restructuring and creation of SAMHSA, efforts to use a public health model with community treatment options for mental health issues were slowly being included in state health plans for services. Efforts also evolved to move services, particularly in mental health, from institutional models to community-based care. In addition, a core value in the creation of SAMHSA was to link services more closely to the results of research models validating an evidence-based framework for service delivery.

Structure and Function

SAMHSA is organized into three centers and an office. The units are the Center for Mental Health Services (CMHS), the Center for Substance Abuse Treatment (CSAT), the Center for Substance Abuse Prevention (CSAP), and the Office of Applied Studies (OAS).

Specifically, the CMHS is charged with improving the quality of and access to mental health services, particularly for those who are underserved. The CSAT promotes the quality and availability of community-based substance abuse treatment services for individuals and families. The CSAP works with states and communities to develop comprehensive prevention systems that create healthy communities in which people enjoy a high quality of life. The OAS serves as a focal point for data collection and analysis and for dissemination of critical public health data to assist policymakers, providers, and the public in making informed decisions regarding the prevention and treatment of mental and substance abuse disorders.

The CMHS leads government efforts to treat mental illnesses by promoting mental health and by preventing the development or the worsening of mental illnesses if at all possible. The center currently has initiatives in the areas of adults with severe mental illnesses, including those who are homeless; services to children and adolescents; emergency mental health and traumatic stress services; and work with jail and prison populations. It also works collaboratively with the other two SAMHSA centers to study the impact of managed care on services to individuals with substance-abuse-related needs. Public health education, advocacy, and data collection and analysis round out the scope of initiatives that are the primary responsibility of the center.

The CSAT works with states and community-based groups to improve and expand existing substance abuse treatment services under the Substance Abuse Prevention and Treatment Block Grant Program. The center supports a free treatment referral service to link people with the community-based substance abuse services they need. Programs and initiatives supported by the center embrace the philosophy that treatment and recovery work best in a community-based, coordinated system of comprehensive services. This philosophy is based on research and a consensus of experts in the addiction-care field. The center also supports the nation's effort to provide multiple treatment modalities, evaluate treatment effectiveness, and use evaluation results to enhance treatment and recovery approaches so as to reach the greatest number of individuals in need of services.

The CSAP provides leadership in the federal effort to prevent alcohol, tobacco, and other drug problems. The center has developed a model for prevention called the Strategic Prevention Framework (SPF), which aims to promote youth development, reduce risk-taking behaviors, build assets and resilience, and prevent problem behaviors across the individual's life span. The SPF is a five-step process—assessment, capacity, planning, implementation, and evaluation—and is designed to create sustainable and culturally relevant prevention services. Programs supported by the center's funds must use the SPF and be based on or adapted from recognized model programs.

Last, the OAS is responsible for providing data to the public related to the incidence of alcohol and drug use, drug-related emergency department treatment and deaths, and the treatment network of services. The data provided help support planning and budget efforts and validate the outcomes of efforts by SAMHSA-funded programs.

Linda F. Samson

See also Disease; Epidemiology; Mental Health; Mental Health Epidemiology; Pharmacy; Prescription and Generic Drug Use; Public Health; Vulnerable Populations

Further Readings

Center for Mental Health Services. *Developing a Stigma Reduction Initiative: Event Planning, Partnership Development, Outreach to Schools and Businesses, Mental Health Resources, Marketing to the General Public, Grassroots Outreach.* Rockville, MD: U.S. Department of Health and Human Services, Substance Abuse and Mental Health Services Administration, Center for Mental Health Services, 2007.
Colliver, James D. *Misuse of Prescription Drugs: Data From the 2002, 2003, and 2004 National Survey on Drug Use and Health.* Rockville, MD: U.S. Department of Health and Human Services, Substance Abuse and Mental Health Services Administration, Office of Applied Studies, 2006.
Office of Applied Studies. *Drug Abuse Warning Network, 2004: National Estimates of Drug Related Emergency Department Visits.* Rockville, MD: U.S. Department of Health and Human Services, Substance Abuse and Mental Health Services Administration, Office of Applied Studies, 2006.

Web Sites

National Clearinghouse for Alcohol and Drug Information (NCADI): http://ncadi.samhsa.gov
Substance Abuse and Mental Health Services Administration (SAMHSA): http://www.samhsa.gov

SUPPLIER-INDUCED DEMAND

Traditional economic theory assumes that the market for health services is characterized by an upward-sloping supply curve and a downward-sloping demand curve. Patients are assumed to be rational consumers who make informed utility-maximizing choices, while physicians are profit maximizers. The theory predicts that an excess supply of physicians in relation to the population will result in an outward shift of the physician supply curve, lower fees charged for services, and lower revenues. To avoid the loss of revenues, most economists believe that physicians exploit the information asymmetry (a result of patients' lack of clinical knowledge) in the market for their services and shift the demand curve up, resulting in higher revenues. This phenomenon is termed supplier-induced demand. It occurs when a physician has a financial incentive to recommend treatments whose medical benefits are outweighed by the costs. Supplier-induced demand is equated with unethical behavior because of the social welfare loss associated with inefficient treatment. Due to the prominent role physicians play in the healthcare industry, cost control measures will be difficult to implement under supplier-induced demand. By studying this phenomenon, policymakers will be able to design and develop relevant tools to minimize waste and improve access to healthcare.

Traditional economic theory predicts that when physicians have mixed patient caseloads (Medicare, Medicaid, and privately insured patients), a decrease in the fees charged to Medicare and Medicaid patients will result in substitution and income effects. Under the substitution effect, physicians will reduce their Medicare patient caseload and treat more privately insured patients. The income effect will result in the delivery of more services to both the Medicare and the privately insured patients to make up the income lost from the reduction in fees paid by Medicare patients. The observed increase in services to privately insured patients is consistent with both physicians' profit-maximizing behavior and demand inducement.

Why is demand inducement an interesting problem for economists to study? In addition to the waste involved, the existence of demand inducement contradicts the predictions of neoclassical economic theories of demand and supply, where the excess supply of physicians should lead to fee reductions. Proponents believe that if the market does not work as expected for physician services, the practitioners must be inducing demand. While this observation may be true, it does not consider the uncertainties involved in medical decision making.

The Demand Inducement Literature

Under the competitive model, physicians are expected to be perfect agents for their patients and should not induce demand for personal financial gains. An increase in physician density relative to population must result in decreased fees and utilization. Researchers have investigated the impacts of physician density, fee changes, physician monopoly power, and target income on the existence of supplier-induced demand.

Impact of Physician Density on Demand Inducement

The evidence of demand inducement using physician density has been ambiguous. Most of the researchers did not control for quality in their studies. If physician density increases, physicians could respond to market competition by differentiating the services delivered based on quality. Under normal circumstances, quality of care is an increasing function of time spent per patient during visits. Patients who value quality must be willing to pay more for higher-quality care. Using time per patient visit as a proxy for quality care, some researchers found that physicians react to increased competition by increasing the time spent per patient visit. Patients were also willing to pay more for longer time spent during visits. This result is attributable to improvements in the quality of care under competition rather than demand inducement. One study found that as the number of competing physicians increases in a given location, fees decline if quality is not controlled for. However, physicians reduce the time spent seeing Medicaid patients (substitution effect) when there is increased competition, while spending more time with the privately insured patients. In general, to survive in physician-dense areas, providers must deliver higher-quality care at higher fees and earnings per patient. This evidence is consistent with nonprice (quality) competition and does not necessarily reflect demand inducement.

Impact of Fees on the Supply of Services

An alternative method of testing for demand inducement relies on the relationship between the fees paid to physicians and the supply of services. Traditional economic theory predicts that when payments to physicians are reduced, they should not induce or create unnecessary demand in order to maintain their previous income levels. Supply of services must be reduced as predicted by the competitive-market model (upward-sloping supply curve). Here too, the evidence on demand inducement according to physician payments has been mixed. One study found that when California froze Medicaid payments in the early 1970s, physicians reacted by increasing the quality of services delivered. The same evidence of demand inducement was found among physicians in urban areas of Colorado in response to Medicare fee reductions. Health services researchers also found that Canadian physicians responded to slow raises in physician payments by increasing the quantity and intensity of the services they delivered. However, other researchers using Canadian data found no significant relationship between fees and the utilization of certain medical procedures. The major critique of using fee reductions to test demand inducement is that fee reductions simultaneously result in lower patient copayments. A utility-maximizing consumer must react to reduced out-of-pocket payments by increasing service utilization.

The physician is assumed to be a utility maximizer where utility is a function of income. However, if leisure is an additional argument in the physician's utility function, the joint optimization of income and leisure will result in a backward-bending supply curve. This implies that depending on the level of fees, payment reductions could lead to increased delivery of services. Therefore, the evidence from using physician payments to test demand inducement is consistent with both supplier-induced demand and predictions of traditional economic theory. It is likely that physicians, acting as agents, make their decisions based on their assessment of patients' utility from treatment. The uncertainty involved in physicians' assessment of patients' utility from treatment may explain some of the lack of consensus in clinical decision making.

After controlling for fees, income, gender, and other socioeconomic factors, some researchers found a wide variation in the use of well-known medical procedures between small geographic locations. For example, in some studies, the actual variation exceeded the predicted utilization of total hip replacement by a factor of 110%; and in the case of colonoscopy, the actual variation exceeded the predicted utilization by 2,000%. The argument is that practice patterns may not strictly reflect an established set of well-defined clinical guidelines. These patterns may instead depend on the multiplicity of factors that influence clinical decision making, such as training, peer behavior, location, conference attendance, direct-to-consumer advertising, use of the Internet by patients, personal temperament and experience, financial incentives, time, age, and infrastructural capacity. Without a clear appreciation of the uncertainties involved in medical decision making, it will be inappropriate to base cost-control or reimbursement policies on the estimated magnitude of demand inducement.

Target Income and Monopoly

The target income hypothesis postulates that physicians use their monopoly power to induce demand in order to satisfy a predetermined target income. Physicians are capable of exercising monopoly power because reputation, location, treatment style, patient preferences, and payment types combine to produce strong bonds among patients and their physicians. These bonds make it difficult for patients to easily substitute one physician for another and provide physicians with some degree of monopoly power. The target income hypothesis implies that an individual physician's behavior may be influenced by relative income. When physician density relative to population increases, physicians may exercise monopoly power by increasing their fees to achieve a target income. Since insured consumers pay only a small fraction of the cost of their treatment, physicians can raise prices without losing their patients. This behavior is aided by the fact that medical care is a credence good, where the utility impact is difficult to ascertain even after consumption. Reputation and price are possible indicators of quality for credence goods. Physicians with established reputations can exercise monopoly power and raise fees and utilization. Critics of the target income hypothesis argue that it has no foundation in economic theory. In addition, it is not known how these targets are set. Results of studies of the effects of target income on physician pricing decisions are mixed.

Future Implications

Studies aimed at identifying supplier-induced demand have resulted in contradictory or mixed results. Critics of these studies have based their arguments on the misspecification of the econometric models used in many of them. The outcomes from these studies can oftentimes be justified by supplier-induced demand behavior, rational utility, and profit maximization models and by uncertainties in medical decision making. The only study that controlled for quality found that when physician density in relationship to population increases, physicians react by differentiating their products based on quality improvements.

Few studies have addressed the uncertainties involved in medical decision making. Is there a set of gold standard guidelines that physicians have to strictly adhere to under all circumstances? If a physician's treatments deviate from the guidelines, is he or she necessarily a biased and unethical agent? Under supplier-induced demand, physicians recommend treatments whose benefits are outweighed by the costs. Medical decision making is characterized by uncertainty, and practice patterns reflect economic and noneconomic factors, including motivation, judgments, altruism, and professionalism. Therefore, there will be significant variability in observed treatment patterns and outcomes based partly on noneconomic factors. Health services researchers have documented wide variances in outcomes within specific locations after controlling for socioeconomic factors.

It has been proposed that an alternative test of the availability of supplier-induced demand is to observe the health services utilization of well-informed patients, namely, physicians. However, the findings by some researchers that physicians and their families do not use fewer medical services than their patients suggest that physicians also self-induce demand. If inducement is for private gains, then this result contradicts the accepted definition of supplier-induced demand. The ambiguity in supplier-induced demand research suggests that physicians, so as to do the best for their patients and themselves based on their medical knowledge, may overtreat or consume excessive amounts of medical services. While some physicians may exploit the gap in information for private gains, there is little evidence that this behavior is pervasive.

Membership in social networks embedded in healthcare-purchasing groups, as well as health literacy education, may diminish the information asymmetry between physicians and patients and lead to more optimal utilization of health services. Future research on supplier-induced demand must include the factors that motivate physicians to deliver excessive healthcare services to their patients. Governments should not base cost-control policies on the concept of supplier-induced demand without understanding the uncertainties involved in medical decision making. In addition, governments must control direct-to-consumer advertising of drugs to prevent consumer-induced demand from being a confounding factor in supplier-induced demand research.

Edward Mensah and Dennis Cesarotti

See also Cost of Healthcare; Healthcare Markets; Health Economics; Health Insurance; Market Failure; Moral Hazard; Physicians; Public Policy

Further Readings

Carlsen, Fredrik, and Grytten Jostein. "Consumer Satisfaction and Supplier Induced Demand," *Journal of Health Economics* 19(5): 731–53, September 2000.

Peacock, Stuart, and Jeffrey Richardson. "Supplier-Induced Demand: Re-Examining Identification and Misspecification in Cross-Sectional Analysis," *European Journal of Health Economics* 8(3): 267–77, September 2007.

Rice, Thomas H. *The Economics of Health Reconsidered.* 2d ed. Chicago: Health Administration Press, 2002.

Van de Voorde, Carine, Eddy Van Doorslaer, and Erik Schokkaert. "Effects of Cost Sharing on Physician Utilization Under Favorable Conditions for Supplier-Induced Demand," *Health Economics* 10(5): 457–71, July 2001.

Xirasagar, Sudha, and Herng-Ching Lin. "Physician Supply, Supplier-Induced Demand and Competition: Empirical Evidence From a Single-Payer System," *International Journal of Health Planning and Management* 21(2): 117–31, April–June 2006.

Web Sites

American Economic Association (AEA): http://www.vanderbilt.edu/AEA
American Society of Health Economists (ASHE): http://healtheconomics.us
International Health Economics Association (iHEA): http://www.healtheconomics.org

T

TARLOV, ALVIN R.

Alvin R. Tarlov is a physician, educator, and researcher whose vision and leadership have influenced physician workforce structure and training, thinking about what constitutes effectiveness in healthcare, and theory and research on the relationships between and among health and its multiple determinants.

Tarlov earned a bachelor's degree at Dartmouth College (1951) and a medical degree from the University of Chicago (1956). He completed a residency in Internal Medicine at the University of Chicago and spent 5 years conducting hematologic research.

Tarlov joined the faculty of the University of Chicago in 1964. As chairman of the Department of Medicine (1968–1981), he established the first academic division of general internal medicine in the country to address the growing problem of fragmented medical care caused by overspecialization of the physician workforce. In 1978, the Secretary of the U.S. Department of Health Education and Welfare appointed Tarlov chairman of the Graduate Medical Education National Advisory Committee (GMENAC) to advise the secretary on the most desirable number, specialty distribution, and geographic placement of physicians in each specialty. GMENAC's report stirred controversy because it refuted the commonly held belief that the geographic maldistribution of physicians and the poor health of large segments of the population could be effectively addressed by increasing the physician supply.

Struck by the lack of evidence comparing the effectiveness of medical specialists, surgical specialists, and generalists in treating specific conditions, Tarlov cofounded the Medical Outcomes Study to develop and apply measures of patients' functional capacity, well-being, and quality of life as the principal indicators of the effectiveness of medical services. This work became a bellwether in health services research as it led to a paradigm shift in thinking about the aims of medical care, the establishment of outcomes as the centerpiece of health services research, and spawned new fields of inquiry, including methodological research on functional status and quality-of-life measurement.

As President of the Henry J. Kaiser Family Foundation in Menlo Park, California (1984–1990), Tarlov developed a national program on community-based health education and disease prevention. Questioning the assumption that the substandard health of disadvantaged Americans could be explained by inadequate access to medical care, Tarlov began an interdisciplinary collaboration with sociologists, economists, psychologists, neuroscientists, and other scholars to explore the question of how social factors influence health. He convened an international conference on the social determinants of health, which led to the first book published on this topic.

Moving to Boston, Tarlov was appointed professor of medicine at Tufts University and professor of health promotion at the Harvard School of Public Health (1990–1999). He was director of The Health Institute at the New England Medical Center, devoted to research on the outcomes of medical care and on the relationship of societal characteristics to population health. At Harvard University, he was chairman of the Mind/Brain/Behavior Society and Health Interfaculty Initiative. During this time, he developed and published a theoretical framework to describe the relationship between social inequality and social, psychological, and biological responses.

Tarlov served as director of the multiuniversity Texas Program for Society and Health in Houston (1999–2005) where he also was a professor in the University of Texas School of Public Health, professor of medicine at the Baylor College of Medicine, and Sid Richardson and Taylor and Robert H. Ray Senior Fellow in Health Policy at the James A. Baker III Institute for Public Policy, Rice University. While there, he received three statewide awards from community organizations in Texas for contributions to public policies to enhance early-childhood development and education.

Tarlov is a former Markle Foundation Scholar and National Institutes of Health (NIH) Research Career Development Awardee. He served as president of the Association of Professors of Medicine. He was elected to the national Institute of Medicine (IOM) and selected a master of the American College of Physicians. In 1992, Tarlov received from the Society for General Internal Medicine the Robert Glaser Award for Distinguished Contributions to the Advancement of General Internal Medicine. He was named Distinguished Internist of 1997 by the American Society of Internal Medicine. In May 2000, he was made an honorary fellow of University College London.

Tarlov, who is currently a professor of medicine at the University of Chicago, is completing as editor a book examining the evidence that public investment in early childhood development has greater promise and cost-effectiveness for improving population health, reducing health disparities, enhancing human capital formation, and promoting economic development than other public policy interventions designed for those purposes.

Elizabeth Tarlov

See also Health Disparities; Health Workforce; Kaiser Family Foundation; Outcomes Movement; Primary-Care Physicians; Public Policy; Short-Form Health Surveys (SF-36, -12, -8)

Further Readings

Amick, Benjamin, Sol Levine, Alvin R. Tarlov, et al., eds. *Society and Health.* New York: Oxford University Press, 1995.

Read, Jennan, Michael Emerson, and Alvin Tarlov. "Implications of Black Immigrant Health for U.S. Racial Disparities in Health," *Journal of Immigrant Health* 7(3): 205–212, July 2005.

Public Health Service, Health Resources Administration. *Report of the Graduate Medical Education National Advisory Committee,* Alvin R. Tarlov, Chairman, to the Secretary, Department of Health and Human Services. 7 vols. Washington, DC: Health Resources Administration, September 1980.

Tarlov, Alvin R. "Social Determinants of Health: The Socio-Biological Translation," In *Health and Social Organization: Towards a Health Policy for the 21st Century,* edited by David Blane, Eric Brunner, and Richard Wilkinson, 71–93. London: Routledge, 1996.

Tarlov, Alvin R., John E. Ware, Jr., S. Greenfield, et al. "The Medical Outcomes Study: An Application of Methods for Monitoring the Results of Medical Care," *Journal of the American Medical Association* 262(7): 925–30, August 18, 1989.

TAX SUBSIDY OF EMPLOYER-SPONSORED HEALTH INSURANCE

One explanation for the structure of health insurance in the United States is the federal tax code. The nation's tax code excludes from taxation compensation received by employees in the form of employer-sponsored health insurance. This implicit subsidy encourages people to purchase insurance through their employers and to buy more health insurance coverage than they otherwise would. Thus, the tax treatment encourages both broader and deeper coverage by individuals. A case can also be made that the tax treatment, by encouraging generous health insurance coverage, increases healthcare utilization and prices. This leads to higher health insurance premiums and to many people forgoing private health insurance coverage.

History

Private health insurance in the United States essentially began with the Great Depression and grew through the 1930s and into the early years of World War II. However, the federal tax code was silent on whether employer-provided health insurance was to be considered income that was subject to income tax. Employers increasingly used health insurance as a means of attracting and paying scarce workers during the war years. In 1943, the Internal Revenue Service (IRS) issued a private ruling holding that employer-sponsored health insurance benefits were not subject to federal income or payroll taxation. Over the years, a series of contradictory private rulings emerged, and in 1954, the U.S. Congress passed legislation making employer-sponsored coverage exempt from federal income taxes. With the enactment of Medicare in 1965, the exemption was expanded. The states have also followed the federal lead in the definition of income subject to state income taxes and similarly exclude employer-sponsored health insurance.

Impact of the Exclusion

The tax exclusion of employer-sponsored health insurance is not a trivial matter. It was estimated that in 2006, the combined federal and state income tax and federal payroll tax exclusions reduced tax collections by $208.6 billion. Nearly 54% were the result of exclusion from the federal income tax, and more than 35% were from the exclusion of Social Security and Medicare payroll taxes. To put these values in context, in 2006, total Medicare spending was $402 billion. The tax subsidy for employer-sponsored health insurance is slightly over one half as much as was spent on Medicare.

The tax exclusion provides strong incentives for workers and their employers to shift the form of employee compensation. From the employer's perspective, the tax exclusion is largely irrelevant. Whether the employer compensates its employees with money wages or with health insurance, both are legitimate business expenses, and both are deducted from revenue before computing the employer's tax liability.

From the worker's perspective, the form of compensation matters. Consider a single individual, who after claiming one exemption and taking the standard deduction has a taxable income of $45,000. Under the federal tax laws and assuming

a 5% state income tax, the individual faces a marginal tax rate of 32.64%. That is, on the last $100 earned, the individual owes combined taxes of $32.64. Suppose that instead of taking all the compensation as money income, the individual took some as employer-sponsored health insurance. For every $100 of coverage the individual took through his or her employer, the individual would reduce the tax liability by $32.64. Stated another way, the $100 of insurance coverage effectively cost the individual only $67.36. If the individual had taken the average insurance bundle offered to insured workers in 2006, he or she would have effectively "purchased" $4,248 worth of coverage for only $2,860.60. The individual can be viewed as purchasing the coverage because he or she gave up money wages that would otherwise have been received as compensation for labor.

It is worth noting that this example is in no way extreme. It is estimated that the average tax subsidy for employer-sponsored health insurance is approximately 35% of the premium.

The tax subsidy for employer-sponsored health insurance provides incentives for people to buy insurance coverage that they otherwise might have ignored. They would do this by seeking out jobs that offered health insurance and lower wages rather than just higher wages. In addition, the tax subsidy provides incentives for people to take jobs that offer more generous health insurance packages than would otherwise be the case. They might do this by seeking out employers who offer better benefits or by encouraging their employers to expand the health benefits offered.

Empirical Evidence

A number of studies have attempted to estimate the effects of differences in tax rates on the prevalence and generosity of employer-sponsored health insurance. The difficulty is in marshalling data that contain information on the relevant household tax rate and the nature of the coverage available.

One study, by Jonathan Gruber and Michael Lettau, provides the most exhaustive analysis to date. It used wage and nonwage compensation data from the 1983 to 1995 Bureau of Labor Statistic's Employment Cost Index (ECI), augmented with data on individual workers from the Bureau of the Census's Current Population Survey

(CPS) and data on family taxes from the Department of the Treasury's Statistics of Income (SOI). The ECI provided information on some 203,000 jobs in more than 48,000 firms. The compensation data were the average for all workers holding the sampled type of job. The average worker could be single or married and file an itemized or nonitemized tax return. For each of these possibilities, the study imputed the average spousal and unearned income based on the state in which the firm was located, its industry, the occupation classification of the job, and the wage rate using data from the CPS and SOI. Given these characteristics and family incomes, the study computed the relevant marginal tax rate for the household. Then, using the proportions of married people and itemizing deductions, married and not itemizing, and single itemizing and nonitemizing, it was able to compute the marginal tax and the marginal "tax price" of health insurance for the average worker in each firm. The tax rate is analogous to the 32.64% marginal rate in the example above; the tax price is the 67.36% of the insurance premium that the employee would pay after the tax exclusion. The computation of the tax price allowed the study to estimate whether or not a firm offered coverage, based on the tax status of their average employee and the generosity of the coverage, if offered.

The study concluded that a 10% increase in the tax price (a cut in taxes) reduced the probability of a firm offering coverage by 3.1%. This is in the lower tail of the range of prior estimates. Thus, the tax subsidy does encourage firms to offer coverage. The study estimates suggest that it is the workers in small firms who are the most tax-price sensitive to buying coverage through their employers.

The effects of the generosity of coverage were much larger. The study estimated that the same 10% increase in the tax price would lead firms that currently offer coverage to reduce their expenditures on that coverage by approximately 11%. This is in the middle of the earlier estimates. Based on insurance theory, such reductions would likely be achieved by eliminating coverage on things that are of lesser value to employees, such as first-dollar coverage of physician services and prescription drugs and perhaps the elimination of dental- and vision-care coverage.

The tax treatment of employer-sponsored health insurance stands in marked contrast to the treatment afforded to individually purchased coverage. Individuals are allowed to deduct for federal income tax, but not payroll tax purposes, the portion of their health insurance premiums (plus other medical expenses) that are in excess of 7.5% of adjusted gross income. This is a very modest subsidy compared to that afforded by employer-sponsored coverage.

Consider again the individual with $45,000 in taxable income and a marginal tax rate of 32.64%. If the individual bought insurance directly from a broker and paid the same average premium of $4,248 as in the original example, the individual would receive a tax subsidy of less than $300, compared with nearly $1,400 for employer-sponsored coverage. In addition, the individual would get this only if he or she itemized the tax return.

Self-employed individuals can do somewhat better. They can deduct all their health insurance premiums prior to computing their adjusted gross income. However, the deduction may not exceed their profits, and they are not eligible to claim the deduction in any month in which they or their spouse was eligible for employer-sponsored coverage.

Proposed Changes

A number of approaches have been proposed to change the nature of the tax treatment of employer-sponsored health insurance. Of course, one could simply abolish the exclusion and treat employer-sponsored health insurance as taxable employee compensation. The study described above suggested that a total elimination would reduce spending on employer-sponsored coverage by 45%, combining both the reduction in the probability that coverage was offered and the reduced generosity. However, healthcare spending likely would be reduced by considerably less than that amount because many people would pay higher deductibles and copays out of pocket.

In 2007, the Bush administration proposed a standard deduction of $7,500 for individuals and $15,000 for families in place of unlimited tax exclusion of employer-sponsored coverage. This deduction was to apply whether one purchased health insurance directly or through an employer. The amount of the deduction would be fixed each year regardless of how much was actually spent on insurance as long as they bought a qualified health plan. However, no action was taken on the proposed plan.

Such a plan could change health insurance incentives in several ways. First, by limiting the size of the deduction, it would provide incentives for those with very generous plans to cut back on their health plans. Effectively, anyone with insurance premiums above the size of the deduction would receive no further tax subsidy. Second, because the size of the deduction would be available to anyone who had a qualified health plan, it would provide incentives for people to consider reducing their benefit package even if the premium was below the size of the deduction. The tax on the difference between the deduction and the premium would be a tax refund. The individual with the $45,000 in taxable income who took the least costly insurance plan, a health maintenance organization (HMO), offered by the employer would receive a tax refund of approximately $450. Third, because the standard deduction applied on any qualified health plan, the tax subsidy would apply to those who purchased individual coverage as well as those who purchased coverage through an employer. Thus, there would be a new tax subsidy for non-employer-based coverage. Finally, if the standard deduction were tied to general inflation rather than medical-care inflation, it would gradually reduce the tax subsidy relative to the costs of medical care.

Both before and after the Bush proposal, a number of policy experts had proposed that the tax exclusion be replaced with a refundable individual tax credit. Under the current exclusion and under the Bush proposal, the value of the tax subsidy depends on one's marginal tax rate. Those with higher taxable incomes face higher tax rates and therefore receive higher tax subsidies for purchasing health insurance through their employers. A tax credit fundamentally changes this. The recipient of a tax credit receives a reduction in tax liability in the amount of the credit. Thus, a $1,000 tax credit reduces one's tax liability by $1,000 regardless of one's marginal tax rate. A refundable tax credit allows one to receive the full tax credit even if one's tax liability is less than $1,000. Moreover, because the tax credit would not be tied to employer-based coverage, it would be available to those who purchased nongroup coverage.

Advocates tend to favor such a general tax credit for several reasons. First, because it expands the tax subsidy for purchasing coverage to all individuals, not just those with employer-sponsored coverage, more people would be likely to buy coverage. Second, because the tax subsidy does not increase with income, it reduces the incentive for those in higher tax brackets to shift more of their income into more generous health insurance plans. Third, in principle, a tax credit could be tailored to the health status of recipients, thereby providing larger subsidies to those with substantial health problems.

In addition to the replacement of the tax exclusion with a general tax credit for the purchase of health insurance, some have proposed targeted refundable tax credits for those with incomes below some level. The argument is one of providing a subsidy to the targeted group to allow them to buy coverage in the private market.

Changes in the tax treatment of employer-sponsored health insurance are not without challenges. First, if nothing else is changed, eliminating its exclusion would constitute a substantial increase in taxes that would be felt by virtually all income tax payers who have employer-sponsored coverage. Second, replacement of the tax exclusion with a standard deduction or a tax credit implies potentially large numbers of winners and losers. Such shifts are always politically difficult. Finally, the introduction of a generous standard deduction or tax credit implies that the tax subsidy will be larger than the current subsidy, suggesting substantial increases in domestic governmental spending. Nonetheless, while politically challenging, reform of the tax treatment of employer-sponsored health insurance offers the potential for both a more efficient and a fairer tax and insurance system.

Michael A. Morrisey

See also America's Health Insurance Plans (AHIP); Blue Cross and Blue Shield; Coinsurance, Copays, and Deductibles; Compensation Differentials; Health Insurance; Moral Hazard; Public Policy; Regulation

Further Readings

Gruber, Jonathan, and Michael Lettau. "How Elastic is the Firm's Demand for Insurance?" *Journal of Public Economics* 88(7–8): 1273–93, July 2004.

Gruber, Jonathan, and Larry Levitt. "Tax Subsidies for Health Insurance: Costs and Benefits," *Health Affairs* 19(1): 72–85, January–February 2000.

Morrisey, Michael A. *Health Insurance*. Chicago: Health Administration Press, 2008.

Pipes, Sally C. *Miracle Cure: How to Solve America's Health Care Crisis and Why Canada Isn't the Answer*. San Francisco: Pacific Research Institute, 2004.

Seldon, Thomas M., and Bradley M. Gray. "Tax Subsidies for Employment-Related Health Insurance: Estimates for 2006," *Health Affairs* 25(6): 1568–79, November–December, 2006.

Web Sites

America's Health Insurance Plans (AHIP): http://www.hiaa.org

Internal Revenue Service (IRS): http://www.irs.gov

Tax Policy Center: http://www.taxpolicycenter.org

TECHNOLOGY ASSESSMENT

Technology assessment is a form of policy analysis and evaluation that poses the question "What will be the social, economic, environmental, ethical, and political impacts of the introduction of a new technology?" In this sense, it is an analytic tool that is designed to provide decision makers with scientific information about the potential impacts of technology that might be introduced in the future. A technology assessment consists of three parts: (1) identification of problems, issues, and applicable technologies; (2) identification of relevant effects and impacts; and (3) development and evaluation/assessment of policy and decision alternatives. In the United States, one of the most important federal agencies to conduct technology assessment was the former Office of Technology Assessment (OTA). Today, several government agencies and private organizations conduct healthcare technology assessment.

History

The technology assessment movement of the 1970s grew out of the history of trying to link the research and policy-making communities.

Technology assessment is a form of systems analysis that attempts to apply rational, systematic approaches to an area of public policy. Specifically, technology assessment represents a class of policy studies that systematically examines the effects on society that may occur when a technology is introduced, extended, or modified, with special emphasis on those consequences that are unintended, indirect, and delayed.

Technology assessment is known for its focus on not limiting impact studies to first-order consequences (e.g., the effect of canceling the Clinch River project on the nuclear power industry) but, instead, concentrating on discovering and predicting as many second- and larger-order effects as possible (e.g., environmental impacts of breeder reactors, the effects of research and development on the other breeder reactor technologies).

In other words, technology assessment represents a new form of evaluation that will allow officials to estimate (forecast) what the consequences of their potential actions are likely to be; as such, technology assessment represents an especially attractive source of expertise within a political environment in which decisions are made through bargaining and minimization of risks.

Office of Technology Assessment

Future-oriented systems analysis became very popular in scientific and government circles in the 1960s and 1970s. In recognition of the importance of this type of analysis, the U.S. Congress created the OTA in 1972 (PL 92–484). This office was designed to provide the Congress with the best scientific and technical information available on emerging technologies. This information was to be presented in a form that was understandable to lay audiences. During its 24 years of existence, the OTA produced 750 studies on a wide range of topics, including healthcare, acid rain, global climate change, and many new technologies that were being introduced (e.g., imaging medical equipment such as CAT scanners, and MRIs).

When the original bill was being drafted for the creation of the OTA, the staff of the House Science and Technology Committee took the tenets of technology assessment methodology quite seriously. The board overseeing the operations of the OTA would consist of citizens, representatives of industry, scientists, and members of the U.S. Congress. However, Congress would not maintain the majority of votes on this board. The theory was that all stakeholders should have equal representation; and Congress was simply one stakeholder.

Clearly, as the history of the OTA indicates, this plan was fine in theory but inconsistent with the realities of politics. This original bill was not acceptable to Congress. If Congress was to have full trust and confidence in this body, then it should also control it. Furthermore, Congress argued that if the results of the OTA studies were to be useful to it, then Congress should also set and control the research agenda. Citizens, and other public representation, were important, but they should be on agency advisory councils or on project advisory committees.

When Harold Brown (then President of the California Institute of Technology) resigned as the first chairman of the OTA's Advisory Council, the strains between researchers/technicians and politicians over the creation of the OTA were evident. In his letter of resignation, Brown noted that few members on the council were satisfied with what had been accomplished, compared with what was hoped for and possible. Specifically, Brown felt that the OTA had failed to provide an early warning system for Congress so that it could consider the social and other impacts of technological advances. He blamed this failure on the tendency of the OTA to squander its energies on routine tasks for congressional committees. The OTA, according to Brown, should be in the position of turning down committee requests, particularly those that did not call for technology assessment but rather sought technical feasibility studies, reviews of existing programs, and literature searches—jobs that might be better performed by other research agencies with greater resources.

Presumably, the tendency to respond to short-term committee needs would not have been as prevalent under the original conception of the OTA first proposed by the House Science and Technology Committee staff. At the same time, Congress would not have supported this version of an OTA. In 1972, when the OTA was created, Congress was concerned with creating some of its own analytic capabilities that would provide information independent of the executive branch. However, Congress did not want to be responsible

for creating large, unwieldy bureaucracies. For example, Texas Democratic Congressman Olin E. Teague, Chairman of the House Science and Technology Committee and one-time chairman of the OTA board, indicated that the OTA was always supposed to be a contract operation with a small but highly capable in-house staff. Teague believed that OTA would not have been created without these assurances.

When the 104th U.S. Congress withdrew funding for the OTA, it had a full-time staff of 143 employees with an annual budget of $21.9 million. The OTA closed on September 29, 1995.

At the time when the OTA was most active, there was also the creation of technology assessment capabilities within many executive branch agencies—most notably with the U.S. Departments of Commerce, Agriculture, and Energy, as well as the creation of the National Science Foundation Program designed to sponsor and develop technology assessment methodology.

The Professionalization of Technology Assessment

The development of technology assessment as a methodology was accompanied by the creation of several professional associations and groups of researchers and technicians who were promoting the technology assessment movement.

From a strictly methodological perspective, technology assessment represents an information resource that, by design, requires the following: boundary spanning and coordination among various disciplines; multidisciplinary work; a coordinated, planned, exploratory approach that is structured to acknowledge the uncertainty of the task; and the conscious and planned involvement of all parties who might be affected (stakeholders) by the adoption of the technology under study.

Each of these facets of technology assessment raises fundamental questions about control, institutional responsibility, and coordination; yet, from the perspectives of researchers, each is critical for attempting to provide the comprehensive analyses at the heart of the technology assessment movement. If they are to be translated into institutional terms, technology assessments would seem to implicitly require coordination at the inter- and intra-organizational levels. However, bureaucrats traditionally have resisted this form of coordination. There have been attempts made at creating lead agencies, which are responsible for coordinating a particular substantive task in government (e.g., coordinating career-planning research). Interagency task forces have also been experimented with. Except for times of crisis, this type of coordination has encountered severe problems, which ultimately have led to failure.

However, as already outlined, the technology assessment movement represented a potentially powerful and useful tool for government officials. This is especially true given the pressure that is being put on government officials to reform their day-to-day operations by being more rational—in a formal, scientific sense of the term; using scientific information—or at least using the results of research funded through public funds; and relying considerably less on intuition than officials have been inclined to do in the past.

Technology Assessment as a System of Analysis

As it evolved, technology assessment was not just another form of research output or a bit of social science knowledge but is instead a system of analysis designed to inform the public-policy-making process.

System of analysis can be thought of as both formal and informal. The critical (essential) distinction between systems of analysis and more routine knowledge or information is that a system of analysis is associated with a set of general rules, procedures, and processes that guide the production of the end product. In recent history, examples of these kinds of systems have included the Program-Planning-Budgeting System (PPBS), the Environmental Impact Statement system, and the attempts by some federal agencies to build a routinized survey capacity into their policy-making process.

Technology assessment, as a system of analysis, is based on a general process that provides a systematic and rational input to societal decision making and management. These particularized policy studies attempt to account for direct and indirect effects as well as indirect and delayed impacts involved with technological change. To this end, technology assessment brings together multidisciplinary approaches, recommendations, and the perspectives related to a new technological development. Although there is no single methodology common to all technology assessments, there are a number of common or generic elements involved in the creation of virtually every comprehensive technology assessment. When a decision maker reads a technology assessment, he or she can expect that each of these elements or perspectives has been taken into account and is documented in the technology assessment study.

It is important to distinguish systems of analysis from other, more routine information, whether generated in-house or sent to the organization free of charge, because the process that accompanies the creation of a technology assessment, which ensures the introduction and reporting of many different perspectives, may be just as important in understanding the ultimate impact of this class of policy studies on decision makers as the substance of the study itself.

Other Systems of Analysis

Technology assessment is not the only form of policy analysis or evaluation that represents a system of analysis. At the same time that technology assessments were becoming popular, environmental impact statements were also being developed and were also seen as attractive by government officials, because they know what to expect; they know the form (generally defined) in which they will receive the information; each environmental impact statement contains specific kinds of information and/or covers (accounts for) a set of perspectives; and there are few unexpected results that emerge from an environmental impact statement because of the process that was followed (i.e., set of procedures predetermined by the bureaucracy) in creating the environmental impact statement.

Future Implications

In the future, technology assessments, especially in healthcare, will likely increase and become a more important factor in evaluation. As new, enormously expensive medical equipment and drugs are introduced, federal and state governments, insurance companies, and consumers are increasingly questioning their value. Although the federal OTA no longer exists, other federal government agencies currently conduct healthcare technology assessments (e.g., National Institutes of Health [NIH] and the Food and Drug Administration [FDA]). Furthermore, several private associations (e.g., Blue Cross Blue Shield Association [BCBSA], and the University HealthSystem Consortium [UHC] also conduct technology assessments for their members. Outside the United States, the best-known organization that conducts healthcare technology assessments is the United Kingdom's National Institute for Health and Clinical Excellence (NICE).

Robert F. Rich

See also Cost-Benefit and Cost-Effectiveness Analysis; Cost of Healthcare; Genetics; Health Economics; Public Policy; Quality of Healthcare; Rationing Healthcare; United Kingdom's National Institute for Health and Clinical Excellence (NICE)

Further Readings

Deckler, Michael, ed. *Interdisciplinarity in Technology Assessment: Implementation and Its Chances and Limits.* New York: Springer-Verlag, 2002.

Kraemet, Sylvia. *Science and Technology Policy in the United States: Open Systems in Action.* New Brunswick, NJ: Rutgers University Press, 2006.

Niewohner, Jorg, and Christof Tannert, eds. *Gene Therapy: Prospective Technology Assessment in Its Societal Context.* Amsterdam: Elsevier, 2006.

Spekowius, Gerhard, and Thomas Wendler, eds. *Advances in Healthcare Technology: Shaping the Future of Medical Care.* Dordrecht, the Netherlands: Springer, 2006.

Webster, Andrew, ed. *New Technologies in Health Care: Challenge, Change and Innovation.* New York: Palgrave Macmillan, 2006.

Web Sites

Blue Cross Blue Shield Association (BCBS), Technology Evaluation Center (TEC): http://www.bcbs.com/blueresources/tec

National Information Center on Health Services Research and Health Care Technology (NICHSR): http://www.nlm.nih.gov/nichsr

United Kingdom's National Institute for Health and Clinical Excellence (NICE): http://www.nice.org.uk

U.S. Office of Technology Assessment Archives: http://fas.org/ota

TELEMEDICINE

Telemedicine is the application of clinical medicine through the the exchange of medical information from one site to another via electronic networks to improve patients' health. The number of existing telemedicine networks in the United States is approximately 200, and it involves nearly 2,000 medical institutions throughout the nation. Furthermore, it is estimated that about half, or nearly 100, of the telemedicine programs are actively providing patient care services on a routine daily basis. The American Telemedicine Association (ATA) reports that the total amount of federal grants and contracts for telemedicine is about $270 million. More than one third of these funds are for research contracts with the U.S. Department of Defense (DOD), which allow for equipment and service delivery.

Overview

An elderly female patient presents at a rural hospital with cardiac problems and depression. The medical staff at this hospital prescribes a course of therapy for her heart troubles, and the patient is seen for regular, routine follow-up visits with a cardiologist. However, there is no psychiatrist on staff at this small facility. To ensure that the patient's depression, a serious comorbidity which can exacerbate the heart problems, is properly treated, the physicians connect her with a home-monitoring service. Every quarter, the service rings the patient and administers a telephone-based, interactive voice recording (IVR) screening using a health questionnaire as a way to monitor the patient's mental status.

A study by Carolyn Turvey and colleagues at the University of Iowa, whose parameters were outlined above, indicated that 90% of patients completed this telemedicine screening. The researchers found that a regular telephone IVR screen for depression could be used in a standard illness protocol. This program could potentially serve as a model for incorporating technology in the management of chronic illness with comorbid depression.

Chronic illnesses, like depression, account for most of the healthcare expenses in the United

States. Cutting-edge telemedicine projects like the one described above are increasingly being developed to decrease the burden of these illnesses on the medical system, to treat comorbidities, and to improve patient care and outcomes.

The term *telemedicine* appears frequently in news media reports and is often mentioned at medical conferences. Although telemedicine is not yet recognized as a separate medical specialty, technologies used for telemedicine are often part of a larger investment by healthcare institutions in either information technology or the delivery of clinical care. The new technologies involved in the practice of telemedicine include IVR, videoconferencing, transmission of still images over the Internet, online patient portals, remote monitoring of vital signs, and continuing medical education delivered online.

For clinical care, there are several applications of telemedicine that are becoming well established. Some of the applications include referral to a specialist, consultation with a patient, remote monitoring, networking hospitals, continuing education, and consumer education.

Referral to a specialist typically occurs when a specialist assists a general practitioner in arriving at a diagnosis. This often involves a patient seeing a specialist over a live network. But it can also happen with transmission of diagnostic images and/or video along with patient data, for later viewing by the specialist. Radiologists make the greatest use of telemedicine, with thousands of images read by remote providers each year. Other major specialties that rely on telemedicine include dermatology, ophthalmology, psychiatry, cardiology, and pathology. According to reports and studies, almost 50 different medical subspecialties have successfully used telemedicine.

Using telecommunications, which includes audio, still or live images, or the Internet, a primary-care health professional can consult with a patient to render a diagnosis and develop an appropriate treatment plan. Devices can be used to remotely collect and send data to a monitoring station for interpretation. The home-based applications may include the collection of vital signs, blood pressure, and blood glucose levels, an EKG, or an array of other health indicators. These services can be used to supplement visiting nurses.

Networking hospitals involves linking urban hospitals and clinics with clinics and community health centers in suburban and rural areas. These networks include dedicated high-speed lines or the Internet for telecommunication links between sites. Additionally, this involves linking primary-care providers, specialists, and nurses with remote patients over single-line telephone-video systems for interactive clinical consultations. This can be used for monitoring of cardiac, pulmonary, or fetal signs. Generally, conventional telephone lines are used to communicate directly between the patient and the center. Using point-to-point private networks, hospitals and clinics also deliver services directly or contract out specialty services to independent medical service providers at ambulatory-care sites. These include specialties such as radiology, psychiatry, and even intensive-care services.

Using the Internet, physicians and other healthcare professionals can receive continuing medical education credits. For example, Harvard Medical School offers courses online for physicians for $20 or less per class.

In terms of consumer education, using online access, consumers may seek out specialized health information and participate in online discussion groups that provide peer-to-peer support for conditions such as cancer and cancer aftercare.

Investment in Telemedicine

Spending on telemedicine in the United States involves both the private and the public sector. The expenditures for telemedicine are composed of three segments: grants for demonstrations and research, direct telemedicine services by federal agencies for covered populations, and reimbursement for remote medical services under Medicare. Although the amount of spending on telemedicine services provided directly by federal agencies is not tracked, the Veterans Health Administration (VA), the largest provider of remote medical services, delivers annually approximately 350,000 patient services remotely. Other federal providers of direct services include the Department of Defense, the Indian Health Service (IHS), and the Bureau of Prisons in the Department of Justice.

Medicare spending for telemedicine is also not accurately tracked. According to the ATA, the largest source of Medicare expenditures for telemedicine is for teleradiology. A Medicare program supporting videoconference-based patient services in nonmetropolitan areas is rapidly growing, but it reimburses less than $1 million a year. Medicare reimburses services for remote cardiac monitoring services, and in some areas for telepathology, and remote screening for diabetic retinopathy. Home telehealth applications fall under Medicare's prospective payment system (PPS) and may be used as part of a patient's plan of care, although no specific Medicare funds may be used to pay for home telehealth delivery.

Limited Growth and Acceptance

Telemedicine has slowly emerged from the fringes of medicine to mainstream use. However, there are still concerns among advocates about its pace of growth and general acceptance. Studies have clearly shown that telemedicine can increase the availability of healthcare services, decrease the amount of travel and related expenses, and enhance patient outcomes. Thus, with all these advantages, the slow take-up of telemedicine poses a dilemma.

Despite a 40-year history and the past 10 years of intensive activity, telemedicine is neither a household word nor secure in clinical use. It is estimated that less than 300 nonradiology programs are in use, with some ceasing operation each year.

Several factors contribute to the slow growth of telemedicine. First, there are reimbursement issues, concerns over whether physicians will be paid for their services rendered online rather than in person. This issue could be remedied if the patients paid for these services. However, there are other issues as well. There are concerns in the medical community about practicing virtual medicine across state lines and whether or not this is legal. Finally, the technology for telemedicine is somewhat complicated. Although physicians are technical specialists, they may not be computer specialists, which may limit the acceptance of telemedicine.

It has been noted that the slow pace of change in medicine is not unusual. The adoption of electronic health records has also been a slow process, despite its touted utility and long history.

There are several possible ways to facilitate the adoption of telemedicine technology. For example, standardization of the technologies and applications could be required by the federal government through regulation, perhaps through additions to the Health Insurance Portability and Accountability Act of 1996 (HIPAA), which mandates privacy of personal health records. There could also be federal and state financial incentives for hospitals and healthcare providers to adopt the technology, including tax reductions. Last, the Medicare program could announce a major spending program on telemedicine technologies, which would influence technology markets in the nation. Ultimately, the use and transformation of telemedicine may be a public policy decision even broader in scope than those envisioned. Some researchers have indicated that the public health benefits of telemedicine are so great that they justify a massive expansion of the investment in the field. The public health concerns raised by the global war on terror and homeland security concerns are becoming drivers of spending in this area. This is particularly salient with the concerns about domestic biological or dirty bomb attacks on American civilian populations.

Currently, most disease reports received by state public health departments originate from clinical laboratories. It has long been recognized that the paper reporting methods used in public health surveillance are unreliable and tremendously slow, which leads to late submission of reports and substantial underreporting of communicable diseases. A recent project undertaken by researchers at the Indiana University medical school automated the reporting of diseases to local public health authorities from clinical laboratories. Reports are sent out overnight and disseminated much more quickly than paper or fax-based transmissions. When an outbreak of shigella occurred in Indianapolis, the electronic reporting system was able to notify public health officials much earlier with greater information.

Imagine the implications of such a telemedicine system in the event of a terrorist biological attack on a major urban public transportation system. The information about this occurrence could be disseminated quickly, including information on the type of attack, the means of detonation, and the type of biological agent involved—and it could be used to prevent further attacks using the same techniques.

Gene J. Koprowski

See also Access to Healthcare; E-Health; Electronic Clinical Records; Emergency and Disaster Preparedness; Health Communication; Health Informatics; Rural Health; Vulnerable Populations

Further Readings

Kumar, Sajeesh, and Jacques Marescaux, eds. *Telesurgery*. New York: Springer, 2008.

Latifi, Rifat, ed. *Current Principles and Practices of Telemedicine and E-Health*. Washington, DC: IOS Press, 2008.

Martinez, Lucia, and Carla Gomez, eds. *Telemedicine in the 21st Century*. New York: Nova Science, 2008.

Turvey, Carolyn, Deborah Willyard, David H. Hickman, et al. "Telehealth Screen for Depression in a Chronic Illness Care Management Program," *Telemedicine and e-Health* 13(1): 51–56, February 2007.

Xiao, Yang, and Hui Chen, eds. *Mobile Telemedicine: A Computing and Networking Perspective*. Boca Raton, FL: CRC Press, 2008.

Web Sites

American Telemedicine Association (ATA): http://www.atmeda.org

Association of Telehealth Service Providers (ATSP): http://www.atsp.org

Canadian Society of Telehealth (CST): http://www.cst-sct.org/en

International Society for Telemedicine and eHealth (ISFTEH): http://www.isft.net

TERRORISM

See Bioterrorism

THOMPSON, JOHN DEVEREAUX

Familiarly known as Tommy, John Devereaux Thompson was a nurse, health administration educator, and health services researcher. Thompson along with Robert B. Fetter developed Diagnosis Related Groups (DRGs) as a tool to standardize hospital cases for studies of quality and cost, subsequently changing the way the nation's hospitals were reimbursed when Medicare adopted DRGs for its prospective payment system (PPS). Thompson's passions for studying the history of hospital operations as well as nursing resulted in a creative and respected book that focused on the social and architectural history of hospitals.

Born in Franklin, Pennsylvania, Thompson was raised in Canton, Ohio. Thompson's stepmother, a nurse, encouraged him to also become a nurse. Following her advice, he completed his nurse training program in 1939. With World War II imminent, he enlisted in the U.S. Navy and served as a pharmacist's mate, eventually achieving the rank of warrant officer. After the war, he enrolled in the City College of New York in 1948, working nights as a nurse riding ambulances and doing psychiatric nursing. Thompson received his bachelor's degree with distinction in business. Subsequently, he enrolled in the new hospital administration program at Yale University and undertook the required administrative residency training at Montefiore Hospital in New York City. Thompson completed this praxis experience in 1950 and remained at Montefiore Hospital for 6 years, becoming one of the hospital's assistant directors. Albert W. Snoke, then director of the hospital administration program at Yale and senior administrator at the then Grace-New Haven Hospital, had received a federal Hill-Burton grant to study hospital function and design, and he was successful in recruiting Thompson back to Yale in 1956.

Thompson's directorship of the hospital administration program at Yale University was novel in its emphasis on public health, yielding students who recognized that their actions as health services managers must be related to improving the health status of communities. He was beloved as a teacher and mentor.

Much of Thompson's research was based on his underlying philosophy that clinical and administrative data must be brought together to identify and solve both operational and financial problems. Thompson was instrumental in creating the Connecticut Hospital Information Management Exchange (CHIME), one of the first of 34 statewide databases built from hospital billing systems that form the foundation of large data sets, which are often used for health services research.

Thompson studied operations research with Russell A. Nelson and Charles D. Flagle at the Johns Hopkins University School of Engineering. This interest in data and their use for management decision making as well as for policy formulation and analysis led Thompson to develop a research and teaching relationship with Robert B. Fetter, then in Yale University's Department of Administrative Sciences. With others, they were important in developing the Center for Health Services Research in Yale University's Institute for Social and Policy Studies; the Center was among the first in the country.

Thompson's published articles include topics such as hospital operations, including nursing services and nursing intensity, hospital function and design, application of operations research to hospital studies, costs of care, economics of care, education for health services administration, emergency medical services, chronic hemodialysis, the role of schools of public health, hospital architecture, case-mix cost accounting, regulation, DRGs and hospital prospective-based payment, quality appraisal, and cost funding.

Thompson epitomized the adage "He who dares to teach must never cease to learn" (Anonymous). Thompson received numerous awards and honors. He shared the Baxter Prize (now the William B. Graham Prize for Health Services Research) with Robert B. Fetter in 1992; this award is the highest distinction that health services researchers can achieve. Various awards have also been named in his honor, including the John D. Thompson Prize for Young Investigators, sponsored by the Association of University Programs in Health Administration (AUPHA), and the John D. Thompson Distinguished Visiting Fellow at the Yale University School of Public Health. In addition, the teaching arm of the Connecticut Hospice was named after him—the John D. Thompson Hospice Institute for Education, Training, and Research.

David A. Pearson

See also Association of University Programs in Health Administration (AUPHA); Diagnostic Related Groups (DRG); Medicare; National Association of Health Data Organizations (NAHDO); Payment Mechanisms; Prospective Payment

Further Readings

Flagle, Charles D. "Some Origins of Operations Research in the Health Services," *Operations Research* 50(1): 52–60, January–February 2002.

Mays, Rick. "The Origins, Development, and Passage of Medicare's Revolutionary Prospective Payment System," *Journal of the History of Medicine and Allied Sciences* 62(1): 21–55, 2007.

Thompson, John D. "DRG and Prepayment: Its Purpose and Performance," *Bulletin of the New York Academy of Medicine* 64(1): 25–51, January–February 1988.

Thompson, John D., and Grace Goldin. *The Hospital: A Social and Architectural History.* New Haven, CT: Yale University Press, 1975.

White, William D. *Compelled by Data: John D. Thompson, Nurse, Health Services Researcher, and Health Administration Educator.* New Haven, CT: Yale University, Department of Epidemiology and Public Health, 2003.

Web Sites

Yale School of Epidemiology and Public Health: http://www.med.yale.edu/library/exhibits/publichealth

TIMELINESS OF HEALTHCARE

Timeliness is one of the six key dimensions of healthcare quality identified by the National Academy of Sciences, Institute of Medicine (IOM). Timeliness can be defined as the healthcare system's capacity to provide care quickly after a need is recognized. Timeliness is a measure of a continuum ranging from an intervention that is too early, in which the diagnosis cannot be made, through a delayed intervention, in which treatment may no longer be effective. There are may reasons why timeliness as a quality measure is critical to the effectiveness of a well-functioning healthcare system, and a great deal of research exists showing its positive and negative repercussions on emergent, urgent, and chronic conditions as well as preventive services. There are also many direct and indirect factors that play a significant role in the aspect of timeliness, including cost, proper access to medical resources, and even individual patient attributes.

There has been increasing attention given to this topic in recent years, and thus, there has been a shift in ideology and the organization of hospitals, primary-care offices, and public health departments to continually improve the timeliness of healthcare.

Benchmarks

Many benchmarks are valuable in the evaluation of timeliness of healthcare, including morbidity, mortality, cost, and patient satisfaction. Quality assurance programs in ambulatory-care and emergency department settings are increasingly implemented and used to monitor timeliness assessments. This is important not only to observe and improve patient outcome data but also to give attention to the service aspects of the healthcare industry. For example, patient visits may be evaluated by the length of wait times, and no-show rates. Wait times, in particular, may be monitored closely as patient satisfaction decreases as perceived wait times increase. Many benefits such as the shorter duration of illness, the decreased likelihood of complications, reduced anxiety on the part of the patient, and reduced activity limitation are linked to receiving timely care.

Contributing Factors

Many contributing factors may affect the aspect of the timeliness of healthcare on multiple levels and points of intervention. These contributing factors, in turn, could have, separately, or in conjunction, large ramifications on the outcomes of care. For example, transportation to and between medical facilities can have a large impact. Ease of scheduling an appointment within a given target time is also essential. In addition, patient individual characteristics such as age, gender, and race may play a role in the diagnosis of some chronic conditions. Attributes such as good communication skills, motivation, positive attitude, good learning capacity, and willingness to seek timely care may be critical factors that result in the early diagnosis of illnesses. The significance of provider judgments in accurately assessing the severity of the presenting problem and patient prognosis has been shown to affect outcomes. After diagnosis, efficient communication within and among providers and medical establishments also play a decisive role in outcomes of care.

These aspects include timely documentation, reliable physician orders, ease of referral, clear prescriptions, and assurance of patient follow-up. Communication between the medical establishment and the public health system is paramount. Timely physician reporting of communicable diseases, obviously, could have far-reaching consequences. Articulation of established clinical practice guidelines and public health initiatives to medical practitioners is also very important. Of course, there are a vast number of contributing factors that should be considered in the evaluation of timeliness within the medical and health systems; however, all influence, ultimately, efficiency, precision, and patient flow.

Range of Medical Settings

The critical nature of the timeliness of healthcare spans the range of care provided within the United States, including emergency department visits, surgical procedures, primary-care visits, specialty-care visits, and public health initiatives. Some research has shown that as many as half of all hospital emergency department visits in the nation are for nonurgent care. This is notable as it illustrates the possibility of emergency department congestion threatening timely care for urgent cases and demonstrates the importance of access to healthcare services. Studies have found that Medicaid patients in urban areas (who are often not accepted by many primary-care offices) are more likely than others to seek nonurgent care at hospital emergency departments.

Timeliness is also a critical aspect in primary healthcare. However, a growing number of individuals are delaying their care because of its cost. The National Center for Health Statistics (NCHS) estimates that about 7.7% of the nation's population in 2005–2006 delayed receiving care because of its cost, up from 6.9% of the population in 1997–1998. This can have devastating effects on patient care, especially in consideration of chronic disease states for which proper care also involves timely specialist referral and ready access to care. For example, a late evaluation by nephrologists of patients with chronic kidney disease results in a significantly greater burden and severity of comorbid disease and a shorter duration of survival. Lack of health insurance plays an important role in individuals delaying care.

As increasing attention is placed on the significance of timeliness, healthcare organizations are changing to address it. In particular, clinical practices are converting to more flexible scheduling systems that allow for a greater number of walk-in appointments and same-day scheduling. These alternative models are sometimes referred to as the carve-out model and the advanced-access model and are being shown to provide more patient satisfaction, shorter wait times, and lower no-show rates. The advanced-access model also creates the possibility for the preservation of the continuity of care. This is of note as the ability of the provider and patient to establish a consistent and reliable relationship has a great impact on the quality of care, in particular the measure of timeliness.

Future Implications

Timeliness is critical to the effectiveness of a well-functioning healthcare system, in particular emergent, urgent, and chronic conditions as well as preventive measures at multiple levels of intervention. There is increasing attention being given to this topic, including major shifts in ideology and organizations to continually improve this measure as the nation strives toward improving the quality of care within the healthcare system.

J. Andrew Dykens

See also Emergency Medical Services (EMS); Equity, Efficiency, and Effectiveness in Healthcare; Joint Commission; National Healthcare Quality Report (NHQR); Patient Safety; Quality Management; Quality of Healthcare; Transportation

Further Readings

Barry, Daniel W., Trisha V. Melhado, Karen M. Chacko, et al. "Patient and Physician Perceptions of Timely Access to Care," *Journal of General Internal Medicine* 21(2): 130–33, February 2006.

Clark, Karen, and Loretta Brush Normile. "Influence of Time-to-Interventions for Emergency Department Critical Care Patients on Hospital Mortality," *Journal of Emergency Nursing* 33(1): 6–13, February 2007.

Longo, Daniel R., Jake Young, David Mehr, et al. "Barriers to Timely Care of Acute Infections in Nursing Homes: A Preliminary Qualitative Study," *Journal of the American Medical Directors Association* 5(2 Suppl.): S4–S10, March–April 2004.

Luman, Elizabeth, Lawrence E. Barker, Mary Mason McCauley, et al. "Timeliness of Childhood Immunization: A State-Specific Analysis," *American Journal of Public Health* 95(8): 1367–74, August 2005.

Williams, Marian E., James Latta, and Persila Conversano. "Eliminating the Wait for Mental Health Services," *Journal of Behavioral Health Services and Research* 35(1): 107–14, January 2008.

Web Sites

Agency for Healthcare Research and Quality (AHRQ): http://www.ahrq.gov

Center for Studying Health System Change (HSC): http://www.hschange.org

Institute for Healthcare Improvement (IHI): http://www.ihi.org

Joint Commission: http://www.jointcommission.org

National Quality Forum (NQF): http://www.qualityforum.org

TOBACCO USE

Tobacco use is one of the biggest public health challenges of the 21st century. It is the single most preventable cause of disease and death. It is estimated that worldwide tobacco use causes about 4 million deaths a year. And the number of deaths caused by tobacco use is expected to rise to about 8.4 million by 2020.

Tobacco use imposes a significant burden on society. People who use tobacco in its various forms face multiple health risks. Moreover, they impose a heavy burden on society by increasing the nation's medical expenditures of treating many costly tobacco-related diseases as well as through an enormous loss in productivity. Sustained public policy efforts, as well as the provision of cessation counseling as a part of routine healthcare, may contribute to the decline of tobacco use in the United States.

Background

The use of tobacco as a stimulant goes back many thousands of years. It is estimated that the cultivation of the tobacco plant began as far back as

6000 BCE in the Americas. The indigenous people of the Americas were using leaf-wrapped cigarettes long before the arrival of Columbus, and from the late 1400s onward, tobacco was used in various other forms such as cigars and pipes, snuff, and chewing tobacco. However, it was not until the 1880s, when the first cigarette-making machine was invented in the United States, that natural-leaf cigarettes made from domestic tobacco began to dominate the consumer market. This development led to machine-rolled butts replacing the hand-rolled varieties, consequently making cigarettes more affordable and thereby more accessible. By World War I, cigarettes had become immensely popular, and troops in both World Wars I and II used smoking as a means of relieving the physical and psychological stress of war.

Public Health Challenge

Smoking continued to gain widespread public acceptance until 1964, when the first U.S. Surgeon General's report on smoking and health brought to the fore the many health risks associated with tobacco use. Although tobacco use has declined by more than 50% since the initial Surgeon General's report, there are still more than 40 million smokers in the United States. Tobacco use in the nation generally begins in early adolescence, and the earlier young people begin using tobacco, the more heavily they are likely to use it as adults. The addictive properties of nicotine ensure that many adolescent smokers will become regular users of tobacco as adults, leading to the eventual development of chronic health problems.

In the general population, tobacco use is associated with many diseases such as cancers of the lung, throat, pharynx, and esophagus and contributes to the development of cancers of the pancreas, cervix, kidney, and stomach. It is also associated with chronic bronchitis, emphysema, and chronic obstructive pulmonary disease (COPD). Specific to female smokers are health risks such as primary and secondary infertility and delays in becoming pregnant. With respect to pregnancy outcomes, women who smoke are at increased risk of premature rupture of membranes, low-birth-weight babies, and preterm delivery. Smoking is also a major cause of coronary heart disease among women.

Economic and Social Costs

Tobacco use not only imposes a heavy toll on health, but it also is associated with a significant economic burden by way of medical expenditures and the loss annually of billions of dollars in lost productivity. Coupled with the high medical costs of treating diseases caused by tobacco is the lost productivity from the shortened lifespan of those who use tobacco regularly. Tobacco users are also less productive while they are alive due to increased sickness and absenteeism from work.

Smokers impose costs on society that are distinct from their private costs of using tobacco. These costs include costs borne by families of tobacco users, health costs borne by governments, and the costs of environmental tobacco smoke. Smokers impose direct health costs on nonsmokers, such as low-birth-weight babies born to mothers who smoke during pregnancy. Furthermore, nonsmokers who are chronically exposed to secondhand smoke are at increased risk of diseases such as asthma and lung cancer along with other adverse health effects. Nonsmokers also end up bearing, at least partially, the higher medical costs incurred by smokers through smokers' increased use of medical-care facilities. Most medical care in the United States, specifically care associated with hospital treatment, is financed through public and/or private health insurance programs. Unless smokers contribute to these financing mechanisms by paying differentially higher insurance premiums or taxes, nonsmokers are in effect partly subsidizing medical care for smokers.

Control Measures

While smoking has been identified as a serious health hazard among healthcare professionals, economists and policymakers are still debating the many aspects of tobacco control measures, including the economic costs and benefits of tobacco consumption, the relative merits of different methods of tobacco control, and how efficient and equitable they prove to be. In the past, efforts were focused on individual-level interventions, such as clinical and small-group interventions. However, current tobacco control measures focus more on population-level strategies, such as normative change of the social acceptability of tobacco use, higher taxes on cigarettes, advertising and marketing restrictions, countertobacco marketing, prevention and cessation services, media campaigns, and other policy and legislative actions. The shift from individual- to population-level interventions has occurred not only because of the realization that large-scale change can only be achieved through concerted public policy efforts but also because of the growing awareness of the rights of nonsmokers.

Niranjana Kowlessar

See also Causal Analysis; Epidemiology; Mortality, Major Causes in the U.S.; Preventive Care; Public Health; Public Health Policy Advocacy; Public Policy; World Health Organization (WHO)

Further Readings

Boyle, Peter, Nigel Gray, Jack Henningfield, et al. eds. *Tobacco: Science, Policy and Public Health*. New York: Oxford University Press, 2004.

Ferrence, Roberta, John Slade, Robin Room, et al. eds. *Nicotine and Public Health*. Washington, DC: American Public Health Association, 2000.

Fiore, Michael C., William C. Bailey, Stuart J. Cohen, et al. eds. *Treating Tobacco Use and Dependence: Quick Reference Guide for Clinicians*. Rockville, MD: U.S. Department of Health and Human Services. Public Health Service, October 2000.

Goodman, Jordan E., ed. *Tobacco in History and Culture: An Encyclopedia*. New York: Charles Scribner's Sons, 2004.

Jha, Prabhat, and Frank J. Chaloupka. *Curbing the Epidemic: Governments and the Economics of Tobacco Control*. Washington, DC: World Bank, 1999.

Orleans, C. Tracy, and John Slade, eds. *Nicotine Addiction: Principles and Management*. New York: Oxford University Press, 1993.

U.S. Department of Health, Education, and Welfare, U.S. Public Health Service, Center for Disease Control. *Smoking and Health. Report of the Advisory Committee to the Surgeon General of the Public Health Service*. Washington, DC: Center for Disease Control, 1964.

Warner, Kenneth E., ed. *Tobacco Control Policy*. San Francisco: Jossey-Bass, 2006.

Web Sites

American Lung Association: http://www.lungusa.org

American Public Health Association (APHA): http://www.apha.org

Centers for Disease Control and Prevention (CDC): http://www.cdc.gov

World Health Organization (WHO) History of Tobacco: http://www.who.int/tobacco/en/atlas2.pdf

TRANSPORTATION

There are many forms of transportation available to transport the ill, the injured, and the disabled to and from various healthcare facilities. Medi-vans, helicopters, and ambulances are some of the ways by which patients are transported to receive needed healthcare. The lack of access to reliable individual and public transportation, however, continues to be one of the largest and most widely recognized barriers to receiving healthcare in the United States. Although patients no longer have to rely on physicians to make routine house calls, rural residents, minorities, the elderly, children, and the indigent are more likely to experience travel burden or transportation barriers to healthcare.

Overview

Studies have shown that people with a driver's license have two and a half times more visits for chronic care and almost two times more visits for regular check-up care than those who do not have a driver's license. Additionally, people with access to affordable public transportation have four more chronic-care visits annually than those who do not. Transportation barriers have also been linked to lower rates of preventive care, compliance with treatment regimens, and accessing emergency care. In 2006, it was estimated that 3.2 million people (4% of the population) either missed a scheduled visit or did not schedule a visit to a healthcare provider because of transportation issues. This estimate increased to 7% for families with an income of less than $50,000 per year.

Urban areas in the United States have tremendously benefited from the vast amounts of healthcare resources available, ranging from ambulatory and air transportation to a choice of medical facility.

Although efficient transportation services in urban areas allow those with an emergent condition to choose from various acute-care facilities, many more individuals fail to receive adequate transportation to even primary healthcare. Urban health departments are using multi-million-dollar government grants to coordinate emergency transportation for thousands of people to receive medical care in the event of a mass casualty; however, more than half of some rural residents cannot find any transportation to receive immediate medical care. Furthermore, if transportation becomes available, many still cannot afford to pay for it.

Inaccessibility

While transportation has certainly eased the suffering of many, it is still an inaccessible resource to many—namely, the elderly, children, minorities, the indigent, and the rural population. The elderly use a variety of transportation methods to access the healthcare system, including driving themselves, depending on someone else, or using public transportation. Due to health problems with aging, the elderly may be unable to access healthcare because of travel burdens.

For children, the lack of transportation may mean missing out on routine medical care such as immunizations and well-child care, in addition to the increased suffering from chronic illness. Because children miss out on routine medical care, they are often transported to emergency rooms when the need for care is urgent—resulting in an increased use of emergency rooms and hospitalizations. These emergency room visits may be prevented with better access to transportation to primary care. As late as 2001, one in five children living in families at or below the poverty level in the United States was unable to access routine medical care due to the lack of transportation. (Though Medicaid recipients are entitled to transportation to receive care, many are unaware of this benefit.) Additionally, almost 50% of families reported that public transportation was not a viable option to travel to medical facilities. In rural areas, this figure was almost 75%.

Racial and ethnic minorities also have a greater likelihood of experiencing transportation barriers to healthcare. Minorities are more likely to use public transportation and travel longer distances than Whites.

The lack of transportation is not merely an option for people without any means of accessing medical care. Transportation becomes a large barrier for people with few financial resources. For the indigent, timely, reliable, and affordable transportation to healthcare can be difficult.

Rural residents are more likely than urban residents to experience travel burden or transportation barriers. This is the case because there are not as many healthcare facilities located in rural areas, and therefore residents must generally travel farther to receive their care. It is not uncommon for families to travel 20 miles or more to receive their primary care in rural areas. Rural areas also typically lack public transportation systems. It has been shown that as the distance traveled increases, healthcare utilization decreases. Because of transportation barriers, people in rural areas access healthcare at later stages of illness and, as a result, have poorer outcomes. Furthermore, many individuals in rural areas are unable to access any care, or they have to wait for a long period of time, resulting in a decline of health status. Public health and medical prevention and intervention efforts rarely reach rural areas because they are so difficult to get to. Additionally, even when present, healthcare providers have limited access to needed resources to modify lifestyles.

Future Implications

Transportation options are pivotal in opening up channels of access to healthcare. Adequate transportation to healthcare is a vital factor in access to care for a large portion of the population. If proper transportation options are not provided, it may not only make it more difficult for patients to access care, but it may also ultimately prove to be more costly for the U.S. healthcare system.

Amy Sulkin

See also Access to Healthcare; Economic Barriers to Healthcare; Emergency Medical Services (EMS); Geographic Barriers to Healthcare; Patient Transfers; Rural Health; Timeliness of Healthcare; Vulnerable Populations

Further Readings

Ahmed, Syed M., Jeanne P. Lemkau, Nichol Nealeigh, et al. "Barriers to Healthcare Access in a Non-Elderly

Urban Poor American Population," *Health and Social Care in the Community* 9(6): 445–53, November 2001.

Arcury, Thomas A., Wilbert M. Gesler, John S. Preisser, et al. "The Effects of Geography and Spatial Behavior on Health Care Utilization Among the Residents of a Rural Region," *Health Services Research* 40(1): 135–56, February 2005.

Arcury, Thomas A., John S. Preisser, Wilbert M. Gesler, et al. "Access to Transportation and Health Care Utilization in a Rural Region," *Journal of Rural Health* 21(1): 31–38, Winter 2005.

Beckman, Ursula, Donna M. Gillies, Sean M. Berenholtz, et al. "Incidents Relating to the Intra-Hospital Transfer of Critically Ill Patients," *Intensive Care Medicine* 30(8): 1579–85, August 2004.

Canto, John G., Robert J. Zalenski, Joseph P. Oranato, et al. "Use of Emergency Medical Services in Acute Myocardial Infarction and Subsequent Quality of Care," *Circulation* 106(24): 3018–3023, December 10, 2002.

Frank, Lawrence D., Peter O. Engelke, and Thomas L. Schmid. *Health and Community Design: The Impact of the Built Environment on Physical Activity.* Washington, DC: Island Press, 2003.

Onega, Tracy, Eric J. Duell, Xun Shi, et al. "Geographic Access to Cancer Care in the U.S." *Cancer* 112(4): 909–18, February 15, 2008.

Web Sites

American Public Transportation Association: http://www.publictransportation.org
Association of Air Medical Services (AAMS): http://www.aams.org
National Association of Emergency Medical Technicians (NAEMT): http://www.naemt.org
National Association of Healthcare Transport Management (NAHTM): http://www.nahtm.org
National Rural Health Association (NRHA): http://www.nrharural.org

TRICARE, MILITARY HEALTH SYSTEM

TRICARE is the U.S. Department of Defense's (DOD's) medical entitlement program that covers eligible uniformed services beneficiaries for medically necessary care. Eligible beneficiaries may receive care either at a DOD military treatment facility or from a TRICARE authorized civilian provider. TRICARE is the health benefit for all seven uniformed services: Army, Navy, Marine Corps, Air Force, Coast Guard, Public Health Service, and National Oceanic Atmospheric Administration.

The TRICARE healthcare program serves active-duty service members, retirees and their families, survivors, and certain family spouses worldwide. As a major component of the Military Health System (MHS), TRICARE brings together the healthcare resources of the uniformed services and supplements them with networks of civilian healthcare professionals, institutions, pharmacies, and suppliers to provide access to healthcare services while maintaining the capability to support military operations.

The plan comprises insurance and care services. The TRICARE Management Activity (TMA) unit of the DOD administers the program. Currently, the system serves 9.2 million beneficiaries at an annual cost of $39 billion.

History

Since 1956, the DOD has been permitted to provide civilian healthcare to dependents of military service members as a result of the U.S. Congress passing the Medical Care Act. Over the years, that Act was amended, and the Civilian Health and Medical Program of the Uniformed Services (CHAMPUS) was created. As of October 1, 1966, only the family members of active-duty personnel were eligible. On January 1, 1967, retired service members and their dependents became eligible. Thus, since 1967, the DOD has funded care by civilian providers to dependents, retirees, and dependents of retirees who are under age 65 and unable to obtain access in a military health facility.

After several demonstration projects in the 1980s, the U.S. Congress and the DOD made numerous changes to the CHAMPUS Program. TRICARE was organized as a separate office under the Assistant Secretary of Defense and replaced CHAMPUS in 1994. Benefits covered under CHAMPUS are now covered under TRICARE Standard.

After 1991, the DOD began, with congressional support, moving toward managed-care arrangements under the TRICARE program that include greater use of civilian healthcare providers even for active-duty personnel. Since then, TRICARE has undergone several restructuring initiatives, including realignment of contract regions, base realignment and closure, and the addition of TRICARE for Life benefits in 2001 for those who are eligible and TRICARE Reserve Select in 2005.

Options

For eligible persons under age 65, TRICARE consists of TRICARE Prime, a managed-care option; TRICARE Extra, a preferred provider option (PPO); and TRICARE Standard, a fee-for-service option. TRICARE partners with civilian companies, Health Net Federal Services, Inc., Humana Military Healthcare Services, Inc., and TriWest Healthcare Alliance, Corp., as well as military hospitals and clinics, to provide healthcare services and support.

TRICARE Prime is a plan similar to a civilian HMO that provides the lowest out-of-pocket cost, in return for the requirement that enrollees use only physicians, hospitals, and other healthcare providers that are part of the TRICARE network. Enrollees are assigned a primary-care physician, known generally as a "gatekeeper," who supervises all medical care and is the one who authorizes referrals for specialty care. Active-duty and reserve service members are automatically enrolled in TRICARE Prime. However, military dependents and retirees must choose the TRICARE option that best suits their needs. Active-duty service members and their dependents have no enrollment fee. Retirees pay an annual enrollment fee and enroll for 1 year at a time.

Eligibility

TRICARE Prime is available to the following beneficiaries as long as they are not entitled to Medicare Part A and Part B due to age (65 years of age or older): active-duty service members and their families; retired service members and their families; eligible former spouses; National Guard and reserve members and their families when the National Guard or reserve member is activated for more than 30 consecutive days; retired National Guard and reserve members and their families; and Medal of Honor recipients and their families.

TRICARE Extra is the PPO. It offers choices of civilian physicians and specialists from a network of healthcare providers. It is often chosen by individuals and families whose regular physician lives too far away from a military hospital. The government shares the costs of healthcare. For using this network of preferred physicians and specialists, the government will pay an additional 5% of medical costs incurred (85% for dependents of active duty). There is no annual enrollment fee to participate in TRICARE Extra.

TRICARE Standard is the healthcare option formerly known as CHAMPUS. Eligible beneficiaries have the greatest flexibility in choosing a healthcare provider, and the government will pay a percentage of the cost. It is chosen most often by individuals and families having established relationships they wish to maintain with civilian physicians. There is no annual enrollment fee to participate in TRICARE Standard.

TRICARE for Life (TFL)

On October 1, 2001, a new TRICARE entitlement for Medicare-eligible uniformed-service retirees, eligible family members, and survivors referred to as TFL came into effect. TFL is TRICARE's Medicare-wraparound coverage available to *all* Medicare-eligible TRICARE beneficiaries, regardless of age, provided they have Medicare Parts A and B. TRICARE acts as a second payer to Medicare. TRICARE pays the remaining out-of-pocket expenses (Medicare deductibles and cost shares) for services paid by Medicare and covered by TRICARE. Under TFL, a beneficiary will currently not pay more than $3,000 per family per year in TRICARE-allowable expenses. After that, TRICARE pays 100%. In most cases, TFL-eligible beneficiaries have little need for other health insurance besides Medicare and TFL.

Other Coverage

The TRICARE senior pharmacy benefit provides Medicare-eligible retirees of the uniformed services, their family members, and survivors the same pharmacy benefit as retirees who are under age 65. It includes access to prescription drugs not only at military treatment facilities but also at retail pharmacies and through the TRICARE mail order pharmacy program. The current pharmacy cost-share structure—meaning the percentage of fixed amount that the beneficiary pays toward the cost of the medication—is based on whether a prescription medication is a generic, formulary, or nonformulary pharmaceutical. The copayment is the same for all TRICARE beneficiaries (except active-duty service members, who receive medications free of charge) depending on where the beneficiaries choose to fill their prescription.

Vision Care

TRICARE vision benefits vary depending on beneficiary status (i.e., active-duty member, active-duty family member, retired service member, or retired family member) and enrollment in TRICARE Prime. TRICARE Prime enrollees aged 3 and older are authorized a comprehensive eye examination once every 2 years. Prime enrollees may receive the services from any TRICARE network provider without a referral or authorization from the primary-care manager, healthcare finder, or any other authority. If the beneficiary receives services from a nonnetwork provider that has not been authorized, the beneficiary is responsible for the entire amount of the bill. Pediatric vision screening is available at birth and at approximately 6 months of age. Diabetic patients, at any age, are allowed annual comprehensive eye examinations.

Behavioral and Mental Health

The behavioral health program now provides a locator and assistance service, which is especially helpful for those who may find it hard to locate a behavioral healthcare provider in the network. Active-duty service members must have a referral from their primary-care physician for behavioral healthcare. TRICARE Prime active-duty family members can receive the first eight outpatient behavioral healthcare visits per fiscal year without a referral, but they must receive the care from TRICARE network providers to avoid point-of-service cost-sharing charges.

Skilled Nursing

Skilled-nursing coverage typically covers the following: medically necessary skilled nursing care, rehabilitative therapies, room and board, prescription drugs, laboratory work, supplies, appliances, and medical equipment. There are four admission criteria for skilled nursing care. First, the beneficiary must be treated in a hospital for at least 3 consecutive days, not including the day of discharge. Second, he or she must be admitted within 30 days of hospital discharge (with some exceptions) to a skilled-nursing facility. Next, a physician's treatment plan must demonstrate the need for medically necessary rehabilitation and skilled services. And finally, the facility must be Medicare certified and a participating provider.

Hospice

Hospice is available for terminally ill patients expected to live 6 months or less if the illness runs its normal course. A Medicare-approved program must provide the hospice care.

Funding and Cost Containment

In addition to revisions in military planning, nationwide changes in the practice of medicine have also affected the DOD. In particular, managed-care initiatives and capitated budgeting that are widely adopted in the civilian community are being implemented in the DOD's TRICARE program. TRICARE is also designed to coordinate the medical-care efforts of the three military departments in three geographical regions, each under a single military commander known as a lead agent. The lead agents are responsible for managing care provided by all military medical facilities in their respective regions and for contracting for additional care from civilian providers. These competitively bid, regionwide contracts represent a significant change in the delivery of defense healthcare and will, it is anticipated, result in cost savings.

The U.S. Congress, as is the case with all federal entitlement programs, determines the funding of TRICARE in the National Defense Authorization Act. The dollar amounts allocated to healthcare in the budget of the DOD have doubled during the past 5 years, from $19 billion in FY2001 to more than $37 billion in FY2006, even as the size of the active-duty force has remained relatively steady. The DOD's projections for healthcare indicate that even further growth can be realistically anticipated, perhaps reaching $64 billion in 2015. In 1990, according to the DOD estimates, healthcare expenses constituted 4.5% of its budget; by 2015 it could reach 12%. This growth in healthcare costs could have a substantial effect on spending for other defense programs and/or the overall size of defense spending within the federal budget.

There are complex considerations with regard to any of the various approaches to dealing with the growth of military medical spending. To some extent, they reflect larger healthcare issues affecting the entire country. In the case of retired service members and their dependents, most recognize a special responsibility for the nation to provide healthcare after retirement, which is an important incentive for those who follow a difficult and often dangerous career.

Bernard H. Baum

See also Congressional Budget Office (CBO); Health Insurance; Health Maintenance Organizations (HMOs); Managed Care; Medicare; Preferred Provider Organizations (PPO); Primary Care

Further Readings

Kress, Amii M., Michael C. Hartzell, Michael R. Peterson, et al. "Status of U.S. Military Retirees and Their Spouses Toward Achieving Healthy People 2010 Objectives," *American Journal of Health Promotion* 20(5): 334–41, May–June 2006.

Mangelsdorff, David A., Ken Finstuen, Stephen D. Larsen, et al. "Patient Satisfaction in Military Medicine: Model Refinement and Assessment of Department of Defense Effects," *Military Medicine* 170(4): 309–14, April 2005.

Mulkey, Shonna L., L. Harrison Hassell, and Kevin G. LaFrance. "The Implications of TRICARE on Medical Readiness," *Military Medicine* 169(1): 16–22, January 2004.

Tieman, Jeff. "Marching Orders. TRICARE Restructuring, Rebidding Designed to Cut Costs, Improve Quality," *Modern Healthcare* 33(20): 52, 54, May 19, 2003.

Web Sites

Military Benefits: http://www.military.com/benefits/tricare

Office of the Assistant Secretary of Defense (Health Affairs), TRICARE: http://www.tricare.mil

U.S. Department of Defense (DOD), Military Health System: http://mhs.osd.mil

U

UNCOMPENSATED HEALTHCARE

Uncompensated healthcare is care provided by physicians, hospitals, and other medical personnel pro bono, a shortened form of *pro bono publico*, a Latin phrase meaning "for the public good." In 2008, about 47 million Americans lack health insurance coverage, and many of the uninsured are indigent. Their only health services come from physicians, hospitals, and other medical personnel who provide uncompensated healthcare pro bono. Public debate concerning the uninsured continues, so it is important to examine why medical personnel provide uncompensated healthcare, its role in American politics and beliefs about healthcare for the poor, issues in defining uncompensated care, how to estimate the amount of uncompensated care, and the future implications of uncompensated healthcare.

History

Uncompensated healthcare, and the general issue of how to care for the poor, has been an important issue in America since colonial times. Reflecting English practice and law, such as the 1601 Statute of Charitable Uses, some colonies emphasized public support for the poor. However, other colonies placed greater emphasis on each community's need to take care of its own poor, the efforts of voluntary charities and mutual benevolent societies, and the private efforts of individual providers. The need for uncompensated healthcare grew during the 19th century, as urbanization and immigration separated many of the poor from traditional sources of support, such as extended families, while exposing them to the health risks of concentrated urban poverty. These developments continued into the 20th century and became part of the new problem of the "uninsured" and "underinsured."

While other nations adopted universal, government-supported medicine, the United States provided healthcare for the poor through private charity, either through institutions such as charitable hospitals or through the charity care provided by physicians and other medical providers who otherwise would be paid for their services. Throughout much of the 19th century, Americans who could afford care paid a physician to come to their home, while the poor went to hospitals or clinics (almost all of which were charitable). Hospitals were founded as charitable institutions, and many held that physicians had an ethical requirement to provide charity care, as part of their accepting the Hippocratic Oath.

Throughout, the 19th century governmental activities were limited primarily to local government (especially cities) establishing public hospitals and clinics. Many of these facilities became part of the safety net of facilities that continue to provide care to the indigent. The federal government did not expand its role in healthcare beyond providing care to merchant seamen, military personnel, and American Indians until the 20th century, when it partnered with states to pay for care to the categorically needy, such as the poor elderly. States administered these programs with financial support from the federal government. While these programs were expanded during the Great Depression, the federal government did not assume a major role in healthcare until these categorical programs became part of Medicare and Medicaid in 1965.

The reliance on the private sector to provide charity care had several sources. American tradition since the Revolutionary War emphasized each person's responsibility to take care of himself or herself ("the rugged individual") and the belief that local governments and private charities, rather than the national government, should care for those who needed and deserved help ("the deserving needy"). The national government's role was seen during most of the 19th century as dealing with issues that involved more than one state—interstate issues rather than local or intrastate issues such as healthcare. During the latter part of the 19th century, the emphasis on private charity, donated services, and local government assumed new importance as an alternative to socialism, especially the Marxism espoused by some immigrant groups and workers' organizations.

After slowly expanding health-related programs during the Great Depression, the U.S. Congress passed the Hospital Survey and Construction Act, commonly called the Hill-Burton Act (PL 725), in 1946. This act provided federal funds to help states construct and modernize nonprofit hospitals, nursing homes, and other health facilities. These facilities were then obligated to provide a reasonable amount of charity care for 20 years afterward. The last Hill-Burton grants were awarded in 1997, and approximately 300 hospitals and nursing homes still have Hill-Burton obligations.

More recently, some states have attempted to require nonprofit hospitals to provide charity care in order to retain their tax-exempt status. Since 1986, the federal government through the Emergency Medical Treatment and Active Labor Act (42 USC 1935), commonly called EMTALA, requires that the hospitals that participate in the Medicare program provide pro bono emergency care to all patients, even if they are not Medicare beneficiaries.

Definitions

Uncompensated healthcare has many definitions, depending on the perspective of the observer. It can be defined narrowly to mean totally uncompensated healthcare (charity or pro bono care) given by those who normally charge for their services. The American Institute of Certified Public Accountants (AICPA) requires that financial statements use this definition, and the Healthcare Financial Management Association (HFMA) recommends it. The American Hospital Association's definition of uncompensated healthcare comes close to this definition, although it includes bad debt as well as charity care. On the other hand, uncompensated healthcare has also been defined to include services provided at less than full charges, such as services to Medicaid recipients, and even services provided on a sliding scale.

The definition of the cost of uncompensated healthcare also can be restricted to the marginal cost to provide that care—the additional cost that the provider incurred by treating that additional patient, or it can be defined to include the full cost of that care, which includes the marginal cost and a share of the fixed cost. This distinction is especially important because healthcare has a substantial fixed cost, which makes the marginal cost much less than the total cost. The marginal cost of 1 day of hospital care is mainly food, linen, drugs, and the marginal cost of a physician's visit. Those costs are much less than the full cost of a day of care, which includes capital costs, salary costs, and maintenance costs. The marginal cost of an outpatient visit to a physician's office can be almost zero, compared with the full cost, which includes physician's capital costs, practice expenses, and so forth. From an accounting perspective, valuing charity care at its marginal cost is more logical when it is only a small percentage of total expenses, such as 3% (or less), versus when it is a larger percentage of total expenses, such as 10%.

These differences in definition determine not only how to measure uncompensated healthcare but also its significance in the American healthcare system. Charity care represents a true cost to the provider, a cost that represents a contribution to society. Including all services provided at less than regular charges can include services that reflect a business decision as much as good intent. A hospital might accept Medicaid recipients because they can serve as patients for its residency programs or because Medicaid's limited payments will still contribute to the hospital's total profits or surplus if it has already covered its fixed costs. Measuring uncompensated healthcare at its marginal cost makes the care burden much smaller than measuring the care at its full cost.

Amount of Uncompensated Healthcare

The American Hospital Association (AHA) reports that community hospitals provided $28.8 billion of uncompensated care in 2005, about 5.6% of total expenses, compared with $3.9 billion in 1980. This change is an increase of 638% unadjusted for inflation and an increase of about 100% adjusting for general inflation. Community hospitals include both nonprofit and for-profit hospitals but exclude long-term hospitals and hospitals that provide only one type of healthcare, such as psychiatric care, rehabilitation care, or orthopedic care. Between 1980 and 2005, uncompensated healthcare ranged between 5.1% and 6% of total expenses. The percentage was constant despite economic fluctuations during this period, which included recessions and changes in the percentage of managed care. The Federation of American Hospitals reported that in 2005, the average acute-care for-profit hospital provided $15.4 million in uncompensated healthcare.

Using data from the Center for Studying Health System Change's Community Tracking Study (CTS), which included a telephone survey of physicians, researchers found that during 2004–2005, 68% of responding physicians had provided charity care during the month prior to their participating in the survey. This estimate is conservative, however, since it includes only the charity care provided during the previous month. During that month, these physicians had provided an average of 10.6 hours of charity care, which represented 6.3% of their practice time. Surgical specialists were more likely to have provided charity care than other physicians, because they were assigned charity care by the hospitals where they have admitting privileges. Physicians in solo practice or in other physician-owned practices were also more likely to have provided charity care than physicians such as those working in hospital-owned practices. The percentage of group practice physicians who provided charity care declined with the size of the practice. In small-group practices, 78% of physicians provided charity care, compared with 62% of physicians in practices with more than 50 physicians.

Using cost survey data from the Medical Group Management Association (MGMA), the researchers also found that 43% of group practices reported having given charity care during 2005, and the average amount of charity care was 1.7% of gross charges, or a median of $180,000 per practice. Preliminary research by the MGMA indicates that this estimate understates the amount of charity care since some practices that reported no charity care actually provided free services but did not include the services in their financial or billing records.

In 2005, the Pharmaceutical Research and Manufacturers of America (PhRMA) helped organize the Partnership for Prescription Assistance (PPA), which provides prescription medications to patients either at no cost or at reduced cost. The American Academy of Family Physicians (AAFP), American Autoimmune Related Diseases Association (AARDA), Lupus Foundation of America (LFA), National Association for the Advancement of Colored People (NAACP), National Alliance for Hispanic Health (NAHH), and National Medical Association (NMA) also collaborate with this program. The PPA directs patients to other sources of pharmaceutical assistance such as Medicaid. It also helps consolidate assistance programs sponsored by individual drug manufacturers, some of which had been in existence for 50 years. Since 2005, the program has helped approximately 3.6 million people, and PhRMA estimates that the program has already provided billions of dollars in pharmaceuticals.

In 1999, the American Dental Association (ADA) reported that 69.7% of dentists provided free or discounted charity care. The ADA also has described the charity care individual dentists have provided and has called attention to the need to enable indigent patients to afford dental care.

The American Health Care Association (AHCA), which represents long-term care facilities, has studied the differences between Medicaid payments and the cost to provide healthcare to Medicaid patients. That study estimated that unreimbursed nursing home Medicaid allowable costs were $4.5 billion in 2006, a 4% increase over the previous year.

Trends in Supply and Demand

As noted above, the percentage of hospital revenue allocated to charity care has remained stable over the past 20 years. However, there is evidence that charity care is becoming more concentrated in a smaller number of hospitals. Some hospitals, especially those that are not a part of the safety net of hospitals that provide healthcare to the indigent, are trimming services commonly used by indigent patients. However, safety net hospitals, especially publicly owned hospitals, will likely face increased financial pressures, while at the same time local governments may seek to avoid tax increases.

The number of physicians providing charity care also appears to be declining. Researchers have found that the percentage of physicians who provide charity care declined from 76% during 1996–1997 to 68% in 2004–2005. They attribute this decrease primarily to the decline in physicians' practice income during the period. MGMA data also show that the percentage of medical groups reporting charity care appears to be declining.

The demand for uncompensated healthcare, however, will almost certainly continue to increase. The reasons include the continued increase in the number of uninsured, increased deductibles and copayments among insured patients, and the increasing age of the nation's population. People with chronic diseases such as diabetes and HIV/AIDS are living longer, and others (especially members of the baby boomer generation) expect to be healthier longer.

Future Implications

A number of factors will likely shape the future of uncompensated healthcare in America. These factors include economic, life style, and health insurance trends, changes among healthcare providers, and the increasing use of nonphysician providers.

Economic Trends

General economic trends will be a major factor in uncompensated healthcare. The adage "It's the economy, stupid" applies to uncompensated care as well. Economic downturns increase the number of unemployed (and therefore uninsured), increase the number of jobs that do not provide health insurance, and increase the number of workers in low-paying jobs who cannot pay for healthcare. Downturns also increase the number of people living in poverty, especially urban poverty, and the health risk factors that poverty brings. The links between poverty and illness are well established.

Life Style Trends

Preventable illnesses are becoming an increasingly large percentage of all illnesses, especially among the poor, who are the most likely to need uncompensated care. Increasing exercise alone could reduce illnesses such as heart disease and diabetes, which are costly to treat and are becoming more frequent. Yet the poor have the least access to opportunities for exercise, including health clubs and parks. Changing lifestyles, especially among vulnerable populations, can do much to reduce the need for uncompensated healthcare.

Health Insurance Trends

While the current health insurance system emphasizes choice, including the choice to have no insurance coverage, it creates coverage gaps that uncompensated healthcare is asked to fill. In recent years, deductibles (the amount that the individual must pay before the insurance starts) and copays (the amount or percentage the individual must pay after the insurance starts) have increased, and a smaller percentage of employers offer health insurance coverage. The current system leaves many poor and low-income people with no health insurance. The Medicaid system covers only the "deserving needy," such as dependent children, and in most states, Medicaid does not pay enough to encourage a large number of physicians, dentists, and therapists to accept Medicaid recipients. The uninsured poor present a substantial burden to safety net providers and to all providers of charity care. Because of this, there have been calls for universal coverage, either through a single-payer system, such as the Canadian system, or through a multipayer/universal enrollment system, such as the one found in Ireland, Japan, and the Netherlands. The poor can be included in a universal health system, or they can be included in community-based programs. Such efforts to change the American health insurance system to a universal system have not succeeded in the past.

Changes Among Healthcare Providers

Changes among healthcare providers may also affect the amount of charity care. Physicians are moving out of solo practice into groups, which are less likely to provide charity care, and the percentage of medical practices not owned by physicians is increasing. Both of these practices are much less likely to offer charity care than physician-owned practices. Whether these trends continue will affect how much uncompensated healthcare is provided. Additionally, hospitals are increasingly becoming part of multihospital systems, although it is too early to tell what these changes mean for the provision of charity care. Not-for-profit hospitals will continue to face debates on whether their tax-exempt status requires charity care or general community benefit.

Use of Nonphysician Providers

Nonphysician providers, especially therapists, are becoming increasingly important in patient care. For example, stroke patients may need physical, speech, and occupational therapy in addition to physician and hospital care to return to normal life. Many patients also need laboratory and diagnostic procedures. Hospitals and physicians have long traditions of providing charity care. In the past, many therapists and laboratory technicians were employed by hospitals and therefore provided charity care as part of the hospital's charitable activities. However, they are increasingly practicing outside hospitals in settings without a strong charity care tradition and no legal charity care obligation. Nonphysician providers may face similar charity care decisions in the future to those hospitals and physicians already face.

Uncompensated care will likely remain an important issue as medical care continues to expand and the categories of personnel providing healthcare continue to increase. Hospitals, physicians, dentists, therapists, and other providers will have to decide how much charity care to provide, society will have to decide how much care to provide to those who cannot afford to pay, and patients who cannot afford to pay will have to find providers that will treat them pro bono.

Steven Andes and David N. Gans

See also Charity Care; Cost of Healthcare; Free Clinics; Healthcare Financial Management; Health Insurance Coverage; Hospitals; Safety Net; Uninsured Individuals

Further Readings

Evans, Melanie. "Uncompensated Care Spikes by 8.3%: AHA. Medicare Losses at General Hospitals Also Up 20% to $18.6 Billion, Association Says," *Modern Healthcare* 37(43): 8–9, October 29, 2007.

Gruber, Jonathan, and David Rodriguez. "How Much Uncompensated Care Do Doctors Provide?" In *NBER Working Paper Series*, no. 13585. Cambridge, MA: National Bureau of Economic Research, 2007.

Lo Sasso, Anthony T., and Dorian G. Seamster. "How Federal and State Policies Affected Hospital Uncompensated Care Provision in the 1990s," *Medical Care Research and Review* 64(6): 731–44, December 2007.

MacKelvie, Charles, Michael Apolskis, and James J. Unland. "Recent Hospital Charity Care Controversies Highlight Ambiguities and Outdated Features of Government Regulations," *Journal of Health Care Finance* 31(4): 14–30, Summer 2005.

Pagan, Jose A., Lakshmi Balasubramanian, and Mark V. Pauly. "Physicians' Career Satisfaction, Quality of Care and Patients' Trust: The Role of Community Uninsurance," *Health Economics, Policy, and Law* 2(pt. 4): 347–62, October 2007.

Schuhmann, Thomas M. "National Trends in Uncompensated Care and Profitability," *Healthcare Financial Management* 62(9): 110–16, 118, September 2008.

Sigmond, Robert M. "Doing Away With Uncompensated Care of the Uninsured," *Inquiry* 41(4): 365–75, Winter 2004–2005.

Weiner, Saul J., Jonathan Van Geest, Richard I. Abrams, et al. "Managing the Unmanaged: A Case Study of Intra-Institutional Determinants of Uncompensated Care at Healthcare Institutions With Differing Ownership Models," *Medical Care* 46(8): 821–28, August 2008.

Web Sites

American Hospital Association (AHA): http://www.aha.org

Center for Studying Health System Change (HSC):
    http://www.hschange.com
Healthcare Financial Management Association (HFMA):
    http://www.hfma.org
Partnership for Prescription Assistance (PPA):
    http://www.pparx.org

UNINSURED INDIVIDUALS

The number of people who do not have any type of health insurance—that is, they are not covered by private policies or public programs such as Medicare and Medicaid—has been steadily increasing since the late 1970s, when the first federal surveys began asking about the coverage of individuals rather than just the head of a household. The uninsured as a percentage of the population has also been increasing. In 2006, the most recent year for which data are available, 47 million Americans did not have any type of health insurance. This was 2.2 million more people than in 2005, and it was the largest 1-year increase in the number of uninsured since the U.S. Census Bureau started collecting insurance status data in 1979. The fraction of the nation's population who were uninsured in 2006 stood at 15.8%, and among the population under age 65, 17.8%—one in six people—are uninsured.

Being without health insurance places a person at risk for potentially catastrophic expenses if he or she develops a disease, such as cancer, or a chronic medical condition, such as multiple sclerosis, or survives a major car accident or stroke. Such expenses can cause families to declare bankruptcy. Equally concerning is that the lack of health insurance can limit a person's access to healthcare. Many physicians and hospitals will not provide nonemergency services to people who are uninsured. Furthermore, people without health insurance who are treated often are not given the newer, most effective treatments, including newer pharmaceuticals, because they cost more. Thus, being uninsured involves serious risks.

Because private health insurance coverage is strongly tied to having an employer that sponsors group coverage and Medicaid coverage is tied to meeting eligibility criteria that include a low income, there are dynamic aspects to being uninsured.

Losing a job is often a trigger for losing health insurance, and likewise, changing jobs to one with a company that offers insurance can enable a person to gain coverage. Similarly, individuals can work in low-wage jobs and qualify for Medicaid, but if their employer asks them to work overtime, they can earn too much to still be eligible for Medicaid. These scenarios play out every day—people lose and gain jobs, and some lose or gain health insurance coverage, and some people lose eligibility for Medicaid, while others become eligible because of some misfortune.

These dynamics mean that over a period of time—say a year—there are people who are uninsured for part of the year while others are uninsured the entire year. Research on the dynamic aspects of health insurance coverage shows that although the median length of time that people are uninsured is about 6 months, a significant fraction (between 25% and 30%) of uninsured spells last more than a year. The implication of these studies is that surveys that ask about people's insurance situation at a point in time are not capturing the full extent to which being uninsured is a problem for people over a year or several years' time. Over the course of 2 years, the number of people who have at least 1 month without health insurance is perhaps one and a half times the number of people who are uninsured in any given week during the year when a survey may occur. Thus, the estimate of 47 million people without health insurance in any given week in 2006 could indicate that between 2005 and 2006, closer to 70 million people spent at least a month without health insurance coverage.

The dynamics of health insurance coverage point up a third risk that uninsured people face even if they are uninsured for only a short time: They may have a medical problem while they are uninsured, and then they are in trouble if they ever want to obtain self-purchased health insurance coverage. Insurers in the individual (or nongroup) market are very wary of adverse selection. In many states, insurers can reject applicants who have had medical problems, place restrictions on what medical services will be covered, or medically underwrite (i.e., increase the usual premium based on the medical history) the premium a person would have to pay. Thus, even being uninsured for a short time creates a risk for people.

Descriptions of the uninsured generally rely on annual surveys of the general population and do not include the dynamic aspects of health insurance coverage. This discussion of the uninsured follows that convention, but it is important to note that many people change their health insurance status over the course of a year.

Major Subgroups

People without health insurance coverage do not fit a single description—and the composition of the uninsured in terms of large subgroups of people has changed considerably since the late 1970s. The reasons for these changes are discussed in a separate section below. Before examining why people are uninsured, however, it is useful to know where the uninsured live and the characteristics that describe major subgroups of the uninsured. Using U.S. Census data from 2006, only slightly more than half are poor by official federal poverty standards, and the uninsured include a substantial number of middle-class people. Certain subgroups stand out: 20% are children, and another 40% are younger adults, 25 to 44 years old. One fifth are foreign-born, legal residents who are noncitizens. The primary reason these people are uninsured is that they lack access to employer-sponsored health insurance and most cannot afford to buy it in the individual market. The doubling of healthcare spending in the past decade has driven premiums to the point that an increasing number of companies are limiting their insurance costs and even individuals with middle-class incomes cannot afford individual coverage.

Where the Uninsured Live

As Figure 1 and Table 1 show, the uninsured are concentrated in the South and Western regions of the nation. More than half live in the South Atlantic, West South Central, and Pacific states. The regions with the highest proportions of their population who are uninsured are the West South Central (26%), Mountain (21%), South Atlantic (20%), and Pacific (19%). In contrast, New England has the lowest proportion of its population who are uninsured (11%). The fact that there is such variation in the proportion of the regions' populations who are uninsured is important because those areas with the higher proportions of uninsured face a more difficult financial situation in their efforts to expand health insurance coverage to their residents.

The Poor and the Middle Class

It is commonly believed that everyone who has an income below the federal poverty level ($10,294 for a single individual and $20,614 for a family of four in 2006) is covered by Medicaid. However, Medicaid covers many of the poor but not all: 11.5 million people—a quarter of all the uninsured younger than 65 years of age—had family incomes in 2006 that were officially in poverty. Another 13.5 million people (29% of the uninsured) were near poor, with incomes between the poverty level and two times the poverty level. Together, just over half of the uninsured—25 million people—had incomes that were poor or near poor by official standards. In terms of simple chances of being uninsured, one third of the people with incomes below two times the poverty level were uninsured in 2006.

Figure 2 shows the family incomes of the uninsured in dollars rather than in comparison with the federal poverty level. Half of the uninsured have family incomes less than $30,000. But almost 30% of the uninsured are middle-class people. The middle class can be defined as anyone with a family income above the median household income (i.e., the income level above which half the households in the nation have incomes). In 2006, the median household income was $48,201. By this definition, 13.5 million uninsured people were middle class.

The simple probability of being uninsured for a working-age adult (23–64 years of age) has increased significantly during the past 25 years. In 2006, a third of all working-age adults with incomes below the middle-class threshold were uninsured. This fraction is again half as large as it was in 1979, when a fifth of lower-income adults were uninsured. For middle-class adults, the simple probability of being uninsured is significantly lower. However, it has increased from just 6% in 1979 and throughout the 1980s to between 10% and 11% in 2005 and 2006. The fact that 1 in 10 working-age middle-class adults is uninsured signals a significant problem with health insurance for a substantial portion of the middle class.

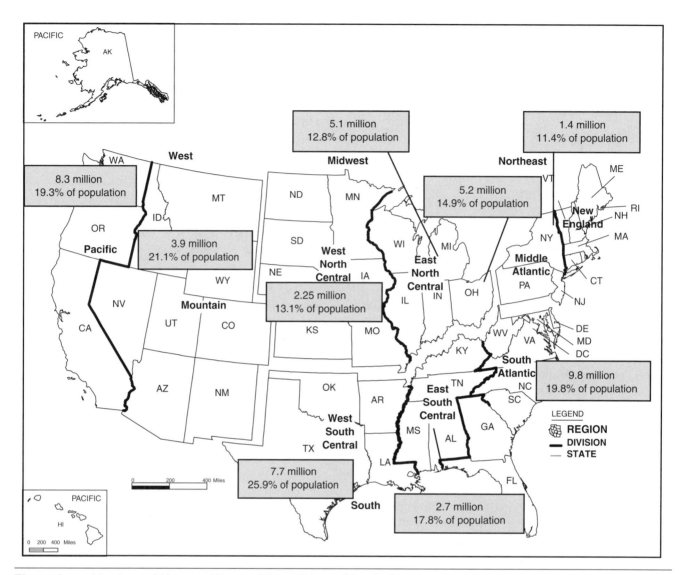

Figure 1   Numbers of Uninsured Younger Than 65 Years of Age by Regions of the United States and Percentage of Each Region's Nonelderly Population That Is Uninsured, 2006

Source: U.S. Census Bureau, Current Population Survey, March 2007.

Table 1   Regions of the United States Where the Uninsured Younger Than 65 Years of Age Live, 2006

Region	Number of Uninsured (Millions)	Percentage of Uninsured	Uninsured as Percentage of Region
New England	1.396	3.0	11.4
Middle Atlantic	5.158	11.1	14.9
East North Central	5.137	11.1	12.8
West North Central	2.253	4.9	13.1
South Atlantic	9.842	21.2	19.8
East South Central	2.711	5.8	17.8
West South Central	7.701	16.6	25.9
Mountain	3.939	8.5	21.1
Pacific	8.301	17.9	19.3
Total United States	46.438	100	17.8

Source: U.S. Census Bureau, Current Population Survey, March 2007.

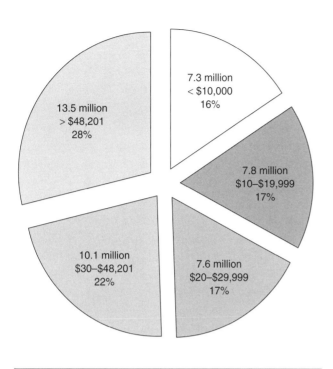

Figure 2   Family Income of the Nonelderly
              Uninsured, 2006

Source: U.S. Census Bureau, Current Population Survey,
March 2007.

Adults 25 to 44 Years of Age and Children

As can be seen in Figure 3, two out of five uninsured in 2006 are 25 to 44 years old. More significantly, as Figure 4 shows, the percentages of all people in these age cohorts who are uninsured are at all-time highs: More than a quarter of all 25- to 34-year-olds and a fifth of all 35- to 44-year-olds were uninsured in 2006. These fractions of each cohort are twice what they were in 1979.

Twenty percent of the uninsured in 2006 were children younger than 19 years of age. This fraction of the uninsured is half what it was in 1979, when 40% of the nonelderly uninsured were children. The major explanation for the drop in the percentage of the uninsured who were children is that the Medicaid income eligibility cap for children was raised starting in the late 1980s and in 1997 the State Children's Health Insurance Program (SCHIP) for near-poor children was implemented. In the early 2000s, the number of uninsured children stopped falling, and between

2005 and 2006, the number increased by 700,000, so that in 2006, 9.4 million children were uninsured. The fraction of all children who were uninsured was 12.1%, which was a slight increase over the past few years.

People With Less Formal Education and Occupations

Having low levels of formal education is a significant handicap for finding a job with employer-sponsored health insurance, and it is a major predictor of someone being uninsured. As Figure 5 shows, almost two thirds of uninsured adults 23 to 64 years of age have not gone past high school for formal education. Among adults who have not completed high school, 44% were uninsured; and a quarter of all adults who have high school diplomas but no further formal education were uninsured. This is a shift from a generation ago, when high school graduates could find well-paying jobs with large manufacturers. In 2006, five of the eight occupations that had the largest numbers of workers did not have high education requirements, and more than a

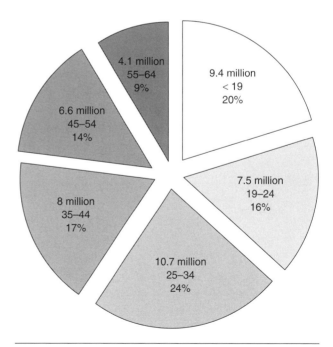

Figure 3   Age Distribution of the Nonelderly
              Uninsured, 2006

Source: U.S. Census Bureau, Current Population Survey,
March 2007.

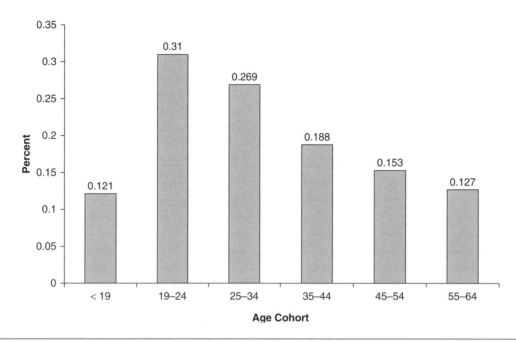

Figure 4   Fraction of People Without Health Insurance by Age Cohort, 2006

Source: U.S. Census Bureau, Current Population Survey, March 2007.

fifth of the people in each of these occupations were uninsured.

Foreign-Born Status

Immigrants who respond to U.S. Census surveys are almost all legally in the country; undocumented immigrants tend to hide from census interviewers. Immigrants are now a large subgroup of the uninsured. Just over a fifth of the uninsured in 2006—10 million people—were not born in the country and were not citizens. Another 2.3 million uninsured were foreign-born and were naturalized citizens. To see these numbers from another angle, not quite half (46.6%) of the foreign-born population who were not yet citizens were uninsured. This is in contrast to 15% of Americans born in the country and 19.8% of naturalized citizens who were uninsured.

The foreign-born who are not citizens include people who have not yet lived here long enough to apply for citizenship and people who may expect to return to their country of origin sometime in the future. Foreign-born residents who have been in the country for longer periods of time are less

likely to be uninsured than people who immigrated within the past 5 years.

A majority of foreign-born noncitizens are younger adults with low levels of formal education, earn low wages, and do not have employer-sponsored insurance at their jobs. Most of these uninsured immigrants live in the three regions of the country with the highest rates of uninsured. But even middle-class and well-educated foreign-born noncitizens are more likely to be uninsured than their native-born counterparts. Two out of five noncitizens have middle-class incomes, yet 28% of middle-class noncitizens are uninsured.

It is too simple to say that the immigrants from Latin America (which is where half the foreign-born population in 2000 came from) are uneducated and that explains the increase in the number of uninsured. Instead, the growth in the number of less educated immigrants in the past 20 years has to be seen as contributing to the imbalance between the demand for and supply of unskilled workers, enabling firms to hire low-wage workers without offering employer-sponsored health insurance.

To sum up, the 47 million people without health insurance coverage are a group of people with

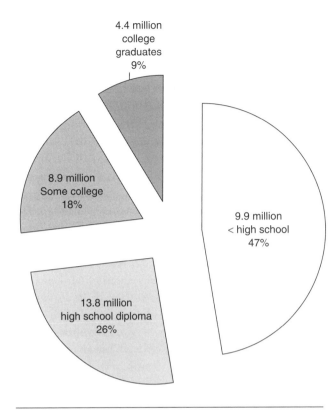

4.4 million
college
graduates
9%

8.9 million
Some college
18%

9.9 million
< high school
47%

13.8 million
high school diploma
26%

Figure 5   Education of Uninsured Adults (19–64 Years Old), 2006

Source: U.S. Census Bureau. Current Population Survey, March 2007.

many characteristics. Although it is tempting to say that many uninsured have several of the characteristics described above, that is not the case. In 2006, there were 3.1 million adults 19 through 34 years of age who had incomes below the poverty level, had not gone beyond high school for formal education, and were uninsured, but they accounted for only 17% of all uninsured adults 19 to 34 years of age. Thus, it is important to understand why an increasing fraction of the population are uninsured and why the uninsured today consist of different types of people compared with 25 years ago.

Reasons People Are Uninsured

Decline in Employer-Sponsored Health Insurance

The large increase in the number of uninsured between 2005 and 2006 reflects a now almost decade-old decline in the percentage of people with employer-sponsored insurance. In 2000, 68.3% of

the population younger than 65 years of age had employer-sponsored coverage, in 2006, the fraction was 62.9%. During the same time period, there was a steady decline in the fraction of firms that sponsored health insurance (from 69% in 2000 to 61% in 2006). In practice, the shrinking of employer-sponsored group coverage is greater than these statistics suggest. Firms that offer health insurance to "regular" employees are increasingly using workers hired through contract houses (often known as contract workers) and temporary agencies, and other self-employed people who work on specific tasks for long periods of time. When companies hire workers in these ways, the workers are not technically employees and are not included in the fringe benefit plans the firms offer. Younger adults are particularly likely to be employed as contract workers, which helps explain their significant representation among the uninsured.

The decline in the proportion of firms offering health insurance and the increased use of contract workers indicates the extent to which companies are moving to limit their financial risk of increases in healthcare costs over which they do not have direct control. For employers, the fastest rising labor cost has been health insurance. Since 1996, premiums for employer-sponsored coverage (both actual policies purchased from insurers and premium-equivalent costs for self-insured plans) have grown every year; the increases reflect the doubling of healthcare spending since 1996. Between 2001 and 2007, premiums for firms with more than three employees increased 78%—outpacing general inflation, which rose 17%. These increases occurred in spite of most employers shifting more out-of-pocket costs onto the workers in the form of higher deductibles and copayments and implementing more restrictions on pharmaceuticals and mental health benefits. In addition, although the average employee share of premiums has remained constant since 1999, there is great variation in the share of premiums paid by employees. A major survey of employer-sponsored health insurance premiums found that workers in firms with a high proportion of low-wage workers (i.e., firms where 35% or more of the workers earn less than $21,000 a year) pay a higher share of family policy premiums than do workers in firms with lower proportions of low-wage workers. Although the rate of increase in premiums between 2006 and 2007 (6.1%) was the smallest since 1999, it is still larger than the rate of inflation.

Employer attitudes toward the costs of employer-sponsored coverage also reflect the labor markets in which they hire workers. Most of the growth in employment over the past two decades has been in the services sector, in particular healthcare services, professional business services, and leisure-hospitality-entertainment services. Many of the companies in these industries are small and employ large numbers of low-wage, less skilled workers. Immigrant labor is particularly prevalent in these markets. As long as the supply of workers willing to work in these service jobs is much larger than the demand for them, the firms can keep wages low and not offer health insurance to attract or keep the workers. Moreover, the demand for the services provided by these industries is very price sensitive, so firms are not in a position to charge higher prices in order to provide higher wages and group health insurance coverage.

High Premiums for Individual Insurance

People who do not have access to employer-sponsored coverage have only one choice for purchasing health insurance: the individual insurance market in their state—the market in which insurers sell policies covering individuals (and their dependents) rather than policies covering groups of people. Individual insurance is far more expensive than is employer-group coverage because insurers face the risk that a disproportionate number of people who want to purchase individual policies are at higher risk of having high medical costs than the general population. This risk is known as adverse selection. As a result, premiums for family policies in individual markets typically cost more than $700 per month and have a deductible of $5,000 or more.

In spite of the fact that many younger adults do not have employer-sponsored coverage and are good candidates to purchase individual coverage, the growth in healthcare costs has driven up premiums and the risk of adverse selection in the individual market. Increasingly, the people who purchase individual insurance are 45 and older— ages when healthcare spending tends to increase. It is not uncommon for those who are older or have medical conditions to face premiums in the individual market of $12,000 or more per year or to be offered policies that do not include care related to their conditions. Those who are younger and healthy also generally face premiums that are higher relative to what they think healthcare costs are likely to be because insurers expect that adverse selection is occurring also among the younger adults. The result is that individual policies are unattractive and unaffordable to younger adults. Even younger adults who are earning middle-class incomes may decide that any "normal" medical care they might use would cost less than the premiums they would face in the individual market.

Low Income

The third major reason why many people are uninsured is that they have low income. A little more than half of the uninsured have family incomes below $30,000, and people with incomes below $30,000 (or below three times the federal poverty level) cannot afford insurance in the individual market. To have an income above the poverty level, a person must be working (or be a dependent of someone who is working). Thus, a majority of the low-income uninsured are employed or dependents of someone who is employed, but they do not have access to employer-sponsored coverage, and they cannot afford to purchase insurance on their own.

Future Implications

People without health insurance are at risk for a financial catastrophe and for not obtaining medical care that could save their lives and improve the quality of their lives if they have chronic medical conditions. One in six nonelderly people in the nation now faces such risks, and a fifth of them are children who do not have a choice in their insurance status. Furthermore, almost 80% of the uninsured are younger than 45 years of age. They would be relatively inexpensive to insure since the vast majority of them are healthy and use little medical care. The fact that more than a quarter of 25- to 34-year-olds and a fifth of 35- to 44-year-olds are uninsured is not good for them or the nation's private health insurance system. Insurers need younger, healthy people among their insured to counterbalance the risks of higher medical costs of older people. For these reasons, many believe that a new strategy for reducing the number of uninsured in the United States is needed.

Katherine Swartz

See also Access to Healthcare; Adverse Selection; Coinsurance, Copays, and Deductibles; Economic Barriers to Healthcare; Healthcare Reform; Health Disparities; Health Insurance; Medicaid

Further Readings

Cassedy, Amy, Gerry Fairbrother, and Paul W. Newacheck, "The Impact of Insurance Instability on Children's Access, Utilization, and Satisfaction with Health Care," *Ambulatory Pediatrics* 8(5): 321–28, September–October 2008.

Chesneys, James D., Herbert C. Smitherman, Cynthia Tareg, et al. *Taking Care of the Uninsured: A Path to Reform.* Detroit, MI: Wayne State University, 2008.

Cohen, Robin A., and Diane M. Makuc, "State, Regional, and National Estimates of Health Insurance Coverage for People Under 65 Years of Age: National Health Interview Survey, 2004–2006," *National Health Statistics Reports* 1: 1–23, June 19, 2008.

Hadley, Jack, John Holahan, Teresa Coughlin, et al. "Covering the Uninsured in 2008: Current Costs, Sources of Payment, and Incremental Costs," *Health Affairs* 27(5): w399–w415, September–October, 2008.

Jost, Timothy Stoltzfus. "Health Care Access in the United States: Conflicting Concepts of Justice and Little Solidarity," *Medicine and Law* 27(3): 605–16, September 2008.

Newton, Manya F., Carla C. Keirns, Rebecca Cunningham, et al. "Uninsured Adults Presenting to U.S. Emergency Departments: Assumptions vs. Data," *Journal of the American Medical Association* 300(16): 1914–24, October 22, 2008.

Rutledge, Matthews S., and Catherine G. McLaughlin. "Hispanics and Health Insurance Coverage: The Rising Disparity," *Medical Care* 46(10): 1086–1092, October 2008.

Web Sites

Agency for Healthcare Research and Quality (AHRQ): http://www.ahrq.gov

Commonwealth Fund: http://www.commonwealthfund.org

Employee Benefits Research Institute (EBRI): http://www.ebri.org

Henry J. Kaiser Family Foundation (KFF): http://www.kff.org

U.S. Census Bureau: http://www.census.gov

UNITED KINGDOM'S NATIONAL HEALTH SERVICE (NHS)

One of the most contentious and complex issues in health services research is defining and assessing the appropriate role of government in delivering healthcare. Great Britain has developed what is widely recognized as the most advanced system of healthcare based on management and delivery by the government through tax financing. The history and experience of the healthcare system in post–World War II Great Britain is a robust example of state control and delivery of healthcare services based on the premise of universal coverage and access. Recently, the National Health Service (NHS) in England has embarked on a program of reform and modernization that is being observed with interest by researchers concerned with questions of access, implementation of technology, health outcomes, and cost controls. The NHS comprises separate organizations in England, Scotland, Wales, and Northern Ireland, but each operates on the same principles of universal access and essentially free care, funded by national tax revenues. This entry focuses on the English NHS.

History

The NHS was created in 1948 (implementation of the NHS Act occurred in 1946), but there were a number of policy debates and developments in the preceding half-century that laid the groundwork for the comprehensive system launched following the end of World War II. In the decades preceding the war, public hospitals grew to be the major treatment centers in the United Kingdom. Although there were few public general hospitals, a diverse collection of specialty public hospitals focused on infectious diseases, mental health, and maternity services, resulting in two thirds of patients being treated at public hospitals by the late 1930s.

Voluntary (not-for-profit) hospitals—originally charity societies—began to charge for services in the two decades before the war, which paralleled the development of health insurance, beginning with the National Health Insurance (NHI) plan created in 1911. This compulsory system provided sickness benefits to the employed working class, including primary care and drugs. By 1939, the NHI, despite excluding the unemployed, married women who did not work, and children, covered 43% of the population. Ninety percent of general-practice physicians participated in the NHI, although specialist services were not covered.

Although there were a number of studies and proposals made with regard to reforming the fragmented British healthcare system in the decade prior to the creation of the NHS, the 1942 Report to Parliament on Social Insurance and Allied Services provided the impetus for the creation of a nationalized healthcare system. Known as the Beveridge Report, after its author Lord William Beveridge, the document proposed a comprehensive social security system, including a national health service to provide tax-funded comprehensive medical care for everyone in the United Kingdom. The Beveridge report became the Labor Party's platform for a social welfare state following the war.

The NHS came into existence in 1948 as the centerpiece of the Labor Party's plan for rebuilding the British economy. There was little opposition at the time, in part because of the clear victory of the Labor Party in the 1945 parliamentary elections and a national consensus that some type of social security program was necessary for rebuilding a stable workforce following the trials of the war.

Evolving Structure

The original structure of the NHS was designed in part to overcome the objections of several important interest groups to a nationalized system of healthcare. The most significant objections came from the medical profession, particularly general practitioners, who feared the loss of their professional autonomy, restrictions on practice, and inadequate compensation. The Minister of Health, Aneurin Bevan, agreed to a number of provisions designed to overcome those objections. Many of

the objections mirrored the Labor Party's internal debate over whether to focus on providing comprehensive health services based on local authority control or whether there should be a national system of healthcare controlled by the central government. Bevan insisted on nationalization of the entire hospital sector, as one element of a tripartite system of providing healthcare services. The social element was the creation of local health authorities to provide primary and specialized services, including mental health clinics, ambulance services, and related public health and social services.

A third element was intended to overcome the objections of the most vocal critics of a national health service, the general-practice physicians. Bevan agreed that these physicians would be independent contractors, rather than salaried employees, and would provide services based on contracts negotiated with representatives of their profession, primarily the British Medical Association. The contracts would be administered by separate administrative units, called executive councils, which would include representatives of the medical profession. The principle that primary-care physicians are contractors, rather than employees, has survived to this day.

The nationalization of hospitals themselves was less contentious than other issues, largely because of the support of specialty physicians and surgeons, called consultants in the United Kingdom. Unlike general practitioners, specialists were largely supportive of the NHS even though they would practice primarily in the newly nationalized hospitals. Their professional organizations, including the Royal College of Physicians and the Royal College of Surgeons, supported the creation of the NHS after Bevan made some important concessions relating to hospital structure and operations, particularly with regard to teaching hospitals. Hospitals would be co-coordinated by regional hospital boards and would be operated by local hospital management committees, including representation from the medical profession. In addition, teaching hospitals, at which many of the top consultants practiced, would have separate boards of governors, again with representation from the medical profession. In addition, consultants could continue to have private practices and would benefit from generous compensation plans.

The NHS began operation in 1948 based on this tripartite model of separate structures for hospitals, physicians, and local health services, all reporting ultimately to the national Minister of Health. This structure remained largely intact until the mid-1970s, when problems that were evident from the earliest days of the NHS reached a critical stage. Through its many changes over the past 60 years, the principle on which the NHS was founded continues to guide the system today: universal and comprehensive healthcare services based on clinical need, not on the ability to pay.

The 1974 Reorganization

At the time the NHS was created, it was assumed that there would be heavy demands on its services for the first few years of operation as patients used services that were unavailable or inaccessible prior to the creation of the nationalized system. It was suggested that the demands on the services would decrease over time as these deferred health issues were addressed. In fact, demand was heavy and did not diminish over time.

Although the NHS enjoyed great public support from its creation, it soon became apparent that there were problems with duplication and overlap of management and coordination functions within the three-part structure that were affecting the ability of the NHS to respond to demands on its operations. The NHS Act of 1974 was intended to address these concerns by reorganizing the NHS to provide a more coordinated system of regional planning and local administration of all health services. At the top level, regional health authorities were created to provide overall planning. Ninety area health authorities were created with responsibility for overall coordination of health services, and several hundred districts were created to manage the actual health services provided.

Unfortunately, it soon became clear that these additional layers of management were not resulting in more efficient utilization of resources and delivery of services. There were several other reorganizations between the mid-1970s and 2002, when the current structure of the NHS was adopted.

Current Structure

The NHS Reform and Health Care Professions Act of 2002 marked the beginning of a major modernization effort for the English NHS and its

constituent units. Twenty-eight regional strategic health authorities (SHAs), serving populations of between 1.5 and 2.4, million people were created. The number of SHAs was reduced to 10 in 2006. The SHAs report directly to the Department of Health. The SHAs are responsible for allocating budgets, strategic planning, and oversight of services within their particular region, but they do not have operating responsibilities. Reporting to each SHA is a range of agencies, called trusts, that provide the actual healthcare and ancillary services. The principal trust types are primary-care trusts (PCTs), NHS (hospital) trusts, and NHS foundation trusts. The SHAs and trusts have a similar structure. They are public corporations governed by a board, which consists of operating executives and outside nonexecutive members appointed through a Department of Health selection process. Each authority and trust is headed by a nonexecutive director, who is appointed after public advertisement and selection by the respective board.

Primary-Care Trusts (PCTs)

Most health services are provided by PCTs. Originally, there were 303, but these were consolidated into 152 PCTs in 2006. The PCTs have responsibility for outpatient services, dental services, mental health services, pharmacies, ambulance and emergency services (through contracts with separate NHS Ambulance trusts), and, through contracts with separate NHS trusts, most hospitals within their defined geographic region. More than 80% of the NHS budget is controlled by the PCTs. The PCTs are also responsible for contracting for primary-care services with general practitioners. Patients select their general practitioner from a list provided by their PCT. Other healthcare services are selected by the general practitioner in consultation with the patient, although this is changing with the Patient Choice initiative discussed below.

NHS (Hospital) Trusts

The NHS trusts operate the majority of hospitals in England. There are approximately 150 hospital trusts that operate several hundred hospitals. These geographically designated hospital trusts contract with the PCTs to provide services for patients within a defined area. They employ physicians for hospital-based care as well as contracting for specialists (consultants). Until recently, patients were required to use a hospital within their geographic region. This will change dramatically with the full implementation of the NHS Choice Plan announced in 2005.

The possibility of competition among hospitals because of the recent NHS initiatives has focused attention on the question of quality differences within the NHS. Until the 1980s, allocation of NHS budgets to local authorities was based almost solely on the previous year's budget allocation. Since that time, there have been a number of attempts to tie budgets to medical needs within a region, but inequities continue to exist. Therefore, there is concern that with choice there will be underutilization of hospitals that are perceived as having lower quality than higher-quality hospitals (which include most of the country's university-related teaching hospitals).

A quality measurement program is being implemented that will financially reward hospitals with better clinical outcomes in the hope that such an incentive will promote quality improvements in the worst-performing hospitals. However, it is acknowledged that this may not be sufficient within the current financing structure, in which there is limited capital for investment in equipment and facilities. One solution has been the creation of NHS foundation trusts.

NHS Foundation Trusts

Beginning in 2004, hospital trusts have had the option to convert to foundation trusts, which have a unique legal status within the NHS. Foundation trust hospitals are independent legal entities, owned by their members (who are patients, staff, and any local individuals who desire to be members). A foundation trust hospital is governed by an independent board of governors elected by the membership and is licensed by an independent regulator outside the NHS and the Department of Health. Unlike other NHS hospitals, a foundation trust hospital may borrow from private-sector financial sources, retain surpluses and proceeds from the sale of assets, contract with NHS entities and private providers for services, and provide pay and benefits different from the NHS schedules.

The most significant change is that the foundation trust hospitals may charge for treatment of private pay patients. The private health insurance market covers almost 15% of the healthcare expenditures in England, and foundation trust hospitals, like private hospitals, are permitted to treat privately insured patients. There is a cap on the percentage of income permitted to be derived from private pay patients. Essentially, the hospitals are required to maintain the level of NHS services provided at the time of conversion to foundation trust status.

The foundation trust program started in 2004 with 10 hospitals. In 2007, more than 70 hospitals had converted to foundation trusts. The government's plan is to have all NHS hospitals convert to foundation trust status within a decade. The government's expectation is that with greater access to private capital, greater operational autonomy, and accountability to its staff and patients, hospitals will be able to overcome the limitation on resources that has plagued them since the creation of the NHS. In addition, the government is no longer financially and operationally responsible for the hospitals that are foundation trusts.

Financing the NHS

Since its inception, the NHS has been funded through a combination of general taxation and a separate national insurance tax contribution from employers and employees. The national insurance funds a range of social benefits, including the NHS and the pension system. In 2007, more than 80% of the NHS budget comes from general taxation and about 12% from the national insurance funds. The balance of revenues comes from fees (less than 3%) and debt instruments. In recent years, the NHS has accounted for about 85% of healthcare expenditures in the United Kingdom. A growing private insurance sector has fostered the growth of private physician practices and private healthcare facilities.

In 2006, government expenditures for the NHS approached $200 billion. The per capita expenditure on healthcare in 2004 was about $2,500, about average for the 30 nations that are members of the Organization for Economic Cooperation and Development (OECD) and substantially less than the $6,100 per capita for the United States. For the same year, healthcare spending in the United

Kingdom was 8.1% of the gross domestic product (GDP), while it was 15.3% in the United States. The median among OECD members was 8.8%.

One of the criticisms of the NHS's financing system is that there is little transparency since taxpayers do not readily know what percentage of their taxes actually goes to the NHS. In addition, each PCT has broad authority to use its devolved budget as it determines, with the principal government control being that the PCTs are not permitted to incur deficits.

The Modernization Initiative

Reacting to criticisms about perceived declining service and lack of investment in the NHS, Prime Minister Tony Blair commissioned a reform program for the NHS that was announced in 2000 ("The NHS Plan"). The plan called for a number of measures to modernize the NHS and improve its services. Central to the implementation of the plan was a promise made in 2002 to increase the expenditures on the NHS from 7.7% of GDP to 9.4% by 2008. Three of the most important initiatives relate to patient waiting times, modernization of information technology, and providing patients with greater control over their healthcare through choice of providers.

Patient Waiting Times

By 1997 the waiting time for treatment after diagnosis was as long as 18 months because of the lack of personnel, equipment, and facilities. One result of this was increased patient dissatisfaction with the NHS. A 1999 poll found that 42% of the British public were fairly or very dissatisfied with the NHS. The long patient waiting times became a primary political issue in successive parliamentary elections. The Blair administration made waiting times the most critical improvement promised in the NHS Plan. The wait time for treatment fell to a maximum of 9 months by 2004, with the government's goal being 18 weeks, from the first appointment with a general practitioner through treatment by 2008. Although it appears that such an ambitious goal may not be met, there has been decreased public attention directed at the NHS waiting times in recent years as they have noticeably decreased.

Modernization of Information Technology

The most ambitious element of the NHS Plan was to increase substantially its investment in information technology, with the goal of creating the most modern infrastructure in healthcare. The Blair administration proposed a national program estimated to cost more that $32 billion over 10 years for electronic medical records, electronic imaging archives, and patient appointment and management systems, along with the necessary infrastructure improvements. By 2007, the actual expenditures were more than $20 billion, but none of the major initiatives had been fully implemented. Technical issues and cost overruns have delayed the program, which is the largest information technology program ever attempted in the country. However, it appears likely that the effort to implement electronic medical records across the NHS will be completed by 2012.

Patient Choice

A major element of the NHS Plan is to increase patient options for treatment. Called Patient Choice, this program has become the major visible change in the NHS over the past 5 years. In addition to the creation of the NHS foundation trust program, the government's plan is to allow patients to choose among several treatment facilities within the country, whether or not part of the NHS. If the facility meets NHS quality and performance standards and the charges do not exceed the maximum price that the NHS pays for such treatments, a patient may choose care at an independent treatment center for specified procedures. To date, approved procedures include many outpatient surgical procedures. In some cases, foundation trusts have entered into contracts with privately operated outpatient treatment centers to provide such services. Several non-British companies, including at least one U.S. healthcare provider, have opened treatment centers in England. Patients can now choose any NHS foundation trust hospital for treatment; in addition to the approved private-sector treatment centers, there are at least four local NHS hospitals that have contracts with the patient's PCT. Before Patient Choice, a patient was assigned to the closest local hospital that provided the prescribed treatment.

To assist patients with making choices, the Department of Health requires the collection of patient outcome data on specified medical conditions, which are published. Patients may use this information to select their treatment center or hospital.

Future Implications

The NHS is one of the most cherished of British institutions. The NHS Plan recognizes that a number of problems need to be addressed if public support and confidence are to be maintained. Foremost among these is the pressing need for modern facilities and improved access to medical technologies. Although the NHS has technologies available that rival those of any health system in the world, the dispersal of those technologies varies depending on the region and other factors that are not based on medical need.

In addition, many parts of the country depend on hospitals with outdated facilities. Although capital investment has tripled in the past 5 years, there is a need for substantial upgrading of facilities in many parts of the country. This is an area in which the NHS's efforts to develop public/private partnerships will likely be most visible. Rather than assuming the entire burden of building new facilities, it is probable that the successful experience with private independent treatment centers will provide the impetus for more ambitious partnerships to develop healthcare facilities.

Finally, there is general recognition both inside the NHS and within the government that the NHS has not developed a culture that encourages innovation in operations. Although a network of NHS innovation centers has been created to help promote the development of innovative approaches to healthcare delivery, critics have suggested that there has been little evidence of an impact to date.

Frank S. Phillips

See also Access to Healthcare; Comparing Health Systems; Healthcare Reform; Health Services Research in the United Kingdom; International Health Systems; National Health Insurance; Rationing Healthcare; United Kingdom's National Institute for Health and Clinical Excellence (NICE)

Further Readings

Aaron, Henry J., William B. Schwartz, and Melissa Cox. *Can We Say No?: The Challenge of Rationing Health Care.* Washington, DC: Brookings Institute Press, 2005.

Baggott, Rob. *Health and Health Care in Britain.* 3d ed. New York: Palgrave Macmillian, 2004.

Edwards, Brian, and Margaret Fall. *The Executive Years of the NHS: The England Account 1985–2003.* Abingdon, UK: Radcliffe, 2005.

Hann, Alison, ed. *Health Policy and Politics.* Burlington, VT: Ashgate, 2007.

Klein, Rudolf. *The New Politics of the NHS: From Creation to Reinvention.* 5th ed. Seattle, WA: Radcliffe, 2006.

Marks, John. *The NHS: Beginning, Middle, and End?: The Autobiography of Dr. John Marks.* New York: Radcliffe Press, 2008.

Newdick, Christopher. *Who Should We Treat?: Rights, Rationing, and Resources in the NHS.* 2d ed. New York: Oxford University Press, 2005.

Player, Stewart, and Colin Leys. *Confuse and Conceal: The NHS and Independent Sector Treatment Centers.* Monmouth, Wales, UK: Merlin Press, 2008.

Smith, Ian. *Building a World-Class NHS.* New York: Palgrave Macmillan, 2007.

Tempest, Michelle, ed. *The Future of the NHS.* St. Albans, UK: XPL Publishing, 2006.

Web Sites

National Health Service (NHS): http://www.nhs.uk
National Institute for Health and Clinical Excellence (NICE): http://www.nice.org.uk

UNITED KINGDOM'S NATIONAL INSTITUTE FOR HEALTH AND CLINICAL EXCELLENCE (NICE)

Within the United Kingdom's National Health Service (NHS), the National Institute for Health and Clinical Excellence (NICE) is the agency charged with the task of developing and disseminating clinical, public health, and healthcare technology guidelines to be followed by all NHS providers and provider organizations. Its objective is to develop ways to standardize treatment approaches at the highest levels among NHS providers in order to try to ensure uniformly good-quality healthcare.

Background

NICE came into being on April 1, 1999, as part of an initiative designed to eliminate perceived historical inequities in access to the best in healthcare. The present agency is an outgrowth of the National Institute for Clinical Excellence (also known as NICE), with an expanded role and mission. In April 2005, another NHS agency, the Health Development Agency, was folded into NICE, expanding the latter agency's scope to include public health. NICE's jurisdiction extends to all NHS providers. Providers that do not belong to the NHS generally meet the standards and guidelines as well, although they are not required to do so.

Organizational Structure

A 15-member board governs NICE. The board's standing committees are the Audit Committee, the Citizen's Council Committee, and the Remuneration and Terms of Service Committee. In addition, NICE calls on the expertise of the NHS and the broad healthcare community to assist in its work. It relies on several independent advisory committees, including those on interventional procedures, public health interventions, research and development, and technology appraisal.

Role

National standards ("frameworks") that essentially define access to and eligibility for specified types of care and services are formulated by the National Service Frameworks (NSFs) body. Typically, the NSFs set up one new framework per year. While frameworks have some resemblance to clinical pathways, they are less detailed. In their annual process called the annual health check, the healthcare commissions serve as the system regulators. The commissions evaluate the system's performance against the core standards that apply to existing performance and the developmental standards that reflect the capacity to

improve. The role of NICE is to develop the working guidelines (guidances) that will be followed by the NHS provider organizations in complying with the frameworks. Currently, NICE's guidance on health technologies and clinical practice only applies to England and Wales, while its guidance on the safety and efficacy of interventional procedures applies to England, Wales, and Scotland. NICE's guidance on public health practices applies to England alone.

In evaluating technology and technological approaches, NICE works with a wide variety of consultative and advisory bodies, including several independent academic centers representing universities and other academic groups. In developing clinical guidelines, the royal medical and nursing colleges, professional bodies, and provider organizations work with NICE. When more information is needed before guidance can be developed on an interventional procedure, NICE convenes an advisory committee composed of experts in the aspect of care being studied. This development process is funded by the NHS Department of Health, which commissions NICE to develop guidelines applying to clinical practice, public health, and healthcare technology.

NICE guidelines reflect and embody the principles of evidence-based medicine as well as cost-effectiveness. Guidelines on a particular subject are developed in response to needs as perceived and articulated by the public, the healthcare community, and professional and technology-oriented organizations and proposed by them to NICE for action. NHS providers to whom a NICE guideline, or guidance, applies are then expected to follow this guideline in their practice, taking it fully into account when deciding what treatments to give people. The healthcare commissions survey and evaluate provider performance with reference to the guidance.

In one sense, the NICE guidances show a superficial resemblance to the advisories published by the U.S. Agency for Healthcare Research and Quality (AHRQ), although NICE publishes specific implementation templates to support its guidances, listing the steps in the implementation process.

When NICE issues a guidance covering a treatment measure addressed in a core standard, the budget provisions needed by the NHS member organization to support practitioner and provider compliance with that guidance must be in place within 3 months. In the case of a guidance reflecting a developmental standard, provider organizations are allowed more than 3 months for implementation.

Jean Gayton Carroll

See also Clinical Practice Guidelines; Cost-Benefit and Cost-Effectiveness Analyses; International Health Systems; Outcomes Movement; Quality of Healthcare; Rationing Healthcare; Technology Assessment; United Kingdom's National Health Service (NHS)

Further Readings

Buxton, Martin. "Implications of the Appraisal Function of the National Institute for Clinical Excellence (NICE)," *Value in Health* 4(3): 212–16, May–June 2001.

Drummond, Michael F., Cynthia P. Inglesias, and Nicola J. Cooper. "Systematic Reviews and Economic Evaluations Conducted for the National Institute for Health and Clinical Excellence in the United Kingdom: A Game of Two Halves?" *International Journal of Technology Assessment in Health Care* 24(2): 146–50, April 2008.

National Health Service. *A Guide to NICE.* London: National Health Service, 2005.

National Health Service. *National Institute for Health and Clinical Excellence Annual Report, 2007/08.* London: The Stationery Office, 2008.

Web Sites

United Kingdom's National Health Service (NHS): http://www.nhs.uk

United Kingdom's National Institute for Health and Clinical Excellence (NICE): http://www.nice.org.uk

University HealthSystem Consortium (UHC)

Established in 1984, the University HealthSystem Consortium (UHC) is a nonprofit alliance of more than 100 academic medical centers and 170 of their affiliated hospitals, representing approximately 90% of the nation's nonprofit academic medical centers. Based in Oak Brook, Illinois, the consortium offers its members specific programs and services to improve clinical, operational, financial, and patient safety performance.

Mission and Vision

The mission of the UHC is to advance knowledge, foster collaboration, and promote change in order to help members succeed in their respective markets. Its vision is to be a catalyst for change, accelerating the achievement of clinical and operational excellence.

Products and Services

The UHC's various products and services provide support and resources for effective and efficient management of clinical, operational, and financial performance of an academic health system's enterprise through comparative data analytics, implementation assistance, educational and developmental resources, and networking and collaboration opportunities. Easy-to-use online reports and other Web-based tools blend clinical, operational, administrative, and financial data, enabling UHC members to benchmark and compare their performance with that of their peers and act on opportunities to improve. Product examples include the Funds Flow Collaborative, a database and reporting system of the economic interdependencies of academic medical centers, schools of medicine, and faculty practice plans; the UHC Patient Safety Net, an online data collection tool for reporting, tracking, and trending of adverse medical events; the Faculty Practice Solution Center, a database used to examine clinical productivity, plan physician incentive compensation, perform workforce analysis, and promote revenue cycle improvement; and the Managed Care Contracting Compass, an interactive database and packaged pricing model that compares various managed care contracts on a regional or national basis. Additionally, the consortium provides a variety of other services and products in areas including quality and risk, technology assessment, business strategy and tactics, and value analysis.

The UHC's supply chain optimization program is another exclusive, integrated offering of services designed to help its members make the best possible decisions when addressing their organizations' supply chains. Novation, LLC, is the group purchasing organization for consortium's participants.

Membership

There are two categories of UHC membership: member and related organizations. For the membership category, an applicant for membership in the consortium must be a nonfederal teaching hospital or health system that has a documented affiliation agreement with a medical school by the Liaison Committee on Medical Education and fulfils one of the following conditions: (a) it is under common ownership with a medical school; (b) the majority of the medical school department chairs serve as the hospital's chiefs of service, or the chairman is responsible for appointing the hospital chief of service; or (c) it has a reputation for excellence in service, teaching, and research as determined at the discretion of the UHC Member Board of Directors, or its designee, based on consideration of clinical support of undergraduate medical education and an employed clinical faculty with a centralized practice plan.

System membership has two or more clinical entities that serve the same medical school and independently meet the criteria for full membership. Each category contains several classes of participation, with the following designations: (a) associate—an acute-care hospital that is sponsored by a consortium member or organizational member; (b) organization—an affiliated organization invited by the consortium's Governing Board to join the UHC (e.g., National Association of Public Hospitals); (3) international—a non-U.S. alliance of teaching hospitals (like the UHC) or a teaching hospital that meets the above membership criteria; (4) faculty practice plan—a faculty group practice organization associated with a medical school and organized with a unified corporate governance structure, which provides identifiable and functionally integrated practice management services and is accountable for the clinical, financial, and operational performance of its member physicians.

In addition, full UHC members and associate members may sponsor entities that provide healthcare services (other than an acute-care hospital) as an affiliate or an alternate shipping location. Other consortium member-sponsored providers, including faculty practice plans, ambulatory clinics, medical schools, universities, and others can access the power of group purchasing through the consortium's affiliate purchasing program.

Implications for Health Services Research

The UHC's major contribution to health services research is its provision of data to researchers from member organizations. Data from the consortium enable researchers to compare clinical practice patterns and the outcomes of care at academic medical centers across the nation. Because of such a large number of medical centers and the large number of patients they treat, data from the consortium can be used to study critical and emerging issues of clinical and strategic importance. Data from the consortium have been used to study the outcomes of bariatric, colon, and other surgeries; various pharmaceutical and disease state evaluations; intensivist physician staffing patterns; and outcomes of various medical education programs, including nurse residency programs.

Karl Matuszewski

See also Academic Medical Centers; Benchmarking; Hospitals; Patient Safety; Quality of Healthcare; Safety Net; Technology Assessment

Further Readings

Bonk Mary Ellen, Heather Krown, Karl Matuszewski, et al. "Potentially Inappropriate Medications in Hospitalized Senior Patients," *American Journal of Health-System Pharmacy* 63(12): 1161–65, June 15, 2006.

Cummings, Joe, Cathy Krsek, Kathy Vermoch, et al. "Intensive Care Unit Telemedicine: Review and Consensus Recommendations," *American Journal of Medical Quality* 22(4): 239–50, 2007.

Flegal, Theresa. *Legal and Risk Management Issues Associated With Informed Consent.* Oak Brook, IL: University HealthSystem Consortium, 2000.

Hinojosa, Marcelo W., Viken R. Konyalian, Zuri A. Murrell, et al. "Outcomes of Right and Left Colectomy at Academic Centers," *American Surgeon* 73(10): 945–48, October 2007.

Kahn, Jeremy M., Helga Brake, and Kenneth P. Steinberg. "Intensivist Physician-Staffing and the

Process of Care in Academic Medical Centers," *Quality and Safety in Health Care* 16(5): 329–33, October 2007.

Khorana, Alok A., Charles W. Francis, Eva Culakova, et al. "Frequency, Risk Factors, and Trends for Venous Thromboembolism Among Hospitalized Cancer Patients," *Cancer* 110(10): 2339–46, November 15, 2007.

Matuszewski, Karl, Robert Schoenhaus, Mary Ellen Bonk, et al. "Use and Outcomes of Antifibrinolytic Therapy in Patients Undergoing Cardiothoracic Surgery at 20 Academic Medical Centers in the U.S.," *Pharmacy and Therapeutics (P&T)* 33(2): 98–1006, 2008.

Nguyen, Ninh T., Michael Silver, Malcolm Robinson, et al. "Results of a National Audit of Bariatric Surgery Performed at Academic Centers: A 2004 University HealthSystem Consortium Benchmarking Project," *Archives of Surgery* 141(5): 445–49, May 2006.

Web Sites

University HealthSystem Consortium (UHC): http://www.uhc.edu

URBAN INSTITUTE

The Urban Institute is a nonprofit, nonpartisan policy research and educational organization established in Washington, D.C., in 1968. Its multidisciplinary staff investigates the social, economic, and governance problems confronting the nation, evaluates the public and private means to alleviate them, and helps other countries build local government capacity, improve public service delivery, and nurture civil society.

Through work that ranges from broad conceptual studies to administrative and technical assistance, Institute researchers contribute to the knowledge available to guide decision making in the public interest and strive to deepen citizens' understanding of the issues and trade-offs policymakers face.

The Institute's genesis came in the mid-1960s, when many U.S. cities were in turmoil and tatters. President Lyndon B. Johnson, seeing the need for independent, unbiased analysis of the problems facing urban America, created a blue-ribbon commission of civic leaders who recommended chartering a center to do that work. The Urban Institute became that center.

Today, the Urban Institute is home to 10 policy centers and more than 230 economists, demographers, statisticians, sociologists, political scientists, educators, and other researchers and analysts. Its Health Policy Center, inaugurated in 1977 and now one of the Institute's largest research centers, uses rigorous methods to bring objective evidence to the panoply of health service concerns, including community-based care, disabilities, health insurance, hospital and physician payments, long-term care, Medicaid, Medicare, the State Children's Health Insurance Program (SCHIP), and uninsured and uncompensated care. Center scholars also address cost containment, managed care, liability and tort reform, the financing and delivery of health services, and their quality and appropriateness, among other issues.

Much of the Health Policy Center's work is on who gets needed health coverage, who doesn't, what the ramifications are of not having health insurance, and what can be done to secure access to care. A review of a quarter-century of studies found strong evidence that the uninsured receive fewer preventive and diagnostic services, tend to be more severely ill when diagnosed, and receive less therapeutic care, resulting in poorer health outcomes and higher mortality rates. Research on why 46 million people lack health insurance found that nearly all of them believe that they need coverage but more than half say that they can't afford it. Perceptions about cost matter, the study determined, whether the uninsured individual is old or young, healthy or disabled, with high income or income well below the poverty level.

Another analysis determined that the number of nonelderly people without health insurance climbed by 1.3 million between 2004 and 2005, bringing this group's uninsurance rate to nearly 18%. Eighty-five percent of this increase was among those with family incomes below 200% of the federal poverty level. The analysis showed that job-based insurance is dropping because of significant increases in premium costs; job shifts away from medium and large firms and those in the manufacturing, finance, and government sectors, employment environments that traditionally have high rates of employer-based insurance coverage; and population movement toward the South and the West, regions with lower rates of employer-based health insurance coverage.

At the 10th anniversary of the SCHIP in 2007, the Institute estimated that the program had signed up close to 70% of its target population, but 1.8 million eligible children nationwide were yet to be enrolled. Federal funding for SCHIP, which was enacted in 1997 to expand health coverage to low-income uninsured children who do not qualify for Medicaid, will have to increase substantially, the study noted, if these children are to join the approximately 3.9 million children with SCHIP coverage.

Health Policy Center researchers also analyze local and regional healthcare circumstances and services, gleaning data, lessons, and insights that are often useful across the country. Legislation enacted in Massachusetts in 2006 aimed at bringing near-universal healthcare coverage to the state. The bipartisan legislation drew partly on the center's extensive analysis and practical policy recommendations on costs and mechanisms for covering the state's 530,000 uninsured residents. As healthcare costs soar nationwide and more businesses trim employee coverage, Institute staff are working with other states to define their range of policy options.

New York State's medical providers cared for 2.5 million uninsured individuals in 2005, a Health Policy Center research team found. Federal, state, and local governments transferred billions of dollars to hospitals and other providers in a number of complex ways, of which $3.5 billion was deemed to relate to uninsured care. After Hurricane Katrina devastated the Gulf Coast, a Health Policy Center white paper examined what happened in New Orleans's hospitals, especially the 11 flood-bound institutions in the most desperate circumstances, why experiences varied for the hospitals and their patients, and how to avoid the most serious shortcomings in planning by hospital and public authorities.

The U.S. Congress, executive branch agencies, and state officials often call on the Urban Institute researchers to present their research or testify on legislative matters. At a U.S. House subcommittee hearing, for instance, legislators were told that developing meaningful universal health insurance coverage within a private insurance system requires four elements: (1) comprehensive subsidized insurance benefits for low- and modest-income individuals, (2) a guaranteed source of coverage for all potential purchasers, (3) a mechanism for spreading across a broad population the costs of covering those with the greatest need for healthcare services, and (4) either a mandate for individuals to obtain coverage or that mandate combined with a "light" employer mandate.

Health policy researchers frequently call on the expertise of other Institute centers. The Transfer Income Model (TRIM), maintained and developed by the Income and Benefits Policy Center under primary funding from the U.S. Department of Health and Human Services (HHS), can illuminate the effects of changes in Medicaid, SCHIP, or employer-sponsored health insurance as well as assess participation rates and cross-program interactions. With the nation spending more than $250 billion annually on tax incentives for workers to buy health insurance, the Urban-Brookings Tax Policy Center investigates how income tax deductions, vouchers, and similar mechanisms can meet healthcare challenges.

Health policy has been a cornerstone of the Institute's biggest research project ever. Started in 1996, Assessing the New Federalism monitored and analyzed the well-being of American children and families as states assumed major responsibility for healthcare, income security, social services, and job-training programs for low-income Americans. Caseloads dropped precipitously after 1996's landmark welfare overhaul, but the Institute research revealed that 1 year later, 49% of mothers who had left the rolls and 29% of their children had no health insurance.

Looking ahead, the Institute's projects will report on the condition of and changes in the healthcare delivery system throughout the United States; estimate the risk, timing, and amount of lifetime disability and long-term care, including both nursing home care and care at home; model health insurance costs and the impact of reinsurance, with technical assistance to states considering health reforms with a reinsurance component; and look at the path from the Food Stamp and school meal programs and family food behavior to child obesity.

Stuart Kantor

See also Access to Healthcare; Cost of Healthcare; Health Insurance Coverage; Medicaid; Medicare; Public Policy; State-Based Health Coverage Initiatives; Uninsured Individuals; State Children's Health Insurance Program (SCHIP)

Further Readings

Blumberg, Linda. J. "Expanding Health Insurance Coverage to the Uninsured: Rationale, Recent Proposals, and Key Considerations." In *Testimony Before the Subcommittee on Health, Employment, Labor, and Pensions, U.S. House Education and Labor Committee.* Washington, DC: Urban Institute, 2007.

Bovbjerg, Randall R., Stan Dorn, Jack Hadley, et al. *Caring for the Uninsured in New York.* Washington, DC: Urban Institute, 2006.

Graves, John A., and Sharon K. Long. *Why Do People Lack Health Insurance?* Washington, DC: Urban Institute, 2006.

Gray, Bradford, and Kathy Hebert. *Hospitals in Hurricane Katrina: Challenges Facing Custodial Institutions in a Disaster.* Washington, DC: Urban Institute, 2006.

Hadley, Jack. "Sicker and Poorer—The Consequences of Being Uninsured: A Review of the Research on the Relationship Between Health Insurance, Medical Care Use, Health, Work, and Income," *Medical Care Research and Review* 60(2 Suppl.): 3S–75S, 2003.

Holahan, John, Linda J. Blumberg, Alan Weil, et al. *Roadmap to Coverage: Synthesis of Findings.* Washington, DC: Urban Institute, 2006.

Holahan, John, and Allison Cook. *Why Did the Number of Uninsured Continue to Increase in 2005?* Menlo Park, CA: Henry J. Kaiser Family Foundation, 2006.

Holahan, John, Alan Weil, and Joshua M. Wiener, eds. *Federalism and Health Policy.* Washington, DC: Urban Institute Press, 2003.

Kenney, Genevieve M., and Allison Cook. *Coverage Patterns Among SCHIP-Eligible Children and Their Parents.* Washington, DC: Urban Institute, 2007.

McLaughlin, Catherine. *Health Policy and the Uninsured.* Washington, DC: Urban Institute Press, 2004.

Moon, Marilyn. *Medicare: A Policy Primer.* Washington, DC: Urban Institute Press, 2006.

Web Sites

Urban Institute: http://www.urban.org
Urban Institute's Health Policy Center: http://www.urban.org/center/hpc

U.S. DEPARTMENT OF VETERANS AFFAIRS (VA)

The U.S. Department of Veterans Affairs (VA) operates the nation's largest integrated healthcare system providing services and benefits to veterans, active-duty military personnel, and their dependents through a nationwide network of 155 hospitals, 881 outpatient clinics, 135 nursing homes, 46 residential rehabilitation treatment programs, 207 readjustment counseling centers, 57 veterans benefits regional offices, and 125 national cemeteries. In 2006, it provided care to nearly 5 million unique patients and 54 million outpatient visits.

Established in 1930 as the Veterans Administration, it was elevated to U.S. Cabinet–level status in 1989, becoming the U.S. Department of Veterans Affairs. Today, the VA is the second largest Cabinet department, employing more than 235,000 individuals. It is composed of a Central Office (VACO), which is located in Washington, D.C., and field facilities throughout the nation administered by its three line organizations: (1) Veterans Health Administration (VHA), which provides healthcare services; (2) Veterans Benefits Administration (VBA), which determines eligibility-level and benefits; and (3) the National Cemetery Administration (NCA), which provides burial services for veterans.

The VA plays a major role in improving the public's health as well as conducting clinical research. Additionally, it is the nation's largest provider of healthcare education and training for medical residents and other trainees and is one of the 10 largest research and development agencies in the federal government. In FY2006, the VA's appropriated budget was $73.6 billion.

History

The early tradition of caring for our nation's veterans can be traced back to colonial times. For more than 140 years, care for the country's veterans was provided by a patchwork of various federal agencies. In 1930, however, the U.S. Congress authorized the President to consolidate all government activities that affected war veterans, combining the Veterans Bureau, the Bureau of Pensions of the Department of Interior, and the National Home for Disabled Volunteer Soldiers within the new Veterans

Administration. After World War II, a large number of veterans needing medical care inundated the VA's rudimentary healthcare capabilities. As a result, in 1946, the U.S. Congress formally authorized a healthcare system for veterans, creating the VA Department of Medicine and Surgery.

Additionally, the VA was given the responsibility of administering the GI Bill, which was passed in 1944. The GI Bill provided education and training for all veterans. Since its passage, more than 21 million veterans, service members, and their dependents have received nearly $27 billion in benefits. In 1973, the VA also assumed the primary responsibility for the National Cemetery System from the Department of the Army. As a result of its increasing responsibility and importance, in 1989, the VA was elevated to an executive-level department with membership in the President's Cabinet.

Today, the VA provides a comprehensive and coordinated system of assistance for all the nation's veterans and their families. It operates national programs providing healthcare, financial assistance, and burial benefits, as well as supporting a large research program. Approximately 63 million individuals are potentially eligible to receive VA benefits and services because they are veterans, dependents, or survivors of veterans.

Medical Care

Because all veterans are potentially eligible for care at the VA, providing access to healthcare and other benefits has long been a challenge. To meet the healthcare needs of America's veterans, the VHA provides a broad range of primary-care, specialized-care, and related medical and social support services. The VHA healthcare facilities provide a broad spectrum of medical-surgical and rehabilitative care. Beginning with a system of 54 hospitals in 1930, the VHA has expanded to 155 medical centers—with at least one medical center in each state, Puerto Rico, and the District of Columbia. It also operates ambulatory care and community-based outpatient clinics, nursing homes, residential rehabilitation treatment programs, veterans centers, and comprehensive home care programs.

To ensure that veterans continue to receive needed medical care in the future, the U.S Veterans Administration runs the largest medical education and health professions training program in the nation. More than one half of the physicians practicing in the United States had some of their professional education in the VHA healthcare system. VHA facilities are affiliated with 107 medical schools, 55 dental schools, and more than 1,200 other schools across the country.

Costs

The annual spending of the VA in FY2005 was $71.2 billion. A total of $31.5 billion was allocated for healthcare, with the largest portion of the budget used for benefit payments. In FY2006, the budget was increased by $1.8 billion for additions in healthcare and disability compensation.

The President's proposed budget for FY2008 seeks funding for an expansion of the services provided to veterans, including $36.6 billion for medical care, $1.3 billion for more prosthetics and sensory aids, $3 billion for needed mental healthcare, and $750 million for the construction of medical facilities. Much of the rapidly increasing budget costs of funding the VA are attributable to national increases in healthcare costs.

Quality

The quality of healthcare given by the VHA has been examined very closely. Recent studies conducted by Harvard Medical School concluded that federal hospitals, including those operated by the VHA, provided superior care for some of the most common medical conditions, including heart attack, heart failure, and pneumonia. The researchers found that patients who were treated in federal facilities were more likely to receive high-quality care than those in for-profit hospitals. Another study conducted by the RAND Corporation found that the VHA outperformed all other sectors of healthcare in the United States across a spectrum of 294 measures of quality in disease prevention and treatment.

Research

The U.S. Veterans Administration is one of the 10 largest research and development agencies in the federal government. Specifically, it has the eighth largest research and development portfolio in the FY2008 budget. The entire research and development budget is allocated to a nationwide network of VHA hospitals and Centers of Excellence (COE).

The VHA advances medical research and development in ways that support veterans' needs by pursuing research in areas that most directly address the diseases and conditions that affect veterans, including combat-related trauma. The knowledge gained from research conducted at the VHA contributes to the public good through improving the understanding of diseases and disabilities. The advances in technologies from research at the VHA, intended primarily for veterans, also lead to gains in medical education, patient care, and public health. Some notable research conducted at the VHA includes construction of the first artificial kidney, development of the cardiac pacemaker, the first successful liver transplant, and development of prosthetic devices such as hydraulic knees and the robotic arm.

The major areas of research and development at the VHA include biomedical laboratory science, clinical science, rehabilitation research, and health services research. The biomedical laboratory science is the largest budgeted area of research, and it focuses on aging, chronic disease, and environmental exposures. Clinical science research funds clinical trials and other medical research using the large patient population in VHA medical facilities. Rehabilitation research focuses on improving the quality of life of veterans with disabilities, such as developing improved prosthetics. Health services research focuses on improving the effectiveness and efficiency of healthcare services and translating research into clinical practice. The objectives of health services research at the VHA include improving clinical decision making and care, informing VHA policy making, evaluating changes in the healthcare system, measuring health outcomes, and informing patients and the public interested in healthcare research.

One of the most significant transformations in the research portfolio at the VHA is the development of the COE, established by the VHA Health Services Research and Development (HSR&D), which provides for 15 centers across the country. Each center, which is affiliated with a VHA medical center, develops its own research agenda and collaborates with local universities and schools of public health to fulfill its mission. The research at each center serves to energize the facility and network with which it is affiliated and is designed to provide a constant source of innovation.

Women Veterans' Healthcare

Of the nation's 27 million veterans, about 6% are women, with the number expected to rise to 10% by 2010. And women constitute the fastest growing segment of eligible VHA healthcare users. Women veterans have their own unique healthcare needs, and the VHA seeks to make sure that they receive the best available care to meet those needs. Research studies conducted or funded by the VHA are mandated to include women veterans as a way of ensuring that their specific health needs are taken into consideration. In the past decade, there has been an expansion of biomedical, clinical, health services and rehabilitation research with the goal of improving the health status of women veterans. Recent initiatives through the VHA Women's Health Research and Development (ORD) commenced a VHA Women's Health Research Planning Group to develop a comprehensive research agenda for women veterans and to position the VHA as a national leader in women's health research.

Organizational Transformation

With the rapid changes in the nation's healthcare system and the aging of the nation's population, the U.S. Department of Veterans Affairs found itself in need of change. In 1995, the VA underwent a significant organizational transformation. The overarching goals of the reorganization were to optimize the value of VHA healthcare and to ensure the consistent and predictable provision of high-quality care throughout its system.

Among the major changes that took place were that the VHA went from a centralized system to a decentralized national network of facilities and 21 Veterans Integrated Service Networks (VISN) were established. These decentralized regional networks of care were created to better focus the needs of veterans in a specific region of the country. Under this new system, each network of providers and facilities assumes responsibility for the health of a specific population of eligible veterans.

Another significant change was the move to increase access to care through ambulatory settings. During this period of restructuring, 28,886 (55%) of inpatient acute-care beds closed, while the outpatient capacity increased with the opening of 302 community-based outpatient clinics.

A shift in the management style also occurred during the VA's organizational transformation with the creation of a performance management program that emphasized quality improvement and quality innovation. Managers were held contractually accountable to achieving predefined targets within a specified time frame. In addition, several best practices were implemented to improve clinical care.

Another major innovation at the VA was the implementation of a systemwide electronic health record called the Veterans Health Information Systems and Technology Architecture (VISTA). The VISTA system is designed to network the health records at all the VHA's inpatient and outpatient healthcare facilities nationwide. Because of VISTA, a wealth of information is available to conduct clinical and health services research studies on the VHA. The VHA also implemented the Quality Enhancement Research Initiative (QUERI), a systemized quality innovation program that links the aspects of clinical care, teaching, research, and the continuous measurement of outcomes to ultimately improve patient care.

Current and Future Direction

The VA has extraordinary responsibilities to meet the healthcare needs of veterans and their families and undertakes research to improve healthcare services. The VA, by necessity, meets new standards of care, the rising drug costs, technological innovations, and labor concerns. Through its radical reengineering and transformation, the VA has become a pioneer in coordinating and systematizing healthcare. Today, the VA continues its legacy of caring for our nation's veterans, conducting research that improves their healthcare, and providing vital education and training to medical professionals. The VA will continue its mandate of serving veterans and their families in the future.

Robert C. Good

See also Cost of Healthcare; Health Services Research at the Veterans Health Administration (VHA); Multihospital Healthcare Systems; Nursing Homes; Public Policy; Quality Enhancement Research Initiative (QUERI) of the Veterans Health Administration (VHA); Quality of Healthcare

Further Readings

Ashton, Carol M., Julianne Soucheck, Nancy J. Peterson, et al. "Hospital Use and Survival Among Veterans Affairs Beneficiaries," *New England Journal of Medicine* 349(17): 1637–46, October 23, 2003.

Kizer, Kenneth W., John G. Demakis, and John R. Feussner. "Reinventing VA Health Care: Systematizing Quality Improvement and Quality Innovation," *Medical Care* 38(6, Suppl. I): I-7–I-16, June 2000.

Klein, R. E. *The Changing Veteran Population, 1990–2020.* Washington, DC: U.S. Department of Veterans Affairs, 2001.

Kolodner, Robert M., ed. *Computerizing Large Integrated Health Networks: The VA Success.* New York: Springer-Verlag, 1997.

Landon, Bruce E., Sharon T. Lise-Normand, Adam Lessler, et al. "Quality of Care for the Treatment of Acute Medical Conditions in U.S. Hospitals," *Archives of Internal Medicine* 166: 2511–17, December 11, 2006.

Longman, Phillip. *Best Care Anywhere: Why VA Health Care Is Better Than Yours.* Sausalito, CA: Polipoint Press, 2007.

Morgan, Robert D, Cayla R. Teal, Siddharta G. Reddy, et al. "Measurement in Veteran's Affairs Health Services Research: Veterans as a Special Population" *Health Services Research* 40(5 pt. 2): 1573–83, October 2005.

U.S. Department of Veterans Affairs, Office of Human Resources and Administration. *Department of Veterans Affairs, 2007 Organization Briefing Book.* Washington, DC: Office of Human Resources and Administration, 2007.

Web Sites

U.S. Department of Veterans Affairs (VA): http://www.va.gov

U.S. Department of Veterans Affairs, Health Services Research and Development: http://www.hsrd.research.va.gov

U.S. FOOD AND DRUG ADMINISTRATION (FDA)

The U.S. Food and Drug Administration (FDA) is an agency of the Department of Health and Human Services (HHS) with massive and broad-ranging consumer protection responsibilities. The mission of the FDA is to protect the public's health through the provision of information and regulation (including the manufacturing, importing, transporting, and sale) of human and veterinary drug products, biological products, medical devices, food products (other than traditional meat, poultry, and egg products, which are regulated by the U.S. Department of Agriculture), cosmetics, and radiation-emitting electronic products. The average American consumer spends more than 20 cents of every dollar in the purchase of FDA-regulated products, which total more than $1 trillion in annual sales. The FDA's far-reaching authority and global influence rank it as among the most influential regulatory agencies in the world. Yet the FDA faces critical challenges in meeting its mission because of leadership transitions and lack of funding.

History

The evolution of the FDA has been described as a series of crisis-legislation-adaptation cycles. A consistent pattern marks historical milestones in societal and governmental responses that affected the FDA: crisis mode following public outcry from a well-publicized public health tragedy, passage of congressional legislation in response to public pressures, and adaptation by the FDA or its predecessors to implement new laws.

Prior to the 20th century, states and local governments were the primary regulatory authorities for foods and drugs, and there were loose oversight and many problems pertaining to the adulteration (contamination) and misbranding (mislabeling) of foods and drugs. The U.S. Congress passed a small number of individual laws pertaining to specific foodstuffs sold in interstate commerce, but these laws were of very limited scope. Early federal legislative efforts that influenced the later establishment of the FDA included the following: the Vaccine Act of 1813, which was enacted to prevent fraudulent marketing of smallpox vaccine and provided for the preservation of a reference standard of smallpox vaccine against which other purported vaccines could be compared (the act was repealed in 1822, after an outbreak of smallpox thought to be related to a contaminated lot supplied for the reference standard and the belief that vaccine regulation should be locally based rather

than federally based); the Drug Importation Act of 1848, which prohibited the importation of adulterated drugs following suspected mortality of U.S. soldiers from contaminated quinine and other drugs imported during the U.S.-Mexican War; and the Biologics Control Act of 1902, which required licensing of establishments that produced and marketed vaccines and antitoxins, following the deaths of almost two dozen children who were inoculated with a diphtheria antitoxin that was later found to be contaminated with tetanus bacillus.

A series of events, based on actuality and hyperbole, revealed disturbing problems of food adulteration in the 1800s and early 1900s, when advances in chemistry enabled increased detection of contamination. The origins of the FDA date back to President Lincoln's appointment of Charles M. Wetherill (as a one-man staff) in the Division of Chemistry of the U.S. Department of Agriculture in 1862. His appointment began the scientific foundations for activities now under the jurisdiction of the FDA, although commensurate regulatory authority was not established for decades to come. Later, Harvey W. Wiley was appointed Chief Chemist from 1883 until 1912 for the Division, which became the Bureau of Chemistry in 1901. In 1927, the Bureau changed its name to the Food, Drug, and Insecticide Administration, and in 1930, it shortened it to the Food and Drug Administration (FDA).

With political acumen, a knack for sensationalizing events and garnering media attention, the ability to form alliances, and an unwavering tenacity, Wiley spearheaded efforts to revolutionize the power of his office. His initiatives included the highly publicized 1902 Poison Squad, which consisted of noncontrolled experiments to assess the effects of chemical preservatives on healthy volunteers and other tactics. Wiley's efforts coincided with accounts of fraudulent and toxic medicines in many magazines, and the publication of Upton Sinclair's novel *The Jungle*, a horrifying and outrageous exposé on the nation's meatpacking industry. This provided the impetus for enactment of the 1906 Pure Food and Drugs Act (nicknamed the Wiley Act). The Pure Food and Drugs Act prohibited the interstate transport of misbranded and contaminated foods, drinks, and drugs; required labeling of a select list of ingredients (if included) and their amounts in patent medicines; and prohibited false and misleading advertising of the ingredients (but not therapeutic claims) of patent medicines on product labeling. Loopholes in the act included the exclusion of advertising materials as part of product labeling and enforcement difficulties due to lack of funding and onerous legal requirements to prove adulteration and misbranding.

Several bills were introduced in the U.S. Congress in an attempt to remedy the shortcomings of the 1906 Pure Food and Drugs Act, but there was no change until another public health crisis occurred. In 1937, in an attempt to improve the flavor, the S. E. Massengill Company of Bristol, Tennessee, added the solvent diethylene glycol to lots of the antibiotic Elixir Sulfanilamide. Given the toxic properties of the solvent (similar to antifreeze), 107 individuals (mostly children) died as the result of ingesting the formulation before the problem was contained. Public uproar prompted congressional passage of the 1938 Food, Drug, and Cosmetic Act. This act provided for the following: requirement of scientific testing to establish drug safety (with the burden imposed on the product manufacturers) prior to marketing; regulation of cosmetics and devices used for therapeutic purposes; authorization of the FDA to inspect manufacturing facilities; virtual prohibition of poisonous additives in foods; authorization to stop false drug claims; and expanded legal options that the FDA could pursue, including product seizures, criminal prosecutions, and federal court injunctions. The 1938 act and its amendments underpin the FDA's current regulatory authority, including amendments regarding pesticides (Miller Pesticide Amendment of 1954), additives (1958 Food Additives Amendment and the Color Additive Amendment of 1960), and drugs. Of note, the 1951 Durham-Humphrey Amendment to the 1938 act specified the FDA classification of prescription drugs (or legend drugs) and nonprescription or over-the-counter drugs; previously, drugs could be purchased much like any other commodity. Attempted legislative efforts that called for the FDA to establish drug product safety and efficacy were unproductive until the thalidomide tragedies.

Thalidomide was marketed in Germany as a sedative and antinausea medicine from 1957 until 1961, during which time it was found to cause thousands of congenital birth defects and malformations, disabilities, and deaths of babies whose mothers took the drug during pregnancy. While the United States experienced only 17 confirmed birth defects from thalidomide, the incident helped bring about the enactment of the Kefauver-Harris Drug Amendments to the 1938 act. The 1962 Kefauver-Harris Drug Amendments mandated demonstration of drug product safety and substantial evidence of efficacy (including review of drug products approved between 1938 and 1962 solely on the basis of safety), FDA authority over well-controlled drug trials, regulation of prescription drug advertising, and establishment of good manufacturing practices. The Medical Device Amendments of the 1938 act were enacted in 1976, based on the findings of more than 10,000 injuries and 731 deaths from faulty devices, such as contraceptive intrauterine devices.

Another legislative milestone was the 1984 Drug Price Competition and Patent Term Restoration Act (also known as the Waxman-Hatch Act), which enabled the FDA to accept abbreviated new-drug applications (ANDAs) for generic drug products and increased the effective patent term of drug products, which had been eroded by the length of the drug approval process. More federal laws were passed pertaining to foods, drugs, devices, or cosmetics over the past 25 years, including the 1990 Nutrition Labeling and Education Act, which required uniform labeling information of nutritional content and allowed for validated scientific health claims, and the 1994 Dietary Supplement Health and Education Act (DSHEA), which greatly restricted the FDA's jurisdiction in regulating dietary supplements (e.g., orally administered vitamins, minerals, herbs, amino acids, metabolites, and other substances) unless the agency found them to be unsafe after marketing them.

One of the more controversial statutes affecting the FDA in recent years was the 1992 Prescription Drug User Fee Act (PDUFA) and its subsequent amendments in 1997 (PDUFA II), 2002 (PDUFA III), and 2007 (PDUFA IV), as well as the 2002 Medical Device User Fee and Modernization Act and its subsequent amendment. The PDUFA legislation established user fees for human drug and biologic products on submission of an application and fees on an annual basis. The additional funding from user fees was designed to enable the hiring of additional FDA staff, which would shorten review times for product approval. Enactment of the PDUFA provisions, however, was met with controversy (accusations of conflict of interest between the FDA and its regulated industries that paid the user fees), increased FDA staff reviewer workloads, compromised staff morale and increased staff turnover, and unresolved questions about increased withdrawal rates of marketed drug products under the tighter product approval times.

Organization and Staffing

The FDA was transferred to different cabinet-level departments throughout the 20th century (from the U.S. Department of Agriculture to the former Federal Security Agency in 1940, which became the U.S. Department of Health, Education, and Welfare [DHEW] in 1953; FDA was reorganized as part of the U.S. Public Health Service [USPHS] within the DHEW in 1968). DHEW was renamed the Department of Health and Human Services (HHS) in 1980, and the FDA remains based in that department.

Under the leadership of the FDA commissioner, the agency has a staff of more than 9,000 employees with about two thirds in the Washington, D.C., area headquarters (i.e., Rockville, Maryland, with an anticipated consolidation of FDA facilities located at a Silver Spring, Maryland, site by 2009). FDA's headquarter staff focus on product review, regulatory policy, and consumer information. The other third of FDA staff are located in field offices and laboratories across the nation, and their responsibilities are concentrated more on inspections, surveillance, and education. Globally, the FDA works with foreign governments to help ensure the safety and quality of imported products.

The FDA employs staff in the physical sciences, medicine, public health, and many other areas. Its professional staff includes physicians, biologists, chemists, veterinarians, animal scientists, toxicologists, pharmacologists, biomedical engineers, nurses, pharmacists, epidemiologists, statisticians, communications experts, business people, consumer safety officers, and public affairs specialists.

Major FDA Centers

The FDA is organized into the Office of the Commissioner (leadership, management, and operations), the Office of Chief Counsel (litigators and counselors), the Office of Regulatory Affairs (Food, Drug, and Cosmetic Act compliance, and field agent activities), and five major centers, described below. Some regulated products are referred to as "combination products" (e.g., a combination of drugs and devices, or a biologic and a device). Assignment of combination products to one of the centers may first require referral from staff in the Office of Combination Products.

Center for Drug Evaluation and Research

The FDA's Center for Drug Evaluation and Research (CDER) reviews, approves, and monitors the safety and efficacy of prescription and nonprescription drug products that are marketed in the United States. More than 10,000 drug products are currently being marketed in the nation. The FDA assumes enormous responsibility in the paradoxical duty of benefit-to-risk judgments regarding timely approval of drug products (especially for serious or life-threatening conditions where no therapeutic options are available) and continued market availability when serious problems are noted.

The drug development and approval process in the United States involves a series of rigorous steps that can take from 11 to 12 years (FDA estimate) to 15 years (industry estimate) to go from initial laboratory testing to product approval. These processes start with preclinical testing of biological activity and safety evaluations for the compound (laboratory tests, animal studies, and computer models). After promising preclinical testing, the sponsor can file an application (i.e., Investigational New Drug Application, or IND) to begin three phases of clinical testing in people (with greater numbers of subjects in each subsequent stage). If the data demonstrate safety and effectiveness, a New Drug Application, or NDA, can be submitted to the FDA for review and possible approval of the product for commercial availability as a new molecular entity. However, very few compounds—estimated to be as few as 1 out of 10,000—make it through the process from preclinical testing to final market approval at costs to the sponsors of hundreds of millions of dollars. Regulatory agencies may also call for postmarketing surveillance and additional studies after drug product approval to evaluate the long-term effects.

Generic drug applications undergo an ANDA process. For approval, the generic product must contain the same active ingredient as the innovator product; be identical in strength, dosage form, and route of administration; list the same indications for treatment; and demonstrate bioequivalence. The median ANDA approval is about 16.6 months.

Center for Biologics Evaluation and Research

The FDA's Center for Biologics Evaluation and Research (CBER) regulates biological products such as blood and blood products, vaccines, allergenic products, and protein-derived bioengineered drug products (e.g., monoclonal antibodies, cytokines, and enzymes). The biotechnology pharmaceutical industry has a product approval process similar to other research-intensive pharmaceutical products, including discovery; preclinical studies; IND and Phase I (safety), Phase II (safety and efficacy), and Phase III (large controlled studies on safety and efficacy) clinical trials; NDA and FDA review; drug product approval; and postapproval monitoring. The approval time for a biopharmaceutical ranges between 7 and 12 years from development to approval. The center also regulates human gene therapies, xenotransplantation of organs from animals to humans, cellular and tissue transplants (including stem cell therapy) and other products derived from living organisms.

Center for Devices and Radiological Health

The FDA's Center for Devices and Radiological Health (CDRH) regulates new medical devices and provides for postmarketing surveillance. A few examples of medical devices include tongue depressors, thermometers, contact lenses, glucose level monitors, blood pressure monitors, surgical robotic-arm tools, laboratory tests, and technologically complex devices such as pacemakers, heart defibrillators, and dialysis machines. The center classifies medical devices based on proposed risk and intended use. Class I medical devices (e.g., examination gloves, bandages) represent the least risk, Class II devices (e.g., X-ray machines, electronic wheelchairs) intermediate risk, and Class III devices (e.g., heart valves, breast implants) the highest risk. With some exceptions, premarket approval is generally required for Class III medical devices. In the majority of cases where premarket approval is not required, medical devices are regulated subject to premarket notification requirements from Section 510(k) of the Food, Drug, and Cosmetic Act. The U.S. Government Accountability Office (GAO) is currently reviewing whether there is a need for revising the 510(k) process in consideration of the possible need for more evaluation of clinical safety.

Additionally, the center establishes performance safety standards for radiation-emitting electronic products such as microwave ovens, television sets, cellular telephones, X-ray equipment and systems (including airport-scanning equipment), laser products, medical imaging techniques, sunlamps, and other products. It also provides accreditation of mammography facilities.

Center for Food Safety and Applied Nutrition

The FDA's Center for Food Safety and Applied Nutrition (CFSAN) regulates the safety and labeling of foods (except meats, poultry, and egg products) and bottled water. The center strives to ensure that food products are uncontaminated, approves food additives, and regulates the contents of medical foods and infant formulas. Within the limits of the 1994 DSHEA, the center is responsible for regulating the safety of dietary supplements. It also monitors the safety and labeling of cosmetics, which do not require premarket approval (with the exception of color additives). The agency cannot require safety testing of cosmetics. The FDA is authorized, however, to pursue enforcement actions when product violations are found regarding the adulteration and misbranding of cosmetics.

Center for Veterinary Medicine

The FDA's Center for Veterinary Medicine (CVM) regulates the safety of animal food products and the improvement of the health and productivity of food-producing animals. Drugs administered to livestock must meet safety standards for the animals and humans who may eat such animal products. Specifically, the center regulates pet food production, feeds for livestock, and the approval and marketing of drug products (prescription and over the counter) used to treat animals. It also regulates the safety, effectiveness, and labeling of veterinary devices, which do not require preapproval before marketing, unlike human medical devices.

National Center for Toxicological Research

The FDA's National Center for Toxicological Research (NCTR) conducts scientific research and provides technical expertise on mechanisms of toxicities, human exposure, susceptibility and risk involving chemicals and pharmaceuticals, food contamination, and biomarkers for chemical and biological terrorism.

Information Provision

Much information from the FDA is provided on its Web pages, which receive more than 1 million hits per day. The FDA publishes numerous consumer resources (e.g., magazines, brochures, fact sheets, and other materials) providing product and health information. It also administers two drug information centers, one in the CDER and the other in the CBER, to provide FDA-approved prescribing information on products and regulatory guidance. Inquiries come from a range of diverse constituents, including patients, consumers, health professionals, trade associations, insurance companies, regulated industries and other sponsors, advertising agencies, attorneys, investment companies, academia, law enforcement, government agencies, and the media. Information is provided by FDA staff on clinical information, adverse events, clinical investigations and trials, electronic regulatory application submissions, review processes, regulations pertaining to imports and exports, patents and exclusivity, product recalls and shortages, and product identification.

Challenges

The FDA faces a number of major challenges, including leadership, funding, and improving the nation's drug safety system. Each is discussed below.

Leadership

The FDA commissioner is appointed by the President of the United States on confirmation by the U.S. Senate. A major challenge to the agency is the lack of stable leadership, highlighted by the fact that no commissioner has served longer than 2 years since 1997. And the position of commissioner has been vacant for many months at various times.

Funding

With small increases in congressional appropriations, the FDA budget has increasingly become dependent on user fees. Its FY2009 budget requested almost $2.4 billion, representing about $1.77 billion in appropriations and $628 million generated from industry-provided user fees. Many researchers and policy analysts believe that the FDA budget is inadequate given its comprehensive regulatory authority and that more public funding is needed. While user fees increased the funding available for drugs and biologics reviews under the PDUFA mechanisms, programs that were not supported by the PDUFA fees (including drug, food, and medical device initiatives) lost about 1,000 FDA staff members since 1992 as the result of diminished funding.

Drug Safety System

In a 2007 report, the National Academy of Sciences, Institute of Medicine (IOM) summarized some of the FDA challenges and needed improvements in the nation's drug safety system. In addition to recommendations for increased funding, the report identified organizational problems in the FDA culture that contribute to the inadequate integration of premarket and postmarket safety review data; technical limitations in the ability of the current passive postmarketing surveillance system to detect signals and analyze safety systems adequately; and unclear regulatory authority over manufacturers postapproval. The report recommended more joint authority for postapproval regulatory actions within the FDA; systematic approaches in benefit-risk judgments; and the establishment of private-public partnerships and collaborative efforts among federal agencies, pharmaceutical and biotechnology companies, and managed-care organizations to consolidate stakeholder data that can support postapproval drug safety monitoring.

Stephanie Y. Crawford

See also Direct-to-Consumer Advertising (DTCA); Pharmaceutical Industry; Pharmacoeconomics; Pharmacy; Prescription and Generic Drugs; Public Health; Randomized Controlled Trials (RCT); Regulation

Further Readings

Borchers, Andrea T., Frank Hagie, Carl L. Keen, et al. "The History and Contemporary Challenges of the U.S. Food and Drug Administration," *Clinical Therapeutics* 29(1): 1–16, January 2007.

Daemmrich, Arthur, and Joanna Radin, eds. *Perspectives on Risk and Regulation: The FDA at 100.* Philadelphia: Chemical Heritage Foundation, 2008.

"FDA Milestones," *FDA Consumer* 40(1): 36–38, January–February 2006.

Glantz, Leonard H., and George J. Annas. "The FDA, Preemption, and the Supreme Court," *New England Journal of Medicine* 358(18): 1883–85, May 1, 2008.

Hickmann, Meredith A. *The Food and Drug Administration (FDA).* New York: Nova Science, 2003.

Hilts, Philip J. *Protecting America's Health: The FDA, Business, and One Hundred Years of Regulation.* New York: Alfred A. Knopf, 2003.

Pray, Leslie, and Sally Robinson. *Challenges for the FDA: The Future of Drug Safety.* Workshop Summary. Washington, DC: National Academies Press, 2007.

Sinclair, U. *The Jungle.* Tucson, AZ: See Sharp Press, 2003.

Web Sites

U.S. Food and Drug Administration (FDA): http://www.fda.gov

U.S. Public Health Service (USPHS): http://www.usphs.gov

World Health Organization (WHO), Drug Regulation: http://www.who.int/medicines/areas/quality_safety/regulation_legislation/en

U.S. GOVERNMENT ACCOUNTABILITY OFFICE (GAO)

The U.S. Government Accountability Office (GAO) is an independent, nonpartisan agency that works for the U.S. Congress. Often called the "congressional watchdog," the GAO investigates how the federal government spends taxpayer dollars. GAO's mission is to support the U.S. Congress in meeting its constitutional responsibilities and to help improve the performance and ensure the accountability of the federal government. This includes performance and accountability related to federal health programs and spending in areas including public health, Medicare and Medicaid, defense healthcare, veterans health, long-term care, disaster preparedness, and pandemic health issues.

The GAO advises the U.S. Congress and the heads of executive agencies about ways to make government more efficient, effective, ethical, equitable, and responsive. The GAO's work is done at the request of congressional committees or subcommittees or is mandated by public laws or committee reports. The agency also undertakes research under the authority of the head of the GAO, the Comptroller General of the United States. The President appoints the Comptroller General to a 15-year term from a slate of candidates the U.S. Congress proposes. The Comptroller General cannot be reappointed and has a mandatory retirement age of 70. However, the President cannot remove the Comptroller General; only the U.S. Congress can through impeachment or joint resolution for specific reasons. GAO's main headquarters is located in Washington, D.C., and it maintains 11 field offices in various cities throughout the nation. It employees more than 3,100 individuals and has an annual budget of approximately $490 million.

History

The GAO has focused on governmental accountability from the time it began operations. Signed into law by President Warren G. Harding in 1921, the GAO was created by the Budget and Accounting Act (Pub. L. 67–13, 42 Stat. 20), which was aimed at improving federal financial management after World War I. The statute transferred to GAO the auditing, accounting, and claims functions previously carried out by the Department of the Treasury; made GAO independent of the executive branch; and gave it a broad mandate to investigate how federal funds are spent. While the agency always has worked for good government, its mission and organization have changed over time to keep up with congressional and national needs. In July 2004, the agency changed its official name from the U.S. General Accounting Office to the U.S. General Accountability Office. The name change better reflects the agency's modern organizational purpose while retaining its well-recognized acronym—GAO.

Health Research

The GAO supports congressional oversight of federal healthcare programs by reporting on how well programs and policies are meeting their objectives; performing policy analyses and outlining options for congressional consideration; auditing agency operations to determine whether federal funds are being spent efficiently and effectively; investigating allegations of illegal and improper activities; and issuing legal decisions and opinions, such as bid protest rulings and reports on agency rules.

Much of the GAO's work on federal healthcare programs relates to the agency's Strategic Goal No. 1: to provide timely, quality service to the U.S. Congress and the federal government to address current and emerging challenges to the well-being and financial security of the American people. For example, in FY2007, the GAO provided information that helped highlight ways to address problems affecting the delivery of health and disability services for injured soldiers and veterans, improve the U.S. Food and Drug Administration's (FDA's) process for removing dangerous drugs from the marketplace, and identify inefficient physician practice patterns to improve performance of the Medicare program.

The agency's best-known products include reports, testimonies, correspondence, and legal decisions and opinions, which are all available to the press and the public from GAO's Web site. The GAO also produces special publications to assist the U.S. Congress and executive branch agencies by recommending corrections to problems in government programs and operations, identifying long-term trends, and raising concerns about the nation's fiscal status. Among its recent special reports is *21st Century Challenges: Reexamining the Base of the Federal Government*. This report is intended to help the U.S. Congress in reviewing and reconsidering the base of federal spending and tax programs, including healthcare-related spending.

The GAO's work also seeks to analyze and monitor changes in the long-term fiscal outlook, including the effects of demographics and health-care costs, as well as other federal fiscal commitments. As the baby boomer generation (those individuals born between 1946 and 1964 who make up about 75 million individuals) retires, federal spending on retirement and health programs—Social Security, Medicare, and Medicaid—will grow dramatically. A long-term model of the federal budget and the economy, maintained by the GAO, simulates the effect of such changes. This model was adapted from work done at the Federal Reserve Bank of New York. For over a decade, the GAO has published the results of its long-term budget simulations in reports, testimonies, and other products. The model's results dramatically illustrate the need for action sooner rather than later to address the long-term fiscal imbalance.

Medicare Payment Advisory Commission

The Comptroller General of the United States and head of the GAO is responsible for appointing individuals to serve as members of the Medicare Payment Advisory Commission (MedPAC). The commission, which was established by the Balanced Budget Act of 1997, is an independent congressional agency that advised the U.S. Congress on issues affecting the Medicare program. The commission consists of 17 members who serve 3-year terms (subject to renewal). Its commissioners include actuaries, lawyers, physicians, and policy experts.

Mary F. Giffin

See also Congressional Budget Office (CBO); Cost of Healthcare; Fraud and Abuse; Medicaid; Medicare; Medicare Payment Advisory Commission (MedPAC); Public Policy; Regulation

Further Readings

Mosher, Frederick C. *The GAO: The Quest for Accountability in American Government.* Boulder, CO: Westview Press, 1979.
Tidrick, Donald E. *The Comptrollers General of the United States and a Conversation With the Surviving CGs.* Alexander, VA: Association of Government Accountants, 2006.

Trask, Roger R. *GAO History: 1921–1991*. Washington, DC: U.S. General Accounting Office, 1991.

Trask, Roger R. *Defender of the Public Interest: The General Accounting Office, 1921–1966*. Washington, DC: Government Printing Office, 1996.

U.S. Government Accountability Office. *21st Century Challenges: Reexamining the Base of the Federal Government*. Washington, DC: U.S. Government Accountability Office, 2005.

U.S. Government Accountability Office. *Serving the Congress and the Nation: Forces That Will Shape America's Future: Themes From GAO's Strategic Plan: 2007–2012*. Washington, DC: U.S. Government Accountability Office, 2007.

Web Sites

Association of Government Accountants (AGA): http://www.agacgfm.org

Medicare Payment Advisory Commission (MedPAC): http://www.medpac.gov

U.S. Government Accountability Office (GAO): http://www.gao.gov

U.S. House of Representatives: http://www.house.gov

U.S. Senate: http://www.senate.gov

U.S. National Health Expenditures

Published yearly by the National Health Statistics Group of the Office of the Actuary at the Centers for Medicare and Medicaid Services (CMS), the U.S. National Health Accounts (NHA) is the definitive source on the nation's past, current, and future healthcare expenditures. The NHA describes the total national amount spent on healthcare by type of services (e.g., hospital care, physician services, and prescription drugs), source of funds (e.g., private health insurance, Medicare, Medicaid, and out-of-pocket costs), and type of sponsors (e.g., businesses, households, and governments). Finally, the NHA presents trends in healthcare expenditures, and it makes various projections and estimates of the future healthcare expenditures.

Historical Trends

Using data from the NHA, Figure 1 shows the annual national health expenditures, the nation's gross domestic product (GDP), and the percentage of the GDP spent on healthcare for the period 1960 through 2005. During the period, the percentage of the nation's GDP spent on healthcare increased dramatically. In 1960, healthcare accounted for 5.2% of the nation's GDP, but by 2006 it had grown to 16.0%. In 1960, total healthcare spending was $27.6 billion, or $143 per person, but by 2006, total healthcare spending had increased to $2.1 trillion, or $7,026 per person.

Types of Services Delivered

Hospitals accounted for the largest share of the nation's health expenditures. In 2006, they accounted for 30.8% of the total spending, down from a peak of 40.6% in 1982. Physician and clinical services accounted for 21.3% of the total spending in 2006, with a peak of 22.4% in 1991. Prescription drug spending reached a peak of 10.1% in 2006 from a low of 4.5% in 1982. Nursing home care accounted for 5.9% of the total spending in 2006, down from a peak of 7.3% in 1978.

Sources of Funds

The distribution of health expenditures by source of funds during the period 1960 through 2005 is shown in Figure 2. In 2006, private payers paid 54% of the nation's total health expenditures compared with 46% paid for by public payers (i.e., federal, state, and local governments). In the period 1960 through 1965, before the federal Medicare and the federal/state Medicaid programs started, private payers paid for 75% of the nation's total health expenditures. Since then, the private share has gradually declined to 54% in 2006. The actual private share may be lower because the calculation does not include the tax subsidy for private health insurance and healthcare spending. The subsidy takes the form of business and individuals deducting health insurance and healthcare spending from their taxable incomes.

The decline of the private share of expenditures was primarily due to the falling share of out-of-pocket spending. The share of out-of-pocket spending declined from nearly half the total healthcare expenditures in 1960 to 12% in 2006. While out-of-pocket spending fell, private

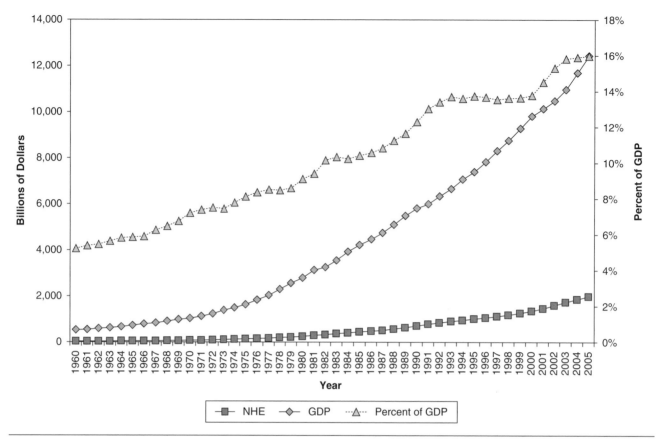

Figure 1   U.S. National Health Expenditure Figures, 1960 to 2005

Source: Centers for Medicare and Medicaid Services, National Health Expenditure Accounts.

health insurance expenditures as a share of total healthcare expenditures grew steadily over the decades.

The public share of healthcare expenditures, which includes Medicare, Medicaid, and the State Children's Health Insurance Program (SCHIP), has grown over the decades. In 2006, the public share totaled $725 billion, accounting for 34% of the nation's healthcare expenditures.

Type of Sponsors

Categorizing healthcare expenditures by source of funds—such as private health insurance, Medicare, Medicaid, and so forth—does not identify the true payers of healthcare costs. In the late 1980s, the NHA started presenting data to identify the underlying entity financing the

healthcare bill—households, businesses, and governments. This structure allows a better understanding of who pays the healthcare bills and what burdens these costs are placing on each sponsor.

Individual households pay healthcare costs in various ways, including private health insurance premiums, payroll taxes such as the Medicare tax, and out-of-pocket costs. Private businesses pay for employer-sponsored health insurance premiums and part of employees' Medicare tax. The federal government pays for healthcare through federal employee health insurance premiums; Medicare taxes; and the Medicare, Medicaid, and other programs. Likewise, state and local governments pay similar taxes and premiums, and state governments pay their portion of the Medicaid program. In 2006, the total amount paid by private sponsors

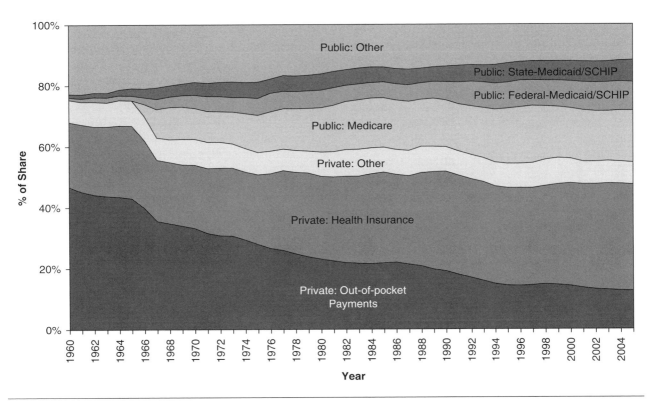

Figure 2   National Healthcare Expenditure by Source of Funding, 1960–2005

Source: U.S. National Health Accounts, 2007.

accounted for 60% of health services and supplies spending, compared with 40% by the combined federal, state, and local governments.

As implied by the spending categorized by sponsor, Medicare is not financed solely by the federal government but by all sponsors—households, businesses, and governments. For example, in 2006, households paid 36% of Medicare spending. The combined households and businesses paid 56% of Medicare spending, and the remaining 44% was paid mostly by the federal government (38%). Unlike Medicare, the Medicaid program does not have its own dedicated tax as a funding source. In 2006, using general revenue funds, the federal government's contribution accounted for 56% of total Medicaid spending, with the remaining 44% being paid for by the states.

Employers have faced rapid increases in healthcare costs. Between 1987 and 1993, the growth rate of health insurance premiums, the largest component of business healthcare costs, averaged 11% per year. Beginning in 1998, the growth in employer-sponsored healthcare premiums accelerated, largely

because managed-care plans tried to cover benefit-cost increases and boost profit margins by increasing premiums.

The Burden of Healthcare Costs

The burden of healthcare costs faced by sponsors can be more adequately measured by comparing healthcare costs relative to income revenues. The share of federal revenues funding healthcare has almost doubled, from 17.3% in 2000 to 32.5% in 2004. In 2005, the burden decreased slightly to 30.0% as overall federal spending decelerated from 9.8% to 7.1%.

For state and local governments, healthcare spending as a percentage of revenues rose from 14% in 1987, to 22% in 2000, to almost 25% in 2005. Much of the increase was driven by increases in Medicaid expenditures.

For households, the share of spending compared with personal income increased from 4.9% in 1987, to 5.3% in 2000, to 6.0% in 2005. This increase appears to be mainly due to increases in insurance premiums and out-of-pocket healthcare spending. It should be noted that there are important disparities among households in overall spending on healthcare as a share of income. The poor and the elderly tend to spend a larger share of their income on healthcare.

Projected Healthcare Expenditures

National Health Expenditures

According to the latest NHA projections for the time period 2007 through 2017, national health expenditures are expected to average a growth rate of 6.7% per year. In 2017, the projected total healthcare expenditures will be about $4.3 trillion and will constitute 19.5% of the nation's GDP.

Public-Private Share

It is expected that the public-private share of national healthcare expenditures will be significantly altered in the future by the Medicare Part D prescription drug program. The program, which was implemented in 2006, lessens the burden that households face in paying for prescription drugs. Employers and state governments may also benefit from the program. Employers may not have to pay the costs of prescription drugs for their retired employees. States can reduce their contributions for prescription drugs for Medicaid recipients. These changes will shift more costs to the federal government. These additional costs may hurt the long-term sustainability of the entire Medicare program.

The growth in public personal healthcare spending is projected to greatly increase, while the growth of private personal healthcare is expected to slow. Specifically, public personal healthcare spending is projected to grow at an average of 7.2% per year compared with 6.5% for private personal care spending during the period 2007 through 2017. The acceleration in public spending will largely be driven by faster growth in Medicare enrollment as the baby boomer generation becomes eligible for coverage. Also, overall out-of-pocket spending growth is expected to slow, flattening out below 10.9% by 2017.

Medicare

The annual reports of the Medicare Board of Trustees to the U.S. Congress represent the federal government's official evaluation of the financial status of the Medicare program. According to the 2007 report, Medicare expenditures are expected to increase at a faster rate than workers' income. As a result, the Hospital Insurance Trust Fund used to pay for Medicare Part A services (i.e., hospital, home health, skilled-nursing facility, and hospice care) will not be adequately financed. Taxes paid into the fund are projected to fall short of expenditures in future years. Between 2007 and 2016, the trust fund's assets are projected to decrease from $305 billion to $221 billion. Because this amount is less than the recommended minimum level of 1 year's expenditures, both the 2006 and 2007 reports issued a "Medicare funding warning."

The second Medicare fund, Supplementary Medical Insurance (SMI), pays for Medicare Part B and D services. Medicare Part B pays for physician, outpatient hospital, and home healthcare, as well as other services. Medicare Part D pays for prescription drugs. Medicare Parts B and D are both voluntary programs, and enrollees pay for them through premiums. The SMI trust fund is financed by beneficiary premiums and general government revenue funds. According to intermediate projections, Medicare Part B's growth rate will average about 8% to 9%, and Medicare Part D's annual growth rate will average 12.6% through 2016. Thus, Medicare Part B and D expenditures will grow significantly faster than the nation's economy, which is projected to grow at 4.8% on average during the same time period.

Future Implications

In the future, the nation's healthcare expenditures will likely continue to grow at a faster pace than the general economy. This growth will be driven by increases in the nation's population, the growth of the elderly, inflation within the healthcare sector, and new medical technology. This growth will continue to strain the nation's Medicare and state Medicaid programs. Taxes may have to be increased in order to pay for the growing expenditures, and new public policies will have to be developed and implemented in order to control healthcare costs.

Kyusuk Chung

See also Cost Containment Strategies; Cost of Healthcare; Healthcare Financial Management; Health Economics; Health Insurance; Medicaid; Medicare; Medicare Part D Prescription Drug Benefit

Further Readings

Fairbank, Alan. *National Health Accounts Interim Estimation Model.* Bethesda, MD: Partners for Health Reformplus/Abt Associates, 2006.
Hilsenrath, Peter, James Hill, and Samuel Levey, "Private Finance and Sustainable Growth of National Health Expenditures," *Journal of Health Care Finance* 30(4): 14–20, Summer 2004.
Huskamp, Haiden A., Anna D. Sinaiko, and Joseph P. Newhouse, "Future Directions for the National Health Expenditure Accounts: Conference Overview," *Health Care Financing Review* 28(1): 1–8, Fall 2006.
Poisal, John A., Christopher Truffer, Sheila Smith, et al., "Health Spending Projections Through 2016: Modest Changes Obscure Part D's Impact," *Health Affairs* 26(2): w242–w253, March–April 2007.
Sensenig, Arthur L., "Refining Estimates of Public Health Spending as Measured in National Health Expenditures Accounts: The United States Experience," *Journal of Public Health Management and Practice* 13(2): 103–14, March–April 2007.

Web Sites

America's Health Insurance Plans (AHIP): http://www.ahip.org
Centers for Medicare and Medicaid Services (CMS): National Health Expenditure Accounts: http://www.cms.hhs.gov/NationalHealthExpendData
Congressional Budget Office (CBO): http://www.cbo.gov

V

VOLUME-OUTCOME RELATIONSHIP

The volume-outcome relationship refers to the association between the number of patients with a specific diagnosis or surgical procedure treated at a hospital or by a surgeon and the outcomes experienced by those patients. Outcomes typically refer to mortality, but they can include other quality measures such as complications or health status. Although high volume has been shown to be associated with better outcomes across a wide range of conditions and procedures, the magnitude and nature of this association are highly variable. Moreover, the reasons for the observed associations are often unclear, and the policy and clinical implications of these studies are often confounded by important methodological issues regarding volume-outcome research.

Background

Training and repetition are necessary to learn the skills needed to expertly accomplish a surgical procedure or become familiar with protocols and organizational nuances in any particular hospital setting. However, the "practice makes perfect" hypothesis raises a series of questions when applied to the real world. How high is the threshold necessary to acquire competency? Once one achieves that threshold, for example, through rigorous training, do the skills deteriorate over time if not maintained? Does quality continue to get better with experience (or volume) above the threshold—that is, should one seek out the highest-volume provider or just avoid those below a threshold level? For surgical procedures, is it just the volume of the primary surgeon, or do the skills of the anesthesiologist and other members of the team matter? In a set of procedures, such as coronary artery bypass graft (CABG), does volume matter for all cases or just for a subset of cases, such as the most risky patients or cases when an unexpected event occurs? An entirely different perspective on the simple association between volume and outcome is that the conventional wisdom is backward. That is, perhaps some physicians are just better than others and receive more referrals because of their better outcomes and thus have higher volumes; this is known as the selective-referral hypothesis. If so, are there subtle techniques and protocols that can be taught so that others with lower case volumes can also achieve better outcomes? There is no reason, moreover, to believe that both practice makes perfect and selective referral may not occur simultaneously, perhaps with differential importance for various conditions and procedures.

Harold Luft and colleagues' 1979 article in the *New England Journal of Medicine* was the first to examine the volume-outcome relationship across a series of surgical procedures. This study examined the 1974–1975 discharge data from 1,498 hospitals on 12 surgical procedures. A volume-outcome relationship was observed for certain procedures, including open-heart surgery, coronary artery bypass, and vascular surgery, in which high-volume (defined as more than 200 procedures per year) hospitals were associated with significantly lower mortality. However, for other services, such as colectomy and hip replacement, mortality also decreased with increasing hospital volume but stabilized at a much lower volume, between 10 and 50 procedures per year. Other procedures, such as cholecystectomy and vagotomy, showed no relation between volume and outcome.

Over the next 30 years, hundreds of studies in the health services research and clinical literature surfaced confirming the volume-outcome relationship for both hospitals and individual providers, although the evidence is stronger for the former. Those procedures and conditions that have been most studied include vascular surgery, cancer, and cardiac care. Important questions have surfaced regarding the volume-outcome relationship: What constitutes adequate volume, and how is this determined? Which procedures are the most sensitive to volume? To what extent is hospital volume—as opposed to physician volume—the key variable? How does one account for severity of illness of patients? Might there be selective biases in referral patterns? To what extent does accumulated experience, versus volume (or "throughput") at a given point in time, account for good outcomes? What are the clinical and other implications of various policies potentially derived from the observed relationship? After three decades of work, these questions remain at the heart of volume-outcome research.

In 2000, Ethan Halm and colleagues conducted a literature review of 135 studies covering 27 different procedures. They found that the hospital-volume relationship was strongest for pancreatic cancer surgery, esophageal cancer, pediatric cardiac surgery, the treatment of AIDS, and abdominal aortic aneurysms. Weaker volume-outcome relationships were found for coronary artery bypass surgery (CABG), coronary angioplasty, orthopedic surgery, and some forms of cancer. In the largest volume-outcome study, published in 2002, John Birkmeyer and colleagues reviewed the experience of 2.5 million Medicare patients who had 1 of 14 procedures between 1994 and 1999. Mortality and volume were inversely related; however, there were large differences between high- and low-volume settings for esophagectomy and pancreatectomy and smaller differences for CABG and carotid endartectomy. While the volume-outcome relationship has been confirmed by many studies, the relationship varies significantly by clinical situation. Methodological issues, however, greatly influence the results and implications of the studies.

Methodological Issues

Various methodological issues are central to both understanding the volume-outcome relationship and drawing valid policy and clinical recommendations from the available studies. Such recommendations need to be based on a comprehensive assessment of the causal linkages (not just correlations) between volume and outcome, of the separate effects of hospital and physician volume, and of their effects over time as volumes change. Without an understanding of the potential weaknesses of studies, it is easy to overinterpret reported findings.

One of the most fundamental issues in assessing the volume-outcome relationship is that it is about outcomes—typically rare ones such as death—rather than quality as measured by process—that is, measuring whether the right thing was done for each patient in each circumstance. Health professionals rarely know the optimal processes of care and the mix of skills required to achieve the best outcomes, but instead they are seeking to identify the characteristics of physicians or hospitals—such as volume—that are associated with the best outcomes for their patients and then attempt to understand why or how they achieve those differentially better outcomes.

The focus on outcomes has several important implications for the underlying methods and approaches. Patient care is not like manufacturing; the results of an episode of care or treatment reflect not only the processes and skills of the providers and organizations but also the exact nature of the clinical problem (severity), what other medical problems the patient may have (comorbidities), and how that person reacts to treatment. These are issues commonly faced in the assessment of new drugs, for example, but the methodological solution there is to take a large number of reasonably similar patients and randomly assign them to the new drug and an alternative. Assuming that the samples are large enough, and in theory replicated, the randomization ensures that differences in the exact nature of the clinical problem, comorbidities, and patient-specific effects are balanced between the two groups and any residual differences observed must be due to the effects of the drugs. There are no large-scale volume-outcome studies that have applied randomization techniques (it is difficult to imagine how one would do so), so statistical adjustments are needed to account for potential alternative explanations.

The last component—individual variability in response to identical treatment—controlling for all the potential measurable risk factors—is a problem of random variation that raises the statistical problems discussed later. The first two categories of problems, severity and comorbidities, are often addressed through what is termed *risk adjustment*. Risk adjustment involves the inclusion of various measures of disease severity and preexisting conditions to account for differences in outcomes apart from volume-related effects. There is a large literature on how to do risk adjustment, but statistical risk adjustment will most likely not be good enough to satisfy those who see randomization as the gold standard. Most volume-outcome studies are based on large numbers of patients and hospitals (or physicians), so the real concern is not the precision of the risk adjustment but the potential for the failings of risk adjustment to be plausibly associated with the key variable of interest—volume.

For an example of how this bias might occur, consider the following situation. Patients in teaching hospitals tend to have more thorough workups and documentation of their comorbidities simply because workups are a part of house-staff training. A patient admitted for a surgical procedure to a teaching hospital is likely to have more comorbidities coded than if admitted to a community hospital, where only the diagnoses directly related to the procedure may be recorded. Most risk adjustment models depend on the conditions coded, so this differential coding will make the patient appear to be sicker based on the information reported by the teaching hospital. With a higher expected risk of a bad outcome, the ratio of observed to expected outcomes across many such patients would be better in teaching hospitals than in community hospitals even if the bad-outcome rates were identical. As teaching hospitals tend to have higher volumes than community hospitals, this simple bias in reporting and coding could lead to the spurious observation of a volume-outcome effect.

The potential for biased estimates of the volume-outcome effects is heightened if one takes into consideration the selection of providers or patients. In many healthcare situations, the patient (or his or her referring physician) has a choice of specialists and sometimes hospitals to provide care. It is plausible that given the opportunity, some patients will seek out the most skilled clinicians; this would yield the observation of higher volume among the best providers, even if volume itself had nothing to do with the outcomes—the selective referral effect. However, when the risk factors of patients are assessed, it sometimes appears that the low-volume hospitals attract a mix of sicker patients—precisely the ones who would benefit the most from the expertise. This seems inexplicable until one realizes that the observed behavior may reflect the selective choice by those patients well enough to have the time to choose a facility. They will seek out the sites with the best reputations, leaving the low-volume ones with the sickest patients, who are not able to "shop." If the risk adjustment models are not perfect, then the low-volume sites may appear to have worse risk-adjusted outcomes than they warrant.

These examples are not intended to suggest that there is no evidence for a true relationship between volume and outcome (although the causality may be unclear) but that inattention to careful risk adjustment and the potential for selection may overestimate the true relationship. Careful testing of the risk models and searching for hints of selection are important. Likewise, one should be sensitive to when these issues are likely to be problematic. For example, treatment of patients for heart attack, when emergency medical teams typically take the patient to the nearest hospital, is not likely to be subject to a great deal of selective referral. Surgical treatment of advanced cancer, however, may be highly sensitive to both selective referral by patients and even refusals by specialists, who may argue that there is little that can be usefully done.

Turning to the implementation of the studies, assessing the impact of volume on rare events such as death creates straightforward, yet often overlooked, statistical issues. Suppose that death occurs 5% of the time after a surgical procedure—actually a rather high mortality rate for most volume-outcome studies. With 20 patients, one would expect 1 death if quality was just average. This "average figure," however, is the result of some hospitals with 20 patients having 0 deaths, some having 1, and some having as much as 2, 3, or 4 deaths. The observed death rates are 0, 5%, 10%, 15%, and 20%, yet all are consistent with a true average quality of 5%. The deviations are simply due to chance, just as a fair coin when flipped 10 times will not always produce exactly 5 "heads." Unfortunately, some observers point to the observation of 0 deaths in low-volume hospitals as evidence that "some low-volume hospitals have very good outcome rates." This may be true, but it cannot be inferred by the observation of 0 deaths when only a small number are expected.

Another problem when examining the volume-outcome relationship is assessing the independent effects of physician (usually surgeon) and hospital volume. High-volume hospitals may have both high- and low-volume surgeons, and some high-volume surgeons may spread their patients over two or more hospitals. Overall, however, surgeon and hospital volume are probably highly correlated at the low end; low-volume hospitals are probably staffed mostly by low-volume surgeons, but there are many ways high-volume hospitals can achieve their patient loads.

The nature of the volume-outcome relationship is often subjected to only minimal testing. Some researchers simply test whether outcomes are better for patients using high-volume providers, but it is more important to understand the "shape of the relationship." That is, if one were to plot mortality on the vertical axis and volume on the horizontal, does the curve look like a \, an L, or a U? If mortality continues to fall as volume increases over the relevant range, only then will the highest-volume providers have the best outcomes. On the other hand, if outcomes cease improving after a certain point, it is critical to know that point. Even worse, there may be volumes above which outcomes actually get worse, and it is critical to know whether that is the case and also the volumes at which the best outcomes occur. Few studies use methods that allow the assessment of which of these alternative explanations best fit the data, yet the methods used often determine the findings.

Policy and Clinical Implications

Many studies assess the presence of a volume-outcome relationship, but this work is primarily of interest because of the potential clinical relevance and policy implications. Are there particular processes or techniques that can be learned from the high-volume settings that can be transferred to those with lower volume? Should patients seek the hospital or physician with the highest volume, or should they simply avoid providers with less than a certain threshold of procedures? Should volume be used as a criterion in the development of preferred referral networks? What are the potential risks and benefits of regionalization? Should there be policies requiring a minimum volume of procedures or cases?

There are several approaches to disseminating volume-outcome data. Insurers and consumer groups have recently taken an interest in public dissemination of data on hospital volumes for specific surgical procedures, recommending that health plans and consumers use the data to choose high-quality hospitals. As discussed above, however, only some procedures have a significant volume-outcome relationship, and volume per se is hardly the optimal measure because it may lead providers to increase the number of cases done even if the care is unnecessary. It is far better to report risk-adjusted outcomes, but reporting outcomes can be quite complicated and controversial.

Physician education about the volume-outcome association is another option. Few physicians really know about the outcome rates (risk adjusted) of their own patients, let alone the outcomes of the specialists to whom they refer. A better understanding of the volume-outcome relationship may lead them to consider referring their patients to high-volume centers or at least ask about the quality of care of their colleagues. The Leapfrog Group advocates volume-based referral strategies, partially because other methods of improving quality of care are impractical or have other restrictions. For instance, process measures are unclear or controversial, regulatory approaches are unpopular, and health report cards have not been very successful in altering consumer behavior. Others, such as R. Dudley and colleagues, support referral strategies to either mandate or encourage the use of designated hospitals, guide professional training, justify restrictive licensing and certification of referral centers, and take a lead in the diffusion of new services.

Last, some view the volume-outcome relationship as suggesting minimum procedure volumes.

Minimum volume regulations, however, may result in more liberal surgical policies in hospitals that are at the fringe of meeting minimums or may be used as a rationale to preclude entry of competing providers. Insurers may also opt to engage in selective contracting to high-volume hospitals, which could have broader implications for low-volume hospitals because they may lose patients not only in the targeted procedure areas but in others as well.

Regionalizing specialty services is often justified by the volume-outcome relationship. High-volume hospitals, however, may be unable to sufficiently increase capacity to maintain capacity, and low-volume hospitals may suffer from being given a bad reputation, closing related services, or struggling with financial viability. In urban areas with many hospitals capable of offering services, concentrating care may not be problematic. In more sparsely served areas, however, regionalization may imply long travel times, and patients may delay or avoid care. Regionalization may lead to better outcomes for cases that can be scheduled but may actually worsen outcomes for emergencies because of the travel time needed to reach a "capable" site.

In summary, volume-based referral strategies have been advocated for procedures with the greatest outcome differences between low- and high-volume providers and for certain high-risk patient subgroups. Thirty years of research have shown that better outcomes are associated with higher volumes among hospitals and physicians, albeit varying greatly with condition and procedure. Methodological issues, however, are central to better understanding these questions and drawing meaningful policy and clinical implications. The volume-outcome relationship is best seen not as an end in itself but as an intermediate step toward better understanding how to achieve improved patient outcomes.

Harold S. Luft and Beth Newell

See also Health Planning; Health Report Cards; Hospitals; Leapfrog Group; Outcome Movement; Physicians; Quality of Healthcare; Structure-Process-Outcome Quality Measures

Further Readings

Birkmeyer, John D., Andrea E. Siewers, Emily V. A. Finlayson, et al. "Hospital Volume and Surgical Mortality in the United States," *New England Journal of Medicine* 346(15): 1128–37, April 11, 2002.

Dudley, R. Adams, Kirsten L. Johansen, Richard Brand, et al. "Selective Referral to High-Volume Hospitals: Estimating Potentially Avoidable Deaths," *Journal of the American Medical Association* 283(9): 1159–66, March 1, 2000.

Halm, Ethan A., Clara Lee, and Mark R. Chassin. "Is Volume Related to Outcome in Health Care? A Systematic Review and Methodological Critique of the Literature," *Annals of Internal Medicine* 137(6): 511–20, September 17, 2002.

Luft, Harold S., John P. Bunker, and Alain C. Enthoven. "Should Operations Be Regionalized? The Empirical Relation Between Surgical Volume and Mortality," *New England Journal of Medicine* 301(25): 1364–69, December 20, 1979.

Luft, Harold S., Deborah W. Garnick, David H. Mark, et al. *Hospital Volume, Physician Volume, and Patient Outcomes: Assessing the Evidence.* Ann Arbor, MI: Health Administration Press Perspectives, 1990.

Shahian, David M., and Sharon-Lise T. Normand. "The Volume-Outcome Relationship: From Luft to Leapfrog," *Annals of Thoracic Surgery* 75(3): 1048–1058, March 2003.

Web Sites

Agency for Healthcare Research and Quality (AHRQ): http://www.ahrq.gov

American Health Planning Association (AHPA): http://www.ahpanet.org

California Hospital Assessment and Reporting Taskforce (CHART): http://www.calhospitalcompare.org

Joint Commission: http://www.jointcommission.org

VULNERABLE POPULATIONS

Vulnerable populations are groups of people whose health needs are not addressed by conventional service providers. Vulnerable populations can include the very young; the elderly; women; racial minorities; those of low socioeconomic status; those experiencing geographic, lingual, or cultural isolation; limited- or non-English–speaking people, those who are incarcerated; immigrants, refugees, and those with undetermined legal status; transient and homeless people; the uninsured; people with disabilities; people with psychiatric, cognitive, or developmental disorders; substance/alcohol abusers; those who have to deal with abusive families; and people living with HIV/AIDS. This list is not all-inclusive, as society is in a constant state of flux. However, vulnerable populations are usually composed of people who have been marginalized by society. It is because of their inability to access, understand, and/or act on health information or obtain medical treatment that is available to the general population that these populations are considered vulnerable.

The aging process leads to mental, physical, hearing, and vision impairments, as well as a decline in physical mobility. Women are slightly more prone to physical, emotional, or mental limitations than men, and they are nearly twice as likely to require help with personal care as men after age 65. Rural residents are disadvantaged by virtue of having higher rates of reported poor health, physical activity limitations, and remoteness from healthcare than metropolitan residents. Those with transportation challenges include the disabled, the elderly, the poor, and those living in remote areas. Vulnerable populations are more likely to live and work where environmental factors expose them to a higher risk of poor health. Vulnerabilities are often compound, leading to additional unmet needs.

The federal Healthy People 2010 initiative earmarked the elimination of health disparities as second on its list of goals, drawing attention to the stark reality that despite the great strides made in improving population health, a void still exists in providing equitable healthcare to all segments of the nation's population. When compared with their more privileged counterparts, disadvantaged or vulnerable populations have higher prevalence, morbidity, and mortality rates for most conditions. Rising healthcare costs in the 1990s led to increased health disparities and raised political interest in healthcare reform.

The aftermath of Hurricanes Katrina and Rita exposed the disparities faced by vulnerable populations in accessing healthcare and emergency medical relief in times of environmental disasters. It fueled an interest in public health preparedness to avoid such disasters. In 2005, the U.S. Environmental Protection Agency (USEPA) defined *vulnerability* as susceptibility or sensitivity, different exposure, differential preparedness, and/or differential ability to recover. The National Environmental Justice Advisory Council (NEJAC) of 2006 recommended that, to avoid such contingencies in the future, vulnerable populations need to be identified and their environmental and/or public health needs assessed through the use of tools such as the Environmental Justice Geographic Assessment Tool. It recommended greater coordination of all resources, including the vulnerable groups, in planning and implementing new disaster response procedures.

The Office of Minority Health and Health Disparities (OMHD) is responsible for eliminating health disparities and improving the health of all ethnic and racial minority populations, who largely constitute vulnerable populations. Fifteen special programs, administered by the U.S. Department of Agriculture (USDA), cater to the health and nutritional needs of vulnerable populations, especially children, pregnant women, the elderly, rural residents, and the poor. Nearly 20% of Americans use at least one food assistance program per year. About half of all infants and 25% of children between the ages 1 and 4 participate in the Special Supplemental Nutrition Program for Women, Infants, and Children (known as the WIC program), and school nutrition programs provide healthy meals to about 30 million children nationwide. The Food Stamp program assists about 30 million low-income Americans in meeting their nutritional needs.

Vulnerability in Healthcare Research

Vulnerable populations are particularly susceptible to exploitation in healthcare research, exemplified by the horrendous experiments conducted by the Nazis on Jews in concentration camps in World War II. The Nuremberg Code of 1947 was established to prevent such exploitation: It laid down the code of informed consent, whose critical components were that all participants must have adequate knowledge of, and comprehend, the proposed research and must be enrolled without duress. Subsequently, the Belmont Report, the National Research Act, and the National Bioethics Advisory Commission (NABC) have created mandatory rules to protect all segments of society from harmful inclusion in research protocols. Institutional review boards (IRBs) are responsible for ensuring that the tenets of American biomedical ethics—autonomy, nonmaleficence, beneficence, and respect for persons in the research context—are followed in all research protocols. The 2001 NABC report identified six groups as "caution areas" for inclusion in health research: those with institutional, deferential, medical, economic, or social vulnerability and people with communication/cognition problems.

The 2007 *National Healthcare Disparities Report* points out persistent, even increasing, disparities in healthcare among all minority populations, even after accounting for demographic and insurance factors. And nearly half of the nation's population is predicted to consist of "minority groups" by 2050. A large percentage is composed of people who have limited skills in understanding and/or speaking English. The elderly population is expected to rise briskly as longevity increases, bringing in its wake vulnerability to disability, disease, and dependence. The number of uninsured, illegal residents, and refugees continues to increase annually. These factors will add to the number of people considered vulnerable to inequitable healthcare. It is imperative that policymakers consider steps to improve healthcare provision to this growing segment of the nation's population. The use of community-based, culturally and linguistically appropriate, interventions is thought to be the most effective approach in improving the health of vulnerable populations.

*Karen Peters, Benjamin C. Mueller,
Marcela Garces, and Sergio Cristancho*

See also Disability; Epidemiology; Ethnic and Racial Barriers to Healthcare; Health Disparities; Healthy People 2010; National Healthcare Disparities Report (NHDR); Public Health; Risk

Further Readings

Aday, LuAnn. *At Risk in America: The Health and Health Care Needs of Vulnerable Populations in the United States.* 2d ed. San Francisco: Jossey-Bass, 2001.

Agency for Healthcare Research and Quality. *National Healthcare Disparities Report.* Rockville, MD: Agency for Healthcare Research and Quality, 2007.

Burbank, Patricia M., ed. *Vulnerable Older Adults: Health Care Needs and Interventions.* New York: Springer, 2006.

Shi, Leiyu, and Gregory D. Stevens. *Vulnerable Populations in the United States.* San Francisco: Jossey-Bass, 2005.

U.S. Department of Health and Human Services. *Healthy People 2010.* Washington, DC: Office of Disease Prevention and Health Promotion, 2000.

Web Sites

Agency for Healthcare Research and Quality (AHRQ): http://www.ahrq.gov
Healthy People 2010: http://www.healthypeople.gov
Office of Minority Health (OMHD): http://www.cdc.gov/omhd
Robert Wood Johnson Foundation (RWJF): http://www.rwjf.org

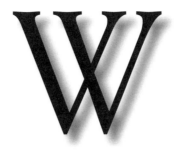

WARE, JOHN E.

John E. Ware, Jr. is a pioneer in the area of quality-of-life assessment and an internationally recognized expert in the field. Ware is noted for being the principal developer of the Short Form 36 (SF-36) Health Survey, one of the most widely used quality-of-life assessment tools in healthcare research. Ware is the founder and president and chief scientific officer of Quality Metric, Inc., an Internet-based healthcare technology company that uses the latest innovations in measurement technology to monitor health outcomes of consumers. Ware is also executive director of the Health Assessment Laboratory and a research professor at the Tufts University School of Medicine.

Ware received his bachelor's and master's degrees in psychology from Pepperdine University in California and completed his doctoral degree in educational measurement and statistics at Southern Illinois University in 1974. While working toward his doctorate, Ware became director of the Measuring Health Concepts Research Project at the University of Southern California School of Medicine and director of the Postgraduate Division in the Department of Psychiatry. In 1972, Ware was appointed assistant professor at the Southern Illinois University School of Medicine, and in 1975, he became a senior research psychologist at the RAND Corporation in the Behavioral Sciences Department and Health Sciences Program. Following this, Ware joined the faculty at Pepperdine University as an instructor and was an

adjunct professor and research advisor for the Clinical Scholars Program at the University of California, Los Angeles, Schools of Medicine and Public Health. In 1988, Ware became senior scientist at the Health Institute at Tufts New England Medical Center in Boston, and eventually, he took on the role of director of the International Quality of Life Assessment Project at Tufts University.

As a result of a research program at the Health Institute of New England Medical Center, the Health Assessment Laboratory was founded in 1988 as a nonprofit organization, located in Waltham, Massachusetts, where Ware is the executive director. The Health Assessment Laboratory conducts basic research on patient-reported outcomes and works in close association with the Health Institute.

Ware was the principal investigator for the Medical Outcomes Study (MOS), which developed the SF-36 Health Survey as well as other widely used health assessment tools. The experience of the SF-36 Health Survey has been cited in nearly 7,500 publications and used in approximately 1,000 clinical studies, and it was judged to be the most widely evaluated patient-assessed health outcome measure.

Ware is a member of many advisory groups, including the Social Security Administration's Disability Evaluation Study, the Joint Commission's Council on Performance Measurement, and the National Committee for Quality Assurance's Technical Advisory Group. He is an elected member of the National Academy of Sciences, Institute of Medicine (IOM). In 2003, he received the

International Society for Quality of Life Research President's Award for his pioneering and tireless work in advancing the ability to assess health-related quality of life.

Ware has made transformative contributions to the field of health related to psychometric theory and improving the measurement of patient outcomes. He is currently developing computer software and Internet applications to assess risk and monitor the health outcomes of patients.

Gregory Vachon

See also Disease; Health; Health Indicators, Leading; Measurement in Health Services Research; Morbidity; Mortality; Quality of Life, Health-Related; Short-Form Health Surveys (SF-36, -12, -8)

Further Readings

McDowell, Ian. *Measuring Health: A Guide to Rating Scales and Questionnaires.* 3d ed. New York: Oxford University Press, 2006.

Ware, John E., Jr. "Improvements in Short-Form Measures of Health Status: Introduction to a Series," *Journal of Clinical Epidemiology* 61(1): 17–33, January 2008.

Web Sites

Quality Metric: http://www.qualitymetric.com

WENNBERG, JOHN E.

John E. Wennberg is a pioneering health services researcher who is perhaps best known for his focus on geographic variations in medical care. He was one of the first researchers to document that geographic variations in medical care, which affect the cost and quality of patient care, are primarily due to physician treatment styles. His work is best exemplified in his major ongoing project, *The Dartmouth Atlas of Health Care.* By attracting the U.S. Congress's attention to outcomes research, Wennberg also helped shape the federal legislation that established the Agency for Health Care Policy and Research (now the Agency for Healthcare Research and Quality [AHRQ]).

Wennberg earned his bachelor's degree from Stanford University (1956) and his medical degree from McGill University (1961). He trained in internal medicine, followed by a fellowship in nephrology, at Johns Hopkins University. While there, he became interested in epidemiology, which led him to earn a master of public health degree from the Johns Hopkins University School of Hygiene and Public Hygiene (1966).

In the early 1970s, Wennberg along with Alan Gittelson developed the methodology of small-area analysis for analyzing healthcare utilization based on population and geographic area. Anecdotally, he was able to refine his research questions on seeking care for his son's tonsillitis: His local Vermont pediatrician recommended tonsillectomy, while the one in a neighboring town across the state border into New Hampshire counseled "watchful waiting." Wennberg was puzzled why medical practice could vary so dramatically over such a short distance. When he compared data on other medical procedures in other locales, other startling differences emerged: Not only does medical intervention and thus spending vary by region, but Wennberg's analyses also showed that different hospitals within the same region often have drastically different healthcare utilization patterns. Most strikingly, what at first seemed heretical has now been well accepted: More medical spending and more healthcare services are not associated with better patient outcomes.

Wennberg has been a professor in the Department of Community and Family Medicine at Dartmouth University since 1980 and in the Department of Medicine since 1989. In 1988, he became the founding director of the Center for the Evaluative Clinical Sciences, now called the Dartmouth Institute for Health Policy and Clinical Practice. In 1989, Wennberg cofounded the Foundation for Informed Medical Decision Making, based on the idea that a better-educated patient will have a safer and more positive experience in the healthcare system when engaged in shared decision making with his or her physician. In 1994, he became the Peggy Y. Thomson Professor of the Evaluative Clinical Sciences, the nation's first endowed chair in clinical evaluative sciences, the field he created. In 1996, Wennberg published the inaugural *Dartmouth Atlas of Health Care.* Updated every 2 years, the *Atlas* is a compendium of color-coded thematic maps dividing the United States into geographic regions based on relative rates of health service utilization in a given time period.

During his distinguished career, Wennberg has received many awards and honors in recognition of his work. He is an elected member of the national Institute of Medicine (IOM). He has received the Association for Health Services Research's Distinguished Investigator Award, the Baxter Foundation's Health Services Research Prize, the Richard and Hinda Rosenthal Foundation Award in Clinical Medicine, and the Picker Institute Award for Career Achievement in Patient-Centered Care. In 2007, he was named the most influential health policy researcher of the past 25 years by the journal *Health Affairs*, and he received the Joint Commission's Ernest Amory Codman Award for his leadership in using outcome measures to improve healthcare quality.

John Henning Schumann

See also Agency for Healthcare Research and Quality (AHRQ); Epidemiology; Geographic Barriers to Healthcare; Geographic Information Systems (GIS); Geographic Variations in Healthcare; Outcomes Movement; Public Health; Quality of Healthcare

Further Readings

Wennberg, John E. "On the Appropriateness of Small-Area Analysis for Cost Containment," *Health Affairs* 15(4): 164–67, Winter 1996.

Wennberg, John E. *The Dartmouth Atlas of Health Care in the United States*. Chicago: American Hospital Association, 1998.

Wennberg, John E. *Variation in Use of Medicare Services Among Regions and Selected Academic Medical Centers: Is More Better?* Pub. No. 874. New York: Commonwealth Fund, 2005.

Wennberg, J. E., and Elliott S. Fisher, eds. *The Care of Patients With Severe Chronic Illness: A Report on the Medicare Program by the Dartmouth Atlas Project*. Hanover, NH: Center for the Evaluative Clinical Sciences, Dartmouth Atlas Project, 2006.

Wennberg, John E., and Alan Gittelsohn. "Small Area Variations in Health Care Delivery: A Population-Based Health Information System Can Guide Planning and Regulatory Decision-Making," *Science* 182(4117): 1102–1108, 1973.

Web Sites

Dartmouth Atlas of Health Care: http://www.dartmouthatlas.org
Dartmouth Institute for Health Policy and Clinical Practice: http://www.dartmouth.edu/~cecs

WHITE, KERR L.

Kerr L. White is arguably the founder of the discipline of health services research in the United States. Throughout his long and distinguished career as a researcher, university professor, and government and foundation administrator, he developed the conceptual framework of health services research, established and shaped government health services research programs, and funded the emerging discipline of health services research.

White was born in Winnipeg in 1917, and he grew up in Ottawa, Canada. His father was a foreign correspondent for the London *Times* and the *Economist,* and his mother operated a lending library that emphasized various medical topics. He majored in economics and political science at McGill University, followed by graduate study in economics at Yale University. During World War II, he interrupted his graduate studies to serve in the Royal Canadian Army. After the war, he undertook medical training at McGill University, graduating in 1949. White completed his residency in internal medicine at Dartmouth College's Hitchcock Clinic and Hospital and a fellowship at McGill's Royal Victoria Hospital in the departments of medicine and psychiatry. He then joined the Department of Internal Medicine at the University of North Carolina–Chapel Hill as an assistant professor of medicine and preventive medicine. In 1962, White was appointed chair of the Department of Epidemiology and Community Medicine at the University of Vermont. In 1965, he moved to Johns Hopkins University to establish the Division of Hospitals and Medical Care, which later became the Department of Health Care Organization. In 1978, he became the deputy director for health sciences at the Rockefeller Foundation. White retired in 1984, remaining active in the health research community as a thought leader and as a mentor.

White's professional legacy can be divided into three domains: (1) scholarship, which defined the field of health services research; (2) training and mentoring leaders in this new field; and (3) the development of programs and other initiatives that have a sustained impact on the research on healthcare quality and the delivery of quality medical care.

While he was a 2nd-year medical student in 1947, White published his first article, which predicted many of the methodological and substantive domains of health services research and their relation to what would eventually be known as evidence-based medicine. At the University of North Carolina, White formulated the key ideas, which he expounded in 1961 in a seminal *New England Journal of Medicine* article that he coauthored, "The Ecology of Medical Care." White stressed, in addition to the appropriate use of methodological tools to conduct health care research, that society has an obligation to allocate healthcare resources as efficiently and effectively as possible to improve the quality of medical outcomes, benefiting both patients and providers. Moreover, he stressed that healthcare research was concerned with medicine as a social institution. White has authored or coauthored some 250 publications, including 11 books.

White proved instrumental in institutionalizing health services research, both through his editorial influence in journals such as *Medical Care* and *Health Services Research* and ensuring funding for the *International Journal of Health Services*, and through his vision in developing the organizational framework for the National Center for Health Services Research (NCHSR), which eventually became a federal agency and in 1999 was reauthorized as the Agency for Healthcare Research and Quality (AHRQ).

In recognition of White's role in establishing the field of health services research, Emory University dedicated a new center, the Kerr L. White Institute for Health Services Research, in his honor in 1996, and the Agency for Healthcare Research and Quality (AHRQ) established the Kerr White Visiting Scholars Program in 2000.

David J. Ballard and Robert S. Hopkins, III

See also Agency for Healthcare Research and Quality (AHRQ); Brook, Robert H.; Epidemiology; Evidence-Based Medicine (EBM); Health; Health Services Research, Origins; Public Health; Wennberg, John E.

Further Readings

Brook, Robert H. "Having a Foot in Both Camps: The Impact of Kerr White's Vision," *Health Services Research* 32(1): 32–6, April 1997.

Haritos, Rosa, and Thomas R. Konrad. "A Timely Partnership: Sociology and Health Services Research," *Contemporary Sociology* 28(5): 529–36, September 1999.

White, Kerr L. "Recent Advances in the Science of Health," *McGill Medical Journal* 16(3): 359–89, 1947.

White, Kerr L. "Health Care Research: Old Wine in New Bottles," *Pharos of Alpha Omega Alpha* 56: 12–16, Summer 1993.

White, Kerr L. "The Ecology of Medical Care: Origins and Implications for Population-Based Healthcare Research," *Health Services Research* 32(1): 11–21, April 1997.

White, Kerr L., Julio Frenk, Cosme Ordonez, et al., eds. *Health Services Research: An Anthology.* Washington, DC: Pan American Health Organization, 1992.

White, Kerr L., T. Franklin Williams, and Bernard G. Greenberg. "The Ecology of Medical Care," *New England Journal of Medicine* 265: 885–92, November 2,1961.

Williamson, John W. "A Personal Tribute to Kerr L. White, M.D., My Career Mentor, Colleague, and Friend," *Health Services Research* 32(1): 22–31, April 1997.

Web Sites

University of Virginia, Kerr White Healthcare Collection: http://historical.hsl.virginia.edu/Kerr

WILENSKY, GAIL R.

Gail R. Wilensky is a well-known and highly respected health economist. She has been associated with Project HOPE (Health Opportunities for People Everywhere) for many years, she was the administrator of the Health Care Financing Administration (HCFA), and she serves on many important national and international healthcare committees.

Born in 1943 in Detroit, Michigan, Wilensky attended the University of Michigan, where she earned a bachelor's degree in psychology (1964), a master's degree (1965), and a doctoral degree in economics (1968).

After graduation, Wilensky served as a staff economist on the President's Commission on Income Maintenance Programs until 1969, when she became executive director of the Maryland Council of Economic Advisers. In 1971, she served as a senior research associate at the Urban Institute until 1973, when she accepted the position of visiting assistant professor and associate research scientist at the University of Michigan. In 1975, she worked for the National Center for Health Services Research (now the Agency for Healthcare Research and Quality), where she was a health service fellow and senior research manager. In 1983, she joined Project HOPE as vice president of health affairs. In 1990, President George H. W. Bush appointed her administrator of the Health Care Financing Administration (HFMA) (now the Centers for Medicare and Medicaid Services [CMS]). In 1992, she became deputy assistant to the President for policy development at the White House. She returned to Project HOPE in 1993 as the John M. Olin Senior Fellow, where she continues to analyze and develop healthcare policies, advise government and private-sector agencies, and write and lecture on various healthcare topics.

Wilensky has served on a number of important healthcare committees, including the Advisory Committee on Health of the General Accounting Office (GAO), the Physician Payment Review Commission (PPRC), the Medicare Payment Advisory Commission (MedPAC), and the President's Task Force to Improve Health Care Delivery for Our Nation's Veterans. She also has served on many committees of the National Academy of Sciences, Institute of Medicine (IOM).

Currently, she serves as a member of the President's Commission on Care for America's Returning Wounded Warriors; Commissioner of the World Health Organization (WHO) Commission on Social Determinants of Health; vice chair of the Maryland Health Care Commission; member of the Board of Trustees of the University of the Sciences in Philadelphia; member of the National Campaign to Prevent Teen Pregnancy; director of the American Heart Association; trustee of the National Mineworkers of America's Combined Benefits Fund; trustee of the National Opinion Research Center (NORC) at the University of Chicago; director, chair, and vice chair of AcademyHealth; cochair of the Task Force on the Future Health Care at the U.S. Department of Defense; and member of the board of directors for Cephalon Corporation.

Wilensky has received numerous awards and honors, including the Darrel J. Mase Distinguished Leadership Award from the University of Florida (2000), the Latiolais Honor Medal from the American Managed Care Pharmacy Association (1996), the Dean Conley Award from the American College of Healthcare Executives (1989), and the Alumna in Residence Award from the University of Michigan (1989). She has received honorary degrees from the University of the Sciences (2002), Rush University (1997), and Hahnemann University (1993). She was named Marshall J. Seidman Lecturer at Harvard Medical School (2003), John D. Thompson Distinguished Visiting Fellow at the Yale Health Management Program (2003), TeKolste Scholar at the Indiana Hospital and Health Association (1997), and Flinn Foundation Distinguished Scholar in Health Policy and Management (1986). Additionally, Wilensky is listed in *Who's Who in America* and *Who's Who in American Women*. She was named as one of the 100 most powerful people in healthcare in 2003 and 2004, and in 2005, she was named as one of the top 25 women in healthcare by *Modern Healthcare*.

Amie Lulinski Norris

See also Centers for Medicare and Medicaid Services (CMS); Health Economics; Medicaid; Medicare; Project HOPE; Public Policy

Further Readings

Wilensky, Gail R. "Consumer-Driven Health Plans: Early Evidence and Potential Impact on Hospitals," *Health Affairs* 25(1): 174–85, January–February 2006.

Wilensky, Gail R. "Developing a Center for Comparative Effectiveness Information," *Health Affairs* 25(6): 572–85, November–December 2006.

Wilensky, Gail R. "Implementing the Medicare Drug Benefit: The First 90 Days," *Healthcare Financial Management* 60(6): 42–3, June 2006.

Wilensky, Gail R. "Pay for Performance and Physicians: An Open Question," *Healthcare Financial Management* 61(2): 40, 42, February 2007.

Wilensky, Gail R., Nicholas Wolter, and Michelle M. Fischer. "Gain Sharing: A Good Concept Getting a Bad Name?" *Health Affairs* 26(1): 58–67, January–February 2007.

Web Sites

Project HOPE: http://www.projecthope.org

WILLIAMS, ALAN H.

Alan H. Williams (1927–2005) was an eminent health economist in the United Kingdom. Williams was a professor of economics at the University of York. At York, he was instrumental in establishing the university's Centre for Health Economics and its graduate program in health economics. During his long and distinguished career, he studied two broad research areas: ways of valuing health and the equity of health and healthcare. Williams is perhaps best known as the originator of the concept of quality-adjusted life years, or QALYs, a measure of health benefits. Today, QALYs are widely used by researchers to measure and compare healthcare technology and treatments.

Williams was born in Birmingham, England, in 1927. He was educated at the Birmingham King Edward's School. After graduation in 1945, he served in the Royal Air Force for 3 years. In 1948, Williams attended the University of Birmingham, where he graduated in 1951 with a bachelor's degree in economics. He continued his education doing graduate work at the Universities of Uppsala and Stockholm. From 1954 to 1963, Williams was a lecturer in economics at the University of Exeter, where he taught courses in public finance. During sabbaticals he taught at the Massachusetts Institute of Technology (MIT) and Princeton University. In 1964, he moved to the newly established University of York, where he was appointed a senior lecturer and reader in economics. Williams would teach and conduct research at that university for more than 40 years.

Besides his academic career, Williams also worked occasionally for the government. From 1966 to 1968, he was seconded (a temporary move or loan of an employee to another organization) to Her Majesty's Treasury as the director of economic studies. At the Treasury, he developed courses in economics for civil servants. He also worked with the Ministry of Health, where he investigated its hospital building program. In 1976, Williams was appointed to the Royal Commission on the National Health Service (NHS). However, in 1978, he resigned over a dispute on the role of researchers working for the commission.

In 1987, Williams convened a meeting in Rotterdam, The Netherlands, of his colleagues and challenged them to determine how the value of health might be measured and how such values might be studied across nations. The group eventually became the EuroQol Group, which developed the EQ-5D, a series of health status measures that are widely used throughout the world.

In his later years, Williams became increasingly interested in the ethical issues determining priorities in healthcare. He expounded the concept of "fair innings." The concept reflects the general belief that everyone should achieve a long life and that if someone dies at a young age, the person is somehow cheated—death at 20 is clearly viewed very differently from death at 80. Williams argued that entitlement to healthcare ought to take into account such differences in perspectives. And more resources should be given to the young who have not had their fair innings.

Williams died in 2005 at the age of 77. In 2006, the University of York's Centre for Health Economics established the Alan Williams Health Economics Fellowships as a lasting tribute to his work and achievements.

Ross M. Mullner

See also Health Economics; Public Policy; Quality-Adjusted Life Years (QALYs); Rationing Healthcare; Technology Assessment; United Kingdom's National Health Service (NHS); United Kingdom's National Institute for Health and Clinical Excellence (NICE)

Further Readings

Culyer, A. J., and Alan Maynard, eds. *Being Reasonable About the Economics of Health: Selected Essays by Alan Williams.* Cheltenham, UK: Edward Elgar, 1997.

Mason, Anne, and Adrian Towse, eds. *The Ideas and Influence of Alan Williams: Be Reasonable: Do It My Way!* Abingdon, UK: Radcliffe, 2008.

Williams, Alan. "Health Economics: The End of Clinical Freedom?" *British Medical Journal* 297(6654): 1183–86, 1988.

Williams, Alan, and Richard Cookson. "Equity in Health." In *Handbook of Health Economics*, Vol. 1A, edited by A. J. Culyer and J. P. Newhouse, 1863–1910. New York: North-Holland, 2000.

Web Sites

EuroQoL Group: http://www.euroqol.org

United Kingdom's National Institute for Health and Clinical Excellence (NICE): http://www.nice.org.uk

University of York, Centre for Health Economics (CHE): http://www.york.ac.uk/inst/che

WOMEN'S HEALTH ISSUES

Women are often the healthcare takers and decision makers of their family's health. During the past several decades, women's health issues have broadened from a focus primarily on reproductive and social issues to include research on gender differences in disease prevention and response to treatment. Although many advances have been made in improving women's healthcare and in understanding women's unique role in the healthcare system, there are significant gaps in areas such as access to healthcare, ability to pay for care, and healthcare outcomes. Several key issues for women's health remain, including the need for further studies, changes in public policy, and increased advocacy.

Health Maintenance

There is overwhelming evidence that preventive healthcare services, particularly among women, favorably affect health outcomes. However, many women often underuse the preventive services. Screening tests are an important tool for the early detection and treatment of various diseases, yet the use of some screening tests by women is declining. A national survey conducted by the Kaiser Family Foundation in 2004 indicates that screening rates for mammograms, pap smears, and blood pressure have decreased slightly since 2001.

Additionally, reproductive care is a significant part of healthcare for women. One of the goals of the Healthy People 2010 initiative of the U.S. Department of Health and Human Services (HHS) is to increase the proportion of pregnant women who receive early and adequate prenatal care to 90% of all pregnancies in the nation. While there has been an overall steady improvement, statistics show a slower rate of increase among minority women, particularly in obtaining early prenatal care.

Being overweight or obese increases adverse health risks, including high blood pressure, diabetes, heart disease, stroke, arthritis, cancer, and poor reproductive health. According to the Centers for Disease Control and Prevention (CDC), 61.5% of all women and 69.6% of men in the nation were overweight or obese in 2003–2004. Furthermore, regular physical activity has been shown to promote health, prevent disease, and facilitate maintenance of a healthy body weight. In 2005, only 50.9% of women reported engaging in at least 10 minutes of moderate leisure-time physical activity per week, and only 32.0% reported at least 10 minutes of vigorous activity, which was significantly less than that reported by men. In contrast, smoking was less common among women 12 years of age or older (22.5%) compared with men of the same age group (27.4%). In addition, women were more likely than men to try to quit smoking (44.8% vs. 40.7%).

Access to Healthcare

Access to quality healthcare services directly affects many aspects of women's health. Numerous studies have found that women who have a usual source of healthcare are more likely to receive preventive care, to have access to care, to receive continuous care, and to have lower rates of hospitalization and lower healthcare costs than those who do not have a usual source of care. Women of all racial and ethnic groups are more likely than men to have a usual source of care. However, access to healthcare is a greater challenge for women who are members of racial or ethnic minority groups with low incomes and who are uninsured. Regardless of family structure, women are more likely than men to live in poverty. Uninsured women consistently fare worse on multiple measures of access to care, including contact with providers, obtaining timely care, access to specialists, and utilization of screen tests.

Many studies have also shown that women who lack economic resources or are from racial or ethnic minorities are more likely to report poor health status and greater chronic health problems and are more likely to confront obstacles to receiving adequate and timely care. Women not only have financial barriers to accessing healthcare but also may experience logistical barriers, such as problems with transportation, childcare, and lack of free time. Among women with family incomes at 300% or more above the federal poverty level (FPL), 73% reported excellent or very good health status compared with 42% of those with family incomes below 100% of the FPL. Women who are Latinas, of low economic status, single, and young are particularly at risk of being uninsured.

Healthcare Costs

There is a significant gender gap in health insurance coverage and the ability to afford medical care in the United States. Women are disadvantaged by greater healthcare needs and lower incomes than men. Men are more likely than women to be uninsured in every age group; however, there are an estimated 16 million uninsured women in the nation. Many studies have shown that women are more likely than men to go without healthcare services because of the costs of healthcare and also because they have higher out-of-pocket expenses. A 2005 survey by the Kaiser Family Foundation indicates that 33% of insured women and 68% of uninsured women do not get the healthcare they need because they cannot afford it as opposed to 23% of insured and 49% of uninsured men who avoid care because of the costs. Researchers also found that 16% of women are underinsured, meaning they have high out-of-pocket costs compared with their income, while only 9% of men are underinsured. Among workers, women are less likely than men to be eligible for and to participate in their employer's health insurance plans. The overall take-up rate for employer-sponsored coverage is 80% for women workers compared with 89% for men. This is in part because women are more likely to work part-time, have lower incomes, and rely more on spousal coverage.

Uninsured women are more likely to suffer serious health problems, partly because they tend to wait too long to seek treatment or preventive care. The lack of health insurance can even be deadly, as research has shown that uninsured adults are more likely to die earlier than those who have insurance. According to the Kaiser Family Foundation survey, in 2004, one in six women nationwide who had health insurance delayed or went without needed care. Reproductive healthcare services accounted for much of this discrepancy. Thirty-nine percent of women with insurance reported difficulty paying their medical bills compared with 29% of men. The gender gap in healthcare insurance coverage and access to care has other contributing factors: For instance, women are more likely to purchase coverage in the more expensive and less comprehensive individual health insurance market and are more likely than men to take prescription drugs.

Quality of Healthcare

The report *Making the Grade for Women's Health: A National and State-by-State Report Card*, published in 2007 by the National Women's Law Center, on the status of women's healthcare in the United States, based on the goals set by Healthy People 2010, gave the nation an overall grade of "unsatisfactory" because it met only 3 of the 23 benchmarks for women's health. The report found that no state met the goal for access to health insurance. Additionally, the report highlighted the many regional differences in the health status of women. In 2005, fewer women were satisfied with how well their physicians communicated with them (81.0%), compared with men (84.3%). Men were also more likely than women (67.0% vs. 62.5%) to be satisfied with their ability to get necessary care from physicians or specialists, including obtaining treatments and tests.

Cardiovascular disease is the leading cause of death for women in the United States. Despite advances in the evaluation and management of heart disease, it is estimated that more than 240,000 women die annually from this condition. In 2005, adult women below 45 years of age had a higher rate of heart disease than men of the same age (50.9 vs. 35.2 per 1,000 adults, respectively), but men had a higher overall rate of heart disease than women. The highest rate of heart disease was among non-Hispanic White women (128.7 per

1,000), followed by non-Hispanic Black women (107.1 per 1,000). Asian women had the lowest rate (51.1 per 1,000) of heart disease among all ethnic groups. Although non-Hispanic White women experience the highest rates of heart disease, deaths from heart disease are highest among non-Hispanic Black women.

According to the Kaiser Family Foundation survey of 2005, women largely underused preventive healthcare measures, such as lifestyle modifications. Although major risk factors for heart disease can often be prevented or controlled through lifestyle changes, physicians are less likely to counsel women than men about diet, exercise, and weight reduction.

In 2004, the American Heart Association (AHA) released the first evidence-based guidelines for cardiovascular disease prevention for women. Embedded in its recommendations are lifestyle interventions that have become the cornerstone of many preventive programs. The current prevention efforts have shifted away from individual disease-specific targets to assessment of "global," or overall, risk. The lifestyle interventions have received the highest level of recommendation from the AHA (Class 1) and include the following: (a) encouraging cessation of cigarette smoking; (b) encouraging daily physical activity for a minimum of 30 minutes at moderate intensity; (c) consumption of a heart-healthy diet—restriction of intake of trans-fatty acids and saturated fat to less than 10% of calories; and (d) weight maintenance/reduction with a target body mass index (BMI) between 18.5 and 24.9 kg/m^2 and a waist circumference of less than 35 inches.

Cancer is the second leading cause of death of women in the United States. Furthermore, the most common cause of cancer deaths in women is lung cancer. It is estimated that more than 70,000 women in the nation die of lung cancer each year, with the majority of these deaths linked to cigarette smoking. Breast cancer is the second leading cause of cancer death in U.S. women, resulting in nearly 40,000 deaths each year, but it is the most common type of cancer among women. For each of the sex-specific cancers, such as breast, uterine, and ovarian cancer, survival rates are higher for White women than for Black women.

Stroke is a major cause of morbidity and mortality and the third leading cause of death of women in the United States. Nearly 160,000 people in the country die of stroke each year, and almost two thirds of them are women. There are important racial and ethnic disparities in the incidence, severity, and mortality of stroke. Minority ethnic groups have higher rates of more severe strokes. In addition to the roles of primary and secondary prevention, it has been suggested that to address these disparities in stroke outcomes, initiatives that foster cultural competence must be a prominent component of a targeted approach. Primary prevention of stroke includes adequate blood pressure control and the reduction and treatment of elevated cholesterol.

In 2005, the CDC estimated there were 10,774 new cases of AIDS in the United States among adolescent and adult women, compared with 29,766 new cases among males of the same age group. AIDS has disproportionately affected men, but the rate among women is increasing at a faster pace. Since 2001, new AIDS cases have increased by 7.2% among women compared with a 6.7% increase among men. Women are biologically more susceptible to HIV infection during sexual intercourse and experience different clinical symptoms and complications. Many studies have shown that women with HIV not only face limited access to care but also experience disparities in access compared with men. Women with HIV are less likely to receive combination drug therapy and fare more poorly on other access measures than men. Compared with men, women with HIV are more likely to postpone care because of lack of transportation and more likely to be too sick to go to the physician.

Minority women also are disproportionately affected by a number of diseases and health conditions, including HIV/AIDS, sexually transmitted infections, diabetes, and overweight or obesity. In 2004, HIV/AIDS was the leading cause of death among non-Hispanic Black women 25 to 34 years of age.

Mental health is an often overlooked but critical aspect of women's healthcare. One of the biggest threats to a woman's overall health is impairment of her mental health. Studies have shown a positive relationship between the frequency and severity of negative social factors and occurrences and the frequency and severity of mental health problems experienced by women.

Despite the increasing prevalence of mental illness among both men and women, there are remarkable gender differences in patterns of mental illness. Slightly less than a quarter of women (23%) in the nation report having been diagnosed with depression or anxiety, over twice the rate of men (11%). Women attempt suicide three times more often than men, but men are much more likely to be successful in taking their lives. Risk factors for the more common mental disorders include the following: gender-based violence, socioeconomic factors, low income and income inequality, inferior social standing, and unalleviated responsibility for the welfare of others. Women now have the highest rates of post-traumatic stress disorders, a direct result of the increasing prevalence of sexual violence against women. The lifetime prevalence rate of violence against women ranges from 16% to 50%.

Healthcare Utilization and Outcomes

Over the course of a woman's life, her use of the healthcare system mirrors her changing healthcare needs, from reproductive health in the younger years to a surfacing of chronic illness during middle age and increased rates of physical limitations with advanced age. Most women in the nation are in good health, with 8 in 10 reporting excellent, very good, or good health, according to a 2005 Kaiser Family Foundation survey. There are, however, racial and ethnic disparities in these statistics. In 2005, 62.3% of non-Hispanic White women reported themselves to be in excellent or very good health, compared with only 53.6% of Hispanic women and 51.6% of non-Hispanic Black women. Men were more likely than women to report being in excellent or very good health (63.0% vs. 59.9%), and this result holds across every racial and ethnic group. However, a considerable number of women—nearly 20%—are in fair or poor health. The proportion of women reporting that they are in fair to poor health increases with age to nearly one third of women 65 years of age or older. Slightly more than a third of women reported a chronic condition requiring ongoing medical attention compared with 30% of men. As women age, there is an associated increase in the incidence of chronic conditions.

Medical outcomes research has determined that women are disproportionately affected by chronic diseases for which clinical data are not easily generalized and traditional medical measures are inadequate. Historically, women have faced unequal treatment, with numerous studies reporting that women on average have fewer medical interventions than their male counterparts. There is evidence in the medical outcomes literature to suggest increasing ethnic disparities in incidence, severity, and mortality for a number of prevalent diseases. In the past decade, there has been a move from defining outcomes using traditional measures of morbidity and mortality to a greater emphasis on quality of life, function, patient satisfaction, and health status. The use of gender-sensitive outcome measures is essential to bridge the discrepancy between quality initiatives at the global level and what actually works at the grassroots level for improving women's healthcare. Such a shift is empowering for women and should translate into comparable health outcomes between men and women in the future.

Future Implications

It is important to understand the current issues concerning women's health and the unique role women play not only as consumers of healthcare but also as leaders in their families in healthcare decision making, as these have salient implications for public health and public policy advocacy. Significant strides have been made in recent decades in understanding not only the physiological but also the sociological health issues faced by women. Despite these advances, however, there is more work to be done in reducing the gender gap in access to healthcare, ability to pay for care, and quality of healthcare outcomes.

Valerie A. Dobiesz and Heather M. Prendergast

See also Access to Healthcare; Acute and Chronic Diseases; Health Disparities; Life Expectancy; Obesity; Quality of Healthcare; Uninsured Individuals; Vulnerable Populations

Further Readings

American College of Obstetricians and Gynecologists. *Special Issues in Women's Health*. Washington, DC: American College of Obstetricians and Gynecologists, 2005.

Berlin, Michelle. *Making the Grade on Women's Health: A National and State-by-State Report Card.* 4th ed. Washington, DC: National Women's Law Center, 2007.

Clouse, Amy L., and Katherine Sherif, eds. *Women's Health in Clinical Practice: A Handbook for Primary Care.* Totowa, NJ: Humana Press, 2008.

Collins, Catherine Fisher, ed. *African American Women's Health and Social Issues.* 2d ed. Westport, CT: Praeger, 2006.

Elit, Laurie, and Jean Chamberlain Froese, eds. *Women's Health in the Majority World: Issues and Initiatives.* New York: Nova Science, 2007.

Kolander, Cheryl A., Danny Ramsey Ballard, and Cynthia K. Chandler. *Contemporary Women's Health: Issues for Today and the Future.* 3d ed. New York: McGraw-Hill, 2007.

National Women's Law Center. *Making the Grade for Women's Health: A National and State-by-State Report Card.* Washington, DC: National Women's Law Center, 2007.

Worcester, Nancy, and Marianne H. Whatley, eds. *Women's Health: Readings in Social, Economic, and Political Issues.* 3d ed. Dubuque, IA: Kendall 2000.

Web Sites

Agency for Healthcare Research and Quality (AHRQ): http://www.ahrq.gov

Henry J. Kaiser Family Foundation (KFF): http://www.kff.org

National Institutes of Health (NIH), Office of Research on Women's Health (ORWH): http://orwh.od.nih.gov

National Women's Law Center (NWLC): http://www.nwlc.org

U.S. Department of Health and Human Services (HHS), National Women's Health Information Center: http://www.hrsa.gov/WomensHealth

U.S. Food and Drug Administration (FDA), Office of Women's Health: http://www.fda.gov/womens

WORLD HEALTH ORGANIZATION (WHO)

The World Health Organization (WHO) is the directing and coordinating authority for health within the United Nations (UN). The WHO was officially constituted at the International Health Conference held in New York City from June 19 to July 22, 1946. WHO began operating on April 7, 1948.

The WHO is an intergovernmental organization (IGO), and its members are the states (countries) recognized by the UN. The 193 member states of the UN pay regulated contribution fees, which partially fund the WHO. In addition, many member states also pay voluntary contributions to fund regular or extrabudgetary programs. Member states also contribute technical expertise either through personnel quotas or through work carried out by national collaborating centers or experts who take active roles in research and technical or advisory committees and extrabudgetary activities.

The total biennial budget for the WHO in 2006–2007 was approximately $3.3 billion. Those funds were allocated into four major areas: (1) about half of the funds (53%) are spent on essential health interventions (i.e., HIV/AIDS prevention and treatment, child and adolescent health, communicable disease prevention and control, malaria control and prevention, mental health and substance abuse programs, reproductive health, tuberculosis control and prevention, and emergency and epidemic preparedness programs); (2) about one fifth of the funds (21%) are spent on effective support for member states (i.e., WHO's core presence in countries, direction, external relations, governing bodies, planning resource and coordination, knowledge, budget and financial management, and infrastructure and logistics); (3) about 1/10 of the funds (13%) are spent on health policies, systems, and products (i.e., health financing and social protection, health information, evidence and research policy, essential health technologies, health systems policies and service delivery, human resources for health, policy making for health, and essential medicines); and (4) about 1/10 of the funds (11%) are spent on the determinants of health (i.e., food safety, women and health, health and environment, health promotion, nutrition, violence prevention, injuries and disabilities, and communicable disease research).

Through its globally recognized functions, the WHO provides leadership on health matters worldwide, and it sets norms and standards on health issues. The WHO's organizational structure allows it to perform a major global role in shaping a health research agenda, articulating evidence-based policy options, and channeling technical support to countries, as well as monitoring and assessing global health trends.

In the 21st century, the WHO performs a critical role in an effort to ensure that health becomes a genuinely shared responsibility, involving equitable access to essential healthcare and a collective defense against transnational threats to health. Traditionally, the WHO's collective knowledge expressed through officially supported research results has been the reference base for member states to establish regulatory measures.

The Concept of Health

In conformity with the Charter of the United Nations, the WHO constitution proposes that to attain basic happiness, harmonious relations, and security for all people in the world, the principles that determine health are essential. Thus, for the WHO, health is a state of complete physical, mental, and social well-being and not merely the absence of disease or infirmity.

Furthermore, WHO constituents affirm that the accomplishment of the highest possible standard of health is one of the fundamental rights of every human being regardless of race, religion, political belief, and economic or social condition. In addition, the health of all people is fundamental to the attainment of peace and security and depends on the fullest cooperation of individuals and countries. The WHO constitution states that the achievement of any country in the promotion and protection of health is of value to all and that unequal development in different countries in the promotion of health and control of disease, especially communicable disease, is a danger for all.

The WHO constituents also affirm that the healthy development of the child is of basic importance and that people's ability to live harmoniously in a changing total environment is essential to such development.

In addition, they affirm that the benefits of medical, psychological, and related knowledge are essential for the fullest attainment of health, but only if extended to all people, and that informed opinion and active cooperation on the part of the public are of utmost importance in the improvement of the health of the people.

The WHO constitution concludes that countries have a responsibility for the health of their people, which can be fulfilled only by the provision of adequate health and social measures. All countries that become members of the WHO accept these principles for the purpose of cooperation among themselves and with others to promote and protect the health of all peoples.

World Health Assembly

All member states are represented in the World Health Assembly. Each member has one vote but may send three delegates. According to the WHO constitution, the delegates are to be chosen for their technical competence and preferably should represent national health administrations. Delegations may include alternates and advisers. The assembly meets annually, usually in May, for approximately 3 weeks. Most assemblies are held at WHO's headquarters in Geneva, Switzerland.

The World Health Assembly determines the policies of the organization and deals with budgetary and administrative questions. By a two-third vote, the assembly may adopt conventions or agreements. While these are not binding on member governments until accepted by them, the member state must take action leading to their acceptance within 18 months of their adoption, even if its delegation voted against a convention in the assembly, by submitting the convention to its legislature for ratification, and it must notify the WHO of the action taken. If the action is unsuccessful, it must notify the WHO of the reasons for nonacceptance.

In addition, the assembly has quasi-legislative powers to adopt regulations on important technical matters specified in the WHO constitution. Once the assembly adopts a regulation, it applies to all WHO member countries (including those whose delegates voted against it, except those whose governments specifically notify WHO that they reject the regulation or accept it only with certain reservations).

The WHO is empowered to introduce uniform technical regulations on the following matters: (a) sanitary and quarantine requirements and other procedures designed to prevent international epidemics; nomenclature with respect to disease, causes of death, and public health practices; (b) standards with respect to diagnostic procedures for international use; (c) standards with respect to the safety, purity, and potency of biological, pharmaceutical, and similar products in international commerce; and (d) advertising and labeling of biological, pharmaceutical, and similar products in international commerce.

Current Role

Currently, the WHO fulfils its objectives through its core functions, which are (a) providing leadership on matters critical to health and engaging in partnerships where joint action is needed; (b) shaping the research agenda and stimulating the generation, translation, and dissemination of valuable knowledge; (c) setting norms and standards and promoting and monitoring their implementation; articulating ethical and evidence-based policy options; (d) providing technical support, catalyzing change, and building sustainable institutional capacity; and (e) monitoring the health situation and assessing health trends.

These core functions are set out in the 11th General Programme of Work, which provides the framework for the organization-wide program of work, its budget, resources, and results. Titled *Engaging for Health,* it covers the 10-year time period 2006–2015.

Scientific Conferences and the World Health Assembly

The WHO supports or sponsors numerous scientific conferences throughout the world. Each year, the World Health Assembly also sponsors a scientific conference on a specific topic of worldwide health interest. Discussions at this conference are held in addition to assembly business. They enable the delegates, who as a rule are top-ranking public health experts, to discuss common problems more thoroughly than formal committee debates would permit. Governments are asked to contribute special working papers and studies to these discussions and, if practicable, to send experts on the matters that are discussed.

Executive Board

The World Health Assembly may elect any 32 member countries to participate in the Executive Board for 3-year terms as long as the representation complies with equitable geographic distribution. Each of the elected countries must designate one person "technically qualified in the field of health" as a member of the Executive Board. The countries are elected by rotation, one third of the membership being replaced every year, and members may succeed themselves. Board members serve as individuals and not as representatives of their governments.

The Executive Board meets twice a year for sessions of a few days to several weeks, but the board may convene a special meeting at any time. One of the board's functions is to prepare the agenda for the World Health Assembly. The WHO constitution authorizes the board to take emergency measures within the functions and financial resources of the organization in order to deal with events requiring immediate action. In particular, it may authorize the Director-General to take the necessary steps to combat epidemics and to participate in the organization of health relief to victims of a calamity.

Structure and Areas of Work

Much of the WHO's work is concentrated on supporting research and providing technical advice to governments. The WHO and its staff work and interact with ministries of health, health-related academia, research centers, the private healthcare sector, and pharmaceutical manufacturers.

The WHO's staff consists of more than 8,000 health experts, including physicians, epidemiologists, scientists, managers, administrators, and other professionals. The staff provides services from the WHO's global headquarters, located in Geneva, Switzerland, and six regional offices—namely, (1) WHO Regional Office for Africa (AFRO), located in Brazzaville, Republic of the Congo; (2) WHO Regional Office for the Americas (AMRO)/Pan American Health Organization (PAHO), located in Washington, D.C.; (3) WHO Regional Office for the Eastern Mediterranean (EMRO), located in Cairo, Egypt; (4) Regional Office for Europe (EURO), located in Copenhagen, Denmark; (5) WHO Regional Office for South-East Asia (SEARO), located in New Delhi, India; and (6) WHO Regional Office for the Western Pacific (WPRO), located in Manila, the Philippines.

In addition, the WHO has local offices located in 147 countries.

The WHO's organizational structure is very dynamic as it has to rapidly adapt to ever changing health conditions around the world. The WHO's regional offices and local country offices tend to follow changes in structure from the organization's headquarters, adapting them to the existing health situations and needs of their own geographical areas.

The WHO headquarters structure consists of the Director General's Office, which includes the Deputy Director General, the Executive Director, advisers, governing bodies, internal oversight services, legal counsel, communications, ombudsmen, official institutional links with other international structures and partnerships, operational links with regional offices, and a special unit for polio eradication. WHO's headquarters also includes (a) organizational and operational structures for health security and environment; (b) HIV/AIDS, tuberculosis, malaria, and neglected tropical diseases; (c) health systems and services; health technology and pharmaceuticals; (d) health action in crises; information, evidence, and research; (e) family and community health; (f) noncommunicable diseases and mental health; and (g) general management.

Milestones in the History of the WHO

The WHO has continuously adapted to changes in scientific, medical advances and world healthcare needs. It has provided the background support for the improvement of health around the world, contributing either directly or indirectly to major achievements in health that include the following:

1948	The WHO takes on the responsibility of developing and implementing the International Classification of Diseases (ICD), which has become the standard clinical and epidemiological tool used worldwide.
1952	Jonas Salk in the United States develops the first successful polio vaccine.
1952–1964	The WHO/UNICEF Global Yaws Control Program reduces the prevalence of the crippling disease, yaws, from 50 million in 1950 to approximately 2.5 million cases in 1965.
1967	South African surgeon Christian Bernard succeeds in conducting the first heart transplant.
1967–1979	The WHO coordinates the smallpox eradication campaign, and for the first time in the history of humankind, a major infectious disease that killed millions is eradicated from the world.
1974	The World Health Assembly creates the Expanded Program for Immunization to bring basic vaccines to all children worldwide.
1974–2004	The WHO's Onchocerciasis Control Program prevents 600,000 cases of river blindness, and 18 million children are spared from the disease. And 25 million hectares of abandoned river land becomes productive again.
1977	The WHO publishes the first *Essential Medicines List*, providing countries with a national list of essential medicines.
1978	The WHO's International Conference on Primary Care in Alma-Ata, Kazakhstan, sets the historic goal of "Health for All."
1983	The Pasteur Institute in France identifies the human immunodeficiency virus (HIV), the causative agent of acquired immunodeficiency syndrome (AIDS).
1988	The WHO's Global Polio Eradication Initiative is established. As a result, 5 million children are prevented from suffering from disability, and 1.5 million childhood deaths are averted.
2003	Severe acute respiratory syndrome (SARS) is first identified and controlled.
2004	The WHO adopts the Global Strategy on Diet, Physical Activity and Health.
2005	The World Health Assembly revises the International Health Regulations.

In the near and distant future, the WHO will continue to promote and protect the health of all the peoples of the world.

Luis L. Zegers-Febres

See also Comparing Health Systems; Health; International Classification for Patient Safety (ICPS); International Classification of Diseases (ICD); Pan American Health Organization (PAHO); Preventive Care; Public Health

Further Readings

Brodsky, J., J. Habib, and M. Hirschfeld, eds. *Key Policy Issues in Long-Term Care.* Geneva, Switzerland: World Health Organization, 2003.

Lee, Kelley. *Historical Dictionary of the World Health Organization (Historical Dictionaries of International Organizations,* no. 15. Lanham, MD: Scarecrow Press, 1998.

Lee, Kelley. *World Health Organization (Global Institutions).* New York: Routledge, 2008.

Murry, C. J. L., and D. B. Evans. *Health Systems Performance Assessment: Debates, Methods, and Empiricism.* Geneva, Switzerland: World Health Organization, 2003.

World Health Organization. *The World Health Report 2005. Make Every Mother and Child Count.* Geneva, Switzerland: World Health Organization, 2005.

World Health Organization. *The World Health Report 2006. Working Together for Health.* Geneva, Switzerland: World Health Organization, 2006.

World Health Organization. *International Travel and Health.* Geneva, Switzerland: World Health Organization, 2007.

World Health Organization. *The World Health Report 2007. A Safer Future: Global Public Health Security in the 21st Century.* Geneva, Switzerland: World Health Organization, 2007.

World Health Organization. *World Health Statistics 2007.* Geneva, Switzerland: World Health Organization, 2007.

Zawide, Firdu, and Hilary Bassett. *Victims of Ineptitude: An Insider's Account of Injustice Within the World Health Organization.* Bloomington, IN: AuthorHouse, 2007.

Web Sites

Directory of nongovernmental organizations working officially with the WHO: http://www.who.int/civilsociety

Directory of the United Nations (UN): http://www.unsystem.org

World Health Organization (WHO) Headquarters: http://www.who.int

World Health Organization (WHO), Regional Office for Africa (AFRO): http://www.afro.who.int

World Health Organization (WHO), Regional Office for Europe (EURO): http://www.euro.who.int

World Health Organization (WHO), Regional Office for South-East Asia (SEARO): http://www.searo.who.int

World Health Organization (WHO), Regional Office for the Americas (AMRO)/Pan-American Health Organization (PAHO): http://www.paho.org

World Health Organization (WHO), Regional Office for the Eastern Mediterranean (EMRO): http://www.emro.who.int/index.asp

World Health Organization (WHO), Regional Officefor the Western Pacific (WPRO): http://www.wpro.who.int

Annotated Bibliography

This bibliography contains a list of core articles and books covering selected topics of health services research.

I. Health Services Research

Health services research is the emerging field that addresses the complex issues related to the healthcare system and informs health policy and practice. Health services research examines important issues such as access, costs, quality, and outcomes of healthcare.

1. *General Works*

Academy Health. *Federal Funding for Health Services Research.* Washington, DC: Academy Health, 2005.

Academy Health. *Placement, Coordination, and Funding of Health Services Research Within the Federal Government.* Washington, DC: Academy Health, 2005.

Black, Nick, and Duncan Neuhauser. "Books That Have Changed Health Services and Health Care Policy," *Journal of Health Services Research and Policy* 11(3): 180–83, July 2006.

Burrows, C., and K. Brown. *Eliciting Values in Health Services Research: Philosophies, Disciplines and Paradigms.* Fairfield, Victoria, Australia: National Centre for Health Program Evaluation, 1991.

Buxton, M., and S. Hanney. "How Can Payback From Health Services Research Be Assessed?" *Journal of Health Services Research and Policy* 1(1): 35–43, January 1996.

Choi, Thomas, and Jay N. Greenberg, eds. *Social Science Approaches to Health Services Research.* Ann Arbor, MI: Health Administration Press, 1982.

Committee on the Role of Institutional Review Boards in Health Services Research Data Privacy Protection, Division of Health Care Services, Institute of Medicine. *Institutional Review Boards and Health Services Research Data Privacy: A Workshop Summary.* Washington, DC: National Academy Press, 2000.

Committee on the Role of Institutional Review Boards in Health Services Research Data Privacy Protection, Division of Health Care Services, Institute of Medicine. *Protecting Data Privacy in Health Services Research.* Washington, DC: National Academy Press, 2000.

Davis, Karen, and Cathy Schoen. *Health Services Research and the Changing Health Care System.* New York: Commonwealth Fund, 1996.

Division of Health Care Services, Institute of Medicine. *Health Services Research: Report of a Study.* Washington, DC: National Academy of Sciences, 1979.

Eagar, K., D. Cromwell, A. Owen, et al. "Health Services Research and Development in Practice: An Australian Experience," *Journal of Health Services Research and Policy* 8(4 Suppl. 2): 7–13, October 2, 2003.

Field, Marilyn, Robert E. Tranquada, and Jill C. Feasley, eds., and Committee on Health Services Research: Training and Work Force Issues, Division of Health Care Services, Institute of Medicine. *Health Services Research: Work Force and Educational Issues.* Washington, DC: National Academy Press, 1995.

Flook, E. Evelyn, and Paul J. Sanazaro, eds. *Health Services Research and R & D in Perspective.* Ann Arbor, MI: Health Administration Press, 1973.

Fracchia, G. N., and M. Theofilatou, eds. *Health Services Research.* Washington, DC: IOS Press, 1993.

Ginzberg, Eli, ed. *Health Services Research: Key to Health Policy.* Cambridge, MA: Harvard University Press, 1991.

Golder, Su, Kate Light, and Kath Wright. "Promoting Public Involvement in Health Services Research," *Journal of Health Services Research and Policy* 11(3): 187–88, July 2006.

Gray, Gerda L. *Health Services Research and Development Abroad: A Selected Bibliography.* Springfield, VA: Capital Systems Group, 1971. (Available through the National Technical Information Service, PB-207 847)

Haas, Marion. "Health Services Research in Australia: An Investigation of Its Current Status," *Journal of Health Services Research and Policy* 9(4 Suppl. 2): 3–9, October 2004.

Hershey, John C., and William P. Pierskalla. *Health Services Research and Health Policy: An Analysis.* Philadelphia: University of Pennsylvania, National Health Care Management Center, 1979.

Mainland, Donald, ed. *Health Services Research,* vols. 1–2. New York: Milbank Memorial Fund, 1967. (Reprinted from the *Milbank Memorial Fund Quarterly* 44(3), July 1966 and 44(4), October 1966)

McKinlay, John B., ed. *Health Services Research: Planning, and Change.* Cambridge: MIT Press, 1981.

Ong, Bie Nio. *The Practice of Health Services Research.* New York: Chapman and Hall, 1993.

Peacock, Stuart, Jane Pirkis, and Jackie Cumming. "Health Services Research, Policy and Practice in Australia and New Zealand: A Coming of Age," *Journal of Health Services Research and Policy* 9(4 Suppl. 2): 1–2, October 2004.

Slaughter, P. M., E. M. Meslin, and C. D. Naylor. *Ethics and Health Services Research: A Resource Bibliography.* Toronto, Ontario, Canada: Institute for Clinical Evaluation Sciences in Ontario, 1994.

Sobo, Elisa J., and Paul S. Kurtin, eds. *Child Health Services Research: Applications, Innovations, and Insights.* San Francisco: Jossey-Bass, 2003.

Taube, Carl A., David Mechanic, and Ann A. Hohmann, eds. *The Future of Mental Health Services Research.* Rockville, MD: U.S. Department of Health and Human Services, Public Health Service, Alcohol, Drug Abuse, and Mental Health Administration, National Institute of Mental Health, Division of Biometry and Applied Sciences, 1989.

Thaul, Susan, Kathleen N. Lohr, and Robert E. Tranquada, eds., and Committee on Health Services Research: Training and Work Force Issues, Division of Health Care Services, Institute of Medicine. *Health Services Research: Opportunities for an Expanding Field of Inquiry.* Washington, DC: National Academy Press, 1994.

Thompson, John D. *Applied Health Services Research.* Lexington, MA: Lexington Books, 1977.

Van Hoek, Robert. *Health Care and the Role of Health Services Research*. Michael M. Davis Lecture Series. Chicago: University of Chicago, Center for Health Administration Studies, 1973.

White, Kerr L., Julio Frenk, Cosme Ordonez, et al., eds. *Health Services Research: An Anthology*. Washington, DC: Pan American Health Organization, Pan American Sanitary Bureau, Regional Office of the World Health Organization, 1992.

2. Definitions, Scope, and Importance

Aday, Lu Ann. "Establishment of a Conceptual Base for Health Services Research," *Journal of Health Services Research and Policy* 6(3): 183–85, July 2001.

Bice, Thomas W. "Social Science and Health Services Research: Contributions to Public Policy," *Milbank Memorial Fund Quarterly/Health and Society* 58(2): 173–200, 1980.

Brook, Robert H. "Health Services Research: Is It Good for You and Me? *Academic Medicine* 64(3): 124–30, March 1989.

Clancy, Carolyn M. "Health Services Research: From Galvanizing Attention to Creating Action," *Health Services Research* 38(3): 777–82, June 2003.

Field, Marilyn J., and Kathleen N. Lohr. "Health Services Research: An Expanding Field of Inquiry," *Journal of Evaluation in Clinical Practice* 1(1): 61–65, September 1995.

Lohr, Kathleen N., and Donald M. Steinwachs. "Health Services Research: An Evolving Definition of the Field," *Health Services Research* 37(1): 15–17, February 2002.

Mechanic, David. "Prospects and Problems in Health Services Research," *Milbank Memorial Fund Quarterly* 56(2): 136–49, 1978.

Shortell, Steven M., and J. P. LoGerfo. "Health Services Research and Public Policy: Definitions, Accomplishments, and Potential," *Health Services Research* 13: 230–37, Fall 1978.

Spitzer, W. O., and B. Starfield. "Health Services Research Can Make a Difference!" *New England Journal of Medicine* 297(25): 1046, December 22, 1977.

3. History

Anderson, Odin W. *The Evolution of Health Services Research: Personal Reflections on Applied Social Science*. San Francisco: Jossey-Bass, 1991.

Bonner, Thomas Neville. *Iconoclast: Abraham Flexner and a Life in Learning*. Baltimore: Johns Hopkins University Press, 2002.

Clinton, Jarrett J., and G. Hernandez. "AHCPR [Agency for Health Care Policy and Research] Background and History," *Decubitus* 4(2): 22–26, May 1991.

Codman, Ernest A. *A Study in Hospital Efficiency: The First Five Years*. Boston: Thomas Todd, 1916.

Flexner, Abraham. *Medical Education in the United States and Canada: A Report to the Carnegie Foundation, 1910*. New York: Carnegie Foundation, 1910.

Flook, E. Evelyn, and Paul J. Sanazaro. "Health Services Research: Origins and Milestones." In *Health Services Research and R&D in Perspective*, edited by E. Evelyn Flook and Paul J. Sanazaro, 1–81. Ann Arbor, MI: Health Administration Press, 1973.

Maynard, Alan, and Iain Chalmers, eds. *Non-Random Reflections on Health Services Research: On the 25th Anniversary of Archie Cochrane's Effectiveness and Efficiency*. London: BMJ Books, 1997.

Naylor, David. "Humility, Perspective and Provocation: Reflecting on Codman," *Journal of Health Services Research and Policy* 6(4): 249–50, October 2001.

Savedoff, W. D. "Kenneth Arrow and the Birth of Health Economics," *Bulletin of the World Health Organization* 82(2): 139–40, February 2004.

White, William D. *Compelled by Data, John D. Thompson: Nurse, Health Services Researcher, and Health Administration Educator*. New Haven, CT: Yale University, Yale School of Medicine, Department of Epidemiology and Public Health, 2003.

4. Methods and Data

Black, Charlyn. *Data, Data, Everywhere: Improving Access to Population Health and Health Services Research Data in Canada, Final Report*. Vancouver, British Columbia, Canada: University of British Columbia, Centre for Health Services and Policy Research, 2005.

Black, Nick, John Brazier, Ray Fitzpatrick, et al., eds. *Health Services Research Methods: A Guide to Best Practice*. London: BMJ Books, 1998.

Boca, Del, and J. A. Noll. "Truth or Consequences: The Validity of Self-Report Data in Health Services Research on Addictions," *Addiction* 95(Suppl. 3–11): 347–60, November 2000.

Crombie, I. K., and H.T.O. Davies. *Research in Health Care: Design, Conduct, and Interpretation of Health Services Research*. New York: Wiley, 1996.

DeFriese, Gordon H., Thomas C. Ricketts, and Jane S. Stein, eds. *Methodological Advances in Health Services Research*. Ann Arbor, MI: Health Administration Press, 1989.

Herman, P. M., K. D'Huyvetter, and M. J. Mohler. "Are Health Services Research Methods a Match for CAM [Complementary and Alternative Medicine]," *Alternative Therapies in Health and Medicine* 12(3): 78–83, May–June 2006.

Huston, Patricia, and C. David Naylor. "Health Services Research: Reporting on Studies Using Secondary Data Sources," *Canadian Medical Association Journal* 155(12): 1697–702, December 15, 1996.

Pope, Catherine, and Nick Mays. "Qualitative Research: Reaching the Parts Other Methods Cannot Research: An Introduction to Qualitative Methods in Health and Health Services Research," *British Medical Journal* 311(6996): 42–45, July 1, 1995.

Richetts, Thomas C., ed. *Geographic Methods for Health Services Research: A Focus on the Rural-Urban Continuum*. Lanham, MD: University Press of America, 1994.

Romeis, James C., Rodney M. Coe, and John E. Morley, eds. *Applying Health Services Research to Long-Term Care.* New York: Springer, 1996.

Shi, Leiyu. *Health Services Research Methods.* Albany, NY: Delmar, 1997.

Sibbald, William J., Julian F. Bion, and Jean-Louis Vincent, eds. *Evaluating Critical Care: Using Health Services Research to Improve Quality.* New York: Springer, 2002.

Stange, Kurt C., Stephen J. Zyzanski, Tracy Fedirko, et al. "How Valid Are Medical Records and Patient Questionnaires for Physician Profiling and Health Services Research? A Comparison With Direct Observation of Patient Visits," *Medical Care* 36(6): 851–67, June 1998.

Von Korff, Michael, Mark P. Jensen, and Paul Karoly. "Assessing Global Pain Severity by Self-Report in Clinical and Health Services Research," *Spine* 25(24): 3140–151, December 15, 2000.

II. Access to Healthcare

Access to healthcare is the ability to establish contact with and use the healthcare system and its services. There are about 47 million uninsured individuals in the United States, many of whom are unable to afford health insurance coverage and thus are unable to access the healthcare system.

5. General Works

Aday, Lu Ann, and Ronald Andersen. *Development of Indices of Access to Medical Care.* Ann Arbor, MI: University Microfilms International, 1978.

Aday, Lu Ann, Gretchen V. Fleming, and Ronald M. Andersen. *Access to Medical Care in the U.S.: Who Has It, Who Doesn't.* Chicago: Pluribus, 1984.

Andersen, Ronald M. "Revisiting the Behavioral Model and Access to Medical Care: Does It Matter?" *Journal of Health and Social Behavior* 36(1): 1–10, March 1995.

Center for Health Economics Research. *Access to Health Care.* Princeton, NJ: Robert Wood Johnson Foundation, 1993.

Davis, Karen. "Inequality and Access to Health Care," *Milbank Quarterly* 69(2): 253–73, 1991.

Donatelle, Rebecca J. *Access to Health.* Reading, MA: Benjamin-Cummings, 2005.

Eichhorn, Robert L., and Lu Ann Aday. *The Utilization of Health Services: Indices and Correlates: A Research Bibliography.* Lafayette, IN: Purdue University, 1972.

Gaskin, Darrell J. *Access to Health Care in a Managed Care Environment.* Washington, DC: Joint Center for Political and Economic Studies, 1999.

Gulliford, Martin, J. Figueroa-Munoz, M. Morgan, et al. "What Does 'Access to Health Care' Mean?" *Journal of Health Services Research and Policy* 7(3): 186–88, July 2002.

Gulliford, Martin, and Myfanwy Morgan, eds. *Access to Health Care.* New York: Routledge, 2003.

Jeffords, James M., ed. *Ensuring Access to Affordable Health Care: Hearing Before the Committee on Labor and Human Resources, U.S. Senate.* Collingdale, PA: Diane, 2000.

Kronenfeld, Jennie Jacobs, ed. *Access, Quality and Satisfaction With Care: Concerns of Patients, Providers and Insurers.* New York: JAI Press, 2007.

Lillie-Blanton, Marsha, and Ana Alfaro-Correa. *In the Nation's Interest: Equity in Access to Health Care Summary Report.* Collingdale, PA: Diane, 1995.

Lurie, Nicole, and Martha Ross. *Health Status and Access to Care Among Low-Income Washington, DC Residents. A Research Brief for the DC Primary Care Medical Homes Project.* Washington, DC: Brookings Institution/RAND, October 2006.

Millman, Michael, ed., and Committee on Monitoring Access to Personal Health Care Services, Institute of Medicine. *Access to Health Care in America.* Washington, DC: National Academy Press, 1993.

Rank, Mark Robert. *One Nation, Underprivileged: Why American Poverty Affects Us All.* New York: Oxford University Press, 2004.

Ricketts, T. C., and L. J. Goldsmith. "Access to Health Services Research: The Battle of the Frameworks," *Nursing Outlook* 53(6): 274–80, November–December 2005.

Secombe, Karen, and Kim A. Hoffman. *Just Don't Get Sick: Access to Health Care in the Aftermath of Welfare Reform.* New Brunswick, NJ: Rutgers University Press, 2007.

Sossin, Lorne Mitchell, ed. *Access to Care, Access to Justice: The Legal Debate Over Private Health Insurance in Canada.* Toronto, Ontario, Canada: University of Toronto Press, 2005.

Weinick, Robin M., Samuel Zuvekas, and Susan K. Drilea. *Access to Health Care: Sources and Barriers, 1996.* AHCPR Pub. No. 98-001. Rockville, MD: Agency for Health Care Policy and Research, 1997.

6. Cultural Competency

Anand, Rohini. *Cultural Competence in Health Care: A Guide for Trainers.* 2d ed. Washington, DC: National MultiCultural Institute (NMCI), 1999.

Betancourt, Joseph R., Alexander R. Green, and J. Emilio Carrillo. *Cultural Competence in Health Care: Emerging Frameworks and Practical Approaches.* New York: Commonwealth Fund, Quality of Care for Underserved Populations, 2002.

Constantine, Madonna G., and Derald Wing Sue, eds. *Addressing Racism: Facilitating Cultural Competence in Mental Health and Educational Settings.* Hoboken, NJ: Wiley, 2006.

Jandt, Fred E. *An Introduction to Intercultural Communication.* 5th ed. Thousand Oaks, CA: Sage, 2007.

Jeffreys, Marianne R. *Teaching Cultural Competence in Nursing and Health Care: Inquiry, Action, and Innovation.* New York: Springer, 2006.

Keefe, Susan E., ed. *Appalachian Cultural Competency: A Guide for Medical, Mental Health, and Social Service Professionals.* Knoxville: University of Tennessee Press, 2005.

Lattanzi, Jill Black, and Larry D. Purnell. *Developing Cultural Competence in Physical Therapy Practice.* Philadelphia: F. A. Davis, 2006.

MacLachian, Malcolm. *Culture and Health: A Critical Perspective Towards Global Health.* 2d ed. San Francisco: Jossey-Bass, 2006.

Morales, Leo S., Juan Antonio Puyol, and Ron D. Hays. *Improving Patient Satisfaction Surveys to Assess Cultural Competence in Health Care.* Oakland: California Health Care Foundation, 2003.

Neuliep, James W. *Intercultural Communication: A Contextual Approach.* 3d ed. Thousand Oaks, CA: Sage, 2006.

Purnell, Larry D., and Betty J. Paulanka. *Guide to Culturally Competent Health Care.* Philadelphia: F. A. Davis, 2005.

Rees, Countney, Sonia Ruiz, Marsha Lillie-Blanton, et al. *Compendium of Cultural Competence Initiatives in Health Care.* Menlo Park, CA: Henry J. Kaiser Family Foundation, 2003.

Rundie, Anne, Maria Carvalho, and Mary Robinson, eds. *Cultural Competence in Health Care: A Practical Guide.* San Francisco: Jossey-Bass, 2002.

U.S. Health Resources and Services Administration. *Cultural Competence in the Delivery of Services Through Medicaid Managed Care.* Merrifield, VA: Health Resources and Services Administration, 2001.

7. Health Disparities

Agency for Healthcare Research and Quality. *The National Healthcare Disparities Report.* Rockville, MD: Agency for Healthcare Research and Quality, 2005. (This is an annual report)

Aizer, Anna, Adriana Lleras-Muney, and Mark Stabile. *Access to Care, Provider Choice, and Racial Disparities in Infant Mortality.* NBER Working Paper No. 10445. Cambridge, MA: National Bureau of Economic Research, 2004.

Allen, Carol Easley, et al. *Eliminating Health Disparities: Conversations With Blacks in America.* Santa Cruz, CA: ETR Associates, 2005.

Applied Research Center. *Closing the Gap: Solutions to Race-Based Health Disparities.* Oakland, CA: Applied Research Center, 2005.

Capitman, John A., Sarita Bhalotra, and Mathilda Ruwe. *Cancer and Elders of Color: Opportunities for Reducing Health Disparities: Evidence Review and Recommendations for Research and Policy.* Burlington, VT: Ashgate, 2005.

Casper, Michele, and Centers for Disease Control and Prevention. *Atlas of Stroke Mortality: Racial, Ethnic, and Geographic Disparities in the United States.* Atlanta, GA: U.S. Department of Health and Human Services, Centers for Disease Control and Prevention, National Center for Chronic Disease Prevention and Health Promotion, 2003.

Chandra, Amitabh, and Jonathan Skinner. *Geography and Racial Health Disparities.* NBER Working Paper No. 9513. Cambridge, MA: National Bureau of Economic Research, 2003.

Curtis, Andrew, and Michael Leitner. *Geographic Information Systems and Public Health: Eliminating Perinatal Disparity.* Hershey, PA: IRM Press, 2006.

Decker, Sandra L., and Dahlia K. Remler. *How Much Might Universal Health Insurance Reduce Socioeconomic Disparities in Health? A Comparison of the U.S. and Canada.* NBER Working Paper No. 10715. Cambridge, MA: National Bureau of Economic Research, 2004.

Fogel, Robert W. *Changes in the Disparities in Chronic Disease During the Course of the Twentieth Century.* NBER Working Paper No. 10311. Cambridge, MA: National Bureau of Economic Research, 2004.

Keppel, Kenneth G. *Methodological Issues in Measuring Health Disparities.* Vital and Health Statistics, Series 2, no. 141. Hyattsville, MD: U.S. Department of Health and Human Services, Centers for Disease Control and Prevention, National Center for Health Statistics, 2005.

Klick, Jonathan, and Sally L. Satel. *The Health Disparities Myth: Diagnosing the Treatment Gap.* Washington, DC: AEI Press, 2006.

LaVeist, Thomas A. *Minority Populations and Health: An Introduction to Health Disparities in the United States.* San Francisco: Jossey-Bass, 2005.

Livingston, Ivor Lensworth, ed. *Praeger Handbook of Black American Health: Policies and Issues Behind Disparities in Health.* 2d ed. 2 vols. Westport, CT: Praeger, 2004.

Metrosa, Elene V., ed. *Racial and Ethnic Disparities in Health and Health Care.* New York: Nova Science, 2006.

Satcher, David, Rubens J. Pamies, and Nancy N. Woelfl, eds. *Multicultural Medicine and Health Disparities.* New York: McGraw-Hill, 2006.

Shin, Peter, Karen Jones, and Sara Rosenbaum. *Reducing Racial and Ethnic Health Disparities: Estimating the Impact of High Health Center Penetration in Low-Income Communities.* Washington, DC: George Washington University Medical Center, Center for Health Services Research and Policy, 2003.

Smedley, Brian D., Adrienne Y. Stith, and Alan R. Nelson, eds., and Committee on Understanding and Eliminating Racial and Ethnic Disparities in Health Care, Board on Health Sciences Policy, Institute of Medicine. *Unequal Treatment: Confronting Racial and Ethnic Disparities in Health Care.* Washington, DC: National Academies Press, 2002.

Swift, Elaine K., ed., and Committee on Guidance for Designing a National Healthcare Disparities Report, Institute of Medicine. *Guidance for the National Healthcare Disparities Report.* Washington, DC: National Academies Press, 2002.

Thomson, Gerald E., Faith Mitchell, and Monique B. Williams, eds., and Committee on the Review and Assessment of the NIH's Strategic Research Plan and Budget to Reduce and Ultimately Eliminate Health Disparities, Board on Health Sciences Policy, Institute of Medicine. *Examining the Health Disparities Research Plan of the National Institutes of*

Health: Unfinished Business. Washington, DC: National Academies Press, 2006.

Weinick, Robin M., Samuel H. Zuvekas, and Joel W. Cohen. "Racial and Ethnic Differences in Access to and Use of Health Care Services, 1977 to 1996," *Medical Care Research and Review* 57(Suppl. 1): 36–54, 2000.

8. Inner-City Health

Andrulis, Dennis P., and Betsy Carrier. *Managed Care in the Inner City: The Uncertain Promise for Providers, Plans, and Communities*. San Francisco: Jossey-Bass, 1999.

Commonwealth Fund, Task Force on Academic Health Centers. *A Shared Responsibility: Academic Health Centers and the Provision of Care to the Poor and Uninsured: A Report of the Task Force on Academic Health Centers*. New York: Commonwealth Fund, 2001.

Boger, John Charles, and Judith Welch Wegner, eds. *Race, Poverty and American Cities*. Chapel Hill: University of North Carolina Press, 1996.

Galea, Sandro, and David Vlahov. *Handbook of Urban Health: Populations, Methods, and Practice*. New York: Springer, 2005.

Ginzberg, Eli, Howard Berliner, Mariam Ostow, et al., eds. *Teaching Hospitals and the Urban Poor*. New Haven, CT: Yale University Press, 2000.

National Center for Health Statistics. *Health, United States, 2001: With Urban and Rural Health Chartbook*. Hyattsville, MD: U.S. Department of Health and Human Services, Centers for Disease Control and Prevention, National Center for Health Statistics, 2001.

Rodwin, Victor, and Michael K. Gusmano, eds. *Growing Older in World Cities: New York, London, Paris, and Tokyo*. Nashville, TN: Vanderbilt University Press, 2006.

Vlahov, D., E. Gibble, N. Freudenberg, et al. "Cities and Health: History, Approaches, and Key Questions," *Academic Medicine* 79(12): 1133–38, December 2004.

9. Rural Health

Anson, Roberto. *State Offices of Rural Health: 50 Success Stories: A Sourcebook and Overview of Their Accomplishments*. Rockville, MD: Health Resources and Services Administration, Federal Office of Rural Health Policy, 2000.

Casey, Michelle, Jill Klingner, and Ira S. Moscovice. *Access to Rural Pharmacy Services in Minnesota, North Dakota, and South Dakota*. Minneapolis: University of Minnesota, School of Public Health, Division of Health Services Research and Policy, Rural Health Research Center, 2001.

Committee on the Future of Rural Health Care, Board on Health Care Services, Institute of Medicine. *Quality Through Collaboration: The Future of Rural Health*. Washington, DC: National Academies Press, 2005.

Coward, Raymond T., Lisa A. Davis, Carol H. Gold, et al., eds. *Rural Women's Health: Mental, Behavioral, and Physical Issues*. New York: Springer, 2006.

Farley, Donna O., Lisa R. Shugarman, Pat Taylor, et al. *Trends in Special Medicare Payments and Service Utilization for Rural Areas in the 1990s*. Santa Monica, CA: RAND Corporation, 2002.

Gale, John, and Andrew Coburn. *The Characteristics and Roles of Rural Health Clinics in the United States: A Chartbook*. Portland: University of Southern Maine, Edmund S. Muskie School of Public Service, 2003.

Gamm, Larry. *Rural Healthy People 2010: A Companion Document to Healthy People 2010*. College Station: Texas A&M University System Health Science Center, School of Rural Public Health, Southwest Rural Health Research Center, 2003.

Gesler, Wilbert M., Donna J. Rabiner, and Gordon H. DeFriese, eds. *Rural Health and Aging Research: Theory, Methods, and Practical Applications*. Amityville, NY: Baywood, 1998.

Glasgow, Nina, Lois Wright Morton, and Nan E. Johnson, eds. *Critical Issues in Rural Health*. Ames, IA: Blackwell, 2004.

Grey, Michael R. *New Deal Medicine: The Rural Health Programs of the Farm Security Administration*. Baltimore: Johns Hopkins University Press, 2002.

Lee, Helen J., and Charlene A. Winters, eds. *Rural Nursing: Concepts, Theory, and Practice*. New York: Springer, 2006.

Loue, Sana, and Beth E. Quill, eds. *Handbook of Rural Health*. New York: Springer, 2006.

Martin, Philip, Michael Fox, and J. Edward Taylor. *The New Rural Poverty: Agriculture and Immigration in California*. Washington, DC: Urban Institute Press, 2006.

Merchant, James, Christine Coussens, and Dalia Gilbert, eds., and Roundtable on Environmental Health Sciences, Research, and Medicine, Board on Population Health and Public Health Practice, Institute of Medicine. *Rebuilding the Unity of Health and the Environment in Rural America: Workshop Summary*. Washington, DC: National Academies Press, 2006.

Mosocovice, Ira S. *Rural Health Networks: Evolving Organizational Forms and Functions*. Minneapolis: University of Minnesota, School of Public Health, Division of Health Services Research and Policy, Rural Health Research Center, 2003.

Office of Rural Health. *Rural Health Dictionary of Terms, Acronyms, and Organizations*. Rockville, MD: U.S. Department of Health and Human Services, Health Resources and Services Administration, Public Health Service, Office of Rural Health, 1997.

Phillips, Charles D., Catherine Hawes, and Malgorzata Leyk Williams. *Nursing Homes in Rural and Urban Areas, 2000*. College Station, TX: Southwest Rural Health Research Center, 2003.

Ricketts, Thomas C. *Arguing for Rural Health in Medicare: A Progressive Rhetoric for Rural America*. Chapel Hill: University of North Carolina, Cecil G. Sheps Center for

Health Services Research, North Carolina Rural Health Research and Policy Analysis Center, 2002.

Ricketts, Thomas C., ed. *Rural Health in the United States.* New York: Oxford University Press, 1999.

Stensland, Jeffrey, and Ira S. Moscovice. *Rural Hospitals' Ability to Finance Inpatient, Skilled Nursing, and Home Health Care.* Minneapolis: University of Minnesota, School of Public Health, Division of Health Services Research and Policy, 2001.

Teevans, James W. *Forming Rural Health Networks: A Legal Primer.* Washington, DC: Alpha Center, 1999.

Wakefield, Mary K. *Linking Rural Health Services Research With Health Policy.* Rockville, MD: Agency for Healthcare Research and Quality, Center for Research Dissemination and Liaison, 2000.

10. Safety Net

Billings, John, and Robin M. Weinick. *Monitoring the Health Care Safety Net.* Rockville, MD: U.S. Department of Health and Human Services, Public Health Service, Agency for Health Care Policy and Research, 2003.

Burt, Catharine W., and Irma E. Arispe. *Characteristics of Emergency Departments Serving High Volumes of Safety-Net Patients.* HHS Pub. No. (PHS) 2004-1726. Hyattsville, MD: U.S. Department of Health and Human Services, Centers for Disease Control and Prevention, National Center for Health Statistics, 2004.

Fishman, Linda E., and James D. Bentley. "The Evolution of Support for Safety-Net Hospitals," *Health Affairs* 16(4): 30–47, July–August 1997.

Hartley, David, Erika C. Ziller, and Caroline MacDonald. *Diabetes and the Rural Safety Net.* Portland: University of Southern Maine, Edmund S. Muskie School of Public Services, Maine Rural Health Research Center, 2002.

Lewin, Marion Ein, and Stuart Altman, eds., and Committee on the Changing Market, Managed Care, and the Future Viability of Safety Net Providers, Institute of Medicine. *America's Health Care Safety Net: Intact but Endangered.* Washington, DC: National Academy Press, 2000. (The report defines safety net providers as "those providers that organize and deliver a significant level of health care and other related services to the uninsured, Medicaid, and other vulnerable patients.")

National Advisory Committee on Rural Health. *A Targeted Look at the Rural Health Care Safety Net: A Report to the Secretary, U.S. Department of Health and Human Services.* Washington, DC: National Advisory Committee on Rural Health, 2002.

Ormond, Barbara A., Susan Wallin, and Susan M. Goldenson. *Supporting the Rural Health Care Safety Net.* Washington, DC: Urban Institute, 2000.

Richardson, L. D., and U. Hwang. "America's Health Care Safety Net: Intact or Unraveling?" *Academic Emergency Medicine* 8(11): 1056–1063, November 1, 2001.

Singer, Ingrid, James Kuzner, and Lynne Fagani. *America's Safety Net Hospitals and Health Systems, 2000: Results of the 2000*

Annual NAPH Member Survey. Washington, DC: National Association of Public Hospitals and Health System, 2002.

Spillman, Brenda C., Stephen Zuckerman, and Bowen Garrett. *Does the Health Care Safety Net Narrow the Access Gap?* Washington, DC: Urban Institute, 2003.

Weinick, Robin M., and Peter Shin. *Monitoring the Health Care Safety Net: Developing Data-Driven Capabilities to Support Policymaking.* AHRQ Pub. No. 04-0037. Rockville, MD: U.S. Department of Health and Human Services, Public Health Service, Agency for Healthcare Policy and Research, 2004.

Weissman, Joel S., and Arnold M. Epstein. *Falling Through the Safety Net: Insurance Status and Access to Health Care.* Baltimore: Johns Hopkins University Press, 1994.

11. Uninsured Individuals

Committee on the Consequences of Uninsurance, Board on Health Care Services, Institute of Medicine. *Coverage Matters: Insurance and Health Care.* Washington, DC: National Academy Press, 2001.

Committee on the Consequences of Uninsurance, Board on Health Care Services, Institute of Medicine. *Care Without Coverage: Too Little, Too Late.* Washington, DC: National Academy Press, 2002.

Committee on the Consequences of Uninsurance, Board on Health Care Services, Institute of Medicine. *Health Insurance Is a Family Matter.* Washington, DC: National Academy Press, 2002.

Committee on the Consequences of Uninsurance, Board on Health Care Services, Institute of Medicine. *A Shared Destiny: Community Effects of Uninsurance.* Washington, DC: National Academy Press, 2003.

Committee on the Consequences of Uninsurance, Board on Health Care Services, Institute of Medicine. *Insuring America's Health: Principles and Recommendations.* Washington, DC: National Academy Press, 2004.

Commonwealth Fund, Task Force on Academic Health Centers. *A Shared Responsibility: Academic Health Centers and the Provision of Care to the Poor and Uninsured: A Report of the Commonwealth Fund Task Force on Academic Health Centers.* New York: Commonwealth Fund, 2001.

Geyman, John P. *Falling Through the Safety Net: Americans Without Health Insurance.* Monroe, ME: Common Courage Press, 2005.

Holahan, John, and Brenda Spillman. *Health Care Access for Uninsured Adults: A Stronger Safety Net Is Not the Same as Insurance.* Washington, DC: Urban Institute, 2002.

Meyer, Jack A., and Elliot K. Wicks. *Covering America: Real Remedies for the Uninsured.* Washington, DC: Economic and Social Research Institute, 2002.

Norton, E. C., and D. O. Staiger. "How Hospital Ownership Affects Access to Care for the Uninsured," *Rand Journal of Economics* 25(1): 171–85, 1994.

Polsky, Daniel, Jalpa Doshi, Jose Escarce, et al. *The Health Effects of Medicare for the Near-Elderly Uninsured.* NBER Working Paper No. 12511. Cambridge, MA: National Bureau of Economic Research, 2006.

Sered, Susan Starr, and Rushika Fernandopulle. *Uninsured in America: Life and Death in the Land of Opportunity.* Berkeley: University of California Press, 2005.

Stoll, Kathleen. *Paying a Premium: The Added Cost of Care for the Uninsured.* Washington, DC: Families USA, 2005.

Swartz, Katherine. *Reinsuring Health: Why More Middle-Class People Are Uninsured and What Government Can Do.* New York: Russell Sage Foundation, 2006.

U.S. Congressional Budget Office. *The Uninsured and Rising Health Insurance Premiums.* CBO Testimony Statement of Douglas Holtz-Eakin Before the Subcommittee on Health, Committee on Ways and Means, U.S. House of Representatives, March 9, 2004.

12. *Vulnerable Populations*

Aday, Lu Ann. *At Risk in America: The Health and Health Care Needs of Vulnerable Populations in the United States.* 2d ed. San Francisco: Jossey-Bass, 2002.

Aguirre-Molina, Marilyn, Carlos W. Molina, and Ruth Enid Zambrana, eds. *Health Issues in the Latino Community.* San Francisco: Jossey-Bass, 2001.

Braithwaite, Ronald L., and Sandra E. Taylor, eds. *Health Issues in the Black Community.* 2d ed. San Francisco: Jossey-Bass, 2001.

Chesnay, Mary de. *Caring for the Vulnerable: Perspectives in Nursing Theory, Practice, and Research.* Sudbury, MA: Jones and Bartlett, 2005.

Edleman, Peter, Harry J. Holzer, and Paul Offner. *Reconnecting Disadvantaged Young Men.* Washington, DC: Urban Institute Press, 2006.

Hattery, Angela, and Earl Smith. *African American Families: Issues of Health, Wealth, and Violence.* Thousand Oaks, CA: Sage, 2007.

Hogue, Carol J. R., Martha A. Hargraves, and Karen Scott Collins, eds. *Minority Health in America: Findings and Policy Implications From the Commonwealth Fund Minority Health Survey.* Baltimore: Johns Hopkins University Press, 2000.

Iezzoni, Lisa I. *More Than Ramps: A Guide to Improving Health Care Quality and Access for People With Disabilities.* New York: Oxford University Press, 2006.

King, Talmadge E., and Margaret B. Wheeler, eds. *Medical Management of Vulnerable and Underserved Patients: Principles, Practice, and Populations.* New York: McGraw-Hill, 2007.

LaVeist, Thomas A. *Race, Ethnicity, and Health: A Public Health Reader.* San Francisco: Jossey-Bass, 2002.

Levin, Bruce Lubotsky, John Petrila, and Kevin D. Hennessy, eds. *Mental Health Services: A Public Health Perspective.* New York: Oxford University Press, 2004.

Loue, Sana. *Assessing Race, Ethnicity, and Gender in Health.* New York: Springer, 2006.

Melnick, Daniel, and Edward Perrin, eds., and Panel on HHS Collection of Race and Ethnicity Data, Committee on National Statistics, Division of Behavioral and Social Sciences and Education, National Research Council. *Improving Racial and Ethnic Data on Health: Report of a Workshop.* Washington, DC: National Academies Press, 2003.

Mincy, Ronald B., ed. *Black Males Left Behind.* Washington, DC: Urban Institute Press, 2006.

Rank, Mark Robert. *One Nation, Underprivileged: Why American Poverty Affects Us All.* New York: Oxford University Press, 2004.

Reed, Wornie, William Darity Sr., and Norma L. Roberson. *Health and Medical Care of African-Americans.* Westport, CT: Auburn House, 1993.

Rhoades, Everett R., ed. *American Indian Health: Innovations in Health Care, Promotion, and Policy.* Baltimore: Johns Hopkins University Press, 2001.

Sandefur, Gary D., Ronald R. Rindfuss, and Barney Cohen, eds., and Committee on Population, Commission on Behavioral and Social Sciences and Education, National Research Council. *Changing Numbers, Changing Needs: American Indian Demography and Public Health.* Washington, DC: National Academy Press, 1996.

Schulz, Amy J., and Leith Mullings, eds. *Gender, Race, Class and Health: Intersectional Approaches.* San Francisco: Jossey-Bass, 2005.

Shi, Leiyu, and Gregory D. Stevens. *Vulnerable Populations in the United States.* San Francisco: Jossey-Bass, 2004.

III. Costs, Economics, and Financing of Healthcare

Costs, economics, and financing of healthcare refer to the expenditures, scarcity in the allocation of healthcare resources, and the way healthcare is paid for. Economic principles are a useful tool to better understand how to control rising healthcare costs and how to finance healthcare.

13. *General Works*

Arrow, Kenneth J. "Uncertainty and the Welfare Economics of Medical Care," *American Economic Review* 53(3): 941–73, December 1963.

Culyer, Anthony J. *The Dictionary of Health Economics.* Northhampton, MA: Edward Elgar, 2005.

Culyer, Anthony J., and Joseph P. Newhouse, eds. *Handbook of Health Economics.* Handbooks in Economics Series, no. 17, vols. 1A–2A. New York: Elsevier, 2000.

Cutler, David M., and Ernst R. Berndt, eds. *Medical Care Output and Productivity.* National Bureau of Economic Research Studies in Income and Wealth (NBER-IW). Chicago: University of Chicago Press, 2001.

Drummond, Michael F., and Alistair McGuire, eds. *Economic Evaluation in Health Care: Merging Theory With Practice.* New York: Oxford University Press, 2002.

Frank, Richard G., and Willard G. Manning, eds. *Economics and Mental Health.* Chicago: University of Chicago Press, 1992.

Fuchs, Victor R. *The Health Economy.* Cambridge, MA: Harvard University Press, 1986.

Getzen, Thomas E. *Health Care Economics.* San Francisco: Jossey-Bass, 2007.

Hammer, Peter J., Deborah Haas-Wilson, Mark A. Peterson, et al., eds. *Uncertain Times: Kenneth Arrow and the Changing Economics of Health Care.* Durham, NC: Duke University Press, 2003.

Jacobs, Phillip, and John Rapoport. *The Economics of Health and Medical Care.* 5th ed. Sudbury, MA: Jones and Bartlett, 2004.

Jones, Andrew M., ed. *The Elgar Companion to Health Economics.* Northhampton, MA: Edward Elgar, 2006.

Klarman, H. E. *The Economics of Health.* New York: Columbia University Press, 1965.

Laxminarayan, Ramanan, ed. *Battling Resistance to Antibiotics and Pesticides: An Economic Approach.* Baltimore: Johns Hopkins University Press, 2002.

Lee, Robert H. *Economics for Healthcare Managers.* Chicago: Health Administration Press, 2000.

Marcinko, David E., and Hope R. Hetico, eds. *Dictionary of Health Economics and Finance.* New York: Springer, 2006.

Morreim, E. Haavi. *Balancing Act: The New Medical Ethics of Medicine's New Economics.* Washington, DC: Georgetown University Press, 1995.

Murphy, Kevin M., and Robert H. Topel, eds. *Measuring the Gains From Medical Research.* Chicago: University of Chicago Press, 2003.

Newhouse, Joseph P. *Pricing the Priceless: A Health Care Conundrum.* Cambridge: MIT Press, 2002.

Pizzi, Laura T., and Jennifer H. Lofland, eds. *Economic Evaluation in U.S. Health Care: Principles and Applications.* Sudbury, MA: Jones and Bartlett, 2006.

Rice, Thomas. *The Economics of Health Reconsidered.* 2d ed. Chicago: Health Administration Press/Academy Health, 2003.

Sloan, Frank. *Valuing Health Care.* New York: Cambridge University Press, 1995.

Wise, David A. *Advances in the Economics of Aging.* Chicago: University of Chicago Press, 1996.

Wonderling, David, Reinhold Gruen, and Nick Black. *Introduction to Health Economics.* Maidenhead, UK: Open University Press, 2005.

14. *Competition and Markets*

Arnould, Richard J., Robert F. Rich, and William D. White, eds. *Competitive Approaches to Health Care Reform.* Washington, DC: Urban Institute Press, 1993.

Bovbjerg, R. R., and J. A. Marsteller. *Health Care Market Competition in Six States: Implications for the Poor.* Washington, DC: Urban Institute, 1998.

Cannon, Michael F., and Michael D. Tanner. *Healthy Competition: What's Holding Healthcare Back and How to Free It.* Washington, DC: Cato Institute, 2006.

Casalino, L. P. "Markets and Medicine: Barriers to Creating a 'Business Case for Quality,'" *Perspectives in Biology and Medicine* 46(1): 38–51, Winter 2003.

Chiappori, Pierre-Andre, and Christian Gollier, eds. *Competitive Failure in Insurance Markets: Theory and Policy Implications.* Cambridge: MIT Press, 2006.

Coddington, Dean C., Keith D. Moore, and Elizabeth A. Fischer. *Strategies for the New Health Care Marketplace: Managing the Convergence of Consumerism and Technology.* San Francisco: Jossey-Bass, 2001.

Escarce, Jose J., Arvind K. Jain, and Jeannette Rogowski. *Hospital Competition, Managed Care, and Mortality After Hospitalization for Medical Conditions: Evidence From Three States.* NBER Working Paper No. 12335. Cambridge, MA: National Bureau of Economic Research, 2006.

Federal Trade Commission and the U.S. Department of Justice. *Improving Health Care: A Dose of Competition: A Report by the Federal Trade Commission and the Department of Justice, July, 2004.* Washington, DC: GPO, 2004.

Frech, H. E. *Competition and Monopoly in Medical Care.* Washington, DC: AEI Press, 1996.

Gaynor, Martin. *What Do We Know About Competition and Quality in Health Care Markets?* NBER Working Paper No. 12301. Cambridge, MA: National Bureau of Economic Research, 2006.

Ginzberg, Eli. "The Potential and Limits of Competition in Health Care," *Bulletin of the New York Academy of Medicine* 73(2): 224–36, Winter 1996.

Greenberg, Warren, ed. "Competition in the Health Care Sector: Past, Present, and Future." In *Proceedings of a Conference Sponsored by the Bureau of Economics, Federal Trade Commission (March 1978).* Germantown, MD: Aspen Systems, 1978.

Greenberg, Warren, ed. *Competition, Regulation, and Rationing in Health Care.* Ann Arbor, MI: Health Administration Press, 1991.

Greenberg, Warren, ed. *The Health Care Marketplace.* New York: Springer, 1998.

Institute of Medicine. *Preparing for a Changing Healthcare Marketplace: Lessons From the Field.* The Richard and Hinda Rosenthal Lectures, 1993–1994. Washington, DC: National Academy Press, 1995.

Kessler, Daniel D., and Jeffrey J. Geppert. *The Effects of Competition on Variation in the Quality and Cost of Medical Care.* NBER Working Paper No. 11226. Cambridge, MA: National Bureau of Economic Research, 2006.

Luke, Roice D., Stephen L. Walston, and Patrick Michael Plummer. *Healthcare Strategy: In Pursuit of Competitive Advantage.* Chicago: Health Administration Press, 2003.

McDonough, Mary. *Can a Health Care Market Be Moral: A Catholic Vision.* Washington, DC: Georgetown University Press, 2007.

Musgrave, Frank W. *The Economics of U.S. Health Care Policy: The Role of Market Forces.* Armonk, NY: M. E. Sharpe, 2006.

Ohsfeldt, Robert L., and John E. Schneider. *The Business of Health: The Role of Competition, Markets, and Regulation.* Washington, DC: AEI Press, 2006.

Pauly, Mark V. "Competition in Medical Services and the Quality of Care: Concepts and History," *International Journal of Health Care Finance and Economics* 4(2): 113–30, June 2004.

Peterson, Mark A., ed. *Healthy Markets? The New Competition in Medical Care.* Durham, NC: Duke University Press, 1998.

Porter, Michael E., and Elizabeth Olmsted Teisberg. *Redefining Health Care: Creating Value-Based Competition on Results.* Boston: Harvard Business School Press, 2006.

Robinson, James C. *The Corporate Practice of Medicine: Competition and Innovation in Health Care.* Los Angeles: University of California Press/Milbank Memorial Fund, 1999.

Smith, P. C., ed. *Reforming Markets in Health Care: An Economic Perspective.* State of Health Series. Philadelphia: Open University Press, 2000.

White, William D. "Market Forces, Competitive Strategies, and Health Care Regulation," *University of Illinois Law Review* 1: 137–66, 2004.

Wieners, Walter W., ed. *Global Health Care Markets: A Comprehensive Guide to Regions, Trends, and Opportunities Shaping the International Health Arena.* San Francisco: Jossey-Bass, 2000.

Zuckerman, Alan M. *Improve Your Competitive Strategy: A Guide for the Healthcare Executive.* Chicago: Health Administration Press, 2002.

Zuckerman, Alan M., and Russell C. Coile. *Competing on Excellence: Healthcare Strategies for a Consumer-Driven Market.* Chicago: Health Administration Press, 2003.

15. *Cost-Benefit and Cost-Effectiveness Analysis*

Brent, Robert J., ed. *Cost-Benefit Analysis and Health Care Evaluation.* Northampton, MA: Edward Elgar, 2003.

Drummond, Michael F., and Alistair McGuire, eds. *Economic Evaluation in Health Care: Merging Theory With Practice.* New York: Oxford University Press, 2002.

Drummond, Michael F., Mark J. Sculpher, George W. Torrance, et al., eds. *Methods for the Economic Evaluation of Health Care Programmes.* 3d ed. New York: Oxford University Press, 2005.

Haddix, Anne C., Steven M. Teutsch, and Phaedra S. Corso, eds. *Prevention Effectiveness: A Guide to Decision Analysis and Economic Evaluation.* New York: Oxford University Press, 2002.

Harwood, Henrick J. *Cost Effectiveness and Cost Benefit Analysis of Substance Abuse Treatment: A Bibliography.* Rockville, MD: Substance Abuse and Mental Health Services Administration, Center for Substance Abuse Treatment, 2002.

Harwood, Henrick J. *Cost Effectiveness and Cost Benefit Analysis of Substance Abuse Treatment: A Literature Review.* Rockville, MD: Substance Abuse and Mental Health Services Administration, Center for Substance Abuse Treatment, 2002.

Miller, Wilhelmine, Lisa A. Robinson, and Robert S. Lawrence, eds. *Valuing Health for Regulatory Cost-Effectiveness Analysis.* Washington, DC: National Academies Press, 2006.

Morris, Stephen, Nancy J. Devlin, and David Parkin. *Economic Analysis in Health Care.* Hoboken, NJ: Wiley, 2007.

Muennig, Peter. *Designing and Conducting Cost-Effectiveness Analyses in Medicine and Health Care.* San Francisco: Jossey-Bass, 2002.

Neumann, Peter J. *Using Cost-Effectiveness Analysis to Improve Health Care: Opportunities and Barriers.* New York: Oxford University Press, 2005.

Olsen, Jan Abel, and Jeffrey Ralph James Richardson. *Production Gains From Health Care: What Should Be Included in Cost-Effectiveness Analysis.* West Heidelberg, Victoria, Australia: National Centre for Health Program Evaluation, 1999.

Petitti, Diana B. *Meta-Analysis, Decision Analysis, and Cost-Effectiveness Analysis.* 2d ed. New York: Oxford University Press, 1999.

Sloan, Frank A., and Chee-Ruey Hsieh, eds. *Pharmaceutical Innovation: Incentives, and Cost-Benefit Analysis in International Perspective.* New York: Cambridge University Press, 2007.

Willan, Andrew R., and Andrew H. Briggs. *Statistical Analysis of Cost-Effectiveness Data.* San Francisco: Jossey-Bass, 2006.

16. *Cost of Healthcare and Illness*

Akobundu, E., J. Ju, L. Blatt, et al. "Cost-of-Illness Studies: A Review of Current Methods," *Pharmacoeconomics* 24(9): 869–90, 2006.

Australian Institute of Health and Welfare. *Health Care Expenditure and the Burden of Disease Due to Asthma in Australia.* Canberra, Australian Capital Territory, Australia: Australian Institute of Health and Welfare, 2005.

Bodenheimer, Thomas. "High and Rising Health Care Costs. Part 1: Seeking an Explanation," *Annals of Internal Medicine* 142(10): 847–54, May 17, 2005.

Bodenheimer, Thomas. "High and Rising Health Care Costs. Part 2: Technologic Innovation," *Annals of Internal Medicine* 142(11): 932–37, June 7, 2005.

Bodenheimer, Thomas. "High and Rising Health Care Costs. Part 3: The Role of Health Care Providers," *Annals of Internal Medicine* 142(12): 996–1002, June 21, 2005.

Bodenheimer, Thomas, and Alicia Fernandez. "High and Rising Health Care Costs. Part 4: Can Costs Be Controlled While Preserving Quality?" *Annals of Internal Medicine* 143(1): 26–31, July 5, 2005.

17. *Developing Countries*

Baah, Asamoah. *Health Economics: Identification of Needs in Health Economics in Developing Countries.* Geneva, Switzerland: WHO Task Force on Health Economics, 1995.

Carrin, Guy. *The Role of Health Economics in Developing Countries, With a Focus on Project Evaluation and Health*

Care Finance. Antwerp, Belgium: University of Antwerp, Centre for Development Studies, 1986.

Jamison, Dean T., Joel G. Bremen, Anthony R. Measham, et al., eds. *Disease Control Priorities in Developing Countries*. 2d ed. New York: Oxford University Press, 2006.

Mills, Anne, and Kenneth Lee, eds. *Health Economics Research in Developing Countries*. New York: Oxford University Press, 1993.

Preker, Alexander S., Richard M. Scheffler, and Mark C. Bassett, eds. *Private Voluntary Health in Development: Friend or Foe?* Washington, DC: World Bank, 2007.

Sorkin, Alan L. *Health Economics in Developing Countries*. Lexington, MA: Heath, 1976.

William, Jack. *Principles of Health Economics for Developing Countries*. Washington, DC: World Bank, 1999.

18. *Healthcare Financial Management*

Aaron, Henry J. *Serious and Unstable Condition: Financing America's Health Care*. Washington, DC: Brookings Institution Press, 1991.

Baker, Judith J., and R. W. Baker. *Health Care Finance: Basic Tools for Nonfinancial Managers*. 2d ed. Sudbury, MA: Jones and Bartlett, 2006.

Berger, Steven. *Fundamentals of Health Care Financial Management: A Practical Guide to Fiscal Issues and Activities*. 2d ed. San Francisco: Jossey-Bass, 2002.

Berger, Steven. *The Power of Clinical and Financial Metrics: Achieving Success in Your Hospital*. Chicago: Health Administration Press, 2005.

Cleverley, William O., and Andrew E. Cameron. *Essentials of Health Care Finance*. 6th ed. Sudbury, MA: Jones and Bartlett, 2006.

Committee on Public Financing and Delivery of HIV Care, Board on Health Promotion and Disease Prevention, Institute of Medicine. *Public Financing and Delivery of HIV/AIDS Care: Securing the Legacy of Ryan White*. Washington, DC: National Academies Press, 2004.

Donaldson, Cam, Karen Gerard, Stephen Jan, et al. *Economics of Health Care Financing: The Visible Hand*. 2d ed. New York: Palgrave Macmillan, 2005.

Eastaugh, Steven R. *Health Care Finance and Economics*. Sudbury, MA: Jones and Bartlett, 2004.

Finkler, Steven A., and David M. Ward. *Accounting Fundamentals for Health Care Management*. Sudbury, MA: Jones and Bartlett, 2006.

Finkler, Steven A., David M. Ward, and Judith J. Baker. *Essentials of Cost Accounting for Healthcare Organizations*. 3d ed. Sudbury, MA: Jones and Bartlett, 2007.

Gapenski, Louis C. *Healthcare Finance: An Introduction to Accounting and Financial Management*. 3d ed. Chicago: Health Administration Press, 2004.

Gapenski, Louis C. *Cases in Healthcare Finance*. 3d ed. Chicago: Health Administration Press, 2005.

Gapenski, Louis C., and George H. Pink. *Understanding Healthcare Financial Management*. 5th ed. Chicago: Health Administration Press, 2006.

Hankins, Robert W., and Judith J. Baker. *Management Accounting for Health Care Organizations: Tools and Techniques for Decision Support*. Sudbury, MA: Jones and Bartlett, 2004.

Kaufman, Kenneth. *Best Practice Financial Management: Six Key Concepts for Healthcare Leaders*. 3d ed. Chicago: Health Administration Press, 2006.

Nowicki, Michael. *The Financial Management of Hospitals and Healthcare Organizations*. 3d ed. Chicago: Health Administration Press and the Healthcare Financial Management Association, 2004.

Nowicki, Michael. *Practice Problems and Case Study to Accompany the Financial Management of Hospitals and Healthcare Organizations*. 3d ed. Chicago: Health Administration Press, 2004.

Nowicki, Michael. *HFMA's Introduction to Hospital Accounting*. 5th ed. Chicago: Health Administration Press and the Healthcare Financial Management Association, 2006.

Pointer, Dennis D., and Dennis M. Stillman. *Essentials of Health Care Organization Finance: A Primer for Board Members*. San Francisco: Jossey-Bass, 2004.

Wang, XiaoHu. *Financial Management in the Public Sector*. Armonk, NY: M. E. Sharpe, 2006.

Wiener, Joshua M., Steven B. Clauser, and David L. Kennell, eds. *Persons With Disabilities: Issues in Health Care Financing and Service Delivery*. Washington, DC: Brookings Institution, 1995.

Young, David W. *Management Accounting in Health Care Organizations*. San Francisco: Jossey-Bass, 2003.

19. *International Comparisons*

Aaron, Henry J., William B. Schwartz, and Melissa Cox. *Can We Say No? The Challenge of Rationing Health Care*. Washington, DC: Brookings Institution Press, 2005.

Decker, Sandra L., and Dahlia K. Remler. *How Much Might Universal Health Insurance Reduce Socioeconomic Disparities in Health? A Comparison of the U.S. and Canada*. NBER Working Paper No. 10715. Cambridge, MA: National Bureau of Economic Research, 2004.

Roth, Julius A., ed. *International Comparisons of Health Services*. Greenwich, CT: JAI Press, 1987.

Wise, David A., and Naohiro Yashiro, eds. *Health Care Issues in the United States and Japan*. National Bureau of Economic Research Conference Report (NBER-C). Chicago: University of Chicago Press, 2006.

20. *Payment Mechanisms*

Abood, Sheila, and David Keepnews. *Understanding Payment for Advanced Practice Nursing Services*. Washington, DC: American Nurses Publishing, 2002.

Carter, Lucy R., and Sara S. Lankford. *Physician's Compensation: Measurement, Benchmarking, and Implementation*. New York: Wiley, 2000.

Committee on Redesigning Health Insurance Performance Measures, Payment, and Performance Improvement Programs, Board on Health Care Services, Institute of Medicine. *Rewarding Provider Performance: Aligning Incentives in Medicare*. Washington, DC: National Academies Press, 2007.

Kling, Arnold. *Crisis of Abundance: Rethinking How We Pay for Health Care*. Washington, DC: Cato Institute, 2006.

Mays, Rick, and Robert A. Berenson. *Medicare Prospective Payment and the Shaping of U.S. Health Care*. Baltimore: Johns Hopkins University Press, 2006.

Miraldo, Marisa, Maria Goddard, and Peter C. Smith. *The Incentive Effects of Payment by Results*. CHE Research Paper 19. York, UK: University of York, Centre for Health Economics, 2006.

Moreno, Jonathan D. *Paying the Doctor: Health Policy and Physician Reimbursement*. New York: Auburn House, 1991.

Newhouse, Joseph P. "Medicare's Challenges in Paying Providers," *Health Care Financing Review* 27(2): 35–44, Winter 2005–2006.

Sood, Neeraji, Melinda Beeuwkes Buntin, and Jose J. Escarce. *Does How Much and How You Pay Matter?* NBER Working Paper No. 12556. Evidence From the Inpatient Rehabilitation Care Prospective Payment System. Cambridge, MA: National Bureau of Economic Research, 2006.

U.S. Congressional Budget Office. *Medicare's Physician Payment Rates and the Sustainable Growth Rate*. Statement of Donald B. Marron, Acting Director, Before the Subcommittee on Health, Committee on Energy and Commerce, U.S. House of Representatives. Washington, DC: U.S. Congressional Budget Office, 2006.

U.S. Congressional Budget Office. *The Sustainable Growth Rate Formula for Setting Medicare's Physician Payment Rates*. Washington, DC: U.S. Congressional Budget Office, 2006.

Vogenberg, F. Randy, ed. *Understanding Pharmacy Reimbursement*. Bethesda, MD: American Society of Health-System Pharmacists, 2006.

Waters, Joanne M., and L. Lamar Blount. *Mastering the Reimbursement Process*. 4th ed. Chicago: American Medical Association, 2006.

21. *Supply and Demand*

Esposito, Domenico. *Copayments and the Demand for Prescription Drugs*. New York: Routledge, 2006.

Grossman, Michael. *The Demand for Health: A Theoretical and Empirical Investigation*. New York: Columbia University Press, 1972.

Kissick, William. *Medicine's Dilemmas: Infinite Needs Versus Finite Resources*. New Haven, CT: Yale University Press, 1994.

Patrick, Donald L., and Pennifer Erickson. *Health Status and Health Policy: Quality of Life in Health Evaluation and Resource Allocation*. New York: Oxford University Press, 1993.

Richardson, Jeffrey Ralph James. *Supply and Demand for Medical Care: Or, Is the Health Care Market Perverse?* West Heidelberg, Victoria, Australia: National Centre for Health Program Evaluation, 2001.

Richardson, Jeffrey Ralph James, and Stuart Peacock. *Supplier Induced Demand Reconsidered*. West Heidelberg, Victoria, Australia: National Centre for Health Program Evaluation, 1999.

IV. Quality of Healthcare

Quality of healthcare can have different meanings for different people, including healthcare providers, payers, and patients. Generally speaking, quality of healthcare refers to receiving the appropriate amount of care at the right time and in the right amount.

22. *General Works*

Adams, Karen, and Janet M. Corrigan, eds., and Committee on Identifying Priority Areas for Quality Improvement, Board on Health Care Services, Institute of Medicine. *Priority Areas for National Action: Transforming Health Care Quality*. Washington, DC: National Academies Press, 2003.

Agency for Healthcare Research and Quality. *The National Healthcare Quality Report*. Rockville, MD: Agency for Healthcare Research and Quality, 2005. (This is an annual report)

Asch, S. M., E. A. Kerr, J. Keesey, et al. "Who Is at Greatest Risk for Receiving Poor-Quality Health Care?" *New England Journal of Medicine* 354(11): 1147–56, March 16, 2006.

Berwick, Donald M. *Escape Fire: Designs for the Future of Health Care*. San Francisco: Jossey-Bass, 2003.

Berwick, Donald M., A. Blanton Godfray, and Jane Rosessner. *Curing Health Care: New Strategies for Quality Improvement*. San Francisco: Jossey-Bass, 1990.

Bisognano, Maureen A., Paul E. Plsek, and Dan Schummers. *10 More Powerful Ideas for Improving Patient Care*. Chicago: Health Administration Press, 2005.

Bosk, Charles L. *Forgive and Remember: Managing Medical Failure*. 2d ed. Chicago: University of Chicago Press, 2003.

Brennan, Troyen A., and Donald M. Berwick. *New Rules: Regulation, Markets, and the Quality of American Health Care*. San Francisco: Jossey-Bass, 1995.

Donabedian, Avedis. "Evaluating the Quality of Medical Care." In *Health Services Research*, vol. 1, edited by D. Mainland, 166–203. New York: Milbank Memorial Fund, 1967.

Donabedian, Avedis. *Explorations in Quality Assessment and Monitoring*. Vol. 1, *The Definition of Quality and Approaches to Its Assessment*. Ann Arbor, MI: Health Administration Press, 1980.

Donabedian, Avedis. *Explorations in Quality Assessment and Monitoring*. Vol. 2, *The Criteria and Standards of Quality*. Ann Arbor, MI: Health Administration Press, 1982.

Donabedian, Avedis. *Explorations in Quality Assessment and Monitoring.* Vol. 3, *The Methods and Findings of Quality Assessment and Monitoring: An Illustrated Analysis.* Ann Arbor, MI: Health Administration Press, 1985.

Donabedian, Avedis. "The Quality of Care: How Can It Be Assessed?" *Journal of the American Medical Association* 260(12): 1743–48, September 23, 1988.

Donabedian, Avedis. *An Introduction to Quality Assurance in Health Care.* New York: Oxford University Press, 2002.

Donaldson, Molla S., ed., and National Roundtable on Health Care Quality, Division of Health Care Services, Institute of Medicine. *Collaboration Among Competing Managed Care Organizations for Quality Improvement: Summary of a Conference, November 13, 1997.* Washington, DC: National Academy Press, 1999.

Fottler, Myron D., Robert C. Ford, and Cherrill Heaton. *Achieving Service Excellence: Strategies for Healthcare.* Chicago: Health Administration Press, 2002.

Gawande, Atul. *Complications: A Surgeon's Notes on Imperfect Science.* New York: Picador, 2002.

Goonan, Kathleen Jennison. *The Juran Prescription: Clinical Quality Management.* San Francisco: Jossey-Bass, 1995.

Halvorson, George C., and George J. Isham. *Epidemic of Care: A Call for Safe, Better, and More Accountable Health Care.* San Francisco: Jossey-Bass, 2003.

Hurtado, Margarita P., Elaine K. Swift, and Janet M. Corrigan, eds., and Committee on the National Quality Report on Health Care Delivery, Board on Health Care Services, Institute of Medicine. *Envisioning the National Health Care Quality Report.* Washington, DC: National Academy Press, 2000.

Institute of Medicine. *Crossing the Quality Chasm: A New Health System for the 21st Century.* Washington, DC: National Academies Press, 2001.

Institute of Medicine. *Fostering Rapid Advances in Health Care: Learning From System Demonstration.* Washington, DC: National Academies Press, 2002.

Institute of Medicine. *Health Professions Education: A Bridge to Quality.* Washington, DC: National Academies Press, 2003.

Institute of Medicine. *Next Steps Toward Higher Quality Health Care.* The Richard and Hinda Rosenthal Lectures, 2005. Washington, DC: National Academies Press, 2006.

Isenberg, Steven F., and Richard E. Gliklich, eds. *Profiting From Quality: Outcomes Strategies for Medical Practice.* San Francisco: Jossey-Bass, 1999.

Kelly, Diane L. *Applying Quality Management in Healthcare: A Systems Approach.* 2d ed. Chicago: Association of University Programs in Health Administration and the Health Administration Press, 2006.

Lloyd, Robert. *Quality Health Care: A Guide to Developing and Using Indicators.* Sudbury, MA: Jones and Bartlett, 2004.

McGlynn E. A., S. M. Asch, J. Adams, et al. "The Quality of Health Care Delivered to Adults in the United States," *New England Journal of Medicine* 348(26): 2635–45, June 26, 2003.

Mechanic, David. "Improving the Quality of Health Care in the United States of America: The Need for a Multi-Level Approach," *Journal of Health Services Research and Policy* 7(3 Suppl. 1): 35–39, July 2002.

Millenson, Michael L. *Demanding Medical Excellence: Doctors and Accountability in the Information Age.* Chicago: University of Chicago Press, 2002.

Montalvo, Isis, and Nancy Dunton, eds. *Transforming Nursing Data Into Quality Care: Profiles of Quality Improvement in U.S. Healthcare Facilities.* Silver Spring, MD: American Nurses Association, 2007. (Available at http://nursingworld.org)

Nelson, Eugene C., Paul B. Batalden, and Marjorie M. Godfrey. *Quality by Design: A Clinical Microsystem Approach.* San Francisco: Jossey-Bass, 2007.

Ransom, Scott B., Maulik S. Joshi, and David B. Nash, eds. *The Healthcare Quality Book: Vision, Strategy, and Tools.* Chicago: Health Administration Press, 2004.

Reinertsen, James L., and Wim Schellekens. *10 Powerful Ideas for Improving Patient Care.* Chicago: Health Administration Press, 2005.

Sherman, V. Clayton. *Raising Standards in American Health Care: Best People, Best Practices, Best Results.* San Francisco: Jossey-Bass, 1999.

Spath, Patrice L. *Leading Your Healthcare Organization to Excellence: A Guide to Using the Baldrige Criteria.* Chicago: Health Administration Press, 2004.

Walburg, Jan, ed. *Performance Management in Health Care: Improving Patient Outcomes: An Integrated Approach.* New York: Routledge, 2006.

23. Benchmarking and Comparative Data

Barnard, Cynthia. *Benchmarking Basics: A Resource Guide for Healthcare Managers.* Marblehead, MA: HCPro, 2006.

Camp, Robert C. *Benchmarking: The Search for Industry Best Practices That Lead to Superior Performance.* Milwaukee, WI: American Society for Quality Press, 1989.

Carter, Lucy R., and Sara S. Lankford. *Physician's Compensation: Measurement, Benchmarking, and Implementation.* New York: Wiley, 2000.

Center for Substance Abuse Treatment. *Medicaid Managed Behavioral Health Care Benchmarking Project.* Rockville, MD: U.S. Department of Health and Human Services, Substance Abuse and Mental Health Services Administration, Center for Substance Abuse Treatment, 2003.

Joint Commission on Accreditation of Healthcare Organizations. *Benchmarking in Health Care: Finding and Implementing Best Practices.* Oakbrook Terrance, IL: Joint Commission on Accreditation of Healthcare Organizations, 2000.

Schilp, Jull Lenk, and Roy E. Gilbreath. *Health Data Quest: How to Find and Use Data for Performance Improvement.* San Francisco: Jossey-Bass, 2000.

Tweet, Arthur G., and Karol Gavin-Marciano. *The Guide to Benchmarking in Healthcare: Practical Lessons From the Field.* New York: Quality Resources, 1998.

24. Clinical Practice Guidelines and Disease Management

Bartell, Jessica, and Maureen Smith. "U.S. Physicians' Perceptions of the Effect of Practice Guidelines and Ability to Provide High-Quality Care," *Journal of Health Services Research and Policy* 10(2): 69–76, April 2005.

Disease Management Association of America. *Dictionary of Disease Management Terminology: Including Extended Definitions of Frequently-Used Disease Management Terminology.* Washington, DC: Disease Management Association of America, 2004.

Eccles, M., N. Rousseau, and N. Freemantle. "Updating Evidence-Based Clinical Guidelines," *Journal of Health Services Research and Policy* 7(2): 98–103, April 2002.

Forman, Samuel, and Matthew Kelliher. *Status One: Breakthroughs in High Risk Population Health Management.* San Francisco: Jossey-Bass, 1999.

Hewitt-Taylor, Jaqui. *Clinical Guidelines and Care Protocols.* Hoboken, NJ: Wiley, 2006.

Howe, Rufus S. *The Disease Manager's Handbook.* Sudbury, MA: Jones and Bartlett, 2005.

Huber, Diane L., ed. *Disease Management: A Guide for Case Managers.* St. Louis, MO: Elsevier Saunders, 2005.

Margolis, Carmi Z., and Shan Cretin, eds. *Implementing Clinical Practice Guidelines.* Chicago: American Hospital Association, 1999.

McManus, Carolyn A. *Group Wellness Programs for Chronic Pain and Disease Management.* St. Louis, MO: Butterworth-Heinemann, 2003.

Muncey, Tessa, and Alison Parker, eds. *Chronic Disease Management: A Practical Guide.* New York: Palgrave, 2002.

National Governors' Association. *Disease Management: The New Tool for Cost Containment and Quality Care.* Washington, DC: National Governors' Association, Center for Best Practices, Health Policy Studies Division, 2003.

Nuovo, Jim, ed. *Chronic Disease Management.* New York: Springer, 2007.

Patterson, Richard, ed. *Changing Patient Behavior: Improving Outcomes in Health and Disease Management.* San Francisco: Jossey-Bass, 2001.

Randall, Michael D., and Karen E. Neil. *Disease Management.* Chicago: Pharmaceutical Press, 2003.

Skolnik, Neil S., Doron Schneider, Richard Neill, et al., eds. *Handbook of Essential Practice Guidelines in Primary Care.* Totowa, NJ: Humana Press, 2007.

Todd, Warren E., and David Nash. *Disease Management: A Systems Approach to Improving Patient Outcomes.* San Francisco: Jossey-Bass, 2001.

U.S. Congressional Budget Office. *An Analysis of the Literature on Disease Management Programs.* Washington, DC: U.S. Congressional Budget Office, 2004.

Wakley, Gill, and Ruth Chambers, eds. *Chronic Disease Management in Primary Care: Quality and Outcomes.* Seattle, WA: Radcliffe, 2005.

25. Decision Making and Clinical Support Systems

Ankner, Gina M. *Clinical Decision Making: Case Studies in Medical-Surgical Nursing.* Clifton Park, NY: Thomson Delmar Learning, 2007.

Berner, Eta S., ed. *Clinical Decision Support Systems: Theory and Practice.* 2d ed. New York: Springer, 2007.

Eeckhoudt, Louis. *Risk and Medical Decision Making.* Boston: Kluwer Academic, 2002.

Flynn, Darren, et al. *Non-Medical Influences Upon Medical Decision Making and Referral Behavior: An Annotated Bibliography.* Westport, CT: Praeger, 2003.

Freeman, Michael, ed. *Ethics and Medical Decision-Making.* Burlington, VT: Ashgate-Dartmouth, 2001.

Gross, Richard. *Making Medical Decisions: An Approach to Clinical Decision Making for Practicing Physicians.* Philadelphia: American College of Medicine, 1999.

Mack, Ken E., Mary Ann Crawford, and Mary C. Reed. *Decision Making for Improved Performance.* Chicago: Health Administration Press, 2004.

Oster, Nancy, Lucy Thomas, and Doral Joseff. *Making Informed Medical Decisions: Where to Look and How to Use What You Find.* Cambridge, MA: O'Reilly, 2000.

Parmigiani, Giovanni. *Modeling in Medical Decision Making: A Bayesian Approach.* New York: Wiley, 2002.

Rao, Goutham. *Rational Medical Decision Making.* New York: McGraw-Hill, 2007.

Richardson, Betty Kehl. *Clinical Decision Making: Case Studies in Psychiatric Nursing.* Clifton Park, NY: Thomson Delmar Learning, 2007.

Robinson, Denise L. *Clinical Decision Making: A Case Study Approach.* 2d ed. Philadelphia: Lippincott, 2002.

Rothman, David J. *Strangers at the Bedside: A History of How Law and Bioethics Transformed Medical Decision Making.* 2d ed. New York: Aldine de Gruyter, 2003.

26. Evidence-Based Medicine (EBM)

Bland, J. Martin, and Janet Peacock. *Statistical Questions in Evidence-Based Medicine.* New York: Oxford University Press, 2000.

Best Practices: Evidence-Based Nursing Procedures. 2d ed. Philadelphia: Lippincott Williams and Wilkins, 2007.

Boswell, Carol, and Sharon Cannon. *Introduction to Nursing Research: Incorporating Evidence-Based Practice.* Sudbury, MA: Jones and Bartlett, 2007.

Daly, Jeanne. *Evidence-Based Medicine and the Search for a Science of Clinical Care.* Berkeley: University of California Press/Milbank Memorial Fund, 2005.

Gray, Denis Pereira. "Evidence-Based Medicine and Patient-Centered Medicine: The Need to Harmonize," *Journal of Health Services Research and Policy* 10(2): 66–68, April 2005.

Gray, J. A. Muir. *Evidence-Based Healthcare: How to Make Health Policy and Management Decisions.* 2d ed. New York: Churchill Livingstone, 2001.

Greenhalgh, Trisha. *How to Read a Paper: The Basics of Evidence-Based Medicine.* 3d ed. Malden, MA: BMJ Books/ Blackwell, 2006.

Levin, Rona F., and Harriet R. Feldman, eds. *Teaching Evidence-Based Practice in Nursing: A Guide for Academic and Clinical Settings.* New York: Springer, 2006.

Melnyk, Bernadette M., and Ellen Fineout-Overholt. *Evidence-Based Practice in Nursing and Healthcare: A Guide to Best Practice.* Philadelphia: Lippincott Williams and Wilkins, 2005.

Newell, Robert, and Philip Burnard. *Research for Evidence-Based Practice.* Malden, MA: Blackwell, 2006.

Nordenstrom, Jorgen. *Evidence-Based Medicine in Sherlock Holmes' Footsteps.* Malden, MA: Blackwell, 2007.

Pearson, Alan, John Field, and Zoe Jordon. *Evidence-Based Clinical Medicine in Nursing and Health Care: Assimilating Research, Experience, and Expertise.* Malden, MA: Blackwell, 2007.

Roberts, Albert R., and Kenneth R. Yeager, eds. *Evidence-Based Practice Manual: Research and Outcome Measures in Health and Human Services.* New York: Oxford University Press, 2003.

Sackett, David L., Sharon E. Straus, W. Scott Richardson, et al. *Evidence-Based Medicine: How to Practice and Teach EBM.* 2d ed. London: Churchill Livingstone, 2000.

Sackett, David L., William M. C. Rosenberg, J. A. Muir Gray, et al. "Evidence-Based Medicine: What It Is and What It Isn't," *British Medical Journal* 312(7023): 71–72, January 13, 1996.

Stanzak, Richard K. *Bottom Line Medicine: A Layman's Guide to Evidence-Based Medicine.* New York: Algora, 2006.

Wulff, Henrik R., and Peter C. Gotzsche. *Rational Diagnosis and Treatment: Evidence-Based Clinical Decision-Making.* Malden, MA: Blackwell Science, 2000.

27. Health Literacy and Communication

Bennett, Peter, and Kenneth Calman. *Risk Communication and Public Health.* New York: Oxford University Press, 1999.

Cohn, Kenneth H. *Better Communication for Better Care: Mastering Physician–Administrator Collaboration.* Chicago: Health Administration Press, 2005.

Desmond, Joanne, and Lanny R. Copeland. *Communication With Today's Patient: Essentials to Save Time, Decrease Risk, and Increase Patient Compliance.* San Francisco: Jossey-Bass, 2000.

Greene, Jessica, Judith Hibbard, and Martin Tusler. *How Much Do Health Literacy and Patient Activation Contribute to Older Adult's Ability to Manage Their Health?* Washington, DC: AARP, 2005.

Haider, Muhiuddin. *Global Public Health Communication: Challenges, Perspectives, and Strategies.* Sudbury, MA: Jones and Bartlett, 2005.

Hibbard, Judith, Jessica Greene, and Martin Tusler. *Identifying Medicare Beneficiaries With Poor Health Literacy Skills: Is a Short Screening Index Feasible?* Washington, DC: AARP, 2005.

Kickbusch, Ilona, Suzanne Wait, and Daniela Maag. *Navigating Health: The Role of Health Literacy.* London: International Longevity Centre, Alliance for Health and the Future, 2005.

Kiefer, Kristen M. *Health Literacy: Responding to the Need for Help.* Washington, DC: Center for Medicare Education, 2001.

Kraemer, Helena Chmura, Karen Kraemer Lowe, and David J. Kupfer. *To Your Health: How to Understand What Research Tells Us About Risk.* New York: Oxford University Press, 2005.

Mayer, Gloria G., and Michael Villaire. *Health Literacy in Primary Care: A Clinician's Guide.* New York: Springer, 2007.

Nielsen-Bohlman, Lynn, Allison M. Panzer, and David A. Kindig, eds., and Committee on Health Literacy, Board on Neuroscience and Behavioral Health, Institute of Medicine. *Health Literacy: A Prescription to End Confusion.* Washington, DC: National Academies Press, 2004.

Osborne, Helen. *Health Literacy From A to Z: Practical Ways to Communicate Your Health Message.* Sudbury, MA: Jones and Bartlett, 2005.

Ray, Eileen Berlin, ed. *Health Communication in Practice: A Case Study Approach.* Mahwah, NJ: Lawrence Erlbaum, 2005.

Schwartzberg, Jonathan B., Jonathan Van Geest, and Claire Wang, eds. *Understanding Health Literacy: Implications for Medicine and Public Health.* Chicago: American Medical Association, 2005.

Thomas, Richard K. *Health Communication.* New York: Springer, 2006.

Whitten, Pam, and David Cook. *Understanding Health Communication Technologies.* San Francisco: Jossey-Bass, 2004.

Woods, James R., and Fay A. Rozovsky. *What Do I Say? Communicating Intended or Unanticipated Outcomes in Obstetrics.* San Francisco: Jossey-Bass, 2003.

Zarcadoolas, Christina, Andrew F. Pleasant, and David S. Geer. *Advancing Health Literacy: A Framework for Understanding and Action.* San Francisco: Jossey-Bass, 2006.

28. Health Report Cards

Atlantic Information Services. *Health Care Report Cards: Profiles of All Major Report Cards, Performance Reports, Shopping Guide, and Consumer Satisfaction Surveys.* 3d ed. Washington, DC: Atlantic Information Services, 1997.

Chernew, Michael, Gautam Gowrisankaran, and Dennis P. Scanlon. *Learning and the Value of Information: The Case of Health Plan Report Cards.* NBER Working Paper No. 8589. Cambridge, MA: National Bureau of Economic Research, 2001.

Committee on Redesigning Health Insurance Performance Measures, Payment, and Performance Improvement Programs, Board on Health Care Services, Institute of Medicine. *Performance Measurement: Accelerating Improvement. Pathways to Quality Health Care.* Washington, DC: National Academies Press, 2005.

Dafny, Leemore S., and David Dranove. *Do Report Cards Tell Consumers Anything They Don't Already Know? The Case of Medicare HMOs*. NBER Working Paper No. 11420. Cambridge, MA: National Bureau of Economic Research, 2005.

Dranove, David, Daniel Kessler, Mark McClellan, et al. *Is More Information Better? The Effects of "Report Cards" on Health Care Providers*. NBER Working Paper 8697. Cambridge, MA: National Bureau of Economic Research, 2002.

Ferris, Timothy G., Denise Dougherty, David Blumenthal, et al. "A Report Card on Quality Improvement for Children's Health Care," *Pediatrics* 107(1): 143–55, January 2001.

Fielding, Jonathan E., and Carol Sutherland. *National Directory of Community Health Report Cards*. Chicago: Health Research and Educational Trust, 1998.

Hanes, Pamela P., and Merwyn R. Greenlick. *Grading Health Care: The Science and Art of Developing Consumer Scorecards*. San Francisco: Jossey-Bass, 1998.

Kenkel, Paul J. *Report Cards: What Every Health Provider Needs to Know About HEDIS and Other Performance Measures*. Gaithersburg, MD: Aspen, 1995.

Laschober, Mary. *Hospital Compare Highlights Potential Challenges in Public Reporting for Hospitals*. Princeton, NJ: Mathematica Policy Research, 2006.

Marshall, M., and H. Davies. "Public Release of Information on Quality of Care: How Are Health Services and the Public Expected to Respond?" *Journal of Health Services Research and Policy* 6(3): 158–62, July 2001.

Mukamel, D. B., and A. I. Mushlin. "The Impact of Quality Report Cards on Choice of Physicians, Hospitals, and HMOs: A Midcourse Evaluation," *Joint Commission Journal of Quality Improvement* 27(1): 20–27, January 2001.

New York State Health Accountability Foundation. *New York State HMO Report Card*. New York: New York State Health Accountability Foundation, 2004.

"The Public Uses Health System Report Cards to Make Decisions About Their Health Care," *Journal of Health Services Research and Policy* 10(2): 126–27, April 2005.

RAND Corporation. *The First National Report Card on Quality of Health Care in America. RAND Health Research Highlights*. Santa Monica, CA: RAND Corporation, 2006.

Spath, Patrice L., ed. *Provider Report Cards: A Guide for Promoting Health Care Quality to the Public*. San Francisco: Jossey-Bass, 1999.

U.S. General Accounting Office. *Physician Performance: Report Cards Under Development but Challenges Remain: Report to Congressional Requesters*. Washington, DC: U.S. General Accounting Office, 1999.

29. Medical Errors

Aspden, Philip, Julie A. Wolcott, J. Lyle Bootman, et al., eds., and Committee on Identifying and Preventing Medication Errors, Board on Health Care Services, Institute of Medicine. *Preventing Medication Errors*. Washington, DC: National Academies Press, 2006.

Banja, John. *Medical Errors and Medical Narcissism*. Sudbury, MA: Jones and Bartlett, 2005.

Berlinger, Nancy. *After Harm: Medical Error and the Ethics of Forgiveness*. Baltimore: Johns Hopkins University Press, 2005.

Bogner, Marilyn Sue, ed. *Human Error in Medicine*. Mahwah, NJ: Lawrence Erlbaum, 1994.

Dhillon, B. S. *Human Reliability and Error in Medical System*. River Edge, NJ: World Scientific, 2003.

Gibson, Rosemary, and Janardan P. Singh. *Wall of Silence: The Untold Story of the Medical Mistakes That Kill and Injure Millions of Americans*. Washington, DC: LifeLine Press, 2003.

Kohn, Linda T., Janet M. Corrigan, and Molla S. Donaldson, eds., and Committee on Quality of Health Care in America. *To Err Is Human: Building a Safer Health System*. Washington, DC: National Academies Press, 2000.

Kralewski, John, and Bryan E. Dowd. *Drug Errors in Medical Practice: It's Dangerous Out There*. Minneapolis: University of Minnesota, Division of Health Services Research and Policy, 2005.

Merry, Allan, and Alexander McCall Smith. *Errors, Medicine, and the Law*. New York: Cambridge University Press, 2003.

Rosenthal, Marilynn M., and Kathleen M Sutcliffe, eds. *Medical Error: What Do We Know? What Do We Do?* San Francisco: Jossey-Bass, 2002.

Rubin, Susan B., and Laurie Zoloth, eds. *Margin of Error: The Ethics of Mistakes in the Practice of Medicine*. Hagertown, MD: University Publishing Group, 2000.

Sharon, Thomas A. *Protecting Yourself in the Hospital: Insider Tips for Avoiding Hospital Mistakes for Yourself or Someone You Love*. New York: McGraw-Hill, 2004.

Spath, Patrice L., ed. *Error Reduction in Health Care: A System Approach to Improving Patient Safety*. San Francisco: Jossey-Bass, 2000.

Wachter, Robert, and Kaveh G. Shojania. *Internal Bleeding: The Truth Behind America's Terrifying Epidemic of Medical Mistakes*. New York: Rugged Land, 2004.

30. Medical Malpractice

Acerbo-Kozuchowski, Nancy, and Kathleen Ashton. *Medical Malpractice Claims Investigation*. 2d ed. Sudbury, MA: Jones and Bartlett, 2007.

American College of Legal Medicine. *The Medical Malpractice Survival Handbook*. Philadelphia: Mosby-Elsevier, 2007.

Anderson, Richard E., ed. *Medical Malpractice: A Physician's Sourcebook*. Totowa, NJ: Humana Press, 2005.

Baker, Tom. *The Medical Malpractice Myth*. Chicago: University of Chicago Press, 2005.

Black, Carrie E. *Academic Health Centers: Responses to the Malpractice Insurance Crisis*. Washington, DC: Association of Academic Health Centers, 2005.

Sage, William M., and Rogan Kersh, eds. *Medical Malpractice and the U.S. Health Care System*. New York: Cambridge University Press, 2006.

Tan, S. Y. *Medical Malpractice: Understanding the Law, Managing the Risk*. Hackensack, NJ: World Scientific, 2006.

Youngson, Robert M., and Ian Schott. *Medical Blunders: Amazing True Stories of Mad, Bad, and Dangerous Doctors*. New York: New York University Press, 1996.

31. Medical Practice Variations

Andersen, Tavs Folmer, and Gavin Mooney, eds. *Challenges of Medical Practice Variations*. London: Macmillian, 1990.

Ashton, Carol M., Nancy J. Petersen, Julianne Souchek, et al. "Geographic Variations in Utilization Rates in Veterans Affairs Hospitals and Clinics," *New England Journal of Medicine* 340(1): 32–39, January 7, 1999.

Davis, P., B. Gribben, A. Scott, et al. "The 'Supply Hypothesis' and Medical Practice Variation in Primary Care: Testing Economic and Clinical Models of Inter-Practitioner Variation," *Social Science and Medicine* 50(3): 407–418, February 2000.

Dranove, David, and William P. Rogerson. *Geographic Variations in Medical Practice, External Efficiencies, and the Role of Practice Guidelines*. Working Paper 95-15. Evanston, IL: Northwestern University, Center for Urban Affairs and Policy Research, 1995.

Elixhauser, A., D. R. Harris, and R. M. Coffey. *Trends in Hospital Diagnoses: Regional Variations, 1980–87*. Rockville, MD: Agency for Health Care Policy and Research, 1995.

Gold, Marsha. *Geographic Variation in Medicare Per Capita Spending: Should Policy-Makers Be Concerned?* Princeton, NJ: Robert Wood Johnson Foundation, 2004.

Miller, Mark E., John Holahan, and W. Pete Welch. *Geographic Variations in Physician Service Utilization and Implications for Health Reform*. Washington, DC: Urban Institute, Health Policy Center, 1993.

Wennberg, John E., and Megan M. Cooper, eds. *The Dartmouth Atlas of Health Care in the United States, 1998*. Chicago: American Hospital Association Press, 1998.

32. Pain Management

Abrahm, Janet L. *A Physician's Guide to Pain and Symptom Management in Cancer Patients*. 2d ed. Baltimore: Johns Hopkins University Press, 2005.

Bonica, J. J. "History of Pain Concepts and Pain Therapy," *Mount Sinai Journal of Medicine* 58(3): 191–202, May 1991.

Dormandy, Thomas. *The Worst of Evils: The Fight Against Pain*. New Haven, CT: Yale University Press, 2006.

Ferrari, Lynne R., ed. *Anesthesia and Pain Management for the Pediatrician*. Baltimore: Johns Hopkins University Press, 1999.

Grahek, Nikola. *Feeling Pain and Being in Pain*. Cambridge: MIT Press, 2007.

Jay, Gary W., ed. *Chronic Pain*. New York: Informa Healthcare USA, 2007.

Lee, John, and Andrew Baranowski, eds. *Long-Term Pain: A Guide to Practical Management*. New York: Oxford University Press, 2007.

Macintyre, Pamela E., and Stephen A. Schug. *Acute Pain Management: A Practical Guide*. 3d ed. New York: Elsevier Saunders, 2007.

Schofield, Patricia A., ed. *The Management of Pain in Older People*. Hoboken, NJ: Wiley, 2007.

Waldman, Steven D., ed. *Pain Management*. Philadelphia: Saunders/Elsevier, 2007.

33. Patient-Centered Care

Brown, Judith Belle, Moira Stewart, and W. Wayne Weston, eds. *Challenges and Solutions in Patient-Centered Care: A Case Book*. Abingdon, UK: Radcliffe Medical Press, 2002.

Couch, James B., ed. *The Health Care Professional's Guide to Disease Management: Patient-Centered Care for the 21st Century*. Gaithersburg, MD: Aspen, 1998.

Earp, Joanne L., Elizabeth A. French, and Melissa B. Gilkey, eds. *Patient Advocacy for Healthcare Quality: Strategies for Achieving Patient-Centered Care*. Sudbury, MA: Jones and Bartlett, 2007.

Frampton, Susan B., Laura Gilpin, and Patrick A. Charmel, eds. *Putting Patients First: Designing and Practicing Patient-Centered Care*. San Francisco: Jossey-Bass, 2003.

Gerteis, Margaret, Thomas L. Delbanco, and Jennifer Daley, eds. *Through the Patient's Eyes: Understanding and Promoting Patient-Centered Care*. San Francisco: Jossey-Bass, 1993.

Gray, Denis Pereira. "Evidence-Based Medicine and Patient-Centered Medicine: The Need to Harmonize," *Journal of Health Services Research and Policy* 10(2): 66–68, April 2005.

Parsons, Mickey L., and Carolyn L. Murdaugh, eds. *Patient-Centered Care: A Model for Restructuring*. Gaithersburg, MD: Aspen, 1994.

Rantz, Marilyn J., and Marcia K. Flesner. *Person Centered Care: A Model for Nursing Homes*. Washington, DC: American Nurses Association, 2004.

Risner, Phyllis B., Claire Blust Rodehaver, and Robin G. Bashore, eds. *Setting the PACE: Managing Transition to Patient-Centered Care*. Ann Arbor, MI: Health Administration Press, 1995.

Smith, James Monroe, ed. *Producing Patient-Centered Health Care: Patient Perspectives About Health and Illness and the Physician/Patient Relationship*. Westport, CT: Auburn House, 1999.

St. Joseph Hospital. *Patient-Centered Care Manual for the Nursing Service Department, St. Joseph Hospital, Flint, Michigan*. St. Louis, MO: Catholic Hospital Association, 1977.

Stewart, Moira, Judith Belle Brown, W. Wayne Weston, et al., eds. *Patient-Centered Medicine: Transforming the Clinical Method*. 2d ed. Abingdon, UK: Radcliffe Medical Press, 2003.

34. Patient Safety

Aspden, Philip, Janet M. Corrigan, Julie Wolcott, et al., eds., and Committee on Data Standards for Patient Safety, Board on Health Care Services, Institute of Medicine. *Patient Safety: Achieving a New Standard for Care.* Washington, DC: National Academies Press, 2004.

Baciu, Alina, Kathleen Stratton, and Sheila P. Burke, eds., and Committee on the Assessment of the U.S. Drug Safety System, Board on Population Health and Public Health Practice, Institute of Health. *The Future of Drug Safety: Promoting and Protecting the Health of the Public.* Washington, DC: National Academies Press, 2006.

Byers, Jacqueline Fowler, and Susan V. White, eds. *Patient Safety: Principles and Practice.* New York: Springer, 2004.

Dankelman, Jenny, Cornelis A. Grimbergen, and Henk G. Stassen, eds. *Engineering for Patient Safety: Issues in Minimally Invasive Procedures.* Mahwah, NJ: Lawrence Erlbaum, 2004.

Lambert, Matthew. *Leading a Patient-Safe Organization.* Chicago: Health Administration Press, 2004.

Leonard, Michael, Allan Frankel, and Terri Simmonds, et al. *Achieving Safe and Reliable Healthcare: Strategies and Solutions.* Chicago: Health Administration Press, Institute for Healthcare Improvement, and the American Organization of Nurse Executives, 2004.

Lewis, Russell F., ed. *The Impact of Information Technology on Patient Safety.* Chicago: Healthcare Information and Management Systems, 2002.

Morath, Julianne M., and Joanne E. Turnbull. *To Do No Harm: Ensuring Patient Safety in Health Care Organizations.* San Francisco: Jossey-Bass, 2004.

Newhouse, Robin P., and Stephanie Poe, eds. *Measuring Patient Safety.* Sudbury, MA: Jones and Bartlett, 2005.

Rozovsky, Fay A., and James R. Woods, eds. *The Handbook of Patient Safety Compliance: A Practical Guide for Health Care Organizations.* San Francisco: Jossey-Bass, 2005.

Sandars, John, and Gary Cook, eds. *ABC of Patient Safety.* Malden, MA: Blackwell, 2007.

Sharpe, Virginia A., ed. *Accountability: Patient Safety and Policy Reform.* Washington, DC: Georgetown University Press, 2004.

Tamuz, M., and M. I. Harrison. "Improving Patient Safety in Hospitals: Contributions of High-Reliability Theory and Normal Accident Theory," *Health Services Research* 41(4 pt. 2): 1654–76, August 2006.

35. Patient Satisfaction

Atlantic Information Services. *A Guide to Patient Satisfaction Survey Instruments: Profiles of Patient Satisfaction Measurement Instruments and Their Use by Health Plans, Employers, Hospitals, and Insurers.* Washington, DC: Atlantic Information Services, 1996.

Bell, Ralph, and Michael J. Krivich. *How to Use Patient Satisfaction Data to Improve Healthcare Quality.* Milwaukee, WI: American Society for Quality Press, 2000.

Cohen-Mansfield, Jiska, Farida K. Ejaz, and Perla Werner, eds. *Satisfaction Surveys in Long-Term Care.* New York: Springer, 2000.

Morales, Leo S., Juan Antonio Puyol, and Ron D. Hays. *Improving Patient Satisfaction Surveys to Assess Cultural Competence in Health Care.* Oakland: California Health Care Foundation, 2003.

Press, Irwin. *Patient Satisfaction: Understanding and Managing the Experience of Care.* Chicago: Health Administration Press, 2006.

Sherman, Stephanie G., and V. Clayton Sherman. *Total Customer Satisfaction: A Comprehensive Approach for Health Care Providers.* San Francisco: Jossey-Bass, 1998.

36. Quality Management

Clark, Gary B. *Continuous Quality Improvement: Integrating Five Key Quality System Components: Approved Guideline.* 2d ed. Wayne, PA: National Committee for Clinical Laboratory Standards, 2004.

Harrigan, Mary Lou. *Quest for Quality in Canadian Health Care: Continuous Quality Improvement.* 2d ed. Ottawa, Ontario, Canada: Health Canada, 2000.

Lighter, Donald, and Douglas C. Fair. *Quality Management in Health Care: Principles and Methods.* 2d ed. Sudbury, MA: Jones and Bartlett, 2004.

McLaughlin, Curtis P., and Arnold D. Kaluzny. *Continuous Quality Improvement in Health Care.* 3d ed. Sudbury, MA: Jones and Bartlett, 2006.

Opus Communications. *Continuous Quality Improvement for Long-Term Care.* Marblehead, MA: Opus Communications, 2000.

Sloan, M. Daniel. *How to Lower Health Care Costs by Improving Health Care Quality: Results-Based Continuous Quality Improvement.* Milwaukee, WI: American Society for Quality Control Quality Press, 1994.

Wick, Gail S., ed. *Continuous Quality Improvement: From Concept to Reality.* Pitman, NJ: American Nephrology Nurses' Association, 1995.

37. Volume-Outcome Relationship

Freeman, Jenny, Jon Nicholl, and Janette Turner. "Does Size Matter? The Relationship Between Volume and Outcome in the Care of Major Trauma," *Journal of Health Services Research and Policy* 11(2): 101–105, April 2006.

Hewitt, Maria, and Diana Petitti, eds., National Cancer Policy Board, Institute of Medicine, and Division on Earth and Life Studies, National Research Council. *Interpreting the Volume–Outcome Relationship in the Context of Cancer Care.* Washington, DC: National Academy Press, 2000.

Institute of Medicine. *Interpreting the Volume–Outcome Relationship in the Context of Health Care Quality: Workshop Summary.* Washington, DC: National Academies Press, 2000.

1216 Annotated Bibliography

Luft, Harold S., J. P. Bunker, and Allan C. Enthoven. "Should Operations Be Regionalized? The Empirical Relationship Between Surgical Volume and Mortality." *New England Journal of Medicine* 301(25): 1364–69, December 20, 1979.

Luft, Harold S., Deborah W. Garnick, David H. Mark, et al. *Hospital Volume, Physician Volume, and Patient Outcomes: Assessing the Evidence.* Ann Arbor, MI: Health Administration Press, 1990.

Shahian, D. M., and S. L. T. Normand. "The Volume–Outcome Relationship: From Luft to Leapfrog," *Annals of Thoracic Surgery* 75(3): 1048–1058, March 2003.

Urbach, D. R., R. Croxford, N. L. MacCallum, et al. "How are Volume–Outcome Associations Related to Models of Health Care Funding and Delivery? A Comparison of the United States and Canada," *World Journal of Surgery* 29(10): 1230–33, October 2005.

V. Organizational Behavior and Structure of Healthcare

Organizational behavior and the structure of healthcare provide a theoretical basis for understanding the dynamic relationships between individuals and groups in healthcare organizational settings and how they operate within the structural components of an organization.

38. General Works

Aldrich, Howard E., and Martin Ruef. *Organizations Evolving.* 2d ed. Thousand Oaks, CA: Sage, 2006.

Barton, Phoebe Lindsey. *Understanding the U.S. Health Services System.* 3d ed. Chicago: Health Administration Press, 2006.

Borkowski, Nancy. *Organizational Behavior in Health Care.* Sudbury, MA: Jones and Bartlett, 2006.

Buchanan, David A., Louise Fitzgerald, and Diane Ketley, eds. *The Sustainability and Spread of Organizational Change: Modernizing Healthcare.* New York: Routledge, 2006.

Clarke, Aileen, Pauline Allen, Stuart Anderson, et al., eds. *Studying the Organisation and Delivery of Health Services: A Reader.* Abingdon, UK: Routledge/Taylor and Francis Group, 2004.

Fulop, Naomi, eds. *Studying the Organisation and Delivery of Health Services: Research Methods.* Abingdon, UK: Routledge/Taylor and Francis Group, 2001.

Garber, Kim M., ed. *The U.S. Health Care Delivery System: Fundamental Facts, Definitions, and Statistics.* Chicago: Health Forum, AHA Press, 2006.

Marszalek-Gaucher, Ellen, and Richard J. Coffey. *Transforming Healthcare Organizations.* San Francisco: Jossey-Bass, 1990.

McNulty, Terry, and Ewan Ferlie. *Reengineering Health Care: The Complexities of Organizational Transformation.* New York: Oxford University Press, 2004.

Shi, Leiyu, and Douglas A. Singh. *Delivering Health Care in America: A Systems Approach.* 3d ed. Sudbury, MA: Jones and Bartlett, 2004.

Shi, Leiyu, and Douglas A. Singh. *Essentials of the U.S. Health Care System.* Sudbury, MA: Jones and Bartlett, 2005.

Sultz, Harry A., and Kristina M. Young. *Health Care USA: Understanding Its Organization and Delivery.* 5th ed. Sudbury, MA: Jones and Bartlett, 2006.

Williams, Stephen J. *Essentials of Health Services.* 3d ed. Clifton Park, NY: Thomson Delmar Learning, 2005.

39. Clinical Coordination, Integration of Care, and Continuum of Care

Center for Healthcare Information Management. *Integrating Clinical Information Across the Continuum of Care.* Ann Arbor, MI: Center for Healthcare Information Management, 1996.

Ebeling, Toni. *Nursing and the Continuum of Care.* Chicago: American Hospital Publishing, 1998.

Evashwick, Connie. *Seamless Connections: Refocusing Your Organization to Create a Successful Continuum of Care.* Chicago: American Hospital Publishing, 1997.

Joint Commission on Accreditation of Healthcare Organizations. *Ethical Issues and Patient Rights Across the Continuum of Care.* Oakbrook Terrace, IL: Joint Commission on Accreditation of Healthcare Organizations, 1998.

Joint Commission Resources. *Assessing Cognitive and Emotional Functioning Across the Continuum of Care.* Oakbrook Terrace, IL: Joint Commission Resources, 2003.

Shepperd, S., and S. Richards. "Continuity of Care: A Chameleon Concept," *Journal of Health Services Research and Policy* 7(3): 130–32, July 2002.

Stout, Chris E. *The Continuum of Care Clinical Documentation Sourcebook: A Comprehensive Collection of Inpatient, Outpatient, and Partial Hospitalization Forms, Handouts, and Records.* New York: Wiley, 2000.

Stout, Chris E., and Arthur E. Jongsma Jr. *The Continuum of Care Treatment Planner.* New York: Wiley, 1998.

Tonges, Mary, ed. *Clinical Integration: Strategies and Practices for Organized Delivery Systems.* San Francisco: Jossey-Bass, 1998.

40. Managed Care

Altman, Stuart H., Uwe E. Reinhardt, and David Shactman. *Regulating Managed Care: Theory, Practice, and Future Options.* San Francisco: Jossey-Bass, 1999.

Andrulis, Dennis P., and Betsy Carrier. *Managed Care in the Inner City: The Uncertain Promise for Providers, Plans, and Communities.* San Francisco: Jossey-Bass, 1999.

Birenbaum, Arnold. *Managed Care: Made in America.* Westport, CT: Praeger, 1997.

Donaldson, Molla S., ed., and National Roundtable on Health Care Quality, Division of Health Care Services, Institute of Medicine. *Collaboration Among Competing Managed Care Organizations for Quality Improvement: Summary of a Conference, November 13, 1997.* Washington, DC: National Academy Press, 1999.

Edmunds, Margaret, Richard Frank, Michael Hogan, et al., eds., and Committee on Quality Assurance and Accreditation Guidelines for Managed Behavioral Health Care, Division of Neuroscience and Behavioral Health, Division of Health Care Services, Institute of Medicine. *Managing Managed Care: Quality Improvement in Behavioral Health.* Washington, DC: National Academy Press, 1997.

Greenrose, Karen, Garry Carneal, and Kashmira Makwana, eds. *Rise in Prominence: The PPO Story.* Arlington, VA: American Association of Preferred Provider Organizations/URAC, 2000.

Jacobson, Peter D. *Strangers in the Night: Law and Medicine in the Managed Care Era.* New York: Oxford University Press, 2002.

Kongstvedt, Peter R. *The Managed Health Care Handbook.* 4th ed. Sudbury, MA: Jones and Bartlett, 2001.

Kongstvedt, Peter R. *Essentials of Managed Health Care.* 4th ed. Sudbury, MA: Jones and Bartlett, 2003.

Kongstvedt, Peter R. *Managed Care: What It Is and How It Works.* 2d ed. Sudbury, MA: Jones and Bartlett, 2004.

Makover, Michael E. *Mismanaged Care: How Corporate Medicine Jeopardizes Your Health.* Amherst, NY: Prometheus Books, 1998.

Veeder, Nancy W., and Wilma Peebles-Wilkins. *Managed Care Services: Policy, Programs, and Research.* New York: Oxford University Press, 2001.

Wilkerson, John D., Kelly J. Devers, and Ruth S. Given. *Competitive Managed Care: The Emerging Health Care System.* San Francisco: Jossey-Bass, 1997.

Wrightson, Charles William. *Financial Strategy for Managed Care Organizations: Rate Setting, Risk Adjustment, and Competitive Advantage.* Chicago: Health Administration Press, 2002.

41. Organizational Theory and Behavior

Borkowski, Nancy. *Organizational Behavior in Health Care.* Sudbury, MA: Jones and Bartlett, 2005.

Mick, Stephen S., and Mindy E. Wyttenbach, eds. *Advances in Health Care Organization Theory.* San Francisco: Jossey-Bass, 2003.

Miner, John B. *Organizational Behavior 1: Essential Theories of Motivation and Leadership.* Armonk, NY: M. E. Sharpe, 2005.

Miner, John B. *Organizational Behavior 2: Essential Theories of Process and Structure.* Armonk, NY: M. E. Sharpe, 2006.

Miner, John B. *Organizational Behavior 3: Historical Origins, Theoretical Foundations, and the Future.* Armonk, NY: M. E. Sharpe, 2006.

Scott, W. Richard, Martin Ruef, Peter J. Mendel, et al. *Institutional Change and Healthcare Organizations: From Professional Dominance to Managed Care.* Chicago: University of Chicago Press, 2000.

Vibert, Conor. *Theories of Macro-Organizational Behavior: A Handbook of Ideas and Explanations.* Armonk, NY: M. E. Sharpe, 2004.

42. Ownership

Crampton, Peter, Peter Davis, Roy Lay-Yee, et al. "Comparison of Private For-Profit With Private Community-Governed Not-For-Profit Primary Care Services in New Zealand," *Journal of Health Services Research and Policy* 9(4 Suppl. 2): 17–22, October 2004.

Duckett, S. "Does It Matter Who Owns Health Facilities?" *Journal of Health Services Research and Policy* 6(1): 59–62, January 2001.

Eggleston, Karen. *Hospital Ownership and Quality of Care: What Explains the Different Results?* NBER Working Paper No. 12241. Cambridge, MA: National Bureau of Economic Research, 2006.

Gray, Bradford H., ed. *The New Health Care for Profit: Doctors and Hospitals in a Competitive Environment.* Washington, DC: National Academy Press, 1983.

Gray, Bradford H., ed. *The Profit Motive and Patient Care: The Changing Accountability of Doctors and Hospitals.* Cambridge, MA: Harvard University Press, 1991.

Gray, Bradford H., ed., and Committee on Implications of For-Profit Enterprise in Health Care, Institute of Medicine. *For-Profit Enterprise in Health Care.* Washington, DC: National Academy Press, 1986.

Maynard, Alan, ed. *The Public–Private Mix for Health.* Oxford, UK: Nuffield Trust/Radcliffe Publishing, 2005.

Needleman, Jack. "The Role of Nonprofits in Health Care." In *Uncertain Times: Kenneth Arrow and the Changing Economics of Health Care*, edited by Peter J. Hammer, Deborah Haas-Wilson, and Mark A. Peterson, 243–58. Durham, NC: Duke University Press, 2003.

Potter, Sharyn J. *Can Efficiency and Community Service Be Symbiotic? A Longitudinal Analysis of Not-for-Profit and For-Profit Hospitals in the United States.* New York: Garland, 2000.

Robinson, James C. *The Corporate Practice of Medicine: Competition and Innovation in Health Care.* Berkeley: University of California Press, 1999.

Schlesinger, Mark, Shannon Mitchell, and Bradford H. Gray. "Public Expectations of Nonprofit and For-Profit Ownership in American Medicine: Clarifications and Implications," *Health Affairs* 23(6): 181–91, November–December 2004.

Silverman, Elaine, Jonathan S. Skinner, and Elliott S. Fisher. "The Association Between For-Profit Hospital Ownership and Increased Medicare Spending," *New England Journal of Medicine* 341(6): 420–26, August 5, 1999.

U.S. Congressional Budget Office. *Nonprofit Hospitals and the Provision of Community Benefits.* Washington, DC: U.S. Congressional Budget Office, 2006.

Weiss, Lawrence D. *Private Medicine and Public Health: Profits, Politics, and Prejudice in the American Health Care Enterprise.* Boulder, CO: Westview Press, 1997.

VI. Health Measurements, Methods, and Outcomes

Health measurements and methods are the tools and techniques that are used to obtain information about the end results or outcomes of an individual's health and health status.

43. General Works

Berger, Steven. *The Power of Clinical and Financial Metrics: Achieving Success in Your Hospital.* Chicago: Health Administration Press, 2005.

Block, Dale. *Health Care Outcomes Management: Strategies for Planning and Evaluation.* Sudbury, MA: Jones and Bartlett, 2006.

DiIorio, Colleen Konicki. *Measurement in Health Behavior: Methods for Research and Evaluation.* San Francisco: Jossey-Bass, 2005.

Dlugacz, Yosef. *Measuring Health Care: Using Quality Data for Operational, Financial, and Clinical Improvement.* San Francisco: Jossey-Bass, 2006.

Institute of Medicine. *Performance Measurement: Accelerating Improvement.* Washington, DC: Institute of Medicine, 2007.

Kane, Robert L., and Rosalie A. Kane, eds. *Assessing Older Persons: Measures, Meaning, and Practical Applications.* New York: Oxford University Press, 2000.

Kemm, John, Jayne Parry, and Stephen Palmer, eds. *Health Impact Assessment: Concepts, Theory, Techniques and Applications.* New York: Oxford University Press, 2004.

Lloyd, Robert. *Quality Health Care: A Guide to Developing and Using Indicators.* Sudbury, MA: Jones and Bartlett, 2004.

Nesbitt, Lori A. *Clinical Research: What It Is and How It Works.* Sudbury, MA: Jones and Bartlett, 2004.

Ozcan, Yasar A. *Quantitative Methods in Health Care Management: Techniques and Applications.* San Francisco: Jossey-Bass, 2005.

Ulin, Priscilla R., Elizabeth T. Robinson, and Elizabeth E. Tolley. *Qualitative Methods in Public Health: A Field Guide for Applied Research.* San Francisco: Jossey-Bass, 2004.

44. Community-Based Participatory Research

Israel, Barbara A., Eugenia Eng, Amy J. Schulz, et al., eds. *Methods in Community-Based Participatory Research for Health.* San Francisco: Jossey-Bass, 2005.

Minkler, Meredith, and Nina Wallerstein, eds. *Community-Based Participatory Research for Health.* San Francisco: Jossey-Bass, 2003.

Viswanathan, Meera. *Community-Based Participatory Research: Assessing the Evidence.* Rockville, MD: Agency for Healthcare Research and Quality, 2004.

45. Epidemiology

Ahrens, Wolfgang, and Iris Pigeot. *Handbook of Epidemiology.* New York: Springer, 2004.

Aschengrau, Ann, and George R. Seage. *Essentials of Epidemiology in Public Health.* Sudbury, MA: Jones and Bartlett, 2003.

Berkman, Lisa F., and Ichiro Kawachi, eds. *Social Epidemiology.* New York: Oxford University Press, 2000.

Bhopal, Raj. *Concepts of Epidemiology: An Integrated Introduction to the Ideas, Theories, Principles and Methods of Epidemiology.* New York: Oxford University Press, 2002.

Brownson, Ross C., and Diana B. Petitti, eds. *Applied Epidemiology: Theory and Practice.* 2d ed. New York: Oxford University Press, 2006.

Cwikel, Julie G. *Social Epidemiology: Strategies for Public Health Activism.* New York: Columbia University Press, 2006.

Dever, G. E. Alan. *Managerial Epidemiology: Practice, Methods and Concepts.* Sudbury, MA: Jones and Bartlett, 2006.

Fleming, Steven T., F. Douglas Scutchfield, and Thomas C. Tucker. *Managerial Epidemiology.* Chicago: Health Administration Press, 2000.

Fos, Peter J., David J. Fine, Brian W. Amy, et al. *Managerial Epidemiology for Health Care Organizations.* 2d ed. San Francisco: Jossey-Bass, 2005.

Friedman, Daniel J., Edward L. Hunter, and R. Gibson Parish II. *Health Statistics: Shaping Policy and Practice to Improve the Population's Health.* New York: Oxford University Press, 2005.

Gail, Mitchell H., and Jacques Benichou, eds. *Encyclopedia of Epidemiologic Methods.* New York: Wiley, 2000.

Gerstman, B. Burt. *Epidemiology Kept Simple: An Introduction to Traditional and Modern Epidemiology.* 2d ed. San Francisco: Jossey-Bass, 2003.

Gordis, Leon. *Epidemiology.* 4th ed. New York: W. B. Saunders, 2008.

Gregg, Michael B. *Field Epidemiology.* 2d ed. New York: Oxford University Press, 2002.

Hebel, J. Richard, and Robert J. McCarter. *Study Guide to Epidemiology and Biostatistics.* 6th ed. Sudbury, MA: Jones and Bartlett, 2006.

Holford, Theodore R. *Multivariate Methods in Epidemiology.* New York: Oxford University Press, 2002.

Klein, John P., and Melvin L. Moeschberger. *Survival Analysis: Techniques for Censored and Truncated Data.* 2d ed. New York: Springer, 2003.

Kleinbaum, David G., Kevin Sullivan, and Nancy Barker. *A Pocket Guide to Epidemiology.* New York: Springer, 2007.

Kleinbaum, David G., Mitchell Klein Emory, and E. Rihl Pryor. *Logistic Regression: A Self-Learning Text.* 2d ed. New York: Springer, 2002.

Koepsell, Thomas D., and Noel S. Weiss. *Epidemiologic Methods: Studying the Occurrence of Illness.* New York: Oxford University Press, 2003.

Last, John M., ed. *A Dictionary of Epidemiology.* 4th ed. New York: Oxford University Press, 2000.

Merrill, Ray M., and Thomas C. Timmreck. *Introduction to Epidemiology.* 4th ed. Sudbury, MA: Jones and Bartlett, 2006.

Oakes, J. Michael, and Jay S. Kaufman, eds. *Methods in Social Epidemiology.* San Francisco: Jossey-Bass, 2006.

Oleske, Denise M., ed. *Epidemiology and the Delivery of Health Care Services: Methods and Applications.* 2d ed. New York: Springer, 2001.

Rothman, Kenneth J. *Epidemiology: An Introduction.* New York: Oxford University Press, 2002.

Savitz, David A. *Interpreting Epidemiologic Evidence: Strategies for Study Design and Analysis.* New York: Oxford University Press, 2003.

Selvin, Steve. *Epidemiologic Analysis: A Case-Oriented Approach.* New York: Oxford University Press, 2001.

Selvin, Steve. *Statistical Analysis of Epidemiologic Data.* 3d ed. New York: Oxford University Press, 2004.

Ziegler, Andreas, and Inke R. Konig. *A Statistical Approach to Genetic Epidemiology: Concepts and Applications.* Weinheim, Germany: Wiley-VCH, 2006.

46. Geographic Information Systems (GIS)

Briggs, David J., Pip Forer, Lars Jarup, et al., eds. "GIS for Emergency Preparedness and Health Risk Reduction." In *Proceedings of the NATO Advanced Research Workshop, Budapest, Hungary (April 22–25, 2001).* Dordrecht, The Netherlands: Kluwer Academic, 2002.

Cromley, Ellen K., and Sara L. McLafferty. *GIS and Public Health.* New York: Guilford Press, 2002.

Curtis, Andrew, and Michael Leitner. *Geographic Information Systems and Public Health: Eliminating Perinatal Disparity.* Hershey, PA: IRM Press, 2006.

Gatrell, Anthony, and Markku Loytonen, eds. *GIS and Health.* GISDATA 6. Philadelphia: Taylor and Francis, 1998.

Khan, Omar A., and Ric Skinner, eds. *Geographic Information Systems and Health Applications.* Hershey, PA: Idea Group, 2003.

Koch, Tom. *Cartographies of Disease: Maps, Mapping, and Medicine.* Redlands, CA: ESRI Press, 2005.

Lang, Laura. *GIS for Health Organizations.* Redlands, CA: ESRI Press, 2000.

Melnick, Alan L. *Introduction to Geographic Information Systems in Public Health.* Sudbury, MA: Jones and Bartlett, 2002.

North American Association of Central Cancer Registries. *Using Geographic Information Systems Technology in the Collection, Analysis, and Presentation of Cancer Registry Data: A Handbook of Basic Practices.* Springfield, IL: North American Association of Central Cancer Registries, 2002.

47. Health Measurement Scales

Bowling, Ann. *Measuring Disease: A Review of Disease-Specific Quality of Life Measurement Scales.* Maidenhead, UK: Open University Press, 2001.

McDowell, Ian. *Measuring Health: A Guide to Rating Scales and Questionnaires.* 3d ed. New York: Oxford University Press, 2006.

Streiner, David L., and Geoffrey R. Norman. *Health Measurement Scales: A Practical Guide to Their Development and Use.* 3d ed. New York: Oxford University Press, 2003.

48. Health Surveys

Aday, Lu Ann, and Llewellyn J. Cornelius. *Designing and Conducting Health Surveys: A Comprehensive Guide.* 3d ed. San Francisco: Jossey-Bass, 2006.

Andersen, Ronald, Judith Kasper, Martin R. Frankel, et al. *Total Survey Error: Applications to Improve Health Surveys.* San Francisco: Jossey-Bass, 1979.

Cohen-Mansfield, Jiska, Farida K. Ejaz, and Perla Werner, eds. *Satisfaction Surveys in Long-Term Care.* New York: Springer, 2000.

Czaja, Ron, and Johnny Blair. *Designing Surveys: A Guide to Decisions and Procedures.* 2d ed. Thousand Oaks, CA: Sage, 2005.

DiIorio, Colleen Konicki. *Measurement in Health Behavior: Methods for Research and Evaluation.* San Francisco: Jossey-Bass, 2005.

Korn, Edward Lee, and Barry I. Graubard. *Analysis of Health Surveys.* New York: Wiley, 1999.

Nosikov, Anatoliy, and Claire Gudex, eds. *EUROHIS: Developing Common Instruments for Health Surveys.* Tokyo, Japan: IOS Press, 2003.

Sethi, Dinesh, S. Habibula, K. McGee, et al., eds. *Guidelines for Conducting Community Surveys on Injuries and Violence.* Geneva, Switzerland: World Health Organization, 2004.

49. Informatics

Aalseth, Patricia. *Codebusters Coding Connection: A Documentation Guide for Compliant Coding.* 2d ed. Sudbury, MA: Jones and Bartlett, 2005.

Aalseth, Patricia. *Medical Coding: What It Is and How It Works.* Sudbury, MA: Jones and Bartlett, 2006.

Austin, Charles J., and Stuart B. Boxerman. *Information Systems for Healthcare Management.* 6th ed. Chicago: Health Administration Press, 2003.

Brown, Gordon D., Tamara T. Stone, and Timothy B. Patrick. *Strategic Management of Information Systems in Healthcare.* Chicago: Health Administration Press, 2005.

Burke, Lillian, and Barbara Weill. *Information Technology for the Health Professions.* 2d ed. Upper Saddle River, NJ: Pearson Prentice Hall, 2005.

Committee on Data Standards for Patient Safety, Board on Health Care Services, Institute of Medicine. *Key Capabilities of an Electronic Health Record System: Letter Report.* Washington, DC: National Academies Press, 2003.

DeLuca, Joseph M., and Rebecca Enmark. *The CEO's Guide to Health Care Information Systems.* 2d ed. San Francisco: Jossey-Bass, 2001.

DeLuca, Joseph M., and Rebecca Enmark Cagan. *Investing for Business Value: How to Maximize the Strategic Benefits of Health Care Information Technology.* San Francisco: Jossey-Bass, 1996.

Friedman, Charles P. *Evaluation Methods in Biomedical Informatics.* 2d ed. New York: Springer, 2006.

Gartee, Richard. *Electronic Health Records: Understanding and Using Computerized Medical Records.* Upper Saddle River, NJ: Pearson Prentice Hall, 2007.

Goldstein, Douglas E., Suniti Ponkshe, Peter J. Groen, et al. *Medical Informatics 20/20: Quality and Electronic*

Health Records Through Collaboration, Open Solutions, and Innovation. Sudbury, MA: Jones and Bartlett, 2006.

Hannah, Kathryn J., Marion J. Ball, and Margaret J. Edwards. *Introduction to Nursing Informatics.* 3d ed. New York: Springer, 2006.

Hanson, C. William. *Healthcare Informatics.* New York: McGraw-Hill, 2006.

Harman, Laurinda Beebe. *Ethical Challenges in the Management of Health Information.* 2d ed. Sudbury, MA: Jones and Bartlett/American Health Information Management Association, 2006.

Lehmann, Harold P., Patricia A. Abbott, Nancy K. Roderer, et al., eds. *Aspects of Electronic Health Record Systems.* New York: Springer, 2006.

Lewis, Deborah. *Consumer Health Informatics: Informing Consumers and Improving Health Care.* New York: Springer, 2005.

Lewis, Russell F., ed. *The Impact of Information Technology on Patient Safety.* Chicago: Healthcare Information and Management Systems, 2002.

Lombardo, Joseph S., and David Buckeridge, ed. *Disease Surveillance: A Public Health Informatics Approach.* Hoboken, NJ: Wiley-Interscience, 2007.

Osborn, Carol E. *Statistical Applications for Health Information Management.* 2d ed. Sudbury, MA: Jones and Bartlett/American Health Information Management Association, 2006.

Roach, William H., Robert G. Hoban, Bernadette M. Broccolo, et al. *Medical Records and the Law.* 4th ed. Sudbury, MA: Jones and Bartlett/American Health Information Management Association, 2006.

Skurka, Margaret A., ed. *Health Information Management: Principles and Organization for Health Information Services.* 5th ed. San Francisco: Jossey-Bass, 2003.

Sullivan, Frank. "What Is Health Informatics?" *Journal of Health Services Research and Policy* 6(4): 249–50, October 2001.

Sullivan, Frank M., and Jeremy Wyatt. *ABC of Health Informatics.* Malden, MA: Blackwell, 2006.

Tan, Joseph K. H. *Health Management Information Systems: Methods and Practical Applications.* 2d ed. Sudbury, MA: Jones and Bartlett, 2001.

Taylor, Paul. *From Patient Data to Medical Knowledge: The Principles and Practice of Health Informatics.* Malden, MA: Blackwell, 2006.

Wager, Karen A., Frances Wickham Lee, and John P. Glaser. *Managing Health Care Information Systems: A Practical Approach for Health Care Executives.* San Francisco: Jossey-Bass, 2005.

Warner, Homer R. *Knowledge Engineering in Health Informatics.* New York: Springer, 1997.

50. Longitudinal Analysis

Fitzmaurice, Garrett M., Nan M. Laird, and James H. Ware. *Applied Longitudinal Analysis.* Hoboken, NJ: Wiley-Interscience, 2004.

Hedeker, Donald, and Robert D. Gibbons. *Longitudinal Data Analysis.* San Francisco: Jossey-Bass, 2006.

Weiss, Robert E. *Modeling Longitudinal Data.* New York: Springer, 2005.

51. Meta-Analysis

American Nurses Association. *A Meta-Analysis of Process of Care, Clinical Outcomes, and Cost Effectiveness of Nurses in Primary Care Roles: Nurse Practitioners and Nurse-Midwives.* Washington, DC: American Nurses Association, 1993.

Eddy, David M., Victor Hasselblad, and Ross D. Shachter. *Meta-Analysis by the Confidence Profile Method: The Statistical Synthesis of Evidence.* Boston: Academic Press, 1992.

Egger, Matthias, George Davey Smith, and Douglas G. Altman, eds. *Systematic Reviews in Health Care: Meta-Analysis in Context.* London: BMJ Books, 2001.

Hunt, Morton M. *How Science Takes Stock: The Story of Meta-Analysis.* New York: Russell Sage Foundation, 1997.

Leandro, Gioacchino. *Meta-Analysis in Medical Research: The Handbook for the Understanding and Practice of Meta-Analysis.* Malden, MA: BMJ Books/Blackwell, 2005.

Pang, Francis, Michael Drummond, and Fujian Song. *The Use of Meta-Analysis in Economic Evaluation.* York, UK: University of York, Centre for Health Economics, 1999.

Paterson, Barbara L. *Meta-Study of Qualitative Health Research: A Practical Guide to Meta-Analysis and Meta-Synthesis.* Thousand Oaks, CA: Sage, 2001.

Petitti, Diana B. *Meta-Analysis, Decision Analysis, and Cost-Effectiveness Analysis: Methods for Quantitative Synthesis in Medicine.* 2d ed. New York: Oxford University Press, 2000.

Rothstein, Hannah, Alexander J. Sutton, and Michael Borenstein, eds. *Publications Bias in Meta-Analysis: Prevention, Assessment, and Adjustments.* Hoboken, NJ: Wiley, 2005.

Schulze, Ralf, Heinz Holling, and Dankmar Bohning, eds. *Meta-Analysis: New Developments and Applications in Medical and Social Sciences.* Cambridge, MA: Hogrefe and Huber, 2003.

Selden, Catherine. *Meta-Analysis: January 1980 Through December 1992: 337 Citations.* Bethesda, MD: U.S. Department of Health and Human Services, Public Health Service, National Institutes of Health, National Library of Medicine, 1992.

Stangl, Dalene K., and Donald A. Berry, eds. *Meta-Analysis in Medicine and Health Policy.* New York: Marcel Dekker, 2000.

Sutton, Alex J., Keith R. Abrams, David R. Jones, et al. *Methods for Meta-Analysis in Medical Research.* New York: Wiley, 2000.

Whitehead, Anne. *Meta-Analysis of Controlled Clinical Trials.* Chichester, UK: Wiley, 2002.

Wolf, F. M. *Meta-Analysis: Quantitative Methods for Research Synthesis.* Beverly Hills, CA: Sage, 1986.

52. Outcomes Research

Chumney, Elinor C. G., and Kit N. Simpson, eds. *Methods and Designs for Outcomes Research*. Bethesda, MD: American Society of Health-System Pharmacists, 2006.

Fayers, Peter M., and David Machin, eds. *Quality of Life: The Assessment, Analysis, and Interpretation of Patient-Reported Outcomes*. 2d ed. Hoboken, NJ: Wiley, 2007.

Kaplan, Sandra L. *Outcome Measurement and Management: First Steps for the Practicing Clinician*. Philadelphia: F. A. Davis, 2007.

Kane, Robert L. *Understanding Health Care Outcomes Research*. 2d ed. Sudbury, MA: Jones and Bartlett, 2006.

Lee, Stephanie J., Craig C. Earle, and Jane C. Weeks. "Outcomes Research in Oncology: History, Conceptual Framework, and Trends in the Literature," *Journal of the National Cancer Institute* 92(3): 195–204, February 2, 2000.

Rodriguez-Garcia, Rosalia, James A. Macinko, and William F. Waters, eds. *Microenterprise Development for Better Health Outcomes*. Westport, CT: Greenwood, 2001.

Weiss, Noel S. *Clinical Epidemiology: The Study of the Outcome of Illness*. 3d ed. New York: Oxford University Press, 2006.

53. Randomized Controlled Trials (RCT) and Research

Aungst, Jessica, Amy Haas, Alexander Ommaya, et al., eds., and Clinical Research Roundtable, Board on Health Sciences Policy, Institute of Medicine. *Exploring Challenges, Progress, and New Models for Engaging the Public in the Clinical Research Enterprise: Clinical Research Roundtable Workshop Summary*. Washington, DC: National Academies Press, 2003.

Barnett, Anthony H. *Applying the Evidence: Clinical Trials in Diabetes*. Chicago: Remedica, 2005.

Beech, Bettina M., and Maurine Goodman, eds. *Race and Research: Perspectives on Minority Participation in Health Studies*. Washington, DC: American Public Health Association, 2004.

Berlin, Jesse A. *Randomized Trial Comparing Masked/Unmasked Meta-Analysis*. Rockville, MD: Agency for Health Care Policy and Research, Center for Research Dissemination and Liasion, 1996.

Chow, Shein-Chung, and Jen-Pei Lin. *Design and Analysis of Clinical Trials: Concepts and Methodologies*. 2d ed. San Francisco: Jossey-Bass, 2003.

Committee on Clinical Trial Registries, Board on Health Sciences Policy, Institute of Medicine. *Developing a National Registry of Pharmacologic and Biologic Clinical Trials: Workshop Report*. Washington, DC: National Academies Press, 2006.

D'Agostino, Ralph B., Lisa Sullivan, and Joseph Massaro, eds. *Wiley Encyclopedia of Clinical Trials*. 6 vols. Hoboken, NJ: Wiley, 2007.

DeMets, David L., and Lawrence M. Friedman. *Data Monitoring in Clinical Trials*. New York: Springer, 2006.

Doshi, J. A., H. A. Glick, and D. Polsky. "Analyses of Cost Data in Economic Evaluations Conducted Alongside Randomized Controlled Trials," *Value in Health* 9(5): 334–40, September–October 2006.

Duley, Lelia, and Barbara Farrell, eds. *Clinical Trials*. London: Blackwell/BMJ Books, 2001.

Elwood, J. Mark. *Critical Appraisal of Epidemiological Studies and Clinical Trials*. 2d ed. New York: Oxford University Press, 1998.

Fayers, Peter, and Ron Hayes. *Assessing Quality of Life in Clinical Trials: Methods and Practice*. 2d ed. New York: Oxford University Press, 2005.

Friedman, Lawrence M., Curt D. Furberg, and David L. DeMets. *Fundamentals of Clinical Trials*. New York: Springer, 1998.

Good, Phillip I. *A Manager's Guide to the Design and Conduct of Clinical Trials*. 2d ed. San Francisco: Jossey-Bass, 2006.

Hu, Feifang, and William F. Rosenberger. *The Theory of Response-Adaptive Randomization in Clinical Trials*. Hoboken, NJ: Wiley-Interscience, 2006.

Kalfoglou, Andrea L., Douglas A. Boenning, and David Korn, and Board on Health Sciences Policy, Institute of Medicine. *Exploring the Map of Clinical Research for the Coming Decade: Symposium Summary, Clinical Research Roundtable, December 2000*. Washington, DC: National Academy Press, 2001.

Kalfoglou, Andrea L., Douglas A. Boenning, and Mary Woolley, and Board on Health Sciences Policy, Institute of Medicine. *Public Confidence and Involvement in Clinical Research: Symposium Summary, Clinical Research Roundtable, September 2000*. Washington, DC: National Academy Press, 2001.

Liu, Margaret B., and Kate Davis. *Lessons From a Horse Named Jim: A Clinical Trials Manual From the Duke Clinical Research Institute*. Durham, NC: Duke Clinical Research Institute, 2001.

Mastroianni, Anna C., Ruth Faden, and Daniel Federman, eds., and Committee on the Ethical and Legal Issues Relating to the Inclusion of Women in Clinical Studies, Division of Health Sciences Policy, Institute of Medicine. *Women and Health Research: Ethical and Legal Issues of Including Women in Clinical Studies*, vols. 1–2. Washington, DC: National Academy Press, 1994.

Matthew, J. N. S. *An Introduction to Randomized Controlled Clinical Trials*. London: Arnold, 2000.

Meinert, Curtis L. *Clinical Trials: Design, Conduct, and Analysis*. New York: Oxford University Press, 1986.

Moye, Lemuel A. *Statistical Monitoring of Clinical Trials: Fundamentals for Investigators*. New York: Springer, 2006.

Piantadosi, Steven. *Clinical Trials: A Methodologic Perspective*. Hoboken, NJ: Wiley-Interscience, 2005.

Pocock, Stuart J. *Clinical Trials: A Practical Approach*. New York: Wiley, 2002.

Proschan, Michael A., K. K. Gordon Lan, and Janet Turk Wittes. *Statistical Monitoring of Clinical Trials: A Unified Approach.* New York: Springer, 2006.

Rozovsky, Fay A., and Rodney K. Adams. *Clinical Trials and Human Research: A Practical Guide to Regulatory Compliance.* San Francisco: Jossey-Bass, 2003.

Spilker, Bert. *Guide to Clinical Trials.* New York: Raven Press, 1991.

Stewart, Derek, ed. *Clinical Trials Explained.* Abingdon, UK: BMJ Books/Blackwell, 2006.

Technology Evaluation Center. *Special Report: Measuring and Reporting Pain Outcomes in Randomized Controlled Trials.* Chicago: Blue Cross and Blue Shield Association, 2006.

Wang, Duolao, and Ameet Bakhai, eds. *Clinical Trials: A Practical Guide to Design, Analysis, and Reporting.* Chicago: Remedica, 2006.

Whitehead, Anne. *Meta-Analysis of Controlled Clinical Trials.* Chichester, UK: Wiley, 2002.

54. Risk- and Case-Mix Adjustment

Cucciare, M. A., and W. O'Donohue. "Predicting Future Healthcare Costs: How Well Does Risk-Adjustment Work?" *Journal of Health Organization and Management* 20(2–3): 150–62, 2006.

Geenwald, L. M., A. Esposito, M. J. Ingber, et al. "Risk Adjustment for the Medicare Program: Lessons Learned From Research and Demonstrations," *Inquiry* 35(2): 193–209, 1998.

Iezzoni, Lisa I., ed. *Risk Adjustment for Measuring Healthcare Outcomes.* 3d ed. Chicago: Health Administration Press, 2003.

Ingber, M. J. "Implementation of Risk Adjustment for Medicare," *Health Care Financing Review* 21(3): 119–26, 2000.

Weissman, J. S., M. Wachterman, and D. Blumenthal. "When Methods Meet Politics: How Risk Adjustment Became Part of Medicare Managed Care," *Journal of Health Politics, Policy, and Law* 30(3): 475–504, June 2005.

55. Small-Area Analysis

Diehr, Paula, Kevin Cain, Frederick Connell, et al. "What Is Too Much Variation? The Null Hypothesis in Small-Area Analysis," *Health Services Research* 24(6): 741–71, February 1990.

Gittelsohn, Alan, and N. R. Powe. "Small Area Variations in Health Care Delivery in Maryland," *Health Services Research* 30(2): 295–317, June 1995.

Goodman, D. C., and G. R. Green. "Assessment Tools: Small Area Analysis," *American Journal of Medical Quality* 11(1): S12–S14, Spring 1996.

Paul-Shaheen, Pamela, and Daniel Williams. "Small Area Analysis: A Review and Analysis of the North American Literature," *Journal of Health Politics, Policy and Law* 12: 741–809, Winter 1987.

Shah, Gutzar H. *A Guide to Designating Geographic Areas for Small Area Analysis in Public Health: Using Utah's Example.* Guidelines and Resources for Health Data Organizations. Salt Lake City, UT: National Association of Health Data Organizations, 2005.

Wennberg, John E. "Understanding Geographic Variations in Health Care Delivery," *New England Journal of Medicine* 340(1): 52–53, January 7, 1999.

Wennberg, John E., and Alan Gittelsohn. "Small Area Variations in Health Care Delivery," *Science* 182(117): 1102–1108, December 14, 1973.

Wennberg, John E., and Alan Gittelsohn. "Variation in Medical Care Among Small Areas," *Scientific American* 246: 120–34, April 1982.

56. Statistical Process Control and Six Sigma Quality

Berry, Robert. *NAN: A Six Sigma Mystery.* Chicago: Health Administration Press, 2003.

Berry, Robert. *NAN'S Arsonist: A Six Sigma Mystery.* Chicago: Health Administration Press, 2004.

Berry, Robert, Amy Murcko, and Clifford E. Brubaker. *The Six Sigma Book for Healthcare: Improving Outcomes by Reducing Errors.* Chicago: Health Administration Press, 2002.

Carey, Raymond, and Robert C. Lloyd. *Measuring Quality Improvement in Healthcare: A Guide to Statistical Process Control Applications.* Milwaukee, WI: American Society for Quality, 2001.

Chassin, Mark R. "Is Health Care Ready for Six Sigma Quality?" *Milbank Quarterly* 76(4): 565–91, 1998.

57. Statistics

Armitage, Peter, and Theodore Colton, eds. *Encyclopedia of Biostatistics.* 2d ed. 8 vols. Hoboken, NJ: Wiley, 2005.

Bolstad, William M. *Introduction to Bayesian Statistics.* San Francisco: Jossey-Bass, 2004.

Daniel, Wayne W. *Biostatistics: A Foundation for Analysis in the Health Sciences.* 8th ed. Hoboken, NJ: Wiley, 2005.

Forthofer, Ronald N., Eun Sul Lee, and Mike Hernandez. *Biostatistics: A Guide to Design, Analysis, and Discovery.* 2d ed. San Diego, CA: Academic Press, 2007.

Gerstman, B. Burt. *Basic Biostatistics: Statistics for Public Health Practice.* Sudbury, MA: Jones and Bartlett, 2008.

Kirkwood, Betty R., and Jonathan A. C. Sterne. *Essential Medical Statistics.* 2d ed. Malden, MA: Blackwell Science, 2003.

Kotz, Samuel, Campbell B. Read, N. Balakrishnan, et al. *Encyclopedia of Statistical Sciences.* 2d ed. 16 vols. San Francisco: Jossey-Bass, 2005.

Kuzma, Jan W., and Stephen E. Bohnenblust. *Basic Statistics for the Health Sciences.* Boston: McGraw-Hill, 2005.

Le, Chap T. *Introductory Biostatistics.* San Francisco: Jossey-Bass, 2005.

Lu, Ying, and Ji-Qian Fang, eds. *Advanced Medical Statistics.* Hackensack, NJ: World Scientific, 2003.

Matthews, David E., and Vernon T. Farewell. *Using and Understanding Medical Statistics.* 4th ed. New York: Karger, 2007.

Moye, Lemuel A. *Statistical Reasoning in Medicine: The Intuitive P-Value Primer.* 2d ed. New York: Springer, 2006.

Riffenburgh, R. H. *Statistics in Medicine.* 2d ed. Burlington, MA: Elsevier Academic Press, 2006.

VII. Health Policy

Health policy is the stance of the government that is aimed at improving health and healthcare. Many researchers, organizations, and advocacy groups work to shape health policy by using evidence-based studies and various resources to aid in policy guidance.

58. General Works

Aday, Lu Ann, Charles E. Begley, David R. Lairson, et al. *Evaluating the Healthcare System: Effectiveness, Efficiency, and Equity.* 3d ed. Chicago: Health Administration Press, 2004.

Altman, Stuart H., and David I Shactman, eds. *Policies for an Aging Society.* Baltimore: Johns Hopkins University Press, 2002.

Almgren, Gunnar Robert. *Health Care Politics, Policy, and Services: A Social Justice Analysis.* New York: Springer, 2007.

Andersen, Ronald M., Thomas H. Rice, and Gerald F. Kominski. *Changing the U.S. Health Care System: Key Issues in Health Services Policy and Management.* 3d ed. San Francisco: Josssey-Bass, 2007.

Barondess, Jermiah A., David E. Rogers, and Kathleen N. Lohr, eds., and Institute of Medicine. *Care of the Elderly Patient: Policy Issues and Research Opportunities.* Report of a Forum of the Council on Health Care Technology. Washington, DC: National Academy Press, 1989.

Barr, Donald A. *Introduction to U.S. Health Policy: The Organization, Financing, and Delivery of Health Care in America.* 2d ed. Baltimore: Johns Hopkins University Press, 2007.

Binstock, Robert H., Leighton E. Cluff, and Otto von Mering, eds. *The Future of Long-Term Care: Social and Policy Issues.* Baltimore: Johns Hopkins University Press, 1996.

Budrys, Grace. *Our Unsystematic Health Care System.* 2d ed. Lanham, MD: Rowman and Littlefield, 2005.

Caldwell, Donald H. *U.S. Health Law and Policy 2001: A Guide to the Current Literature.* 2d ed. San Francisco: Jossey-Bass, 2001.

Calkins, David, Rushika J. Fernandopulle, and Bradley S. Marino, eds. *Health Care Policy.* Cambridge, MA: Blackwell Science, 1995.

Callahan, Daniel, and Angela A. Wasunna. *Medicine and the Market: Equity v. Choice.* Baltimore: Johns Hopkins University Press, 2006.

Cookson, Richard. "Evidence-Based Policy Making in Health Care: What It Is and What It Isn't," *Journal of Health Services Research and Policy* 10(2): 118–21, April 2005.

Cutler, David M. *Your Money or Your Life: Strong Medicine for America's Health Care System.* New York: Oxford University Press, 2004.

Danis, Marion, Carolyn Clancy, and Larry R. Churchill, eds. *Ethical Dimensions of Health Policy.* New York: Oxford University Press, 2005.

Evans, Timothy, Margaret Whitehead, Finn Diderichsen, et al. *Challenging Inequities in Health: From Ethics to Action.* New York: Oxford University Press, 2001.

Feldstein, Paul J. *The Politics of Health Legislation: An Economic Perspective.* 3d ed. Chicago: Health Administration Press, 2006.

Feldstein, Paul J. *Health Policy Issues: An Economic Perspective.* 4th ed. Chicago: Health Administration Press, 2007.

Frank, Richard G., and Sherry A. Glied. *Better But Not Well: Mental Health Policy in the United States Since 1950.* Baltimore: Johns Hopkins University Press, 2006.

Fuchs, Victor R. *The Future of Health Policy.* Cambridge, MA: Harvard University Press, 1993. (Chapter 2 of the book provides a very concise summary of the history of health economics)

Fuchs, Victor R. *Who Shall Live? Health, Economics, and Social Choice.* 2d ed. River Edge, NJ: World Scientific, 1998.

Gingrich, Newt, Diana Pavey, and Anne Woodbury. *Saving Lives and Saving Money: Transforming Health and Healthcare.* Arlington, VA: Alexis de Toqueville Institution, 2003.

Ginzberg, Eli, ed. *The Medical Triangle: Physicians, Politicians, and the Public.* Cambridge, MA: Harvard University Press, 1990.

Ginzberg, Eli, ed. *Health Services Research: Key to Health Policy.* Cambridge, MA: Harvard University Press, 1991.

Gunn, S. W. B., P. B. Mansourian, Anthony Piel, et al. *Understanding the Global Dimensions of Health.* New York: Springer, 2005.

Hacker, Jacob S. *The Great Risk Shift: The Assault on American Jobs, Families, Health Care and Retirement and How You Can Fight Back.* New York: Oxford University Press, 2006.

Hofrichter, Richard, ed. *Health and Social Justice: Politics, Ideology, and Inequity in the Distribution of Disease.* San Francisco: Jossey-Bass, 2003.

Hudson, Robert B., ed. *The New Politics of Old Age Policy.* Baltimore: Johns Hopkins University Press, 2005.

Institute of Medicine. *Unintended Consequences of Health Programs and Policies: Workshop Summary.* Washington, DC: National Academy Press, 2001.

Jost, Timothy Stoltzfus. *Disentitlement? The Threats Facing Our Public Health Care Programs and a Right-Based Response*. New York: Oxford University Press, 2003.

Kleinke, J. D. *Oxymorons: The Myth of a U.S. Health Care System*. San Francisco: Jossey-Bass, 2001.

Kronenfeld, Jennie Jacobs. *Health Care Policy: Issues and Trends*. Westport, CT: Praeger, 2002.

Levine, Carol, and Thomas H. Murray, eds. *The Cultures of Caregiving: Conflict and Common Ground Among Families, Health Professionals, and Policy Makers*. Baltimore: Johns Hopkins University Press, 2004.

Longest, Beaufort B., Jr. *Health Policymaking in the United States*. 4th ed. Chicago: Health Administration Press, 2006.

Marcus, Alan I., and Hamilton Cravens, eds. *Health Care Policy in Contemporary America*. University Park: Pennsylvania State University Press, 1997.

Marmor, Theodore R. *Fads, Fallacies and Foolishness in Medical Care Management and Policy*. Hackensack, NJ: World Scientific, 2007.

Moniz, Cynthia, and Stephen H. Gorin. *Health and Mental Health Care Policy: A Biopsychosocial Perspective*. 2d ed. Boston: Allyn and Bacon, 2007.

Mullan, Fitzhugh, Ellen Ficklen, and Kyna Rubin, eds. *Narrative Matters: The Power of the Personal Essay in Health Policy*. Baltimore: Johns Hopkins University Press, 2006.

Ornstein, Norman J., and Thomas E. Mann, eds. *Intensive Care: How Congress Shapes Health Policy*. Washington, DC: Brookings Institution, 1995.

Patel, Kant, and Mark Rushefsky. *Health Care Politics and Policy in America*. 3d ed. Armonk, NY: M. E. Sharpe, 2006.

Porzsolt, Franz, and Robert M. Kaplan, eds. *Optimizing Health: Improving the Value of Healthcare Delivery*. New York: Springer, 2007.

Powers, Madison, and Ruth R. Faden. *Social Justice: The Moral Foundations of Public Health and Health Policy*. New York: Oxford University Press, 2006.

Rhodes, Rosamond, Margaret P. Battin, and Anita Silvers, eds. *Medicine and Social Justice: Essays on the Distribution of Health Care*. New York: Oxford University Press, 2002.

Rich, Robert F., and Christopher T. Erb, eds. *Consumer Choice: Social Welfare and Health Policy*. New Brunswick, NJ: Transaction Publishers, 2005.

Rovner, Julie. *Health Care Policy and Politics A to Z*. Washington, DC: CQ Press, 2000.

Smith, Peter C., Laura Ginnelly, and Mark Sculpher, eds. *Health Policy and Economics: Opportunity and Challenges*. New York: Open University Press, 2005.

Starr, Paul. *The Social Transformation of American Medicine*. New York: Basic Books, 1982.

Stevens, Rosemary, Charles E. Rosenberg, and Lawton R. Burns, eds. *History and Health Policy in the United States: Putting the Past Back In*. New Brunswick, NJ: Rutgers University Press, 2006.

Stewart, Charles T. *Healthy, Wealthy, or Wise? Issues in American Health Care Policy*. Armonk, NY: M. E. Sharpe, 1995.

Verheijde, Joseph L. *Managing Care: A Shared Responsibility*. New York: Springer, 2006.

Weissert, Carol S., and William G. Weissert. *Governing Health: The Politics of Health Policy*. 3d ed. Baltimore: Johns Hopkins University Press, 2006.

59. *Healthcare Reform*

Bloche, M. Gregg, ed. *The Privatization of Health Care Reform: Legal and Regulatory Perspectives*. New York: Oxford University Press, 2002.

Carter, Larry E. *Health Care Reform: Policy Innovations at the State Level in the United States*. New York: Garland, 1998.

Emery, Douglas W. *Customer-Directed Healthcare Reform With Episode Pricing*. Mason, OH: Thomson, 2006.

Engstrom, Timothy H., and Wade L. Robison. *Health Care Reform: Ethics and Politics*. Rochester, NY: University of Rochester Press, 2006.

Fuchs, Victor R., and Ezekiel J. Emanuel. "Health Care Reform: Why? What? When?" *Health Affairs* 24(6): 1399–414, November–December 2005.

Ginzberg, Eli, ed. *Critical Issues in U.S. Health Reform*. Boulder, CO: Westview Press, 1994.

Harrington, Charlene, and Carroll L. Estes. *Health Policy: Crisis and Reform in the U.S. Health Care Delivery System*. 4th ed. Sudbury, MA: Jones and Bartlett, 2004.

Institute of Medicine. *Changing the Health Care System: Models From Here and Abroad*. The Richard and Hinda Rosenthal Lectures. Washington, DC: National Academy Press, 1994.

Lynn, Joanne. *Sick to Death and Not Going to Take It Anymore! Reforming Health Care for the Last Years of Life*. Los Angeles: University of California Press/Milbank Memorial Fund.

Marmor, Theodore R. *Understanding Health Care Reform*. New Haven, CT: Yale University Press, 1994.

Mechanic, David. *The Truth About Health Care: Why Reform Is Not Working in America*. Piscataway, NJ: Rutgers University Press, 2006.

O'Rourke, Thomas W., and Nicholas K. Iammarino. "Future of Healthcare Reform in the USA: Lessons From Abroad," *Expert Review of Pharmacoeconomics and Outcomes Research* 2(3): 279–91, June 2002.

Relman, Arnold S. *A Second Opinion: How to Prevent the Collapse of America's Healthcare*. New York: Century Foundation, PublicAffairs, 2007.

Roberts, Marc J., William Hsiao, Peter Berman, et al. *Getting Health Reform Right: A Guide to Improving Performance and Equity*. New York: Oxford University Press, 2003.

Terry, Ken. *Rx for Health Care Reform*. Nashville, TN: Vanderbilt University Press, 2007.

Twaddle, Andrew C., ed. *Health Care Reform Around the World*. Westport, CT: Auburn House, 2002.

Zhou, Huizhong, ed. *The Political Economy of Health Care Reforms*. Kalamazoo, MI: W. E. Upjohn Institute for Employment Research, 2001.

60. Health Insurance

America's Health Insurance Plans, Center for Policy and Research. *Small Group Health Insurance in 2006: A Comprehensive Survey of Premiums, Consumer Choice, and Benefits.* Washington, DC: America's Health Insurance Plans, 2006.

Chiappori, Pierre-Andre, and Christian Gollier, eds. *Competitive Failures in Insurance Markets: Theory and Policy Implications.* Cambridge: MIT Press, 2006.

Green, Michelle A., and Jo Ann C. Rowell. *Understanding Health Insurance: A Guide to Billing and Reimbursement.* 8th ed. Clifton Park, NY: Thomson Delmar Learning, 2006.

Marcinko, David E. *Insurance and Risk Management Strategies for Physicians and Advisors.* Sudbury, MA: Jones and Bartlett, 2005.

Marcinko, David E., and Hope R. Hetico, eds. *Dictionary of Health Insurance and Managed Care.* New York: Springer, 2006.

Monheit, Alan C., Renate Wilson, and Ross A. Arnett. *Informing American Health Care Policy: The Dynamics of Medical Expenditure and Insurance Surveys, 1977–1996.* San Francisco: Jossey-Bass, 1996.

Pauly, Mark V. *Health Benefits at Work: An Economic and Political Analysis of Employment-Based Health Insurance.* Ann Arbor: University of Michigan Press, 1997.

RAND Corporation. "Consumer Decision Making in the Insurance Market," *RAND Health Research Highlights.* Santa Monica, CA: RAND Corporation, 2006.

Vaughan, Emmett J., and Therese Vaughan. *Fundamentals of Risk and Insurance.* 9th ed. New York: Wiley, 2003.

61. Law and Ethics

American Bar Association. *The American Bar Association Complete and Easy Guide to Health Care Law: Your Guide to Protecting Your Rights as a Patient, Dealing With Hospitals, Health Insurance, Medicare, and More.* New York: Three Rivers Press, 2001.

Annas, George J. *American Bioethics: Crossing Human Rights and Health Law Boundaries.* New York: Oxford University Press, 2004.

Baker, Robert B., Arthur L. Caplan, Linda L. Emanuel, et al., eds. *The American Medical Ethics Revolution: How the AMA's Code of Ethics Has Transformed Physicians' Relationships to Patients, Professionals, and Society.* Baltimore: Johns Hopkins University Press, 1999.

Boyle, Philip J., Edwin R. DuBose, Stephen J. Ellingson, et al. *Organizational Ethics in Health Care: Principles, Cases, and Practical Solutions.* San Francisco: Jossey-Bass, 2001.

Danis, Marion, Carolyn Clancy, and Larry R. Churchill, eds. *Ethical Dimensions of Health Policy.* New York: Oxford University Press, 2002.

Eckenwiler, Lisa A., and Felicia G. Cohn, eds. *The Ethics of Bioethics: Mapping the Moral Landscape.* Baltimore: Johns Hopkins University Press, 2007.

Emanuel, Ezekiel J., Robert A. Crouch, John D. Arras, et al., eds. *Ethical and Regulatory Aspects of Clinical Research: Readings and Commentary.* Baltimore: Johns Hopkins University Press, 2003.

Gillett, Grant R. *Bioethics in the Clinic: Hippocratic Reflections.* Baltimore: Johns Hopkins University Press, 2004.

Goodman, Richard A., Mark A. Rothstein, Richard E. Hoffman, et al., eds. *Law in Public Health Practice.* New York: Oxford University Press, 2002.

Harman, Laurinda Beebe. *Ethical Challenges in the Management of Health Information.* 2d ed. Sudbury, MA: Jones and Bartlett/American Health Information Management Association, 2006.

Harris, Dean M. *Contemporary Issues in Healthcare Law and Ethics.* 2d ed. Chicago: Health Administration Press, 2003.

Hofmann, Paul B., and William A. Nelson, eds. *Managing Ethically: An Executive's Guide.* Chicago: Health Administration Press, 2001.

King, Nancy M. P., Gail Henderson, and Jane S. Stein, eds. *Beyond Regulations: Ethics in Human Subjects Research.* Chapel Hill: University of North Carolina Press, 1999.

Mastroianni, Anna C., Ruth Faden, and Daniel Federman, eds., and Committee on the Ethical and Legal Issues Relating to the Inclusion of Women in Clinical Studies, Division of Health Sciences Policy, Institute of Medicine. *Women and Health Research: Ethical and Legal Issues of Including Women in Clinical Studies,* vol. 2. Workshop and Commissioned Papers. Washington, DC: National Academy Press, 1994.

May, Thomas. *Bioethics in a Liberal Society: The Political Framework of Bioethics Decision Making.* Baltimore: Johns Hopkins University Press, 2002.

Mezey, Mathy D., Christine K. Cassel, Melissa M. Bottrall, et al., eds. *Ethical Patient Care: A Casebook for Geriatric Health Care Terms.* Baltimore: Johns Hopkins University Press, 2002.

Miller, Robert D. *Problems in Health Care Law.* 9th ed. Sudbury, MA: Jones and Bartlett, 2006.

Moody, Harry R. *Ethics in an Aging Society.* Baltimore: Johns Hopkins University Press, 1996.

Morrison, Eileen E. *Ethics in Health Administration: A Practical Approach for Decision Makers.* Sudbury, MA: Jones and Bartlett, 2006.

Perry, Frankie. *The Tracks We Leave: Ethics in Healthcare Management.* Chicago: Health Administration Press, 2002.

Pierce, Jessica, and Andrew Jameton. *The Ethics of Environmentally Responsible Health Care.* New York: Oxford University Press, 2003.

Post, Linda Farber, Jeffery Blustein, and Nancy Neveloff Dubler. *Handbook for Health Care Ethics Committees.* Baltimore: Johns Hopkins University Press, 2006.

Post, Stephen G., ed. *Encyclopedia of Bioethics.* 3d ed. 5 vols. New York: Macmillan Reference USA, 2004.

Pozgar, George D. *Legal Aspects of Health Care Administration.* 10th ed. Sudbury, MA: Jones and Bartlett, 2004.

Pozgar, George D., and Nina Santucci. *Legal and Ethical Issues for Health Professionals*. Sudbury, MA: Jones and Bartlett, 2005.

Ramsey, Paul. *The Patient as Person: Explorations in Medical Ethics*. 2d ed. New Haven, CT: Yale University Press, 2002.

Rhodes, Rosamond, Leslie Francis, and Anita Silvers, eds. *The Blackwell Guide to Medical Ethics*. Malden, MA: Blackwell, 2007.

Roach, William H., Robert G. Hoban, Bernadette M. Broccolo, et al. *Medical Records and the Law*. 4th ed. Sudbury, MA: Jones and Bartlett/American Health Information Management Association, 2006.

Sales, Bruce Dennis, and Susan Folkman, eds. *Ethics in Research With Human Participants*. Washington, DC: American Psychological Association, 2000.

Showalter, J. Stuart. *The Law of Healthcare Administration*. 4th ed. Chicago: Health Administration Press, 2003.

Spencer, Edward M., Ann E. Mills, Mary V. Rorty, et al. *Organization Ethics in Health Care*. New York: Oxford University Press, 2000.

Steiner, John. *Handbook of Clinical Research Law and Compliance*. Sudbury, MA: Jones and Bartlett, 2006.

Stevens, M. L. Tina. *Bioethics in America: Origins and Cultural Politics*. Baltimore: Johns Hopkins University Press, 2003.

Trotter, Griffin. *The Ethics of Coercion in Mass Casualty Medicine*. Baltimore: Johns Hopkins University Press, 2007.

Walter, Jennifer K., and Eran P. Klein, eds. *The Story of Bioethics: From Seminal Works to Contemporary Explorations*. Washington, DC: Georgetown University Press, 2003.

Wing, Kenneth R., and Benjamin Gilbert. *The Law and the Public's Health*. 7th ed. Chicago: Health Administration Press, 2006.

Zussman, Robert. *Intensive Care: Medical Ethics and the Medical Profession*. Chicago: University of Chicago Press, 1994.

62. Medicaid and the State Children's Health Insurance Program (SCHIP)

Aizer, Anna, Janet M. Currie, and Enrico Moretti. *Competition in Imperfect Markets: Does It Help California's Medicaid Mothers?* NBER Working Paper No. 10429. Cambridge, MA: National Bureau of Economic Research, 2004.

Alliance for Health Reform. *SCHIP and Medicaid Environment: What's Next?* Washington, DC: Alliance for Health Reform, 2006.

Berkowitz, Edward. "Medicare and Medicaid: The Past as Prologue," *Health Care Financing Review* 27(2): 11–23, Winter 2005–2006.

Brown, Randall, and Arnold Chen. *Disease Management Options: Issues for State Medicaid Programs to Consider*. Princeton, NJ: Mathematica Policy Research, 2004.

Cuellar, Alison Evans, and Sara Markowitz. *Medicaid Policy Changes in Mental Health Care and Their Effect on Mental Health Outcomes*. NBER Working Paper No. 12232. Cambridge, MA: National Bureau of Economic Research, 2006.

Engel, Jonathan. *Poor People's Medicine: Medicaid and American Charity Care Since 1965*. Durham, NC: Duke University Press, 2006.

Fong, T. "Assessing Four Decades of Medicare, Medicaid," *Modern Healthcare* 35(29): 6–7, 24, 42, 1, July 18, 2005.

Gilman, Jean Donovan. *Medicaid and the Costs of Federalism, 1984–1992*. New York: Garland, 1998.

Grannemann, Thomas W., and Mark V. Pauly. *Controlling Medicaid Costs: Federalism, Competition, and Choice*. Washington, DC: American Enterprise Institute, 1983.

Holahan, John F., and Joel W. Cohen. *Medicaid: The Trade-Off Between Cost Containment and Access to Care*. Washington, DC: Urban Institute Press, 1986.

Hynes, Margaret M. *Who Cares for Poor People? Physicians, Medicaid, and Marginality*. New York: Garland, 1998.

"Key Milestones in Medicare and Medicaid History, Selected Years: 1965–2003," *Health Care Financing Review* 27(2): 1–3, Winter 2005–2006.

Leibowitz, Arleen, and Earl S. Pollack, eds., and Panel for the Workshop on the State Children's Health Insurance Program, Committee on National Statistics, Division of Behavioral and Social Sciences and Education, National Research Council. *Data Needs for the State Children's Health Insurance Program*. Washington, DC: National Academy Press, 2002.

Mann, Cindy, and Robin Rudowitz. *Financing Health Coverage: The State Children's Health Insurance Program Experience*. Menlo Park, CA: Henry J. Kaiser Family Foundation, 2005.

Moore, Judith D., and David G. Smith. "Legislating Medicaid: Considering Medicaid and Its Origins," *Health Care Financing Review* 27(2): 45–52, Winter 2005–2006.

Moses, Stephen A. *Aging America's Achilles' Heel: Medicaid Long-Term Care*. Washington, DC: Cato Institute, 2005.

National Health Policy Forum. *Medicaid Financing: The Basics*. Washington, DC: George Washington University, National Health Policy Forum, 2006.

Rader, Anya, Cynthia Pernice, and Trish Riley. *State and Federal Health Data Sources: An Inventory for CHIP Evaluators*. Portland, ME: National Academy for State Health Policy, 1998.

Rich, Robert F., Cinthia L. Deye, and Elizabeth Mazur. "The State Children's Health Insurance Program: An Administrative Experiment in Federalism," *University of Illinois Law Review* (1): 107–135, 2004.

Rosenbaum, Sara, Alexandra Stewart, and Colleen Sonosky. *Negotiating the New Health System: Findings From a Nationwide Study of Medicaid Primary Care Case Management Contracts*. Lawrenceville, NJ: Center for Health Care Strategies, 2002.

Rowland, Diane. "Medicaid at Forty," *Health Care Financing Review* 27(2): 63–77, Winter 2005–2006.

Rowland, Diane, and James R. Tallon Jr. "Medicaid: Lessons From a Decade," *Health Affairs* 22(1): 138–44, January–February 2003.

Shenkman, Elizabeth. *Using Administrative Data to Assess Quality of Care in the State Children's Health Insurance*

Program. Portland, ME: National Academy for State Health Policy, 2003.

Shirk, Cynthia. *Rebalancing Long-Term Care: The Role of the Medicaid HCBS [Home and Community-Based Services] Waiver Program.* Washington, DC: National Health Policy Forum, 2006.

Smith, Vernon K., Terrisca, Des Jardins, and Karin A. Peterson. *Exemplary Practices in Primary Care Case Management: A Review of State Medicaid PCCM Programs.* Princeton, NJ: Center for Health Care Strategies, 2000.

Sparer, Michael J. *Medicaid and the Limits of State Health Reform.* Philadelphia: Temple University Press, 1996.

Ubokudom, Sunday E. *Physician Participation in Medicaid Managed Care.* New York: Garland, 1997.

U.S. Government Accountability Office. *Medicaid Fraud and Abuse: CMS's Commitment to Helping States Safeguard Program Dollars Is Limited: Testimony Before the Committee on Finance, U.S. Senate.* Washington, DC: U.S. Government Accountability Office, 2005.

Williams, Claudia. *Medicaid Disease Management: Issues and Promises.* Washington, DC: Henry J. Kaiser Family Foundation, 2004.

63. Medicare

Acemoglu, Daron, et al. *Did Medicare Induce Pharmaceutical Innovation?* NBER Working Paper No. 11949. Cambridge, MA: National Bureau of Economic Research, 2006.

Berkowitz, Edward. "Medicare and Medicaid: The Past as Prologue," *Health Care Financing Review* 27(2): 11–23, Winter 2005–2006.

Blevins, Sue A. *Medicare's Midlife Crisis.* Washington, DC: Cato Institute, 2001.

Cassel, Christine K. *Medicare Matters: What Geriatric Medicine Can Teach American Health Care.* Los Angeles: University of California Press/Milbank Memorial Fund, 2007.

Center for Rural Health Policy Analysis. *Redesigning Medicare: Considerations for Rural Beneficiaries and Health Systems.* Omaha, NE: Rural Policy Research Institute, Center for Rural Health Policy Analysis, 2001.

Committee on Redesigning Health Insurance Performance Measures, Payment, and Performance Improvement Programs, Board on Health Care Services, Institute of Medicine. *Medicare's Quality Improvement Organization Program: Maximizing Potential.* Pathways to Quality Health Care Series. Washington, DC: National Academies Press, 2006.

Committee on Redesigning Health Insurance Performance Measures, Payment, and Performance Improvement Programs, Board on Health Care Services, Institute of Medicine. *Rewarding Provider Performance: Aligning Incentives in Medicare.* Washington, DC: National Academies Press, 2007.

Davis, Karen, and Sara R. Collins. "Medicare at Forty," *Health Care Financing Review* 27(2): 53–62, Winter 2005–2006.

Finkelstein, Amy. *The Aggregate Effects of Health Insurance: Evidence From the Introduction of Medicare.* NBER

Working Paper No. 11619. Cambridge, MA: National Bureau of Economic Research, 2005.

Fong, T. "Assessing Four Decades of Medicare, Medicaid," *Modern Healthcare* 35(29): 6–7, 24, 42, July 18, 2005.

Foote, Susan Bartlett, Rachel Halpern, and Douglas R. Wholey. *Variation in Medicare's Local Coverage Policies: Content Analysis of Local Medical Review Policies.* Minneapolis: University of Minnesota, Division of Health Services Research and Policy, 2005.

Gold, Marsha. *Geographic Variation in Medicare per Capita Spending: Should Policy-Makers Be Concerned?* Princeton, NJ: Robert Wood Johnson Foundation, 2004.

Hyman, David A. *Medicare Meets Mephistopheles.* Washington, DC: Cato Institute, 2006.

"Key Milestones in Medicare and Medicaid History, Selected Years: 1965–2003," *Health Care Financing Review* 27(2): 1–3, Winter 2005–2006.

Lawlor, Edward F. *Redesigning the Medicare Contract: Politics, Markets, and Agency.* Chicago: University of Chicago Press, 2003.

Lohr, Kathleen N., ed., and Committee to Design a Strategy for Quality Review and Assurance in Medicare, Division of Health Care Services, Institute of Medicine. *Medicare: A Strategy for Quality Assurance.* Vol. 2, *Sources and Methods.* Washington, DC: National Academy Press, 1990.

Marmor, Theodore R. *The Politics of Medicare.* 2d ed. New York: Aldine de Gruyter, 2000.

Mayes, Rick, and Robert A. Berenson. *Medicare Prospective Payment and the Shaping of U.S. Health Care.* Baltimore: Johns Hopkins University Press, 2006.

Mebane, Felicia E. *Medicare Politics: Exploring the Roles of Media Coverage, Political Information, and Political Participation.* New York: Garland, 2000.

Medicare Payment Advisory Commission. *Report to the Congress: Increasing the Value of Medicare.* Washington, DC: Medicare Payment Advisory Commission, 2006.

Milgate, Karen, and Glenn Hackbarth. "Quality in Medicare: From Measurement to Payment and Provider to Patient," *Health Care Financing Review* 27(2): 91–101, Winter 2005–2006.

Moon, Marilyn. *Medicare: A Policy Primer.* Washington, DC: Urban Institute Press, 2006.

Newhouse, Joseph P. "Medicare's Challenges in Paying Providers," *Health Care Financing Review* 27(2): 35–44, Winter 2005–2006.

Oberlander, Jonathan. *The Political Life of Medicare.* Chicago: University of Chicago Press, 2003.

Oliver, T. R., P. R. Lee, and H. L. Lipton, "A Political History of Medicare and Prescription Drug Coverage," *Milbank Quarterly* 82(2): 283–354, 2004.

Polsky, Daniel, Jalpa Doshi, Jose Escarce, et al. *The Health Effects of Medicare for the Near-Elderly Uninsured.* NBER Working Paper No. 12511. Cambridge, MA: National Bureau of Economic Research, 2006.

Potetz, Lisa A., and Thomas H. Rice. *Medicare Tomorrow: The Report of the Century Foundation Task Force on Medicare Reform.* New York: Century Foundation Press, 2001.

Rettenmaier, Andrew J., and Thomas R. Saving. *The Diagnosis and Treatment of Medicare.* Washington, DC: AEI Press, 2007.

Ricketts, Thomas C. *Arguing for Rural Health in Medicare: A Progressive Rhetoric for Rural America.* Chapel Hill: University of North Carolina at Chapel Hill, Cecil G. Sheps Center for Health Services Research, North Carolina Rural Health Research and Policy Analysis Center, 2002.

Shaviro, Daniel. *Who Should Pay for Medicare?* Chicago: University of Chicago Press, 2004.

White, Joseph. *False Alarm: Why the Greatest Threat to Social Security and Medicare Is the Campaign to "Save" Them.* Baltimore: Johns Hopkins University Press, 2003.

64. National Health Insurance

Armstrong, Pat, Hugh Armstrong, and Claudia Fegan. *Universal Healthcare: What the United States Can Learn From the Canadian Experience.* New York: New Press, 1998.

Botsman, Peter. *USACare: A National Health Insurance Strategy for the USA.* Chicago: Midwest Center for Labor Research, 1992.

Cummings, Nicholas A., William T. O'Donohue, and Michael A. Cucciare, eds. *Universal Healthcare: Readings for Mental Health Professionals.* Reno, NV: Context Press, 2005.

Davis, K. "Universal Coverage in the United States: Lessons From Experience of the 20th Century," *Journal of Urban Health* 78(1): 46–58, March 2001.

Decker, Sandra L., and Dahlia K. Remler. *How Much Might Universal Health Insurance Reduce Socioeconomic Disparities in Health? A Comparison of the U.S. and Canada.* NBER Working Paper 10715. Cambridge, MA: National Bureau of Economic Research, 2004.

Derickson, Alan. *Health Security for All: Dreams of Universal Health Care in America.* Baltimore: Johns Hopkins University Press, 2005.

Enthoven, Alain C. *Theory and Practice of Managed Competition in Health Care Financing.* New York: North-Holland, 1988.

Feder, Judith, John Holahan, and Theodore Marmor, eds. *National Health Insurance: Conflicting Goals and Policy Choices.* Washington, DC: Urban Institute, 1980.

Goodman, John C., Gerald L. Musgrave, and Devon M. Herrick. *Lives at Risk: Single-Payer National Health Insurance Around the World.* Lanham, MD: Rowman and Littlefield, 2004.

Hall, George M. *A Tide in the Affairs of Medicine: National Health Insurance as the Augury of Medicine.* St. Louis, MO: Warren H. Green, 2004.

Kooijman, Jaap. *And the Pursuit of National Health: The Incremental Strategy Toward National Health Insurance in the United States of America.* Atlanta, GA: Rodopi, 1999.

Laham, Nicholas. *A Lost Cause: Bill Clinton's Campaign for National Health Insurance.* Westport, CT: Praeger, 1996.

Marmor, Theodore R., and Jonathan Oberlander. "Paths to Universal Health Insurance: Progressive Lessons From the Past for the Future," *University of Illinois Law Review* (1): 205–230, 2004.

Mayes, Rick. *Universal Coverage: The Elusive Quest for National Health Insurance.* Lanham, MD: Lexington Books, 2001.

Pauly, Mark V., ed. *National Health Insurance: What Now, What Later, What Never?* Washington, DC: American Enterprise Institute, 1980.

Pauly, Mark V., Patricia Danzon, Paul J. Feldstein, et al. *Responsible National Health Insurance.* Washington, DC: American Enterprise Institute, 1992.

Quadagno, Jill. *One Nation, Uninsured: Why the U.S. Has No National Health Insurance.* New York: Oxford University Press, 2005.

Terris, M. "National Health Insurance in the United States: A Drama in Too Many Acts," *Journal of Public Health Policy* 20(1): 13–35, 1999.

U.S. Congress. *Health Security Act.* 103rd Congress 1st Session. Washington, DC: U.S. GPO, 1993.

White House Domestic Policy Council. *Health Security: The President's Report to the American People.* Washington, DC: U.S. GPO, 1993.

65. Rationing Healthcare

Aaron, Henry J., and William B. Schwartz. *The Painful Prescription: Rationing Hospital Care.* Washington, DC: Brookings Institution, 1984.

Aaron, Henry J., William B. Schwartz, and Melissa Cox. *Can We Say No? The Challenge of Rationing Health Care.* Washington, DC: Brookings Institution Press, 2005.

Barry, Robert L., and Gerard V. Bradley, eds. *Set No Limits: A Rebuttal to Daniel Callahan's Proposal to Limit Health Care for the Elderly.* Champaign: University of Illinois Press, 1991.

Blank, Robert K. *Rationing Medicine.* New York: Columbia University Press, 1988.

Callahan, Daniel. *Setting Limits: Medical Goals in an Aging Society.* New York: Simon and Schuster, 1987.

Daniels, Norman, and James Sabin. *Settings Limits Fairly: Can We Learn to Share Medical Resources?* New York: Oxford University Press, 2002.

Dranove, David. *What's Your Life Worth? Health Care Rationing . . . Who Lives? Who Dies? Who Decides?* New York: Financial Times/Prentice Hall, 2003.

Ham, C., and A. Coulter. "Explicit and Implicit Rationing: Taking Responsibility and Avoiding Blame for Health Care Choices," *Journal of Health Services Research and Policy* 6(3): 163–69, July 2001.

Menzel, Paul T. *Strong Medicine: The Ethical Rationing of Health Care.* New York: Oxford University Press, 1990.

Rice, Charles L. "Rationing Revisited," *University of Illinois Law Review* (1): 197–203, 2004.

Schulenburg, Johann-Matthias, and Michael Blanks, eds. *Rationing of Medical Services in Europe: An Empirical Study.* Amsterdam: IOS Press, 2004.

66. Regulation

Abbott, Thomas A. *Health Care Policy and Regulation.* Boston: Kluwer Academic, 1995.

American Accreditation HealthCare Commission, URAC. *Survey of State Health Utilization Review Laws and Regulations*. Washington, DC: American Accreditation HealthCare Commission, URAC, 1998.

Bradley, Herring, and Mark V. Pauly. *The Effect of State Community Rating Regulations on Premiums and Coverage in the Individual Health Insurance Market*. NBER Working Paper No. 12504. Cambridge, MA: National Bureau of Economic Research, 2006.

Carneal, Garry, ed. *The PPO Guide: State Laws and Regulations, Market Trends, Legal Analysis, Accreditation Issues*. Washington, DC: American Accreditation HealthCare Commission, URAC, 1999.

CCH Incorporated. *Nursing Home Regulations: Medicare and Medicaid: Explanation, Law, Regulations*. Chicago: CCH Incorporated, 1995.

Field, Robert I. *Health Care Regulation in America: Complexity, Confrontation, and Compromise*. New York: Oxford University Press, 2007.

Fischbeck, Paul S., and R. Scott Farrow, eds. *Improving Regulation: Cases in Environment, Health, and Safety*. Washington, DC: Resources for the Future, 2001.

Greaney, Thomas L., and Robert L. Schwartz. *Health Law: Selected Statutes and Regulations*. St. Paul, MN: Thomas West, 2003.

Hackey, Robert B. *Rethinking Health Care Policy: The New Politics of State Regulation*. Washington, DC: Georgetown University Press, 1998.

Jones, Nancy Lee. *The Americans With Disabilities Act (ADA): Overview, Regulations and Interpretations*. New York: Nova Science, 2003.

Lass, Gene, and JoAnn Petaschnick, eds. *State-by-State Health Care Collection Laws and Regulations*. Gaithersburg, MD: Aspen, 2000.

Maynard, A., and R. Cookson. "Money or Your Life? The Health–Wealth Trade-Off in Pharmaceutical Regulation," *Journal of Health Services Research and Policy* 6(3): 186–89, July 2001.

Nielsen, Ronald P. *OSHA Regulations and Guidelines: A Guide for Health Care Providers*. Albany, NY: Delmar/Thomson Learning, 2000.

World Health Organization. *Global Crises—Global Solutions: Managing Public Health Emergencies of International Concern Through the Revised International Health Regulations*. Geneva, Switzerland: World Health Organizations, 2002.

World Health Organization. *International Health Regulations: Working Paper for Regional Consultations*. Geneva, Switzerland: World Health Organization, 2004.

VIII. Health Professionals and Healthcare Organizations

Health professionals are the individuals who work to ensure the smooth functioning and operation of the healthcare system, and they are the primary deliverers of healthcare services. Healthcare organizations are the entities that provide essential healthcare services.

67. *General Works*

Lee, Philip R., and Carroll L. Estes. *The Nation's Health*. 7th ed. Sudbury, MA: Jones and Bartlett, 2003.

Mullan, Fitzhugh. *Big Doctoring in America: Profiles in Primary Care*. Los Angeles: University of California Press/ Milbank Memorial Fund, 2002.

Shi, Leiyu, and Douglas A. Singh. *Delivering Health Care in America: A Systems Approach*. 3d ed. Sudbury, MA: Jones and Bartlett, 2005.

Shi, Leiyu, and Douglas A. Singh. *Essentials of the U.S. Health Care System*. Sudbury, MA: Jones and Bartlett, 2005.

Sultz, Harry A., and Kristina M. Young. *Health Care USA: Understanding Its Organization and Delivery*. 5th ed. Sudbury, MA: Jones and Bartlett, 2006.

Wicks, Robert J. *Overcoming Secondary Stress in Medical and Nursing Practice: A Guide to Professional Resilience and Personal Well-Being*. New York: Oxford University Press, 2005.

68. *Academic Medical Centers*

Black, Carrie E. *Academic Health Centers: Responses to the Malpractice Insurance Crisis*. Washington, DC: Association of Academic Health Centers, 2005.

Ginzberg, Eli, Howard Berliner, Miriam Ostow, et al., eds. *Teaching Hospitals and the Urban Poor*. New Haven, CT: Yale University Press, 2000.

Kohn, Linda T., ed., and Committee on the Roles of Academic Health Centers in the 21st Century, Board on Health Care Services, Institute of Medicine. *The Roles of Academic Health Centers in the 21st Century: A Workshop Summary*. Washington, DC: National Academy Press, 2002.

Souba, W. W., M. R. Weitekamp, and J. F. Mahon. "Political Strategy, Business Strategy, and the Academic Medical Center: Linking Theory and Practice," *Journal of Surgical Research* 100(1): 1–10, September, 2001.

Task Force on Academic Health Centers. *A Shared Responsibility: Academic Health Centers and the Provision of Care to the Poor and Uninsured: A Report of the Commonwealth Fund Task Force on Academic Health Centers*. New York: Commonwealth Fund, 2001.

Task Force on Academic Health Centers. *Training Tomorrow's Doctors: The Medical Education of Academic Health Centers: A Report of the Commonwealth Fund Task Force on Academic Health Centers*. New York: Commonwealth Fund, 2002.

Task Force on Academic Health Centers. *Envisioning the Future of Academic Health Centers: Final Report of the Commonwealth Fund Task Force on Academic Health Centers*. New York: Commonwealth Fund, 2003.

69. Dentistry

American Dental Education Association. *ADEA Official Guide to Dental Schools*. Washington, DC: American Dental Education Association, 2004. (This directory is published annually)

Burt, Brian A., and Stephen A. Eklund. *Dentistry, Dental Practice, and the Community*. St. Louis, MO: Elsevier Saunders, 2005.

Christensen, Gordon J. *A Consumer's Guide to Dentistry*. 2d ed. St. Louis: MO, Elsevier 2001.

Devlin, Hugh. *Operative Dentistry: A Practical Guide to Recent Innovations*. New York: Springer, 2006.

Kulacz, Robert, and Thomas E. Levy. *The Roots of Disease: The Connection Between Dentistry and Medicine*. Victoria, British Columbia, Canada: Trafford, 2002.

Mitchell, David A., Laura Mitchell, and Paul A. Brunton. *Oxford Handbook of Clinical Dentistry*. 4th ed. New York: Oxford University Press, 2005.

Rattan, Ray, and George Manolescue. *The Business of Dentistry*. Chicago: Quintessence, 2002.

Weinberger, Bernhard Wolf. *An Introduction to the History of Dentistry: With Medical and Dental Chronology and Bibliographic Data*. Mansfield Centre, CT: Martino, 2005.

70. Emergency Care and Intensive-Care Units

Committee on the Future of Emergency Care in the United States Health System. *Emergency Care for Children: Growing Pains*. Future of Emergency Care Series. Washington, DC: Institute of Medicine, Board on Health Care Services, Committee on the Future of Emergency Care in the United States Health System, 2007.

Committee on the Future of Emergency Care in the United States Health System. *Emergency Medical Services: At the Crossroads*. Future of Emergency Care Series. Washington, DC: Institute of Medicine, Board on Health Care Services, Committee on the Future of Emergency Care in the United States Health System, 2007.

Committee on the Future of Emergency Care in the United States Health System. *Hospital-Based Emergency Care: At the Breaking Point*. Future of Emergency Care Series. Washington, DC: Institute of Medicine, Board on Health Care Services, Committee on the Future of Emergency Care in the United States Health System, 2007.

Corke, C. F. *Practical Intensive Care Medicine: Problem Solving in the ICU*. Boston: Butterworth-Heinemann, 2000.

Curtis, J. Randall, and Gordon D. Rubenfeld, eds. *Managing Death in the ICU: The Transition From Cure to Comfort*. New York: Oxford University Press, 2001.

DeVita, Michael A., Ken Hillman, and R. Bellomo, eds. *Medical Emergency Teams: Implementation and Outcome Measurement*. New York: Springer, 2006.

Joint Commission Resources. *Accreditation Issues for Emergency Departments*. Oakbrook Terrace, IL: Joint Commission Resources, 2003.

Joint Commission Resources. *Improving Care in the ICU: Improving Health Care Quality and Safety*. Oakbrook Terrace, IL: Joint Commission Resources, 2004.

Marcucci, Lisa, Elizabeth A. Martinez, Elliott R. Haut, et al. *Avoiding Common ICU Errors*. Philadelphia: Lippincott Williams and Wilkins, 2007.

Marino, Paul L., and Kenneth M. Sutin. *The ICU Book*. 3d ed. Philadelphia: Lippincott Williams and Wilkins, 2007.

Mistovich, Joseph J., Brent Q. Hafen, Keith J. Karren, et al., eds. *Prehospital Emergency Care*. 8th ed. Upper Saddle River, NJ: Pearson Education, 2008.

Ridley, Saxon A., ed. *The Psychological Challenges of Intensive Care*. Malden, MA: BMJ Books/Blackwell, 2005.

Rosenblatt, R. A., G. E. Wright, L. M. Baldwin, et al. "The Effect of the Doctor-Patient Relationship on Emergency Department Use Among the Elderly," *American Journal of Public Health* 90(1): 97–102, January 2000.

Schoeni, Patricia Q., Whitney Lindahl, and Christina A. Lau, eds. *Care in the ICU: Profiles of Individuals and Institutions That Have Made a Commitment to Quality in Intensive Care Units*. Washington, DC: National Coalition on Health Care, 2002.

Smeby, L. Charles. *Fire and Emergency Services Administration: Management and Leadership Practices*. Sudbury, MA: Jones and Bartlett, 2006.

Society of Critical Care Medicine. *The Case for the Intensivist-Directed Model: Making the Transition to an Intensivist-Directed ICU*. Des Plaines, IL: Society of Critical Care Medicine, 2002.

U.S. General Accounting Office. *Hospital Emergency Departments: Crowded Conditions Vary Among Hospitals and Communities: Report to the Ranking Minority Member, Committee on Finance, U.S. Senate*. Washington, DC: U.S. General Accounting Office, 2003.

71. Healthcare Administration and Management

Alemi, Farrokh, and David H. Gustafson. *Decision Analysis for Healthcare Managers*. Chicago: Health Administration Press, 2006.

Broyles, Robert W. *Fundamentals of Statistics in Health Administration*. Sudbury, MA: Jones and Bartlett, 2006.

Buchbinder, Sharon B., and Nancy Shanks. *Introduction to Health Care Management*. Sudbury, MA: Jones and Bartlett, 2007.

Charns, Martin P., and Laura J. Smith Tewksbury. *Collaborative Management in Health Care: Implementing the Integrative Organization*. San Francisco: Jossey-Bass, 1992.

Cohn, Kenneth H. *Collaborate for Success: Breakthrough Strategies for Engaging Physicians, Nurses, and Hospital Executives*. Chicago: Health Administration Press, 2006.

Dunn, Rose T. *Haimann's Healthcare Management*. 8th ed. Chicago: Health Administration Press, 2006.

Goldsmith, Seth B. *Principles of Health Care Management: Compliance, Consumerism, and Accountability in the 21st Century*. Sudbury, MA: Jones and Bartlett, 2005.

Griffith, John R., and Kenneth R. White. *The Well-Managed Healthcare Organization.* 6th ed. Chicago: Health Administration Press, 2006.

Hofmann, Paul B., and Frankie Perry, eds. *Management Mistakes in Healthcare: Identification, Correction, and Prevention.* Chicago: Health Administration Press, 2005.

Kelly, Diane L. *Applying Quality Management in Healthcare: A System Approach.* 2d ed. Chicago: Health Administration Press and the Association of University Programs in Health Administration, 2006.

Kovner, Anthony R., and Duncan Neuhauser. *Health Services Management: Readings, Cases, and Commentary.* 8th ed. Chicago: Health Administration Press, 2004.

Liebler, Joan Gratto, and Charles R. McConnell. *Management Principles for Health Professionals.* 4th ed. Sudbury, MA: Jones and Bartlett, 2004.

Lombardi, Donald N. *Handbook for the New Health Care Manager.* 2d ed. San Francisco: Jossey-Bass, 2001.

Longest, Beaufort B. *Managing Health Programs and Projects.* San Francisco: Jossey-Bass, 2004.

McConnell, Charles R. *Managing the Health Care Professional.* Sudbury, MA: Jones and Bartlett, 2004.

McConnell, Charles R. *Umiker's Management Skills for the New Health Care Supervisor.* 4th ed. Sudbury, MA: Jones and Bartlett, 2006.

Pozgar, George D. *Legal Aspects of Health Care Administration.* 9th ed. Sudbury, MA: Jones and Bartlett, 2004.

Ronen, Boaz, Joseph S. Pliskin, Shimeon Pass, et al. *Focused Operations Management for Health Services Organizations.* San Francisco: Jossey-Bass, 2006.

Stahl, Michael J., ed. *Encyclopedia of Health Care Management.* Thousand Oaks, CA: Sage, 2004.

Wolper, Lawrence F. *Health Care Administration: Planning, Implementing, and Managing Organized Delivery Systems.* 4th ed. Sudbury, MA: Jones and Bartlett, 2004.

72. Hospitals

Abraham, Jean, Martin Gaynor, and William B. Vogt. *Entry and Competition in Local Hospital Markets.* NBER Working Paper No. 11649. Cambridge, MA: National Bureau of Economic Research, 2005.

American Hospital Association. *Hospital Statistics.* Chicago: American Hospital Association, 2007. (This is an annual publication)

Berger, Steven. *The Power of Clinical and Financial Metrics: Achieving Success in Your Hospital.* Chicago: Health Administration Press, 2005.

Biggs, Errol. *The Governance Factor: 33 Keys to Success in Healthcare.* Chicago: Health Administration Press, 2003.

Dranove, David, and William D. White. *How Hospitals Survived: Competition and the American Hospital.* Washington, DC: AEI Press, 1999.

Gaynor, Martin, and William B. Vogt. *Competition Among Hospitals.* NBER Working Paper No. 9471. Cambridge, MA: National Bureau of Economic Research, 2003.

Geisler, Eliezer, Koos Krabbendam, and Roel Schuring, eds. *Technology, Health Care, and Management in the Hospitals of the Future.* Westport, CT: Praeger, 2003.

Ginzberg, Eli. *Tomorrow's Hospital: A Look to the Twenty-first Century.* New Haven, CT: Yale University Press, 1996.

Gowrisankaran, Gautam, and Robert J. Town. *Competition, Payers, and Hospital Quality.* NBER Working Paper No. 9206. Cambridge, MA: National Bureau of Economic Research, 2002.

Griffin, Don. *Hospitals: What They Are and How They Work.* 3d ed. Sudbury, MA: Jones and Bartlett, 2006.

Kastor, John A. *Governance of Teaching Hospitals: Turmoil at Penn and Hopkins.* Baltimore: Johns Hopkins University Press, 2003.

Kastor, John A. *Specialty Care in the Era of Managed Care: Cleveland Clinic Versus University Hospitals of Cleveland.* Baltimore: Johns Hopkins University Press, 2005.

Kaufman, Sharon R. *And a Time to Die: How American Hospitals Shape the End of Life.* Chicago: University of Chicago Press, 2005.

McCauley, Bernadette. *Who Shall Take Care of Our Sick? Roman Catholic Sisters and the Development of Catholic Hospitals in New York City.* Baltimore: Johns Hopkins University Press, 2005.

Reynolds, Max M. *Hospital Joint Ventures Legal Handbook.* Sudbury, MA: Jones and Bartlett, 2004.

Risse, Guenter B. *Mending Bodies, Saving Souls: A History of Hospitals.* New York: Oxford University Press, 1999. (This book is a very detailed history of the evolution of hospitals from antiquity to the present)

Rosenberg, Charles E. *The Care of Strangers: The Rise of America's Hospital System.* Baltimore: Johns Hopkins University Press, 1995.

Rundall, Thomas G., David B. Starkweather, and Barbara R. Norrish. *After Restructuring: Empowerment Strategies at Work in America's Hospitals.* San Francisco: Jossey-Bass, 1998.

Schwartz, James R., and H. Chester Horn. *Health Care Alliances and Conversions: A Handbook for Nonprofit Trustees.* San Francisco: Jossey-Bass, 1998.

Stevens, Rosemary. *In Sickness and in Wealth: American Hospitals in the Twentieth Century.* Baltimore: Johns Hopkins University Press, 1999.

73. Nursing

Anderson, Elizabeth T., and Judith M. McFarlane. *Community as Partner: Theory and Practice in Nursing.* 5th ed. Philadelphia: Lippincott Williams and Wilkins, 2008.

Blais, Kathleen Koenig. *Professional Nursing Practice: Concepts and Perspectives.* 5th ed. Upper Saddle River, NJ: Pearson Prentice Hall, 2006.

Catalano, Joseph T. *Nursing Now: Today's Issues, Tomorrow's Trends.* Philadelphia: F. A. Davis, 2006.

Cherry, Barbara, and Susan R. Jacob, eds. *Contemporary Nursing: Issues, Trends, and Management.* 3d ed. St. Louis, MO: Mosby-Elsevier, 2005.

Ellis, Janice Rider, and Celia Love Hartley. *Managing and Coordinating Nursing Care.* 4th ed. Philadelphia: Lippincott Williams and Wilkins, 2005.

Hawkins, Joellen W., and Janice A. Thibodeau. *The Advanced Practice Nurse: Issues for the New Millennium.* 5th ed. New York: Tiresias Press, 2000.

Hood, Lucy J., Susan K. Leddy, and J. Mae Pepper. *Leddy and Pepper's Conceptual Bases of Professional Nursing.* Philadelphia: Lippincott Williams and Wilkins, 2006.

Ian, Peate. *Becoming a Nurse in the 21st Century.* Hoboken, NJ: Wiley, 2006.

Jones, C. B., and B. A. Mark. "The Intersection of Nursing and Health Services Research: An Agenda to Guide Future Research," *Nursing Outlook* 53(6): 324–32, November– December 2005.

Jones, Rebecca Patronis. *Nursing Leadership and Management: Theories, Processes, and Practice.* Philadelphia: F. A. Davis, 2007.

Lee, Helen J., and Charlene A. Winters, eds. *Rural Nursing: Concepts, Theory, and Practice.* New York: Springer, 2006.

Longe, Jacqueline L., ed. *The Gale Encyclopedia of Nursing and Allied Health.* 2d ed. 5 vols. Detroit, MI: Thomson Gale, 2007.

Masters, Kathleen, ed. *Role Development in Professional Nursing Practice.* Sudbury, MA: Jones and Bartlett, 2005.

Polifko-Harris, Karin. *Concepts of the Nursing Profession.* Clifton Park, NY: Thomson Delmar Learning, 2007.

Potter, Patricia Ann, and Anne Griffin Perry, eds. *Basic Nursing: Essentials for Practice.* 6th ed. St. Louis, MO: Mosby-Elsevier, 2007.

Rubenfeld, M. Gaie, and Barbara K. Scheffer. *Clinical Thinking Tactics for Nurses: Tracking, Assessing, and Cultivating Thinking to Improve Competency-Based Strategies.* Sudbury, MA: Jones and Bartlett, 2006.

Spouse, Jenny, Carol Lynn Cox, and Michael J. Cook, eds. *Common Foundation Studies in Nursing.* 4th ed. New York: Elsevier/Churchill Livingstone, 2007.

Stellenberg, Ethelwynn L., and Judith C. Bruce, eds. *Nursing Practice: Hospitals and Community.* New York: Elsevier, Churchill Livingstone, 2007.

Timofeeva, A. A., ed. *The Nursing Profession: Description and Issues.* New York: Novinka Books, 2002.

Warren, Mame, ed. *Our Shared Legacy: Nursing Education at Johns Hopkins, 1889–2006.* Baltimore: Johns Hopkins University Press, 2006.

Brown, Thomas R. *Handbook of Institutional Pharmacy Practice.* Bethesda, MD: American Society of Hospital Pharmacists, 2006.

Dally, Joseph D., ed. *Good Manufacturing Practices for Pharmaceuticals.* 6th ed. New York: Informa Healthcare, 2007.

Epstein, Richard A. *Overdose: How Excessive Government Regulations Stifles Pharmaceutical Innovation.* New Haven, CT: Yale University Press, 2006.

Greene, Jeremy A. *Prescribing by Numbers: Drugs and the Definition of Disease.* Baltimore: Johns Hopkins University Press, 2006.

Kelly, William N. *Pharmacy: What It Is and How It Works.* 2d ed. Boca Raton, FL: Taylor and Francis, 2007.

Petryna, Adriana, Andrew Lakoff, and Arthur Kleinman, eds. *Global Pharmaceuticals: Ethics, Markets, Practices.* Durham, NC: Duke University Press, 2006.

Remington, Joseph P., and Paul Beringer. *Remington: The Science and Practice of Pharmacy.* 21st ed. Philadelphia: Lippincott Williams and Wilkins, 2006.

Rovers, John P., and Jay D. Currie. *A Practical Guide to Pharmaceutical Care: A Clinical Skills Primer.* 3d ed. Washington, DC: American Pharmacists Association, 2007.

Santoro, Michael A., and Thomas M. Gorrie, eds. *Ethics and the Pharmaceutical Industry.* New York: Cambridge University Press, 2005.

Schacter, Bernice Zeldin. *The New Medicines: How Drugs are Created, Approved, Marketed, and Sold.* Westport, CT: Praeger, 2006.

Sloan, Frank A., and Chee-Ruey Hsieh, eds. *Pharmaceutical Innovation: Incentives, and Cost-Benefit Analysis in International Perspective.* New York: Cambridge University Press, 2007.

Smith, Michael Ira, Albert I. Wertheimer, and Jack E. Fincham, eds. *Pharmacy and the U.S. Health Care System.* 3d ed. New York: Pharmaceutical Products Press, 2005.

Strom, Brian L., ed. *Pharmacoepidemiology.* 4th ed. Chichester, UK: Wiley, 2005.

Vogel, Ronald J. *Pharmaceutical Economics and Public Policy.* New York: Pharmaceutical Products Press, 2007.

Wick, Jeannette Y. *Pharmacy Practice in an Aging Society.* New York: Pharmaceutical Products Press, 2006.

Wiffen, Philip, Marc Mitchell, Melanie Snelling, et al. *Oxford Handbook of Clinical Pharmacy.* New York: Oxford University Press, 2007.

74. *Pharmacists and Pharmacy*

Abood, Richard R. *Pharmacy Practice and the Law.* 4th ed. Sudbury, MA: Jones and Bartlett, 2005.

Baciu, Alina, Kathleen Stratton, and Sheila P. Burke, eds., and Committee on the Assessment of the U.S. Drug Safety System, Board on Population Health and Public Health Practice, Institute of Medicine. *The Future of Drug Safety: Promoting and Protecting the Health of the Public.* Washington, DC: National Academies Press, 2006.

75. *Physicians*

American Medical Association. *Directory of Physicians in the United States.* 40th ed. 4 vols. Chicago: American Medical Association, 2006.

American Medical Association. *Physician Characteristics and Distribution in the U.S. 2007.* Chicago: American Medical Association, 2006.

Chisolm, Stephanie. *The Health Professions: Trends and Opportunities in U.S. Health Care.* Sudbury, MA: Jones and Bartlett, 2007.

Gevitz, Norman. *The DOs: Osteopathic Medicine in America*. 2d ed. Baltimore: Johns Hopkins University Press, 2004.

Keagy, Blair, and Marci Thomas, eds. *Essentials of Physician Practice Management*. San Francisco: Jossey-Bass, 2004.

Millenson, Michael L. *Demanding Medical Excellence: Doctors and Accountability in the Information Age*. Chicago: University of Chicago Press, 2002.

Prather, Stephen E. *The New Health Partners: Renewing the Leadership of Physician Practice*. San Francisco: Jossey-Bass, 1999.

Reckless, Ian, John Reynolds, and Ali Raghib, eds. *An Insider's Guide to the Medical Specialties*. New York: Oxford University Press, 2006.

Starr, Paul. *The Social Transformation of American Medicine*. New York: Basic Books, 1982.

U.S. General Accounting Office. *Physician Workforce: Physician Supply Increased in Metropolitan and Nonmetropolitan Areas but Geographic Disparities Persisted*. Washington, DC: U.S. General Accounting Office, 2003.

76. Prepaid Group Practice

Banthin, Jessica S., and Amy K. Taylor. *HMO Enrollment in the United States: Estimates Based on Household Reports, 1996*. Rockville, MD: Agency for Healthcare Research and Quality, 2001.

Coombs, Jan G. *The Rise and Fall of HMOs: An American Health Care Revolution*. Madison: University of Wisconsin Press, 2005.

Donabedian, A. "An Evaluation of Prepaid Group Practice," *Inquiry* 6: 3–27, September 1969.

Enthoven, Alain C., and Laura A. Tollen, eds. *Toward a 21st Century Health System: The Contributions and Promise of Prepaid Group Practice*. San Francisco: Jossey-Bass, 2004.

Freeborn, Donald K., and Clyde R. Pope. *Promise and Performance in Managed Care: The Prepaid Group Practice Model*. Baltimore: Johns Hopkins University Press, 2000.

Markovich, Martin. *The Rise of HMOs*. Santa Monica, CA: RAND Corporation, 2003.

Wrightson, Charles William. *Financial Strategy for Managed Care Organizations: Rate Setting, Risk Adjustment, and Competitive Advantage*. Chicago: Health Administration Press, 2002.

77. Primary Care

Bodenheimer, Thomas, and Kevin Grumbach. *Improving Primary Care: Strategies and Tools for a Better Practice*. New York: Lange Medical Books/McGraw-Hill, 2007.

Isaacs, Stephen L., and James R. Knickman, eds. *Generalist Medicine and the U.S. Health System*. San Francisco: Jossey-Bass, 2004.

Mullan, Fitzhugh. *Big Doctoring in America: Profiles in Primary Care*. Berkeley: University of California Press/ Milbank Memorial Fund, 2002.

Showstack, Jonathan, Arlyss Anderson Rothman, and Sue Hasmiller, eds. *The Future of Primary Care*. San Francisco: Jossey-Bass, 2004.

Skolnik, Neil S., Doron Schneider, Richard Neill, et al., eds. *Handbook of Essential Practice Guidelines in Primary Care*. Totowa, NJ: Humana Press, 2007.

Starfield, Barbara. *Primary Care: Balancing Health Needs, Services, and Technology*. New York: Oxford University Press, 1998.

Sweeney, Kieran. *Complexity in Primary Care: Understanding Its Value*. Seattle, WA: Radcliffe, 2006.

Wakley, Gill, and Ruth Chambers, eds. *Chronic Disease Management in Primary Care: Quality and Outcomes*. Seattle, WA: Radcliffe, 2005.

78. Veterans Administration (VA)

Baker, Rodney R., and Wade E. Pickren. *Psychology and the Department of Veterans Affairs: A Historical Analysis of Training, Research, Practice, and Advocacy*. Washington, DC: American Psychological Association, 2006.

Barbour, Galen L., ed. *Redefining a Public Health System: How the Veterans Health Administration Improved Quality Measurement*. San Francisco: Jossey-Bass, 1996.

Barbour, Galen L., Larry Malby, Richard R. Lussier, et al., eds. *Quality in the Veterans Health Administration: Lessons From the People Who Changed the System*. San Francisco: Jossey-Bass, 1996.

Figley, Charles R., and William P. Nash, eds. *Combat Stress Injury: Theory, Research, and Management*. New York: Routledge, 2007.

Gerber, David A., ed. *Disabled Veterans in History*. Ann Arbor: University of Michigan Press, 2000.

Henry, Lesley M., and Gregory C. Gray. *Topical Bibliography of Published Works Regarding the Health of Veterans of the Persian Gulf War*. San Diego, CA: Naval Health Research Center, 1999.

McMurray-Avila, Marsha. *Homeless Veterans and Health Care: A Resource Guide for Providers*. Nashville, TN: National Health Care for the Homeless Council, 2001.

Roche, John D. *The Veteran's Survival Guide: How to File and Collect on VA Claims*. 2d ed. Washington, DC: Potomac Books, 2006.

Tick, Edward. *War and the Soul: Healing Our Nation's Veterans From Post-Traumatic Stress Disorders*. Wheaton, IL: Quest Books, 2005.

U.S. Congressional Budget Office. *The Potential Cost of Meeting Demand for Veterans' Health Care*. Washington, DC: U.S. Congressional Budget Office, 2005.

IX. Public Health

Public health is the discipline that is aimed at promoting health, preventing and treating diseases, and improving the quality of life of populations. Public health provides the essential social function of keeping populations healthy.

79. General Works

Aday, Lu Ann, ed. *Reinventing Public Health: Policies and Practices for a Healthy Nation.* San Francisco: Jossey-Bass, 2005.

Breslow, Lester, Bernard Goldstein, Lawrence W. Green, et al., eds. *Encyclopedia of Public Health.* 4 vols. New York: Thomson Gale/Macmillan Reference USA, 2002.

Carney, Jan K. *Public Health in Action: Practicing in the Real World.* Sudbury, MA: Jones and Bartlett, 2006.

Davis, Jonathan R., and Joshua Lederberg, eds., and Division of Health Sciences Policy, Institute of Medicine. *Public Health Systems and Emerging Infections: Assessing the Capabilities of the Public and Private Sectors. Workshop Summary.* Washington, DC: National Academy Press, 2000.

Detels, Roger, James McEwen, Robert Beaglehole, et al., eds. *Oxford Textbook of Public Health.* 4th ed. New York: Oxford University Press, 2002.

Duffy, John. *The Sanitarians: A History of American Public Health.* Champaign: University of Illinois Press, 1992.

Fallon, L. Fleming, Jr., and Eric J. Zgodzinski, eds. *Essentials of Public Health Management.* Sudbury, MA: Jones and Bartlett, 2005.

Gebbie, Kristine, Linda Rosenstock, and Lyla M. Hernandez, eds., and Committee on Educating Public Health Professionals for the 21st Century, Board on Health Promotion and Disease Prevention, Institute of Medicine. *Who Will Keep the Public Healthy? Educating Public Health Professionals for the 21st Century.* Washington, DC: National Academies Press, 2003.

Knight, Joseph A. *A Crisis Call for New Preventive Medicine: Emerging Effects of Lifestyle on Morbidity and Mortality.* Hackensack, NJ: World Scientific, 2004.

Levy, Barry S., and Victor W. Sidel, eds. *Social Injustice and Public Health.* New York: Oxford University Press, 2005.

Novick, Lloyd F., and Glen P. Mays, eds. *Public Health Administration: Principles for Population-Based Management.* Sudbury, MA: Jones and Bartlett, 2005.

Patel, Kant, and Mark E. Rushefsky. *The Politics of Public Health in the United States.* Armonk, NY: M. E. Sharpe, 2005.

Pencheon, David, Charles Guest, David Melzer, et al., eds. *Oxford Handbook of Public Health Practice.* New York: Oxford University Press, 2001.

Schneider, Mary-Jane. *Introduction to Public Health.* 2d ed. Sudbury, MA: Jones and Bartlett, 2006.

Tulchinksy, Theodore H., and Elena A. Varavikova. *The New Public Health: An Introduction for the 21st Century.* San Diego, CA: Academic Press, 2000.

Turnock, Bernard J. *Public Health: What It Is and How It Works.* 3d ed. Sudbury, MA: Jones and Bartlett, 2004.

Turnock, Bernard J. *Public Health: Career Choices That Make a Difference.* Sudbury, MA: Jones and Bartlett, 2006.

Ward, John W., and Christian Warren, eds. *Silent Victories: The History and Practice of Public Health in Twentieth-Century America.* New York: Oxford University Press, 2007.

80. Community and Population Health

Brookmeyer, Ron, and Donna F. Stroup, eds. *Monitoring the Health of Populations: Statistical Principles and Methods for Public Health Surveillance.* New York: Oxford University Press, 2003.

Butterfoss, Frances Dunn. *Coalitions and Partnerships in Community Health.* San Francisco: Jossey-Bass, 2007.

Heller, Richard. *Evidence for Population Health.* New York: Oxford University Press, 2005.

Johnson, Kathryn, Wynne Grossman, and Anne Cassidy, eds. *Collaborating to Improve Community Health: Workbook and Guide to Best Practices in Creating Healthier Communities and Populations.* San Francisco: Jossey-Bass, 1997.

Marmot, Michael, and Richard Wilkinson, eds. *Social Determinants of Health.* 2d ed. New York: Oxford University Press, 2006.

McAlearney, Ann S. *Population Health Management: Strategies to Improve Outcomes.* Chicago: Health Administration Press, 2003.

McKenzie, James F., Robert R. Pinger, and Jerome E. Kotecki. *An Introduction to Community Health.* 5th ed. Sudbury, MA: Jones and Bartlett, 2005.

Novick, Lloyd F., and Glen P. Mays. *Public Health Administration: Principles for Population-Based Management.* Sudbury, MA: Jones and Bartlett, 2005.

Palta, Mari. *Quantitative Methods in Population Health: Extensions of Ordinary Regression.* San Francisco: Jossey-Bass, 2003.

Richards, Ronald W. *Building Partnerships: Educating Health Professionals for the Communities They Serve.* San Francisco: Jossey-Bass, 1995.

Smith, Marcia Bayne, Yvonne Graham, and Sally Guttmacher. *Community-Based Health Organizations: Advocating for Improved Health.* San Francisco: Jossey-Bass, 2005.

Stoto, Michael A., Cynthia Abel, and Anne Dievler, eds., and Institute of Medicine. *Healthy Communities: New Partnerships for the Future of Public Health. A Report of the First Year of the Committee on Public Health.* Washington, DC: National Academy Press, 1996.

Wurzbach, Mary Ellen. *Community Health Education and Promotion: A Guide to Program Design and Evaluation.* 2d ed. Sudbury, MA: Jones and Bartlett, 2002.

Young, T. Kue. *Population Health: Concepts and Methods.* New York: Oxford University Press, 2004.

81. Disaster Preparedness, Emergency Management, and Relief

Cohen, Raquel E., and Frederick L. Ahrens. *Handbook for Mental Health Care of Disaster Victims.* Baltimore: Johns Hopkins University Press, 2001.

Committee on Using Information Technology to Enhance Disaster Management, Computer Science and Telecommunications Board, National Research Council.

Summary of a Workshop on Using Information Technology to Enhance Disaster Management. Washington, DC: National Academies Press, 2005.

Few, Roger, and Franziska Matthies, eds. *Flood Hazards and Health: Responding to Present and Future Risks.* Sterling, VA: Earthscan, 2006.

Hooke, William H., and Paul G. Rogers, eds., Institute of Medicine, and National Research Council. *Public Health Risks of Disasters: Communication, Infrastructure, and Preparedness. Workshop Summary.* Washington, DC: National Academies Press, 2005.

Khardori, Nancy, ed. *Bioterrorism Preparedness: Medicine, Public Health, Policy.* Weinheim, Germany: Wiley-VCH, 2006.

Pepper, Lewis, Kathryn Brinsfield, Kirsten Levy, et al. *Public Health Preparedness: Handbook for Disaster Response.* Sudbury, MA: Jones and Bartlett, 2007.

Pilch, Richard F., and Raymond A. Zilinskas, eds. *Encyclopedia of Bioterrorism Defense.* New York: Wiley, 2005.

Rodriguez, Havidan, Enrico L. Quarantelli, and Russell Dynes. *Handbook of Disaster Research.* New York: Springer, 2006.

Ronan, Kevin, and David Johnston. *Promoting Community Resilience in Disasters: The Role of Schools, Youth, and Families.* New York: Springer, 2005.

Rosner, David, and Gerald Markowitz. *Are We Ready? Public Health Since 9/11.* Los Angeles: University of California Press/Milbank Memorial Fund, 2006.

Trotter, Griffin. *The Ethics of Coercion in Mass Casualty Medicine.* Baltimore: Johns Hopkins University Press, 2007.

Waugh, William L., ed. *Shelter From the Storm: Repairing the National Emergency Management System After Hurricane Katrina.* Annals of the American Academy of Political and Social Science, vol. 604. Thousand Oaks, CA: Sage, 2006.

82. *Environmental Health*

Aron, Joan L., and Jonathan A. Patz, eds. *Ecosystem Change and Public Health: A Global Perspective.* Baltimore: Johns Hopkins University Press, 2001.

Friis, Robert H. *Essentials of Environmental Health.* Sudbury, MA: Jones and Bartlett, 2007.

Frumkin, Howard, ed. *Environmental Health: From Global to Local.* San Francisco: Jossey-Bass, 2005.

Goldman, Lynn, and Christine M. Coussens, eds., and Roundtable on Environmental Health Sciences, Research, and Medicine, Board on Health Sciences Policy, Institute of Medicine. *Environmental Health Indicators: Bridging the Chasm of Public Health and the Environment. Workshop Summary.* Washington, DC: National Academies Press, 2004.

Goldstein, Bernard D., Baruch Fischhoff, Steven J. Marcus, et al., eds., and Roundtable on Environmental Health Sciences, Research, and Medicine, Board on Health Sciences Policy, Institute of Medicine. *Ensuring Environmental Health in Postindustrial Cities: Workshop Summary.* Washington, DC: National Academies Press, 2003.

Hilgenkamp, Kathryn. *Environmental Health: Ecological Perspectives.* Sudbury, MA: Jones and Bartlett, 2006.

Johnson, Barry L. *Environmental Policy and Public Health.* Boca Raton, FL: Taylor and Francis, 2007.

Lichter, S. Robert, and Stanley Rothman. *Environmental Cancer: A Political Disease?* New Haven, CT: Yale University Press, 1999.

Lippmann, Morton, Beverly S. Cohen, and Richard B. Schlesinger. *Environmental Health Science: Recognition, Evaluation, and Control of Chemical and Physical Health Hazards.* New York: Oxford University Press, 2003.

Wigle, Donald T. *Child Health and the Environment.* New York: Oxford University Press, 2003.

Yassi, Annalee, Tord Kjellstrom, Theo de Kok, et al. *Basic Environmental Health.* New York: Oxford University Press, 2001.

83. *Evidence-Based Public Health*

Brownson, Ross C., Elizabeth A. Baker, Terry L. Leet, et al. *Evidence-Based Public Health.* New York: Oxford University Press, 2002.

Jenicek, Milor. *Clinical Case Reporting in Evidence-Based Medicine.* New York: Oxford University Press, 2001.

Perrin, Edward B., and Jeffrey J. Koshel, eds., and Committee on National Statistics, Commission on Behavioral and Social Sciences and Education, National Research Council. *Assessment of Performance Measures for Public Health, Substance Abuse, and Mental Health.* Washington, DC: National Academy Press, 1997.

84. *Global Health*

Airhihenbuwa, Collins O. *Healing Our Differences: The Crisis of Global Health and the Politics of Identity.* Lanham, MD: Rowman and Littlefield, 2006.

Bashford, Alison, ed. *Medicine at the Border: Disease, Globalization and Security, 1850 to the Present.* New York: Palgrave Macmillian, 2006.

Beaglehole, Robert, ed. *Global Public Health: A New Era.* New York: Oxford University Press, 2003.

Bennett, Belinda, and George F. Tomossy. *Globalization and Health: Challenges for Health Law and Bioethics.* New York: Springer, 2006.

Bryant, John H., and Polly F. Harrison, eds., and Board on International Health, Institute of Medicine. *Global Health in Transition: A Synthesis: Perspectives From International Organizations.* Washington, DC: National Academy Press, 1996.

Foege, William H., Nils M. P. Daulaire, Robert E. Black, et al., eds. *Global Health Leadership and Management.* San Francisco: Jossey-Bass, 2005.

Fried, Bruce J., and Laura M. Gaydos, eds. *World Health Systems: Challenges and Perspectives.* Chicago: Health Administration Press, 2002.

Frumkin, Howard, ed. *Environmental Health: From Global to Local.* San Francisco: Jossey-Bass, 2005.

Gunn, S. W. A., P. B. Mansourian, Anthony Piel, et al. *Understanding the Global Dimensions of Health.* New York: Springer, 2005.

Heymann, Jody, ed. *Global Inequalities at Work: Work's Impact on the Health of Individuals, Families, and Societies.* New York: Oxford University Press, 2003.

Kawachi, Ichiro, and Sarah P. Wamala, eds. *Globalization and Health.* New York: Oxford University Press, 2007.

Koop, C. Everett, Clarence E. Pearson, and M. Roy Schwarz, eds. *Critical Issues in Global Health.* San Francisco: Jossey-Bass, 2002.

MacLachian, Malcolm. *Culture and Health: A Critical Perspective Towards Global Health.* 2d ed. San Francisco: Jossey-Bass, 2006.

McQueen, David, and Pekka Puska. *Global Behavioural Risk Factor Surveillance.* New York: Springer, 2003.

Merson, Michael H., Robert E. Black, and Anne J. Mills. *International Public Health: Diseases, Programs, Systems, and Policies.* 2d ed. Sudbury, MA: Jones and Bartlett, 2006.

Muhiuddin, Haider. *Global Public Health Communication: Challenges, Perspectives, and Strategies.* Sudbury, MA: Jones and Bartlett, 2005.

Mullan, Fitzhugh, Claire Panosian, and Patricia Cuff, eds., and Committee on the Options for Overseas Placement of U.S. Health Professionals, Board on Global Health, Institute of Medicine. *Healers Abroad: Americans Responding to the Human Resource Crisis in HIV/AIDS.* Washington, DC: National Academies Press, 2005.

Skolnik, Richard. *Essentials of Global Health.* Sudbury, MA: Jones and Bartlett, 2007.

U.S. Government Accountability Office. *Global Health: Spending Requirement Presents Challenges for Allocating Prevention Funding Under the President's Emergency Plan for AIDS Relief: Report to Congressional Committees.* Washington, DC: U.S. Government Accountability Office, 2006.

Wieners, Walter W., ed. *Global Health Care Markets: A Comprehensive Guide to Regions, Trends, and Opportunities Shaping the International Health Arena.* San Francisco: Jossey-Bass, 2000.

World Health Organization. *Global Crises—Global Solutions: Managing Public Health Emergencies of International Concern Through the Revised International Health Regulations.* Geneva, Switzerland: World Health Organization, 2002.

85. Health Promotion and Disease Prevention

Andreasen, Alan R. *Marketing Social Change: Changing Behavior to Promote Health, Social Development, and the Environment.* San Francisco: Jossey-Bass, 1995.

Bartholomew, L. Kay, Guy S. Parcel, Gerjo Kok, et al., eds. *Planning Health Promotion Programs: An Intervention Mapping Approach.* 2d ed. San Francisco: Jossey-Bass, 2006.

Blonna, Richard, and Dan Watter. *Health Counseling: A Microskills Approach.* Sudbury, MA: Jones and Bartlett, 2005.

Board on Population Health and Public Health Practices, Institute of Medicine. *Estimating the Contributions of Lifestyle-Related Factors to Preventable Death: Workshop Summary.* Washington, DC: National Academies Press, 2005.

Cottrell, Randall R., and James F. McKenzie. *Health Promotion and Education Research Methods: Using the Five Chapter Thesis/Dissertation Model.* Sudbury, MA: Jones and Bartlett, 2005.

Crosby, Richard A., Ralph J. DiClemente, and Laura F. Salazar, eds. *Research Methods in Health Promotion.* San Francisco: Jossey-Bass, 2006.

DiClemente, Ralph J., Richard A. Crosby, and Michelle C. Kegler. *Emerging Theories in Health Promotion Practice and Research: Strategies for Improving Public Health.* San Francisco: Jossey-Bass, 2002.

Gilmore, Gary D., and M. Donald Campbell. *Needs and Capacity Assessment Strategies for Health Education and Health Promotion.* 3d ed. Sudbury, MA: Jones and Bartlett, 2005.

Gunn, S. William A., P. B. Mansourian, A. M. Davies, et al., eds. *Understanding the Global Dimensions of Health.* New York: Springer, 2005.

Johnson, James A. *Managing Health Education and Promotion Programs: Leadership Skills for the 21st Century.* 2d ed. Sudbury, MA: Jones and Bartlett, 2007.

L'Abate, Luciano, ed. *Low-Cost Approaches to Promote Physical and Mental Health: Theory, Research and Practice.* New York: Springer, 2006.

Leddy, Susan Kun. *Integrative Health Promotion: Conceptual Bases for Nursing Practice.* 2d ed. Sudbury, MA: Jones and Bartlett, 2006.

Marmot, Michael, and Richard G. Wilkinson, eds. *Social Determinants of Health.* 2d ed. New York: Oxford University Press, 2006.

McQueen, David. *Health and Modernity: The Role of Theory in Health Promotion.* New York: Springer, 2007.

Modeste, Naomi, and Teri Tamayose. *Dictionary of Public Health Promotion and Education: Terms and Concepts.* 2d ed. San Francisco: Jossey-Bass, 2004.

Perkins, Elizabeth R., Ina Simnett, and Linda Wright, eds. *Evidence-Based Health Promotion.* San Francisco: Jossey-Bass, 1999.

Sheinfeld-Gorin, Sherri, and Joan Arnold. *Health Promotion in Practice.* San Francisco: Jossey-Bass, 2006.

Thorogood, Margaret, and Yolande Coombes, eds. *Evaluating Health Promotion: Practice and Methods.* New York: Oxford University Press, 2000.

Valente, Thomas W. *Evaluating Health Promotion Programs.* New York: Oxford University Press, 2002.

Wurzbach, Mary Ellen. *Community Health Education and Promotion: A Guide to Program Design and Evaluation.* 2d ed. Sudbury, MA: Jones and Bartlett, 2002.

Zaza, Stephanie, Peter A. Briss, and Kate W. Harris, eds. *The Guide to Community Preventive Services: What Works to Promote Health?* New York: Oxford University Press, 2005.

86. Maternal and Child Health

Besharov, Douglas J., ed. *Family and Child Well-Being After Welfare Reform*. Somerset, NJ: Transaction Publishers, 2003.

Board on Children, Youth, and Families, Commission on Behavioral and Social Sciences and Education, Board on Health Promotion and Disease Prevention, National Research Council and Institute of Medicine. *Paying Attention to Children in a Changing Health Care System: Summaries of Workshops*. Washington, DC: National Academy Press, 1996.

Freeman, Michael, ed. *Children's Health and Children's Rights*. Boston: Martinus Nijhoff, 2006.

Health Resources and Services Administration. *Child Health USA 2005*. Rockville, MD: U.S. Department of Health and Human Services, 2005.

Kotch, Jonathan. *Maternal and Child Health: Programs, Problems, and Policy in Public Health*. 2d ed. Sudbury, MA: Jones and Bartlett, 2005.

Mahy, Mary. *Childhood Mortality in the Developing World: A Review of Evidence From the Demographic and Health Surveys*. Calverton, MD: ORC Macro, Measure DHS+, 2003.

Morewitz, Stephen J. *Domestic Violence and Maternal and Child Health*. New York: Springer, 2004.

Palfray, Judith S. *Child Health in America: Making a Difference Through Advocacy*. Baltimore: Johns Hopkins University Press, 2006.

Parens, Erik, ed. *Surgically Shaping Children: Technology, Ethics, and the Pursuit of Normality*. Baltimore: Johns Hopkins University Press, 2006.

Turkington, Carol, and Albert Tzell, eds. *The Encyclopedia of Children's Health and Wellness*. New York: Facts on File, 2004.

Wigle, Donald T. *Child Health and the Environment*. New York: Oxford University Press, 2003.

X. Selective Diseases and Conditions

Selective diseases and conditions include a host of acute, chronic, and infectious diseases and health conditions. These diseases and conditions can be caused by various sources, including microbial pathogens, the environment, and genetics.

87. Acute and Infectious Diseases

Abraham, Thomas. *Twenty-First Century Plague: The Story of SARS*. Baltimore: Johns Hopkins University Press, 2007.

Apostolopoulos, Yorghos, and Sevil Sonmez, eds. *Crossing Boundaries, Compounding Infections: The Impact of Population Migration and Infectious Diseases*. New York: Springer, 2006.

Arias, Kathleen Meehan, and Barbara M. Soule, eds. *The APIC/JCAHO Infection Control Workbook*. Oakbrook Terrace, IL: APIC/Joint Commission Resources, 2006.

Berger, Stephen A., and John S. Marr. *Human Parasitic Diseases Sourcebook*. Sudbury, MA: Jones and Bartlett, 2006.

Bourdelais, Patrice. *Epidemics Laid Low: A History of What Happened in Rich Countries*. Baltimore: Johns Hopkins University Press, 2006.

Callahan, Gerald N. *Infection: The Uninvited Universe*. New York: St. Martin's Press, 2006.

Casman, Elizabeth A., and Hadi Dowlatabadi, eds. *Contextual Determinants of Malaria*. Baltimore: Johns Hopkins University Press, 2002.

Chan, Voon L., Philip M. Sherman, and Billy Bourke, eds. *Bacterial Genomes and Infectious Diseases*. Totowa, NJ: Humana Press, 2006.

Cliff, Andrew, Peter Haggett, and Matthew Smallman-Raynor. *World Atlas of Epidemic Diseases*. New York: Oxford University Press, 2004.

Colgrove, James. *State of Immunity: The Politics of Vaccination in Twentieth-Century America*. Los Angeles: University of California Press/Milbank Memorial Fund, 2006.

Giesecke, Johan. *Modern Infectious Disease Epidemiology*. 2d ed. New York: Oxford University Press, 2002.

Goudsmit, Jaap. *Viral Fitness: The Next SARS and West Nile in the Making*. New York: Oxford University Press, 2004.

Gualde, Norbert. *Resistance: The Human Struggle Against Infection*. New York: Dana Press, 2006.

Heymann, David L., ed. *Control of Communicable Diseases Manuel*. 18th ed. Washington, DC: American Public Health Association, 2005.

Institute of Medicine. *Microbial Threats to Health: The Threat of Pandemic Influenza*. Washington, DC: National Academies Press, 2005.

Knobler, Stacey L., Alison Mack, Adel Mahmoud, et al., eds., and Forum on Microbial Threats, Board on Global Health, Institute of Medicine. *The Threat of Pandemic Influenza: Are We Ready? Workshop Summary*. Washington, DC: National Academies Press, 2004.

Knobler, Stacey L., Thomas Burroughs, Adel Mahmoud, et al., and Forum on Microbial Threats, Board on Global Health, Institute of Medicine. *Ensuring an Infectious Disease Workforce: Education and Training Need for the 21st Century. Workshop Summary*. Washington, DC: National Academies Press, 2007.

Laxminarayan, Ramanan, ed. *Battling Resistance to Antibiotics and Pesticides: An Economic Approach*. Baltimore: Johns Hopkins University Press, 2002.

Magnus, Manya. *Essentials of Infectious Disease Epidemiology*. Sudbury, MA: Jones and Bartlett, 2007.

McLean, Angela R., Robert M. May, John Pattison, et al., eds. *SARS: A Case Study in Emerging Infections*. New York: Oxford University Press, 2005.

National Academies Keck Futures Initiative. *The Genomic Revolution: Implications for Treatment and Control of Infectious Disease: Working Group Summaries*. Conference held at the Arnold and Mabel Bechman Center of the National Academies, Irvine, CA (November 10–13, 2005). Washington, DC: National Academies Press, 2006.

Nelson, Kenrad, and Carolyn Masters Williams. *Infectious Disease Epidemiology: Theory and Practice.* 2d ed. Sudbury, MA: Jones and Bartlett, 2007.

Playfair, John. *Living With Germs: In Sickness and in Health.* New York: Oxford University Press, 2005.

Podolsky, Scott H. *Pneumonia Before Antibiotics: Therapeutic Evolution and Evaluation in Twentieth-Century America.* Baltimore: Johns Hopkins University Press, 2006.

Roberts, Jennifer A., ed. *The Economics of Infectious Disease.* New York: Oxford University Press, 2006.

Sleigh, Adrian, Chee Heng Leng, Brenda S. A. Yeoh, et al., eds. *Population Dynamics and Infectious Disease in Asia.* Hackensack, NJ: World Scientific, 2006.

Thomas, James C., and David J. Weber, eds. *Epidemiologic Methods for the Study of Infectious Diseases.* New York: Oxford University Press, 2001.

Tibayrenc, Michel. *Encyclopedia Guide to Infectious Disease Research: Modern Methodologies.* Hoboken, NJ: Wiley-LISS, 2006.

Turkington, Carol, and Bonnie Lee Ashby. *The Encyclopedia of Infectious Diseases.* 3d ed. New York: Facts on File, 2007.

Webber, Roger. *Communicable Disease Epidemiology and Control: A Global Perspective.* 2d ed. New York: Oxford University Press, 2005.

Yoshikawa, Thomas T., and Joseph G. Ouslander, ed. *Infection Management for Geriatrics in Long-Term Care Facilities.* 2d ed. New York: Informa Healthcare, 2007.

88. AIDS/HIV

Baldwin, Peter. *Disease and Democracy: The Industrialized World Faces AIDS.* Los Angeles: University of California Press/Milbank Memorial Fund, 2005.

Barnett, Tony, and Alan Whiteside. *AIDS in the Twenty-First Century: Disease and Globalization.* New York: Palgrave Macmillan, 2006.

Bartlett, John G., and Ann K. Finkbeiner. *The Guide to Living With HIV Infection: Developed at the Johns Hopkins AIDS Clinic.* 6th ed. Baltimore: Johns Hopkins University Press, 2006.

Bowser, Benjamin P., Ernest Quimby, and Merrill Singer, eds. *When Communities Assess Their AIDS Epidemics: Results of Rapid Assessment of HIV/AIDS in Eleven U.S. Cities.* Lanham, MD: Lexington Books, 2007.

Braithwaite, Ronald L., Theodore M. Hammett, and Robert M. Mayberry. *Prisons and AIDS: A Public Health Challenge.* San Francisco: Jossey-Bass, 1996.

Clark, Rebecca A., Robert T. Maupin, and Jill Hayes Hammer. *A Woman's Guide to Living With HIV Infection.* Baltimore: Johns Hopkins University Press, 2004.

Committee on Public Financing and Delivery of HIV Care, Board on Health Promotion and Disease Prevention, Institute of Medicine. *Public Financing and Delivery of HIV/AIDS Care: Securing the Legacy of Ryan White.* Washington, DC: National Academies Press, 2004.

Committee on Reviewing the HIVNET 012 Perinatal HIV Prevention Study, Board on Population Health and Public Health Practice, Institute of Medicine. *Review of the HIVNET 012 Perinatal HIV Prevention Study.* Washington, DC: National Academies Press, 2005.

Engel, Jonathan. *The Epidemic: A Global History of AIDS.* New York: Smithsonian Books/Collins, 2006.

Essex, Max, Souleymane Mboup, Phyllis J. Kanki, et al. *AIDS in Africa.* New York: Springer, 2002.

Falola, Toyin, and Matthew M. Heaton, eds. *HIV/AIDs, Illness, and African Well-Being.* Rochester, NY: University of Rochester Press, 2007.

Farber, Celia. *Serious Adverse Events: An Uncensored History of AIDS.* Hoboken, NJ: Melville House, 2006.

Feldman, Eric, and Ronald Bayer, eds. *Blood Feuds: AIDS, Blood, and the Politics of Medical Disaster.* New York: Oxford University Press, 1999.

Friedman, Samuel R., Richard Curtis, Alan Neaigus, et al. *Social Networks, Drug Injectors' Lives, and HIV/AIDS.* New York: Springer, 1999.

Gibney, Laura, Ralph J. DiClemente, and Sten H. Vermund. *Preventing HIV in Developing Countries.* New York: Springer, 1999.

Gill, Peter. *Body Count: Fixing the Blame for the Global AIDS Catastrophe.* New York: Thunder's Mouth Press, 2006.

Holtgrave, David R. *Handbook of Economic Evaluation of HIV Prevention Programs.* New York: Springer, 1998.

Institute of Medicine. *Confronting AIDS: Directions for Public Health, Health Care, and Research.* Washington, DC: National Academy Press, 1986.

International Labour Organization on HIV/AIDS. *HIV/AIDS and Work in a Globalizing World, 2005.* Geneva, Switzerland: International Labour Organization, World of Work, 2006.

Kalichman, Seth C. *Positive Prevention: Reducing HIV Transmission Among People Living With HIV/AIDS.* New York: Springer, 2005.

Klitzman, Robert, and Ronald Bayer. *Mortal Secrets: Truth and Lies in the Age of AIDS.* Baltimore: Johns Hopkins University Press, 2005.

Knox, Michael D., and Caroline H. Sparks, eds. *HIV and Community Mental Healthcare.* Baltimore: Johns Hopkins University Press, 1997.

Letona, Maria Elena. *State Government Provision of HIV/AIDS Prevention Programs: Towards a Partnership Model of the Contractual Relationship Between State Governments and Community Agencies.* New York: Garland, 2000.

Loue, Sana. *Sexual Partnering, Sexual Practices, and Health.* New York: Springer, 2005.

Lu, Yichen, and Max Essex. *AIDS in Asia.* New York: Springer, 2004.

Mullan, Fitzhugh, Claire Panosian, and Patricia Cuff, eds., and Committee on the Options for Overseas Placement of U.S. Health Professionals, Board on Global Health, Institute of Medicine. *Healers Abroad: Americans Responding to the Human Resource Crisis in HIV/AIDS.* Washington, DC: National Academies Press, 2005.

O'Leary, Ann. *Beyond Condoms: Alternative Approaches to HIV Prevention.* New York: Springer, 2002.

Ostrow, David, and Seth C. Kalichman. *Psychosocial and Public Health Impacts of New HIV Therapies*. New York: Springer, 1999.

Peterson, John L., and Ralph J. DiClemente. *Handbook of HIV Prevention*. New York: Springer, 2000.

Seckinelgin, Hakan. *International Politics of HIV/AIDS: Global Disease—Local Pain*. New York: Routledge, 2007.

Shelling, Gene M., ed. *AIDS Policies and Programs*. New York: Nova Science, 2006.

Stillwaggon, Eileen. *AIDS and the Ecology of Poverty*. New York: Oxford University Press, 2006.

Treisman, Glenn J., and Andrew F. Angelino. *The Psychiatry of AIDS: A Guide to Diagnosis and Treatment*. Baltimore: Johns Hopkins University Press, 2004.

U.S. Government Accountability Office. *Global Health: Spending Requirement Presents Challenges for Allocating Prevention Funding Under the President's Emergency Plan for AIDS Relief Report to Congressional Committees*. Washington, DC: U.S. Government Accountability Office, 2006.

Valdiserri, Ronald O., ed. *Dawning Answers: How the HIV/AIDS Epidemic Has Helped to Strengthen Public Health*. New York: Oxford University Press, 2002.

Watstein, Sarah B., and Stephen E. Stratton. *The Encyclopedia of HIV and AIDS*. New York: Facts on File, 2003.

Wollmann, Emmanuelle E. *Legal and Ethical Aspects of HIV-Related Research*. New York: Springer, 1995.

89. Asthma

Australian Institute of Health and Welfare. *Health Care Expenditure and the Burden of Disease Due to Asthma in Australia*. Canberra, Australian Capital Territory, Australia: Australian Institute of Health and Welfare, 2005.

Bellenir, Karen, ed. *Asthma Sourcebook: Basic Consumer Health Information About the Causes, Symptoms, Diagnosis, and Treatment of Asthma in Infants, Children, Teenagers, and Adults*. 2d ed. Detroit, MI: Omnigraphics, 2006.

Blaser, Kurt, Reto Crameri, and R. C. Aalberse, eds. *Allergy and Asthma in Modern Society: A Scientific Approach*. New York: Karger, 2006.

Busse, William W., and Robert F. Lemanske, eds. *Asthma Prevention*. Boca Raton, FL: Taylor and Francis, 2005.

Chung, Fan, and George C. Kassianos. *Best Medicine: Asthma*. Long Hanborough, UK: CSF Medical Communications, 2005.

Fanta, Christopher H., Elaine L. Carter, Elisabeth S. Stieb, et al. *The Asthma Educator's Handbook*. New York: McGraw-Hill Medical, 2007.

Gershwin, M. Eric, and Timothy E. Albertson, eds. *Bronchial Asthma: A Guide for Practical Understanding and Treatment*. Totowa, NJ: Humana Press, 2006.

Gibson, Peter, ed. *Monitoring Asthma*. Boca Raton, FL: Taylor and Francis, 2005.

Ho, Kare, Rosanna M. Coffey, and Donna Rae Castillo. *Asthma Care Quality Improvement: A Workbook for State*

Action. Rockville, MD: Agency for Healthcare Research and Quality, 2006.

Institute for Clinical Systems Improvement. *Health Care Guideline: Diagnosis and Outpatient Management of Asthma*. Bloomington, MN: Institute for Clinical Systems Improvement, 2005.

Institute for Clinical Systems Improvement. *Health Care Guideline: Emergency and Inpatient Management of Asthma*. Bloomington, MN: Institute for Clinical Systems Improvement, 2006.

Li, James T. C., ed. *Pharmacotherapy of Asthma*. New York: Taylor and Francis, 2006.

Miller, Amy P., ed. *New Developments in Asthma Research*. New York: Nova Biomedical Books, 2006.

Navarra, Tova. *The Encyclopedia of Asthma and Respiratory Disorders*. New York: Facts on File, 2003.

Postma, Dirkje S., and Scott T. Weiss, eds. *Genetics of Asthma and Chronic Obstructive Pulmonary Disease*. New York: Informa Healthcare, 2007.

Rees, John, and Dipak Kanabar. *ABC of Asthma*. 5th ed. Malden, MA: BMJ Books/Blackwell, 2006.

Sepiashvili, Revaz, ed. "Advances in Research and Management of Asthma." In *Proceedings of the 3rd European Asthma Congress: Athens, Greece (October 20–23, 2005)*. Bologna, Italy: Medimond International Proceedings, 2005.

Szefler, Stanley J., and Soren Pedersen, eds. *Childhood Asthma*. New York: Taylor and Francis, 2006.

Tersa, Miroslav, ed. *Trends in Asthma Research*. Hauppauge, NY: Nova Biomedical Books, 2005.

90. Cancer

Abrahm, Janet L. *A Physician's Guide to Pain and Symptom Management in Cancer Patients*. 2d ed. Baltimore: Johns Hopkins University Press, 2005.

Adami, Hans-Olov, David Hunter, and Dimitrios Trichopoulos, eds. *Textbook of Cancer Epidemiology*. New York: Oxford University Press, 2002.

Altman, Arnold J., ed. *Supportive Care of Children With Cancer: Current Therapy and Guidelines From the Children's Oncology Group*. 3d ed. Baltimore: Johns Hopkins University Press, 2004.

Bertino, Joseph R. *Encyclopedia of Cancer*. 2d ed. 4 vols. San Diego, CA: Academic Press, 2002.

Capitman, John A., Sarita Bhalotra, and Mathilda Ruwe. *Cancer and Elders of Color: Opportunities for Reducing Health Disparities: Evidence Review and Recommendations for Research and Policy*. Burlington, VT: Ashgate, 2005.

Coleman, C. Norman. *Understanding Cancer: A Patient's Guide to Diagnosis, Prognosis, and Treatment*. Baltimore: Johns Hopkins University Press, 2006.

Columbus, Frank H., ed. *Trends in Cancer Prevention Research*. New York: Nova Science, 2006.

Eden, Jill, and Joseph V. Simone, eds., Committee on Assessing Improvement in Cancer Care in Georgia, National Cancer Policy Board, Institute of Medicine, and National Research

Council. *Assessing the Quality of Cancer Care: An Approach to Measurement in Georgia.* Washington, DC: National Academies Press, 2005.

Feuerstein, Michael. *Handbook of Cancer Survivorship.* New York: Springer, 2007.

Foley, Kathleen M., and Hellen Gelband, eds., National Cancer Policy Board, Institute of Medicine, and National Research Council. *Improving Palliative Care for Cancer: Summary and Recommendations.* Washington, DC: National Academy Press, 2001.

Ganz, Patricia A. *Cancer Survivorship: Today and Tomorrow.* New York: Springer, 2007.

Grossman, S. A., E. M. Dunbar, and S. A. Nesbit, "Cancer Pain Management in the 21st Century," *Oncology* 20(11): 1333–39, October 2006.

Halvorson-Boyd, Glenna, and Lisa K. Hunter. *Dancing in Limbo: Making Sense of Life After Cancer.* San Francisco: Jossey-Bass, 1995.

Herdman, Roger, and Leonard Lichtenfeld, eds., National Cancer Policy Board, Institute of Medicine, and National Research Council. *Fulfilling the Potential of Cancer Prevention and Early Detection: An American Cancer Society and Institute of Medicine Symposium.* Washington, DC: National Academies Press, 2000.

Hewitt, Maria, and Joseph V. Simone, eds., National Cancer Policy Board, Institute of Medicine, and Commission on Life Sciences, National Research Council. *Ensuring Quality Cancer Care.* Washington, DC: National Academy Press, 1999.

Kedrowski, Karen M., and Marilyn S. Sarow. *Cancer Activism: Gender, Media, and Public Policy.* Urbana: University of Illinois Press, 2007.

Lichter, S. Robert, and Stanley Rothman. *Environmental Cancer: A Political Disease?* New Haven, CT: Yale University Press, 1999.

Longe, Jacqueline L. *The Gale Encyclopedia of Cancer: A Guide to Cancer and Its Treatments.* 2d ed. 2 vols. Detroit, MI: Thomson Gale, 2005.

Montz, F. J., Robert E. Bristow, and Paula J. Anastasia. *A Guide to Survivorship for Women With Ovarian Cancer.* Baltimore: Johns Hopkins University Press, 2005.

Nasca, Phillip C., and Harris Pastides. *Fundamentals of Cancer Epidemiology.* Sudbury, MA: Jones and Bartlett, 2001.

Olopade, Olufunmilayo I., Carla I. Falkson, and Christopher Kwesi Williams, eds. *Breast Cancer in Women of African Descent.* New York: Springer, 2006.

Olson, James S. *Bathsheba's Breast: Women, Cancer, and History.* Baltimore: Johns Hopkins University Press, 2005.

Patlak, Margie, and Sharyl J. Nass, and National Cancer Policy Forum, Institute of Medicine. *Developing Biomarker-Based Tools for Cancer Screening, Diagnosis, and Treatment: The State of the Science, Evaluation, Implementation, and Economics. Workshop Summary.* Washington, DC: National Academies Press, 2006.

Patlak, Margie, Sharyl J. Nass, I. Craig Henderson, et al., eds., Committee on the Early Detection of Breast

Cancer, National Cancer Policy Board, Institute of Medicine, and Commission on Life Sciences, National Research Council. *Mammography and Beyond: Developing Technologies for the Early Detection of Breast Cancer: A Non-Technical Summary.* Washington, DC: National Academy Press, 2000.

Schottenfeld, David, and Joseph F. Fraumeni, eds. *Cancer Epidemiology and Prevention.* 3d ed. New York: Oxford University Press, 2006.

Seligman, Linda. *Promoting a Fighting Spirit: Psychotherapy for Cancer Patients, Survivors, and Their Families.* San Francisco: Jossey-Bass, 1996.

Siminoff, L. A., and L. Ross. "Access and Equity to Cancer Care in the USA: A Review and Assessment," *Postgraduate Medical Journal* 81(961): 674–79, November 2005.

Spingarm, Natalie Davis. *The New Cancer Survivors: Living With Grace, Fighting With Spirit.* Baltimore: Johns Hopkins University Press, 1999.

Turkington, Carol, and William LiPera. *The Encyclopedia of Cancer.* New York: Facts on File, 2005.

91. *Chronic Diseases*

Fogel, Robert W. *Changes in the Disparities in Chronic Disease During the Course of the Twentieth Century.* NBER Working Paper No. 10311. Cambridge, MA: National Bureau of Economic Research, 2004.

Fraser, Gary E. *Diet, Life Expectancy, and Chronic Disease.* New York: Oxford University Press, 2003.

Kane, Robert L., Reinhard Priester, and Annette M. Totten. *Meeting the Challenge of Chronic Illness.* Baltimore: Johns Hopkins University Press, 2005.

Kuh, Diana, and Yoav Ben Shlomo, eds. *A Life Course Approach to Chronic Diseases Epidemiology.* 2d ed. New York: Oxford University Press, 2004.

Lubkin, Ilene Morof, and Pamala D. Larsen, eds. *Chronic Illness: Impact and Interventions.* 6th ed. Sudbury, MA: Jones and Bartlett, 2006.

Morewitz, Stephen J. *Chronic Diseases and Health Care: New Trends in Diabetes, Arthritis, Osteoporosis, Fibromyalgia, Low Back Pain, Cardiovascular Disease and Cancer.* New York: Springer, 2006.

Nuovo, Jim, ed. *Chronic Disease Management.* New York: Springer, 2007.

Van Zwanenberg, Patrick, and Erik Millstone. *BSE: Risk, Science, and Governance.* New York: Oxford University Press, 2005. (BSE stands for bovine spongiform encephalopathy, or mad cow disease.)

Wakley, Gill, and Ruth Chambers, eds. *Chronic Disease Management in Primary Care: Quality and Outcomes.* Seattle, WA: Radcliffe, 2005.

Webster, Barbara D. *All of a Piece: A Life With Multiple Sclerosis.* Baltimore: Johns Hopkins University Press, 1998.

Zazworsky, Donna, Jane Nelson Bolin, and Vicki Gaubeca. *Handbook of Diabetes Management.* New York: Springer, 2005.

92. Diabetes

American Diabetes Association. *Diabetes 411: Facts, Figures, and Statistics at a Glance.* Alexandria, VA: American Diabetes Association, 2005.

American Pharmacists Association. *Pharmacist Disease Management: Diabetes.* 3d ed. Washington, DC: American Pharmacists Association, 2005.

Barnett, Anthony H. *Applying the Evidence: Clinical Trials in Diabetes.* Chicago: Remedica, 2005.

Diabetes Mellitus: A Guide to Patient Care. Philadelphia: Lippincott Williams and Wilkins, 2007.

Fonseca, Vivian A. *Clinical Diabetes: Translating Research Into Practice.* Philadelphia: Saunders Elsevier, 2006.

Hartley, David, Erika C. Ziller, and Caroline MacDonald. *Diabetes and the Rural Safety Net.* Portland: University of Southern Maine, Edmund S. Muskie School of Public Services, Maine Rural Health Research Center, 2002.

Mantzoros, Christos S., ed. *Obesity and Diabetes.* Totowa, NJ: Humana Press, 2006.

Mazze, R. S., et al. *Staged Diabetes Management: A Systematic Approach.* Hoboken, NJ: Wiley, 2007.

McDowell, Joan R. S., David M. Matthews, and Florence J. Brown, eds. *Diabetes: A Handbook for the Primary Care Healthcare Team.* New York: Elsevier, Churchill Livingstone, 2007.

Mertig, Rita G. *The Nurse's Guide to Teaching Diabetes Self-Management.* New York: Springer, 2007.

Petit, William A., and Christine Adamec. *The Encyclopedia of Diabetes.* New York: Facts on File, 2002.

Ross, Tami, Jackie Boucher, and Belinda O'Connell, eds. *American Dietetic Association Guide to Diabetes Medical Nutrition Therapy and Education.* Chicago: American Dietetic Association, 2005.

Unger, Jeff. *Diabetes Management in Primary Care.* Philadelphia: Wolters Kluwer Health/Lippincott Williams and Wilkins, 2007.

Zazworsky, Donna, Jane Nelson Bolin, and Vicki Gaubeca, eds. *Handbook of Diabetes Management.* New York: Springer, 2005.

93. Emerging Diseases

Abraham, Thomas. *Twenty-First Century Plague: The Story of SARS.* Baltimore: Johns Hopkins University Press, 2007.

Davis, Jonathan R., and Joshua Lederberg, eds., and Division of Health Sciences Policy, Institute of Medicine. *Public Health Systems and Emerging Infections: Assessing the Capabilities of the Public and Private Sectors. Workshop Summary.* Washington, DC: National Academy Press, 2000.

Gualde, Norbert. *Resistance: The Human Struggle Against Infection.* New York: Dana Press, 2006.

Laxminarayan, Ramanan, Anup Malani, David Howard, et al. *Extending the Cure: Policy Responses to the Growing Threat of Antibiotic Resistance.* Washington, DC: Resources for the Future, 2007.

Packard, Randall M., Peter J. Brown, Ruth Berkelman, et al., eds. *Emerging Illnesses and Society: Negotiating the Public Health Agenda.* Baltimore: Johns Hopkins University, 2004.

Tambyah, Paul A., and Ping-Chung Leung. *Bird Flu: A Rising Pandemic in Asia and Beyond?* Hackensack, NJ: World Scientific, 2006.

94. Heart Disease

Jeffrey, Kirk. *Machines in Our Hearts: The Cardiac Pacemaker, the Implantable Defibrillator, and American Health Care.* Baltimore: Johns Hopkins University Press, 2001.

Krumholz, H. M., and F. A. Masoudi. "The Year in Epidemiology, Health Services Research, and Outcomes Research," *Journal of the American College of Cardiology* 48(9): 1886–95, November 7, 2006.

Marmot, Michael, and Paul Elliott, eds. *Coronary Heart Disease Epidemiology: From Aetiology to Public Health.* 2d ed. New York: Oxford University Press, 2005.

Naill, Catherine A., Edward B. Clark, and Carleen Clark. *The Heart of a Child: What Families Need to Know About Health Disorders in Children.* 2d ed. Baltimore: Johns Hopkins University Press, 2001.

Rosendorff, Clive, ed. *Essential Cardiology: Principles and Practice.* 2d ed. Totowa, NJ: Humana Press, 2005.

95. Hypertension

Battegay, Edouard J., Gregory Y. H. Lip, and George L. Bakris, eds. *Hypertension: Principles and Practice.* Boca Raton, FL: Taylor and Francis, 2005.

Beevers, D. Gareth, Gregory Y. H. Lip, and Eoin O'Brien. *ABC of Hypertension.* 5th ed. Malden, MA: BMJ Books, 2007.

Benhagen, Elwood F., ed. *Hypertension: New Research.* New York: Nova Biomedical Books, 2005.

Cheng-Lai, Angela, James Nawarskas, and William H. Frishman. *Hypertension: A Clinical Guide.* Philadelphia: Lippincott Williams and Wilkins, 2007.

Institute for Clinical Systems Improvement. *Health Care Guideline: Hypertension Diagnosis and Treatment.* Bloomington, MN: Institute for Clinical Systems Improvement, 2006.

Kaplan, Norman M., and Joseph T. Flynn. *Kaplan's Clinical Hypertension.* 9th ed. Philadelphia: Lippincott Williams and Wilkins, 2006.

Khatib, Oussama M. N. *Clinical Guidelines for the Management of Hypertension.* Geneva, Switzerland: World Health Organization, 2005.

Korner, Paul I. *Essential Hypertension and Its Causes: Neural and Non-Neural Mechanisms.* New York: Oxford University Press, 2006.

Long, Genia, David M. Cutler, Ernst R. Berndt, et al. *The Impact of Antihypertensive Drugs on the Number and Risk of Death, Stroke and Myocardial Infarction in the United States.* NBER Working Paper No. 12096. Cambridge, MA: National Bureau of Economic Research, 2006.

MacGregor, Graham, and Norman M. Kaplan. *Hypertension.* 3d ed. Abingdon, UK: Health Press, 2006.

Matthews, Dawn D., and Karen Bellenir, eds. *Hypertension Sourcebook.* Detroit, MI: Omnigraphics, 2004.

Miller, G. Edward, and Marc Zodel. *Trends in the Pharmaceutical Treatment of Hypertension: 1997 to 2003.* Rockville, MD: Agency for Healthcare Research and Quality, 2006.

Weir, Matthew R., ed. *Hypertension.* Philadelphia: American College of Physicians, 2005.

96. *Iatrogenic Diseases and Nosocomial Infections*

Baughman, Robert P. *Contemporary Diagnosis and Management of Nosocomial Pneumonias.* Newtown, PA: Handbooks in Health Care, 2005.

D'Arcy, Patrick Francis, and John Parry Griffin, eds. *Iatrogenic Disease.* New York: Oxford University Press, 1986.

Jarvis, William R., ed. *Nosocomial Pneumonia.* New York: Marcel Dekker, 2000.

Paste, Loomis Richie. *Iatrogenic Diseases: Medical Subject Analysis and Research Guide With Bibliography.* Washington, DC: Abbe Publishers Association, 1985.

Preger, Leslie, ed. *Iatrogenic Diseases.* Boca Raton, FL: CRC Press, 1986.

Raje, Ravindra R., and Priscila D. Wong. *Iatrogenic Diseases.* Westbury, NY: PJD, 1999.

Tisdale, James E., and Douglas A. Miller, eds. *Drug-Induced Diseases: Prevention, Detection, and Management.* Bethesda, MD: American Society of Health-System Pharmacists, 2005.

Wenzel, Richard P. *Prevention and Control of Nosocomial Infections.* 4th ed. Philadelphia: Lippincott Williams and Wilkins, 2003.

97. *Injuries and Trauma*

Christoffel, Tom, and Susan Scavo Gallagher. *Injury Prevention and Public Health: Practical Knowledge, Skills, and Strategies.* 2d ed. Sudbury, MA: Jones and Bartlett, 2006.

Doll, Lynda, Sandra Bonzo, James Mercy, et al. *Handbook of Injury and Violence Prevention.* New York: Springer, 2006.

Committee on Trauma Research, Commission on Life Sciences, National Research Council and Institute of Medicine. *Injury in America: A Continuing Public Health Problem.* Washington, DC: National Academy Press, 1985.

Finkelstein, Eric A., Phaedra S. Corso, and Ted R. Miller. *The Incidence and Economic Burden of Injuries in the United States.* New York: Oxford University Press, 2006.

Garrick, Jacqueline, and Mary Beth Williams, eds. *Trauma Treatment Techniques: Innovative Trends.* Binghamton, NY: Haworth Maltreatment and Trauma Press, 2006.

Gielen, Andrea Carlson, David A. Sleet, and Ralph J. DiClemente, eds. *Injury and Violence Prevention: Behavioral Science Theories, Methods, and Applications.* San Francisco: Jossey-Bass, 2006.

Palmer, Sara, Kay Harris Kriegsman, and Jeffery B. Palmer. *Spinal Cord Injury: A Guide for Living.* Baltimore: Johns Hopkins University Press, 2000.

Robertson, Leon S. *Injury Epidemiology: Research and Control Strategies.* 3d ed. New York: Oxford University Press, 2007.

98. *Stroke*

American Medical Directors Association. *Stroke Management and Prevention in the Long-Term Care Setting.* Columbia, MD: American Medical Directors Association, 2005.

Barnes, Michael P., Bruce H. Dobkin, and Julien Bogousslavsky, eds. *Recovery After Stroke.* New York: Cambridge University Press, 2005.

Bhardwaj, Anish, Nabil J. Alkayed, Jeffrey R. Kirsch, et al., eds. *Acute Stroke: Bench to Bedside.* New York: Informa Healthcare, 2007.

Bogousslavsky, Julien, Louis R. Caplan, Helen M. Dewey, et al. *Stroke: Selected Topics.* New York: Demos Medical, 2006.

Brown, Martin M., Hugh Markus, and Stephen Oppenheimer. *Stroke Medicine.* New York: Taylor and Francis, 2006.

Casper, Michele, and Centers for Disease Control and Prevention. *Atlas of Stroke Mortality: Racial, Ethnic, and Geographic Disparities in the United States.* Atlanta, GA: U.S. Department of Health and Human Services, Centers for Disease Control and Prevention, National Center for Chronic Disease Prevention and Health Promotion, 2003.

Gillen, Glen, and Ann Burkhardt, eds. *Stroke Rehabilitation: A Function-Based Approach.* 2d ed. St. Louis, MO: Mosby-Elsevier, 2004.

Hankey, Graeme J. *Stroke Treatment and Prevention: An Evidence-Based Approach.* New York: Cambridge University Press, 2005.

Hennerici, Michael, Michael Daffertshofer, Louis Caplan, et al. *Case Studies in Stroke: Common and Uncommon Presentations.* New York: Cambridge University Press, 2007.

Institute for Clinical Systems Improvement. *Health Care Guidelines: Diagnosis and Initial Treatment of Ischemic Stroke.* 5th ed. Bloomington, MA: Institute for Clinical Systems Improvement, 2006.

Intercollegiate Working Party for Stroke. *National Clinical Guidelines for Stroke.* 2d ed. London: Royal College of Physicians, Clinical Effectiveness and Evaluation Unit, 2004.

Massaro, Lori M. *Stroke Care: The Guide to JCAHO Certification.* Marblehead, MA: HCPro, 2006.

Moon, Lynelle. *Stroke Care in OECD Countries: A Comparison of Treatment, Costs, and Outcomes in 17 Countries.* Paris: Organization for Economic Cooperation and Development, Directorate for Employment, Labor and Social Affairs, Employment, Labor and Social Affairs Committee, 2003.

National Institute of Neurological Disorders and Stroke. *Improving the Chain of Recovery for Acute Stroke in Your Community: Task Force Reports.* Bethesda, MD: U.S. Department of Health and Human Services, National Institutes of Health, National Institute of Neurological

Disorders and Stroke, Office of Communications and Public Liaison, 2003.

Ruper, Garret D., ed. *New Developments in Stroke Research.* Hauppauge, NY: Nova Science, 2006.

Rymer, Marilyn M., Debbie Summers, Pooja Khatri, et al. *The Stroke Center Handbook: Organizing Care for Better Outcomes: A Guide to Stroke Center Development and Operations.* Boca Raton, FL: Informa Healthcare, 2007.

Sharma, Mukul. *Acute Stroke: Evaluation and Treatment.* Rockville, MD: Agency for Healthcare Research and Quality, 2005.

Stein, Joel, Julie Silver, and Elizabeth Pegg Frates. *Life After Stroke: The Guide to Recovering Your Health and Preventing Another Stroke.* Baltimore: Johns Hopkins University Press, 2006.

Torbey, Michel T., and Magdy H. Selim, eds. *The Stroke Book.* New York: Cambridge University Press, 2007.

Virani, Tazim. *Stroke Assessment Across the Continuum of Care.* Toronto, Ontario, Canada: Registered Nurses Association of Ontario, Nursing Best Practice Guidelines Program, 2005.

Wiebers, David O., Valery L. Feigin, and Robert D. Brown. *Handbook of Stroke.* 2d ed. Philadelphia: Lippincott Williams and Wilkins, 2006.

Wityk, Robert J., and Rafael H. Llinas. *Stroke.* Philadelphia: American College of Physicians, 2007.

Guide for Health Care Professionals. Baltimore: Johns Hopkins University Press, 2006.

Moore, Elaine A., and Lisa Moore. *Encyclopedia of Alzheimer's Disease: With Directories of Research, Treatment and Care Facilities.* Jefferson, NC: McFarland, 2003.

Nasso, Jackie, and Lisa Celia. *Dementia Care: Inservice Training Modules for Long-Term Care.* Clifton Park, NY: Thomson Delmar Learning, 2007.

Post, Stephen G. *The Moral Challenge of Alzheimer Disease: Ethical Issues From Diagnosis to Dying.* 2d ed. Baltimore: Johns Hopkins University Press, 2000.

Purtilo, Ruth B., and Henk A. M. J. van Have, eds. *Ethical Foundations of Palliative Care for Alzheimer Disease.* Baltimore: Johns Hopkins University Press, 2004.

Turkington, Carol. *The Encyclopedia of Alzheimer's Disease.* New York: Facts on File, 2003.

Welsh, Eileen M., ed. *Trends in Alzheimer's Disease Research.* New York: Nova Science, 2006.

Whitehouse, Peter J., Konrad Maurer, and Jesse F. Ballenger, eds. *Concepts of Alzheimer Disease: Biological, Clinical, and Cultural Perspectives.* Baltimore: Johns Hopkins University Press, 2003.

Zgola, Jika M. *Care That Works: A Relationship Approach to Persons With Dementia.* Baltimore: Johns Hopkins University Press, 1999.

XI. Mental Health and Behavioral Disorders

Mental health is the level of an individual's cognitive well-being and functioning. Behavioral disorders are a pattern of disruptive, hostile, and potentially aggressive misconduct.

99. Alzheimer's Disease and Dementia

Ballenger, Jesse F. *Self, Senility, and Alzheimer's Disease in Modern America: A History.* Baltimore: Johns Hopkins University Press, 2006.

Binstock, Robert H., Stephen G. Post, and Peter J. Whitehouse, eds. *Dementia and Aging: Ethics, Values and Policy Choices.* Baltimore: Johns Hopkins University Press, 1992.

California Workgroup on Guidelines for Alzheimer's Disease Management. *Guidelines for Alzheimer's Disease Management: Final Report.* Los Angeles: State of California, Department of Health Services, 2002.

Emery, V., Olga B., and Thomas E. Oxman, eds. *Dementia: Presentations, Differential Diagnosis, and Nosology.* Baltimore: Johns Hopkins University Press, 2003.

Harris, Phyllis Braudy, ed. *The Person With Alzheimer's Disease: Pathways to Understanding the Experience.* Baltimore: Johns Hopkins University Press, 2002.

LooboPrabhu, Sheila M., Victor A. Molinari, and James W. Lomax, eds. *Supporting the Caregiver in Dementia: A*

100. Depression

Allen, Jon G. *Coping With Depression: From Catch-22 to Hope.* Washington, DC: American Psychiatric Publishing, 2006.

El-Mallakh, Rif S., and S. Nassir Ghaemi, eds. *Bipolar Depression: A Comprehensive Guide.* Washington, DC: American Psychiatric Publishing, 2006.

Gilliam, Frank G., Andres M. Kanner, and Yvette I. Sheline, eds. *Depression and Brain Dysfunction.* New York: Taylor and Francis, 2006.

Henri, Maurice J., ed. *Trends in Depression Research.* New York: Nova Science, 2006.

Martin, Emily. *Bipolar Expeditions: Mania and Depression in American Culture.* Princeton, NJ: Princeton University Press, 2007.

Mondimore, Francis Mark. *Depression, the Mood Disease.* 3d ed. Baltimore: Johns Hopkins University Press, 2006.

Munoz, Richard F., and Yu-Wen Ying. *The Prevention of Depression: Research and Practice.* Baltimore: Johns Hopkins University Press, 2002.

Pettit, Jeremy W., and Thomas E. Joiner. *Chronic Depression: Interpersonal Sources, Therapeutic Solutions.* Washington, DC: American Psychological Association, 2006.

Steptoe, Andrew, ed. *Depression and Physical Illness.* New York: Cambridge University Press, 2007.

Wasserman, Danuta. *Depression: The Facts.* New York: Oxford University Press, 2006.

101. Mental Health

Ahles, Scott R. *Our Inner World: A Guide to Psychodynamics and Psychotherapy*. Baltimore: Johns Hopkins University Press, 2004.

Arbuckle, Margaret Bordeaux, and Charlotte Herrick. *Child and Adolescent Mental Health: Interdisciplinary Systems of Care*. Sudbury, MA: Jones and Bartlett, 2006.

Avison, William, Jane McLeod, and Bernice Pescosolido, eds. *Mental Health, Social Mirror*. New York: Springer, 2007.

Cohen, Raquel E., and Frederick L. Ahrens. *Handbook for Mental Health Care of Disaster Victims*. Baltimore: Johns Hopkins University Press, 2001.

Findling, Robert L., and S. Charles Schulz, eds. *Juvenile-Onset Schizophrenia: Assessment, Neurobiology, and Treatment*. Baltimore: Johns Hopkins University Press, 2005.

Frank, Richard G., and Sherry A. Glied. *Better but not Well: Mental Health Policy in the United States Since 1950*. Baltimore: Johns Hopkins University Press, 2006.

Frank, Richard G., and Willard G. Manning, eds. *Economics and Mental Health*. Chicago: University of Chicago Press, 1992.

Gedo, John E. *Psychoanalysis as Biological Science: A Comprehensive Theory*. Baltimore: Johns Hopkins University Press, 2004.

Ghaemi, S. Nassir. *The Concepts of Psychiatry: A Pluralistic Approach to the Mind and Mental Illness*. 2d ed. Baltimore: Johns Hopkins University Press, 2007.

Ingleby, David, ed. *Forced Migration and Mental Health: Rethinking the Care of Refugees and Displaced Persons*. New York: Springer, 2005.

Institute of Medicine. *Improving the Quality of Health Care for Mental and Substance-Use Conditions*. Washington, DC: Institute of Medicine, 2006.

Kahn, Ada P., and Jan Fawcett. *The Encyclopedia of Mental Health*. 3d ed. New York: Facts on File, 2007.

Levin, Bruce Lubotsky, John Petrila, and Kevin D. Hennessy. *Mental Health Services: A Public Health Perspective*. 2d ed. New York: Oxford University Press, 2004.

McHugh, Paul R. *The Mind Has Mountains: Reflections on Society and Psychiatry*. Baltimore: Johns Hopkins University Press, 2005.

Moniz, Cynthia, and Stephen H. Gorin. *Health and Mental Health Care Policy: A Biopsychosocial Perspective*. 2d ed. Boston: Allyn and Bacon, 2007.

Perrin, Edward B., and Jeffrey J. Koshel, eds., and Committee on National Statistics, Commission on Behavioral and Social Sciences and Education, National Research Council. *Assessment of Performance Measures for Public Health, Substance Abuse, and Mental Health*. Washington, DC: National Academy Press, 1997.

Sadler, John Z., ed. *Descriptions and Prescriptions: Values, Mental Disorders, and the DSMs*. Baltimore: Johns Hopkins University Press, 2002.

Slade, Mike, and Stefan Priebe, eds. *Choosing Methods in Mental Health Research: Mental Health Research From Theory to Practice*. New York: Routledge, 2006.

Slavney, Phillip R. *Psychotherapy: An Introduction for Psychiatry Residents and Other Mental Health Trainees*. Baltimore: Johns Hopkins University Press, 2005.

Treisman, Glenn J., and Andrew F. Angelino. *The Psychiatry of AIDS: A Guide to Diagnosis and Treatment*. Baltimore: Johns Hopkins University Press, 2004.

Zarit, Steven H., and Judy M. Zarit. *Mental Disorders in Older Adults: Fundamentals of Assessment and Treatment*. New York: Guilford Press, 2007.

102. Obesity, Eating Disorders, and Nutrition

Cassell, Dana K., and David H. Gleaves. *The Encyclopedia of Obesity and Eating Disorders*. 3d ed. New York: Facts on File, 2006.

Crawford, David, and Robert W. Jeffery, eds. *Obesity Prevention and Public Health*. New York: Oxford University Press, 2005.

Flamenbaum, Richard K., ed. *Global Dimensions of Childhood Obesity*. New York: Nova Science, 2006.

Hassink, Sandra Gibson. *A Clinical Guide to Pediatric Weight Management and Obesity*. Philadelphia: Lippincott Williams and Wilkins, 2007.

Hassink, Sandra Gibson. *Pediatric Obesity: Prevention, Intervention, and Treatment Strategies for Primary Care*. Elk Grove Village, IL: American Academy of Pediatrics, 2007.

Institute of Medicine. *Perspectives on the Prevention of Childhood Obesity in Children and Youth*. The Richard and Hinda Rosenthal Lectures, 2004. Washington, DC: National Academies Press, 2005.

Institute of Medicine. *Progress in Preventing Childhood Obesity: Focus on Schools*. Brief Summary: Institute of Medicine Regional Symposium, Wichita, KS (June 27–28, 2005). Washington, DC: National Academies Press, 2005.

Jelalian, Elissa, and Ric G. Steele, eds. *Handbook of Child and Adolescent Obesity*. New York: Springer, 2007.

Kumanyika, Shiriki, and Ross Brownson, eds. *Obesity and Obesity Prevention: A Handbook for Health Professionals*. New York: Springer, 2007.

Kushner, Robert F., and Daniel H. Bessesen, eds. *Treatment of the Obese Patient*. Totowa, NJ: Humana Press, 2007.

Mantzoros, Christos S., ed. *Obesity and Diabetes*. Totowa, NJ: Humana Press, 2006.

Mehler, Philip S., and Arnold E. Andersen, eds. *Eating Disorders: A Guide to Medical Care and Complications*. Baltimore: Johns Hopkins University Press, 2000.

Michel, Deborah M., and Susan G. Willard. *When Dieting Becomes Dangerous: A Guide to Understanding and Treating Anorexia and Bulimia*. New Haven, CT: Yale University Press, 2003.

Oliver, J. Eric. *Fat Politics: The Real Story Behind America's Obesity Epidemic*. New York: Oxford University Press, 2005.

Paxson, Christina, Elisabeth Donahue, Tracy Orleans, et al., eds. *Childhood Obesity*. Washington, DC: Brookings Institution Press, 2006.

Ronzio, Robert A. *The Encyclopedia of Nutrition and Good Health.* 2d ed. New York: Facts on File, 2003.

Rosenthal, Jill, and Deborah Chang. *State Approaches to Childhood Obesity: A Snapshot of Promising Practices and Lessons Learned.* Portland, ME: National Academy for State Health Policy, 2004.

Rubin, Jerome S., ed. *Eating Disorders and Weight Loss Research.* Hauppauge, NY: Nova Science, 2006.

Sattar, Naveed, and Mike Lean, eds. *ABC of Obesity.* Malden, MA: Blackwell, 2007.

Shils, Maurice E., Moshe Shike, A. Catharine Ross, et al., eds. *Modern Nutrition in Health and Disease.* 10th ed. Philadelphia: Lippincott Williams and Wilkins, 2006.

103. Substance Abuse

Acker, Caroline Jean. *Creating the American Junkie: Addiction Research in the Classic Era of Narcotic Control.* Baltimore: Johns Hopkins University Press, 2005.

Armstrong, Elizabeth M. *Conceiving Risk, Bearing Responsibility: Fetal Alcohol Syndrome and the Diagnosis of Moral Disorder.* Baltimore: Johns Hopkins University Press, 2003.

Babor, Thomas. *Alcohol and Public Policy: No Ordinary Commodity.* New York: Oxford University Press, 2003.

Bonnie, Richard J., and Mary Ellen O'Connell, eds., and Committee on Developing a Strategy to Reduce and Prevent Underage Drinking, Board on Children, Youth, and Families, Division of Behavioral and Social Sciences and Education, National Research Council and Institute of Medicine. *Reducing Underage Drinking: A Collective Responsibility.* Washington, DC: National Academy Press, 2004.

Committee on Crossing the Quality Chasm: Adaptation to Mental Health and Addictive Disorders. *Improving the Quality of Health Care for Mental and Substance-Use Conditions.* Washington, DC: Institute of Medicine, Board on Health Care Services, Committee on Crossing the Quality Chasm: Adaptation to Mental Health and Addictive Disorders, 2006.

Galanter, Marc, D. Lagressa, G. Boyd, et al., eds. *Alcohol Problems in Adolescents and Young Adults: Epidemiology, Neurobiology, Prevention, and Treatment.* New York: Springer, 2006.

Miller, Richard Lawrence. *The Encyclopedia of Addictive Drugs.* Westport, CT: Greenwood, 2002.

Mosher, Clayton J., and Scott Akins. *Drugs and Drug Policy: The Control of Consciousness Alteration.* Thousand Oaks, CA: Sage, 2006.

National Center on Addiction and Substance Abuse at Columbia University. *Women Under the Influence.* Baltimore: Johns Hopkins University Press, 2005.

Perrin, Edward B., and Jeffrey J. Koshel, eds., and Committee on National Statistics, Commission on Behavioral and Social Sciences and Education, National Research Council. *Assessment of Performance Measures for Public Health, Substance Abuse, and Mental Health.* Washington, DC: National Academy Press, 1997.

Sloboda, Zili. *Epidemiology of Drug Abuse.* New York: Springer, 2005.

Strain, Eric C., and Maxine L. Stitzer, eds. *The Treatment of Opioid Dependence.* Baltimore: Johns Hopkins University Press, 2005.

Sutton, Amy L., ed. *Alcoholism Source Book: Basic Consumer Health Information About Alcohol Use, Abuse, and Dependence.* Detroit, MI: Omnigraphics, 2006.

Winger, Gail, James H. Woods, and Frederick G. Hofmann. *A Handbook on Drug and Alcohol Abuse: The Biomedical Aspects.* 4th ed. New York: Oxford University Press, 2004.

104. Tobacco Use

Boyle, Peter, Nigel Gray, Jack Henningfield, et al., eds. *Tobacco: Science, Policy and Public Health.* New York: Oxford University Press, 2004.

Forey, Barbara, Jan Hamling, and Peter Lee, eds. *International Smoking Statistics: A Collection of Historical Data From Economically Developed Countries.* New York: Oxford University Press, 2002.

Goodman, Jordan, ed. *Tobacco in History and Culture: An Encyclopedia.* 2 vols. Detroit, MI: Thomson Gale, 2005.

Lynch, Barbara S., and Richard J. Bonnie, eds., and Committee on Preventing Nicotine Addiction in Children and Youths, Division of Biobehavioral Sciences and Mental Disorders, Institute of Medicine. *Growing Up Tobacco Free: Preventing Nicotine Addiction in Children and Youths.* Washington, DC: National Academy Press, 1994.

Pampel, Fred C. *Tobacco Industry and Smoking.* New York: Facts on File, 2004.

U.S. Department of Health and Human Services. *The Health Consequences of Involuntary Exposure to Tobacco Smoke: A Report of the Surgeon General.* Atlanta, GA: U.S. Department of Health and Human Services, Centers for Disease Control and Prevention, Coordinating Center for Health Promotion, National Center for Chronic Disease Prevention and Health Promotion, Office on Smoking and Health, 2006.

Viscusi, W. Kip. *Smoke-Filled Rooms: A Postmortem on the Tobacco Deal.* Chicago: University of Chicago Press, 2002.

Warner, Kenneth E., Stephen L. Isaacs, and James Knickman. *Tobacco Control Policy.* San Francisco: Jossey-Bass, 2006.

XII. Aging, Disability, and Long-Term Care

Aging is the process of getting older, and it is concerned with issues of the elderly. Disability is the lack of ability as compared with a normal group of individuals. Long-term care is the care that is provided to the chronically ill and the disabled.

105. Aging and the Elderly

Aaron, Henry J., and William B. Schwartz, eds. *Coping With Methuselah: The Impact of Molecular Biology on Medicine and Society.* Washington, DC: Brookings Institution Press, 2004.

Achenbaum, W., Andrew. *Older Americans, Vital Communities: A Bold Vision for Societal Aging.* Baltimore: Johns Hopkins University Press, 2005.

Altman, Stuart H., and David I. Shactman, eds. *Policies for an Aging Society.* Baltimore: Johns Hopkins University Press, 2002.

Anderson, Mary Ann, ed. *Caring for Older Adults Holistically.* 4th ed. Philadelphia: F. A. Davis, 2007.

Atchley, Robert C. *Continuity and Adaptation in Aging: Creating Positive Experiences.* Baltimore: Johns Hopkins University Press, 2000.

Binstock, Robert H., and Linda K. George, eds. *Handbook of Aging and the Social Sciences.* 5th ed. San Diego, CA: Academic Press, 2001.

Binstock, Robert H., and Stephen Post. *Too Old for Health Care? Controversies in Medicine, Law, Economics, and Ethics.* Baltimore: Johns Hopkins University Press, 1991.

Bond, John, Sheila M. Peace, Freya Dittmann-Kohli, et al., eds. *Ageing in Society.* 3d ed. Thousand Oaks, CA: Sage, 2007.

Butler, Robert N. *Why Survive? Being Old in America.* Baltimore: Johns Hopkins University Press, 2003.

Conn, P. Michael, ed. *Handbook of Models for Human Aging.* Boston: Elsevier Academic Press, 2006.

Dangour, Alan, Astrid Fletcher, and Emily Grundy, eds. *Ageing Well: Nutrition, Health, and Social Interventions.* Boca Raton, FL: CRC Press, Taylor and Francis, 2007.

Ekerdt, David J. *Encyclopedia of Aging.* 4 vols. New York: Macmillan Reference USA, 2002.

Hickey, Tom, Marjorie A. Speers, and Thomas R. Prohaska, eds. *Public Health and Aging.* Baltimore: Johns Hopkins University Press, 1997.

Kandel, Joseph, and Christine A. Adamec. *The Encyclopedia of Senior Health and Well-Being.* New York: Facts on File, 2003.

Karasek, Michal, ed. *Aging and Age-Related Diseases: The Basics.* New York: Nova Biomedical, 2006.

Kausler, Donald, and Barry C. Kausler, eds. *The Graying of America: An Encyclopedia of Aging, Health, Mind, and Behavior.* 2d ed. Champaign: University of Illinois Press, 2001.

Kemp, Bryan J., and Laura Mosqueda, eds. *Aging With a Disability: What the Clinician Needs to Know.* Baltimore: Johns Hopkins University Press, 2004.

Levine, Martin Lyon, ed. *The Elderly: Legal and Ethical Issues in Health Care Policy.* Aldershot, UK: Ashgate, 2001.

Loue, Sana, and M. Sajatovic, eds. *Encyclopedia of Aging and Public Health.* New York: Springer, 2007.

Markides, Kyriakos S., ed. *Encyclopedia of Health and Aging.* Thousand Oaks, CA: Sage, 2007.

Moody, Harry R. *Aging: Concepts and Controversies.* 5th ed. Thousand Oaks, CA: Sage, 2006.

Morrow-Howell, Nancy, James Hinterlong, and Michael Sherraden, eds. *Productive Aging: Concepts and Challenges.* Baltimore: Johns Hopkins University Press, 2001.

Rattan, Suresh I. S., ed. *Aging Interventions and Therapies.* Hackensack, NJ: World Scientific, 2005.

Romeis, James C., and Rodney M. Coe, eds. *Quality and Cost-Containment in Care for the Elderly: Health Services Research Perspectives.* New York: Springer, 1991.

Satariano, William A. *Epidemiology of Aging: An Ecological Approach.* Sudbury, MA: Jones and Bartlett, 2006.

Schulz, Richard, Linda S. Noelker, Kenneth Rockwood, et al., eds. *The Encyclopedia of Aging: A Comprehensive Resource in Gerontology and Geriatrics.* 4th ed. New York: Springer, 2006.

Schwarz, Benyamin, and Ruth Brent, eds. *Aging, Autonomy, and Architecture: Advances in Assisted Living.* Baltimore: Johns Hopkins University Press, 1999.

Walters, James W. *Choosing Who's to Live: Ethics and Aging.* Champaign: University of Illinois Press, 1996.

Wise, David A. *Advances in the Economics of Aging.* Chicago: University of Chicago Press, 1996.

106. Assisted Living

Allen, James E. *Assisted Living Administration: The Knowledge Base.* 2d ed. New York: Springer, 2004.

Ball, Mary M., Molly M. Perkins, Frank J. Whittington, et al. *Communities of Care: Assisted Living for African American Elders.* Baltimore: Johns Hopkins University Press, 2005.

Marsden, John P. *Humanistic Design of Assisted Living.* Baltimore: Johns Hopkins University Press, 2005.

Schwarz, Benyamin, and Ruth Brent, eds. *Aging, Autonomy, and Architecture: Advances in Assisted Living.* Baltimore: Johns Hopkins University Press, 1999.

Zimmerman, Sheryl, Philip D. Sloane, and J. Kevin Eckart, eds. *Assisted Living: Needs, Practices, and Policies in Residential Care for the Elderly.* Baltimore: Johns Hopkins University Press, 2001.

107. Disability

Albrecht, Gary L. *The Disability Business: Rehabilitation in America.* Thousand Oaks, CA: Sage, 1992.

Albrecht, Gary L., Jerome Bickenbach, Scott Brown, et al., eds. *Encyclopedia of Disability.* 5 vols. Thousand Oaks, CA: Sage, 2005.

Albrecht, Gary L., Katherine D. Seelman, and Michael Bury, eds. *Handbook of Disability Studies.* Thousand Oaks, CA: Sage, 2001.

Davis, Lennard J., ed. *The Disability Studies Reader.* 2d ed. New York: Routledge, 2006.

Iezzoni, Lisa I., and Bonnie L. O'Day. *More Than Ramps: A Guide to Improving Health Care Quality and Access for People With Disabilities.* New York: Oxford University Press, 2006.

Jones, Nancy Lee. *The Americans with Disabilities Act (ADA): Overview, Regulations and Interpretations.* New York: Nova Science, 2003.

Kemp, Bryan J., and Laura Mosqueda, eds. *Aging With a Disability: What the Clinician Needs to Know.* Baltimore: Johns Hopkins University Press, 2004.

Racino, Julie Ann. *Policy, Program Evaluation, and Research in Disability: Community Support for All*. New York: Haworth, 1999.

Resources for Rehabilitation. *Resources for Elders With Disabilities*. 5th ed. Winchester, MA: Resources for Rehabilitation, 2003.

Schultz, Izabela Z., and Robert J. Gatchel. *Handbook of Complex Occupational Disability Claims: Early Risk Identification, Intervention, and Prevention*. New York: Springer, 2005.

Snyder, Sharon L., and David T. Mitchell. *Cultural Locations of Disability*. Chicago: University of Chicago Press, 2005.

Turner, David M., and Kevin Stagg, eds. *Social Histories of Disability and Deformity*. New York: Routledge, 2006.

Wiener, Joshua M., Steven B. Clauser, and David L. Kennell, eds. *Persons With Disabilities: Issues in Health Care Financing and Service Delivery*. Washington, DC: Brookings Institution, 1995.

108. End-of-Life Care

Bearison, David J. *When Treatment Fails: How Medicine Cares for Dying Children*. New York: Oxford University Press, 2006.

Casey, Michelle. *Models for Providing Hospice Care in Rural Areas: Successes and Challenges*. Minneapolis: University of Minnesota, School of Public Health, Division of Health Services Research and Policy, Rural Health Research Center, 2003.

Cassell, Dana K., Robert C. Salinas, and Peter A. S. Winn. *The Encyclopedia of Death and Dying*. New York: Facts on File, 2005.

Chen, Pauline W. *Final Exam: A Young Surgeon's Reflections on Mortality*. New York: Alfred A. Knopf, 2007.

Enck, Robert E. *The Medical Care of Terminally Ill Patients*. 2d ed. Baltimore: Johns Hopkins University Press, 2001.

Field, Marilyn J., and Richard E. Behrman, eds., and Committee on Palliative and End-of-Life Care for Children and Their Families, Board on Health Sciences Policy, Institute of Medicine. *When Children Die: Improving Palliative and End-of-Life Care for Children and Their Families*. Washington, DC: National Academies Press, 2003.

Foley, Kathleen, and Herbert Hendin, eds. *The Case Against Assisted Suicide: For the Right to End-of-Life Care*. Baltimore: Johns Hopkins University Press, 2004.

Gelfand, Donald E., Richard Raspa, Sherylyn H. Briller, et al., eds. *End-of-Life Stories: Crossing Disciplinary Boundaries*. New York: Springer, 2005.

Institute of Medicine. *Working Together: We Can Help People Get Good Care When They Are Dying*. Washington, DC: National Academy Press, 2000.

Kaufman, Sharon R. *And a Time to Die: How American Hospitals Shape the End of Life*. Chicago: University of Chicago Press, 2005.

Kiernan, Stephen P. *Last Rights: Rescuing the End of Life From the Medical System*. New York: St. Martin's Press, 2006.

Lantos, John D. *The Lazarus Case: Life-and-Death Issues in Neonatal Intensive Care*. Baltimore: Johns Hopkins University Press, 2001.

Lewis, Milton James. *Medicine and Care of the Dying: A Modern History*. New York: Oxford University Press, 2007.

Lizza, John P. *Persons, Humanity, and the Definition of Death*. Baltimore: Johns Hopkins University Press, 2005.

Lynn, Joanne, Janice Lynch Schuster, and Andrea Kabcenell. *Improving Care for the End of Life: A Sourcebook for Health Care Managers and Clinicians*. 2d ed. New York: Oxford University Press, 2007.

Mezey, Mathy D., and Nancy Neveloff Dubler, eds. *Voices of Decision in Nursing Homes: Respecting Residents' Preferences for End-of-Life Care*. New York: United Hospital Fund of New York, 2001.

Quill, Timothy E. *A Midwife Through the Dying Process: Stories of Healing and Hard Choices at the End of Life*. Baltimore: Johns Hopkins University Press, 2001.

Quill, Timothy E., and Margaret P. Battin, eds. *Physician-Assisted Dying: The Case for Palliative and Patient Choice*. Baltimore: Johns Hopkins University Press, 2004.

Sankar, Andrea. *Dying at Home: A Family Guide to Caregiving*. Baltimore: Johns Hopkins University Press, 1999.

Wanzer, Sidney H., and Joseph Glenmullen. *To Die Well: Your Right to Comfort, Calm, and Choice in the Last Days of Life*. Cambridge, MA: Da Capo Press, 2007.

Wetle, Terrie Todd, et al., eds. *End of Life in Nursing Homes: Experiences and Policy Recommendations*. Washington, DC: AARP Public Policy Institute, 2004.

Youngner, Stuart J., Robert M. Arnold, and Renie Schapiro, eds. *The Definition of Death: Contemporary Controversies*. Baltimore: Johns Hopkins University Press, 2002.

109. Home Healthcare

Buhler-Wilkerson, Karen. *No Place Like Home: A History of Nursing and Home Care in the United States*. Baltimore: Johns Hopkins University Press, 2003.

Harris, Marilyn D., ed. *Handbook of Home Health Care Administration*. 4th ed. Sudbury, MA: Jones and Bartlett, 2005.

Ladd, Rosalind Ekman, Lynn Pasquerella, and Sheri Smith. *Ethical Issues in Home Health Care*. Springfield, IL: Charles C Thomas, 2002.

Mullner, Ross M., and Mark Jewell. *A Bibliography of Recent Works on Home Health Care*. Lewiston, NY: Edwin Mellen Press, 2000.

Rantz, Marilyn, and Marcia K. Flesner. *Person Centered Care: A Model for Nursing Homes*. Washington, DC: American Nurses Association, 2004.

Rappaport, Meryl Beth. *Remodeling Home Care: Making the Transition From Fee-for-Service to Managed Care*. New York: Garland, 2000.

U.S. General Accounting Office. *Medicare: Utilization of Home Health Care by State*. Washington, DC: U.S. General Accounting Office, 2002.

110. Nursing Homes and Long-Term Care

Allen, James E. *Nursing Home Federal Requirements: Guidelines to Surveyors and Survey Protocols.* 6th ed. New York: Springer, 2007.

Baker, Beth. *Old Age in a New Age: The Promise of Transformative Nursing Homes.* Nashville, TN: Vanderbilt University Press, 2007.

Bartlett, Helen C. *Nursing Homes for Elderly People: Questions of Quality and Policy.* Langhorne, PA: Harwood Academic, 1993.

Binstock, Robert H., Leighton E. Cluff, and Otto von Mering, eds. *The Future of Long-Term Care: Social and Policy Issues.* Baltimore: Johns Hopkins University Press, 1996.

Bostick, J. E., M. J. Rantz, M. K. Flesner, et al. "Systematic Review of Studies of Staffing and Quality in Nursing Homes," *Journal of the American Medical Directors Association* 7(6): 366–76, July 2006.

Burger, Sarah Greene, Virginia Fraser, Sara Hunt, et al., eds. *Nursing Homes: Getting Good Care There.* 2d ed. Atascadero, CA: Impact Publishers, 2002.

Burke, Steven S., and Tessa L. Chenaille. *30 Essential Policies and Procedures for Long-Term Care.* Marblehead, MA: HCPro, 2006.

Cawley, John H., David C. Grabowski, and Richard A. Hirth. *Factor Substitution and Unobserved Factor Quality in Nursing Homes.* NBER Working Paper No. 10465. Cambridge, MA: National Bureau of Economic Research, 2004.

Dalton, Kathleen. *Background Paper: Rural and Urban Differences in Nursing Home and Skilled Nursing Supply.* Chapel Hill: University of North Carolina at Chapel Hill, Cecil G. Sheps Center for Health Services Research, North Carolina Rural Health Research and Policy Analysis Center, 2002.

Evashwick, Connie, and James Riedel. *Managing Long-Term Care.* Chicago: Health Administration Press, 2004.

Freiman, Marc P. *A New Look at U.S. Expenditures for Long-Term Care and Independent Living Services, Settings, and Technologies for the Year 2000.* Washington, DC: AARP Public Policy Institute, 2005.

Gaugler, Joseph E., ed. *Promoting Family Involvement in Long-Term Care Settings: A Guide to Programs That Work.* Baltimore: Health Professions Press, 2005.

Harris, Diana K., and Michael L. Benson. *Maltreatment of Patients in Nursing Homes: There Is No Safe Place.* New York: Haworth Pastoral Press, 2006.

Hegner, Barbara R., and Mary Jo Gerlach, eds. *Assisting in Long-Term Care.* 5th ed. Clifton Park, NY: Thomson Delmar Learning, 2007.

Institute of Medicine. *Toward a National Strategy for Long-Term Care of the Elderly: A Study Plan for Evaluation of New Policy Options for the Future.* Washington, DC: National Academies Press, 1986.

Kane, Robert L., and Joan C. West. *It Shouldn't Be This Way: The Failure of Long-Term Care.* Nashville, TN: Vanderbilt University Press, 2005.

Kane, Rosalie A., Robert L. Kane, and Richard C. Ladd. *The Heart of Long-Term Care.* New York: Oxford University Press, 1998.

Levine, Jeffery M., ed. *Medical-Legal Aspects of Long-Term Care.* Tucson, AZ: Lawyers and Judges Publishing, 2003.

Olson, Laura Katz. *The Not-So-Golden Years: Caregiving, the Frail Elderly, and the Long-Term Care Establishment.* Lanham, MD: Rowman and Littlefield, 2003.

Phillips, Charles D., Catherine Hawes, and Malgorzata Leyk Williams. *Nursing Homes in Rural and Urban Areas, 2000.* College Station, TX: Southwest Rural Health Research Center, 2003.

Pratt, John R. *Long-Term Care: Managing Across the Continuum.* 2d ed. Sudbury, MA: Jones and Bartlett, 2004.

Rhoades, Jeffrey A., D. E. B. Potter, and Nancy Krauss. *Nursing Homes: Structure and Selected Characteristics: 1996.* Rockville, MD: Agency for Health Care Policy and Research, 1998.

Scanlon, William. *Nursing Homes: Prevalence of Serious Quality Problems Remains Unacceptably High, Despite Some Decline: Testimony Before the Committee on Finance, U.S. Senate.* Washington, DC: U.S. General Accounting Office, 2003.

Silin, Peter S. *Nursing Homes: The Family's Journey.* Baltimore: Johns Hopkins University Press, 2001.

Singh, Douglas A. *Effective Management of Long-Term Care Facilities.* Sudbury, MA: Jones and Bartlett, 2005.

U.S. Congressional Budget Office. *Financing Long-Term Care for the Elderly.* Washington, DC: U.S. Congressional Budget Office, 2004.

U.S. Congressional Budget Office. *The Cost and Financing of Long-Term Care Services.* CBO Testimony Statement of Douglas Holtz-Eakin Before the Subcommittee on Health, Committee on Ways and Means, U.S. House of Representatives, April 19, 2005.

U.S. Government Accountability Office. *Nursing Home Deaths: Arkansas Coroner Referrals Confirm Weakness in State and Federal Oversight of Quality of Care: Report to Congressional Requesters.* Washington, DC: U.S. Government Accountability Office, 2004.

Winzelberg, G. S. "The Quest for Nursing Home Quality: Learning History's Lessons," *Archives of Internal Medicine* 163(21): 2552–56, November 24, 2003.

Wood, Erica. *Termination and Closure of Poor Quality Nursing Homes: What Are the Options?* Washington, DC: AARP Public Policy Institute, 2002.

Wunderlich, Gooloo S., and Peter O. Kohler, eds., and Committee on Improving Quality in Long-Term Care, Division of Health Care Services, Institute of Medicine. *Improving the Quality of Long-Term Care.* Washington, DC: National Academy Press, 2000.

Yoshikawa, Thomas T., and Joseph G. Ouslander, eds. *Infection Management for Geriatrics in Long-Term Care Facilities.* 2d ed. New York: Informa Healthcare, 2007.

XIII. Other

This section includes a potpourri of selected topics in health services research and provides an amalgam of informative readings.

111. Bioterrorism

Antosia, Robert E., and John D. Cahill, eds. *Handbook of Bioterrorism and Disaster Medicine*. New York: Springer, 2006.

Butler, Adrienne Stith, Allison M. Panzer, and Lewis R. Goldfrank, eds., and Committee on Responding to the Psychological Consequences of Terrorism, Institute of Medicine. *Preparing for the Psychological Consequences of Terrorism: A Public Health Strategy*. Washington, DC: National Academies Press, 2003.

D'Arcy, Michael, Michael O'Hanlon, Peter Orszag, et al. *Protecting the Homeland 2006/2007*. Washington, DC: Brookings Institution Press, 2006.

Demuth, Julie L. *Countering Terrorism: Lessons Learned From Natural and Technological Disasters: A Summary of the Natural Disasters Roundtable*. National Academy of Sciences Conference, Washington, DC (February 28–March 1, 2002). Washington, DC: National Academies Press, 2002.

Greenberg, Michael I. *Encyclopedia of Terrorist, Natural, and Man-Made Disasters*. Sudbury, MA: Jones and Bartlett, 2006.

Griset, Pamala L., and Sue Mahan. *Terrorism in Perspective*. Thousand Oaks, CA: Sage, 2002.

Henderson, Donald A., Thomas V. Ingelsby, and Tara O'Toole, eds. *Bioterrorism: Guidelines for Medical and Public Health Management*. Chicago: American Medical Association, 2002.

Levy, Barry S., and Victor W. Sidel, eds. *Terrorism and Public Health: A Balanced Approach to Strengthening Systems and Protecting People*. New York: Oxford University Press, 2002.

McGlown, K. Joanne, ed. *Terrorism and Disaster Management: Preparing Healthcare Leaders for the New Reality*. Chicago: Health Administration Press, 2004.

Pilch, Richard F., and Raymond A. Zilinskas, eds. *Encyclopedia of Bioterrorism Defense*. Hoboken, NJ: Wiley-LISS, 2005.

Trotter, Griffin. *The Ethics of Coercion in Mass Casualty Medicine*. Baltimore: Johns Hopkins University Press, 2007.

112. E-Health and Telemedicine

Bashshur, Rashid. *State of the Art: Telemedicine/Telehealth Symposium: An International Persepective: Abstract, Executive and Final Report of Symposium*. Rockville, MD: Agency for Healthcare Research and Quality, Center for Research Dissemination and Liaison, 2001. (The symposium was held at the University of Michigan in 2001)

Demiris, George, ed. *E-Health: Current Status and Future Trends*. Washington, DC: IOS Press, 2004.

Goldsmith, Jeff. *Digital Medicine: Implications for Healthcare Leaders*. Chicago: Health Administration Press, 2003.

Hersh, William R., and James A. Wallace. *Telemedicine for the Medicare Population*. Rockville, MD: U.S. Department of Health and Human Services, Public Health Service, Agency for Healthcare Research and Quality, 2001.

Lingle, Virginia A., and Eric P. Delozier, eds. *World Wide Web and Other Internet Information Services in the Health Sciences: A Collection of Policy and Procedure Statements*. Chicago: Medical Library Association, 1996.

Maheu, Marlene M., Pamela Whitten, and Ace Allen. *E-Health, Telehealth, and Telemedicine: A Guide to Start-Up and Success*. San Francisco: Jossey-Bass, 2001.

Norris, Anthony Charles. *Essentials of Telemedicine and Telecare*. New York: Wiley, 2002.

Schrimsher, Robert H., and T. Harmon Straiton Jr. *Health Data on the Internet: An Annotated Bibliography and Guide*. Chicago: Medical Library Association, 1999.

Tan, Joseph, ed. *E-Health Care Information Systems: An Introduction for Students and Professionals*. San Francisco: Jossey-Bass, 2005.

Telemedicine and Telecommunications: Options for the New Century: Program Book. Bethesda, MD: National Institutes of Health, National Library of Medicine, Lister Hill National Center for Biomedical Communications, Office of High Performance Computing and Communications, 2001.

Whitten, Pamela, and David Cook, eds. *Understanding Health Communication Technologies*. San Francisco: Jossey-Bass, 2004.

Wootton, Richard, John Craig, and Victor Patterson, eds. *Introduction to Telemedicine*. 2d ed. London: Royal Society of Medicine Press, 2006.

113. Fraud and Abuse

Baumann, Linda A., ed. *Health Care Fraud and Abuse: Practical Perspectives*. Washington, DC: Bureau of National Affairs Press, 2002.

Nathanson, Martha Dale, and Carel T. Hedlund. *Home Care Fraud and Abuse: Critical Questions, Essential Answers*. Gaithersburg, MD: Aspen, 1999.

Sparrow, Malcolm K. *License to Steal: How Fraud Bleeds America's Health Care System*. Boulder, CO: Westview Press, 2000.

U.S. Department of Health and Human Services and Department of Justice. *Health Care Fraud and Abuse Control Program Annual Report for FY2005*. Washington, DC: U.S. Department of Health and Human Services/ Department of Justice, 2006.

U.S. General Accountability Office. *Health Care Fraud and Abuse Control Programs: Results of Review of Annual Reports for Fiscal Years 2002 and 2003: Report to*

Congressional Committees. Washington, DC: U.S. Government Accountability Office, 2005.

U.S. General Accountability Office. *Medicaid Fraud and Abuse: CMS's Commitment to Helping States Safeguard Program Dollars Is Limited: Testimony Before the Committee on Finance, U.S. Senate.* Washington, DC: U.S. Government Accountability Office, 2005.

114. *Future Trends*

Berwick, Donald M. *Escape Fire: Designs for the Future of Health Care.* San Francisco: Jossey-Bass, 2003.

Ellis, David. *Technology and the Future of Health Care: Preparing for the Next 30 Years.* San Francisco: Jossey-Bass, 2001.

Enthoven, Alain C., and Laura A. Tollen, eds. *Toward a 21st Century Health System: The Contribution and Promise of Prepaid Group Practice.* San Francisco: Jossey-Bass, 2004.

Geisler, Eliezer, Koos Krabbendam, and Roel Schuring, eds. *Technology, Health Care, and Management in Hospitals of the Future.* Westport, CT: Praeger, 2003.

Institute for the Future. *Health and Health Care 2010: Forecast, the Challenge.* 2d ed. San Francisco: Jossey-Bass, 2003.

Institute of Medicine. *Informing the Future: Critical Issues in Health.* 3d ed. Washington, DC: National Academies Press, 2005.

Institute of Medicine. *2020 Vision: Health in the 21st Century.* Institute of Medicine 25th Anniversary Symposium. Washington, DC: National Academy Press, 1996.

Lutz, Sandy, Woodrin Grossman, and John Bigalke. *Med Inc.: How Consolidation Is Shaping Tomorrow's Healthcare System.* San Francisco: Jossey-Bass, 1998.

Morrison, Ian. *Health Care in the New Millennium: Vision, Values, and Leadership.* San Francisco: Jossey-Bass, 2002.

Showstack, Jonathan, Arlyss Anderson Rothman, and Sue Hasmiller, eds. *The Future of Primary Care.* San Francisco: Jossey-Bass, 2004.

Silberglitt, Richard, Philip S. Anton, David R. Howell, et al. *The Global Technology Revolution 2020: Bio, Nano, Materials, Information Trends, Drivers, Barriers, and Social Implications.* Santa Monica, CA: RAND Corporation, 2006.

Society for Healthcare Strategy and Market Development and American College of Healthcare Executives. *Futurescan: Healthcare Trends and Implications, 2006–2011.* Chicago: Health Administration Press/Society for Healthcare Strategy and Market Development, 2006.

Styring, Willams, and Donald K. Jones. *Health Care 2020: The Coming Collapse of Employer-Provided Health Care.* Washington, DC: Hudson Institute, 1999.

115. *Genetics*

Alper, Joseph S., Catherine Ard, Jon Beckwith, et al., eds. *The Double-Edged Helix: Social Implications of Genetics in a Diverse Society.* Baltimore: Johns Hopkins University Press, 2004.

Chapman, Audrey R., and Mark S. Frankel, eds. *Designing Our Descendants: The Promises and Perils of Genetic Modifications.* Baltimore: Johns Hopkins University Press, 2003.

Childs, Barton. *Genetic Medicine: A Logic of Disease.* 2d ed. Baltimore: Johns Hopkins University Press, 2003.

Davies, Kevin. *Cracking the Genome: Inside the Race to Unlock Human DNA.* Baltimore: Johns Hopkins University Press, 2002.

Guttmacher, Alan E., Francis S. Collins, and Jeffrey M. Drazen, eds. *Genomic Medicine: Articles From the New England Journal of Medicine.* Baltimore: Johns Hopkins University Press, 2004.

Hernandez, Lyla M., ed., and Committee on Genomics and the Public's Health in the 21st Century, Board on Health Promotion and Disease Prevention, Institute of Medicine. *Implications of Genomics for Public Health: Workshop Summary.* Washington, DC: National Academies Press, 2006.

Holtzman, Neil A., and Michael S. Watson, eds. *Promoting Safe and Effective Genetic Testing in the United States: Final Report of the Task Force on Genetic Testing.* Baltimore: Johns Hopkins University Press, 1998.

Jorde, Lynn B., ed. *Encyclopedia of Genetics, Genomics, Proteomics, and Bioinformatics.* Hoboken, NJ: Wiley, 2005.

Khoury, Muin J., Julian Little, and Wylie Burke. *Human Genome Epidemiology: A Scientific Foundation for Using Genetic Information to Improve Health and Prevent Disease.* New York: Oxford University Press, 2003.

Lindee, Susan. *Moments of Truth in Genetic Medicine.* Baltimore: Johns Hopkins University Press, 2005.

Milunsky, Aubrey, ed. *Genetic Disorders and the Fetus: Diagnosis, Prevention, and Treatment.* 5th ed. Baltimore: Johns Hopkins University Press, 2004.

National Academies Keck Futures Initiative. *The Genomic Revolution: Implications for Treatment and Control of Infectious Disease: Working Group Summaries.* Conference held at the Arnold and Mabel Beckman Center of the National Academies, Irvine, CA (November 10–13, 2005). Washington, DC: National Academies Press, 2006.

Ness, Bryan D., ed. *Encyclopedia of Genetics.* 2 vols. Pasadena, CA: Salem Press, 2004.

Nys, Herman. *Genetic Testing: Patient's Rights, Insurance, and Employment: A Survey of Regulations in the European Union.* Luxembourg: Office for Official Publications of the European Communities, 2002.

Ott, Jurg. *Analysis of Human Genetic Linkage.* 3d ed. Baltimore: Johns Hopkins University Press, 1999.

Parens, Erik, Audrey R. Chapman, and Nancy Press, eds. *Wrestling With Behavioral Genetics: Science, Ethics, and Public Conversation.* Baltimore: Johns Hopkins University Press, 2005.

Parthasarathy, Shobita. *Building Genetic Medicine: Technology, Breast Cancer, and the Comparative Politics of Health Care.* Cambridge: MIT Press, 2007.

Peltz, Gary, ed. *Computational Genetics and Genomics: Tools for Understanding Disease*. Totowa, NJ: Humana Press, 2005.

Reilly, Philip. *Is It in Your Genes? The Influence of Genes on Common Disorders and Diseases That Affect You and Your Family*. Cold Spring Harbor, NY: Cold Spring Harbor Laboratory Press, 2004.

Thomas, Duncan C. *Statistical Methods in Genetic Epidemiology*. New York: Oxford University Press, 2004.

Tokar, Brian, ed. *Redesigning Life? The Worldwide Challenge to Genetic Engineering*. New York: Zed Books, 2001.

Wailoo, Keith, and Stephen Pemberton. *The Troubled Dream of Genetic Medicine: Ethnicity and Innovation in Tay-Sachs, Cystic Fibrosis, and Sickle Cell Disease*. Baltimore: Johns Hopkins University Press, 2006.

116. Health Planning

Green, Andrew. *An Introduction to Health Planning in Developing Countries*. New York: Oxford University Press, 1999.

Hayward, Cynthia. *Healthcare Facility Planning: Thinking Strategically*. Chicago: Health Administration Press, 2005.

Hodges, Bonni C., and Donna M. Videto. *Assessment and Planning in Health Programs*. Sudbury, MA: Jones and Bartlett, 2005.

Issel, L. Michele. *Health Program Planning and Evaluation: A Practical, Systematic Approach for Community Health*. Sudbury, MA: Jones and Bartlett, 2004.

Thomas, Richard K. *Health Services Planning*. 2d ed. New York: Springer, 2003.

Zuckerman, Alan M. *Healthcare Strategic Planning*. 2d ed. Chicago: Health Administration Press, 2005.

117. Physician–Patient Relationship

Defining the Patient-Physician Relationship for the 21st Century. Third Annual Disease Management Outcome Summit, Phoenix, AZ (October 30–November 2, 2003). Nashville, TN: American Healthways, 2004.

Katz, Jay. *The Silent World of Doctor and Patient*. Baltimore: Johns Hopkins University Press, 2002.

Levi, Benjamin H. *Respecting Patient Autonomy*. Champaign: University of Illinois Press, 1999.

Ramsey, Paul. *The Patient as Person: Explorations in Medical Ethics*. 2d ed. New Haven, CT: Yale University Press, 2002.

Rosenblatt, R. A., G. E. Wright, L. M. Baldwin, et al. "The Effect of the Doctor-Patient Relationship on Emergency Department Use Among the Elderly," *American Journal of Public Health* 90(1): 97–102, January 2000.

Smith, James Monroe, ed. *Producing Patient-Centered Health Care: Patient Perspectives About Health and Illness and the Physician/Patient Relationship*. Westport, CT: Auburn House, 1999.

Thurston, Jeffrey M. *Death of Compassion: The Endangered Doctor-Patient Relationship*. Waco, TX: WRS, 1996.

Watts, David H. *Bedside Manners: One Doctor's Reflections on the Oddly Intimate Encounters Between Patient and Healer*. New York: Harmony Books, 2005.

118. Privacy, Confidentiality, and the Health Insurance Portability and Accountability Act of 1996 (HIPAA)

Beaver, Kevin, and Rebecca Herold. *The Practical Guide to HIPAA Privacy and Security Compliance*. Boston: Auerbach, 2003.

Black, Nick. "Secondary Use of Personal Data for Health and Health Services Research: Why Identifiable Data Are Essential," *Journal of Health Services Research and Policy* 8(3 Suppl. 1): 36–40, July 1, 2003.

Chaikind, H. R., J. Hearne, B. Lyke, et al. *The Health Insurance Portability and Accountability Act (HIPAA): Overview and Analysis*. New York: Novinka Books, 2004.

Committee on the Role of Institutional Review Boards in Health Services Research Data Privacy Protection, Division of Health Care Services, Institute of Medicine. *Institutional Review Boards and Health Services Research Data Privacy: A Workshop Summary*. Washington, DC: National Academies Press, 2000.

Dennis, Jill Callahan. *Privacy and Confidentiality of Health Information*. San Francisco: Jossey-Bass, 2000.

Herdman, Roger, and Harold Moses, and National Cancer Policy Forum, Institute of Medicine. Effect of the HIPAA Privacy Rule on Health Research. In *Proceedings of a Workshop Presented to the National Cancer Policy Forum*. Washington, DC: National Academies Press, 2006.

Roach, William H. *Medical Records and the Law*. 4th ed. Sudbury, MA: Jones and Bartlett, 2006.

119. Program Evaluation

Aday, Lu Ann, Charles E. Begley, David R. Lairson, et al. *Evaluating the Healthcare System: Effectiveness, Efficiency, and Equity*. 3d ed. Chicago: Health Administration Press, 2004.

Grembowski, David. *The Practice of Health Program Evaluation*. Thousand Oaks, CA: Sage, 2001.

Steckler, Allan, and Laura Linnan, eds. *Process Evaluation for Public Interventions and Research*. San Francisco: Jossey-Bass, 2002.

Telfair, Joseph, Laura C. Leviton, and Jeanne S. Merchant. *Evaluating Health and Human Service Programs in Community Settings: New Directions for Evaluation*. San Francisco: Jossey-Bass, 1999.

Timmreck, Thomas C. *Planning, Program Development, and Evaluation*. 2d ed. Sudbury, MA: Jones and Bartlett, 2003.

Wynn, Barbara O., Arindam Dutta, and Martha I. Nelson. *Challenges in Program Evaluation of Health Interventions in Developing Countries*. Santa Monica, CA: RAND Center for Domestic and International Health Security, 2005.

120. Technology Assessment

Acemoglu, Daron, et al. *Did Medicare Induce Pharmaceutical Innovation?* NBER Working Paper No. 11949. Cambridge, MA: National Bureau of Economic Research, 2006.

Aspden, Philip, ed., Board on Science, Technology, and Economic Policy, Policy and Global Affairs, Board on Health Care Services, Institute of Medicine, and National Research Council. *Medical Innovation in the Changing Healthcare Marketplace: Conference Summary.* Washington, DC: National Academy Press, 2002.

Becker, Karen, and John J. Whyte, eds. *Clinical Evaluation of Medical Devices: Principles and Case Studies.* 2d ed. Totowa, NJ: Humana Press, 2006.

Coddington, Dean C., Keith D. Moore, and Elizabeth A. Fischer. *Strategies for the New Health Care Marketplace: Managing the Convergence of Consumerism and Technology.* San Francisco: Jossey-Bass, 2001.

Duesterburg, Thomas, David Weinshropp, and David Murray. *Health Care Reform, Regulation, and Innovation in the Medical Device Industry: A Study of Competitiveness in a Vital U.S. Industry.* Washington, DC: Hudson Institute, 1996.

Eaton, Margaret L., and Donald L. Kennedy. *Innovation in Medical Technology: Ethical Issues and Challenges.* Baltimore: Johns Hopkins University Press, 2007.

Ellis, David. *Technology and the Future of Health Care: Preparing for the Next 30 Years.* San Francisco: Jossey-Bass, 2001.

Epstein, Richard A. *Overdose: How Excessive Government Regulations Stifles Pharmaceutical Innovation.* New Haven, CT: Yale University Press, 2006.

Garber, Alan M., and Victor R. Fuchs. "The Expanding Role of Technology Assessment in Health Policy," *Stanford Law and Policy Review* 3: 203–209, Fall 1991.

Gedeon, Andras. *Science and Technology in Medicine: An Illustrated Account Based on Ninety-Nine Landmark Publications From Five Centuries.* New York: Springer, 2006.

Geisler, Eliezer, Koos Krabbendam, and Roel Schuring, eds. *Technology, Health Care, and Management in the Hospitals of the Future.* Westport, CT: Praeger, 2003.

Gelijns, Annetine C., and Holly V. Dawkins, eds., and Committee on Technology Innovation in Medicine, Institute of Medicine. *Adopting New Medical Technology.* Washington, DC: National Academy Press, 1994.

Halley, D. *Australian Experience in the Use of Economic Evaluation to Inform Policy on Medical Technology.* West Heidelberg, Victoria, Australia: National Centre for Health Program Evaluation, 1996.

Hanna, Kathi E., Frederick J. Manning, Peter Bouxsein, et al., and Roundtable on Research and Development of Drugs, Biologics, and Medical Devices, Board on Health Sciences Policy, Institute of Medicine. *Innovation and Invention in Medical Devices: Workshop Summary.* Washington, DC: National Academies Press, 2001.

Jeffrey, Kirk. *Machines in Our Hearts: The Cardiac Pacemaker, the Implantable Defibrillator, and American Health Care.* Baltimore: Johns Hopkins University Press, 2001.

Lantos, John D., and William L. Meadow. *Neonatal Bioethics: The Moral Challenges of Medical Innovation.* Baltimore: Johns Hopkins University Press, 2006.

Mohr, Penny E., Curt Mueller, Peter Neumann, et al. *The Impact of Medical Technology on Future Health Care Costs.* Bethesda, MD: Center for Health Affairs, Project HOPE, 2001.

Patlak, Margie, Sharyl J. Nass, I. Craig Henderson, et al., eds., Committee on the Early Detection of Breast Cancer, National Cancer Policy Board, Institute of Medicine, and Commission on Life Sciences, National Research Council. *Mammography and Beyond: Developing Technologies for the Early Detection of Breast Cancer: A Non-Technical Summary.* Washington, DC: National Academy Press, 2000.

Rosenau, R. V. "Managing Medical Technology: Lessons for the United States From Quebec and France," *International Journal of Health Services* 30(3): 617–39, 2000.

Schacter, Bernice Zeldin. *Issues and Dilemmas of Biotechnology: A Reference Guide.* Westport, CT: Greenwood, 1999.

Schlich, Thomas, and Ulrich Trohler, eds. *The Risks of Medical Innovation: Risk Perception and Assessment in Historical Context.* New York: Routledge, 2006.

Silberglitt, Richard, Philip S. Anton, David R. Howell, et al. *The Global Technology Revolution 2020: Bio, Nano, Materials, Information Trends, Drivers, Barriers, and Social Implications.* Santa Monica, CA: RAND Corporation, 2006.

Sloan, Frank A., and Chee-Ruey Hsieh, eds. *Pharmaceutical Innovation: Incentives, and Cost-Benefit Analysis in International Perspective.* New York: Cambridge University Press, 2007.

Spekowius, Gerhard, and Thomas Wendler, eds. *Advances in Healthcare Technology: Shaping the Future of Medical Care.* New York: Springer, 2006.

Stelzer, Irwin, ed. *Innovation in the Medical Technology Industries: Regulation, Competition, Reimbursement, and the Availability of Venture Capital.* Washington, DC: Hudson Institute, 2002.

Turisco, Fran, and Jane Metzger. *Rural Health Care Delivery: Connecting Communities Through Technology.* Oakland: California HealthCare Foundation, 2002.

U.S. Congress, Office of Technology Assessment. *Tools for Evaluating Health Technologies: Five Background Papers.* Washington, DC: U.S. Congress, Office of Technology Assessment, 1995.

Wailoo, Keith. *Drawing Blood: Technology and Disease Identity in Twentieth-Century America.* Baltimore: Johns Hopkins University Press, 1999.

Webster, John G., ed. *Encyclopedia of Medical Devices and Instrumentation.* 2d ed. 6 vols. Hoboken, NJ: Wiley, 2006.

121. Women's Health Issues

Ammer, Christine. *The Encyclopedia of Women's Health.* 5th ed. New York: Facts on File, 2005.

Clark, Rebecca A., Robert T. Maupin, and Jill Hayes Hammer. *A Women's Guide to Living With HIV Infection.* Baltimore: Johns Hopkins University Press, 2004.

Collins, Catherine Fisher, ed. *African American Women's Health and Social Issues.* 2d ed. Westport, CT: Praeger, 2006.

Coward, Raymond T., Lisa A. Davis, Carol H. Gold, et al., eds. *Rural Women's Health: Mental, Behavioral, and Physical Issues.* New York: Springer, 2006.

Gay, Kathlyn. *Encyclopedia of Women's Health Issues.* Westport, CT: Oryx Press, 2002.

Health Resources and Services Administration. *Women's Health USA 2006.* Rockville, MD: U.S. Department of Health and Human Services, 2006.

James, Genie. *Winning in the Women's Health Care Marketplace: A Comprehensive Plan for Health Care Strategists.* San Francisco: Jossey-Bass, 1999.

Kishor, Katherine Neitzel. *The Status of Women: Indicators for Twenty-Five Countries.* Calverton, MD: Macro International, 1996.

Kramer, Elizabeth J., Susan L. Ivey, and Yu-Wen Ying, eds. *Immigrant Women's Health: Problems and Solutions.* San Francisco: Jossey-Bass, 1998.

Kuh, Diana, and Rebecca Hardy, eds. *A Life Course Approach to Women's Health.* New York: Oxford University Press, 2003.

Loue, Sana, and Martha Sajatovic. *Encyclopedia of Women's Health.* New York: Kluwer Academic Press/Plenum Press, 2004.

Mastroianni, Anna C., Ruth Faden, and Daniel Federman, eds., and Committee on the Ethical and Legal Issues Relating to the Inclusion of Women in Clinical Studies, Division of Health Sciences Policy, Institute of Medicine. *Women and Health Research: Ethical and Legal Issues of Including Women in Clinical Studies,* vols. 1–2. Workshop and Commissioned Papers. Washington, DC: National Academy Press, 1994.

Middleberg, Maurice I. *Promoting Reproductive Security in Developing Countries.* New York: Springer, 2003.

Montz, F. J., Robert E. Bristow, and Paula J. Anastasia. *A Guide to Survivorship for Women With Ovarian Cancer.* Baltimore: Johns Hopkins University Press, 2005.

National Center on Addiction and Substance Abuse at Columbia University. *Women Under the Influence.* Baltimore: Johns Hopkins University Press, 2005.

O'Leary, Ann, and Loretta Sweet Jemmott. *Women and AIDS: Coping and Care.* New York: Springer, 1996.

Olson, James S. *Bathsheba's Breast: Women, Cancer, and History.* Baltimore: Johns Hopkins University Press, 2005.

Wallach, Edward E., and Esther Eisenberg. *Hysterectomy: Exploring Your Options.* Baltimore: Johns Hopkins University Press, 2003.

Weisman, Carol S. *Women's Health Care: Activist Traditions and Institutional Change.* Baltimore: Johns Hopkins University Press, 1998.

World Health Organization. Women and Health: Better Health and Welfare Systems, Women's Perspectives. In *Proceedings of a WHO Kobe Centre International Meeting, Awaji Yumebutai International Conference Centre (April 5–7, 2000).* Kobe, Japan: World Health Organization, 2000.

Appendix: Web Resources

This listing contains useful resources that are available on the Internet for selected topics of health services research. It contains a brief description of each topic and links to Web sites based on particular categories of interest. These links are current as of the publication date.

Index

1. Academic Medical Centers

Academic medical centers are teaching hospitals that are generally affiliated with a medical school or university. These hospitals have a broad mission that includes teaching, clinical research, and medical education, and they may offer the latest advancements in medical technologies and treatments.

Alliance of Independent Academic Medical Centers (AIAMC)   http://www.aiamc.org

Association of Academic Health Centers   http://www.ahcnet.org

Association of Canadian Academic Healthcare Organizations (ACAHO)   http://www.acaho.org

University HealthSystem Consortium (UHC)   http://www.uhc.edu

See also Hospitals; Medical Residents and Interns; Physicians

2. Accreditation, Certification, and Licensing

Accreditation, certification, and licensing are ways of credentialing healthcare providers and facilities to ensure that a minimum professional standard has been met. Several private organizations carry out credentialing activities in healthcare.

Accreditation Association for Ambulatory Health Care (AAAHC)   http://www.aaahc.org

Accreditation Canada, formerly known as the Canadian Council on Health Services Accreditation   http://www.accreditation-canada.ca

American Board of Medical Specialties (ABMS)   http://www.abms.org

Association of American Medical Colleges (AAMC)   http://www.aamc.org

Association of Faculties of Medicine of Canada (AFMC)   http://www.afmc.ca

Commission on Accreditation of Rehabilitation Facilities (CARF)   http://www.carf.org

Commission on Dental Accreditation of Canada   http://www.cda-adc.ca/cdacweb

Commission on Osteopathic College Accreditation (COCA), American Osteopathic Association   http://www.osteopathic.org

Council on Accreditation (COA)   http://www.coanet.org

Federation of State Medical Boards of the United States (FSMB)   http://www.fsmb.org

Healthcare Facilities Accreditation Program (HFAP), American Osteopathic Association   https://www.do-online.org/index.cfm?au=D&PageId=edu_main&SubPageId=acc_main

Joint Commission   http://www.jointcommission.org

National Committee for Quality Assurance (NCQA)   http://www.ncqa.org

Royal College of Dentists of Canada (RCDC)   http://www.rcdc.ca

Utilization Review Accreditation Committee (URAC)   http://www.urac.org

See also Health Law; Hospitals; Public Health; Quality of Healthcare; Regulation

3. Adult Day Care

Adult day care is provided at facilities that care for the elderly and/or disabled. Health and social services may also be provided at these facilities.

National Adult Day Services Association (NADSA)   http://www.nadsa.org

See also Aging; Disability; Assisted Living; Gerontology; Nursing Homes

4. Advocacy, Education, and Research Organizations

Advocacy, education, and research organizations are engaged in and inform the public policy debate on relevant health policy issues. These organizations play an important role in educating and raising awareness of the public and policymakers on timely and key issues affecting the healthcare system.

Abt Associates   http://www.abtassociates.com

AcademyHealth   http://www.academyhealth.org

Alliance for Health Reform   http://www.allhealth.org

American Enterprise Institute for Public Policy Research (AEI)   http://www.aei.org

Brookings Institution   http://www.brookings.edu

Caledon Institute of Social Policy (Canada)   http://www.caledoninst.org

Canadian Centre for Policy Alernatives   http://www.policyalternatives.ca

Canadian Council on Social Development (CCSD)   http://www.ccsd.ca

Cato Institute   http://www.cato.org

Center for Budget and Policy Priorities   http://www.cbpp.org

Center for Health Care Strategies, Inc. (CHCS)   http://www.chcs.org

Center for Studying Health System Change (HSC)
   http://www.hschange.com

Employee Benefit Research Institute (EBRI)
   http://www.ebri.org

Families USA   http://www.familiesusa.org

Galen Institute   http://www.galen.org

Health Affairs   http://www.healthaffairs.org

Heritage Foundation   http://www.heritage.org

Institute of Medicine (IOM), National Academy of
   Sciences   http://www.iom.edu

Kaiser Family Foundation   http://www.kaisernetwork.org

Lewin Group   http://www.lewin.com

Mathematica Policy Research, Inc.
   http://www.mathematica-mpr.com

MEDTAP International   http://www.medtap.com

National Academy of Social Insurance (NASI)
   http://www.nasi.org

National Institute for Health Care Management
   (NIHCM)   http://www.nihcm.org

Policy Action Network   http://www.movingideas.org

Public Citizen   http://www.citizen.org

RAND Corporation   http://www.rand.org

Research Triangle Institute International (RTI)   http://www.rti.org

Urban Institute   http://www.urban.org

See also Federal Government; Foundations and Philanthropies;
   Health Policy Organizations

5. African American Health

African American health recognizes the unique healthcare needs and health disparities of this minority racial
group. Several organizations are focused on the particular health needs of African Americans.

African American Family Services (AAFS)   http://www.aafs.net

African-American Health, Medline Plus, National Library of
   Medicine (NLM)   http://www.nlm.nih.gov/medlineplus/
   africanamericanhealth.html

American Sickle Cell Anemia Association (ASCAA)
   http://www.ascaa.org

Black AIDS Institute   http://www.blackaids.org

National Black Alcoholism and Addictions Council
   http://www.nbacinc.org

Waltham Forest Black People's Mental Health
   Association   http://www.bpmha.orgmenu.htm

See also AIDS/HIV; Health Disparities; Minority Health;
   Public Health

6. Aging

A number of organiations are dedicated to promoting
the health and welfare of the elderly and aging. As the
population continues to grow older with life expectancy increasing, these organizations will continue to
serve an important role in our communities.

AARP (formerly the American Association of Retired
   Persons)   http://www.aarp.org

Administration on Aging (AOA)   http://www.aoa.gov

Alliance for Aging Research (AAR)
   http://www.agingresearch.org

American Association of Homes and Services for the Aging
   (AAHSA)   http://www.aahsa.org

American Federation for Aging Research (AFAR)
   http://www.afar.org

American Health Assistance Foundation (AHAF)
   http://www.ahaf.org

American Society on Aging (ASA)   http://www.asaging.org

Center for Healthy Aging
   http://www.centerforhealthyaging.org

Centre on Aging (Canada)
   http://www.umanitoba.ca/centres/aging

Centre on Aging, University of Victoria, Canada
   http://www.coag.uvic.ca

European Federation of Older Persons (EURAG)
   http://www.eurageurope.org

Institute for the Future of Aging Services (IFAS)
   http://www.futureofaging.org

International Institute on Ageing, United Nations (UN)
   http://www.inia.org.mt

National Aging Information and Referral Support Center
   http://www.nasua.org/informationandreferral

National Associations of Area Agencies on Aging (n4a)
   (members are Area Agencies on Aging, established under the
   provisions of the Older Americans Act of 1965)
   http://www.n4a.org

National Association of County Aging Programs
   (NACAP)   http://www.naco.org

National Association of State Units on Aging (NASUA)
   http://www.nasua.org

National Caucus and Center on Black Aged (NCBA)
http://www.ncba-aged.org

National Council on the Aging (NCOA)   http://www.ncoa.org

National Eldercare Locator   http://www.eldercare.gov

National Hispanic Council on Aging (NHCOA)
http://www.nhcoa.org

National Institute on Aging (NIA), U.S. National Institutes of
Health   http://www.nia.nih.gov

National Program on Women and Aging, The Heller School of
Social Policy and Management, Brandeis University,
Waltham, MA   http://iasp.brandeis.edu/womenandaging

National Resource Center on Nutrition, Physical Activity &
Aging, Florida International University, Miami, FL
http://nutritionandaging.fiu.edu

RAND Center for the Study of Aging
http://www.rand.org/labor/aging

Resource Center on Aging, University of California, Berkeley,
CA   http://socrates.berkeley.edu/~aging

Retirement Research Foundation (RRF)   http://www.rrf.org

See also Assisted Living; Disability; Gerontology; Nursing Homes

7. AIDS/HIV

AIDS/HIV cases continue to be reported each year with
those residing in resource poor settings and with
minority groups being disproportionately burdened. As
people with AIDS/HIV live longer with better treatment options available, the quality of life of these individuals remains a concern.

AIDS Alliance for Children, Youth and Families
http://www.aids-alliance.org

AIDS Clinical Trials Group (ACTG)   http://www.aactg.org

AIDS Resource Foundation for Children (ARFC)
http://www.aidsresource.org

American Foundation for AIDS Research (amfAR)
http://www.amfar.org

Association of Nurses in AIDS Care (ANAC)
http://www.anacnet.org

Black AIDS Institute   http://www.blackaids.org

Body Positive   http://www.thebody.com/bp/bp.html

Canadian HIV/AIDS Information Centre
http://www.aidssida.cpha.ca

Elizabeth Glaser Pediatric AIDS Foundation
http://www.pedaids.org

Gay Men's Health Crisis (GMHC)   http://www.gmhc.org

Global AIDS Alliance (GAA)
http://www.globalaidsalliance.org

HIV/AIDS Program, World Health Organization
http://www.who.int/hiv/en

HIV Medicine Association (HIVMA)   http://www.hivma.org

National AIDS Fund   http://www.aidsfund.org

National AIDS Treatment Advocacy Program (NATAP)
http://www.natap.org

National Association of People with AIDS (NAPWA)
http://www.napwa.org

National Center for HIV/AIDS, Viral Hepatitis, STD, and TB
Prevention (NCHHSTP)   http://www.cdc.gov/nchhstp

National Minority AIDS Council (NMAC)
http://www.nmac.org

Student Global AIDS Campaign (SGAC)
http://www.fightglobalaids.org

See also Epidemiology; Minority Health; Public Health

8. Alcoholism

Alcoholism is a serious condition where individuals
persistently use alcohol to the detriment of their health.
The abuse of alcohol results in negative health consequences that can have lasting effects.

Alcohol and Drug Problems Association of North America
(ADPA)   http://www.adpana.com

Alcoholics Anonymous World Service (AA)   http://www.aa.org

Century Council   http://www.centurycouncil.org

Drug and Alcohol Testing Industry Association (DITIA)
http://www.datia.org

National Association of State Alcohol and Drug Abuse
Directors (NASADAD)   http://www.nasadad.org

National Black Alcoholism and Addictions Council
http://www.nbacinc.org

National Institute on Alcohol Abuse and Alcoholism
(NIAAA)   http://www.niaaa.nih.gov

SAMHSA's National Clearinghouse for Alcohol and Drug
Information   http://www.health.org

See also Federal Government; Public Health; Substance Abuse

9. Allied Health

Allied health represents the group of healthcare professionals outside the realm of medicine and nursing. These professionals work together with other healthcare providers to make up the healthcare team and to help ensure the proper functioning of the healthcare system.

American Occupational Therapy Association (AOTA)
http://www.aota.org

American Physical Therapy Association (APTA)
http://www.apta.org

Canadian Association of Occupational Therapists
(CAOT)   http://www.caot.ca

Canadian Physiotherapy Association
http://www.physiotherapy.ca

National Rehabilitation Association
http://www.nationalrehab.org

See also Case Management; Medical Technologists

10. Alzheimer's Disease

Alzheimer's disease is the most common form of dementia and it is an incurable and terminal condition. Several organizations have led efforts to promote research and care for those afflicted with this degenerative disease.

Alzheimer's Association (ALZ)   http://www.alz.org

Alzheimer's Disease Education and Referral (ADEAR)
Center   http://www.nia.nih.gov/alzheimers

Alzheimer Society of Canada   http://www.alzheimer.ca

National Institute on Aging (NIA)   http://www.nia.nih.gov

See also Aging; Disability; Gerontology; Nursing Homes

11. Ambulatory Care

Ambulatory care is medical care that is provided on an outpatient basis. Ambulatory care can be delivered in doctor's offices and clinics, emergency departments, and urgent care centers.

Academic Pediatric Association, formerly known as the
Ambulatory Pediatric Association   http://www.ambpeds.org

Accreditation Association for Ambulatory Health Care
(AAAHC)   http://www.aaahc.org

See also Ambulatory Surgery Centers; Community Health
Centers (CHCs); Physicians

12. Ambulatory Surgery Centers

Ambulatory surgery centers are healthcare facilities that provide same-day surgeries on an outpatient basis that do not require a patient to be hospitalized.

American Association for Accreditation of Ambulatory Surgery
Facilities (AAAASF)   http://www.aaaasf.org

American Association of Ambulatory Surgery Centers
(AAASC)   http://www.aaasc.org

See also Ambulatory Care; Surgery and Surgeons

13. Anesthesiology

Anesthesiology is a medical speciality that focuses on administering anesthesia to patients and monitoring vital bodily functions during a medical procedure such as surgery.

American Society of Anesthesiologists (ASA)
http://www.asahq.org

American Society of Regional Anesthesia and Pain Medicine
(ASRA)   http://www.asra.org

Society of Cardiovascular Anesthesiologists (SCA)
http://www.scahq.org

See also Ambulatory Surgery Centers; Dentistry; Hospitals;
Surgery and Surgeons

14. Antitrust

Antitrust is an area that promotes competition in healthcare to benefit consumers. At its core, competition serves to improve healthcare quality, reduce costs, and increase access.

American Antitrust Institute   http://www.antitrustinstitute.org

Antitrust Coalition for Consumer Choices in Health
Care   http://www.healthantitrust.org

Health Care Antitrust Division, U.S. Department of Justice
http://www.usdoj.gov/atr/public/health_care/health_care.htm

U.S. Federal Trade Commission (FTC)   http://www.ftc.gov/bc

See also Ethics; Health Law; Regulation

15. Arthritis and Rheumatism

Arthritis and rheumatism are common diseases of the bones and joints. These difficult to treat conditions afflict many individuals each year and cause chronic pain.

American College of Rheumatology (ACR)
http://www.rheumatology.org

Arthritis Foundation   http://www.arthritis.org

Arthritis Society (Canada)   http://www.arthritis.ca

National Institute of Arthritis and Musculoskeletal and Skin
Diseases (NIAMS)   http://www.niams.nih.gov

See also Epidemiology; Public Health; Women's Health Issues

16. Assisted Living

Assisted living facilities provide assistance with activities of daily living to individuals and may also assist with personal care and medical supervision.

Consumer Consortium on Assisted Living (CCAL)
http://www.ccal.org

See also Adult Day Care; Aging; Disability

17. Asthma

Asthma is a condition in which the airways of the lungs become blocked or narrowed and results in breathing difficulties. Several organizations are dedicated to education, research, and advocacy efforts for those suffering from asthma.

American Academy of Allergy, Asthma, and Immunology
(AAAAI)   http://www.aaaai.org

American College of Allergy, Asthma and Immunology
(ACAAI)   http://www.acaai.org

Asthma and Allergy Foundation of America (AAFA)
http://www.aafawa.org

Asthma Society of Canada   http://www.asthma.ca

Food Allergy and Anaphylaxis Network
http://www.foodallergy.org

National Institute of Allergy and Infectious Diseases
(NIAID)   http://www3.niaid.nih.gov

World Allergy Organization (WAO)
http://www.worldallergy.org

See also Chronic Diseases; Environmental Health; Public Health;
Tobacco Use

18. Bioterrorism

Bioterrorism is the use of biological, chemical, and other agents as a deliberate means of coercion or intimidation to further an ideology without regard for the well-being of others.

Coordinating Office for Terrorism Preparedness and Emergency
Response, Centers for Disease Control and Prevention
(CDC)   http://www.cdc.gov/maso/pdf/COTPERfs.pdf

U.S. Department of Homeland Security (DHS)
http://www.dhs.gov

See also Disaster Preparedness and Relief; Federal Government;
Public Health

19. Birth Defects

Birth defects are the malformation and abnormalities in a developing fetus that can be caused by a variety of sources, including genetics and the environment.

March of Dimes Birth Defects Foundation (MDBDF)
http://www.marchofdimes.com

National Birth Defects Prevention Network (NBDPN)
http://www.nbdpn.org

National Center on Birth Defects and Developmental
Disabilities (NCBDDD)   http://www.cdc.gov/ncbddd

National Institute of Child Health and Human Development
(NICHD)   http://www.nichd.nih.gov

See also Child Development and Health; Environmental Health;
Genetics; Public Health

20. Blind and Visually Impaired

Blind and visually impaired refers to the condition of having vision loss. More than 10 million individuals in North America are considered to have some visual impairment.

American Council of the Blind (ACB)   http://www.acb.org

American Foundation for the Blind (AFB)   http://www.afb.org

American Printing House for the Blind (APH)
http://www.aph.org

Blind Veterans Association (BVA)   http://www.bva.org

Canadian National Institute for the Blind (CNIB)
http://www.cnib.ca

Foundation Fighting Blindness (FFB)
http://www.fightblindness.org

Guide Dog Foundation for the Blind (GDFB)
http://www.guidedog.org

Guide Dogs of America (GDA)
http://www.guidedogsofamerica.org

Helen Keller International (HKI)   http://www.hki.org

Leader Dogs for the Blind (LDB)   http://www.leaderdog.org

National Consortium on Deaf-Blindness
    http://www.nationaldb.org

National Federation of the Blind (NFB)   http://www.nfb.org

National Library Service for the Blind and Physically
    Handicapped   http://www.loc.gov/nls

Prevent Blindness America
    http://www.preventblindness.org

Recording for the Blind and Dyslexic (RFB&D)
    http://www.rfbd.org

Research to Prevent Blindness (RPB)   http://www.rpbusa.org

The Seeing Eye   http://www.seeingeye.org

See also Disability; Eye Diseases; Ophthalmology; Optometry

21. Blood and Blood Banks

Blood is a bodily fluid that is necessary to sustain life and provide cells with needed substances. Blood banks are centers that receive and store blood from donors to be later used for patients in need of blood transfusions.

American Association of Blood Banks (AABB)
    http://www.aabb.org

American Red Cross   http://www.redcross.org

America's Blood Centers   http://www.americasblood.org

Canadian Blood Services   http://www.bloodservices.ca

Héme Québec (Canada)   http://www.hema-quebec.qc
    .ca/anglais

See also Blood Disorders; Donors and Organ Transplantation

22. Blood Disorders

Blood disorders are conditions that affect blood and its components. Blood disorders may affect blood proteins, blood cells, hemolglobin, or coagulation.

Center for International Blood and Marrow Transplant
    Research (CIBMTR)   http://www.cibmtr.org

National Heart, Lung, and Blood Institute (NHLBI)
    http://www.nhlbi.nih.gov

National Hemophilia Foundation
    http://www.hemophilia.org

See also Blood and Blood Banks; Genetics; Rare Diseases

23. Burn Care

Burn care is the specialized medical care that is given to patients who suffer from serious burns.

American Burn Association (ABA)   http://www.ameriburn.org

See also Cosmetic and Plastic Surgery; Emergency Medicine; Injury

24. Business Coalitions on Health

Business coalitions on health are organizations that represent a group of businesses from both public and private sectors and their interests in healthcare.

National Organizations

Leapfrog Group, Washington, DC
    http://www.leapfroggroup.org

National Business Coalition on Health (NBCH), Washington,
    DC   http://www.nbch.org

Regional and Local Organizations

Alabama

Employers Coalition for Healthcare Options, Inc., Huntsville,
    AL   http://www.echoal.com

Arizona

Southwest Health Alliance, Scottsdale, AZ
    http://www.southwesthealthalliance.org

Arkansas

Employers' Health Coalition, Fort Smith, AR
    http://www.ehcark.org

California

Pacific Business Group on Health, San Francisco, CA
    http://www.pbgh.org

Colorado

Colorado Business Group on Health, Denver, CO
    http://www.coloradohealthonline.com

Florida

Employers Health Coalition, Tampa, FL
    http://www.ehcaccess.org

Florida Health Care Coalition, Orlando, FL
    http://www.flhcc.com

Georgia

Savannah Business Group on Health, Savannah, GA
http://www.savannahbusinessgroup.com

Hawaʻi

Hawaʻi Business Health Council, Honolulu, HI
http://www.hbhc.biz/index.html

Illinois

Employer's Coalition on Health, Rockford, IL
http://www.ecoh.com

Heartland Healthcare Coalition, Morton, IL
http://www.hhco.org

Midwest Business Group on Health, Chicago, IL
http://www.mbgh.org

Tri-State Health Care Coalition, Quincy, IL
http://www.tri-statehealthcare.com

Indiana

Indiana Employers Quality Health Alliance,
Indianapolis, IN   http://www.qualityhealthalliance.org

Tri-State Business Group on Health, New Burgh, IN
http://www.tsbgh.evansville.net

Kentucky

Four Rivers Health Care Purchasing Alliance, Inc., Calvert City,
KY   http://www.fourrivershc.com

Louisiana

Louisiana Business Group on Health, Baton Rouge, LA
http://www.lbgh.org

Maine

Maine Health Management Coalition, Scarborough,
ME   http://www.mhmc.info

Maryland

Mid-Atlantic Business Group on Health, Greenbelt,
MD   http://mabgh.org

Massachusetts

Massachusetts Healthcare Purchaser Group, Boston,
MA   http://www.mhpg.org

Michigan

AFL-CIO Employer Purchasing Coalition, Bloomfield,
MI   http://www.nlahcc.orgmembers/afl_cio_.html

Alliance for Health, Grand Rapids, MI   http://www.afh.org

Greater Detroit Area Health Council, Detroit, MI
http://www.gdahc.org

Michigan Purchasers Health Alliance, Ann Arbor, MI
http://www.michpha.org

REAL Health Association, Grand Rapids, MI
http://www.realhealth.org

Minnesota

Buyers Health Care Action Group, Bloomington, MN
http://www.bhcag.com

Missouri

Mid-America Coalition on Health Care, Kansas
City, MO   http://www.machc.org

Missouri Consolidated Health Care Plan, Jefferson
City, MO   http://www.mchcp.org

St. Louis Area Business Health Coalition, St. Louis,
MO   http://www.stlbhc.org

Montana

Montana Association of Health Care Purchasers, Missoula,
MT   http://www.mahcp.info

Nevada

Nevada Health Care Coalition, Reno, NV
http://www.nhccreno.org

New Jersey

The Health Care Payers Coalition of New Jersey,
Edison, NJ   http://www.hcpc.org

New York

New York Business Group on Health, New York, NY
http://www.nybgh.org

Niagara Health Quality Coalition, Buffalo, NY
http://www.nhqc.com

North Carolina

Piedmont Health Coalition, Inc., Burlington, NC
http://www.piedmonthealthcoalition.org

WNC Health Coalition, Inc., Asheville, NC   http://wnchc.org

Ohio

Employer Health Care Alliance, Cincinnati, OH
http://www.cintiehca.com

Employers Health Purchasing Corporation of Ohio, Canton,
OH   http://www.ehpco.com

Franklin County Cooperative Health Benefits Program,
Columbus, OH   http://www.eelect.com

Front Path Health Coalition, Maumee, OH
  http://www.frontpathcoalition.com

Health Action Council of Northeast Ohio, Cleveland,
  OH   http://www.healthactioncouncil.org

Tri-River Employers Healthcare Coalition, Dayton, OH
  http://www.tri-river.org

Oregon

Oregon Coalition of Health Care Purchasers, Portland,
  OR   http://www.ochcp.org

Pennsylvania

Lancaster County Business Group on Health,
  Lancaster, PA   http://www.lcbgh.org

Northeast Pennsylvania Regional Healthcare Coalition, Inc.,
  Orwigsburg, PA   http://www.nprhcc.com

Pittsburgh Business Group on Health, Ambridge, PA
  http://www.pbghpa.com

Tennessee

Healthcare 21 Business Coalition of East and Middle
  Tennessee, Knoxville, TN   http://www.hc21.org

Memphis Business Group on Health, Memphis, TN
  http://www.memphisbusinessgroup.org

Texas

Dallas/Fort Worth Business Group on Health, Dallas,
  TX   http://www.dfwbgh.org

Virginia

Virginia Business Coalition on Health, Virginia Beach,
  VA   http://www.myVBCH.org

Washington

Puget Sound Health Alliance, Seattle, WA
  http://www.pugetsoundhealthalliance.org

Wisconsin

The Alliance (WI), Madison, WI
  http://www.alliancehealthcoop.com

Business Health Care Group of South East Wisconsin, Franklin,
  WI   http://www.bhcgsw.org

Employers Health Cooperative, Janesville, WI
  http://www.ehchealth.com

Fond Du Lac Area Businesses on Health, Fond
  Du Lac, WI   http://www.faboh.com

Greater Milwaukee Business Foundation on Health, Inc.,
  Sussex, WI   http://www.gmbfh.org

See also Health Insurance; Prevention and Health Promotion

25. Canadian Healthcare Organizations

Canadian healthcare organizations are organizations that are dedicated to the health and healthcare system of Canada.

Association of Canadian Academic Healthcare Organizations
  (ACAHO)   http://www.acaho.org

Association of Faculties of Medicine of Canada
  http://www.afmc.ca

Canada's Health Informatics Association (COACH)
  http://www.coachorg.com

Canadian Association of Blue Cross Plans (CABCF)
  http://www.bluecross.ca

Canadian Association for Health Services and Policy Research
  (CAHSPR)   http://www.cahspr.ca

Canadian Association on Gerontology   http://www.cagacg.ca

Canadian Generic Pharmaceutical Association (CGPA)
  http://www.cdma-acfpp.org

Canadian Healthcare Association (CHA)   http://www.cha.ca

Canadian Health Economics Research Association
  (CHERA)   http://www.chera.ca

Canadian Health Services Research Foundation
  (CHSRF)   http://www.chsrf.ca

Canadian Home Care Association (CHCA)
  http://www.cdnhomecare.ca

Canadian Institutes of Health Research (CIHR)
  http://www.cihr.ca

Canadian Medical Association (CMA)   http://www.cma.ca

Canadian Pain Society (CPS)
  http://www.canadianpainsociety.ca

Canadian Public Health Association (CPHA)
  http://www.cpha.ca

Canadian Women's Health Network (CWHN)
  http://www.cwhn.ca

Chronic Pain Association of Canada (CPAC)
  http://www.chronicpaincanada.com

Health Canada   http://www.hc-sc.gc.ca

Institute of Health Services and Policy Research (IHSPR),
  Canadian Institutes of Health Research (CIHR)
  http://www.cihr.cae/13948.html

Public Health Agency of Canada, Injury
  http://www.phacaspc.gc.cainjury-bles

See also International Health Systems; National Health
  Insurance; World Health Organization (WHO)

26. Cancer

Cancer is a class of disease where the body's cells undergo uncontrolled growth, invade other tissues, and spread to other parts of the body. Cancer can occur at all ages but it predominantly affects individuals as they grow older. Cancer can be caused by genetics, behavioral, and/or environmental factors.

American Association for Cancer Research (AACR)
    http://www.aacr.org

American Cancer Society (ACS)   http://www.cancer.org

American Foundation for Cancer Research (NFCR)
    http://www.nfcr.org

American Institute for Cancer Research (AICR)
    http://www.aicr.org

Association of Cancer Online Resources (ACOR)
    http://www.acor.org/about/about.html

Association of Community Cancer Centers (ACCC)
    http://www.accc-cancer.org

Breast Cancer Network of Strength
    http://www.networkofstrength.org

Canadian Cancer Society   http://www.cancer.ca

Cancer Care (CC)   http://www.cancercare.org

Cancer Information Service (CIS)   http://cis.nci.nih.gov

Coalition of Cancer Cooperative Groups
    http://www.cancertrialshelp.org

Damon Runyon Cancer Research Foundation
    http://www.cancerresearchfund.org

Leukemia and Lymphoma Society   http://www.lls.org

Lymphoma Research Foundation   http://www.lymphoma.org

National Breast Cancer Coalition (NBCC)
    http://www.stopbreastcancer.org

National Cancer Institute (NCI)   http://www.cancer.gov

National Coalition for Cancer Survivorship (NCCS)
    http://www.canceradvocacy.org

OncoLink, Abramson Cancer Center of the University of
    Pennsylvania   http://www.oncolink.com

Skin Cancer Foundation (SCF)   http://www.skincancer.org

Susan G. Komen for the Cure (SGKF)
    http://www.komen.org

Your Disease Risk, Siteman Cancer Center Prevention
    http://www.yourdiseaserisk.wustl.edu

See also Oncology; National Institutes of Health (NIH); Public
    Health; Tobacco Use

27. Cardiology

Cardiology is the field of medicine that studies the heart and blood vessels.

American Association of Cardiovascular and Pulmonary
    Rehabilitation (AACVPR)   http://www.aacvpr.org

American College of Cardiology (ACC)   http://www.acc.org

American College of Chest Physicians (ACCP)
    http://www.chestnet.org

American Society of Echocardiography (ASE)
    http://www.asecho.org

American Society of Nuclear Cardiology (ASNC)
    http://www.asnc.org

National Heart, Lung, and Blood Institute (NHLBI)
    http://www.nhlbi.nih.gov

See also Epidemiology; Heart Disease; Public Health

28. Care Giving

Care giving is done by family or unpaid friends or relatives of who provide care and support to an individual with a disabling condition.

Family Caregiver Alliance   http://www.caregiver.org

National Family Caregivers Association (NFCA)
    http://www.nfcacares.org

See also Aging; Assisted Living; Disability; Nursing Homes

29. Case Management

Case management is a service that is provided to meet the healthcare needs of a patient and it is designed to produce cost-effect outcomes.

Case Management Society of America (CMSA)
    http://www.cmsa.org

Commission for Case Manager Certification (CCMC)
    http://www.ccmcertification.org

See also Allied Health; Care Giving; Chronic Diseases; Disability

30. Centers for Disease Control and Prevention (CDC)

The Centers for Disease Control and Prevention (CDC) is a public health agency of the federal government that works to protect the health and safety of all Americans.

The CDC is based in Atlanta, Georgia, and focuses its efforts on disease prevention and control.

Centers for Disease Control and Prevention (CDC)
http://www.cdc.gov

Director

Office of the Director   http://www.cdc.gov/about/director.htm

Coordinating Centers for Environmental Health and Injury Prevention

Agency for Toxic Substances and Disease Registry (ATSDR)   http://www.atsdr.cdc.gov

National Center for Environmental Health (NCEH)
http://www.cdc.gov/nceh

National Center for Injury Prevention and Control (NCIPC)   http://www.cdc.gov/ncipc

Coordinating Centers for Health Information and Service

National Center for Health Statistics (NCHS)
http://www.cdc.gov/nchs

National Center for Health Marketing (NCHM)
http://www.cdc.gov/healthmarketing

National Center for Public Health Informatics (NCPHI)
http://www.cdc.gov/ncphi

Coordinating Center for Health Promotion

National Center for Chronic Disease Prevention and Health Promotion (NCCDPHP)   http://www.cdc.gov/nccdphp

National Center on Birth Defects and Developmental Disabilities (NCBDDD)   http://www.cdc.gov/ncbddd

Office of Genomics and Disease Prevention
http://www.cdc.gov/genomics

Coordinating Centers for Infectious Diseases

National Center for HIV, Viral Hepatitis, STD, and TB Prevention (NCHHSTP)   http://www.cdc.gov/nchhstp

National Immunization Program (NIP)
http://www.cdc.gov/nip

Other

Coordinating Office for Global Health
http://www.cdc.gov/cogh

Coordinating Office for Terrorism Preparedness and Emergency Response   http://www.bt.cdc.gov

National Institute for Occupational Safety and Health (NIOSH)   http://www.cdc.gov/niosh/homepage.html

See also Emerging Diseases: Epidemiology; Health Surveys; Public Health; World Health Organization (WHO)

31. Centers for Medicare and Medicaid Services (CMS)

The Centers for Medicare and Medicaid Services (CMS) is the federal agency that is responsible for administering the Medicare, Medicaid, and State Children's Health Insurance Program (SCHIP). CMS works to ensure that its beneficiaries are provided with effective and quality healthcare.

Centers for Medicare and Medicaid Services (CMS)
http://www.cms.gov

Health Insurance Portability and Accountability Act of 1996 (HIPAA)   http://cms.hhs.gov/hipaa

Medicaid   http://cms.hhs.gov/medicaid

Medicare   http://cms.hhs.gov/medicare

State Children's Health Insurance Program (SCHIP)
http://cms.hhs.gov/schip

See also Medicaid; Medicare; State Children's Health Insurance Program (SCHIP)

32. Certificate of Need (CON)

Certificate of need is a program that works to control healthcare facility costs through the coordinated planning of services and new construction projects.

American Association of Health Plans (AAHP) (The AAHP publishes an annual directory of state certificate of need programs)   http://www.aahp.org

See also Health Law; Health Planning; Regulation

33. Childbirth

Childbirth is the process of giving birth to a newborn infant.

Lamaze International   http://www.lamaze.org

Maternity Center Association (MCA)
http://www.maternitywise.org

National Association of Birth Centers (NACC)
http://www.birthcenters.org

See also Birth Defects; Child Development and Health;
Obstetrics and Gynecology

34. Child Development and Health

Child development refers to the physiological and psychological changes that occur as a child grows older. Child health refers to the unique health needs of children.

Ambulatory Pediatric Association (APA)
http://www.ambpeds.org

American Academy of Child and Adolescent Psychiatry
(AACAP)   http://www.aacap.org

American Academy of Pediatrics (AAP)   http://www.aap.org

American Pediatric Surgical Association (APSA)
http://www.eapsa.org

American Public Human Services Association (APHSA)
http://www.aphsa.org

Association of Maternal and Child Health Programs
(AMCHP)   http://www.amchp.org

Children's Defense Fund (CDF)
http://www.childrensdefense.org

Children's Health Fund (CHF)
http://www.childrenshealthfund.org

Children's Organ Transplant Association (COTA)
http://www.cota.org

Institute for Child Health Policy (ICHP), University of
Florida   http://www.ichp.ufl.edu

Maternal and Child Health Bureau, Health Resources and
Services Administration (HRSA)   http://mchb.hrsa.gov

Maternal and Child Health Library
http://www.mchb.hrsa.gov/mchirc

Maternal and Child Health Policy Research Center,
Washington, DC   http://www.mchpolicy.org

National Association of Children's Hospitals and Related
Institutions (NACHRI)   http://www.childrenshospitals.net

National Child Care Information Center   http://nccic.org

National Healthy Mothers, Healthy Babies Coalition
http://www.hmhb.org

National Initiative for Children's Healthcare Quality (NICHQ)
http://www.nichq.org

National Institute of Child Health and Human Development
(NICHD)   http://www.nichd.nih.gov

Sidelines National High-Risk Pregnancy Support Networks
http://www.sidelines.org

Women's and Children's Health Policy Center (WCHPC),
School of Public Health, Johns Hopkins University
http://www.jhsph.edu/wchpc

Zero to Three: National Center for Infants, Toddlers, and
Families   http://www.zerotothree.org

See also Birth Defects; Childbirth; Immunization and
Vaccination; Pediatrics; Public Health

35. Chiropractic Care

Chiropractic care involves the care provided to patients that involves the musculoskeletal system and spine. The treatment provided by chiropractors may involve spinal manipulation and manual therapy.

American Chiropractic Association (ACA)
http://www.amerchiro.org

Council on Chiropractic Orthopedics (CCO)
http://www.ccodc.org

Foundation for Chiropractic Education and Research
(FCER)   http://www.fcer.org

International Chiropractors Association (ICA)
http://www.chiropractic.org

See also Chronic Diseases; Injury; Physical Medicine and
Rehabiliation; Physicians; Spinal Disorders and Injuries

36. Chronic Diseases

Chronic diseases are diseases that are persistent or long-lasting in nature. It is estimated that nearly one in two Americans have a chronic disease.

Chronic Disease Prevention Alliance of Canada
(CDPAC)   http://www.cdpac.ca

Improving Chronic Illness Care Program
http://www.improvingchroniccare.org

National Center for Chronic Disease Prevention and Health
Promotion (NCCDPHP)   http://www.cdc.gov/nccdphp

National Institute on Aging (NIA)   http://www.nia.nih.gov

See also Arthritis and Rheumatism; Asthma; Cancer; Diabetes;
Heart Disease; Hypertension

37. Clinical Laboratories

Clinical laboratories are facilities that provide clinical tests and diagnostic services and they play an important role in the healthcare system.

American Clinical Laboratory Association (ACLA)
http://www.clinical-labs.org

American Society for Clinical Laboratory Science (ASCLS)
http://www.ascls.org

Clinical and Laboratory Standards Institute (CLSI) (This organization was formerly the National Committee for Clinical Laboratory Standards [NCCLS])
http://www.nccls.org

Clinical Laboratory Management Association (CLMA)
http://www.clma.org

See also Hospitals; Medical Technologists; Medical Tests and Diagnostics

38. Clinical Practice Guidelines

Clinical practice guidelines are evidence based and serve to provide guidance to providers on the prevention, diagnosis, prognosis, and treatment of medical conditions.

Agency for Healthcare Research and Quality (AHRQ)
http://www.ahrq.gov

Agency for Healthcare Research and Quality (AHRQ) Guidelines   http://www.ahrq.gov/clinic

Alberta (Canada) Medical Association Clinical Practice Guidelines   http://www.topalbertadoctors.org/cpg.html

American Academy of Pediatrics (AAP)   http://www.aap.org

American Association of Clinical Endocrinology (AACE) Guidelines   http://www.aace.com/pub/guidelines

American College of Cardiology (ACC)/American Heart Association (AHA) Clinical Guidelines
http://www.acc.orgclinical/guidelines/index.html

American College of Gastroenterology (ACG) Guidelines   http://www.acg.gi.org

American College of Rheumatology Clinical Guidelines
http://www.rheumatology.org

American Society of Anesthesiology Clinical Guidelines
http://www.asahq.orgpublicationsAndServices/sgstoc.htm

Australian Clinical Guidelines
http://www.mihsr.monash.orgcce/res

Canadian Medical Association (CMA) Clinical Practice Guidelines   http://www.cma.ca/cpgs

Canadian Task Force on Preventive Health Care (CTFPHC)
http://www.ctfphc.org

Cardiac Surgery Clinical Practice Guidelines (Cedars-Sinai)   http://www.csmc.edu/cvs/md/guide.html

Cholesterol Clinical Guidelines   http://www.nhlbi.nih.gov/guidelines/cholesterol/index.htm

Cochrane Library   http://www.cochrane.co.uk

Diabetes Guidelines (American Association of Clinical Endocrinologists)   http://www.aace.com/pub/pdf/guidelines/DMGuidelines2007.pdf

eGuidelines (This Web site contains a comprehensive collection of United Kingdom clinical guidelines and related information)   http://www.eguidelines.co.uk

Health Services/Technology Assessment (HSTAT)
http://text.nlm.nih.gov

National Guideline Clearinghouse (NGC)
http://www.guideline.gov

National Institute for Health and Clinical Excellence (NICE), United Kingdom   http://www.nice.org.uk

National Quality Measures Clearinghouse
http://www.qualitymeasures.ahrq.gov

See also Evidence-Based Medicine EBM; Health Outcomes; Medical Decision Making; Medical Practice Variations; Randomized Controlled Trials (RCT)

39. Community Health Centers (CHCs)

Community health centers are primary care clinics in communities that provide access to healthcare and function as a vital part of the healthcare safety net.

Bureau of Primary Health Care (BPHC), Health Resources and Services Administration (HRSA)   http://www.bphc.hrsa.gov

National Association of Community Health Centers (NACHC)   http://www.nachc.com

See also Ambulatory Care; Health Disparities; Minority Health; Public Health

40. Complementary and Alternative Medicine

Complimentary and alternative medicine are the medical products and practices that fall outside the realm of traditional Western medicine and standards of care. Studies are beginning to be undertaken to better understand the potential benefits of alternative and complimentary medicine.

Acupuncture Foundation of Canada Institute
    http://www.afcinstitute.com

Alternative Medicine Homepage
    http://www.pitt.edu/~cbw/altm.html

American Association of Oriental Medicine (AAOM)
    http://www.aaom.org

American Society of Alternative Therapists (ASAT)
    http://www.asat.org

Entirely On-Line Alternative Medicine Primer
    http://www.veterinarywatch.com/Primer1.htm

HerbMed   http://www.herbmed.org

National Center for Complementary and Alternative Medicine
    (NCCAM) (This center was formed at NIH in 1999)
    http://www.nccam.nih.gov

National Certification Commission for Acupuncture and
    Oriental Medicine (NCCAOM)   http://www.nccaom.org

National Institutes of Health, Office of Dietary
    Supplements   http://dietary-supplements.info.nih.gov

Rosenthal Center for Complementary and Alternative
    Medicine   http://www.rosenthal.hs.columbia.edu

See also Chiropractic Care; National Institutes of Health (NIH)

41. Consumer-Directed Health Plans (CDHPs)

Consumer-directed health plans are a type of arrangement that allows invididuals to use health savings accounts or other products to pay for routine healthcare services. Additionally, a high-deductible health plan protects the individual from catastrophic expenses.

Consumer-Driven Health Care Institute (CDHCI)
    http://www.cdhci.org

Defined Care   http://www.definedcare.com

See also Health Insurance

42. Consumer Health Information

Consumer health information is information that is made available to consumers on health-related questions including such topics as cost, quality, and alternative treatment options.

Center for Medical Consumers
    http://www.medicalconsumers.org

Federal Citizen Information Center   http://www.pueblo.gsa.gov

HospitalWeb   http://neuro-www.mgh.harvard.edu/hospital
    web.shtml

Mayo Clinic   http://www.mayoclinic.com

MedConnect   http://www.medconnect.com

Merck Source   http://www.mercksource.com

My Medicare Matters, The National Council on the
    Aging   http://www.mymedicarematters.org

National Health Information Center (NHIC)
    http://www.health.gov/nhic

NOAH (New York Online Access to Health)
    http://www.noah-health.org

PDR (Physician's Desk Reference) Health
    http://www.pdrhealth.com

Virtual Hospital: Information for Patients
    http://www.uihealthcare.com/vh

WebMD   http://www.webmd.com

Your Disease Risk, Siteman Cancer Center
    http://www.yourdiseaserisk.wustl.edu

See also Centers for Medicare and Medicaid Services (CMS);
    Health Outcomes; Health Report Cards; Quality of Healthcare

43. Cosmetic and Plastic Surgery

Cosmetic and plastic surgery is a surgical specialty that focuses on enhancing one's appearance or correcting the form or function of a body part.

American Academy of Cosmetic Surgery (AACS)
    http://www.cosmeticsurgery.org

American Academy of Facial Plastic and Reconstructive Surgery
    (AAFPRS)   http://www.aafprs.org

American Society of Plastic Surgeons (ASPS)
    http://www.plasticsurgery.org

See also Birth Defects; Burn Care; Injury; Surgery and Surgeons

44. Cost-Benefit and Cost-Effectiveness Analysis

Cost-benefit and cost-effectiveness analysis are types of economic analyses that are done to compare the relative expenditures in relation to outcomes among two or more competing interventions.

Cost Effectiveness Analysis Registry   https://research.tufts-nemc
    .org/cear/default.aspx

See also Health Economics, Academic Centers of; Randomized
    Controlled Trials (RCT); Technology Assessment

45. Critical Care

Critical care is the specialized care provided to patients who are critically ill and require constant monitoring and possibly need life support.

Society of Critical Care Medicine (SCCM)
    http://www.sccm.org

See also Emergency Medicine; Hospitalists; Hospitals; Injury

46. Deafness and Hearing Impairment

Deafness and hearing impairment is a disability that results in partial or total hearing loss in one or both ears. The level of hearing impairment that a person experiences may range from mild to severe.

Alexander Graham Bell Association for the Deaf and Hard of Hearing   http://www.agbell.org

Canadian Hard of Hearing Association (CHHA)
    http://www.chha.ca

Deafness Research Foundation (DRF)   http://www.drf.org

Dogs for the Deaf (DFD)   http://www.dogsforthedeaf.org

Helen Keller National Center for Deaf-Blind Youths and Adults (HKNC)   http://www.hknc.org

International Hearing Society (IHS)   http://www.ihsinfo.org

National Association of the Deaf (NAD)   http://www.nad.org

National Consortium on Deaf-Blindness http://nationaldb.org

National Institutes on Deafness and Other Communication Disorders (NIDCD) Information Clearinghouse http://www.nidcd.nih.gov

Registry of Interpreters for the Deaf (RID)   http://www.rid.org

Self Help for Hard of Hearing People (SHHH)
    http://www.hearingloss.org

See also Disability

47. Dental Research

Dental research involves clinical research that is focused on oral health.

American Association for Dental Research (AADR)
    http://www.aadronline.org

International Association for Dental Research (IADR)
    http://www.iadr.com

National Institute of Dental and Craniofacial Research (NIDCR)   http://www.nidcr.nih.gov

See also Dentistry; Dentistry, Public Health; Oral Health

48. Dentistry

Dentristy is the profession that is focused on the prevention, evaluation, diagnosis, and treatment of conditions of the oral cavity and maxillofacial area. Dentists are a key component in promoting oral health.

Academy of General Dentistry (AGD)   http://www.agd.org

American Academy of Cosmetic Dentistry (AACD)
    http://www.aacd.com

American Academy of Pediatric Dentistry (AAPD)
    http://www.aapd.org

American Academy of Periodontology (AAP)
    http://www.perio.org

American Association of Endodontists (AAE)
    http://www.aae.org

American Association of Orthodontists (AAO)
    http://www.braces.org

American College of Dentists (ACD)   http://www.acd.org

American Dental Assistants Association (ADAA)
    http://www.dentalassistant.org

American Dental Association (ADA)   http://www.ada.org

American Dental Hygienists' Association (ADHA)
    http://www.adha.org

See also Dentistry, Public Health; Oral Health; Public Health

49. Dentistry, Public Health

Public health dentistry is the field of dentristy that focuses on the oral health of a community as opposed to an individual patient. Public health dentists work to promote oral health policy, evaluate the oral health needs of a community, and provide services that improve overall oral health.

Association of State and Territorial Dental Directors (ASTDD)
    http://www.astdd.org

Canadian Association of Public Health Dentistry
    http://www.caphd-acsdp.org

See also Dentistry; Oral Health; Public Health

50. Dermatology

Dermatology is the field of medicine that is focused on the skin and its associated diseases, and includes both medical and surgical aspects.

American Dermatological Association (ADA)
    http://www.amer-derm-assn.org

Society for Investigative Dermatology (SID)
    http://www.sidnet.org

See also Ambulatory Care; Burn Care; Physicians

51. Diabetes

Diabetes is a metabolic disorder and chronic condition that results in the body being unable to break down blood sugar properly. Diabetes can be caused by genetics or the environment.

American Association of Diabetes Educators (AADE)
    http://www.aadenet.org

American Diabetes Association (ADA)
    http://www.diabetes.org

Division of Diabetes Treatment and Prevention, Indian Health Service (IHS)
    http://www.ihs.gov/medicalprograms/diabetes

International Diabetes Federation (IDF)   http://www.idf.org

National Diabetes Information Clearinghouse (NDIC)
    http://www.diabetes.niddk.nih.gov

National Institute of Diabetes and Digestive and Kidney Diseases (NIDDK)   http://www2.niddk.nih.gov

See also Diet and Nutrition; Fitness and Exercise; Genetics; Overweight and Obesity; Public Health

52. Diet and Nutrition

Diet and nutrition refer to the consumption of food and the nutrients required to sustain life.

American Council for Fitness and Nutrition (ACFN)
    http://www.acfn.org

American Dietetic Association (ADA)   http://www.eatright.org

American Society for Parenteral and Enteral Nutrition (ASPEN)   http://www.nutritioncare.org

Center for Food Safety and Applied Nutrition, Outreach and Information Center
    http://www.cfsan.fda.gov/~comm/oic-info.html

Center for Nutrition and Policy Promotion, U.S. Department of Agriculture   http://www.usda.gov/cnpp

Dietary Managers Association (DMA)
    http://www.dmaonline.org

Food and Nutrition Board (FNB)
    http://www.iom.edu/board.asp?id=3788

Food and Nutrition Information Center, U.S. Department of Agriculture   http://fnic.nal.usda.gov

Food Safey and Inspection Service, U.S. Department of Agriculture   http://www.fsis.usda.gov

International Life Sciences Institute   North America (ILSINA)   http://www.ilsina.org

National Resource Center on Nutrition, Physical Activity and Aging, Florida International University, Miami, FL
    http://nutritionandaging.fiu.edu/index.asp

Weight-Control Information Network   http://win.niddk.nih.gov

See also Eating Disorders; Overweight and Obesity; Public Health

53. Digestive Disorders

Digestive disorders are disorders that affect the digestive system and/or its organs.

National Digestive Diseases Information Clearinghouse (NDDIC)   http://www.digestive.niddk.nih.gov

National Institute of Diabetes and Digestive and Kidney Diseases (NIDDK)   http://www2.niddk.nih.gov

See also Diet and Nutrition; Public Health

54. Disability

Disability is having a lack of ability as compared to a normal group of persons.

American Academy of Disability Evaluating Physicians (AADEP)   http://www.aadep.org

Amputee Coalition of America (ACA)
    http://www.amputee-coalition.org

Clearinghouse on Disability Information
    http://www.ed.gov/about/offices/list/osers

Consortium for Citizens with Disabilities   http://www.c-c-d.org

Disability Resources on the Internet
    http://www.disabilityresources.org

International Center for Disability Resources on the Internet (ICDRI)   http://www.icdri.org

National Center for the Dissemination of Disability Research (NCDDR)   http://www.ncddr.org

National Dissemination Center for Children with Disabilities http://www.nichcy.org

National Institute on Aging (NIA)   http://www.nia.nih.gov

World Committee on Disability http://www.worldcommitteeondisability.org

See also Assisted Living; Blind and Visually Impaired; Chronic Diseases; Deafness and Hearing Impairment; Mentally Disabled; Nursing Homes; Physical Medicine and Rehabilitation

55. Disaster Preparedness and Relief

Disaster preparedness and relief is the process of being prepared for a disaster before it strikes and dealing with this event after it occurs. Several agencies and organizations are committed specifically to responding to disasters.

American Disaster Reserve (ADR) http://www.disasterreserve.us

American Red Cross National Headquarters (ARC) http://www.redcross.org

Center for International Disaster Information (CIDI) http://www.cidi.org

Federal Emergency Management Agency (FEMA) http://www.fema.gov

International Association of Emergency Managers (IAEM)   http://www.iaem.com

International Emergency Management Society (TIEMS) http://www.tiems.org

National Voluntary Organizations Active in Disaster (NVOAD)   http://www.nvoad.org

See also Bioterrorism; Federal Government; Influenza Pandemic; Public Health

56. Disease and Procedure Classifications

Disease and procedure classifications is a standardized classification system used to categorize diseases and medical procedures.

ICD9/ICD9CM Codes   http://icd9cm.chrisendres.com

National Center for Health Statistics (NCHS), Classification of Diseases, Functioning and Disability http://www.cdc.gov/nchs/icd9.htm

Physician Outpatient CPT-4 Procedure   http://www .myhealthscore.com/consumer/phyoutcptsearch.htm

World Health Organization (WHO) Classification of Diseases (ICD)   http://www.who.int/classifications/icd

See also Hospitals; Medical Billing; Medical Records; Medical Sociology; Mental Health; World Health Organization (WHO)

57. Disease Management

Disease management is a patient management process that is used to improve the quality of life and control healthcare costs through integrated care for individuals with chronic conditions.

Disease Management Association of America (DMAA) http://www.dmaa.org

See also AIDS/HIV; Case Management; Chronic Diseases; Disability

58. Donors and Organ Transplantation

Donors are individuals who donate their blood or organs to people in need. Organ transplantation is the act of replacing a diseased organ with a functional one from an organ donor. A number of organizations are available to assist with organ donors and transplant recipients.

American Association of Tissue Banks (AATB) http://www.aatb.org

American Bone Marrow Donor Registry (ABNDR) http://www.charityadvantage.com/abmdr/Home.asp

American Society of Transplantation (ASTA) http://www.a-s-t.org

Center for International Blood and Marrow Research (CIBMTR)   http://www.cibmtr.org

Children's Organ Transplant Association (COTA) http://www.cota.org

Eye Bank Association of America (EBAA) http://www.restoresight.org

Eye Bank for Sight Restoration (EBSR) http://www.eyedonation.org

International Society for Heart and Lung Transplantation (ISHLT)   http://www.ishlt.org

Kidney Transplant/Dialysis Association (KT/DA) http://www.ktda.org

Living Bank International (TLBI)   http://www.livingbank.org

National Marrow Donor Program (NMDP)
http://www.marrow.org

National Bone Marrow Transplant Link (NBMTL)
http://www.nbmtlink.org

United Network for Organ Sharing (UNOS)
http://www.unos.org

See also Blood and Blood Banks; Kidney Diseases; Liver
Diseases; Surgery and Surgeons

59. Drugs

Drugs are chemical substances that are used to prevent,
treat, or cure diseases. Drugs may be used intermittently
for acute episodes or on a regular basis to treat chronic
diseases.

American Association of Poison Control Centers
(AAPCC)   http://www.aapcc.org

Drug InfoNet   http://www.druginfonet.com

Drug Information Association (DIA)   http://www.diahome.org

Electronic Orange Book—Approved Drug Products with
Therapeutic Equivalence Evaluations
http://www.fda.gov/cder/ob/default.htm

Food and Drug Administration (FDA)   http://www.fda.gov

Food and Drug Administration (FDA) Drug Approvals List (This
list is updated weekly)   http://www.fda.gov/cder/da/da.htm

Johns Hopkins Antibiotic Guide   http://hopkins-abxguide.org

New Medicines in Development
http://www.phrma.org/medicines_in_development

NewsRx   http://www.newsrx.com

Pharmaceutical Research and Manufacturers of America
(PhRMA)   http://www.phrma.org

Recently Approved Drugs or Indications—Doctors Guide
http://www.docguide.com/news/content.nsf/Drugs-Indications

RxList (This website lists the top 200 drugs prescribed in the
United States)   http://www.rxlist.com

SafeMedication.com   http://www.safemedication.com

U.S. Pharmacopeia   http://www.usp.org

See also Pharmaceuticals; Pharmacists and Pharmacy;
Pharmacoeconomics

60. Drugs, Generic

Generic drugs are pharmaceutical agents that contain
the same active ingredients as a brand name drug and
are produced without a patent protection.

Canadian Generic Pharmaceutical Association (CGPA)
http://www.canadiangenerics.ca

Generic Pharmaceutical Association (GPhA)
http://www.gphaonline.org

European Generic Medicines Association (EGM)
http://www.egagenerics.com

See also Drugs, Prices of; Pharmaceutical Companies, List of;
Pharmacists and Pharmacy; Pharmacoeconomics

61. Drugs, Prices of

Prices of drugs are the charges related to pharmaceutical agents.

National Legislative Association on Prescription Drug Prices
(NLARX)   http://www.nlarx.org

See also Drugs; Pharmacoeconomics

62. Eating Disorders

Eating disorders cause a person to compulsively eat or
avoid eating. Eating disoders may lead to other health
consequences such as hypertension, cardiovascular disease, and morbid obesity, among others.

European Council on Eating Disorders (ECED)
http://www.eced.org.uk

International Association of Eating Disorders Professionals
(IAEDP)   http://www.iaedp.com

National Association of Anorexia Nervosa and Associated
Disorders (ANAD)   http://www.anad.org

National Eating Disorders Association (NEDA)
http://www.nationaleatingdisorders.org

See also Diet and Nutritionl; Overweight and Obesity

63. E-Health

E-health involves the integration of information technology with healthcare to improve the quality, safety,
and efficiency of the system.

e-Health Initiative   http://www.ehealthinitiative.org

Internet Healthcare Coalition
http://www.ihealthcoalition.org

SATELLIFE Global Health Information Network
http://www.satellife.org

See also Informatics; Information Technology (IT); Telemedicine

64. Emergency Medicine

Emergency medicine is the specialty of medicine that focuses on treating patients with acute conditions that require urgent attention.

American Academy of Emergency Medicine (AAEM)
    http://www.aaem.org

American College of Emergency Physicians (ACEP)
    http://www.acep.org

American College of Osteopathic Emergency Physicians (ACOEP)   http://www.acoep.org

American Trauma Society (ATS)   http://www.amtrauma.org

Emergency Nurses Association (ENA)   http://www.ena.org

National Association of Emergency Medical Technicians (NAEMT)   http://www.naemt.org

National Association of EMS Educators
    http://www.naemse.org

National Association of EMS Physicians
    http://www.naemsp.org

National Association of State EMS Officials
    http://www.nasemsd.org

National Registry of Emergency Medical Technicians (NREMT)   http://www.nremt.org

Society for Academic Emergency Medicine (SAEM)
    http://www.saem.org

See also Burn Care; Hospitals; Injury; Occupational Medicine

65. Emerging Diseases

Emerging infections are infectious diseases that are new, emerging, or re-emerging drug-resistant diseases. These infections have recently increased in populations and their incidence is likely to grow.

Center for Infectious Disease Research and Policy (CIDRAP), University of Minnesota, Minneapolis, MN
    http://www.cidrap.umn.edu/cidrap

Center for the Study of Bioterrorism and Emerging Infections, School of Public Health, St. Louis University, St. Louis, MO   http://www.slu.edu/colleges/sph/bioterrorism

Emerging Infectious Diseases   http://www.cdc.gov/ncidod/eid

Infectious Diseases Society of America Emerging Infections Network (IDSAEIN)   http://www.ein.idsociety.org

See also Centers for Disease Control and Prevention (CDC); Hospital Infections and Nosocomial Diseases; Infectious Diseases; Influenza Pandemic; World Health Organization (WHO)

66. Environmental Health

Environmental health is concerned with the physical, biological, and chemical factors that affect a person's health. This field promotes efforts to assess and control environmental factors that may negatively impact one's well-being.

Agency for Toxic Substances and Disease Registry (ATSDR)   http://www.atsdr.cdc.gov

Indoor Air Quality Information Clearinghouse
    http://www.epa.gov/iaq

National Center for Environmental Health (NCEH)
    http://www.cdc.gov/nceh

National Environmental Health Association (NEHA)
    http://www.neha.org

National Institute of Environmental Health Sciences (NIEHS)   http://www.niehs.nih.gov

National Lead Information Center
    http://www.epa.gov/lead/pubs/nlic.htm

National Pesticide Information Center   http://npic.orst.edu

Safe Drinking Water Hotline
    http://www.epa.gov/safewater/hotline

Society of Environmental Toxicology and Chemistry (SETAC)   http://www.setac.org

U.S. Environmental Protection Agency (EPA)
    http://www.epa.gov

U.S. Environmental Protection Agency (EPA) Headquarters Library   http://www.epa.gov/natlibra/hqirc

See also Epidemiology; Public Health

67. Epidemiology

Epidemiology is the study of factors that cause disease or affect health. Epidemiology serves as the foundation for public health and preventive medicine.

American College of Epidemiology   http://acepidemiology2.org

Council of State and Territorial Epidemiologists (CSTE)
    http://www.cste.org

International Clinical Epidemiology Network (INCLEN)
    http://www.inclen.org

Morbidity and Mortality Weekly Report (MMWR)
    http://www.cdc.gov/mmwr

Society for Healthcare Epidemiology of America (SHEA)
    http://www.shea-online.org

Weekly Epidemiological Record (WER)
    http://www.who.int/wer

See also Centers for Disease Control and Prevention (CDC); Disease and Procedure Classifications; Public Health; World Health Organization (WHO)

68. Ethics

Ethics is the branch of philosophy that studies issues related to right conduct. Bioethics more specifically focuses on ethical questions that arise due to the advancements of medicine and biology.

Alden March Bioethics Institute (AMBI), Albany Medical Center   http://www.bioethics.org

American Society of Law, Medicine, and Ethics (ASLME)   http://www.aslme.org

Applied Research Ethics National Association (ARENA)   http://www.arena.org

Association for Practical and Professional Ethics   http://www.indiana.edu/~appe

Bioethics.Net   http://www.bioethics.net

Bioethics for Clinicians   http://www.cmaj.camisc/bioethics_e.shtml

Center for Bioethics, University of Pennsylvania   http://www.bioethics.upenn.edu

Center for Medical Ethics and Health Policy, Baylor College of Medicine   http://www.bcm.edu/ethics

Ethics in Medicine, University of Washington   http://depts.washington.edu/bioethx

Hastings Center (HC)   http://www.thehastingscenter.org

National Reference Center for Bioethics Literature   http://bioethics.georgetown.edu/databases/index.htm

Neiswanger Institute for Bioethics and Health Policy, Stritch School of Medicine, Loyola University, Chicago   http://bioethics.lumc.edu

See also Fraud and Abuse; Health Law; Regulation

69. Evidence-Based Medicine (EBM)

Evidence-based medicine is the application of the best evidence gained from scientific medical studies. Evidence-based medicine is used to make clinical judgments regarding the best course of care for patients.

Bandolier Evidence-Based Health Care   http://www.jr2.0x.ac.uk/bandolier

Canadian Association for Population Therapeutics   http://www.capt-actp.com

Center for Evidence-Based Medicine   http://www.cebm.net/index.asp

Centre for Health Evaluation and Outcome Science (Canada)   http://www.cheos.ubc.camain.html

ECRI: Emergency Care Research Institution (This institution is designated as an Evidence-Based Practice Center by the Agency for Healthcare Quality and Research)   http://www.ecri.org

Institute for Clinical Evaluative Sciences (Canada)   http://www.ices.on.ca

New York Academy of Medicine, Evidence-Based Medicine Resource Center   http://www.ebmny.org

Understanding Medical Information (Evidence-Based)   http://www.noah-health.org/n/ebm

See also Clinical Practice Guidelines; Health Outcomes; Quality of Healthcare; Randomized Controlled Trials (RCT)

70. Eye Diseases

Eye diseases are conditions that cause problems to the eye. These conditions may range from minor issues to permanent vision loss.

Association for Macular Diseases (AMD)   http://www.macula.org

All About Vision   http://www.allaboutvision.com

Glaucoma Foundation (TGF)   http://www.glaucomafoundation.org

Glaucoma Research Foundation   http://www.glaucoma.org

International Eye Foundation (IEF)   http://www.iefusa.org

National Eye Institute (NEI)   http://www.nei.nih.gov

National Glaucoma Research Program, American Health Assistance Foundation (AHAF)   http://www.ahaf.org/glaucoma/about/glabout.htm

See also Blind and Visually Impaired; Epidemiology; Ophthalmology; Optometry; Prevention and Health Promotion; Public Health

71. Federal Government

The federal government is the central governing body of the United States and it is divided into the judicial, legislative, and executive branches. Through its policies, the federal government may have a significant impact both domestically and abroad.

Agency for Healthcare Research and Quality (AHRQ) (AHRQ was formerly the Agency for Health Care Policy and Research)   http://www.ahrq.gov

Bureau of Health Professions (BHPr)   http://www.bhpr.hrsa.gov

Bureau of Labor Statistics (BLS)   http://www.bls.gov

Census Bureau   http://www.census.gov

Centers for Disease Control and Prevention (CDC)
http://www.cdc.gov

Centers for Medicare and Medicaid Services (CMS) (CMS was
formerly the Health Care Financing Administration
(HCFA))   http://www.cms.hhs.gov

Congressional Budget Office (CBO)   http://www.cbo.gov

Congressional Research Service   http://www.loc.gov/crsinfo

Consumer Product Safety Commission (CPSC)
http://www.cpsc.gov

Department of Agriculture (USDA)   http://www.usda.gov

Department of Health and Human Services (HHS)
http://www.hhs.gov

Department of Homeland Security (DHS)   http://www.dhs.gov

Department of Justice   http://www.usdoj.gov

Department of State   http://www.state.gov

Department of Veterans Affairs (VA)   http://www.va.gov

Environmental Protection Agency (EPA)   http://www.epa.gov

Federal Budget   http://www.whitehouse.gov/omb/budget/
fy2006/budget.html

Federal Emergency Management Agency (FEMA)
http://www.fema.gov

Federal Judiciary   http://www.uscourts.gov

Federal Legislation   http://thomas.loc.gov

Federal Register   http://www.gpoaccess.gov/fr

FirstGov (This is a comprehensive portal to government
sites)   http://www.firstgov.gov

Food and Drug Administration (FDA)   http://www.fda.gov

General Accountability Office (GAO)   http://www.gao.gov

Healthfinder (This is a service of the Office of Disease
Prevention and Health Promotion)
http://www.healthfinder.gov

Health Resources and Services Administration (HRSA)
http://www.hrsa.gov

House Committee on Appropriations
http://appropriations.house.gov

House Committee on Energy and Commerce
http://energycommerce.house.gov

House Committee on Ways and Means
http://waysandmeans.house.gov

House of Representatives   http://www.house.gov

House Office of Legislative Counsel
http://legcoun.house.gov/public.htm

Indian Health Service (IHS)   http://www.ihs.gov

Library of Congress (LOC)   http://www.loc.gov

Medicare Payment Advisory Commission (MedPAC)
http://www.medpac.gov

National Center for Health Statistics (NCHS)
http://www.cdc.gov/nchs

National Institutes of Health (NIH)   http://www.nih.gov

National Library of Medicine (NLM) (The NLM's Web-based
databases include PubMed/Medline and Medline Plus)
http://www.nlm.gov/hinfo.html

Occupational Safety and Health Administration (OSHA)
http://www.osha.org

Office of Disease Prevention and Health Promotion (ODPHP)
http://odphp.osophs.hhs.gov

Office of Management and Budget (OMB)
http://www.whitehouse.gov/omb

Organization for Economic Co-operation and Development
(OECD)   http://www.oecd.org

President's Commission to Strengthen Social Security
(CSSS)   http://www.csss.gov

President's Management Agenda   http://www.whitehouse.gov/
omb/budgintegration/pma_index.html

Senate   http://www.senate.gov

Senate Committee on Appropriations
http://appropriations.senate.gov

Senate Committee on Finance   http://finance.senate.gov

Senate Committee on Health, Education, Labor, and
Pensions   http://help.senate.gov

Senate Office of Legislative Counsel
http://slc.senate.gov/index.htm

Social Security Administration (SSA)   http://www.ssa.gov

Substance Abuse and Mental Health Services Administration
(SAMHSA)   http://www.samhsa.gov

U.S. Government Printing Office (GPO) (The GPO publishes
the Federal Register and other government
reports)   http://www.access.gpo.gov

U.S. Public Health Service   http://www.usphs.gov

White House   http://www.whitehouse.gov

See also Centers for Disease Control and Prevention (CDC);
Centers for Medicare and Medicaid Services (CMS); Federal
Health Information Centers and Clearinghouses; National
Institutes of Health (NIH)

72. Federal Health Information Centers and Clearinghouses

Federal health information centers and clearinghouses provide the public with publications and referrals, and answer inquiries on a variety of health-related topics.

ABLEDATA (This site lists assistive devices and rehabilitation equipment products for people with disabilities)
http://www.abledata.com

Alzheimer's Disease Education and Referral Center
http://www.alzheimers.org

Cancer Information Service   http://www.cancer.gov

CDC National Prevention Information Network
http://www.cdcnpin.org

Center for Food Safety and Applied Nutrition, Outreach and Information Center
http://www.cfsan.fda.gov/~comm/oic-info.html

Clearinghouse on Disability Information
http://www.ed.gov/about/offices/list/osers

Drug Policy Information Clearinghouse
http://www.whitehousedrugpolicy.gov/about/clearingh.html

Educational Resources Information Center (ERIC)
http://www.eric.ed.gov

Environmental Protection Agency Headquarters Library
http://www.epa.gov/natlibra/hqirc

Federal Citizen Information Center
http://www.pueblo.gsa.gov

Food and Nutrition Information Center
http://www.nal.usda.gov/fnic

Genetic and Rare Diseases Information Center
http://www.genome.gov/10000409

Health Resources and Services Administration Information Center   http://www.ask.hrsa.gov

Housing and Urban Development User
http://www.huduser.org

Indoor Air Quality Information Clearinghouse
http://www.epa.gov/iaq

Maternal and Child Health Information Resource Center
http://www.mchb.hrsa.gov/mchirc

Maternal and Child Health Library
http://www.mchlibrary.info

National Adoption Information Clearinghouse
http://naic.acf.hhs.gov

National Aging Information and Referral Support Center
http://www.nasua.org/issues/tech_assist_resources/national_aging_ir_support_ctr

National Audiovisual Center at NTIS
http://www.ntis.gov/products/nac.aspx

National Center for Complementary and Alternative Medicine Information Clearinghouse   http://nccam.nih.gov

National Center for the Dissemination of Disability Research
http://www.ncddr.org

National Center on Elder Abuse
http://www.elderabusecenter.org

National Center on Sleep Disorders Research
http://www.nhlbi.nih.gov/sleep

National Child Care Information Center   http://nccic.org

National Clearinghouse on Child Abuse and Neglect Information   http://nccanch.acf.hhs.gov

National Clearinghouse on Families and Youth
http://www.ncfy.com

National Consortium on Deaf-Blindness   http://nationaldb.org

National Criminal Justice Reference Service
http://www.ncjrs.org

National Diabetes Information Clearinghouse
http://diabetes.niddk.nih.gov

National Digestive Diseases Information Clearinghouse
http://digestive.niddk.nih.gov

National Dissemination Center for Children with Disabilities
http://www.nichcy.org

National Eldercare Locator   http://www.eldercare.gov

National Guideline Clearinghouse   http://www.guideline.gov

National Health Information Center
http://www.health.gov/nhic

National Heart, Lung, and Blood Institute Health Information Center   http://www.nhlbi.nih.gov

National Information Center on Health Services Research and Health Care Technology (NICHSR)
http://www.nlm.nih.gov/nichsr

National Injury Information Clearinghouse
http://www.cpsc.gov/about/clrnghse.html

National Institute for Occupational Safety and Health Information Inquiry Service
http://www.cdc.gov/niosh/inquiry.html

National Institute of Arthritis and Musculoskeletal and Skin Diseases Information Clearinghouse
http://www.niams.nih.gov

National Institute of Child Health and Human Development Information Resource Center   http://www.nichd.nih.gov

National Institute of Dental and Craniofacial Research
http://www.nidcr.nih.gov/HealthInformation

National Institute on Aging Information Center
http://www.nia.nih.gov

National Institute on Deafness and Other Communication Disorders
Information Clearinghouse   http://www.nidcd.nih.gov

National Kidney and Urologic Diseases Information
Clearinghouse   http://www.kidney.niddk.nih.gov

National Lead Information Center   http://www.epa.gov/lead

National Library Service for the Blind and Physically
Handicapped   http://www.loc.gov/nls

National Maternal and Child Oral Health Resource
Center   http://www.mchoralhealth.org

National Pesticide Information Center   http://npic.orst.edu

National Quality Measures Clearinghouse
http://www.qualitymeasures.ahrq.gov

National Rehabilitation Information Center
http://www.naric.com

National Resource and Training Center on Homelessness and
Mental Illness   http://www.nrchmi.samhsa.gov

National SIDS/Infant Death Syndrome Resource Center
http://www.sidscenter.org

National Technical Information Service (NTIS)
http://www.ntis.gov

National Women's Health Information Center
http://www.womenshealth.gov

National Youth Violence Prevention Resource Center
http://www.safeyouth.org

NIH Osteoporosis and Related Bone Diseases   National
Resource Center   http://www.osteo.org

Office of Boating Safety   http://www.uscgboating.org

Office of Minority Health Resource Center
http://www.omhrc.gov

Office of Population Affairs Clearinghouse
http://opa.osophs.hhs.gov/clearinghouse.html

Office on Smoking and Health   http://www.cdc.gov/tobacco

Policy Information Center   http://aspe.hhs.gov/pic

Rural Assistance Center   http://www.raconline.org

Rural Information Center   http://www.nal.usda.gov/ric

Safe Drinking Water Hotline
http://www.epa.gov/safewater/hotline

SAMHSA's National Clearinghouse for Alcohol and Drug
Information   http://ncadi.samhsa.gov

SAMHSA's National Mental Health Information
Center   http://www.mentalhealth.samhsa.gov

Weight-Control Information Network
http://win.niddk.nih.gov

See also Federal Government; Health Libraries and Information
Centers; Health Literacy; Health Report Cards

73. Fitness and Exercise

Fitness and exercise refers to workout regimens to keep
people fit, healthy, and strong.

American Council for Fitness and Nutrition (ACFN)
http://www.acfn.org

American Council on Exercise (ACE)   http://www.acefitness.org

Medical Fitness Association   http://medicalfitness.org

National Association for Health and Fitness (NAHF)
http://www.physicalfitness.org

See also Diet and Nutrition; Prevention and Health Promotion;
Self-Help

74. Foundations and Philanthropies

Foundations and philanthropies are organizations that
have a charitable purpose. These organizations may
provide financial support to outside entities or fund
other charitable activities.

Annie E. Casey Foundation   http://www.aecf.org

Bill and Melinda Gates Foundation
http://www.gatesfoundation.org

California Health Care Foundation   http://www.chcf.org

Carnegie Corporation of New York   http://www.carnegie.org

Commonwealth Fund   http://www.cmwf.org

David and Lucile Packard Foundation   http://www.packard.org

Duke Endowment   http://www.dukeendowment.org

Ford Foundation   http://www.fordfound.org

Foundation Center (Publishes an annual list of American
foundations)   http://www.foundationcenter.org

Henry J. Kaiser Family Foundation (KFF)   http://www.kff.org

John A. Hartford Foundation   http://www.jhartfound.org

John D. and Catherine T. MacArthur Foundation
http://www.macfound.org

Josiah Macy, Jr. Foundation
http://www.josiahmacy foundation.org

Milbank Memorial Fund   http://www.milbank.org

Pew Charitable Trusts   http://www.pewtrusts.org

Robert Wood Johnson Foundation (RWJ)   http://www.rwjf.org

Rockefeller Foundation   http://www.rockfound.org

Wellcome Trust, United Kingdom   http://www.wellcome.ac.uk

William T. Grant Foundation
    http://www.wtgrantfoundation.org

W. K. Kellogg Foundation   http://www.wkkf.org

World Bank Group   http://www.worldbank.org

See also Advocacy, Education, and Research Organizations;
    Health Policy Organizations

75. Fraud and Abuse

Fraud and abuse involve activities that may result in misinformation, overpayment, or other deceitful acts that result in harm.

America's Health Insurance Plans (AHIP)
    http://www.avoidfraud.org

MIB Group (The MIB Group was formerly the Medical
    Information Bureau)   http://www.mib.com

National Council Against Health Fraud (NCAHF)
    http://www.ncahf.com

National Health Care Anti-Fraud Association (NHCAA)
    http://www.nhcaa.org

Taxpayers Against Fraud (TAF)   http://www.taf.org

See also Ethics; Health Law; Regulation

76. Genetics

Genetics is the heredity information that is passed on in living organisms. The application of genetics to molecular medicine holds much promise and potential in biotechnology.

American College of Medical Genetics (ACMG)
    http://www.acmg.net

American Society of Gene Therapy (ASGT)   http://www.asgt.org

International Society for Stem Cell Research (ISSCR)
    http://www.isscr.org

National Human Genome Research Institute (NHGRI)
    http://www.genome.gov

National Society of Genetic Counselors (NSGC)
    http://www.nsgc.org

Office of Genomics and Disease Prevention
    http://www.cdc.gov/genomics

See also Blood Disorders; Diabetes; Disease and Procedure
    Classifications

77. Geographic Information Systems (GIS)

Geographic information systems (GIS) is a technology that is used to display trends, patterns, or relationships in geographic data. GIS systems in public health are used to better understand health outcomes, disease prevalence, and other health issues at different geographic levels.

Association of American Geographers (AAG)
    http://www.aag.org

Cancer Mortality Maps and Graphs (Shows various cancer
    rates in the United States for 1950–94)
    http://www3.cancer.gov/atlasplus

Census 2000   http://www.census.gov/main/www/cen2000.html

EPA EnviroMapper   http://www.epa.gov/enviro/html/em

ESRI (Environmental Systems Research Institute)
    http://www.esri.com

FEMA Mapping and Analysis Center
    http://www.gismaps.fema.gov

GIS and Public Health (Public Health GIS News and
    Information is a bimonthly electronic report published by
    the National Center for Health Statistics)   http://www.cdc
    .gov/nchs/about/otheract/gis/gis_publichealthinfo.htm

GIS.com   http://www.gis.com

Interactive Atlas of Reproductive Health (This is a web-based
    GIS dealing with reproductive health issues such as infant
    mortality, fertility, and low birth weight)
    http://www.cdc.gov/reproductivehealth/gisatlas

National Geographic Society
    http://www.nationalgeographic.com

TOXMAP: Environmental Health E-Maps
    http://toxmap.nlm.nih.gov/toxmap/main/index.jsp

University Consortium for Geographic Information Science
    (UCGIS)   http://www.ucgis.org

USGS (U.S. Geological Survey)   http://geography.usgs.gov

Web-Based Injury and Statistics Inquiry System
    http://www.cdc.gov/injury/wisqars

World Health Organization Public Health Mapping
    http://www.who.int/csr/mapping

See also Environmental Health; Health Planning; Medical
    Practice Variations; Population Estimates; Public Health;
    Rural Health

78. Gerontology

Gerontology is the study of the various aspects of aging. Several organizations are committed to better understanding and serving the needs of the elderly.

American Geriatrics Society (AGS)
http://www.americangeriatrics.org

Australian Association of Gerontology (AAG)
http://www.aag.asn.au

British Geriatrics Society (BGS)   http://www.bgs.org.uk

British Society of Gerontology
http://www.britishgerontology.org

Canadian Association on Gerontology   http://www.cagacg.ca

Center for Gerontology and Health Care Research, Brown
University, Providence, RI   http://www.chcr.brown.edu

Gerontological Society of America (GSA)
http://www.geron.org

Institute of Gerontology, Wayne State University, Detroit,
MI   http://www.iog.wayne.edu

International Association of Gerontology and Geriatrics
(IAGG)   http://www.iagg.com.br

International Psychogeriatric Association (IPA)
http://www.ipa-online.org

New England Gerontological Association
http://www.negaonline.org

See also Aging; Disability; Nursing Homes; Physicians

79. Health

Health is the physicial, social, and mental well-being of
an indivdual. Health is shaped by biological, environmental, and behavioral factors as well as access to
healthcare.

American Council on Science and Health (ACSH)
http://www.acsh.org

National Health Council (NHC)   http://www.nhcouncil.org

National Health Information Center
http://www.health.gov/nhic

See also Centers for Disease Control and Prevention (CDC);
National Institutes of Health (NIH); World Health
Organization (WHO)

80. Health Administration,
Association of Academic Programs of

The Association of Academic Programs of Health
Administration is comprised of a number of universities and colleges, faculty, individuals, and organizations that are committed to improving health through
health management education.

Association of University Programs in Health Administration
(AUPHA)   http://www.aupha.org

See also Health Administration, Graduate Programs in; Hospitals

81. Health Administration,
Graduate Programs in

Graduate programs in health administration train students to become healthcare managers and administrators through education, research, and practice.

Alabama

University of Alabama at Birmingham (UAB), Birmingham,
AL   http://www.uab.edu/hsa

Arizona

Arizona State University, Tempe, AZ
http://wpcarey.asu.edu/shmp/index.cfm

Arkansas

University of Arkansas for Medical Sciences, Little Rock,
Arkansas   http://www.ualr.edu/hsadmin

California

California State University, Long Beach, Long Beach,
CA   http://www.csulb.edu/colleges/chhs/departments/hca

Chapman University College, McChord Air Force Base,
CA   http://www.chapman.edu/catalog/current/cuc/mha.html

San Diego State University, San Diego, CA
http://publichealth.sdsu.edu/divisionshsa.php

University of California, Berkeley, Berkeley, CA
http://www.haas.berkeley.edu/advantage/health

University of California, Los Angeles, Los Angeles, CA
http://www.ph.ucla.edu/hs

University of Southern California, Los Angeles, CA
http://www.usc.edu/schools/sppd

Colorado

University of Colorado at Denver, Denver, CO
http://www.cudenver.edu/business

University of Colorado at Denver, Executive MBA in Health
Administration http://business.cudenver.edu/Disciplines/
HealthAdmin/ExecHealthMBA

Connecticut

Yale University, School of Public Health, New Haven, CT
  http://info.med.yale.edu/eph/hpa

District of Columbia

George Washington University, Washington, DC
  http://www.gwumc.edu/sphhs/hsml

Georgetown University, Washington, DC
  http://nhs.georgetown.edu/healthsystems/dept.html

Florida

Barry University, Miami Shores, FL   http://www.barry.edu/hsa

Florida International University, Miami, FL
  http://chua2.fiu.edu/hsa

University of Central Florida, Orland, FL
  http://www.cohpa.ucf.edu/health.pro/hsams.cfm

University of Florida, Gainesville, FL
  http://www.phhp.ufl.edu/hsrmp

University of Miami, Coral Gables, FL
  http://www.miami.edu/grad

University of North Florida, Jacksonville, FL
  http://www.unf.edu/coh/mha.htm

University of South Florida, Tampa, FL
  http://www.publichealth.usf.edu/hpm

Georgia

Armstrong Atlantic State University, Savannah, GA
  http://www.healthscience.armstrong.edu

Georgia State University, Atlanta, GA
  http://robinson.gsu.edu/healthadmin

Illinois

Governors State University, University Park, IL
  http://www.govst.edu/ha

Northwestern University, Chicago, IL
  http://www.kellogg.northwestern.edu/academic/health,

Rush University, Chicago, IL   http://www.rushu.rush.edu/hsm

University of Illinois at Chicago, Chicago, IL
  http://www.uic.edu/sph/mha

Indiana

Indiana University, Indianapolis, IN   http://www.mha.iupui.edu

Iowa

Des Moines University, Des Moines, IA
  http://www.dmu.edu/mha

University of Iowa, Iowa City, IA
  http://www.public-health.uiowa.edu/hmp

Kansas

University of Kansas Medical Center, Kansas City, KS
  http://www.kumc.edu/som/hpm

Kentucky

University of Kentucky, Lexington, KY
  http://www-martin.uky.edu/~web/programs/mha/mha.html

Western Kentucky University, Bowling Green, KY
  http://www.wku.edu/health/graduate.php

Louisiana

Tulane University, New Orleans, LA   http://www.hsm.tulane.edu

Maine

University of Southern Maine, Portland, ME
  https://muskie.usm.maine.edu/academics/hpm.jsp

Maryland

Johns Hopkins University, Baltimore, MD
  http://www.jhsph.edu/Dept/HPM

Massachusetts

Boston University, Boston, MA
  http://management.bu.edu/gpo/fulltime/hsm

Simmons College, Boston, MA
  http://www.simmons.edu/shs/academics/hca/degrees.shtml

Suffolk University, Boston, MA   http://www.suffolk.edu

Michigan

University of Michigan, Ann Arbor, MI
  http://www.sph.umich.edu/hmp

Minnesota

Capella University, Minneapolis, MN   http://www.capella.edu/
  schools_programs/human_services/masters/health_
  management_policy.aspx

University of Minnesota, Minneapolis, MN
  http://www.hsr.umn.edu/mha

Missouri

St. Louis University, St. Louis, MO
http://publichealth.slu.edu/hmp_department.htm

University of Missouri Columbia, MO
http://www.hmi.missouri.edu

Washington University, St. Louis, St. Louis, MO
http://hap.wustl.edu

Nebraska

Bellevue University, Omaha, NE
http://www.bellevue.edu/degrees/mshca_new.asp

New Jersey

Seton Hall University, South Orange, NJ
http://artsci.shu.edu/gdpha

New York

Baruch College and Mt. Sinai School of Medicine, New York,
NY   http://www.healthcaremba.org

Columbia University, New York, NY   http://www.mailman.hs
.columbia.edu/hpm

Cornell University, Ithaca, NY   http://www.sloan.cornell.edu

Hofstra University, Hempstead, NY   http://www.hofstra.edu/mha

New York University, New York, NY   http://wagner.nyu.edu

Union Graduate College, Schenectady, NY   http://www
.uniongraduatecollege.edu/pages/schools/management/
degreePr02.asp

University of Rochester, Rochester, NY
http://www.simon.rochester.edu/centers/HCM.aspx

North Carolina

University of North Carolina at Chapel Hill, Chapel Hill,
NC   http://www.sph.unc.edu/hpaa

University of North Carolina at Charlotte, Charlotte,
NC   http://www.health.uncc.edu

Ohio

Cleveland State University, Cleveland, OH
http://www.csuohio.edu/cba/mba

Ohio State University, Columbus, OH
http://sph.osu.edu/hsmp

Xavier University, Cincinnati, OH   http://www.xavier.edu/mhsa

Oklahoma

University of Oklahoma, Oklahoma City, OK
http://www.ou.edu

Pennsylvannia

Kings College, Wilkes Barre, PA
http://departments.kings.edu/hca/index.htm

Pennsylvania State University, University Park, PA
http://www.hhdev.psu.edu/hpa

Temple University, Philadelphia, PA
http://sbm.temple.edu/dept/rihm/healthcare/grad-hm.html

University of Pittsburgh, Pittsburgh, PA
http://www.hpm.pitt.edu

University of Scranton, Scranton, PA
http://academic.scranton.edu/department/HAHR/mha

South Carolina

Medical University of South Carolina, Charleston, SC
http://www.musc.edu/chp/mha

University of South Carolina, Columbia, SC
http://hspm.sph.sc.edu

Tennessee

University of Memphis, Memphis, TN
http://healthadmin.memphis.edu

Texas

Army-Baylor University, Ft. Sam Houston, TX
http://www.baylor.edu/graduate/mha/index.php

Baylor University, Waco, TX
http://www.baylor.edu/business/mba/index.php?id=4596

Midwestern State University, Wichita Falls, TX
http://hs2.mwsu.edu/healthandpublic

Texas A&M University System, College Station, TX
http://www.srph.tamhsc.edu

Texas Southern University, Houston, TX
http://www.tsu.edu/academics/pharmacy/program/admin.asp

Texas State University, San Marcos, San Marcos, TX
http://www.health.txstate.edu/HA

Texas Tech University, Lubbock, TX   http://www.hom.ba.ttu.edu

Texas Woman's University, Houston, TX
http://www.twu.edu/hs/h-hca

Trinity University, San Antonio, TX
http://www.trinity.edu/departments/healthcare

University of Houston, Clear Lake, Houston, TX
http://www.uhcl.edu

University of North Texas, Fort Worth, TX
http://www.hsc.unt.edu

University of Texas at Arlington, Fort Worth, TX
http://www2.uta.edu/gradbiz/HealthAdmin

Virginia

George Mason University, Fairfax, VA   http://chhs.gmu.edu/
HealthAdministrationPolicyDepartment/index.html

Marymount University, Arlington, VA
http://marymount.edu/academic/business/lahcm/mshcm.html

Virginia Commonwealth University, Richmond, VA
http://www.had.vcu.edu

Washington

University of Washington, Seattle, Seattle, WA
http://depts.washington.edu/mhap

Washington State University, Spokane, WA
http://www.hpa.spokane.wsu.edu

See also Health Administration, Association of Academic
Programs of

82. Health Disparities

Health disparities are the gaps in healthcare across
racial or ethnic groups and/or socioeconomic status.
These disparities may be in terms of access to healthcare, health outcomes, or in the occurrence of disease.

National Center on Minority Health and Health Disparities
(NCMHD) (This center was formed as part of NIH in
1993)   http://www.ncmhd.nih.gov

National Healthcare Disparities Report
http://www.ahrq.gov/qual/measurix.htm#quality

Office of Minority Health
http://www.omhrc.gov

See also Healthy People 2010; Minority Health; Uninsured
Individuals

83. Health Economics, Academic Centers of

Academic centers of health economics apply economic
principles and techniques to health policy analysis and
work to improve the efficiency of the healthcare system.

Center for Health Economics (CHE), Monash University,
Australia   http://www.buseco.monash.edu.au/Centres/che

Center for Health Economics (CHE), University of York,
United Kingdom   http://www.york.ac.uk/inst/che

Center for Health Economics and Policy Analysis (CHEPA),
McMaster University, Canada   http://www.chepa.org

Center for Health Economics Research and Evaluation
(CHERE), University of Technology, Sidney,
Australia   http://www.chere.uts.edu.au

Health Economics Research Center (HERC), University of
Oxford, United Kingdom   http://www.herc.ox.ac.uk

Health Economics Research Program (HERO), University of
Oslo, Norway   http://www.hero.uio.no

Institute of Health Economics (Canada)   http://www.ihe.ab.ca

Leonard Davis Institute of Health Economics (LDI), University
of Pennsylvannia   http://www.upenn.edu/ldi

See also Health Economics, Associations of; Pharmacoeconomics

84. Health Economics, Associations of

Associations of health economics serve as a venue for
health economists to share research findings and as a
forum to discuss health economic applications to
health and the healthcare system.

Canadian Health Economics Research Association (CHERA)
http://www.chera.ca

International Health Economics Association (iHEA)/American
Society of Health Economists (ASHE)
http://www.healtheconomics.org

See also Health Economics, Academic Centers of; Pharmacoeconomics

85. Health Insurance

Health insurance is a form of insurance that covers
healthcare-related expenses. Health benefits refers to
the specific services and procedures that are covered by
the health insurance plan.

American Academy of Actuaries   http://www.actuary.org

American Benefits Council
http://www.americanbenefitscouncil.org

America's Health Insurance Plans (AHIP) (AHIP was formed in
late 2003 following the merger of the American Association
of Health Plans and the Health Insurance Association of
America.)   http://www.ahip.org

Blue Cross and Blue Shield Association (BCBSA)
http://www.bluecares.com

Canadian Association of Blue Cross Plans (CABCP)
http://www.bluecross.ca

Canadian Life and Health Insurance Association
(CLHIA)   http://www.clhia.ca

Employee Benefit Research Institute (EBRI)
http://www.ebri.org

Health Benefits Advisor, U.S. Department of Labor
http://www.dol.gov/elaws/ebsa/health

Health Benefits Coalition for Affordable Choice and
Quality   http://www.hbcweb.com

International Federation of Health Plans (IFHP)
http://www.ifhp.com

National Academy of Social Insurance (NASI)
http://www.nasi.org

Pharmacy Benefit Management Institute (PBMI)
http://www.pbmi.com

See also Health Disparities; Healthcare Financial Management;
Medicaid; Medicare; Uninsured Individuals

86. Health Insurance Portability and Accountability Act of 1996 (HIPAA)

Health Insurance Portability and Accountability Act refers to legislation that was passed in 1996 that protects the health insurance coverage of workers and their families who lose or change their jobs. This law also sets up requirements for national standards of electronic healthcare transactions as well as the security and privacy of health data.

Centers for Medicare and Medicaid Services (CMS)
http://www.cms.hhs.gov/HIPAAGenInfo

HIPAAdvisory, Phoenix Health Systems
http://www.hipaadvisory.com

HIPAA.org   http://www.hipaa.org

Office of Civil Rights   http://www.hhs.gov/ocr/hipaa

See also Federal Government; Health Insurance; Health Law;
Regulation

87. Health Law

Health law refers to the laws, rules, and regulations that affect the healthcare system or the providers, payers, suppliers, and consumers of the system.

American College of Legal Medicine (ACLM)
http://www.aclm.org

American Health Lawyers Association (AHLA)
http://www.healthlawyers.org

American Society of Law, Medicine, and Ethics (ASLME)
http://www.aslme.org

Center for Health Care Rights (CHCR)
http://www.healthcarerights.org

Center for Medicare and Medicaid Services (CMS) Regulations
and Guidance
http://www.cms.hhs.gov/home/regsguidance.asp

Health Law, Findlaw   http://www.findlaw
.com/01topics/19health/index.html

Health Law Section, American Bar Association (ABA)
http://www.abanet.org/health

Legal Information Institute, Cornell Law School, Ithaca, New
York   http://www.law.cornell.edu/topics/health.html

National Senior Citizens Law Center (NSCLC)
http://www.nsclc.org

Office of Civil Rights, Department of Health and Human
Services (HHS)   http://www.hhs.gov/ocr

Washburn Law Library, Washburn University School of Law,
Topeka, Kansas   http://www.washlaw.edu

See also Ethics; Fraud and Abuse; Health Insurance Portability
and Accountability Act of 1996 (HIPAA); Regulation

88. Health Libraries and Information Centers

Health libraries and information centers serve as repositories for resources that include books, journals, reports, and other reference material on medicine and health.

American Hospital Association's Resource Center (AHA)
http://www.aha.org/aha/resource-center/index.html

Association of Academic Health Sciences Libraries (AAHSL)
http://www.aahsl.org

Canadian Health Libraries Association (CHLA)
http://www.chla-absc.ca

Canadian Library Gateway
http://www.collectionscanada.ca/gateway/index-e.html

Cochrane Library   http://www.cochrane.co.uk

Environmental Protection Agency (EPA) Headquarters
Repository Services   http://www.epa.gov/natlibra/hqirc

Federal Citizen Information Center   http://www.pueblo.gsa.gov

Food and Nutrition Information Center
http://www.nal.usda.gov/fnic

Genetic and Rare Diseases Information Center
http://www.genome.gov/10000409

Health and Social Care Information Centre, United
Kingdom's National Health Service (NHS)
http://www.ic.nhs.uk

1286   Appendix: Web Resources

Health Resources and Services Administration (HRSA) Information Center   http://www.ask.hrsa.gov

Library of Congress (LOC)   http://www.loc.gov

Maternal and Child Health Information Resource Center   http://mchb.hrsa.gov/mchirc

Maternal and Child Health Library http://www.mchlibrary.info

Medical Library Association (MLA)   http://www.mlanet.org

National Child Care Information Center   http://nccic.org

National Electronic Library for Health, United Kingdom's National Health Service (NHS)   http://www.library.nhs.uk

National Health Information Center (NHIC) http://www.health.gov/nhic

National Heart, Lung, and Blood Institute Health Information Center   http://www.nhlbi.nih.gov

National Information Center on Health Services Research and Health Care Technology (NICHSR) http://www.nlm.nih.gov/nichsr

National Institute on Aging Information Center http://www.nia.nih.gov

National Library of Medicine (NLM)   http://www.nlm.nih.gov

WHO Library and Information Networks for Knowledge (LNK)   http://www.who.int/library

See also Federal Health Information Centers and Clearinghouses; Health Services Research Journals; Journals, Medical; News Services

89. Health Literacy

Health literacy is the ability of individuals to obtain, process, and understand health information and form appropriate healthcare decisions.

American Medical Association Foundation (AMAF) http://www.ama-assn.org

Ask Me 3   http://www.askme3.org

National Institute for Literacy   http://www.nifl.gov

Roundtable on Health Literacy, Institute of Medicine (IOM) of the National Academies http://www.iom.edu/CMS/3793/31487.aspx

See also Aging; Minority Health; Patient Safety; Quality of Healthcare

90. Health Maintenance Organizations (HMO)

See Managed Care

91. Health Outcomes

Health outcomes are the end results of healthcare; they include a patient's health status, well-being, and satisfaction with healthcare.

Center for Health Policy/Center for Primary Care and Outcomes Research (PCOR/CHP), School of Medicine, Stanford University, Stanford, CA   http://chppcor.stanford.edu

Health Outcomes Core Library Recommendations, 2004 http://www.nlm.nih.gov/nichsr/corelib/houtcomes.html

Health Outcomes Resource Center   http://medconsult.com

See also Evidence-Based Medicine (EBM); Health Report Cards; Quality of Healthcare

92. Health Planning

Health planning includes the strategic process of allocating and utilizing resources to meet the healthcare needs of a community.

American Health Planning Association (AHPA) http://www.ahpanet.org

Policy Information Center, Office of the Assistant Secretary for Planning and Evaluation, Department of Health and Human Services (HHS)   http://aspe.hhs.gov/pic

Prairie Region Health Promotion Research Centre (Canada)   http://www.usask.ca/healthsci/che/prhprc

Western Canada Waiting List Project   http://www.wcwl.org

See also Certificate of Need (CON); Health Law; Hospitals; Public Health; Regulation

93. Health Policy, Academic Centers of

Academic centers of health policy focus on examining policy issues that improve the practice and delivery of healthcare.

Center for Health and Public Policy Studies (CHPPS), School of Public Health, University of California, Berkeley, CA http://chpps.berkeley.edu

Center for Health and Public Service Research (CHPSR), Robert F. Wagner Graduate School of Public Service, New York University, New York, NY http://www.nyu.edu/wagner/chpsr

Center for Health Policy and Primary Care Outcomes Research (CHPPCOR), Stanford University, Stanford, CA http://chppcor.stanford.edu

Center for Health Policy, Duke University, Durham, NC   http://www.hpolicy.duke.edu

Center for Health Policy Research, School of Public Health, University of California, Los Angeles, CA http://www.healthpolicy.ucla.edu

Center for Medical Ethics and Health Policy, Baylor College of Medicine, Houston, TX   http://bcm.edu/ethics

Children's Health Policy Centre, Simon Fraser University, Vancouver, BC (Canada) http://www.childhealthpolicy.sfu.ca

Department of Health Management and Policy, School of Public Health, University of Michigan, Ann Arbor, MI   http://www.sph.umich.edu/hmp

Department of Health Policy, Thomas Jefferson University, Philadelphia, PA   http://www.jefferson.edu/dhp

Department of Health Policy and Management, School of Public Health, Columbia University, New York, NY http://cpmcnet.columbia.edu/dept/sph/hpm/index.html

Department of Health Policy and Management, School of Public Health, Harvard University, Boston, MA http://www.hsph.harvard.edu/Academics/hpm

Health Policy Institute, Georgetown Public Policy Institute http://ihcrp.georgetown.edu

Health Policy, University of the Sciences in Philadelphia, PA   http://www.healthpolicy.usip.edu

Health Policy Institute, School of Public Health, University of Pittsburgh, PA   http://www.healthpolicyinstitute.pitt.edu

Institute for Child Health Policy (ICHP), University of Florida, Gainesville, FL   http://www.ichp.ufl.edu

Institute for Health Research and Policy, University of Illinois at Chicago, Chicago, IL   http://ihrp.uic.edu

Manitoba Centre for Health Policy, University of Manitoba, Winnipeg, MB (Canada) http://umanitoba.ca/medicine/units/mchp

National Health Policy Forum (NHPF), George Washington University, Washington, DC   http://www.nhpf.org

Population Health Institute, University of Wisconsin, Madison, WI http://www.pophealth.wisc.edu/uwphi

Women's and Children's Health Policy Center (WCHPC), School of Public Health, Johns Hopkins University, Baltimore, MD   http://www.jhsph.edu/wchpc

See also Advocacy, Education, and Research Organizations; Health Policy Organizations; Public Health

94. Health Policy Organizations

Health policy organizations conduct research into issues that affect the healthcare system and delivery of care.

American Enterprise Institute (AEI) for Public Policy Research   http://www.aei.org

Brookings Institution (BI)   http://www.brookings.edu

Canadian Policy Research Networks (CPRN) http://www.cprn.org

Center for Health Policy Studies, Heritage Foundation http://www.heritage.org

Center for Studying Health System Change (HSC) http://www.hschange.com

Coalition for Evidence-Based Policy   http://www.excelgov.org/ Programs/ProgramDetail.cfm?ItemNumber=9711

Commonwealth Fund   http://www.commonwealthfund.org

Dialogue on Health Reform (Canada) http://www.utoronto.ca/hpme/dhr/index.html

Galen Institute   http://www.galen.org

Health Council of Canada   http://www.healthcouncilcanada.ca

Heritage Foundation   http://www.heritage.org

Institute of Medicine (IOM)   http://www.iom.edu

Henry J. Kaiser Family Foundation (KFF) http://www.kaisernetwork.org

Mathematica Policy Research, Inc. http://www.mathematica-mpr.com/index.htm

National Health Policy Forum   http://www.nhpf.org

Office of Rural Health Policy, Health Resources and Services Administration (HRSA)   http://ruralhealth.hrsa.gov

Pew Charitable Trusts   http://www.pewtrusts.org

Policy Information Center, Office of the Assistant Secretary for Planning and Evaluation, Department of Health and Human Services (HHS)   http://aspe.hhs.gov/pic

RAND Corporation   http://www.rand.org

Urban Institute   http://www.urban.org

See also Advocacy, Education, and Research Organizations; Foundation and Philanthropies; Health Policy, Academic Centers of; Public Health

95. Health Report Cards

Quality performance indicators is a type of metric that is used to assist healthcare organizations evaluate if they are meeting healthcare quality goals and objectives.

Agency for Health Care Research and Quality (AHRQ)
http://www.ahrq.gov

Health Grades, Inc.   http://www.healthgrades.com

Health Plan Employer Data and Information Set (HEDIS), National Committee for Quality Assurance (NCQA)
http://web.ncqa.org/tabid/59/Default.aspx

Hospital Compare, Hospital Quality Alliance (HQA)
http://www.hospitalcompare.hhs.gov

Medical Outcomes Trust   http://www.outcomes-trust.org

National Centre for Health Outcomes Development (NCHOD)   http://www.nchod.nhs.uk

Performance Data, Department of Health
http://www.performance.doh.gov.uk

Quality Check, Joint Commission   http://www.jointcommission.org/qualitycheck/06_about_qc.htm

U.S. News and World Report Best Hospitals
http://www.usnews.com/besthospitals

See also Centers for Medicare and Medicaid Services (CMS); Health Outcomes; Hospitals; Nursing Homes; Physicians; Quality of Healthcare

96. Health Services Research, Academic and Training Centers of

Academic and training centers of health services research provide training to develop professionals and researchers with a background in health services research and health policy.

Case Western Reserve University School of Medicine, Cleveland, OH   http://mediswww.meds.cwru.edu

Cecil G. Sheps Center for Health Services Research, University of North Carolina, Chapel Hill, NC
http://www.schsr.unc.edu

Center for Health Care Research and Department of Biometry and Epidemiology, Medical University of South Carolina, Charleston, SC   http://www.musc.edu/chcr

Center for Health Policy/Center for Primary Care and Outcomes Research (PCOR/CHP), School of Medicine, Stanford University, Stanford, CA
http://chppcor.stanford.edu

Center for Gerontology and Health Care Research, Brown University, Providence, RI   http://www.chcr.brown.edu

Centre for Health Services and Policy Research, Queens University, Kingston, Ontario (Canada)
http://chspr.queensu.ca

Centre for Health Services and Policy Research, University of British Columbia, Vancouver, BC (Canada)
http://www.chspr.ubc.ca

Center for Health Services Research and Policy, George Washington University, Washington, DC
http://www.gwumc.edu/sphhs/healthpolicy

Center for Outcomes and Effectiveness Research and Education, University of Alabama at Birmingham, Birmingham, AL   http://www.dopm.uab.edu/coere/index.html

Chicago Department of Health Studies, University of Chicago, Chicago, IL   http://harrisschool.uchicago.edu

Cornell University Weill Medical College, New York, NY
http://www.cornellmedicine.com

Dartmouth Medical School, Hanover, NH
http://www.dartmouth.edu/~cecs

Department of Community and Preventive Medicine, University of Rochester, Rochester, NY
http://www.urmc.rochester.edu/cpm

Department of Health Services, University of Washington, Seattle, WA   http://depts.washington.edu/hserv

Department of Population Health Sciences, School of Medicine, University of Wisconsin, Madison, Madison, WI
http://www.pophealth.wisc.edu/HSR/traininggrant.htm

Institute for Clinical Research and Health Policy Studies (ICRHPS), Tufts Medical Center, Boston, MA
http://160.109.101.132/icrhps/default.asp

Duke University Center for Clinical Health Policy Research (CCHPR), Durham, NC
http://www.ahrq.gov/clinic/epc/dukeepc.htm

Harvard Medical School, Boston MA
http://web.hms.harvard.edu/hfdfp/research.htm

Health Services Research and Development Center, School of Public Health, Johns Hopkins University
http://www.jhsph.edu/HSR/index.html

Institute for Health Services Research and Policy Studies (IHSRPS), Northwestern University Feinberg School of Medicine, Chicago, IL
http://www.medschool.northwestern.edu/ihs

Institute of Gerontology, Wayne State University, Detroit, MI   http://www.iog.wayne.edu

Leonard Davis Institute, The Wharton School, University of Pennsylvania, Philadelphia, PA   http://www.wharton.upenn.edu/doctoral/programs/healthcare

Schneider Institute for Health Policy, Heller School of Social Policy and Management, Brandeis University, Waltham, MA   http://www.sihp.brandeis.edu

School of Public Health and Public Policy, University of California, Berkeley, and School of Medicine, University of California, San Francisco   http://ihps.medschool.ucsf.edu

School of Public Health, University of California, Los Angeles/ RAND Corporation, Los Angeles, CA http://www.ph.ucla.edu/hs/degree.html

School of Public Health, University of Michigan, Ann Arbor, MI   http://www.sph.umich.edu/hmp/programs

School of Public Health, University of Minnesota, Minneapolis, MN   http://www.hsr.umn.edu

Vanderbilt University, Nashville, TN http://www.mc.vanderbilt.edu/prevmed/mph

See also Health Services Research, Associations and Foundations of

97. Health Services Research, Associations and Foundations of

Associations and foundations of health services research are dedicated groups of health services researchers, health policy experts, and practitioners who work to advance research, policy, and practice in the field.

AcademyHealth (Established in 2000 following the merger between the Alpha Center and the Association for Health Services Research (AHSR)   http://www.academyhealth.org

American Health Care Association (AHCA), Research and Data http://www.ahcancal.org/research_data/Pages/default.aspx

Canadian Association for Health Services and Policy Research (CAHSPR)   http://www.cahspr.ca

Canadian Health Services Research Foundation (CHSRF)   http://www.chsrf.ca

Health Services Research Association of Australia and New Zealand (HSRAANZ) http://www.chere.uts.edu.au/hsraanz

See also Health Policy Organizations; Health Services Research, Academic and Training Centers of

98. Health Services Research, History of

History of health services research includes the background, stories, and experiences of key leaders and scholars of this growing field.

National Information Center on Health Services Research and Health Care Technology (NICHSR) (NICHSR conducted a History of Health Services Research Project that interviewed many prominent health services researchers)   http://www.nlm.nih.gov/nichsr

See also Federal Government; Health Policy Organizations

99. Health Services Research Journals

Health services research journals are peer-reviewed publications that publish original and innovative work that advances the field of health services and improves the health of individuals.

American Journal of Public Health   http://www.ajph.org

Forum for Health Economics and Policy http://www.bepress.com/fhep

Health Affairs   http://www.healthaffairs.org

Health Care Financing Review http://www.cms.hhs.gov/HealthCareFinancingReview

Health Economics   http://www3.interscience.wiley.com

Health Services Research   http://hsr.org

Inquiry: The Journal of Health Care Organization, Provision, and Financing   http://www.inquiryjournal.org

Journal of Health Economics   http://www.elsevier.com/wps/ find/journaldescription.cws_home/505560/description

Journal of Health Politics, Policy and Law http://jhppl.dukejournals.org

Journal of Health Services Research and Policy http://www.rsmpress.co.uk/jhsrp.htm

Medical Care   http://www.lww-medicalcare.com

Medical Care Research and Review   http://mcr.sagepub.com

Milbank Quarterly   http://www.milbank.org/quarterly.html

Research in Healthcare Financial Management http://www.rhfm.org

See also Journals, Medical; News Services

100. Health Statistics and Data Sources

Sources of health statistics and data include places where researchers, policymakers, and the public can turn to to obtain information on health, disease, and mortality.

Agency for Healthcare Research and Quality (AHRQ) http://www.ahrq.gov

American Hospital Association (AHA) (Conducts an annual survey of the nation's hospitals) http://www.aha.org

American Medical Association (AMA) http://www.ama-assn.org

Area Resource File (ARF): National County-level Health Resource Information Database (The ARF contains population and health data for each county in the United States) http://www.arfsys.com

Bureau of Health Professions (BHPr), Health Resources and Services Administration (HRSA) http://bhpr.hrsa.gov

Canadian Institute for Health Information (CIHI) http://www.cihi.ca

Centers for Medicare and Medicaid Services (CMS) http://www.cms.hhs.gov

Department of Veterans Affairs (VA) http://www.va.gov

Health Statistics, Statistics Canada http://cansim2.statcan.ca

Hospital Episodes Statistics, United Kingdom's National Health Service http://www.dh.gov.uk/PublicationsAndStatistics/Statistics/HospitalEpisodeStatistics/en

National Association of Health Data Organizations (NAHDO) http://www.nahdo.org

National Center for Health Statistics (NCHS) http://www.cdc.gov/nchs

Pan American Health Organization (PAHO) http://www.paho.org

Statistical Abstract of the United States http://www.census.gov/statab/www

Statistics Canada http://www.statcan.ca

U.S. Census Bureau http://www.census.gov

World Health Organization Statistical Information System http://www.who.int/whosis

See also Centers for Disease Control and Prevention (CDC); Health Surveys; State and County Data Sources; Vital Statistics; World Health Organization (WHO)

101. Health Surveys

Health surveys include questionnaires that are conducted across the nation to assess different aspects of health, healthcare, or demographics.

Annual Health Care and Social Assistance Survey (NAICS 62), U.S. Census (NAICS stands for North American Industry Classification System) http://www.census.gov/svsd/www/sas62.html

Annual Survey of Hospitals, American Hospital Association (AHA) http://www.aha.org/aha/resource-center/Statistics-and-Studies/index.html

Healthcare Cost and Utilization Project (HCUP) http://www.ahrq.gov/data/hcup

Inter-University Consortium for Political and Social Research (ICPSR), Institute for Social Research, University of Michigan http://www.icpsr.umich.edu/org/index.html

Longitutional Studies of Aging (LSOA) http://www.cdc.gov/nchs/lsoa.htm

Medical Expenditure Panel Survey (MEPS) http://www.ahrq.gov/data/mepsix.htm

National Ambulatory Medical Care Survey (NAMCS) http://www.cdc.gov/nchs/about/major/ahcd/ahcd1.htm

National Employer Health Insurance Survey (NEHIS) http://www.cdc.gov/nchs/about/major/nehis/nehis.htm

National Health and Nutrition Examination Survey (NHANES) http://www.cdc.gov/nchs/nhanes.htm

National Health Care Survey (NHCS) http://www.cdc.gov/nchs/nhcs.htm

National Health Interview Surveys (NHIS) http://www.cdc.gov/nchs/nhis.htm

National Health Provider Inventory (NHPI) Public-Use Data Files http://www.cdc.gov/nchs/products/elec_prods/subject/nhpi.htm

National Home and Hospice Care Survey (NHHCS) http://www.cdc.gov/nchs/nhhcs.htm

National Hospital Ambulatory Medical Care Survey (NHAMCS) http://www.cdc.gov/nchs/about/major/ahcd/ahcd1.htm

National Hospital Discharge and Ambulatory Surgery Survey (NHDS) http://www.cdc.gov/nchs/about/major/hdasd/nhds.htm

National Immunization Survey (NIS) http://www.cdc.gov/nis

National Medical Expenditures Survey (NMES) http://wonder.cdc.gov/wonder/sci_data/surveys/nmes/nmes.asp

National Nursing Home Survey (NNHS) http://www.cdc.gov/nchs/nnhs.htm

National Survey of Ambulatory Surgery (NSAS) http://www.cdc.gov/nchs/nsas.htm

National Survey of Family Growth (NSFG) http://www.cdc.gov/nchs/nsfg.htm

Service Annual Survey, Health Care and Social Assistance (NAICS 62), U.S. Census Bureau (NAICS stands for the North American Industry Classification System) http://www.census.gov/econ/www/servmenu.html

See also Centers for Disease Control and Prevention (CDC); Health Statistics and Data Sources; Public Health; State and County Data Sources

102. Healthcare Administration and Management

Healthcare administration and management includes professionals who work to ensure the smooth and functional operation of a healthcare facility or system.

American College of Healthcare Executives (ACHE)
http://www.ache.org

American College of Physician Executives (ACPE)
http://www.acpe.org

Canadian College of Health Service Executives (CCHSE)
http://www.cchse.org

Healthcare Financial Management Association (HFMA)
http://www.hfma.org

European Healthcare Management Association (EHMA)
http://www.ehma.org

Management Sciences for Health   http://www.msh.org

National Institute for Health Care Management (NIHCM)
http://www.nihcm.org

See also Health Administration, Association of Academic Programs of; Health Administration Programs, Graduate Programs in

103. Healthcare Financial Management

Healthcare financial management is the technique of using fiscally responsible standards and practices to run a healthcare organization.

Changes in Health Care Financing and Organizations (This program is part of AcademyHealth)   http://www.hcfo.net

Healthcare Financial Management Association (HFMA)
http://www.hfma.org

International Society for Research in Healthcare Financial Management (isRHFM)   http://www.rhfm.org

See also Centers for Medicare and Medicaid Services (CMS); Health Insurance; Medicaid; Medical Billing; Medical Records; Medicare; Regulation

104. Healthy People 2010

Healthy People 2010 is the set of the nation's objectives to identify the most preventable threats to the country's health and to create goals to reduce and eliminate these threats.

Healthy People 2010   http://www.healthypeople.gov

See also Federal Government; Health Disparities; Minority Health; Public Health

105. Heart Disease

Heart disease refers to a number of diseases that relate to the heart. Heart disease remains one of the leading causes of death in the United States.

American Heart Association (AHA)
http://www.americanheart.org

Canadian Adult Congenital Heart Network
http://www.cachnet.org

Congenital Heart Information Network (CHIN)
http://tchin.org

Heart Rhythm Society   http://www.hrsonline.org

National Heart, Lung, and Blood Institute (NHLBI)
http://www.nhlbi.nih.gov

See also Cardiology; Chronic Diseases; Emergency Medicine; Hospitals

106. Hispanic

Hispanic refers to the heterogenous groups of people and cultures who speak Spanish and were once ruled by Spain.

Association of Hispanic Healthcare Executives (AHHE)
http://www.ahhe.org

National Alliance for Hispanic Health (NAHH)
http://www.hispanichealth.org

National Association of Hispanic Nurses (NAHN)
http://thehispanicnurses.org

National Council on La Raza   http://www.nclr.org

National Hispanic Council on Aging (NHCOA)
http://www.nhcoa.org

National Hispanic Medical Association (NHMA)
http://www.nhmamd.org

Office of Minority Health Resource Center
http://www.omhrc.gov

See also Health Disparities; Migrant Health; Minority Health; Rural Health

107. Home Health Care

Home health care is a type of care provided to allow seniors with health conditions to live as independelty as possible. Home health care may involve therapy, nursing, and assistance with daily living.

Canadian Home Care Association (CHCA)
http://www.cdnhomecare.ca

National Association for Home Care and Hospice (NAHC)
http://www.nahc.org

Team in Community Care and Health Human Resources
http://teamgrant.ca

United Kingdom Home Care Association
http://www.ukhca.co.uk

See also Aging; Assisted Living; Disability; Nursing

108. Hospice and Palliative Care

Hospice and palliative care is the specialized comfort care provided to individuals with terminal conditions to alleviate pain and suffering.

Association for Death Education and Counseling (ADEC)
http://www.adec.org

Children's Hospice International (CHI)
http://www.chionline.org

Hospice Association of America (HAA)
http://www.nahc.org/haa

Hospice Education Institute   http://www.hospiceworld.org

International Association for Hospice and Palliative Care (IAHPC)   http://www.hospicecare.com

National Association for Home Care and Hospice (NAHC)
http://www.nahc.org

National Institute for Jewish Hospice   http://www.nijh.org

See also Aging; Gerontology; Health Insurance; Nursing Homes

109. Hospital Infections and Nosocomial Diseases

Hospital infections are infections that are acquired secondarily to a patient's primary medical condition, and acquired during the course of a hospitalization.

National Nosocomial Infections Surveillance System
http://www.cdc.gov/ncidod/dhqp/nnis_pubs.html

See also Emerging Diseases; Hospitals; Infection Control and Prevention; Infectious Diseases; Public Health

110. Hospitalist

Hospitalists are physicians who specialize in the general medical care of hospitalized patients.

Society of Hospital Medicine (SHM)
http://www.hospitalmedicine.org

See also Hospitals; Quality of Healthcare

111. Hospitals

Hospitals are a type of healthcare institution that provides care to patients needing medical treatment. Hospitals house specialized medical equipment and staff and can accomodate patient stays.

American Hospital Association (AHA) (The AHA represents all of the nation's hospitals)   http://www.aha.org

American Hospital Directory (AHD)   http://www.ahd.com

Catholic Health Association of the United States (CHA)
http://www.chausa.org

Council of Teaching Hospitals and Health Systems (COTH)
http://www.aamc.org

Federation of American Hospitals (FAH) (FAH represents the nation's for-profit hospitals)
http://www.americashospital.com

HospitalWeb
http://neuro-www.mgh.harvard.edu/hospitalweb.shtml

National Association of Children's Hospitals and Related Institutions (NACHRI)   http://www.childrenshospitals.net

National Association of Public Hospitals and Health Systems (NAPH)   http://www.naph.org

National Ministries (This organization was formerly the American Baptist Homes and Hospitals Association)
http://www.nationalministries.org

U.S. News and World Report Best Hospitals
http://www.usnews.com/besthospitals

VHA: Voluntary Hospitals of America   http://www.vha.com

Virtual Hospital: Information for Patients
http://www.uihealthcare.com/vh

See also Emergency Medicine; Hospital Infections and Nosocomial Diseases; Hospitalists; Physicians; Nursing

112. Hypertension

Hypertension, also known as high blood pressure, is when a person's blood pressure is chronically elevated.

American Society of Hypertension (ASH)
http://www.ash-us.org

International Society on Hypertension in Blacks (ISHIB)
http://www.ishib.org

Pulmonary Hypertension Association (PHA)
http://www.phassociation.org

World Hypertension League
http://www.worldhypertensionleague.org

See also Chronic Diseases; Heart Disease; Kidney Diseases; Public Health

113. Immunization and Vaccination

Immunization is when a person's immune system is protected against an agent and it is generally done by giving vaccinations.

Immunization Action Coalition (IAC)
    http://www.immunize.org

Vaccines and Immunizations, CDC
    http://www.cdc.gov/vaccines

See also Prevention and Health Promotion; Public Health

114. Infection Control and Prevention

Infection control and prevention is the process of protecting against and reducing the spread of disease within a healthcare setting.

Center for Infectious Disease Research and Policy (CIDRAP), University of Minnesota
    http://www.cidrap.umn.edu/cidrap

Infection Control Guidelines, Centers for Disease Control and Prevention (CDC)
    http://www.cdc.gov/ncidod/dhqp/guidelines.html

National Center for HIV, Viral Hepatitis, STD, and TB Prevention (NCHHSTP)   http://www.cdc.gov/nchhstp

Society for Healthcare Epidemiology of America (SHEA)
    http://www.shea-online.org

See also Emerging Diseases; Hospital Infections and Nosocomial Diseases; Infectious Diseases

115. Infectious Diseases

Infectious diseases are diseases that result from microbial pathogens. Infectious diseases may be spread through a number of ways including airborne transmission, food, liquids, bodily fluids, and vectors.

Center for Infectious Disease Research and Policy (CIDRAP), University of Minnesota
    http://www.cidrap.umn.edu/cidrap

Communicable Disease Review Weekly
    http://www.hpa.org.uk/cdr

Infectious Diseases Society of America (IDSA)
    http://www.idsociety.org

Morbidity and Mortality Weekly Report
    http://www.cdc.gov/mmwr

National Institute of Allergy and Infectious Diseases (NIAID)
    http://www3.niaid.nih.gov

Society of Infectious Diseases Pharmacists (SIDP)
    http://www.sidp.org

See also Centers for Disease Control and Prevention (CDC); Emerging Diseases; Hospital Infections and Nosocomial Diseases; Infection Control and Prevention; Public Health

116. Influenza Pandemic

Influenza pandemic is an outbreak of the flu in which people have little to no natural immunity and for which no vaccine exists. An influenza pandemic would spread rapidly throughout the population and result in serious illness.

Pandemic Flu   http://www.pandemicflu.gov

See also Centers for Disease Control and Prevention (CDC); Disaster Preparedness and Relief; Emerging Diseases; Public Health

117. Informatics

Informatics is the field of information science that includes information processing and the development of information technologies. Informatics is growing in its application to health and medicine.

American Medical Informatics Association (AMIA)
    http://www.amia.org

Canada's Health Informatics Association (COACH)
    http://www.coachorg.com

European Federation for Medical Informatics (EFMI)
    http://www.efmi.org

Health Informatics New Zealand (HINZ)
    http://www.hinz.org.nz

Health Informatics Society of Australia (NISA)
    http://www.hisa.org.au

International Medical Informatics Association (IMIA)
    http://www.imia.org

National Center for Public Health Informatics (NCPHI)
    http://www.cdc.gov/ncphi

UK Health Informatics Society (UKHiS)   http://www.bmis.org

See also E-Health; Information Technology (IT); Telemedicine

118. Information Technology (IT)

Information technology allows for the management and transmission of health data and information between providers and consumers.

Agency for Healthcare Research and Quality (AHRQ)
    http://www.ahrq.gov

American Health Information Management Association
    (AHIMA)   http://www.ahima.org

Commonwealth Fund   http://www.cmwf.org

National Resource Center for Health Information Technology,
    Agency for Healthcare Research and Quality (AHRQ)
    http://www.ahrq.gov

See also E-Health; Informatics; Telemedicine

119. Injury

Injury is bodily damage or harm caused to a structure or part of the body.

Injuries, Illnesses, and Fatalities Bureau of Labor Statistics, U.S.
    Department of Labor   http://www.bls.gov/iif

Injury Control Resource Information Network
    http://www.injurycontrol.com/icrin

National Center for Injury Prevention and Contol (NCIPC),
    Centers for Disease Control and Prevention (CDC)
    http://www.cdc.gov/ncipc

National Highway Traffic Safety Administration (NHTSA)
    http://www.nhtsa.dot.gov

National Injury Information Clearinghouse
    http://www.cpsc.gov/about/clrnghse.html

National Institute for Occupational Safety and Health
    (NIOSH), Centers for Disease Control and Prevention
    (CDC)   http://www.cdc.gov/niosh

Public Health Agency of Canada, Injury
    http://www.phac-aspc.gc.ca/injury-bles

World Health Organization (WHO) Violence and Injury
    Prevention
    http://www.who.int/violence_injury_prevention/en

See also Burn Care; Emergency Medicine; Occupational
    Medicine; Workers' Compensation

120. Internal Medicine

Internal medicine is the speciality of medicine that is focused on the diagnosis, nonsurgical treatment, and management of serious or unusal medical conditions.

American Board of Internal Medicine (ABIM)
    http://www.abim.org

American College of Physicians, American Society of Internal
    Medicine (ACP-ASIM)   http://www.acponline.org

Society of General Internal Medicine (SGIM)
    http://www.sgim.org

See also Hospitals; Physicians

121. International Health Systems

International health systems refers to the public health models used in various countries. Studying them often provides insight into a one's own healthcare system.

Academy for International Health Studies (AIHS)
    http://www.aihs.com

American Association for World Health (AAWH)
    http://www.thebody.com/content/art33029.html

Bill and Melinda Gates Foundation
    http://www.gatesfoundation.org

Canadian Society for International Health (CSIH)
    http://www.csih.org

Fogarty International Center (FIC), National Institutes of
    Health (NIH)   http://www.fic.nih.gov

Global Health Council   http://www.globalhealth.org

International Association for Medical Assistance to Travelers
    (IAMAT)   http://www.iamat.org

Pan American Health Organization (PAHO)
    http://www.paho.org

People-to-People Health Foundation (HOPE)
    http://www.projecthope.org

Project Concern International (PCI)
    http://www.projectconcern.org

Project HOPE   http://www.projecthope.org

U.S. Agency for International Development (USAID)
    http://www.usaid.gov

W. K. Kellogg Foundation   http://www.wkkf.org

World Bank Group   http://www.worldbank.org

World Health Organization (WHO)   http://www.who.int

See also Canadian Healthcare Organizations; United Kingdom
    Healthcare Organizations; World Health Organization (WHO)

122. Journals, Medical

Medical journals are peer-reviewed publications that publish original work on recent health and medical findings.

British Medical Journal (BMJ)   http://www.bmj.com

Free Medical Journals   http://www.freemedicaljournals.com

Journal of Postgraduate Medicine
    http://www.jpgmonline.com

Journal of the American Medical Association
    (JAMA)   http://jama.ama-assn.org

New England Journal of Medicine (NEJM)
    http://www.nejm.org

PubMed (The National Library of Medicine produces this huge database. It lists author, title, and summaries of medical journal articles.)   http://www.pubmed.gov

See also Federal Health Information Centers and Clearinghouses; Health Services Research Journals; News Services

123. Kidney Diseases

Kidney diseases are conditions that affect the kidneys, the organ that is responsible for the removal of waste and fluids from the body. Kidney diseases can be acquired or heredity.

American Association of Kidney Patients (AAKP)
    http://www.aakp.org

American Kidney Fund (AKF)   http://www.kidneyfund.org

Kidney Transplant/Dialysis Association (KT/DA)
    http://www.ktda.org

National Institute of Diabetes and Digestive and Kidney Diseases (NIDDK)   http://www2.niddk.nih.gov

National Kidney Foundation (NKF)   http://www.kidney.org

University Renal Research and Education Association
    http://www.ustransplant.org

See also Donors and Transplantation; Hypertension; Nephrology

124. Latino

See Hispanic

125. Liver Diseases

Liver diseases are conditions that affect the liver, which is responsible for many functions including metabolizing toxic substances, converting nutrients, storing minerals, synthesizing proteins and enzymes, and maintaining hormone levels.

American Association for the Study of Liver Diseases
    (AASLD)   http://www.aasld.org

American Liver Foundation (ALF)
    http://www.liverfoundation.org

Hepatitis Foundation International   http://www.hepfi.org

See also Donors and Organ Transplantation; Internal Medicine

126. Long-Term Care

Long-term care is the care that is provided to the chronically ill and disabled. Long-term care may be provided in a variety of settings including the home, community, or nursing home and it may provide support and assist with activities of daily living.

American Health Care Association (AHCA)
    http://www.ahcancal.org

National Association for the Support of Long Term Care
    (NASL)   http://www.nasl.org

See also Aging; Chronic Diseases; Gerontology; Nursing Homes

127. Lung Diseases

Lung diseases are conditions that affect the lungs and may cause people to experience difficulty in breathing. Many factors that cause lung disease are behavioral, environmental, and biological in nature.

American Lung Association   http://www.lungusa.org

National Heart, Lung, and Blood Institute (NHLBI)
    http://www.nhlbi.nih.gov

See also Asthma; Cancer; Tobacco Use

128. Managed Care

Managed care is the term that is used to refer to the techniques that are designed to control healthcare costs and improve the quality of care through such mechanisms as cost-sharing and financial incentives. Managed care may operate in a variety of forms, including as health maintenance organizations or preferred provider organizations.

Academy of Managed Care Pharmacy (AMCP)
    http://www.amcp.org

Academy of Managed Care Providers (AMCP)
    http://www.academymcp.org

American Association of Managed Care Nurses (AAMCN)
    http://www.aamcn.org

American Board of Managed Care Medicine (ABMCM)
http://www.abmcm.org

Integrated Healthcare Association (IHA)   http://www.iha.org

See also Health Insurnce; Healthcare Financial Management

129. Medicaid

Medicaid is a health program for individuals and families with low income and resources that is jointly funded by the federal government and states. The Medicaid program is means tested and primarily serves the elderly, disabled, and low-income families with children.

Centers for Medicare and Medicaid Services (CMS)
http://www.cms.hhs.gov

National Academy for State Health Policy (NASHP)
http://www.nashp.org

National Association of State Medicaid Directors (NASMD)
http://www.nasmd.org

See also Centers for Medicare and Medicaid Services CMS; Health Insurance; Medicaid, List of State Programs

130. Medicaid, List of State Programs

The list of state programs of Medicaid includes the programs that are run by each state. The specific benefits and eligibility requirements provided by the Medicaid program may vary according to state.

Alabama Medical Agency   http://www.medicaid.state.al.us

Alaska Department of Health and Social Services
http://www.hss.state.ak.us

Arizona Health Care Cost Containment System (AHCCCS)
http://www.ahcccs.state.az.us

Arkansas Department of Human Services
http://www.arkansas.gov/dhs/serv_gr.html

California Department of Health Services
http://www.medi-cal.ca.gov

Colorado Department of Health Care Policy and
Financing   http://www.chcpf.state.co.us

Connecticut Department of Social Services, Medical Care
Administration   http://www.ctmedicalprogram.com

Delaware Department of Health and Social Services
http://www.dhss.delaware.gov/dhss/dph/index.html

Department of Health and Human Services, Office of Medicaid
Business and Policy   http://wwwdhhs.state.nh.us/DHHS

Florida Agency for Health Care Administration
http://www.fdhc.state.fl.us/Medicaid/index.shtml

Georgia Department of Community Health, Medical Assistance
Plans   http://www.dch.georgia.gov

Hawaii Department of Human Services, Med-Quest Division
http://www.state.hi.us/dhs

Idaho Department of Health and Welfare, Division of
Medicaid   http://www.healthandwelfare.idaho.gov

Illinois Department of Healthcare and Family Services,
Medicaid and SCHIP Programs   http://www.hfs.illinois.gov

Indiana Family and Social Services Administration, Office of
Medicaid Policy and Planning   http://www.in.gov/fssa

Iowa Department of Human Services, Division of Medical
Services   http://www.dhs.state.ia.us

Kansas Medical Assistance Program
https://www.kmap-state-ks.us

Kentucky Cabinet for Health and Family Services
http://www.chfs.ky.gov

Louisiana Department of Health and Hospitals, Bureau of
Health Services Financing   http://www.dhh.state.la.us

Maine Department of Health and Human Services, Bureau of
Medical Services   http://www.maine.gov/dhhs/bms

Maryland Department of Health and Mental Hygiene
http://www.dhmh.state.md.us/mma/mmahome.html

Massachusetts Department of Health and Human Services,
Office of Medicaid   http://www.mass.gov

Michigan Department of Community Health
http://www.michigan.gov/mdch

Minnesota Department of Human Services
http://www.dhs.state.mn.us

Mississippi Division of Medicaid   http://www.medicaid.ms.gov/

Missouri Department of Social Services, Division of Medical
Services   http://www.dss.mo.gov/dms

Montana Department of Public Health and Human Services
http://www.dphhs.mt.gov/PHSD

Nebraska Health and Human Services and Support
http://www.hhs.state.ne.us/med/medindex.htm

Nevada Division of Health Care Financing and Policy
http://dhcfp.state.nv.us

New Jersey Department of Human Services, Division of
Medical Assistance and Health   http://www.state.nj.us/
humanservices/dmahs/dhsmed.html

New Mexico Department of Human Services, Medical
Assistance Division   http://www.hsd.state.nm.us/mad

New York Department of Health, Medicaid   http://www
.health.state.ny.us/health_care/medicaid/index.htm

North Carolina Department of Health and Human Services, Division of Medical Assistance http://www.dhhs.state.nc.us/dma

North Dakota Department of Human Services, Medical Services   http://www.nd.gov/dhs/services/medicalserv

Ohio Department of Job and Family Services, Ohio Health Plans   http://www.jfs.ohio.gov

Oklahoma Health Care Authority http://www.ohca.state.ok.us

Oregon Department of Human Resources, Office of Medical Assistance Programs   http://www.oregon.gov/DHS/healthplan/index.shml

Pennsylvania Department of Public Welfare, Medical Assistance Programs   http://www.dpw.state.pa.us

Rhode Island Department of Human Services, Medical Assistance Program http://www.dhs.state.ri.us/dhs/adults/dmadult.htm

South Carolina Department of Health and Human Services http://www.dhhs.state.sc.us/dhhsnew/index.asp

South Dakota Department of Social Services, Medical Services   http://www.dss.sd.gov

Tennessee Bureau of TennCare http://www.state.tn.us/tenncare

Texas Health and Human Services Commission http://www.hhsc.state.tx.us/medicaid

Utah Department of Health   http://health.utah.gov/medicaid

Vermont Department of Social Welfare, Office of Health Access http://ovha.vermont.gov

Virginia Department of Medical Assistance Services http://www.dmas.virginia.gov

Washington, D.C. Department of Health, Medical Assistance Administration http://app.doh.dc.gov/about/index_maa.shtm

Washington Department of Social and Health Services, Medical Assistance Administration http://fortress.wa.gov/dshs/maa/index.html

West Virginia Department of Health and Human Resources, Bureau for Medical Services   http://www.wvdhhr.org/bms

Wisconsin Department of Health and Family Services, Division of Health Care Financing http://www.dhfs.state.wi.us/medicaid

Wyoming Department of Health, Office of Health Care Financing http://wdh.state.wy.us/healthcarefin/equalitycare/index.html

See also Centers for Medicare and Medicaid Services (CMS); Health Insurance; Medicaid

131. Medical Assistants

Medical assistants are healthcare professionals who provide administrative and clinical support. Medical assistants may be employed in both inpatient and outpatient healthcare settings.

American Association of Medical Assistants (AAMA) http://www.aama-ntl.org

See also Allied Health; Clinical Laboratories

132. Medical Billing

Medical billing is the process of submitting claims to payers for healthcare services rendered.

American Academy of Professional Coders (AAPC) http://www.aapc.com

Healthcare Billing and Management Association (HBMA) http://www.hbma.com

Medical Association of Billers (MAB) http://www.e-medbill.com

See also Disease and Procedure Classifications; Fraud and Abuse; Health Insurance; Healthcare Financial Management; Medical Records

133. Medical Colleges, Associations of

Associations of medical colleges represent a group of medical schools that work to improve the healthcare system.

American Association of Colleges of Osteopathic Medicine (AACOM)   http://www.aacom.org

Association of American Medical Colleges (AAMC) http://www.aamc.org

Association of Faculties of Medicine of Canada (AFMC) http://www.afmc.ca

See also Medical Colleges, List of; Physicians

134. Medical Colleges, List of

The list of medical colleges includes all medical colleges, universities, and programs that train professionals to enter the field of medicine.

Alabama

University of Alabama School of Medicine,
Birmingham, AL
http://main.uab.edu/uasom/show.asp?durki=2023

University of South Alabama College of Medicine, Mobile,
AL   http://www.southalabama.edu/com

Arizona

University of Arizona College of Medicine, Tucson, AZ
http://www.medicine.arizona.edu

Arkansas

University of Arkansas for Medical Sciences, College of
Medicine, Little Rock, AR
http://www.uams.edu/com/default.asp

California

Keck School of Medicine of the University of Southern
California, Los Angeles, CA
http://www.usc.edu/schools/medicine/ksom.html

Loma Linda University School of Medicine, Loma Linda,
CA   http://www.llu.edu/llu/medicine

Stanford University School of Medicine, Stanford, CA
http://med.stanford.edu

University of California, Davis, School of Medicine, Davis,
CA   http://www.ucdmc.ucdavis.edu/medschool

University of California, Irvine, College of Medicine, Irvine,
CA   http://www.ucihs.uci.edu

University of California, Los Angeles, David Geffen School of
Medicine, Los Angeles, CA
http://dgsom.healthsciences.ucla.edu

University of California, San Diego, School of Medicine, La
Jolla, CA   http://som.ucsd.edu

University of California, San Francisco, School of Medicine,
San Francisco, CA   http://medschool.ucsf.edu

Colorado

University of Colorado School of Medicine, Denver,
CO   http://www.uchsc.edu/sm/sm/offdean.htm

Connecticut

University of Connecticut School of Medicine, Farmington,
CT   http://www.uchc.edu

Yale University School of Medicine, New Haven, CT
http://info.med.yale.edu/ysm

District of Columbia

Georgetown University School of Medicine, Washington,
DC   http://som.georgetown.edu/index.html

George Washington University School of Medicine and Health
Sciences, Washington, DC   http://www.gwumc.edu

Howard University College of Medicine, Washington,
DC   http://www.med.howard.edu

Florida

Florida State University College of Medicine, Tallahassee,
FL   http://med.fsu.edu

University of Florida College of Medicine, Gainesville,
FL   http://www.med.ufl.edu

University of Miami Leonard M. Miller School of Medicine,
Miami, FL   http://www.med.miami.edu

University of South Florida College of Medicine,
Tampa, FL   http://health.usf.edu/medicine/home.html

Georgia

Emory University School of Medicine, Atlanta, GA
http://www.med.emory.edu/index.cfm

Medical College of Georgia School of Medicine, Augusta,
GA   http://www.mcg.edu

Mercer University School of Medicine, Macon, GA
http://medicine.mercer.edu

Morehouse School of Medicine, Atlanta, GA
http://www.msm.edu

Hawaii

University of Hawaii, John A. Burns School of Medicine,
Honolulu, HI   http://jabsom.hawaii.edu/jabsom

Illinois

Chicago Medical School at Rosalind Franklin University of
Medicine and Science, North Chicago, IL
http://www.rosalindfranklin.edu

Loyola University Chicago Stritch School of Medicine,
Maywood, IL   http://www.meddean.lumc.edu

Northwestern University, Feinberg School of Medicine,
Chicago, IL   http://www.medschool.northwestern.edu

Rush Medical College of Rush University Medical
Center   http://www.rushu.rush.edu/medcol

Southern Illinois University School of Medicine, Springfield,
IL   http://www.siumed.edu

University of Chicago, Division of the Biological Sciences, Pritzker School of Medicine, Chicago, IL
http://pritzker.bsd.uchicago.edu

University of Illinois College of Medicine, Chicago, IL
http://www.uic.edu/depts/mcam

Indiana

Indiana University School of Medicine, Indianapolis, IN
http://www.medicine.iu.edu

Iowa

University of Iowa, Roy J. and Lucille A. Carver College of Medicine, Iowa City, IA   http://www.medicine.uiowa.edu

Kansas

University of Kansas School of Medicine, Kansas City, KS   http://www.kumc.edu/som/index.html

Kentucky

University of Kentucky College of Medicine, Lexington, KY   http://www.mc.uky.edu/medicine

University of Louisville School of Medicine, Louisville, KY   http://www.louisville.edu/medschool

Louisiana

Louisiana State University School of Medicine in New Orleans, New Orleans, LA   http://www.medschool.lsuhsc.edu

Louisiana State University School of Medicine in Shreveport, LA   http://www.sh.lsuhsc.edu/index.html

Tulane University School of Medicine, New Orleans, LA   http://www.som.tulane.edu

Maryland

Johns Hopkins University School of Medicine, Baltimore, MD   http://www.hopkinsmedicine.org

Uniformed Services University of the Health Sciences, F. Edward Herbert School of Medicine, Bethesda, MD
http://www.usuhs.mil

University of Maryland School of Medicine, Baltimore, MD   http://medschool.umaryland.edu

Massachusetts

Boston University School of Medicine, Boston, MA
http://www.bumc.bu.edu

Harvard Medical School, Boston, MA
http://hms.harvard.edu/hms/home.asp

Tufts University School of Medicine, Boston, MA
http://www.tufts.edu/med

University of Massachusetts Medical School, Worcester, MA   http://www.umassmed.edu/index.aspx

Michigan

Michigan State University College of Human Medicine, East Lansing, MI   http://humanmedicine.msu.edu

University of Michigan Medical School, Ann Arbor, MI
http://www.med.umich.edu/medschool

Wayne State University School of Medicine, Detroit, MI
http://www.med.wayne.edu

Minnesota

Mayo Medical School, Rochester, MN
http://www.mayo.edu/mms

University of Minnesota Medical School, Minneapolis, MN
http://www.med.umn.edu

Mississippi

University of Mississippi School of Medicine, Jackson, MS
http://som.umc.edu

Missouri

Saint Louis University School of Medicine, St. Louis, MO
http://medschool.slu.edu/index.phtml

University of Missouri, Columbia, School of Medicine, Columbia, MO   http://www.muhealth.org~medicine

University of Missouri, Kansas City, School of Medicine, St. Louis, MO   http://research.med.umkc.edu

Washington University in St. Louis School of Medicine, St. Louis, MO   http://medinfo.wustl.edu

Nebraska

Creighton University School of Medicine, Omaha, NE
http://www2.creighton.edu/medschool

University of Nebraska College of Medicine, Omaha, NE
http://www.unmc.edu/dept/com/index.cfm

Nevada

University of Nevada School of Medicine, Reno, NV
http://www.unr.edu/med

New Hampshire

Dartmouth Medical School, Hanover, NH
   http://dms.dartmouth.edu

New Jersey

University of Medicine and Dentistry of New Jersey, New
   Jersey Medical School, Newark, NJ   http://njms.umdnj.edu

University of Medicine and Dentistry of New Jersey, Robert
   Wood Johnson Medical School, Piscataway, NJ
   http://rwjms.umdnj.edu

New Mexico

University of New Mexico School of Medicine, Albuquerque,
   NM   http://hsc.unm.edu/som

New York

Albany Medical College, Albany, NY   http://www.amc.edu

Albert Einstein College of Medicine of Yeshiva University,
   Bronx, NY   http://www.aecom.yu.edu/home

Columbia University College of Physicians and Surgeons, New
   York, NY   http://cpmcnet.columbia.edu/dept/ps

Joan and Sanfort I. Weill Medical College of Cornell University,
   New York, NY   http://www.med.cornell.edu

Mount Sinai School of Medicine of New York University, New
   York, NY   http://www.mssm.edu

New York Medical College, Valhalla, NY
   http://www.nymc.edu

New York University School of Medicine, New York, NY
   http://www.med.nyu.edu/education

State University of New York Downstate Medical Center
   College of Medicine, Brooklyn, NY
   http://downstate.edu/college_of_medicine/default.html

State University of New York Upstate Medical University,
   Syracuse, NY   http://www.upstate.edu

Stony Brook University Health Sciences Center School of
   Medicine, Stony Brook, NY
   http://www.stonybrookmedicalcenter.orghsc/index.cfm

University at Buffalo, State University of New York School of
   Medicine and Biomedical Sciences, Buffalo, NY
   http://wings.buffalo.edu/smbs

University of Rochester School of Medicine and Dentistry,
   Rochester, NY   http://www.urmc.rochester.edu/SMD

North Carolina

Brody School of Medicine at East Carolina University,
   Greenville, NC   http://www.ecu.edu/med

Duke University School of Medicine, Durham, NC
   http://medschool.duke.edu

University of North Carolina at Chapel Hill School of
   Medicine, Chapel Hill, NC   http://www.med.unc.edu

Wake Forest University School of Medicine, Winston-Salem,
   NC   http://www1.wfubmc.edu

North Dakota

University of North Dakota School of Medicine and Health
   Sciences, Grand Forks, ND
   http://www.med.und.nodak.edu

Ohio

Case Western Reserve University School of Medicine,
   Cleveland, OH   http://mediswww.meds.cwru.edu

Northeastern Ohio Universities College of Medicine,
   Rootstown, OH   http://www.neoucom.edu

Ohio State University College of Medicine, Columbus,
   OH   http://medicine.osu.edu

University of Cincinnati College of Medicine, Cincinnati,
   OH   http://www.med.uc.edu

University of Toledo College of Medicine, Toledo, OH
   http://hsc.utoledo.edu/med

Wright State University Boonshoft School of Medicine, Dayton,
   OH   http://www.med.wright.edu

Oklahoma

University of Oklahoma College of Medicine, Oklahoma
   City, OK   http://www.medicine.ouhsc.edu

Oregon

Oregon Health and Science University School of Medicine,
   Portland, OR   http://www.ohsu.edu

Pennsylvania

Drexel University College of Medicine, Philadelphia, PA   http://
   www.drexelmed.edu

Jefferson Medical College of Thomas Jefferson University,
   Philadelphia, PA   http://www.jefferson.edu/jmc

Pennsylvania State University College of Medicine, Hershey,
   PA   http://www.hmc.psu.edu/college

Temple University School of Medicine, Philadelphia, PA   http://www.temple.edu/medicine

University of Pennsylvania School of Medicine, Philadelphia, PA   http://www.med.upenn.edu

University of Pittsburgh School of Medicine, Pittsburgh, PA   http://www.medschool.pitt.edu

Rhode Island

Brown Medical School, Providence, RI   http://bms.brown.edu

South Carolina

Medical University of South Carolina College of Medicine, Charleston, SC   http://www.musc.edu/com1

University of South Carolina School of Medicine, Columbia, SC   http://www.med.sc.edu

South Dakota

Sanford School of Medicine of the University of South Dakota, Sioux Falls, SD   http://www.usd.edu/med

Tennessee

East Tennessee State University James H. Quillen College of Medicine, Johnson City, TN   http://com.etsu.edu

Meharry Medical College, Nashville, TN   http://www.mmc.edu

University of Tennessee Health Science Center College of Medicine, Memphis, TN   http://www.utmem.edu

Vanderbilt University School of Medicine, Nashville, TN   http://www.mc.vanderbilt.edu/medschool

Texas

Baylor College of Medicine, Houston, TX   http://www.bcm.edu

Texas A&M University System Health Science Center School of Medicine, College Station, TX   http://medicine.tamhsc.edu

Texas Tech University Health Sciences Center School of Medicine, Lubbock, TX   http://www.ttuhsc.edu/som

University of Texas Medical Branch at Galveston, Galveston, TX   http://www.utmb.edu

University of Texas Medical School at Houston, Houston, TX   http://med.uth.tmc.edu

University of Texas Medical School at San Antonio, San Antonio. TX   http://som.uthscsa.edu

University of Texas Southwestern Medical Center at Dallas, Dallas, TX   http://www8.utsouthwestern.edu/home/education/medicalschool/index.html

Utah

University of Utah School of Medicine, Salt Lake City, UT   http://uuhsc.utah.edu

Vermont

University of Vermont College of Medicine, Burlington, VT   http://www.med.uvm.edu

Virginia

Eastern Virginia Medical School, Norfolk, VA   http://www.evms.edu

University of Virginia School of Medicine, Charlottesville, VA   http://www.healthsystem.virginia.edu/internet/som/home.cfm

Virginia Commonwealth University School of Medicine, Richmond, VA   http://www.medschool.vcu.edu

Washington

University of Washington School of Medicine, Seattle, WA   http://www.uwmedicine.org

West Virginia

Joan C. Edwards School of Medicine at Marshall University, Huntington, WV   http://musom.marshall.edu/index2.asp

West Virginia University School of Medicine, Morgantown, WV   http://www.hsc.wvu.edu/som

Wisconsin

Medical College of Wisconsin, Milwaukee, WI   http://www.mcw.edu

University of Wisconsin School of Medicine and Public Health, Madison, WI   http://www.med.wisc.edu

See also Academic Medical Centers; Medical Colleges, Association of; Physicians

135. Medical Decision Making

Medical decision making involves the systematic approach of making appropriate choices to improve health, healthcare, and policy decisions.

Foundation for Informed Medical Decision Making
http://www.fimdm.org

Society for Medical Decision Making (SMDM)
http://www.smdm.org

See also Clinical Practice Guidelines; Evidence-Based Medicine
EBM; Informatics; Randomized Controlled Trials (RCT)

136. Medical Errors

Medical errors involve the diagnosis or treatment by a
provider that results in injury or harm to a patient.
Medical errors can range from minor to severe and
impose significant costs to the healthcare system.

Med-E.R.R.S.   http://www.med-errs.com

Medication Compliance Institution (MCI)
http://medicationcomplianceinstitute.org

National Council on Patient Information and Education
(NCPIE)   http://www.talkaboutrx.org

National Coordinating Council for Medication Error Reporting
and Prevention (NCCMERP)   http://www.nccmerp.org

See also Health Outcomes; Medical Malpractice; Patient Safety;
Quality of Healthcare

137. Medical Group Practice

Medical group practice is a group of physicians who share
the same office and/or other healthcare resources. About
half of all physician practices are group practices.

Medical Group Management Association (MGMA)
http://www.mgma.com

See also Physicians

138. Medical Malpractice

Medical malpractice is an act of omission or commission by a healthcare provider that does not conform
with the standard of care and results in harm or injury
to a patient.

Anerican Association for Justice, formerly the American Trial
Lawyers of America
http://www.justice.org

American Tort Reform Association (ATRA)
http://www.atra.org

Health Law Section, American Bar Association (ABA)
http://www.abanet.org/health

See also Clinical Practice Guidelines; Health Law; Medical
Errors; Patient Safety

139. Medical Practice Variations

Medical practice variations are differences in healthcare utilization and spending across geographic areas.

Dartmouth Atlas of Healthcare   http://www.dartmouthatlas.org

See also Clinical Practice Guidelines; Geographic Information
Systems (GIS): Quality of Healthcare

140. Medical Records

Medical records include the official documentation of
a patient's medical history and care and they are traditionally maintained by the healthcare provider.

American Academy of Professional Coders (AAPC)
http://www.aapc.com

American Health Information Management Association
(AHIMA)   http://www.ahima.org

Medical Records Institute (MRI)   http://www.medrecinst.com

See also Disease and Procedure Classifications; Health Insurance
Portability and Accountability Act of 1996 (HIPAA);
Informatics; Medical Billing

141. Medical Residents and Interns

Medical residents and interns include physicians who
have completed medical school but are undergoing further
training under the supervision of a fully licensed physician. Residencies allow physicians to gain a more in-depth
experience within a particular specialty of medicine.

American Medical Student Association (AMSA)
http://www.amsa.org

National Association of Residents and Interns (NARI)
http://www.nari-assn.com

National Resident Matching Program (NRMP)
http://www.nrmp.org

Resident Web   http://www.residentweb.com

See also Hospitals; Physicians

142. Medical Sociology

Medical sociology is the study of individuals and
groups within the social context of health, illness, and

healthcare. Medical sociology draws upon a number of different perspectives to understand health and healthcare within the context of sociology.

American Sociological Association (ASA)
    http://www.asanet.org

British Sociological Association
    http://www.britsoc.co.uk/medsoc

Medical Sociology Section of the American Sociological Association (ASA)
    http://dept.kent.edu/sociology/asamedsoc

SocioSite: Sociology of Health   http://www.sociosite.net

See also Disease and Procedure Classifications; Health

143. Medical Technologists

Medical technologists are healthcare professionals who perform clinical tests on bodily fluids and other specimens for diagnostic purposes. Medical technologists work in a variety of settings, including hospitals, physician's offices, and laboratories.

American Medical Technologists (AMT)
    http://www.amt1.com

American Registry of Radiologic Technologists (ARRT)
    http://www.arrt.org

American Society of Radiologic Technologists (ASRT)
    http://www.asrt.org

Association of Surgical Technologists (AST)
    http://www.ast.org

See also Allied Health; Clinical Laboratories; Medical Tests and Diagnostics

144. Medical Tests and Diagnostics

Medical tests and diagnostics are clinical tests that are performed to aid in the diagnosis of a health condition.

Lab Tests Online   http://www.labtestsonline.org

Tests and Procedures, MedlinePlus
    http://www.nlm.nih.gov/medlineplus/tutorial.html

See also Allied Health; Clinical Laboratories; Medical Technologists

145. Medicare

Medicare is a federal health insurance program for those 65 years of age or older and other defined benefits groups. The Centers for Medicare and Medicaid Services (CMS) administer the Medicare program.

Centers for Medicare and Medicaid Services (CMS)
    http://www.cms.hhs.gov

Medicare Rights Center   http://www.medicarerights.org

See also Centers for Medicare and Medicaid Services (CMS); Health Insurance; Hospitals

146. Medicare Prescription Drug Coverage (Medicare Part D)

The Medicare prescription drug coverage program is a program that allows Medicare beneficiaries to receive coverage for their prescription drugs regardless of income, health status, or type of prescription drugs used. This program covers both brand name and generic drugs.

Centers for Medicare and Medicaid Services (CMS)
    http://www.cms.hhs.gov/PrescriptionDrugCovGenIn

MedicareAide.Com   http://www.medicareaide.com/index.html

Medicare.gov
    http://www.medicare.gov/medicarereform/drugbenefit.asp

My Medicare Matters, The National Council on the Aging   http://www.mymedicarematters.org

Policy and Advocacy, American Academy of Family Physicians (AAFP)   http://www.aafp.org/online/en/home/policy/medicare.html

Resources on the Medicare Prescription Drug Benefit, Kaiser Family Foundation (KFF)
    http://www.kff.org/medicare/rxdrugbenefit.cfm

See also Drugs; Drugs, Prices of; Medicare; Pharmacoeconomics

147. Mental Health

Mental health may be referred to as the level of an individual's cognitive and emotion well-being and the absence of any mental condition. Mental health is needed to ensure proper functioning and quality of life.

American Psychiatric Association   http://www.psych.org

American Psychological Association (APA)
    http://www.apa.org

Depression and Bipolar Support Alliance (DBSA)
http://www.dbsalliance.org

National Alliance for Research on Schizophrenia and
Depression (NARSAD)   http://www.narsad.org

National Alliance for the Mentally Ill   http://www.nami.org

National Association of State Mental Health Program Directors
(NASMHPD)   http://www.nasmhpd.org

National Institute of Mental Health (NIMH)
http://www.nimh.nih.gov

National Mental Health Association (NMHA)
http://www.nmha.org

SAMHSA's National Mental Health Information Center
http://www.mentalhealth.samhsa.gov

World Federation for Mental Health (WFMH)
http://www.wfmh.org

See also Disability; Psychiatric Care

148. Mentally Disabled

Mentally disabled refers to the chronic disability that is
caused by a mental disorder(s) and it may also involve
physical impairment. Mental disability also affects an
individual's ability in daily functioning.

American Association on Mental Retardation (AAMR)
http://www.aamr.org

Association for the Help of Retarded Children (AHRC)
http://www.ahrc.org

See also Disability; Mental Health; Psychiatric Care

149. Migrant Health

Migrant health is concerned with promoting the health
of the Mexican border communities and farmworkers.

Migrant Clinicians Network   http://www.migrantclinician.org

Office of Rural Health Policy, Health Resources and Services
Administration (HRSA)   http://ruralhealth.hrsa.gov

Washington Association of Community and Migrant Health
Centers   http://www.wacmhc.org

See also Hispanic; Public Health; Rural Health

150. Military Health Systems

Military health systems refers to the healthcare systems
that serve the members and reitrees of the military and

their families. The military health system also responds
to natural disasters, humanitarian crises, and military
operations.

Office of the Assistant Secretary of Defense (Health Affairs)
http://www.health.mil

TRICARE, Military Health System   http://www.tricare.mil

See also Federal Government; Veterans Health

151. Minority Health

Minority health is concnered with the health issues of
racial and ethnic minority groups and the elimination
of health disparities.

Alliance of Minority Medical Associations
http://www.allamericanhealth.org

American Public Health Association (APHA)
http://www.apha.org

Asian and Pacific Islander American Health Forum
http://www.apiahf.org

Association of American Indian Physicians
http://www.aaip.org

Association of Asian Pacific Community Health
Organizations   http://www.aapcho.org

Health Professionals for Diversity, Association of American
Medical Colleges   http://www.aamc.org/diversity

National Alliance for Hispanic Health
http://www.hispanichealth.org

National Asian Women's Health Organizations
http://www.nawho.org

National Center on Minority Health and Health Disparities
(NCMHD)   http://www.ncmhd.nih.gov

National Hispanic Medical Association
http://www.nhmamd.org

National Indian Health Board   http://www.nihb.org

National Medical Association   http://www.nmanet.org

National Minority AIDS Council   http://www.nmac.org

National Minority Quality Forum
http://www.nmqf.org

Transcultural Nursing Society   http://www.tcns.org

See also African American Health; Hispanic; Native American
Health; Nursing, Minority Associations

152. National Health Insurance

National health insurance is a universal, single-payer health program. A national health insurance program aims to provide healthcare coverage for everyone.

Physicians for a National Health Program (PNHP)
   http://www.pnhp.org

See also Health Insurance; Health Policy Organizations; Uninsured Individuals

153. National Institutes of Health (NIH)

The National Institutes of Health (NIH) is the premier federal agency that conducts cutting-edge biomedical and health-related research in the United States. Through its institutes and centers, the NIH works to prevent, protect, diagnose, and treat diseases.

General

National Institutes of Health (NIH)   http://www.nih.gov

Director

Office of the Director (OD)   http://www.nih.gov/icd/od

Institutes

National Cancer Institute (NCI)   http://www.cancer.gov

National Eye Institute (NEI)   http://www.nei.nih.gov

National Heart, Lung, and Blood Institute (NHLBI)
   http://www.nhlbi.nih.gov

National Human Genome Research Institute (NHGRI)
   http://www.genome.gov

National Institute of Allergy and Infectious Diseases (NIAID)   http://www3.niaid.nih.gov

National Institute of Arthritis and Musculoskeletal and Skin Diseases (NIAMS)   http://www.niams.nih.gov

National Institute of Biomedical Imaging and Bioengineering (NIBIB)   http://www.nibib.nih.gov

National Institute of Child Health and Human Development (NICHD)   http://www.nichd.nih.gov

National Institute of Dental and Craniofacial Research (NIDCR)   http://www.nidcr.nih.gov

National Institute of Diabetes and Digestive and Kidney Diseases (NIDDK)   http://www2.niddk.nih.gov

National Institute of Environmental Health Sciences (NIEHS)
   http://www.niehs.nih.gov

National Institute of General Medical Sciences (NIGMS)
   http://www.nigms.nih.gov

National Institute of Mental Health (NIMH)
   http://www.nimh.nih.gov

National Institute of Neurological Disorders and Stroke (NINDS)   http://www.ninds.nih.gov

National Institute of Nursing Research (NINR)
   http://www.ninr.nih.gov

National Institute on Aging (NIA)   http://www.nia.nih.gov

National Institute on Alcohol Abuse and Alcoholism (NIAAA)   http://www.niaaa.nih.gov

National Institute on Deafness and Other Communication Disorders (NIDCD)   http://www.nidcd.nih.gov

National Institute on Drug Abuse (NIDA)
   http://www.nida.nih.gov

National Library of Medicine (NLM)   http://www.nlm.nih.gov

Centers

Center for Information Technology (CIT)
   http://www.cit.nih.gov

Center for Scientific Review (CSR)   http://cms.csr.nih.gov

John E. Fogarty International Center (FIC)
   http://www.fic.nih.gov

National Center for Complementary and Alternative Medicine (NCCAM)   http://www.nccam.nih.gov

National Center for Research Resources (NCRR)
   http://www.ncrr.nih.gov

National Center on Minority Health and Health Disparities (NCMHD)   http://www.ncmhd.nih.gov

NIH Clinical Center (CC)   http://clinicalcenter.nih.gov

See also Centers for Disease Control and Prevention (CDC); Federal Government; Public Health

154. Native American Health

Native American health refers to the unique health needs of this group.

American Indian Health, National Library of Medicine (NLM)   http://americanindianhealth.nlm.nih.gov

Indian Health Service (HIS), U.S. Department of Health and Human Services (HHS)   http://www.ihs.gov

Medicare and Medicaid Services for American Indian and Alaska Native, Centers for Medicare and Medicaid Services (CMS)   http://www.cms.hhs.gov/aian

National Council of Urban Indian Health (NCUIH) http://www.ncuih.org

See also Health Disparities; Minority Health; Public Health

155. Nephrology

Nephrology is the medical specialty that focuses on diseases and conditions of the kidney.

American Society of Nephrology (ASN) http://www.asn-online.org

Kidney Transplant/Dialysis Association (KT/DA) http://www.ktda.org

National Institute of Diabetes and Digestive and Kidney Diseases (NIDDK)   http://www2.niddk.nih.gov

Renal Physicians Association   http://www.renalmd.org

See also Chronic Diseases; Kidney Diseases

156. Neurological Disorders

Neurological disorders are disorders of the brain and nervous system. Many organizations are dedicated to researching, advocating, and developing policies related to neurological disorders.

American Association of Neuromuscular and Electrodiagnostic Medicine (AANEM)   http://www.aanem.net

American Parkinson Disease Association (APDA) http://www.apdaparkinson.org

Amyotrophic Lateral Sclerosis Association (ALSA) http://www.alsa.org

Children and Adults with Attention Deficit/Hyperactivity Disorders (CHADD)   http://www.chadd.org

Huntington's Disease Society of America (NDSA) http://www.hdsa.org

Multiple Sclerosis Foundation (MSF)   http://www.msfocus.org

Muscular Dystrophy Association (MDA) http://www.mdausa.org

National Institute of Neurological Disorders and Stroke (NINDS)   http://www.ninds.nih.gov

National Multiple Sclerosis Society (NMSS) http://www.nmss.org

National Parkinson Foundation (NPF) http://www.parkinson.org

Parkinson's Disease Foundation (PDF)   http://www.pdf.org

Tourette Syndrome Association (TSA)   http://www.tsa-usa.org

See also Disability; National Institutes of Health (NIH); Neurology; Stroke

157. Neurology

Neurology is the specialty of medicine that deals with the study of the brain and nervous system.

American Academy of Neurology (AAN)   http://www.aan.com

See also Physicians; Neurological Disorders; Neurosurgery; Spinal Disorders and Injuries

158. Neurosurgery

Neurosurgery is the discipline of surgery that focuses on treating disorders of the central and peripheral nervous system and spinal cord. The field of neurosurgery has undergone many advancements with the development of new medical technologies.

American Association of Neurological Surgeons (AANS) http://www.aans.org

See also Neurological Disorders; Neurology; Surgery and Surgeons

159. News Services

News services provide information to the public on recent medical breakthroughs, discoveries, and research findings. News services play an important part in disseminating the latest knowledge.

American Medical News (AMA) http://www.ama-assn.org/amednews

CNN Health   http://www.cnn.com/health/library

MedlinePlus: Health News http://www.nlm.nih.gov/medlineplus/newsbydate.html

Reuters Health Information Services http://www.reutershealth.com

See also Health Services Research Journals; Journals, Medical

160. Nuclear Medicine

Nuclear medicine is the field of medicine and medical imaging that uses nuclear compounds to aide in diagnosis and treatment.

Society of Nuclear Medicine (SNM)   http://www.snm.org

See also Cancer; Medical Tests and Diagnostics; Oncology

161. Nurse Practitioners

Nurse practitioners are registered nurses with advanced training who provide a range of healthcare services. Nurse practitioners are able to diagnose and treat common and some complicated conditions.

American Academy of Nurse Practitioners (AANP)
   http://www.aanp.org

See also Nursing; Rural Health

162. Nursing

Nursing is a healthcare profession that advocates and provides care to individuals, families, and communities. Nursing has been described as an art and science that promotes the quality of life of individuals from birth until death.

American Nurses Association (ANA)
   http://www.nursingworld.org

National League for Nursing (NLN)   http://www.nln.org

See also Nurse Practitioners; Nursing, Collegiate Organizations; Nursing Specialties

163. Nursing, Collegiate Organizations

Collegiate organizations of nursing are organizations that represent the concerns of nursing professionals.

American Association of Colleges of Nursing
   http://www.aacn.nche.edu

American College of Nurse Practitioners
   http://www.acnpweb.org

Canadian Nurses Association (CNA)   http://www.cna-nurses.ca

Commission on Graduates of Foreign Nursing Schools
   (CGFNS International)   http://www.cgfns.org

National Student Nurses' Association, Inc.   http://www.nsna.org

See also Nursing; Nursing, Minority Associations of; Nursing Specialties

164. Nursing, Minority Associations of

Minority associations of nursing are organizations of racial and ethnic nursing professionals.

Aboriginal Nurses Association of Canada   http://www.anac.on.ca

American Assembly for Men in Nursing   http://www.aamn.org

Asian and Pacific Islander Nurses Association
   http://www.aapina.org

Filipino Nurses Online   http://www.filipinonurses.net

National Alaska Native/American Indian Nurses Association
   http://www.nanainanurses.org/

National Association of Hispanic Nurses
   http://www.thehispanicnurses.org

National Black Nurses Association, Inc.   http://www.nbna.org

National Coalition of Ethnic Minority Nurse Association
   http://www.ncemna.org

Philippine Nurses Association of America
   http://www.philippinenursesaa.org

See also Minority Health; Nursing; Nursing, Collegiate Organizations

165. Nursing Homes

Nursing homes are facilities that provide constant nursing care to inviduals who have deficits with activities of daily living. Residents of nursing homes typically include the elderly and disabled.

American College of Health Care Administrators (ACHCA)
   http://www.achca.org

American Association of Homes and Services for the Aging
   (AAHSA) (it represents not-for-profit nursing homes)
   http://www.aahsa.org

American Health Care Association (AHCA) (It represents both
   not-for-profit and for-profit nursing homes.)
   http://www.ahcancal.org

American Medical Directors Association (AMDA)
   http://www.amda.com

Catholic Health Association of the United States (CHA)
   http://www.chausa.org

National Ministries (This organization was formerly the
   American Baptist Homes and Hospitals Association)
   http://www.nationalministries.org

Nursing Home Compare, Centers for Medicare and Medicaid
   Services (CMS)
   http://www.medicare.gov/NHCompare/home.asp

See also Aging; Alzheimer's Disease; Gerontology; Hospice and Palliative Care; Medicaid

166. Nursing Research

Nursing research is focused on research that aims to promote and improve the health of individuals, families, and communities.

National Institute of Nursing Research (NINR)
http://www.ninr.nih.gov

See also National Institutes of Health (NIH); Nursing; Nursing Specialities

167. Nursing Specialties

Nursing specialties include the many different focus areas within nursing that provide specialized care.

American Association of Critical Care Nurses (AACN)
http://www.aacn.org

American Association of Nurse Anesthetists (AANA)
http://www.aana.org

American Association of Occupational Health Nurses (AAOHN)   http://www.aaohn.org

American College of Nurse Midwives (ACNM)
http://www.midwife.org

American Organization of Nurse Executives (AONE)
http://www.aone.org

Association of PeriOperative Registered Nurses (AORN)
http://www.aorn.org

Association of Rehabilitation Nurses (ARN)
http://www.rehabnurse.org

Association of Women's Health, Obstetrics and Neonatal Nurses (AWHONN)   http://www.awhonn.org

Hospice and Palliative Nurses Association (HPNA)
http://www.hpna.org

National Association of Neonatal Nurses (NANN)
http://www.nann.org

National Association of Orthopaedic Nurses (NAON)
http://www.orthonurse.org

National Association of School Nurses (NASN)
http://www.nasn.org

Oncology Nursing Society (ONS)   http://www.ons.org

Pediatric Nursing Certification Board
http://www.pncb.org

See also Nurse Practitioners; Nursing; Nursing Research

168. Obstetrics and Gynecology

Obstretrics and gynecology is the specialty of medicine that focuses on a women's reproductive organs. This specialty provides care to both pregnant and non-pregnant women.

American Board of Obstetrics and Gynecology (ABOG)
http://www.abog.org

American College of Obstetricians and Gynecologists (ACOG)
http://www.acog.org

American College of Osteopathic Obstetricians and Gynecologists (ACOOG)   http://www.acoog.org

See also Childbirth; Child Development and Health; Physicians

169. Occupational Medicine

Occupational medicine is an interdisciplinary specialty of medicine that is concerned with the health, safety, and welfare of individuals at their work site or place of employment.

American College of Occupational and Environmental Medicine (ACOEM)   http://www.acoem.org

American Industrial Hygiene Association (AIHA)
http://www.aiha.org

American Occupational Therapy Foundation (AOTF)
http://www.aotf.org

Canadian Centre for Occupational Health and Safety (CCOHS)
http://www.ccohs.ca

Institute for Work and Health (Canada)
http://www.iwh.on.ca

National Institute for Occupational Safety and Health (NIOSH) Information Inquiry Service
http://www.cdc.gov/niosh/inquiry.html

See also Injury; Physicians; Workers' Compensation

170. Oncology

Oncology is the specialty of medicine that focuses on cancers. The field of oncology deals with the screening, diagnosis, treatment, and follow-up of cancer patients as well as palliative care.

American Society of Clinical Oncology (ASCO)
http://www.asco.org

See also Cancer

171. Ophthalmology

Opthalmology is the medical specialty that is concerned with conditions of the eye as well as surgical procedures dealing with the visual pathway that includes the eye, brain, and areas surrounding the eye.

American Academy of Ophthalmology (AAO)
   http://www.aao.org

American Board of Ophthalmology (ABO)
   http://www.abop.org

American Society of Cataract and Refractive Surgery (ASCRS)   http://www.ascrs.org

Association for Research in Vision and Opthalmology
   http://www.arvo.org

Joint Commission on Allied Health Personnel in Opthalmology (JCAHPO)   http://www.jcahpo.org

See also Blind and Visually Impaired; Eye Diseases; Optometry; Physicians

172. Optometry

Optometry is a healthcare profession that focuses on the eye and surrounding structures, in addition to vision and visual processing.

American Academy of Optometry (AAO)
   http://www.aaopt.org

American Optometric Association (AOA)
   http://www.aoanet.org

National Board of Examiners in Optometry (NBEO)
   http://www.optometry.org

National Optometric Association (NOA)
   http://www.natoptassoc.org/user/default.php

See also Blind and Visually Impaired; Eye Diseases; Ophthalmology

173. Oral Health

Oral health is concerned with the health of the oral cavitiy including the teeth, gums, jawbone, and surrounding tissues. Oral health is necessary for overall good health.

National Institute of Dental and Craniofacial Research
   http://www.nidcr.nih.gov

National Maternal and Child Oral Health Resource Center
   http://www.mchoralhealth.org

See also Dentistry; Dentistry, Public Health; Public Health

174. Orthopedics

Orthopedics is the surgical specialty that focuses on conditions and injuries of the musculoskeletal system.

American Academy of Orthopaedic Surgeons (AAOS)
   http://www.aaos.org

American Orthopaedic Association (AOA)
   http://www.aoassn.org

American Orthopaedic Foot and Ankle Society (AOFAS)
   http://www.aofas.org

Council on Chiropractic Orthopedics (CCO)
   http://www.ccodc.org

Health Volunteers Overseas (OO)   http://www.hvousa.org

See also Chiropractic Care; Injury; Physical Medicine and Rehabilitation

175. Osteopathic Medicine

Osteopathic medicine includes a branch of medicine that trains allopathic physicians. Osteopathic medicine focuses on osteopathic manipulative medicine and alternative medical therapies.

American Academy of Osteopathy (AAO)
   http://www.academyofosteopathy.org

American Association of Colleges of Osteopathic Medicine (AACOM)   http://www.aacom.org

American College of Osteopathic Family Physicians (ACOFP)
   http://www.acofp.org

American Osteopathic Association (AOA)
   http://www.osteopathic.org

See also Hospitals; Physicians

176. Osteoporosis

Osteoporosis is a disease of the bone where individuals have decreased bone mineral density that leads to a greater risk of fractures.

National Institutes of Health Osteoporosis and Related Bone Diseases   National Resource Center
   http://www.osteo.org

National Osteoporosis Foundation (NOF)   http://www.nof.org

See also Public Health; Women's Health Issues

177. Overweight and Obesity

Overweight and obesity is a condition when an individual gains excess body fat. This condition may cause an individual to have negative health consequences and be at greater risk for other health conditions.

American Society for Bariatric Surgery (ASBS)
http://www.asbs.org

Association for the Study of Obesity (ASO)
http://www.aso.org.uk

See also Diabetes; Diet and Nutrition; Eating Disorders; Fitness and Exercise

178. Pain

Pain management is the medical discipline that is concerned with relieving pain through a variety of techniques including pharmacologic, non-pharmacologic, and psychologic interventions.

American Academy of Pain Management
http://www.aapainmanage.org

American Pain Society (APS)   http://www.ampainsoc.org

American Society of Regional Anesthesia and Pain Medicine (ASRA)   http://www.asra.com

Canadian Pain Society (CPS)
http://www.canadianpainsociety.ca

Chronic Pain Association of Canada (CPAC)
http://www.chronicpaincanada.com

International Association for the Study of Pain (IASP)
http://www.iasp-pain.org

See also Health Outcomes; Hospice and Palliative Care; Quality of Healthcare

179. Patient Advocacy

Patient advocacy refers to acting on behalf of patients to protect their rights and assist in obtaining needed services and information. Patient advocacy generally involves liaising between the patient and healthcare provider.

Patient Care Partnership, American Hospital Association (AHA)
http://www.aha.org/aha/issues/Communicating-With-Patients/index.html

See also Health Law; Health Literacy; Medical Errors; Patient Safety

180. Patient Safety

Patient safety is the discipline that deals with reporting, analyzing, and preventing medical errors. Patient safety initiatives are increasing their recognition of the number of medical errors that occur each year.

Canadian Patient Safety Institute
http://www.patientsafetyinstitute.ca

Center for the Advancement of Patient Safety, U.S. Pharmacopeia   http://www.usp.org

Communicating Health Care   http://www.geriamori.com

Consumers Advancing Patient Safety
http://www.patientsafety.org

Doctors in Touch   http://www.doctorsintouch.com

Emergency Medicine Patient Safety Foundation
http://www.empsf.org

FDA Patient Safety News   http://www.accessdata.fda.gov/scripts/cdrh/cfdocs/psn/index.cfm

Institute for Healthcare Improvement   http://www.ihi.org

Institute for Safe Medication Practices (ISMP)
http://www.ismp.org

Joint Commission International, Patient Safety
http://www.jointcommission.org/PatientSafety

National Patient Safety Foundation (NPSF)   http://www.npsf.org

National Safety Council (NSC)   http://www.nsc.org

Partnership for Patient Safety   http://www.p4ps.org

Patient Safety and Quality Healthcare   http://www.psqh.com

Patient Safety First, Association of periOperative Registered Nurses (AORN)   http://www.aorn.org/AboutAORN/WhoWeAre/PatientSafetyFirst

Patient Safety Network, Agency for Healthcare Research and Quality (AHRQ)   http://psnet.ahrq.gov

Premier Patient Safety Institute   http://www.premierinc.com

VA National Center for Patient Safety
http://www.patientsafety.gov

Voice for Patients   http://www.voice4patients.com

World Alliance for Patient Safety, World Health Organization (WHO)   http://www.who.int/patientsafety/en

See also Health Literacy; Medical Errors; Medical Malpractice; Quality of Healthcare

181. Pathology

Pathology is the specialty of medicine that focuses on the diagnosis of disease by examining whole bodies, bodily fluids, organs, and tissues.

American Society for Clinical Pathology (ASCP)
    http://www.ascp.org

College of American Pathologists (CAP)   http://www.cap.org

International Academy of Pathology (IAP)
    http://iaphomepage.org

See also Clinical Laboratories; Hospitals; Medical Tests and
    Diagnostics; Physicians

182. Pediatrics

Pediatrics is the medical specialty that provides medical care to infants, children, and adolescents.

American Academy of Pediatrics (AAP)   http://www.aap.org

See also Child Development and Health; Immunization and
    Vaccination; Prevention and Health Promotion

183. Pharmaceutical Companies, Association of

The association of pharmaceutical companies includes a group that represents the interests of pharmaceutical manufacturers and biotechnology companies.

Pharmaceutical Research and Manufacturers of America
    (PHRMA)   http://www.phrma.org

See also Drugs; Drugs, Prices of; Pharmaceutical Companies,
    List of

184. Pharmaceutical Companies, List of

The list of pharmaceutical companies includes a compilation of pharmaceutical manufacturers who produce medicines and therapies.

3M Pharmaceuticals   http://www.mmm.com

Abbott   http://www.abbott.com

Amgen, Inc.   http://www.amgen.com

Amylin Pharmaceuticals, Inc.   http://www.amylin.com

Astellas US LLC   http://www.astellas.com/en

AstraZeneca LP   http://www.astrazeneca.com

Baxter   http://www.baxter.com

Bayer Healthcare Pharmaceuticals   http://www.pharma.bayer
    .com/scripts/pages/en/index.php

Berlex Laboratories, Inc.   http://www.berlex.bayerhealthcare.com

Boehringer Ingelheim Pharmaceuticals, Inc.
    http://www.boehringer-ingelheim.com

Bristol-Myers Squibb Company
    http://www.bms.com

Celgene Corporation   http://www.celgene.com

Cephalon, Inc.   http://www.cephalon.com

Daiichi Sankyo, Inc.   http://www.sankopharma.com

Eli Lilly and Company   http://www.lilly.com

Genzyme Corporation   http://www.genzyme.com

GlaxoSmithKline   http://www.gsk.com

Hoffman-La Roche, Inc.   http://www.rocheusa.com

Johnson & Johnson   http://www.jnj.com

Merck & Company, Inc.   http://www.merck.com

Millennium Pharmaceuticals, Inc.   http://www.millennium.com

Novartis Corporation   http://www.novartis.com

Organon USA Inc.   http://www.schering-plough.com

Otsuka America, Inc.   http://www.otsuka-us.com

Pfizer, Inc.   http://www.pfizer.com/main

Procter & Gamble Co.   http://www.pgpharma.com/index.shtml

Purdue Pharma L.P.   http://www.purduepharma.com

Sanofi-Aventis U.S.
    http://www.sanofi-aventis.us/live/us/en/index.jsp

Schering-Plough Corporation
    http://www.schering-plough.com

Schwarz Pharma, Inc.   http://www.schwarzpharma.com

Sepracor, Inc.   http://www.sepracor.com

Serono, Inc.   http://www.merckserono.net

Solvay Pharmaceuticals, Inc.
    http://www.solvaypharmaceuticals-us.com

Valeant Pharmaceuticals International
    http://www.valeant.com

Wyeth   http://www.wyeth.com

See also Drugs; Pharmacists and Pharmacy; Pharmacoeconomics

185. Pharmaceuticals

See Drugs

186. Pharmacists and Pharmacy

Pharmacists are healthcare professionals who dispense medication ordered by a healthcare provider and also counsel patients on the proper use and adverse effects. Pharmacy is the healthcare profession of pharmacists that is concerned with the safe and effective use of medications.

Academy of Managed Care Pharmacy (AMCP)
    http://www.amcp.org

American Association of Colleges of Pharmacy (AACP)
    http://www.aacp.org

American College of Clinical Pharmacy (ACCP)
    http://www.accp.com

American Pharmacists Association (APA)
    http://www.pharmacist.com

American Society of Consultant Pharmacists (ASCP)
    http://www.ascp.com

American Society of Health-System Pharmacists (ASHP)
    http://www.ashp.org

National Association of Boards of Pharmacy (NABP)
    http://www.nabp.net

National Pharmaceutical Association (NPhA)
    http://www.npha.net

Society of Infectious Diseases Pharmacists (SIDP)
    http://www.sidp.org

See also Drugs; Drugs, Generic; Pharmacoeconomics

187. Pharmacoeconomics

Pharmacoeconomics is a discipline that compares the relative value of one pharmaceutical agent to another by examining the costs and effects.

International Society for Pharmacoeconomics and Outcomes Research (ISPOR)   http://www.ispor.org

Society for Medical Decision Making (SMDM)
    http://www.smdm.org

See also Drugs; Drugs, Generic; Drugs, Prices of; Pharmacists and Pharmacy

188. Physical Medicine and Rehabilitation

Physical medicine and rehabilition is the field of medicine that is focused on restoring the physical functioning of individuals who have a disability through the use of medicines, exercises, assistive devices and equipment, and other approaches.

American Board of Physical Medicine and Rehabilitation (ABPMR)   http://www.abpmr.org

American Congress of Rehabilitation Medicine (ACRM)
    http://www.acrm.org

Commission on Accreditation of Rehabilitation Facilities (CARF)   http://www.carf.org

Institute for Rehabilitation and Research, The (TIRR)
    http://www.tirr.org

International Society of Physical Medicine and Rehabilitation (ISPRM)   http://www.isprm.org

National Rehabilitation Association (NRA)
    http://www.nationalrehab.org

National Rehabilitation Counseling Association (NRCA)
    http://www.nrca-net.org

National Rehabilitation Information Center
    http://www.naric.com

See also Chiropractic Care; Chronic Diseases; Disability

189. Physicians

Physicians are medical doctors who work to promote and maintain health through the diagnosis and treatment of injuries and disease.

American Academy of Family Physicians (AAFP)
    http://www.aafp.org

American College of Physicians (ACP)
    http://www.acponline.org

American Medical Association (AMA)
    http://www.ama-assn.org

American Medical Students Association (AMSA)
    http://www.amsa.org

American Osteopathic Association (AOA)
    http://www.osteopathic.org

National Medical Association (NMA)
    http://www.nmanet.org

See also Academic Medical Centers; Hospitals; Osteopathic Medicine; Surgery and Surgeons

190. Population Estimates

Population estimates include data on populations and demographic characteristics.

U.S. Census Bureau Population Estimates Data Sets
    http://www.census.gov/popest/datasets.html

See also Federal Government; Health Surveys; Vital Statistics

191. Preferred Provider Organizations (PPO)

Preferred provider organizations are a type of managed care plan where physicians, hospitals, and other healthcare providers are contracted to provide care to a group of patients at a reduced rate. Preferred provider organizations may also allow patients to use healthcare providers outside of the network but at a higher out-of-pocket cost.

American Association of Preferred Provider Organizations (AAPPO)   http://www.aappo.org

See also Health Insurance; Managed Care

192. Prevention and Health Promotion

Prevention and health promotion works to improve the health of individuals by preventing the occurrence of disease and injury.

American Board of Preventive Medicine (ABPM) http://www.abprevmed.org

American College of Preventive Medicine (ACPM) http://www.acpm.org

Canadian Task Force on Preventive Health Care http://www.ctfphc.org

CDC National Prevention Information Network (CDC NPIN)   http://www.cdcnpin.org

Center for Adolescent Health, School of Public Health, Johns Hopkins University   http://www.jhsph.edu/adolescenthealth

Office of Disease Prevention and Health Promotion http://odphp.osophs.dhhs.gov

Partnership for Prevention   http://www.prevent.org

See also Diet and Nutrition; Fitness and Exercise; Immunization and Vaccination; Public Health

193. Psychiatric Care

Psychiatric care works to treat and provide for patients who have mental health conditions.

American Academy of Child and Adolescent Psychiatry (AACAP) http://www.aacap.org

American Association for Geriatric Psychiatry (AAGP) http://www.aagpgpa.org

National Association of Psychiatric Health Systems http://www.naphs.org

See also Mental Health

194. Public Health

Public health is the discipline that works to promote the health and extend the lives of populations through the prevention and treatment of disease.

American Public Health Association (APHA) http://www.apha.org

Association of State and Territorial Dental Directors (ASTDD)   http://www.astdd.org

Association of State and Territorial Health Officials (ASTHO)   http://www.astho.org

Canadian Public Health Association (CPHA) http://www.cpha.ca

European Public Health Association (EUPHA) http://www.eupha.org

National Association of City and County Health Officials (NACCHO)   http://www.naccho.org

Pan American Health Organization (PAHO) http://www.paho.org

Public Health Association of Australia (PHAA) http://www.phaa.net.au

Public Health Agency of Canada http://www.phac-aspc.gc.ca/chn-rcs/index-eng.php

United Kingdom Public Health Association (UKPHA) http://www.ukpha.org.uk

World Health Organization (WHO) http://www.who.int

See also Centers for Disease Control and Prevention (CDC); Environmental Health Epidemiology; World Health Organization (WHO)

195. Public Health, Associations of Schools of

The list of associations of schools of public health includes organizations that represent schools and programs of public health.

Association of Schools of Public Health (ASPH) http://www.asph.org

Council on Education for Public Health (CEPH) http://www.ceph.org

Society of Public Health Education   http://www.sophe.org

See also Public Health; Public Health, Schools of

196. Public Health, Schools of

Schools of Public Health conduct research and provide education and training for students to enter a professional career in public health that leads to a master's or doctoral degree.

Alabama

University of Alabama at Birmingham School of Public Health, Birmingham, AL   http://www.soph.uab.edu

Arizona

University of Arizona Mel and Enid Zuckerman College of Public Health, Tucson, AZ http://www.publichealth.arizona.edu

Arkansas

University of Arkansas for Medical Sciences Fay W. Boozman College of Public Health, Little Rock, AR http://www.uams.edu/coph

California

Loma Linda University School of Public Health, Loma Linda, CA   http://www.llu.edu/llu/sph

San Diego State University Graduate School of Public Health, San Diego, CA   http://publichealth.sdsu.edu

University of California at Berkeley School of Public Health, Berkeley, CA   http://sph.berkeley.edu

University of California at Los Angeles School of Public Health, Los Angeles, CA   http://www.ph.ucla.edu

Connecticut

University of Connecticut Graduate Program in Public Health, Farmington, CT   http://grad.uchc.edu

Yale School of Public Health, New Haven, CT http://publichealth.yale.edu

District of Columbia

George Washington University School of Public Health and Health Services, Washington, DC http://www.gwumc.edu/sphhs

Florida

Florida International University Robert Stempel School of Public Health, Miami, FL   http://chua2.fiu.edu/SSPH

University of Florida College of Public Health and Health Professions, Gainesville, FL   http://www.phhp.ufl.edu

University of South Florida College of Public Health, Tampa, FL   http://publichealth.usf.edu

Georgia

Emory University Rollins School of Public Health, Atlanta, GA   http://www.sph.emory.edu

University of Georgia College of Public Health, Athens, GA   http://www.publichealth.uga.edu

Illinois

University of Illinois at Chicago School of Public Health, Chicago, IL   http://www.uic.edu/sph/index.shtml

Iowa

University of Iowa College of Public Health, Iowa City, IA http://www.public-health.uiowa.edu

Kentucky

University of Kentucky College of Public Health, Lexington, KY   http://www.mc.uky.edu/publichealth

Louisiana

Louisiana State University Health Sciences Center School of Public Health, New Orleans, LA http://publichealth.lsuhsc.edu

Tulane University School of Public Health and Tropical Medicine, New Orleans, LA   http://www.sph.tulane.edu

Maryland

Johns Hopkins Bloomberg School of Public Health, Baltimore, MD   http://www.jhsph.edu

University of Maryland Baltimore School of Public Health, Baltimore, MD   http://www.sph.umaryland.edu

Massachuetts

Boston University School of Public Health, Boston, MA http://www.bu.edu/sph

Harvard School of Public Health, Boston, MA http://www.hsph.harvard.edu

University of Massachusetts School of Public Health and Health Sciences, Amherst, MA http://www.umass.edu/sphhs/index.html

Michigan

University of Michigan School of Public Health, Ann Arbor,
MI   http://www.sph.umich.edu

Minnosota

University of Minnesota School of Public Health, Minneapolis,
MN   http://www.sph.umn.edu

Missouri

Saint Louis University School of Public Health, St. Louis,
MO   http://publichealth.slu.edu

New Jersey

University of Medicine and Dentistry of New Jersey-School of
Public Health, Piscataway, NJ   http://sph.umdnj.edu

New York

Columbia University Mailman School of Public Health, New
York, NY   http://www.mailman.hs.columbia.edu

New York Medical College School of Public Health, Valhalla,
NY   http://www.nymc.edu/sph

University at Albany SUNY School of Public Health,
Rensselaer, NY   http://www.albany.edu/sph

North Carolina

University of North Carolina at Chapel Hill School of Public
Health, Chapel Hill, NC   http://www.sph.unc.edu

Ohio

Ohio State University School of Public Health, Columbus,
OH   http://sph.osu.edu

Oklahoma

University of Oklahoma College of Public Health, Oklahoma
City, OK   http://www.ouhsc.edu

Pennsylvania

Drexel University School of Public Health,
Philadelphia, PA   http://publichealth.drexel.edu

University of Pittsburgh Graduate School of Public Health,
Pittsburgh, PA   http://www.publichealth.pitt.edu

South Carolina

University of South Carolina Arnold School of Public Health,
Columbia, SC   http://www.sph.sc.edu

Tennesse

University of Louisville School of Public Health and
Information Science, Louisville, TN
http://www.louisville.edu/hsc/sphis

Texas

Texas A&M School of Rural Public Health, Bryan, TX
http://www.srph.tamhsc.edu

University of North Texas Health Science Center School of
Public Health, Fort Worth, TX
http://www.hsc.unt.edu/education/sph

University of Texas School of Public Health, Houston, TX
http://www.sph.uth.tmc.edu

Washington

University of Washington School of Public Health and
Community Medicine, Seattle, WA
http://sphcm.washington.edu

See also Public Health; Public Health, State Departments of

197. Public Health, State Departments of

State departments of public health provide a vital function to keep residents of states healthy through health
promotion and disease prevention activities.

Alabama Department of Public Health   http://www.adph.org

Alaska Department of Health and Social Services
http://www.hss.state.ak.us

Arkansas Department of Health
http://www.healthyarkansas.com

Arizona Department of Health Services
http://www.hs.state.az.us

California Department of Health Services
http://www.dhs.ca.gov

Colorado Department of Public Health and Environment
http://www.cdphe.state.co.us/cdphehom.asp

Connecticut Department of Health
http://www.dph.state.ct.us

District of Columbia Department of Health
http://www.dchealth.dc.gov/doh/site/default.asp

Florida Department of Health   http://www.doh.state.fl.us

Georgia Division of Public Health   http://health.state.ga.us

Hawaii Department of Health   http://www.hawaii.gov/health

Idaho Department of Health and Welfare
http://www.healthandwelfare.idaho.gov

Illinois Department of Public Health
http://www.idph.state.il.us

Indiana State Department of Health   http://www.in.gov/isdh

Iowa Department of Health   http://www.idph.state.ia.us

Kansas Department of Health and Environment
http://www.kdheks.gov

Kentucky Department of Public Health
http://www.publichealth.state.ky.us

Louisiana Department of Health and Hospitals, Office of Public
Health   http://www.oph.dhh.state.la.us

Maryland Department of Health and Mental Hygiene
http://www.dhmh.state.md.us

Massachusetts Department of Health
http://www.state.ma.us/dph.dphhome.htm

Michigan Department of Public Health
http://www.michigan.gov/mdch

Minnesota Department of Public Health
http://www.health.state.mn.us

Mississippi Department of Health
http://www.msdh.state.ms.us/msdhsite/index.cfm

Missouri Department of Health   http://www.dhss.mo.gov

Montana Department of Health   http://www.dphhs.state.mt.us

Nebraska Department of Health   http://www.hhs.state.ne.us

Nevada State Health Division   http://www.health2k.state.nv.us

New Hampshire Department of Health and Human Services
http://www.dhhs.state.nh.us

New Jersey Department of Health and Senior Services
http://www.state.nj.us/health

New Mexico Department of Health
http://www.health.state.nm.us

New York State Department of Health
http://www.health.state.ny.us

North Carolina Department of Public Health
http://www.dhhs.state.nc.us/dph

North Dakota Department of Health
http://www.health.state.nd.us

Ohio Department of Health   http://www.odh.state.oh.us

Oklahoma State Department of Health
http://www.health.state.ok.us

Oregon Department of Human Resources
http://www.ohd.hr.state.or.us

Pennsylvania Department of Health
http://www.health.state.pa.us

Rhode Island Department of Health
http://www.health.state.ri.us

South Carolina Department of Health and Environmental
Control   http://www.dhhs.state.sc.us

South Dakota Department of Health
http://www.state.sd.us/doh

Tennessee Department of Health   http://www.state.tn.us

Texas Department of Health   http://www.dshs.state.tx.us

Utah Department of Health   http://www.health.utah.gov

Vermont Department of Health
http://healthvermont.gov

Virginia Department of Health   http://www.vdh.state.va.us

Washington State Department of Health
http://www.doh.wa.gov

Wisconsin Department of Health and Family Services
http://www.dhfs.state.wi.us

Wyoming Department of Health   http://wdh.state.wy.us

See also Public Health; State and County Government
Organizations; Vital Statistics

198. Quality Assurance

Quality assurance is the systematic process of ensuring that
healthcare products and services meet certain standards.

American Board of Quality Assurance and Utilization Review
Physicians (ABQAURP)   http://www.abqaurp.org

American Health Quality Association (AHQA)
http://www.ahqa.org

Michigan Quality Council (MQC)
http://www.michiganquality.org

National Association for Healthcare Quality (NAHQ)
http://www.nahq.org

National Committee for Quality Assurance (NCQA) (The
NCQA publishes the Health Plan Employer Data and
Information Set HEDIS)   http://www.ncqa.org

See also Accreditation, Certification, and Licensing; Hospitals;
Medical Malpractice; Quality of Healthcare

199. Quality of Healthcare

Quality of healthcare can have different meanings to different individuals; however, it broadly refers to receiving appropriate care at the right time in the right amount.

Agency for Healthcare Quality and Research (AHRQ)
http://www.ahrq.gov

Bridges to Excellence   http://www.bridgestoexcellence.org

Consumer Coalition for Quality Health Care
http://www.consumers.org

Doctorquality.com   http://www.doctorquality.com

European Society for Quality in Healthcare (ESQH)
http://www.esqh.net

Foundation for Accountability (FACCT)
http://www.markle.org/resources/facct/index.php

Institute for Clinical Systems Improvement (ICSI)
http://www.icsi.org

Institute for Healthcare Improvement (IHI)   http://www.ihi.org

Irish Society for Quality and Safety in Healthcare (ISQSH)
http://www.isqsh.ie

Joint Commission   http://www.jointcommission.org

National Initiative for Children's Healthcare Quality
(NICHQ)   http://www.nichq.org

National Quality Forum (NQF) (NQF was formerly the
National Forum for Health Care Quality Measurement and
Reporting)   http://www.qualityforum.org

National Quality Measures Clearinghouse (NQMC)
http://www.qualitymeasures.ahrq.gov

See also Health Outcomes; Medical Errors; Pain; Patient Safety

200. Randomized Controlled Trials (RCT)

Randomized controlled trials (sometimes called clinical trials) is a type of study that is conducted to evaluate the safety and efficacy of new drugs or interventions.

AIDS Clinical Trials Group (ACTG)   http://www.aactg.org

American Society for Clinical Investigation (ASCI)
http://www.asci-jci.org

Association for the Accreditation of Human Research
Protection Programs (AAHRPP)   http://www.aahrpp.org

Centerwatch Clinical Trials Listing Service
http://www.centerwatch.com

National Institutes of Health (NIH) and National Library of
Medicine (NLM)   http://www.clinicaltrials.gov

Society for Clinical Trials (SCT)   http://www.sctweb.org

See also Clinical Practice Guidelines; Drugs; Epidemiology;
Evidence-Based Medicine (EBM); Health Outcomes

201. Rare Diseases

Rare diseases are conditions that have a low prevalence. Rare diseases may be caused genetically and can be life threatening or chronically disabling in nature.

National Organization for Rare Disorders (NORD)
http://www.rarediseases.org

See also Epidemiology; Genetics; Health Surveys; National
Institutes of Health (NIH)

202. Regulation

Regulations are legal restrictions that are made by the government and they may include sanctions.

Regulatory Affairs Professionals Society (RAPS)   http://raps.org

See also Centers for Medicare and Medicaid Services (CMS);
Certificate of Need (CON); Health Law

203. Rural Health

Rural health involves the study of the needs and delivery of healthcare in rural areas.

National Advisory Committee on Rural Health and Human
Services, Office of Rural Health Policy, Health Resources
and Services Administration (HRSA)   http://ruralcommittee
.hrsa.gov/index.htm

National Association of Rural Health Clinics (NARHC)
http://www.narhc.org

National Center for Farmworker Health (NCFH)
http://www.ncfh.org

National Rural Health Association (NRHA)
http://www.nrharural.org

Nebraska Center for Rural Health Research, University of
Nebraska Medical Center   http://www.unmc.edu/rural

Office of Rural Health Policy, Health Resources and Services
Administration (HRSA)   http://ruralhealth.hrsa.gov

Rural Assistance Center   http://www.raconline.org

Rural Information Center, U.S. Department of
Agriculture   http://www.nal.usda.gov/ric

See also Federal Government; Hospitals; Physicians; Public
Health

204. Safety Net

Healthcare safety net is the healthcare system that provides care for the poor and vulnerable populations.

Healthcare Safety Net Program, Agency for Healthcare Research and Quality (AHRQ)
http://www.ahrq.gov/data/safetynet/netfact.htm

See also Community Health Centers (CHCs); Hospitals; Physicians

205. Self-Help

Self-help is the self-reliability to gain publicly available information or the use of support groups.

American Self-Help Group Clearinghouse
http://www.selfhelpgroups.org

National Mental Health Consumer's Self-Help Clearinghouse (NSHC)   http://www.mhselfhelp.org

See also Diet and Nutrition; Fitness and Exercise; Prevention and Health Promotion

206. Spinal Disorders and Injuries

Spinal disorders and injuries are conditions that affect the spinal cord.

American Paraplegia Society (APS)   http://www.apssci.org

National Spinal Cord Injury Association (NSCIA)
http://www.spinalcord.org

North American Spine Society (NASS)   http://www.spine.org

Spinal Cord Society (SCS)   http://scsus.org

See also Chronic Diseases; Disability; Physical and Rehabilitation Medicine

207. State and County Data Sources

State and county data sources are sources of health and demographic information at the state or county level.

Area Resource File (ARF)   http://www.arfsys.com

Dartmouth Atlas of Health Care
http://www.dartmouthatlas.org

State Health Facts Online
http://www.statehealthfacts.org

See also Health Statistics and Data Sources; Health Surveys; Vital Statistics

208. State and County Government Organizations

State and county government organizations represent groups of state and county-level government employees.

Association of State and Territorial Dental Directors (ASTDD)
http://www.astdd.org

Association of State and Territorial Health Officials (ASTHO)
http://www.astho.org

Information for State Health Policy
http://www2.umdnj.edu/ishppweb/homepage.htm

National Academy for State Health Policy (NASHP)
http://www.nashp.org

National Association of County and City Health Officials (NACCHO)   http://www.naccho.org

National Association of State Budget Officers (NASBO)
http://www.nasbo.org

National Association of State Medicaid Directors
http://www.nasmd.org

National Conference of State Legislatures (NCSL)
http://www.ncsl.org

National Governors Association (NGA)   http://www.nga.org

State Health Facts Online (This website is produced by the Kaiser Family Foundation)
http://www.statehealthfacts.kff.org

Stateline.org (This site is produced by the Pew Center on the States)   http://www.stateline.org

See also Health Statics and Data Sources; Public Health

209. State Children's Health Insurance Program (SCHIP)

The State Children's Health Insurance Program is a federal health program that provides funding to the states to insure families with children that have a modest income but do not qualify for Medicaid.

Centers for Medicare and Medicaid (CMS)
http://www.cms.hhs.gov/home/schip.asp

Medicaid/SCHIP, Henry J. Kaiser Family Foundation (KFF)   http://www.kff.org/medicaid/index.cfm

National Academy for State Health Policy (NASHP)
CHIPCentral.org   http://www.chipcentral.org

National Conference of State Legislatures (NCSL)
http://www.ncsl.org/programs/health/chiphome.htm

National Health Policy Forum (NHPF)   http://www.nhpf
.org/index.cfm?fuseaction=SearchCatalogue&iissueid=3

SCHIP and Public Health, American Public Health Association
(APHA)   http://www.apha.org/advocacy/priorities/schip

State Access to Children's Health Insurance, American
Academy of Pediatrics (AAP)
http://www.aap.org/advocacy/staccess.htm

U.S. Government Info/Resources   http://usgovinfo.about.com/
od/medicarehealthinsurance/a/schip.htm

See also Centers for Medicare and Medicaid Services (CMS);
Child Development and Health; Health Insurance; Medicaid

210. Stroke

Stroke is a condition when the blood flow to the brain
is disrupted either because of a blockage or hemorrhage of the blood vessels. Stroke can result in the loss
of brain function and paralysis of the body.

American Stroke Association (ASA)
http://www.strokeassociation.org

Division for Heart Disease and Stroke Prevention, Centers for
Disease Control and Prevention (CDC)
http://www.cdc.gov/DHDSP

The Internet Stroke Center, Washington University, St. Louis,
MO   http://www.strokecenter.org

National Institute of Neurological Disorders and Stroke
(NINDS)   http://www.ninds.nih.gov

National Stroke Association (NSA)   http://www.stroke.org

The Stroke Association   http://www.stroke.org.uk

See also Aging; Disability; Chronic Diseases; Hypertension;
Physical Medicine and Rehabilitation

211. Substance Abuse

Substance abuse is the overuse or dependence on a drug
or chemical that results in negative physical or mental
health consequences that may affect the welfare of others. Substance abuse can result in drug addiction and
physiological or behavioral problems.

American Society of Addiction Medicine (ASAM)
http://www.asam.org

Association for Addiction Professionals (NAADAC) (The
association was formerly the National Association of
Alcoholism and Drug Abuse Counselors)
http://www.naadac.org

Center for Substance Abuse Prevention (CSAP)
http://www.prevention.samhsa.gov

National Clearinghouse for Alcohol and Drug Information
(NCADI)   http://www.health.org

National Institute on Drug Abuse   http://www.nida.nih.gov

See also Alcoholism; Federal Government; Public Health;
Tobacco Use

212. Surgery and Surgeons

Surgery is a specialty of medicine that uses both manual
and invasive techniques to treat or explore disease or
injuries to the body, help the body to improve in its
form or function, and other reasons. Surgeons are
healthcare providers who perform surgeries.

American College of Surgeons (ACS)   http://www.facs.org

Accociation for Academic Surgery (AAS)   http://www.aasurg.org

International College of Surgeons (ICS)   http://www.icsglobal.org

Tests and Procedures, MedlinePlus
http://www.nlm.nih.gov/medlineplus/tutorial.html

YourSurgery   http://www.yoursurgery.com

See also Ambulatory Surgery Centers; Cosmetic and Plastic
Surgery; Neurosurgery; Physicians

213. Technology Assessment

Technology assessment is the examination and evaluation of new technologies.

Agency for Healthcare Research and Quality (AHRQ)
http://www.ahrq.gov

Canadian Agency for Drugs and Technologies in Health
(CADTH)   http://www.cadth.ca

Canadian Medical Devices Conformity Assessment System
http://www.hc-sc.gc.ca/dhp-mps/md-im/qualsys/cmdcas_
scecim_syst_pol-eng.php

ECRI Institute   http://www.ecri.org

NIHR Health Technology Assessment Programme
http://www.inahta.org

National Coordinating Centre for Health Technology
Assessment (NCCHTA)   http://www.hta.nhs.uk

National Information Center on Health Services Research and
Health Care Technology (NICHSR)   http://www.nlm.nih
.gov/nichsr

Swedish Council on Technology Assessment in Health Care
http://www.sbu.se

See also Cost-Benefit and Cost-Effectiveness Analysis; Drugs; Randomized Controlled Trials (RCT)

214. Telemedicine

Telemedicine is the application of clinical practices through the use of network systems such as the telephone, Internet, or other technologies.

American Telemedicine Association (ATA)
http://www.americantelemed.org

Association of Telehealth Service Providers (ATSP)
http://www.atsp.org

Office for the Advancement of Telehealth, Health Resources and Services Administration (HRSA)
http://www.hrsa.gov/telehealth

Telemedicine and Telehealth Resources, Indian Health Service (IHS)   http://www.ihs.gov/NonMedicalPrograms/DFEE/telemed/default.cfm?content=resources_page_1.htm

See also E-Health; Informatics; Information Technology (IT)

215. Tobacco Use

Tobacco use includes the smoking and consumption of tobacco products that may be done as part of recreational drug use.

Action on Smoking and Health (ASH)   http://www.ash.org

American Cancer Society   http://www.cancer.org

American Heart Association   http://www.americanheart.org

American Lung Association   http://www.lungusa.org

Americans for Nonsmokers' Rights Foundation (ANR)
http://www.no-smoke.org

Foundation for a Smoke Free America
http://www.notobacco.org

Office on Smoking and Health, Centers for Disease Control and Prevention (CDC)   http://www.cdc.gov/tobacco

See also Cancer; Lung Diseases; Public Health; Substance Abuse

216. Uninsured Individuals

The uninsured include groups of individuals who do not have any health insurance or who have decreased access to approrpiate healthcare services.

Alliance for Health Reform   http://www.allhealth.org

Association of Clinicians for the Underserved (ACU)
http://www.clinicians.org

Center for Studying Health System Change (HSC)
http://www.hschange.com

Covering the Uninsured   http://www.coveringtheuninsured.org

Economic Research Initiative on the Uninsured (ERIU), University of Michigan, Ann Arbor, MI
http://www.umich.edu/~eriu

Henry J. Kaiser Family Foundation (KFF)   http://www.kff.org

State Access to Children's Health Insurance, American Academy of Pediatrics
http://www.aap.org/advocacy/staccess.htm

Urban Institute   http://www.urban.org

See also Health Disparities; Health Insurance; Healthcare Financial Management; National Health Insurance

217. United Kingdom Healthcare Organizations

The United Kingdom (UK) healthcare organizations include organizations in the UK that are related to health and healthcare.

National Electronic Library for Health   http://www.library.nhs.uk

National Health Service (NHS)   http://www.nhs.uk

National Institute for Clinical Excellence (NICE)
http://www.nice.org.uk

Nuffield Trust for Research and Policy Studies in Health Services   http://www.nuffieldtrust.org.uk

The Stroke Association   http://www.stroke.org.uk

UK Health Informatics Society (UKHIS)   http://ukhis.org.uk

See also International Health Systems; World Health Organization (WHO)

218. Veterans Health

Veterans health includes healthcare programs that are targeted to veterans of the military.

Department of Veterans Affairs (VA)   http://www.va.gov

National Association of State Veterans Homes (NASVH)
http://www.nasvh.org

National Center for Health Promotion and Disease Prevention   http://www.prevention.va.gov

VA National Center for Patient Safety http://www.patientsafety.gov

Veterans Health Administration (VHA) http://www1.va.gov/health

See also Federal Government; Hospitals; Military Health Systems

219. Vital Statistics

Vital statistics are the records of births, deaths, marriages, and divorces.

Birth Data   http://www.cdc.gov/nchs/births.htm

Fetal Deaths   http://www.cdc.gov/nchs/about/major/fetaldth/abfetal.htm

Marriage and Divorce   http://www.cdc.gov/nchs/pressroom/96facts/mardiv.htm

Mortality Data   http://www.cdc.gov/nchs/deaths.htm

National Death Index   http://www.cdc.gov/nchs/ndi.htm

National Vital Statistics System, National Center for Health Statistics (NCHS)   http://www.cdc.gov/nchs/nvss.htm

See also Epidemiology; Public Health; Public Health, State Departments of; State and County Data Sources

220. Women's Health Issues

Women's health represents the unique health needs of women and it works to address the disparities in health between men and women.

Association of Women's Health, Obstetric and Neonatal Nurses (AWHONN)   http://www.awhonn.org

Canadian Women's Health Network (CWHN) http://www.cwhn.ca/indexeng.html

Foundation for Women's Health Research and Development (FORWARD)   http://www.forwarduk.org.uk

Global Alliance for Women's Health (GAWH) http://www.gawh.org

Institute for Women's Policy Research (IWPR) http://www.iwpr.org

International Women's Health Coalition (IWHC) http://www.iwhc.org

National Black Women's Health Imperative http://www.blackwomenshealth.org

National Organization for Women (NOW)   http://www.now.org

National Partnership for Women and Families http://www.nationalpartnership.org

National Program on Women and Aging, The Heller School for Social Policy and Management, Brandeis University, Waltham, MA   http://iasp.brandeis.edu/womenandaging/index.html

National Women's Health Information Center http://www.womenshealth.gov

Society for Women's Health Research (SWHR) http://www.womenshealthresearch.org

Women's and Children's Health Policy Center, School of Public Health, Johns Hopkins University http://www.jhsph.edu/wchpc

Women's Health   http://www.womenshealthlondon.org.uk

See also Arthritis and Rheumatism; Childbirth; Child Development and Health; Chronic Diseases; Osteoporosis; Public Health

221. Workers' Compensation

Workers' compensation is a type of state-based insurance that provides compensation and medical care to employees who are injured working on the job.

American Academy of Disability Evaluating Physicians (AADEP) http://www.aadep.org

Office of Workers' Compensation Programs, U.S. Department of Labor   http://www.dol.gov/esa/owcp_org.htm

See also Health Insurance; Health Law; Injury; Occupational Medicine

222. World Health Organization (WHO)

The World Health Organization, based in Geneva, Switzerland, is an agency of the United Nations and it is the leading authority on international public health.

Headquarters

WHO Headquarters, Geneva, Switzerland http://www.who.int

Regional Offices

WHO Regional Office for Africa (AFRO), Brazzaville, Congo   http://www.afro.who.int

WHO Regional Office for the Americas (AMRO), Pan American Health Organization   http://www.paho.org

WHO Regional Office for the Eastern Mediterranean (EMRO), Alexandria, Egypt   http://www.emro.who.int

WHO Regional Office for Europe (EURO), Copenhagen, Denmark   http://www.euro.who.int

WHO Regional Office for South East Asia (SEARO), New Delhi, India   http://www.searo.who.int

WHO Regional Office for the Western Pacific (WPRO), Manila, Philippines   http://www.wpro.who.int

See also Centers for Disease Control and Prevention (CDC); International Health Systems; Public Health

Index

Entry titles and their page numbers are in **bold**.

method of, **2:**764–765
vs. narrative reviews, **2:**767
omnibus methods and, **2:**767
results graphic inspection of, **2:**766–767
sensitivity analysis and, **2:**766
statistical methods for, **2:**765–766
Metaregression, **2:**765, **2:**766
METeOR, **1:**557
*Methods for the Economic Evaluation of Health Care
    Programmes* (Drummond), **1:**322
MetraHealth, **1:**105–106
Metropolitan counties, **2:**1054
Metropolitan Medical Response System, **1:**100
Metropolitan statistical areas (MSA), **1:**472
Michigan Community Health Project (MCHP), **1:**674
Microbes, role in chronic diseases, **1:**26
Microorganisms, **1:**627
Micropolitan counties, **2:**1054
Middle class, uninsured individuals, **2:**1139–1141
Mid-South Delta Initiative, **1:**675
Midtown Manhattan Study, **2:**760
Midwest Business Group on Health (MBGH), 2:768–769
    organizational structure of, **2:**768–769
    products and services of, **2:**769
Midwest Health Purchasers Foundation (MHPF), **2:**769
Migrant Health Act of 1962, **1:**201, **1:**398
Migrant Health Centers, **1:**534
Mikhailov, Alexander I., **1:**501
Milbank, Samuel L., **2:**771
Milbank Memorial Fund, 2:770–771
    future implications of, **2:**771
    history of, **2:**770–771
Milbank Quarterly, **1:**584, **2:**770, **2:**771
Military, electronic patient clinical record system of,
    1:243
Military Health System (MHS), **2:**1129
Military Support to Civil Authorities (MSCA), **1:**100
Mill, John Stuart, **1:**134
Millennium Health Care and Benefits Act of 1999, **2:**692
Milliman, Inc., **2:**705
Mills, Wilbur D., **1:**183
Mind-body medicine, **1:**222–223, **1:**225
Minimal brain dysfunction, **2:**739
Minimum data set (MDS), **1:**283–284, **2:**863–864
    Canada and, **2:**773
    design of, **2:**772
**Minimum data set (MDS) for nursing home resident
    assessment, 2:771–774**
    clinical scales for, **2:**773
    computerized data for, **2:**773
    field testing of, **2:**772–773
    future changes in, **2:**774
    instrument development and, **2:**772
    policy, regulatory and quality improvement use of,
        2:773–774
Minimum necessary, **1:**279

Minimum Standards for Hospitals, **1:**664
Minnesota Care and Basic Health, **2:**1064
Minnesota Heart Health Program, **1:**198
Misfeasance, **2:**700
Mistake-proofing, **2:**1000
Mobile Army Surgical Hospital (MASH), **1:**346
Mobilizing for Action through Planning and Partnership
    (MAPP), **1:**526
Model expectations, **2:**721
Model fit, **2:**721
Moderator variables, **2:**766
Modern Healthcare, **1:**584, **2:**846
Molecular genetic research, **1:**435f
Monopolies. *See also* **Antitrust law**
    market failure and, **2:**709
Monthly Vital Statistics Report, **2:**804
Moore, Harry M., **1:**187
Moral hazard, 1:36, **1:**83, **1:**185–186, **1:**421, **1:**496,
    1:503, **2:**711, **2:775–777**
    asymmetric information and, **2:**775
    ex post, **1:**496
    future implications of, **2:**776
    health insurance and, **2:**775–776
    solutions for, **2:**776
Morbidity, 2:777–779
    of acute and chronic diseases, **1:**25–26
    ADE and, **2:**732
    compression of, **2:**778
    disease's global burden and, **2:**778–779
    drug-related costs, **1:**33
    economic recession and, **1:**327
    future implications of, **2:**779
    geographic differences in, **1:**447
    incidence of, **2:**1037
    increase of, **2:**955–956
    measures of, **2:**777–778, **2:**778
    rates, **1:**366–367
Morbidity and Mortality Weekly Report (MMWR),
    1:142, **2:**781
Morrisey, Michael A., **1:**658
Mortality, 2:779–783
    acute and chronic diseases and, **1:**25–26
    American Indians and, **1:**625
    cancer and, **2:**784
    crude rate of, **2:**779
    data sources for, **2:**781–782
    disease-specific rate of, **2:**780
    drug-related costs, **1:**33
    economic recession and, **1:**327
    fetal rate of, **2:**781
    future implications of, **2:**782
    Harlem and, **1:**638
    heart disease and, **2:**783
    iatrogenic causes of, **2:**992
    incidence of, **2:**1037
    maternal rate of, **2:**780